Clinical Neuropsychology

Clinical Neuropsychology

Fourth Edition

Edited by

KENNETH M. HEILMAN, M.D.

*The James E. Rooks Jr. Distinguished Professor of Neurology
and Clinical and Health Psychology*
University of Florida College of Medicine

EDWARD VALENSTEIN, M.D.

The William L. and Janice M. Neely Professor of Neurology
Chair, Department of Neurology
University of Florida College of Medicine

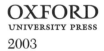

OXFORD
UNIVERSITY PRESS
2003

OXFORD
UNIVERSITY PRESS

Oxford   New York
Auckland   Bangkok   Buenos Aires   Cape Town   Chennai
Dar es Salaam   Delhi   Hong Kong   Istanbul   Karachi   Kolkata
Kuala Lumpur   Madrid   Melbourne   Mexico City   Mumbai
Nairobi   São Paulo   Shanghai   Taipei   Tokyo   Toronto

Published by Oxford University Press, Inc.
198 Madison Avenue, New York, New York, 10016
http://www.oup-usa.org

Library of Congress Cataloging-in-Publication Data

Clinical neuropsychology /
edited by Kenneth M. Heilman, Edward Valenstein.—4th ed.
p. ; cm.
Includes bibliographical references and index.
ISBN 0-19-513367-6 (cloth)
1. Neuropsychiatry. 2. Clinical neuropsychology. I. Heilman, Kenneth M., 1938–II.
Valenstein, Edward, 1942–
[DNLM: 1. Brain Diseases—diagnosis. 2. Neurobehavioral Manifestations.
3. Delirium, Dementia, Amnestic, Cognitive Disorders—diagnosis.
4. Neuropsychology—methods.
WL 340 C641 2003]
RC341 .C693 2003
616.8—dc21   2002070352

9 8 7 6 5 4 3 2 1

Printed in the United States of America
on acid-free paper

We dedicate the fourth edition of this book to our wives,

Patricia Carolyn Phillips Heilman

and

Candace Leavitt Valenstein

Preface to the Fourth Edition

This fourth edition of *Clinical Neuropsychology*, like all the former editions, focuses on the clinical presentation of the major neurobehavioral syndromes. It has been 9 years since the last edition was published and while the major syndromes have remained the same, much has been learned about them. As in prior editions the authors have included clinical descriptions and have addressed neuropsychological mechanisms that might account for these disorders, brain pathology associated with these disorders, and when possible aspects of therapy and management. In our effort to be comprehensive and include the advances that have occurred since our last edition, each of the chapters has been updated and enlarged. We also added chapters on anosognosia and on hallucinations. We deleted the chapter on schizophrenia, because we did not have space in the book to include discussion of the many other psychiatric disorders with neuropsychological deficits, and including only one created an unbalanced view. The chapter on recovery of function has been supplemented by a chapter on pharmacotherapy.

When we first considered editing this book, Arthur Benton was very supportive and put us in touch with Jeffrey House at Oxford University Press. After the first edition was published, some people complained about the title because we (K.M.H. and E.V.) were neurologists, not neuropsychologists. It was actually Arthur who suggested this title and when we told him about these complaints, after he stopped laughing, he said that neuropsychology is both a profession and a discipline and that a book which describes the major neurobehavioral disorders was certainly about the discipline of clinical neuropsychology. Arthur was the primary author of two chapters in each of our three prior editions, Disorders of the Body Schema, and Visuoperceptual, Visuospatial and Visuoconstructive Disorders. Arthur has retired, and we have replaced his chapters (and the separate chapter on acalculia) by chapters on visual-spatial perception and cognition, and the other on acalculia and disorders of the body schema.

We were saddened by the death of D. Frank Benson, who was a fine person and one of the leaders of American behavioral and cognitive neurology. Frank had contributed the chapter on aphasia for our three prior editions. His chapter primarily addressed the classic aphasia syndromes, but our knowledge of the components of aphasia has substantially increased. For the fourth edition we have added to a chapter on aphasic syndromes three chapters covering, respectively, phonologic, syntactic, and lexical-semantic aspects of language.

Writing a chapter is financially unrewarding and is generally not held in as high regard as writing papers for peer-reviewed journals. But it is very difficult for students to learn neuropsychology by reading original papers, and reading review chapters is perhaps the most efficient means of learning. Thus, we are fortunate that the authors of our chapters are also educators and know the importance of their efforts. The editors are deeply indebted to them for producing such excellent chapters.

We would like to thank Fiona Stevens and the staff at Oxford University Press for their considerable help and encouragement. The energy that allowed us to pursue this project comes in part from the professional gratification of working with superb colleagues in a fine institution. It also comes from the unquestioning support and loyalty of our families. We are dedicating this book to our wives, who have endured and supported us through all four editions of this book, and much else.

Gainesville, Florida   K.M.H.
                                                                                                                          E.V.

Preface to the First Edition

The growth of interest in brain–behavior relationships has generated a literature that is both impressive and bewildering. In teaching neuropsychology, we have found that the reading lists necessary for adequate coverage of the subject have been unwieldy, and the information provided in the reading has been difficult to integrate. We therefore set out to provide a text that comprehensively covers the major clinical syndromes. The focus of the text is the *clinical* presentation of human brain dysfunction. The authors who have contributed to this volume have provided clinical descriptions of the major neuropsychological disorders. They have discussed methods of diagnosis, and have described specific tests, often of use at the bedside. They have also commented upon therapy. Since the study of pathophysiological and neuropsychological mechanisms underlying these disorders is inextricably intertwined with the definition and treatment of these disorders, considerable space has been devoted to a discussion of these mechanisms, and to the clinical and experimental evidence which bears on them.

A multi-authored text has the advantage of allowing authorities to write about areas in which they have special expertise. This also exposes the reader to several different approaches to the study of brain-behavior relationships, an advantage in a field in which a variety of theoretical and methodological positions have been fruitful. We therefore have not attempted to impose our own views on the contributing authors, but where there were conflicts in terminology, we have provided synonyms and cross-references. Much of brain activity is integrative, and isolated neuropsychological disturbances are rare. Discussions of alexia or agraphia must necessarily include more than a passing reference to aphasia, and so on. Since we wanted each chapter to stand on its own, with its author's viewpoint intact, we have generally allowed some overlap between chapters.

We wish to thank all of the persons who devoted their time and effort to this book. Professor Arthur Benton not only contributed two outstanding chapters, but was instrumental in advising us about authors and content, and in leading us to Oxford University Press. We are grateful to all the other contributing authors, who promptly provided high quality manuscripts; to our secretary, Ann Tison, who typed our manuscripts so many times; and to the editors at Oxford University Press, who helped to improve our grammar and syntax, and, not infrequently, the clarity of our thought. Not least, we are grateful to our families, who have endured many evenings of work with this volume with patience and understanding.

Gainesville, Florida   K.M.H.
March 1979   E.V.

Contents

Contributors

JOHN C. ADAIR, M.D.
*Neurology Service, Albuquerque VA Medical
Center
Assistant Professor of Neurology
University of New Mexico
Albuquerque, New Mexico*

MARTIN L. ALBERT, M.D., PH.D.
*Professor of Neurology
Director, Harold Goodglass Aphasia Research
Center
Boston University School of Medicine
Veterans Affairs Medical Center
Boston, Massachusetts*

STEVEN W. ANDERSON, PH.D.
*Assistant Professor of Neurology
Executive Director, Benton Neuropsychology
Laboratory
University of Iowa College of Medicine
Iowa City, Iowa*

ANNA M. BARRETT, M.D.
*Assistant Professor of Medicine (Neurology)
University of Pennsylvania State School of
Medicine
Hershey, Pennsylvania*

RUSSELL M. BAUER, PH.D.
*Professor of Clinical and Health Psychology
University of Florida
Gainesville, Florida*

RITA SLOAN BERNDT, PH.D.
*Professor, Department of Neurology
University of Maryland School of Medicine
Baltimore, Maryland*

LEE X. BLONDER, PH.D.
*Associate Professor in the Department of
Behavioral Science
Sanders-Brown Center on Aging
University of Kentucky College of Medicine
Lexington, Kentucky*

JOSEPH E. BOGEN, M.D., PH.D.
*Clinical Professor of Neurological Surgery
USC School of Medicine
Adjunct Professor of Psychology, UCLA
Los Angeles, California
Visiting Professor of Biology
California Institute of Technology
Pasadena, California*

DAWN BOWERS, PH.D.
*Professor of Clinical and Health Psychology
University of Florida
Gainesville, Florida*

DAVID CAPLAN, M.D., PH.D.
Professor of Neurology
Harvard Medical School
Medical Director, Neuropsychology Laboratory,
Massachusetts General Hospital
Boston, Massachusetts

H. BRANCH COSLETT, M.D.
Professor of Neurology
University of Pennsylvania College of Medicine
Philadelphia, Pennsylvania

JEFFREY L. CUMMINGS, M.D.
The Augustus S. Rose Professor of Neurology
Professor of Psychiatry and Biobehavioral Sciences
Director, Alzheimer's Disease Center
David Geffen School of Medicine at UCLA
Los Angeles, California

ANTONIO R. DAMASIO, M.D.
Distinguished Professor and Chair
Department of Neurology
University of Iowa College of Medicine
Iowa City, Iowa

JASON A. DEMERY, M.A.
Department of Clinical and Health Psychology
University of Florida College of Medicine
Gainesville, Florida

NATALIE L. DENBURG, PH.D.
Assistant Professor (Clinical) of Neurology
Division of Behavioral Neurology and Cognitive
  Neuroscience
University of Iowa College of Medicine
Iowa City, Iowa

MARTHA J. FARAH, PH.D.
Professor of Psychology
Director, Center for Cognitive Neuroscience
University of Pennsylvania
Philadephia, Pennsylvania

BRIAN T. GOLD, PH.D.
St. Joseph's Health Centre
Lawson Research Institute
London, Ontario

LAURA GRANDE, PH.D.
Department of Clinical and Health Psychology
University of Florida
Gainesville, Florida

KENNETH M. HEILMAN, M.D.
The James E. Rooks Jr. Distinguished Professor of
  Neurology
University of Florida College of Medicine
Malcolm Randall Veterans Administration Hospital
Gainesville, Florida

MARCO IACOBONI, M.D., PH.D.
Associate Professor, Neuropsychiatric Institute
Director, Transcranial Magnetic Stimulation
  Laboratory
Ahmanson-Lovelace Brain Mapping Center
David Geffen School of Medicine at UCLA
Los Angeles, California

ANDREW KERTESZ, M.D., F.R.C.P. (C)
Professor of Neurology
Director of Cognitive Neurology
Department of Clinical Neurological Sciences
University of Western Ontario
London, Ontario

DAVID KNOPMAN, M.D.
Professor of Neurology
Mayo Clinic
Rochester, Minnesota

PATRICK McNAMARA, PH.D.
Assistant Professor of Psychiatry
Boston University School of Medicine
Boston, Massachusetts

STEPHEN E. NADEAU, M.D.
Co-Director, Rehabilitations Outcome Research
  Center
Malcolm Randall Veterans Administration Hospital
Professor of Neurology
University of Florida College of Medicine
Gainesville, Florida

DAVID P. ROELTGEN, M.D.
Associate Clinical Professor
Pennsylvania State University
Hershey, Pennsylvania

LESLIE J. GONZALEZ ROTHI, PH.D.
Professor of Neurology
Director of the Veterans Administration Brain
  Rehabilitation Research Center
University of Florida College of Medicine
Gainesville, Florida

RONALD L. SCHWARTZ, M.D.
Saint Barnabas Institute of Neurology
Assistant Professor of Neurology
New York University School of Medicine
New York City, New York

OLA SELNES, PH.D.
Associate Professor of Neurology
Johns Hopkins Medical Institutions
Baltimore, Maryland

SIBEL TEKIN, M.D.
UCLA Alzheimer's Disease Center
Reed Neurological Research Center
UCLA School of Medicine
Los Angeles, California

DANIEL TRANEL, PH.D.
Professor of Neurology
Division of Behavioral Neurology and Cognitive
  Neuroscience
University of Iowa College of Medicine
Iowa City, Iowa

EDWARD VALENSTEIN, M.D.
The William L. and Janice M. Neely Professor of
  Neurology
Chair, Department of Neurology
University of Florida College of Medicine
Gainesville, Florida

ROBERT T. WATSON, M.D.
Jules B. Chapman MD Professor in Clinical Care
  and Humaness
Department of Neurology
Senior Associate Dean for Educational Affairs
University of Florida College of Medicine
Gainesville, Florida

DAHLIA W. ZAIDEL, PH.D.
Professor of Psychology
David Geffen School of Medicine at UCLA
Los Angeles, California

ERAN ZAIDEL, PH.D.
Professor of Behavioral Neuroscience and
  Cognition
Department of Psychology
David Geffen School of Medicine at UCLA
Los Angeles, California

Clinical Neuropsychology

1

Introduction

KENNETH M. HEILMAN AND EDWARD VALENSTEIN

Aristotle thought that the mind, with the function of thinking, had no relation to the body or the senses and could not be destroyed. The first attempts to localize mental processes to the brain may nevertheless be traced back to antiquity. In the fifth century B.C., Hippocrates of Croton claimed that the brain was the organ of intellect and the heart the organ of the senses. Herophilus, in the third century B.C., studied the structure of the brain and regarded it as the site of intelligence. He believed that the middle ventricle was responsible for the faculty of cognition and the posterior ventricle was the seat of memory. Galen, in the second century B.C., thought that the activities of the mind were performed by the substance of the brain rather than the ventricles, but it was not until the anatomical work of Vesalius in the sixteenth century A.D. that this thesis was accepted. Vesalius, however, thought that the brains of most mammals and birds had similar structures in almost every respect and differed only in size, attaining the greatest dimensions in humans. In the seventeenth century, Descartes suggested that the soul resided in the pineal. He chose the pineal because of its central location: all things must emanate from the soul.

At the end of the eighteenth century, Gall postulated that various human faculties were localized in different organs, or centers of the brain. He thought that these centers were expansions of lower nervous mechanisms and that, although independent, they were able to interact with one another. Unlike Descartes, Gall conceived brain structures as having successive development, with no central point where all nerves unite. He proposed that the vital forces resided in the brainstem and that the intellectual qualities were situated in various parts of the two cerebral hemispheres. The hemispheres were united by the commissures, the largest being the corpus callosum.

Unfortunately, Gall also postulated that measurements of the skull may allow one to deduce moral and intellectual characteristics, since the shape of the skull is modified by the underlying brain. This hypothesis was the foundation of phrenology. When phrenology fell into disrepute, many of Gall's original contributions were blighted. His teachings, however, are the foundation of modern neuropsychology.

Noting that students with good verbal memory had prominent eyes, Gall suggested that memory for words was situated in the frontal lobes. He studied two patients who had lost their memory for words and attributed their disorder to frontal lobe lesions. In 1825, Bouillard wrote that he also believed cerebral function to be localized. He demonstrated that discrete lesions could produce paralysis in one limb and not others and cited this as proof of localized function. He also believed that the anterior lobe was the center of speech. He observed that the tongue had many functions other than speech and that one function could be disordered (e.g., speech) while others remained intact (e.g., mastication). This observation suggested to him that an effector can have more than one center that controls its actions.

In 1861, Broca heard Bouillaud's pupil Auburtin speak about the importance of the anterior lobe in speech and asked Auburtin to see a patient suffering from right hemiplegia and loss of speech and writing. The patient was able to understand speech but could articulate only one word, "tan." This patient died, and postmortem inspection of the brain revealed that there was a cavity filled with fluid on the lateral aspect of the left hemisphere. When the fluid was drained, there could be seen a large left hemisphere lesion that included the first temporal gyrus, the insula and the corpus striatum, and the frontal lobe, including the second and third frontal convolutions as well as the inferior portion of the transverse convolution. In 1861, Broca saw another patient who had lost the power of speech and writing but could comprehend spoken language. Autopsy again revealed a left hemisphere lesion involving the second and third frontal convolutions.

Broca later saw eight patients who suffered a loss of speech (which he called "aphemia," but which Trousseau later called "aphasia"). All eight had left hemisphere lesions. This was the first demonstration of left hemisphere dominance for language (Broca, 1865).

Broca's observations produced great excitement in the medical world. Despite his clear demonstration of left hemisphere dominance, medical opinion appeared to split into two camps, one favoring the view that different functions are exercised by the various portions of the cerebral hemisphere and the other denying that psychic functions are or can be localized.

Following Broca's initial observations, there was a flurry of activity. In 1868, Hughlings Jackson noted that there were two types of aphasic patients—fluent and nonfluent—and,

in 1869, Bastian argued that there were patients who had deficits not only in the articulation of words but also in the memory for words. Bastian also postulated the presence of a visual and auditory word center and a kinesthetic center for the hand and the tongue. He proposed that these centers were connected and that information, such as language, was processed by the brain in different ways by each of these centers. Lesions in these centers would thus produce distinct syndromes, depending upon which aspect of the processing was disturbed. Bastian thus viewed the brain as a processor. He was the first to describe word deafness and word blindness.

In 1874, Wernicke published his famous *Der Aphasische Symptomenkomplex*. He was familiar with Meynert's work, which demonstrated that sensory systems project to the posterior portions of the hemispheres whereas the anterior portions appear to be efferent. Wernicke noted that lesions of the posterior portion of the superior temporal region produced an aphasia in which comprehension was poor. He thought that this auditory center contained sound images, while Broca's area contained images for speech movements (Fig. 1–1). He also thought that these areas were connected by a commissure and that a lesion of this commissure would disconnect the area for sound images from the area for images of speech movement.

Wernicke's scheme could account for motor, conduction, and sensory aphasia with poor repetition. Lichtheim (1885), however, described patients who were nonfluent but repeated normally and sensory aphasics who could not comprehend but could repeat words. Elaborating on Wernicke's ideas, he devised a complex scheme to explain the mechanism underlying seven types of speech and language disorders. Bastian, Wernicke, and Lichtheim demonstrated that complex behaviors can be fractionated into modular components. They also developed information-processing models by which these components interacted to produce complex behaviors such as speech. These models have had heuristic and clinical value.

Following World War I, the localizationist–information-processing approach was abandoned in favor of a holistic approach. Probably there were many factors underlying the

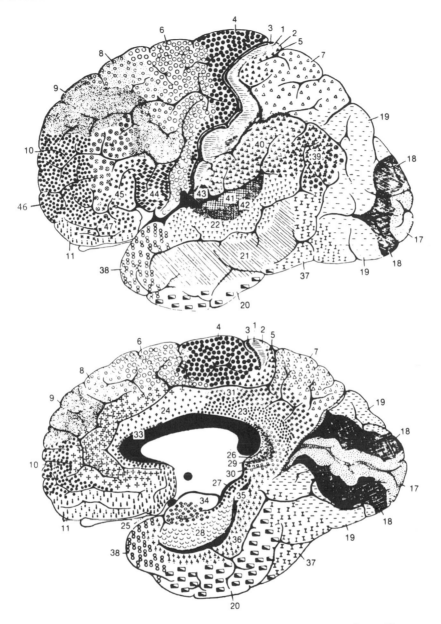

Figure 1–1. Brodmann's cytoarchitectural map of the human brain. The different areas are defined on the basis of subtle differences in cortical cell structure and organiza-tion. Broca's area corresponds roughly to areas 44 and 45 and Wernicke's area to the posterior part of area 22.

change. The localizationist theory was built on the foundation laid by Gall. When phrenology was discredited, other localizationist theories became suspect. Lashley (1938), using experimental methods (as opposed to the case reports of the classical neurologists), found that engrams were not localized in the brain but rather appeared to be diffusely represented. From these observations, he proposed a theory of mass action: the behavioral result of a lesion depends on the amount of brain removed more than on the location of the lesion. Head (1926) studied aphasics' linguistic performance and was not satisfied with the classical neurologists' attempts to deduce schemas from clinical observations. Discussing one of Wernicke's case reports, he wrote, "No better example could be chosen of the manner in which the writers of this period were compelled to lop and twist their cases to fit the Procrustean bed of their hypothetical conceptions" (Vol 1, p. 63). Although Freud studied the relationships between the brain and behavior early in his career, he later provided the scientific world with explanations of behavior based on psychodynamic relationships. The Gestalt psychologists abandoned localization in favor of the holistic approach.

Social and political influences, however, were perhaps more important in changing neuropsychological thought than were the newer scientific theories. The continental European scientific community was strongly influenced by Kant's *Critique of Pure Reason*, which held that even though knowledge cannot transcend experience, it is nevertheless in part a priori. According to Kant, the outer world produces only the matter of sensation while the mental apparatus (the brain) orders this matter and supplies the concepts by means of which we understand experience. After World War I, the influence on science on the continent waned while in English-speaking countries it bloomed. The American and English political and social systems were strongly influenced by Locke, the seventeenth-century liberal philosopher who, unlike Kant, believed that behavior and ideas were not innate but rather derived from experience. This conceptual scheme provides little reason to look at the structure of the brain in order to understand behavior.

In the second half of the twentieth century, there was a reawakening of interest in brain–behavior relationships. Many developments contributed to this. The classical neurologists were rediscovered and their findings replicated. Electronic technology provided researchers with new instruments for observing physiological processes. New statistical procedures enabled them to distinguish random results from significant relationships. New behavioral paradigms, such as dichotic listening and lateral visual half-field viewing, permitted psychologists to explore brain mechanisms in normal individuals as well as in pathological cases. Anatomical studies using new staining methods permitted more detailed mapping of connections, and advances in neurochemistry and neuropharmacology ushered in a new form of neuropsychology in which, in addition to studying behavioral–structural relationships, investigators could study behavioral–chemical relationships. Finally, functional imaging has enabled us to map some correlates of brain activity during specific behaviors in both normal and brain-injured subjects.

METHODS AND CONCEPTS

The attempt to relate behavior to the brain rests on the assumptions that all behavior is mediated by physical processes and that the complex behavior of higher animals depends upon physical processes in the central nervous system. Changes in complex behavior must therefore be associated with changes in the physical state of the brain. Conversely, changes in the physical state of the brain (such as these associated with brain damage) affect behavior. The genetically determined organization of the nervous system sets limits on what can be perceived and learned. This organization also determines to a great extent the nature of the behavioral changes that occur in response to brain injury.

The understanding of brain–behavior relationships is aided most by the study of behaviors that can be clearly defined and are likely to be related to brain processes that can be directly or indirectly observed. Behaviors that can be selectively affected by focal brain lesions or by specific pharmacological agents are therefore most often chosen for neuropsychological study. Conversely, behaviors that are difficult to define or appear unlikely to be correlated with observable anatomical, physiological, or chemical processes in the brain are poor candidates for study. As techniques for studying the brain improve, more kinds of behavior become amenable to study.

Psychodynamic explanations of behavior may be of considerable clinical utility in the evaluation and treatment of certain behavior disorders, but they will be of little interest to neuropsychologists until some correlation with underlying brain processes is demonstrated. Furthermore, psychodynamic explanations of the behavior of brain-damaged patients must be examined critically since the brain damage may have impaired normal emotional mechanisms. Depression, for example, can be seen in brain-damaged persons. The obvious psychodynamic explanation is that depression is a "normal" reaction to the loss of function resulting from the brain injury. Evidence that depression correlates less with the severity of functional loss than with the site of the brain lesion, however, suggests that in some patients depression may be a direct result of the brain injury and that in such cases the psychodynamic explanation may be irrelevant. Similar caveats apply to the better-documented association of apathy and denial of illness with lesions in the frontal lobes or right hemisphere.

There are many valid approaches to the study of brain–behavior relationships, and no morally and intellectually sound approach should be neglected. We will briefly consider the major approaches, emphasizing those that have been used to greatest advantage.

INTROSPECTION

At times, patients' observations of their own mental state may be not only helpful but necessary. How else can one learn of many sensory abnormalities, hallucinations, or emotional changes? It is conceivable that people's insights into their own mental processes may be of importance in delineating brain mechanisms. For example, persons with "photographic" memory not surprisingly report that they rely on visual rather than verbal memory, and experiments suggest that visual memory has a greater capacity than verbal memory. Patients may have similarly useful insights, and clinicians would do well to listen carefully to what their patients say. This does not mean, however, that they must believe everything recounted by their patients. In normal persons, introspection is not always trustworthy; in brain-damaged patients, it may be even less reliable. This is particularly true when the language centers have been disconnected from the region of the brain that processes the information the patient is asked about (Geschwind, 1965). For example, patients with a callosal lesion (separating the left language-dominant hemisphere from the right

hemisphere) cannot name correctly an object placed in their left hand. Curiously, such patients do not say that they cannot name the object nor do they explain that their left hand can feel it but they cannot find the right word. Instead, in nearly every such case recorded, the patient confabulates a name. It is clear that in this situation the patient's language area, which is providing the spoken "insight," cannot even appreciate the presence of a deficit (until it is later brought to its attention), let alone explain the nature of the difficulty. In other situations, it is apparent that patients make incorrect assumptions about their deficits. Patients with pure word deafness (who cannot understand spoken language but nevertheless can speak well and can hear) often assume that people are deliberately being obscure; the result of this introspection is paranoia. Thus, although a patient's introspection at times can provide useful clues for the clinician, this information must always be analyzed critically and used with caution.

THE BLACK BOX APPROACH

Behavior can be studied without any knowledge of the nervous system. Just as the electrical engineer can study the function of an electronic apparatus without taking it apart (by applying different inputs and studying the outputs), the brain can be approached as a "black box." The object of the black box approach is to determine laws of behavior. These laws can then be used to predict behavior, which of course is one expressed aim of the study of psychology.

To the extent that laws of behavior are determined by the "hard-wiring" of the brain, the black box approach also yields information about brain function. In this regard, the systematic study of any behavior or set of behaviors is relevant to the study of brain function. Psychology, linguistics, sociology, aesthetics, and related disciplines may all reveal a priori principles of behavior. The study of linguistics, for example, has indicated a structure common to all languages (Chomsky, 1967). Since there is no logical constraint that gives language this structure and since its generality makes environmental influences unlikely, one can assume that the basic structure of language is hard-wired in the brain. Thus, observations of behavior can constrain theories of brain function without any reference to brain anatomy, chemistry, or physiology (see, for example, Caramazza, 1992).

Although the black box approach yields useful information about brain function, such information is limited because the brain itself is not studied. The study of neuropsychology reflects its origins in nineteenth-century medical science by emphasizing brain anatomy, chemistry, and physiology as relevant variables: purely cognitive studies are but a part of this endeavor.

BRAIN ABLATION PARADIGMS

Lesions in specific areas of the brain change behavior in specific ways. Studies correlating these behavioral changes with the site of lesions yield information that can be used to predict from a given behavioral disturbance the site of the lesions, and vice versa. Such information has great clinical utility.

It is another matter, however, to try to deduce from the behavioral effects of an ablative lesion the normal mechanisms of brain function. As Hughlings Jackson pointed out more than a century ago, the abnormal behavior observed after a brain lesion reflects the functioning of the remaining brain tissue. This remaining brain may react adversely to or compensate for the loss of function caused by the lesion, and thus either add to or minimize the behavioral deficit. Acute lesions often disturb function in other brain areas (termed "diaschisis"); these metabolic and physiological changes may not be detectable by neuropathological methods and may thus contribute to an overestimate of the function of the lesioned area. Lesions may also produce changes in behavior by releasing other brain areas from facilitation or inhibition. Thus it may be difficult to distinguish behavioral effects caused by an interruption of processing normally occurring in the damaged area from effects due to less specific alterations of function in other areas of the brain.

Possible nonspecific effects of a lesion, such as diaschisis, mass action effects, and reactions to disability or discomfort, can be excluded as major determinants of abnormal behavior by the use of "control" lesions. If lesions of comparable size in other brain areas do not produce similar behavioral effects, one cannot ascribe these effects to nonspecific causes. It is especially elegant to be able to demonstrate that such a control lesion has a different behavioral effect. This has been termed "double-dissociation": lesion A produces behavioral change a but not b, while lesion B produces behavioral change b but not a (Teuber, 1955).

Once nonspecific effects have been excluded, one must take into account the various ways in which a lesion may specifically affect behavior. If a lesion in a particular region results in the loss of a behavior, one must not simply ascribe to that region the normal function of performing that behavior. The first step toward making a meaningful statement about brain–behavior relationships is a scrupulous analysis of the behavior in question. If a lesion in a particular area of the brain interferes with writing, that does not mean that the area is the "writing center" of the brain. Writing is a complex process that requires many other functions: sensory and motor control over the limb must be excellent; there must be no praxic disturbances; language function must be intact; the subject must be mentally alert and able to attend to the task; and so on. To fractionate complex behaviors such as writing into components, one must study every aspect of behavior that is directly related to the task of writing and define as closely as possible which aspects of the process of writing are disturbed. It may then be possible to make a correlation between the damaged portion of the brain and the aspect of the writing process that has been disrupted. It is important to distinguish between lesions that destroy areas of the brain that store specific forms of information (representations) and lesions that disconnect such areas from one another, disrupting processes that require coordination between two or more such areas (Geschwind, 1965). When a person is writing, for example, there must be coordination between areas that contain representations of how words are spelled and areas important in programming the movements needed to write letters. Lesions that disconnect these areas produce agraphia even though there may be no other language or motor deficit. A lesion in the corpus callosum, for example, may disconnect the language areas in the left hemisphere from the right-hemisphere motor area, thus producing agraphia in the left hand.

Partial recovery of function often occurs after brain lesions and can be attributed to many factors, including resolution of edema, increase in blood supply to ischemic areas, and resolution of diaschisis (see Chapter 20). In addition, the brain is capable of a limited but substantial amount of reorganization that may enable remaining structures to take over the functions of the damaged portion. Brain plasticity is greatest in the developing organism and decreases with increasing age; however, it is still a factor even in the elderly. This clearly complicates the study of behavioral disorders that follow focal lesions, more so in children. It particularly complicates the study of abnormalities of development of the nervous system both before and after birth. It is difficult to make precise correlations between structural and behavioral abnormalities, since the plasticity of the developing nervous system tends to minimize focal deficits. But there is nevertheless great interest in correlating developmental abnormalities with behavioral syndromes, as evidenced, for example, by the study of brain anomalies in certain children with dyslexia. Another approach is to study the behavioral changes that attend normal development in childhood and to attempt to correlate them with anatomic and physiologic changes in the developing nervous system.

Another disadvantage of the ablative paradigm is that natural lesions, such as strokes or tumors, do not necessarily respect functional neuroanatomical boundaries. Ischemic strokes occur in the distribution of particular vessels, and the vascular territory often overlaps anatomical boundaries. The association of two behavioral deficits may thereby result not from a functional relationship but rather from the fact that two brain regions with little anatomical or physiological relation are supplied by the same vessel. The association of a memory disturbance with pure word blindness (alexia without agraphia) merely indicates that the mesial temporal lobe, the occipital lobe, and the splenium of the corpus callosum are all in the distribution of the posterior cerebral artery. Use of experimental lesions in animals can avoid this problem; even within a specific anatomical region, however, there may be many systems operating, often with contrasting behavioral functions.

Despite all these problems, the study of brain lesions in humans and animals has yielded more information about brain–behavior relationships than any other approach and it has been given renewed impetus by the development of powerful methods of neural imaging. Lesions as small as 2 or 3 mm in diameter can be detected by modern X-ray computerized tomography (CT). Positron emission tomography (PET) has less resolution but can provide images that reflect the metabolic activity of brain regions (see below). Nuclear magnetic resonance imaging (MRI) scanning gives information about brain structure and blood flow and can also provide information about metabolic activity. Because MRI does not expose the subject to X-irradiation, it can be justified in a larger number of persons.

BRAIN STIMULATION PARADIGMS

Brain stimulation has been used to map connections in the brain and to elicit changes in behavior. One attraction of this method has been that stimulation, in contrast to ablation, is reversible. (Reversible methods of ablation, such as cooling, have also been used to study brain–behavior relationships.) The additional claim that stimulation is more like normal physiological function is open to question: it is highly unlikely that gross electrical stimulation of the brain reproduces any normally occurring physiological state. The stimulation techniques that are usually employed cannot selectively affect only one class of neurons. Furthermore, stimulation disrupts ongoing activity, frequently inhibiting it in a way that resembles the effects of ablation. Some of these objections may be overcome by the use of neurotransmitters or drugs with similar properties to stimulate (or inhibit) specific neurotransmitter systems.

NEUROCHEMICAL MANIPULATIONS

Neurochemical and immunological methods have been used to identify groups of neurons in the central nervous system that use specific neurotransmitters. The number of neurotransmitters identified continues to increase, and one neuron may express more than one neurotransmitter. The anatomy of major neurotransmitter pathways has been elucidated, and the molecular mechanisms by which some neurotransmitters function is now known in some detail. Drugs given systemically or applied to specific anatomic areas may stimulate or block specific neurotransmitter receptors. There are also drugs that will selectively destroy neurons containing specific neurotransmitters, and genetic methods are available to produce animals that lack specific enzymes. Through PET studies, specific neurotransmitters such as dopamine can be imaged in humans. Using these and other techniques, it is possible to correlate the behavioral effects of pharmacological agents with dysfunction in anatomical areas defined by chemical criteria.

PHYSIOLOGICAL STUDIES

The Electroencephalograph and Magnetoencephalograph

Electrophysiological studies of human behavior have been attempted during brain surgery, and depth electrode recording may be justified in the evaluation of a few patients (usually in preparation for epilepsy surgery), but most studies rely on the surface-recorded electroencephalogram (EEG). The raw EEG, however, demonstrates changes in amplitude and frequency that are generally nonspecific and poorly localizing. Computer analysis of EEG frequency and amplitude (power spectra) in different behavioral situations (and from different brain regions) has demonstrated correlations between EEG activity and behavior, but only for certain aspects of behavior (such as arousal) or for broad anatomical fields (e.g., between hemispheres). The use of computer averaging has increased our ability to detect electrical events that are time locked to stimuli or responses. Thus, cortical evoked potentials to visual, auditory, and somesthetic stimuli have been recorded, as have potentials that precede muscle activation. Certain potentials appear to correlate with expectancy (the contingent negative variation and the P300 potential). That potentials can be "evoked" by purely mental events is demonstrated by the recording of potentials time linked to the nonoccurrence of expected stimuli. Computer algorithms have been developed to trace the spatial and temporal spread of electrical activity associated with specific single events or with ongoing behaviors, and to assess the coherence of activity from different brain regions.

Changes in magnetic fields can also be measured. Although magnetoencephalography requires much more elaborate equipment than EEG, it is less affected by intervening brain skull and scalp, and can detect signals generated at a greater depth. The principal advantage of these physiologic techniques is their temporal resolution, measured in milliseconds. But their spatial resolution is poor.

Single-unit Recording

Discrete activity of individual neurons can be recorded by inserting microelectrodes into the brain. Obviously, this practice is largely limited to animal experiments. Much has been learned (and remains to be learned) from the use of this technique in alert, responding animals. Responses to well-controlled stimuli can be recorded with precision and analyzed quantitatively. Interpretation of single-unit recording presents its own difficulties. The brain activity related to a behavioral event may occur simultaneously in many cells spatially dispersed over a considerable area. Recording from only one cell may not yield a meaningful pattern. In addition, single-unit recording may be difficult to analyze in relation to complex behaviors.

Functional Neuroimaging

One of the most exciting developments in recent years has been the advent of powerful techniques for imaging changes in brain function in the intact organism. We have already referred to mapping of electrical and magnetic activity. Regional glucose utilization can be mapped using fluorodeoxyglucose (FDG) PET. Changes in regional blood flow related to changes in brain activity can be mapped by several techniques, including single photon emission computed tomography (SPECT), PET (using other ligands), and functional magnetic resonance imaging (fMRI). These studies all lack the temporal resolution of electrophysiologic methods, which is measured in milliseconds; however PET and especially fMRI have much better spatial resolution, and fMRI studies now have temporal resolutions of close to 1 second. These techniques will be very briefly described here (for additional information see Nadeau and Crosson, 1995; D'Esposito 2000; Mazziotta, 2000).

The SPECT studies employing hexamethyl-propylene-amine-oxime (HMPAO) as the radioactive ligand indirectly measure changes in blood flow. The ligand binds to vascular endothelial membranes over a period of about 2 minutes, and has a half-life of 6 hours, so the behavioral task can be performed outside the scanner and the subject scanned afterwards, a distinct advantage over fMRI studies. The spatial resolution of this technique is about 6–7 mm, and the temporal resolution is 3–4 minutes. The dose of radioactivity limits the number of studies that can be done to about three a year.

Positron emission tomographic studies using very-short-half-life radiotracers (such as $H_2^{15}O$) provide measures of absolute blood flow. The short half-life (about 2 minutes) allows for relatively brief behavioral trials, and the low radiation exposure enables multiple trials in one sitting. Because of its short half-life, the tracer must be manufactured close to the experiment, a very costly constraint. Also, the experiment must be performed within the scanner; however, the scanner environment is not as constrained or noisy as with fMRI (see below). The PET blood flow studies have a temporal resolution of about 2 minutes, and a spatial resolution of from 4 to 16 mm. Because data must be acquired over more than 10 seconds, PET studies usually use blocked trials, and responses to a single event are difficult to discern.

Positron emission tomographic studies using FDG are a more direct measure of brain metabolic activity. The FDG is taken up into the brain by the same transporters as glucose, but then is metabolized slowly, so it marks areas of greater metabolic activity for several hours. As with SPECT, the task can be performed outside the scanner, thus there are few constraints on the type of behavior that can be studied. But the uptake of FDG takes 30–40 minutes, so temporal resolution is very poor.

Functional magnetic resonance imaging is faster than PET, and is capable of measuring activity generated by a single behavioral event. The temporal resolution is as little as 1 second. Also, fMRI has much better spatial resolution, as little as 1 mm. The need to acquire data during the task, however, places constraints on the kind of behavior that can be studied. The subject is confined in a very noisy MRI machine, and movement, speech, and electromagnetic signals can seriously interfere with the quality of the image.

Functional imaging studies of cerebral blood flow assume that a local change in blood flow (that results in a change in measured signal) is related to changes in synaptic activity, and changes in synaptic activity are responsible for specific changes in behavior. Even in the absence of stimuli, the brain is active. Thus, to determine how a behavior influences brain activity, one must subtract irrelevant "background" signals. Because "resting" activity is uncontrolled, investigators often use control tasks that resemble the study task in all but a single variable, which then becomes the behavior that is studied.

There are many methodological and theoretic problems with functional imaging. At the most fundamental level, the exact means by which the fMRI signal is generated is not entirely understood. The blood oxygen level–dependent (BOLD) method used in fMRI studies assumes that blood oxygen levels, reflected by the ratio of oxyhemoglobin to deoxyhemoglobin, are related to synaptic activity in the brain. During synaptic activity, oxygen is consumed and the relative concentration of deoxyhemoglobin increases; but within a couple of seconds there is a reactive increase in blood flow and the proportion of oxyhemoglobin actually increases over baseline. It is very difficult to detect the initial dip in oxygen levels, and the BOLD technique has relied upon the reactive increase in blood flow and oxyhemoglobin levels.

The neuroimaging techniques of SPECT, PET, and fMRI have all demonstrated reproducible blood flow changes in primary sensory areas in response to stimuli of the appropriate modality. These responses are an order of magnitude larger than behavior-related blood flow changes in association cortex, especially in polymodal and supramodal cortex. One reason for this is that primary sensory cortex is relatively quiet in the absence of the appropriate sensory stimulus, whereas supramodal cortex is not so dependent upon external stimulation. Therefore, when the control activity is subtracted from the task-related activity, much more of the signal is lost in high-order cortex than in primary sensory cortex. Interpretation of observed changes may be problematic. It is usual to expect that an area that mediates a behavior will become more active and will have greater blood flow with that behavior; however, it is possible that a change in pattern of activity could mediate a behavior without an increase, or perhaps with an overall decrease, in activity. Indeed, task-related reductions in blood flow have been interpreted as reflecting involvement in a behavior. It has been reasoned that a brain region that is adept at a behavior will be less activated than when involved in a behavior at which it is less adept. If this is true, almost any functional imaging result can have two opposite interpretations. Also, many neurons in the cerebral cortex are inhibitory. During a specific behavior, areas of the brain that might interfere with implementing this behavior must be inhibited. Thus, functional imaging might not be able to distinguish whether the observed changes are related to the neuronal assemblies mediating the behavior or to the neurons inhibiting other neuronal assemblies. Hence, interpretation of functional images is often problematic and needs to be confirmed by convergent evidence using other techniques.

COMPUTATIONAL MODELS

The function of the brain is thought to depend principally upon the firing patterns of numerous highly interrelated neurons. This assumption has naturally led to the attempt to describe brain function in terms of computer function, but the typical serially organized computer has not fared well as a model for brain function. Computers that use multiple parallel processors arranged in a network (parallel distributed processors, or PDP networks) have interesting "brainlike" properties, including the ability, without further programming, to "learn" associations between coincident stimuli, to behave as if "rules" are learned despite being exposed only to data, and to continue to function in the face of damage to a portion of the network ("graceful degradation") (Rumelhart et al., 1986). Properties of PDP networks are now often invoked to help explain the nature of neuropsychological deficits occasioned by brain injury, such as interlanguage differences in error rates in aphasics.

Although the brain is highly interconnected, it is not considered to function as a single network, but rather as a collection of many overlapping "modular" networks, each having a specific function. The function of a module depends upon its connections. One can therefore see that network theory can easily be reconciled with the traditional methods of localization of brain function discussed above.

ANIMAL VERSUS HUMAN EXPERIMENTATION

Many of the techniques mentioned above are either not applicable to humans or can be applied only with great difficulty. In detailed anatomical studies, for instance, discrete brain lesions are made and the whole brain is studied meticulously soon after the operation. Other anatomical methods entail the injection of substances into the brain. Advances in neurochemistry and neurophysiology, like those in neuroanatomy, rely heavily on animal work. Despite major differences in anatomy between even the subhuman primates and humans (Fig. 1–2), much of this basic research is of direct relevance to human neurobiology. Behavioral studies in animals have also yielded a great deal of information, but the applicability of this information to the study of complex human behavior is not clear-cut. In 1950, nothing in the

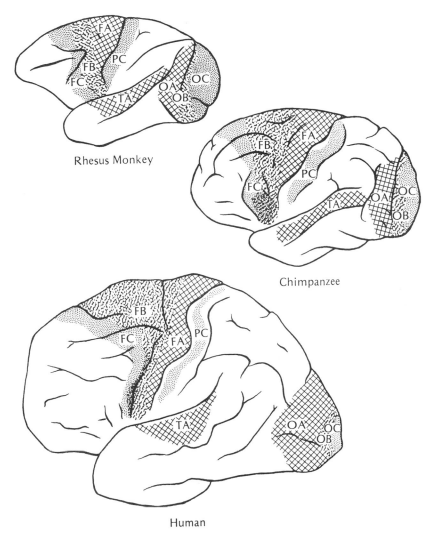

Rhesus Monkey

Chimpanzee

Human

Figure 1–2. The primary motor (FA) and visual (OC) areas and the association areas of the motor, visual, somatosensory (PC), and auditory (TA) systems are compared in these lateral views of the hemispheres of the monkey, chimpanzee, and human. Note the expansion of the unshaded areas of cortex, particularly in the frontal lobe and in the area between TA and OA, as one progresses from monkey to human. The latter area is important for language development (see Chapter 2). The significance of the frontal lobes is discussed in Chapter 15.

literature on temporal lobe lesions in animals would have led to the prediction that bilateral temporal lobectomy in humans would result in permanent impairment of memory; it took 20 years for new testing paradigms to be developed that demonstrated memory impairment in animals with bitemporal ablations (Mishkin, 1978). Conversely, the applicability of behavioral deficits in animals (and especially in nonhuman primates) to syndromes in humans has also recently been systematically investigated, and some parallels are discernible (Oscar-Berman et al., 1982). Studies of the limbic system and hypothalamus in animals have contributed important information about the relevance of these structures to emotional behavior; however, the emotional content of behavior is difficult to study in animals that cannot report how they feel. Most obviously, animals cannot be used to study behavior that is uniquely human, such as language. Studies of nonlinguistic communication in animals may relate to some aspects of speech in humans but they do not elucidate the neural mechanisms underlying language. Studies of linguistic behavior in primates are controversial, and their relevance to the study of language in humans remains unclear.

CONCEPTUAL ANALYSIS

We hear that science proceeds by way of careful observation followed by analysis and then hypothesis on the basis of the observed data (a posteriori hypothesis). In fact, meaningful observations frequently cannot be made without some sort of a priori hypothesis. How else can one decide which observations to make? An observation can be significant only in terms of a conceptual framework.

Some investigators are loathe to put either a priori or posteriori hypotheses in print, feeling that they are too tentative. They report observations with a minimum of interpretation. This may be unfortunate because tentative hypotheses are the seeds of further observations and hypotheses. Other investigators speculate extensively on the basis of only a few observations. These speculations may lead to clearly stated hypotheses that generate further observations, but there is a risk that observations may be honestly and inadvertently distorted to fit the hypotheses. For example, investigators discard "irrelevant" information either intentionally or not; however, an investigator with an alternative hypothesis may find observations presumed irrelevant by others to be of critical importance. It is important to deal with all hypotheses as though they were tentative so that, as Head (1926) warned, we do not invite observations to sleep in the Procrustean bed of our hypotheses.

We are too far from understanding brain–behavior relationships to be able to state hypotheses entirely without the use of metaphorical terms. Diagrams, for example, may be used in a metaphorical way to present a hypothesis. The diagrams found in this book are offered in this spirit: they should not be taken literally. They are meant to be not pictures of the brain, but sketches of hypotheses.

Similarly, when we speak of the function of different areas of the brain, it often appears that we assume that the area under discussion operates entirely independently from other areas. Clearly, this is true only to a limited extent. For the purposes of analysis, however, we must often ignore interactions between brain regions to discuss the distinguishing features of these areas. We do not deny that consideration of the brain as a functioning whole may at times be of equal value in explaining behavioral data, as it is in explaining the concept of diaschisis.

Thus, we support a flexible approach to the study of brain–behavior relationships. We know too little about the subject to limit our methods of investigation. We must be prepared to analyze data from many sources and make new hypotheses and test them with the best methods available. Similarly, behavioral testing and methods of treatment must be tailored to the individual situation. Inflexible test batteries, although necessary for obtaining normative data, limit our view of the nervous system if used exclusively. Rigid formulations of therapy similarly limit progress. Changes in testing and therapy, however, should not be made capriciously but rather according to our current understanding of brain–behavior relationships. In this book, therefore, we do not emphasize standardized tests or treatment batteries; instead, we present the existing knowledge on brain–behavior relationships, which should form the basis of diagnosis and treatment.

REFERENCES

Bastian, H. C. (1869). On the various forms of loss of speech in cerebral disease. *Br. Foreign Medico-Surg. Rev.* 43:470–492.

Bouillaud, J. B. (1825). Récherches cliniques propres a démontrer que la perte de la parole correspond à la lésion de lobules anterieurs du cerveau, et à confirmer l'opinion de M. Gall sur le siege de l'organe du langage articulé. *Arch. Gen. Med.* 8:25–45.

Broca, P. (1865). Sur la faculté du langage articulé. *Bull. Soc. Anthropol. Paris* 6:337–393.

Caramazza, A. (1992). Is cognitive neuropsychology possible? *J. Cogn. Neurosci.* 4:80–95.

Chomsky, N. (1967). The general properties of language. In *Brain Mechanisms Underlying Speech and Language*, C. H. Millikan and F. L. Darley (eds.). New York: Grune and Stratton, pp. 73–88.

D'Esposito, M. (2000). Functional neuroimaging in cognition. *Semin. Neurol.* 20:487–498.

Geschwind, N. (1965). Disconnexion syndrome in animals and men. I and II. *Brain* 88:237–294, 585–644.

Head, H. (1926). *Aphasia and Kindred Disorders of Speech*. Cambridge, UK: Cambridge University Press.

Lashley, K. S. (1938). Factors limiting recovery after central nervous lesions. *J. Nerv. Ment. Dis.* 888:733–755.

Lichtheim, L. (1885). On aphasia. *Brain* 7:433–484.

Mazziotta, J. C. (2000). Imaging: window on the brain. *Arch. Neurol.* 57:1413–1421.

Mishkin, M. (1978). Memory in monkeys severely impaired by combined but not by separate removal of amygdala and hippocampus. *Nature* 273:297–298.

Nadeau, S.E., and Crosson, B. (1995). A guide to the functional imaging of cognitive processes. *Neuropsychiatry Neuropsychol. Behav. Neurol.* 8:143–162.

Oscar-Berman, M., Zola-Morgan, S. M., Oberg, R. G. E., and Bonner, R. T. (1982). Comparative neuropsychology and Korsakoff's syndrome. III: Delayed response, delayed alternation and DRL performance. *Neuropsychologia* 20:187–202.

Rumelhart, D. E., McClelland, J. L., and the PDP Research Group (1986). *Parallel Distributed Processing. Explorations in the Microstructure of Cognition*. Cambridge, MA: MIT Press.

Teuber, H. L. (1955). Physiological psychology. *Annu. Rev. Psychol.* 6:267–296.

Wernicke, C. (1874). *Der Aphasische Symptomenkomplex*. Breslau: Cohn and Weigart.

2

Aphasic Syndromes

DAVID CAPLAN

Webster's Dictionary defines a syndrome as "a number of symptoms occurring together and characterizing a particular disease." Most people would agree that these two features—symptoms that occur together, and symptoms that characterize a particular disease—are the basic features of a medical syndrome. For instance, the symptoms of cold intolerance, lethargy, deepening of the voice, large tongue, pericardial effusion, carpal tunnel entrapment, and lowered body temperature form (part of) a syndrome. They are all related to disease of a single organ, and they all respond to the same treatment.

Not all the symptoms of a syndrome occur in every individual who has the disease. Not all patients with disease of the organ responsible for the symptoms listed above have all the symptoms on the list. There are individual differences in the occurrence of the features of a syndrome across the population, and understanding the reasons for these differences is an important part of understanding the syndrome.

Moreover, there are many symptoms that co-occur with those that constitute a syndrome but that are not part of the syndrome. Many patients with disease of the organ responsible for the symptoms listed above have headaches,

but headaches are not recognized as a part of the syndrome. This is not just because a lot of people who don't have the disease causing these symptoms have headaches, since a lot of people who don't have the disease that causes these symptoms can have symptoms on the list. The most important reason that headaches are not part of the syndrome in question is that they do not pattern with these symptoms. There is no clear pathogenetic link between them and the disease that causes these symptoms, and they do not respond to the same treatment.

The disease refered to is hypothyroidism. As the example of hypothyroidism shows, a syndrome does useful work. It relates symptoms functionally, explains individual variability in symptom occurrence, excludes symptoms that co-occur with those in the syndrome that are not functionally related to those in the syndrome, and predicts natural history. Neurologists and Speech-Language Pathologists often describe language-impaired patients as having one of a number of *aphasic syndromes*, such as Broca's aphasia, Wernicke's aphasia and conduction aphasia. We shall see whether the aphasic syndromes have similar characteristics.

CLASSICAL APHASIC SYNDROMES

The aphasic syndromes were first postulated in 1885 by Lichtheim, who built upon prior work, especially studies by Broca (1861) and Wernicke (1874). We begin with a discussion of these three studies.

Broca (1861) described a patient, Leborgne, with a severe speech output disturbance: Leborgne 's speech was limited to the monsyllable "tan." In contrast, Broca described Leborgne's ability to understand spoken language and to express himself through gestures and facial expressions, as well as his understanding of nonverbal communication, as normal. Broca claimed that Leborgne had lost "the faculty of articulate speech." Broca related this impairment to damage of neural tissue; Leborgne's brain contained a lesion whose center was in the posterior portion of the inferior frontal convolution of the left hemisphere. The lesion extended posteriorly into the parietal lobe. Broca related the most severe part of the lesion to the expressive language impairment. This area became known as "Broca's area." Broca argued that it was the neural site of the mechanism involved in speech production.

Over the ensuing years, many other cases of language impairments were described. In some, speech impairments were related to lesions in the left frontal lobe; other speech impairments were associated with more posterior lesions. In 1874, Wernicke published a paper that appeared to reconcile many of these different findings. He described a patient with a speech disturbance, but one that was very different from that seen in Leborgne. Wernicke's patient was fluent; her speech, however, contained words with sound errors, other errors of word forms, and words that were semantically inappropriate. Also, unlike Leborgne, Wernicke's patient did not understand spoken language. Wernicke related the two impairments—that of speech production and that of comprehension—by arguing that the patient had sustained damage to "the storehouse of auditory word forms." Under these conditions, speech would be expected to contain the types of errors that were seen in this case, and comprehension would be affected. Establishing the

location of the lesion in this case was more problematic, however, as Wernicke did not have the opportunity to perform an autopsy on this patient. He did examine the brain of a second patient, however, whose language had been described by her physician in terms that made Wernicke think she had had a set of symptoms that were the same as those seen in his case. The lesion in this second patient occupied the posterior portion of the first temporal gyrus, also on the left. Wernicke suggested that this region, which came to be known as "Wernicke's area," was the locus of the "storehouse of auditory word forms."

Wernicke's paper was the first to describe an aphasic syndrome, in the sense of a constellation of symptoms. He had found two deficits—fluent paraphasic speech and poor auditory comprehension—and he related them both to a single functional abnormality: abnormal representations of the sound patterns of words. If he was right, these two symptoms ought to pattern together: they ought to improve naturally at similar rates, respond favorably to effective treatments, and worsen in response to the same aggravating conditions such as fatigue or distraction.

Wernicke went a step beyond relating the symptoms he saw in his patient to a single underlying deficit. He related them to the location of the lesion that he thought produced this deficit, in the area of the brain adjacent to the primary auditory cortex (Heschl's gyrus). It made sense to Wernicke that a lesion in this location would affect the long-term storage of the sounds of words, because he thought that auditory stimuli were processed in a special ways (e.g., as language) in the areas of cortex just adjacent to the primary auditory cortex. Wernicke also noted that Broca's area, in which a lesion was thought to produce an impairment of motor speech, was adjacent to the motor cortex. He developed the germ of the general theory that receptive aspects of language processing are localized adjacent to primary sensory cortex and output language processes are adjacent to primary motor cortex. The permanent storage of the sounds of words in a receptive area of the brain was due to children first hearing, and only later producing, the words of their language.

Broca and Wernicke thus gave us the three fundamental principles that underlie the classical aphasic syndromes:

1. Language processors are localized (Broca, 1861).
2. Diverse language symptoms can be due to an underlying deficit in a single language processor (Wernicke, 1874).
3. Language processors are localized in brain regions because of the relationship of the processor to sensory or motor functions (Wernicke, 1874).

It remained for Lichtheim to apply these three principles to a wider range of symptoms. Lichtheim recognized seven syndromes (excluding those that affected reading and writing, which are not dealt with here):

1. *Broca's aphasia:* a severe expressive language disturbance reducing the fluency of speech in all tasks (repetition and reading as well as speaking) and affecting elements of language such as grammatical words and morphological endings, without an equally severe disturbance of auditory comprehension
2. *Wernicke's aphasia:* the combination of fluent speech with erroneous choices of the sounds of words (phonemic paraphasias) and an auditory comprehension disturbance
3. *Pure motor speech disorders:* anarthria, dysarthria, and apraxia of speech: output speech disorders due to motor disorders, in which speech is misarticulated but comprehension is preserved
4. *Pure word deafness:* a disorder in which the patient does not recognize spoken words, but spontaneous speech is normal
5. *Transcortical motor aphasia:* a disorder in which spontaneous speech is reduced but repetition is intact
6. *Transcortical sensory aphasia:* a disorder in which a comprehension disturbance exists without a disturbance of repetition
7. *Conduction aphasia:* a disturbance in spontaneous speech and repetition, con-

sisting of fluent paraphasic speech, without a disturbance in auditory comprehension.

These syndromes are listed in Table 2–1.

Lichtheim argued that these syndromes followed lesions in regions of the brain as depicted in schematic form in Figure 2–1. Before discussing Lichtheim's schema for relating these syndromes to these lesions, however, we need to mention two more aspects of Lichtheim's model. The first is that Lichtheim made the assumption that the meaning of words resided in the superior portion of the parietal lobe, indicated as *C*, for *Concepts*, in Figure 2–1. The second is that he assumed, and then justified on the basis of cases he described, that in speech production word meanings activated both word sounds in Wernicke's area and the motor speech planning mechanism in Broca's area, hence the two arrows originating in the Concept Center (*C*) in Figure 2–1.

With this background, Lichtheim's linking of the seven syndromes to lesion sites is quite straightforward. Broca's aphasia, which affects expressive language alone, is due to lesions in Broca's area, the center for motor speech planning adjacent to the motor strip. Wernicke's aphasia follows lesions in Wernicke's area that disturb the representations of word sounds. Pure motor speech disorders arise from lesions interrupting the motor pathways from the cortex to the brainstem nuclei that control the articulatory system. These disorders differ from Broca's aphasia in that they are not linguistic; they affect articulation itself, not the planning of speech. Pure word deafness affects the transmission of sound input into Wernicke's area. It therefore disrupts word recognition but not speech, since words themselves are intact and accessible for speech production purposes. Transcortical motor aphasia results from the interruption of the pathway from the Concept Center to Broca's area. This affects speech, but not repetition or comprehension. Transcortical sensory aphasia follows lesions between Wernicke's area and the concept center; repetition of words is intact, but comprehension is affected. Finally Conduction aphasia follows

Table 2–1. Aphasic Syndromes Described by Lichtheim (1885)

Syndrome	Clinical Manifestations	Hypothetical Deficit	Classical Lesion Location
Broca's aphasia	Major disturbance in speech production with sparse, halting speech; words, often misarticulated; frequently missing function words and bound morphemes	Disturbances in the speech planning and production mechanisms	Posterior aspects of the 3rd frontal convolution (Broca's area)
Wernicke's aphasia	Major disturbance in auditory comprehension; fluent speech with disturbances of sounds and structures of words (phonemic, morphological, and semantic paraphasias); poor repetition and naming	Disturbances of the permanent representations the sound structures of words	Posterior half of the first temporal gyrus and possibly adjacent cortex (Wernicke's area)
Pure motor speech disorder	Disturbance of articulation; apraxia of speech, dysarthria, anarthria, aphemia	Disturbance of artculatory mechanisms	Outflow tracts from motor cortex
Pure word deafness	Disturbance of spoken word comprehension; repetition often impaired	Failure to access spoken words	Input tracts from auditory system to Wernicke's area
Transcortical motor aphasia	Disturbance of spontaneous speech similar to Broca's aphasia with relatively preserved repetition; comprehension relatively preserved	Disconnection between conceptual representations of words and sentences and the motor speech production system	White matter tracts deep to Broca's area connecting it to parietal lobe
Transcortical sensory aphasia	Disturbance in single word comprehension with relatively intact repetition	Disturbance in activation of word meanings despite normal recognition of auditorily presented words	White matter tracts connecting parietal lobe to temporal lobe or portions of inferior parietal lobe
Conduction aphasia	Disturbance of repetition and spontaneous speech (phonemic paraphasias)	Disconnection between the sound patterns of words and the speech production mechanism	Lesion in the arcuate fasciculus and/or cortico-cortical connections between Wernicke's and Broca's areas

from a lesion between Wernicke's area and Broca's area. Repetition is affected, but comprehension is intact. Speech is also affected, in the same way as in Wernicke's aphasia, because the sound patterns of words, though activated, are not transmitted properly to Broca's area to plan speech.

These syndromes have had a checkered history. They have been criticized on neuroanatomical grounds (Marie, 1906; Moutier, 1908), dismissed as simplifications of reality that are only of help to schoolboys (Head, 1926), and ignored in favor of different approaches to language (Jackson, 1878; Goldstein, 1948). Nonetheless they have endured. Benson and Geschwind (1971) reviewed the major approaches to aphasia as they saw them, and concluded that all researchers recognized the same basic patterns of aphasic impairments, despite using different nomenclature.

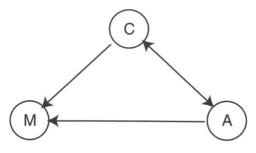

Figure 2–1. The classical Connectionist model (from Lichtheim, 1885). *A* represents the auditory center for the long-term storage of word sounds. *M* represents the motor center for speech planning. *C* represents the concept center. Information flow is indicated by arrows.

Lichtheim's seven original syndromes have been amplified. Three more syndromes have been added by theorists such as Benson (1979), and Lichtheim's model has been rounded out with specific hypotheses about the neuroanatomical bases for several functions that he could only guess at. The three additional syndromes described by Benson (1979) are anomia, global aphasia, and isolation of the speech area. The symptoms and related neural localizations are shown in Table 2–2. Additional neuroanatomical foundation was first suggested in a very influential paper by Geschwind (1965), who argued that the inferior parietal lobe was a tertiary association cor-

tical area that received projections from the association cortex immediately adjacent to the primary visual, auditory, and somesthetic cortices in the occipital, temporal, and parietal lobes. Because of these anatomical connections, the inferior parietal lobe served as a cross-modal association region, associating word sounds with the sensory qualities of objects. This underlay word meaning, in Geschwind's view. Damasio and Tranel (1993) extended this model to actions, arguing that associations between word sounds and memories of actions were created in the association cortex in the inferior frontal lobe. Geschwind (1965) and Damasio and Damasio (1980) also argued that the anatomical link between Wernicke's and Broca's areas (in which a lesion caused conduction aphasia) was the white matter tract known as the "arcuate fasciculus." These extensions and clarifications of Lichtheim's model are shown in Figure 2–2.

These syndromes have defined the domain of aphasia as a description of performances in the usual tasks of language use—speaking, understanding spoken language, reading and writing—in terms of the linguistic elements—words, sounds of words, word endings, classes of words such as function words—that are produced, recognized, or understood. This approach contrasts with other approaches to the description of aphasia. Jackson, Head, Goldstein, and other pioneers in aphasiology concentrated on the conditions under which lan-

Table 2–2. Additional Classical Aphasic Syndromes

Syndrome	Clinical Manifestations	Hypothetical Deficit	Classical Lesion Location
Anomic aphasia	Disturbance in the production of single words, most marked for common nouns; intact comprehension and repetition	Disturbances of concepts and/or of the sound patterns of words	Inferior parietal lobe or connections between parietal lobe and temporal lobe; can follow many lesions
Global aphasia	Major disturbance in all language functions	Disruption of all language-processing components	Large portion of the perisylvian association cortex
Isolation of the language zone	Disturbance of both spontaneous speech (sparce, halting speech) and comprehension, with some preservation of repetition; echolalia is common	Disconnection between concepts and both representations of word sounds and speech production mechanism	Cortex just outside the perisylvian association cortex

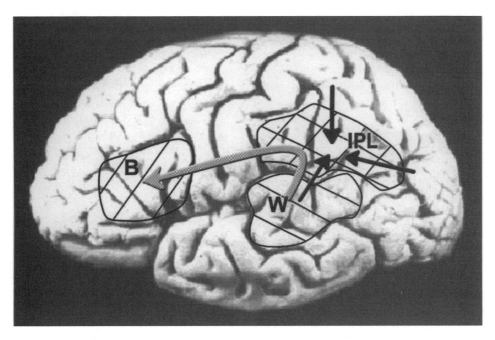

Figure 2–2. The version of the classical model developed by Geschwind (1982). The major addition is that the Concept Center is eliminated and the inferior parietal lobe (IPL) is identified as the locus of associations between word forms and sensory properties W is Wernicke's area; B is Broca's area.

guage is used. In a famous paper, Hughlings Jackson described a patient, a carpenter, who was mute but who mustered up the capacity to say "Master's" in response to his son's question about where his tools were. Jackson's poignant comments convey his emphasis on the conditions that provoke speech, rather than on the form of the speech itself:

The father had left work; would never return to it; was away from home; his son was on a visit, and the question was directly put to the patient. Anyone who saw the abject poverty the poor man's family lived in would admit that these tools were of immense value to them. Hence we have to consider as regards this and other occassional utterances the strength of the accompanying emotional state. (Jackson, 1878, p. 181)

Goldstein (1948) was concerned about whether patients, both those with and those without aphasia, were capable of abstracting away from the immediacy of a situation to consider longer-term goals—a capacity he called the ability to assume "the abstract attitude."

Both Jackson and Goldstein sought a description of language use as a function of mo-

tivational and intellectual states, and tried to describe aphasic disturbances of language in relation to the factors that drive language production and make for depth of comprehension. This is surely a vital aspect of understanding language impairments. In many ways it is more humanly relevant than a description of language impairments that focuses on which phonemes are produced in spontaneous speech or repetition. Unfortunately, Jackson and Goldstein's approach is a very intractable goal, both in terms of psychological descriptions and in terms of relating these specific motivational states to the brain. Wernicke, Lichtheim, Geschwind, and the researchers who conceived and developed the framework of the classical syndromes focused aphasiology on the description of the linguistic representations and psycholinguistic operations that are responsible for everyday language use.

The three and a half decades since publication of Geschwind's paper have brought new evidence for these syndromes and their relationships to brain lesions. Aphasic syndromes have been related to the brain using a series of neuroimaging techniques—first T^{99} scanning, then computed tomography (CT), magnetic resonance (MR), and positron emission tomography (PET). All have confirmed the relationship of the major syndromes to lesion locations. Broca's aphasia is associated with anterior lesions; Wernicke's aphasia is associated with posterior lesions, centered in the temporal–parietal juncture (Hayward et al., 1977; Naeser and Hayward, 1978; Kertesz, 1979; Naeser, 1989). Pure motor deficits of speech are associated with subcortical lesions (Schiff et al., 1983; Alexander et al., 1987; Naeser et al., 1989). Pure word deafness is associated with lesions in the auditory association areas and surrounding white matter tracts, often bilaterally (Denes and Semenza, 1975; Auerbach et al., 1982; Coslett et al., 1984; Metz-Lutz and Dahl, 1984). Transcortical motor aphasia and transcortical sensory aphasia are associated with watershed infarcts between the anterior and middle cerebral arteries (transcortical motor aphasia; Freedman et al., 1984) and between the middle and posterior cerebral arteries (transcortical sensory aphasia; Kertesz et al., 1982). Conduction aphasia is associated with smaller lesions that often appear to affect the arcuate fasciculus (Damasio and Damasio, 1980). When the lesioned brain is imaged by PET, which is sensitive to metabolic, as opposed to its structural abnormalities, damage following stroke is seen to be more widespread and the relationships between syndromes and lesion are less obvious, but even then these relationships are discernable (Metter et al., 1983, 1984, 1986, 1988, 1989, 1990, 1992; Kempler et al, 1988, 1991).

Concepts of how the brain is organized have changed considerably since 1965, let alone since 1885. Neuroscientists no longer use the term "center." Instead, they talk about "systems neuroscience" in which there are "distributed large-scale neurocognitive nets" with "functional specializations" (Mesulam, 1990). There are new models to explain how the elements in the brain accomplish computations (Rumelhart and MacClelland, 1986). There are new classifications of types of cortex (Mesulam, 1998). But despite these changes in both terminology and in our ability to model language processing, the central idea that underlies the classical syndromes—that the brain supports complex psychological functions through a set of connected areas, each related to a set of cognitive operations—is ubiquitous in cognitive neuroscience. Although the term "center" is anathema, the essence of the concept is alive and well and constantly applied, in other terms, to the aphasias. Recent reviews of aphasia in leading medical journals (e.g., Damasio, 1992), while acknowledging the changes in neuroscience, retain the aphasic syndromes and their relationships to the brain.

Besides their localizing value, the syndromes also have prognostic significance. Kertesz and McCabe (1977) have shown that Wernicke's aphasia tends to resolve toward either conduction aphasia or anomia, and global aphasia toward Broca's aphasia. The relation between lesion site and recovery in specific syndromes has been charted (Kertesz et al., 1979, 1993). If we return to the original Webster definition ("a number of symptoms occurring together and characterizing a particular disease") and the requirement that a syndrome be a useful category, and ask if the classical syndromes are a success, the answer is certainly "yes."

Nonetheless, these classical aphasic syndromes are under attack. The dissatisfaction many researchers feel toward these syndromes comes from several quarters. One problem lies with the level of description of language and language functioning that they present. A related problem is that they do not cover all patients' symptoms well. A third problem is that there are many exceptions to the patterns of localization they hypothesize. A fourth is related to the utility of these syndromes in developing approaches to therapy. We shall review these issues in turn.

PROBLEMS WITH THE CLASSICAL APHASIC SYNDROMES

A major limitation of the classical syndromes is that they stay at arm's length from the linguistic details of language impairments. The classical aphasic syndromes basically reflect the relative ability of patients to perform entire language tasks (speaking, comprehension, etc.), not the integrity of specific operations within the language processing system. This is not to say that there are no linguistic or qualitative descriptions of language in the characterizations of the classical aphasic syndromes, but to point out that they are incomplete and unsystematic. For instance, the speech production problem seen in Broca's aphasia can consist of one or more of a large number of impairments. Benson and Geschwind (1971) describe Broca's aphasia as follows:

The language output of Broca's aphasia can be described as nonfluent. It is sparse, dysprosodic, and poorly articulated; it is made up of very short phrases and it is produced with effort, particularly in initiation of speech. The output consists primarily of substantive words, i.e., nouns, action verbs, or significant modifiers. The pattern of short phrases lacking prepositions is often termed "telegraphic speech." . . . Comprehension of spoken language is much better than speech but varies, being completely normal in some cases and moderately disturbed in others. (p. 7)

The abnormalities that determine that a patient is a Broca's aphasic are only related to each other at a very general level of description of the language-processing system—that of speech production. The definition of the syndrome ignores finer distinctions. For instance, the symptoms of "dysprosodic" speech, "poorly articulated" speech, and "short phrases lacking prepositions" are likely to reflect disturbances in the assignment of prosody, specifying the articulatory gestures for phonemes and construction of syntactic forms, respectively. If all we know about a patient is that he or she is a Broca's aphasic, we cannot tell which of these problems the patient has.

The heterogeneity of deficits across patients with the same syndrome is not limited to Broca's aphasia. Patients with Wernicke's aphasia can have deficits affecting either the sounds of words or their meanings or both, as well as any number of other language-processing deficits (Luria, 1947). There are at least two major deficits that underlie conduction aphasia, one affecting word production and one affecting verbal short-term memory (Shallice and Warrington, 1977). Schwartz (1984) pointed out that the actual application of the criteria used to classify aphasic patients into the classical syndromes has led to a grouping to-

gether of many patients with no symptoms in common. At the same time as patients with the same syndrome can have different deficits, identical deficits occur in different syndromes. For instance, certain types of naming problems can occur in any aphasic syndrome (Benson, 1979).

Because of these problems, the classical syndromes do not do a very good job of classifying many aphasic patients. In practice, most applications of the clinical taxonomy result in widespread disagreements over a patient's classification (Holland et al., 1986) and/or in a large number of "mixed" or "unclassifiable" cases (Lecours et al., 1983). The criteria for inclusion in a syndrome are often somewhat arbitrary: how bad must a patient's comprehension be for the patient to be considered Wernicke's aphasic instead of conduction aphasic, or a global aphasic instead of a Broca's aphasic? There have been many efforts to answer this question (see, e.g., Goodglass and Kaplan, 1972, 1982; Kertesz, 1979), but none is satisfactory. As an example, consider the patient whose scores on the Boston Diagnostic Aphasia Examination are shown in Figure 2–3. The patient does not fit the formal criteria set out by Goodglass and Kaplan for any syndrome.

The third problem that the classical aphasic syndromes face is that they are not as well correlated with lesion sites as the theory claims they should be. Several studies above found general correlations between lesion site and syndrome, but a closer look at those studies and at others reveals many discrepancies. First, virtually all studies exclude many types of lesions, such as various sorts of tumors, degenerative diseases, and others. The rule of thumb seems to be that the classical syndromes are only related to lesion sites in cases of rapidly developing lesions, such as stroke. Even with these types of lesions, the syndromes are never applied to acute and subacute phases of the illness. But the situation is worse than that. In the chronic phase of diseases such as stroke, at least 15% of patients have lesions that are not predictable from their syndromes (Basso et al., 1985), and some researchers think this number is much higher—as high as 40% or more, depending on what counts as an exception to the rule (de Bleser, 1988). Also, we now know

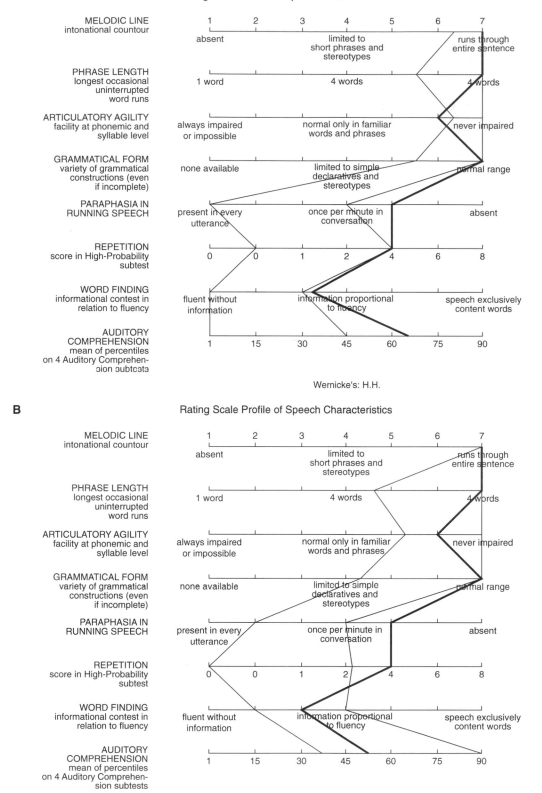

Figure 2–3. Performance of patient H.H. (dark line) on the Boston Diagnostic Aphasia Examination, compared to the range of performances associated with Wernicke's (*A*), conduction (*B*), and anomic (*C*) aphasia (within light lines).

C

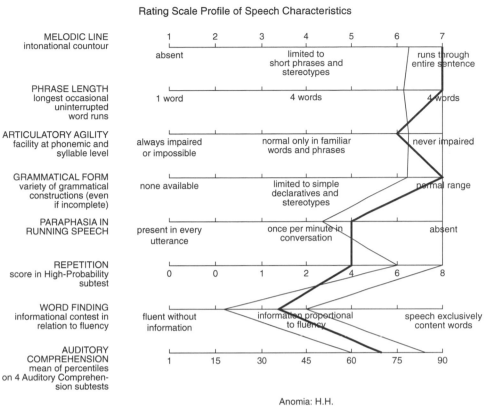

Figure 2–3. *Continued.*

that the relation between lesion location and syndrome is more complex than we had previously thought, even in cases where the classical localization captures part of the picture. Broca's aphasia, for instance, does not usually occur in the chronic state after lesions restricted to Broca's area, but requires much larger lesions (Mohr et al., 1978).

We said at the beginning of this chapter that a good syndrome can account for variability. The variability in lesion–deficit correlations is a challenge to the classical aphasic syndromes. One approach to explaining this variability without abandoning the syndromes is to look for individual differences in the brain regions that can take over language after a lesion occurs. Some of the factors that affect this process are partially understood. For instance, handedness affects lateralization of language, and it is likely that there is more ability of the right hemisphere to take over language functions after a lesion occurs in patients who are

not as strongly right-handed. Age affects recovery from lesions, with much better recovery seen in children than in adults and possibly some effect of age occurring within the adult life span. However, these factors do not explain all the observed variability. Lesions of similar size in similar locations can be associated with very different types and levels of impairments in patients with similar degrees of right-handedness, of similar ages, of the same sex, and with similar educational and socioeconomic backgrounds. The classical syndromes, and the model of language–brain relationships on which they are based, are missing something.

Some theorists have gone farther in their criticisms of the classical syndromes in the area of syndrome–lesion correlations. They have argued that the relationships between the classical syndromes and the locations of lesions are not due to the effects of brain lesions on language but to the effects of lesions in different locations on motor functions. In their view, the localizing value of the classical syndromes reflects the co-occurence of variable combinations of language-processing deficits with motor impairments that affect the fluency of speech (Caplan, 1987; McNeil and Kent, 1991). If a patient has many and/or severe language function deficits, the patient is either a global aphasic, if motor speech mechanisms are affected, or a Wernicke's aphasic, if motor speech mechanisms are not involved. If the patient has only a few and/or minor language function deficits, he or she has one of the "nonfluent" aphasias, such as Broca's aphasia, "aphemia," or transcortical motor aphasia, if there are motor speech impairments, or one of the minor "fluent" aphasias, such as anomia, conduction aphasia, or transcortical sensory aphasia, if there are no motor speech impairments. From this point of view, the localizing value of the classical syndromes is due to the invariant location of the motor system, while language processing components are themselves quite variable in their localization in different individuals. We shall return to this possibility after discussing a different approach to aphasic syndromes.

Finally, the classical syndromes offer very limited help to the clinician planning therapy. This is because they give insufficient information about what is wrong with a patient. For example, knowing that a patient has Broca's aphasia does not tell the therapist what aspects of speech, such as articulation of sound segments, prosody, production of grammatical elements, formulation of syntactic structures, need remediation. Nor does it guarantee that the patient does not need therapy for a comprehension problem; it only implies that any comprehension problem is mild relative to either other aphasics or to the patient's speech problem. Finally, it does not guarantee that the patient does not have other problems, such as anomia or difficulty reading. In practice, most clinicians do not believe that they have adequately described a patient's language problems when they have classified that patient as having one of the classic aphasic syndromes. Rather, they specify the nature of the disturbance found in the patient within each lan-

guage-related task; e.g., they indicate that a patient with Broca's aphasia is agrammatic, or has a mild anomia.

It is a feature of the history of science, and, some think, a tenet of the philosophy of science, that people do not abandon a theory because it has inadequacies. Some philosophers of science think that no theory is ever proven wrong. Theories are abandoned because people get tired of them, and they get tired of them because they develop theories that they think are better. This perspective on science applies to the classical aphasic syndromes as well. They have not been abandoned, but their acceptance is waning and new developments speak to some of their inadequacies. We now turn to these developments.

PSYCHOLINGUISTIC APPROACH TO APHASIC SYNDROMES

Many of the problems with the classical syndromes outlined above would be addressed, and possibly solved, if we described aphasic language impairments in terms of impairments of psycholinguistic operations rather than in terms of tasks. Researchers have included such descriptions in their accounts of syndromes since the beginning of the study of aphasia, but a true revision of the classical syndromes requires a thorough enumeration of all the psycholinguistic operations that are defective in a patient and a taxonomy of aphasic deficits in terms of such impairments. This approach can be seen as a natural extension of the approach that led to the classical syndromes, rather than as an entirely new direction. It adds to the classical approach a greater concern for the details of psycholinguistic processing, while essentially adopting the classical framework for the field as being the description of disorders in the tasks of speaking, auditory comprehension, reading, and writing.

Through the language code particular types of representations are connected to particular aspects of meaning. People use words to connect phonological units with items, actions, properties, and logical connections. In sentences words are related to each other in hier-

Table 2–3. Basic Levels of Language

Level	Form	Associated Semantic Values
Lexical	Words, consisting of sound units (phonemes) organized into higher-order structures (feet, syllables). Syllabic prominence is marked by stress or tone. Words have syntactic catgeories. *Open-class, content* words (noun, verb, adjective) accept new members. *Closed class, function* words (article, auxiliary, pronoun, etc.) are a fixed set.	Content words describe items, actions, or features. Function words make logical connections. Words are primarily denotative and related to categories.
Morphological	Words formed from other words by prefixes, suffixes, and infixes. Morphology can be inflectional or derivational.	Inflectional morphology indicates connections between words (e.g., agreement). Derivational morphology changes syntactic category (e.g., changes adjectives to nouns: *happy → happiness*). Declension, aspect and temporal markings, and other phenomena are also morphological in nature.
Sentential	Syntactic structures: hierarchically arranged sets of syntactic categories over which relations are defined (e.g., subject, object, c-command)	Semantic relations between words, such as thematic roles (agent, theme, beneficiary, etc.), attribution of modification, scope of quantification, etc. These "propositional" aspects of meaning describe events and states of affairs. Propositions can have truth values and be used to update semantic memory, to reason, and for other functions.
Discourse	Position in syntactic structures (e.g., first words play important roles in discourse). Intonational contrastive stress is used to indicate some semantic value.	Relationships between propositions—topic, focus, given information, temporal order, and causation. The intentions of the participants are given in the discourse. Some of these semantic features are provided by inferences that go beyond the verbatim content of the discourse.

archical syntactic structures to determine semantic relationships between them such as who is accomplishing or receiving an action. Table 2–3 attempts to systematically describe the levels of linguistic representations that are basic to language. Tables 2–4 and 2–5 and Figures 2–4 and 2–5 present models of how these forms are processed. Although Tables 2–3 through 2–5 and Figures 2–4 and 2–5 are highly simplified, they present the basic elements of language and the language-processing system.

There are many levels of detail at which one can describe language and language processing. Depending on the level of detail at which language impairments are described, there may be hundreds of primary language-processing impairments. For instance, we may recognize a disturbance of converting the sound waveform into linguistically relevant units of sound—acoustic-to-phonemic conversion—or we may recognize disturbances affecting the ability to recognize subsets of phonemes, such as vowels, consonants, stop consonants, fricatives, and nasals (Saffran et al., 1976). For many clinical purposes, an adequate way to approach a psycholinguistic taxonomy of aphasic impairments is at the level of detail that identifies language-processing impairments in terms of sets of related operations responsible for activating the major forms of the language code and their associated meanings in the usual language tasks

Table 2–4. Summary of Components of Language-Processing System for Simple Words

Component	Input	Operation	Output
Auditory–Oral Modality			
Input side			
Acoustic–phonetic processing	Acoustic waveform	Matches acoustic properties to phonetic features	Phonological segments (phonemes, allophones, syllables)
Auditory lexical access	Phonological units	Activates lexical items in long-term memory on basis of sound; selects best fit to stimulus	Phonological forms of words
Lexical semantic access	Words (represented as phonological forms)	Activates semantic features of words	Word meanings
Output side			
Phonological lexical access	Word meanings ("lemmas")	Activates the phonological forms of words	Phonological forms of words
Phonological output planning	Phonological forms of words (and non-words)	Activates detailed phonetic features of words (and non-words)	Phonetic values of phonological segments; word stress patterns
Articulatory planning	Phonetic values	Specifies articulatory movements	Neural commands for articulation

of speaking, comprehending auditorily presented language, writing, and reading. These levels of the language code are listed in Table 2–3. It needs to be recognized, however, that, for many research purposes and for some clinical purposes, a more detailed taxonomy of linguistic representations and operations is needed.

The psycholinguistic approach to aphasia differs from the classical syndrome approach in recognizing more levels of language. Most (though certainly not all) of the researchers and clinicians who developed the classical syndromes concentrated on single words. In the psycholinguistic approach there is equal concern for disorders of the processes through which words are formed from one another (morphology and compounding) and those through which sentences, syntactic structures, intonation contours, and aspects of discourse structure and meaning are formed or used. For instance, a great deal of attention has focused on deficits in the ability to use syntactic struc-

ture to determine aspects of sentence meaning (Caramazza and Zurif, 1976; Caplan et al., 1985, 1996; Caplan and Hildebrandt, 1988; Grodzinsky, 1990; Berndt et al, 1996), an area of aphasiology that was never discussed in the classical syndromes. Thus progress has been made toward solving the first problem that confronts the classical syndromes—the need for more detail about the psycholinguistic operations affected in a patient.

A second way in which the psycholinguistic approach to aphasia differs from the classical syndromic approach is related to the first difference. In the classical approach to syndromes, each patient has to be classified into one and only one syndrome; a patient cannot be a conduction aphasic and a Wernicke's aphasic at the same time. In the psycholinguistic approach, a patient may have—indeed, is likely to have—more than one deficit. A patient can have an output disorder affecting one aspect of processing and a completely unrelated disturbance of reading. Thus the second major

Table 2–5. Summary of Components of Language-Processing System for Derived Words and Sentences (Collapsed over Auditory–Oral and Written Modalities)

Component	Input	Operation	Output
Processing Affixed Words			
Input side			
Morphological analysis	Word forms	Segments words into structural (morphological) units; activates syntactic features of words	Morphological structure; syntactic features
Morphological comprehension	Word meaning; morphological structure	Combines word roots and affixes	Meanings of morphologically complex words
Output side			
Accessing affixed words from semantics	Word meanings; syntactic features	Activates forms of affixes and function words	Forms of affixes and function words
Sentence-Level Processing			
Input side			
Lexico-inferential comprehension	Meanings of simple and complex words;	Infers aspects of sentence meaning on basis of pragmatic plausibility world knowledge	Aspects of propositional meaning (thematic roles; attribution of modifiers)
Parsing and syntactic comprehension	Word meanings; syntactic features	Constructs syntactic representation and combines it with word meanings	Aspects of propositional meaning
Heuristic sentence comprehension	Syntactic categories of words	Constructs simplified syntactic structures; combines word meanings in these structures	Aspects of propositional meaning
Output side			
Construction of functional level representation	Messages	Activates content words; assigns thematic roles and other aspects of propositional meaning	Content words; thematic roles; other aspects of propositional meaning
Construction of positional level representation	Content words, syntactic frames, discourse features	Activates syntactic frames in conjunction with function words; inserts phonological forms of content words into syntactic frames	Surface forms of sentences
Phonological output planning	Surface forms of sentences	Combines lexical phonological and sentence-level phonological information	Phonetic values; stress and intonation

problem with the classical syndromes, the difficulty in fitting many patients into a single syndrome. This problem essentially evaporates.

We may pose the question of what constitutes a "syndrome" in this approach, if by "syndrome" we mean "a number of symptoms occurring together and characterizing a particular disease." The answer is that disturbances of some components of the language processing system have a number of functional consequences. For instance, most models of word sound production postulate a "phonological output lexicon" in which the sounds of words are represented, and a "phonological output

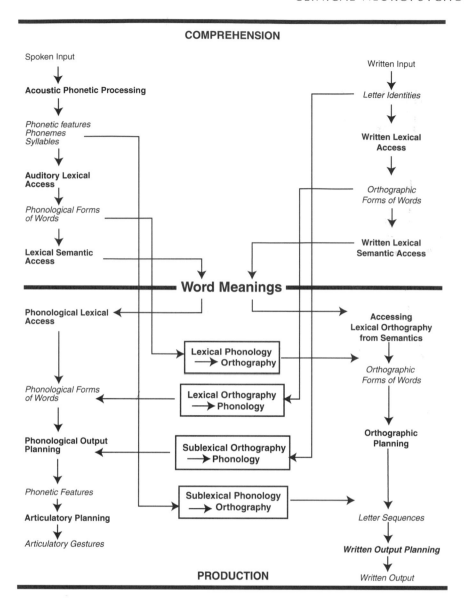

Figure 2–4. Diagrammatic representation of the sequence of activation of components of the processing system for single words. Processing components are presented in boldface; representations are presented in italics. Arrows represent the flow of information (representations) from one processing component to another.

buffer" in which these sounds are used to plan articulatory gestures (see Fig. 2–4). Both these components are needed because the way in which a word is pronounced varies as a function of context while the permanent representation of the sound of a word presumably does not. The phonological output lexicon only deals with words, whereas the phonological output buffer is used for all speech production, including repeating and reading nonwords. A dis-

turbance of the phonological output buffer would result in phonemic errors in all speech production tasks—spontaneous speech, object naming, repetition, and reading—and would affect both words and nonwords. This "syndrome" of the phonological output buffer has been described in many patients (see, e.g., Caplan and Waters, 1995). Disorders of the phonological output lexicon would only affect the activation of words from their meanings as

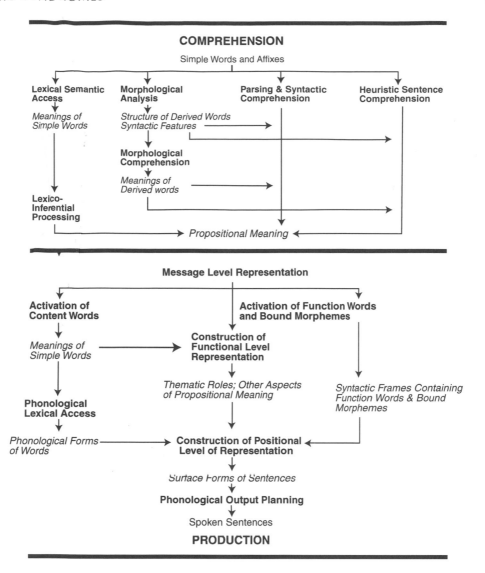

Figure 2–5. Diagrammatic representation of the sequence of operation of components of the language processing system for morphologically complex words and sentences. Processing components are presented in boldface; repre-sentations are presented in italics. Arrows represent the flow of information (representations) from one processing component to another.

in spontaneous speech, naming objects, and providing words from definitions, because both words and nonwords can gain access to the phonological output buffer through a nonlexi-cal route in repetition and reading, as shown in Figure 2–4.

The psycholinguistic approach requires de-tailed study of individual patients to identify their deficits. This has led researchers to use new tasks, some of which are not part of the usual use of language, such as repetition and reading aloud of nonwords. For example, the model in Figure 2–4 would predict that a pa-tient with a disturbance of the phonological output buffer would be able to activate the sounds of words from their meanings, even if the patient could not produce them correctly. Therefore, such a patient should be able to say whether the words for two pictures were the same, a task called "picture homophone match-ing." This is a very useful task for analyzing the speech production disorders seen in aphasia that emerges from the psycholinguistic lab, not from a study of everyday language use. There are also many psycholinguistic tasks that use reaction times as dependent variables (lexical priming, word monitoring, timed judgments of grammaticality or plausibility) that have been helpful in studying aphasic patients. These tasks are particularly useful in describing patients' "on-line" language processing of language—the unconscious processes that go on when subjects speak and comprehend speech. The use of these techniques has shown that some patients retain abilities that would not be suspected through consideration of their performances on standard tasks. For instance, use of priming tasks, in which subjects respond to a word faster if it has been preceded by a semantically related word, has shown that some Wernicke's aphasics retain at least some knowledge of the meanings of words, despite not being able to demonstrate such knowledge on word–picture matching tasks (Milberg and Blumstein, 1981; Blumstein et al., 1982). These findings provide new information that radically changes our ideas about what is wrong with such patients. The importance of this additional information extends beyond characterizing a patient's deficit and therefore being able to fit that patient into a category of aphasia. It is relevant to the issues of localization and therapy as well.

In the psycholinguistic approach to aphasia, the problem of localization of language is addressed by attempting to determine the location of the various language processors. In this enterprise, information from deficit–lesion correlations is used: the deficits are defined in terms of language processing components, not syndromes. It also relies on changes in hemodynamic responses to language processing as measured by PET and functional magnetic resonance imaging (fMRI), electro- and magnetoencephalographic correlates of language processing (evoked response potentials [ERP] and magnetoencephalographic [MEG] studies), direct activation and recording from cortex, and transcranial cortical stimulation. One major advantage of approaching aphasia in terms of deficits in language-processing operations is that it allows the study of aphasia to make contact with this increasingly rich literature in a way that studying the classical syndromes cannot.

By identifying the neural localization of language processing operations, researchers could explain the variability in the relationship of lesion sites to the classical syndromes. If each language processor is localized in a different region of the brain, variability in the lesion sites associated with the classical syndromes may be related to the variability of deficits found across patients with the same syndrome, which we discussed above. However, there is very good evidence that the picture is far more complex. First, many modern studies have identified areas of the brain outside the traditional language area in the perisylvian association cortex as being important to language (e.g., the inferior temporal lobe; see Damasio et al., 1996). This requires some revision of the classical models, though perhaps not revisions that are beyond the spirit of those models. More important is the fact that many studies point to some degree of individual variability in the localization of specific language processing components (see Caplan, 1987; Howard, 1995, for discussion). A psycholingusitically based theory cannot explain such variability any better than the theory on which the classical syndromes are based can, but it differs from the classical theory in that it doesn't have to!

The classical model ties the relationship of language-processing components to sensory and motor areas of the brain, via the functional relationship of language functions to sensory and motor processes. There is no obvious reason that these relationships should vary across individuals. In contrast, in the psycholinguistic approach, language is seen as an abstract code, and language processing as a correspondingly abstract set of operations, and is not placed in the Procrustean bed in which the marriage between language processors and sensory-motor functions is consummated in the classical theory. Variability in localization of language processors, if it exists, though still a challenge for any theory, is thus easier to accomodate in a psycholinguistic approach than in the classical framework.

The psycholinguistic approach also addresses the last problem we discussed for the classical syndromes—use of the description of aphasia that is generated by a diagnostic taxonomy for planning therapy. When aphasic disturbances are characterized as disorders of particular linguistic representations in the tasks of speaking and comprehension, the therapist has something to work on. This is only one step toward developing effective therapy programs. Many patients have multiple impairments, and the therapist must decide which of these are important to address in any individual patient. To plan therapy rationally, diagnosis must be coupled with knowledge about the natural history of impairments and their responses to therapy, as it is very likely that some impairments improve on their own more than others or are particularly resistant to therapy, at least in certain cases. The clinician must decide when to abandon a direct effort to ameliorate a disorder in favor of trying to bypass it with other functions, such as in the use of augmentative communication systems. There are a variety of ways to undertake therapy of most deficits. Characterizing a patient's deficits in psycholinguistic terms does, however, start the process of planning therapeutic interventions.

The newly developing psycholinguistic approach is far from perfect. It does not attempt to deal with the issues that were raised by Jackson, Head, Goldstein, and others regarding the mechanisms that regulate language use. It has not paid much attention to many aspects of aphasia that are not immediately related to psycholinguistic processing, such as a patient's fluency. For instance, most patients with agrammatism, a speech output disorder that affects function words and morphology, speak slowly, while patients whose disturbance affects the choice and ordering of phonemes in content words speak at normal rates. Why does one deficit slow down the speech planning process and the other does not? Is this because of the relationship of the lesions in these disorders to the motor system, or because there is a true functional relationship between the speed of language planning and the level of the language code being planned? Do difficulties in planning function words, morphology, and syntactic structures slow down the speech-planning process, while difficulties in planning the phonemic content words do not? The psycholinguistic approach has not addressed questions such as this.

The psycholinguistic approach has also not fulfilled its promise to add clear information to our knowledge of the relationship of language processors to the brain through deficit–lesion correlations. For instance, there is a raging controversy over the localization of the language processors involved in syntactic comprehension (Grodzinsky, 2000). Progress has been slow in this area, in part because of the difficulty in obtaining adequately detailed measurements of both language and lesions in a large enough set of patients, and in part because of different results in activation studies that may reflect differences in tasks, populations, imaging techniques and methods of analysis across studies.

Finally, the psycholinguistic approach has not yet spawned many diagnostic tests utilized by a large number of clinicians, at least not in the U.S. Its major impact has been felt in research studies of language impairments. But some bench-to-bedside transfer of concepts and methods has occurred, and more of this is likely to take place in the coming years.

CONCLUSION

Syndromes are part and parcel of medicine, and it is only to be expected that the concept of a syndrome would be applied to the study of aphasia by its founders, all of whom were medical men. It is also natural to assume that the neural tissue responsible for speech planning and comprehension would be close to that involved in motor planning and auditory perception, respectively. Finally, it is understandable that an approach to language disorders would have developed that centered on the usual tasks to which language is put and that incorporated descriptions of language features that are obvious "to the naked eye," so to speak—words, their meanings, their sounds, grammatical words and endings, and sentences. Syndromes that incorporated these features have helped clinicians and researchers to describe and classify aphasias for over a century.

Was this effort successful? Let us go back to what we said a successful syndrome does:

It relates symptoms functionally, explains individual variability in symptom occurrence, excludes symptoms that co-occur with those in the syndrome that are not functionally related to those in the syndrome, and predicts natural history.

The classical syndromes had partial success in the first and last of these areas. They relate some symptoms functionally and have some predictive value. However, the approach fails in the areas of explaining individual variability and excluding co-occurring symptoms. Even in the areas in which it has been successful, its success is at best partial: it only deals with some aspects of language, and then quite generally.

As researchers with backgrounds in linguistics and psychology entered the field of aphasiology in greater numbers, beginning in the 1960s, concepts about language structure and processing have had greater impact on the way in which we think about language disorders, the relationship of language to the brain, and the approaches we might take to therapy. This approach has yielded a fair literature, but it is still truly in its infancy. It can be seen as a challenge to the classical syndromes, or as an extension of them. Does it do better than the classical approach to syndromes according to our criteria? Certainly, in the areas of relating symptoms functionally and excluding co-occurring symptoms that are not part of a syndrome, the psycholinguistic approach has proven more successful. It offers promise in the areas of dealing with individual variability and predicting natural history in more detail than the classical approach. But work on the aphasias is far from over.

The current scene is a vibrant one, in which hypotheses about language itself, its processing, its neural basis, and its disorders are all being investigated and debated vigorously. Unlike 20 or so years ago, very little is agreed upon today by experts in most of these areas. The truly encouraging feature of current research is that the combination of the conceptual framework within which aphasia is approached with the behavioral and imaging investigative techniques now available offers unparalleled opportunities to make progress in this area.

ACKNOWLEDGMENTS

This work was supported in part by a grant from NIDCD (DC00942).

REFERENCES

Alexander, M. P., Naeser, M. A., and Palumbo, C. L. (1987). Correlations of subcortical CT lesion sites and aphasia profiles. *Brain* 110:961–991.

Auerbach, S. H., Allard, T., Naeser, M., Alexander, M. P., and Albert, M. L. (1982). Pure word deafness: analysis of a case with bilateral lesions and a defect at the prephonemic level. *Brain* 105:271–300.

Basso, A., Lecours, A. R., Moraschini, S., Vanier, M. (1985). Anatomoclinical correlations of the aphasias as defined through computerized tomography: exceptions. *Brain Lang.* 26:201–229.

Benson, D. F. (1979). *Aphasia, Alexia and Agraphia*. London: Churchill Livingstone.

Benson, D. F., and Geschwind, N. (1971). Aphasia and related cortical disturbances. In *Clinical Neurology*, A. B. Baker and L. H. Baker (eds.). New York: Harper & Row, Chapter 8.

Berndt, R., Mitchum, C., and Haendiges, A. (1996). Comprehension of reversible sentences in "agrammatism": a meta-analysis. *Cognition* 58:289–308.

Blumstein, S. E., Milberg, W., and Shrier, R. (1982). Semantic processing in aphasia: evidence from an auditory lexical decision task. *Brain Lang* 17:301–315.

Broca, P. (1861). Remarques sur le siege de la faculte de la parole articulee, suives d'une observation d'aphemie (perte de parole). *Bull. Soc. Anat.* 36:330–357.

Caplan, D. (1987). Discrimination of normal and aphasic subjects on a test of syntactic comprehension. *Neuropsychologia* 25:173–184.

Caplan, D., Baker, C., and Dehaut, F. (1985). Syntactic determinants of sentence comprehension in aphasia. *Cognition* 21:117–175.

Caplan D., and Hildebrandt N. (1988). *Disorders of Syntactic Comprehension*. Cambridge, MA: M.I.T. Press (Bradford Books).

Caplan, D., Hildebrandt, N., and Makris, N. (1996). Location of lesions in stroke patients with deficits in syntactic processing in sentence comprehension. *Brain* 119:933–949.

Caplan, D. and Waters, G.S. (1995). Phonological output planning and verbal rehearsal: evidence from aphasia. *Brain Lang.* 48:191–220

Caramazza, A., and Zurif, E. B. (1976). Dissociation of algorithmic and heuristic processes in language comprehension: evidence from aphasia. *Brain Lang* 3:572–582.

Coslett, H. B., Brashear, H. R., and Heilman, K. M. (1984). Pure word deafness after bilateral primary auditory cortex infarcts. *Neurology* 34:347–352.

Damasio, A. R. (1992). Aphasia. *N. Engl. J. Med.* 326:531–539.

Damasio, A., and Tranel D. (1993). Nouns and verbs are retrieved with differently distributed neural systems. *Proc. Natl. Acad. Sci. U.S.A.* 90:4957–4960.

Damasio, H., and Damasio, A. R. (1980). The anatomical basis of conduction aphasia. *Brain* 103:337–350.

Damasio, H., Grabowski, T. J., Tranel, D., Hichwa, R. D., and Damasio, A. R. (1996). A neural basis for lexical retrieval. *Nature* 380:499–505.

de Bleser, R. (1988). Localization of aphasia: science or fiction? In *Perspectives on Cognitive Neurology*, D. Denes, C. Semenza, and P. Bisiacchi (eds.). Hove, UK: Lawrence Erlbaum Associates.

Denes, G., and Semenza, C. (1975). Auditory modality-specific anomia: evidence from a case of pure word deafness. *Cortex* 11:401–411.

Freedman, M., Alexander, M. P., Naeser, M. A., and Palumbo, C. (1984). Anatomic basis for transcortical motor aphasia. *Neurology* 34:409–417.

Geschwind, N. (1965). Disconnection syndromes in animals and man. *Brain* 88:237–294, 585–644.

Goldstein, K. (1948). *Language and Language Disturbances*. New York: Grune and Stratton.

Goodglass, H., and Kaplan, E. (1972). Boston Diagnostic Aphasia Examination. *The Assessment of Aphasia and Related Disorders*. Philadelphia: Lea and Febiger.

Goodglass, H., and Kaplan, E. (1982). *The Assessment of Aphasia and Related Disorders, 2nd ed.* Philadelphia: Lea & Febiger.

Grodzinsky, Y. (1990). *Theoretical Perspectives on Language Deficits*. Cambridge, MA: MIT Press.

Grodzinsky, Y. (2000). The neurology of syntax: language use without Broca'a area, *Behav. Brain Sci.* 23:1–71.

Hayward, R., Naeser, M. A., Zatz, L. M., et al. (1977). Cranial computer tomography in aphasia. *Radiology* 123:653–660.

Head, H. (1926). *Aphasia and Kindred Disorders of Speech*. New York: Macmillan Press.

Holland, A. L., Fromm, D., and Swindell, C. S. (1986). The labeling problem in aphasia: an illustrative case. *J. Speech Hear. Disord.* 51:176–180.

Howard, D. (1995). Language in the human brain. In *Cognitive Neuroscience*, M. R. Rugg (ed.). Cambridge, MA: MIT Press, pp. 277–304.

Jackson. H. H. (1878). On affections of speech from disease of the brain. *Brain*, 1:304–330, 203–222, 332–356.

Kempler, D., Curtiss, S., Metter, E., Jackson, C., and Hanson, W. (1991). Grammatical comprehension, aphasic syndromes and neuroimaging. *J. Neurolinguist.* 6:301–318.

Kempler, D., Metter, E., Jackson, C., Hanson, W., Riege, W., Mazziotta, J., and Phelps, M. (1988). Disconnection and cerebral metabolism: the case of conduction aphasia. *Arch. Neurol.* 45:275–279.

Kertesz, A. (1979). *Aphasia and Associated Disorders: Taxonomy, Localization and Recovery*. New York: Grune and Stratton.

Kertesz, A., Harlock, W., and Coates, R. (1979). Computer tomographic localization, lesion size, and prognosis in aphasia and nonverbal impairment. *Brain Lang.* 8:34–50.

Kertesz, A., Lau, W. K., and Polk, M. (1993). The structural determinants of recovery in Wernicke's aphasia. *Brain Lang.* 44.153–164.

Kertesz, A. and McCabe, P. (1977). Recovery patterns and prognosis in aphasia. *Brain* 100:1–18.

Kertesz, A., Sheppard, A., and MacKenzie, R. (1982). Localization in transcortical sensory aphasia. *Arch. Neurol.* 39:475–478.

Lecours, A. R., Lhermitte, F., and Bryans, B. (1983). *Aphasiology*. London: Balliere Tindall.

Lichtheim, L. (1885). On aphasia. *Brain* 7:433–484.

Luria, A. R. (1947). *Traumatic Aphasia* (reprinted in translation 1970, trans.). The Hague: Mouton.

Marie, P. (1906). Revision de la question de l'aphasie: la troisieme circonvolution frontale gauche ne joue aucun role special dans la fonction du langage. *Semaine Med.* 26:241–247.

McNeil, M. R., and Kent, R. D. (1991). Motoric characteristics of adult aphasic and apraxic speakers. In *Advances in Psychology: Cerebral Control of Speech and Limb Movements*, G. R. Hammond (ed.). New York: Elsevier/North Holland, pp. 317–354.

Mesulam, M.-M. (1990). Large-scale neurocognitive networks and distributed processing for attention, language, and memory. *Ann. Neurol.* 28:597–613.

Mesulam, M.-M. (1998). From sensation to cognition. *Brain 121:*1013–1052.

Metter, E. J., Hanson, W. R., Jackson, C. A., Kempler, D., van Lancker, D., Mazziotta, J. C., and Phelps, M. E. (1990). Temporoparietal cortex in aphasia. Evidence from positron emission tomography. *Arch. Neurol. 47:*1235–1238.

Metter, E. J., Jackson, C. A., Kempler, D., and Hanson, W. R. (1992). Temporoparietal cortex and the recovery of language comprehension in aphasia. *Aphasiology 6:*349–358.

Metter, E. J., Kempler, D., Hanson, R., Jackson, C., Mazziotta, J. C., and Phelps, M. E. (1986). Cerebral glucose metabolism: differences in Wernicke's, Broca's and conduction aphasias. *Clin. Aphasiol. 16:*97–104.

Metter, E. J., Kempler, D., Jackson, C. A., Hanson, W. R., Mazziotta, J. C., and Phelps, M. E. (1989). Cerebral glucose metabolism in Wernicke's, Broca's and conduction aphasia. *Arch. Neurol. 46:*27–34.

Metter, E. J., Riege, W. H., Hanson, W. R., Camras, L. R., Phelps, M. E., and Kuhl, D. E. (1984). Correlations of glucose metabolism and structural damage to language function in aphasia. *Brain Lang. 21:*187–207.

Metter, E. J., Riege, W. H., Hanson, W. R., Jackson, C. A., Kempler, D., and VanLancker, D. (1983). Comparison of metabolic rates, language and memory, and subcortical aphasias. *Brain Lang. 19:*33–47.

Metter, E. J., Riege, W. H., Hanson, W. R., Jackson, C. A., Kempler, D., and VanLancker, D. (1988). Subcortical structures in aphasia: an analysis based on (F-18)-fluorodeoxyglucose positron emission tomography and computed tomography. *Arch. Neurol. 45:*1229–1234.

Metz-Lutz, M.-N., and Dahl, E. (1984). Analysis of word comprehension in a case of pure word deafness. *Brain Lang. 23:*13–25.

Milberg, W., and Blumstein, S. E. (1981). Lexical decision and aphasia: evidence for semantic processing. *Brain Lang. 14:*371–385.

Mohr, J. P., Pessin, M. S., Finkelstein, S., Funkenstein, H., Duncan, G. W., and Davis, K. R. (1978). Broca aphasia: pathologic and clinical. *Neurology 28:*311–324.

Moutier, F. (1908). *L'Aphasie de Broca.* Paris: Steinheil.

Naeser, M. (1989). CT scan lesion site analysis and recovery in aphasia. *Brain 112:*1–38.

Naeser, M. A., and R. W. Hayward (1978). Lesion localization in aphasia with cranial computed tomography and the Boston Diagnostic Aphasia Exam. *Neurology 28:*545–551.

Naeser, M. A., Palumbo, C. L., Helm-Estabrooks, N., Stiassny-Eder, D., and Albert, M. L. (1989). Severe nonfluency in aphasia: role of the medial subcallosal fasciculus and other white matter pathology in recovery of spontaneous speech. *Brain 112:*1–38.

Rumelhart, and McClelland, (1986). *Parallel Distributed Processing.* Cambridge, MA: MIT Press.

Saffran, E. M., Marin, O., and Yeni-Komshian, G. (1976). An analysis of speech perception and word deafness. *Brain Lang. 3:*209–228.

Shallice, T., and Warrington, E. K. (1977). Auditory–verbal short-term memory impairment and conduction aphasia. *Brain Lang. 4:*479–491.

Schiff, H. B., Alexander, M. P., Naeser, M. A., and Galaburda, A. M. (1983). Aphemia: clinical–anatomic correlates. *Arch. Neurol. 40:*720–727.

Schwartz, M. (1984). What the classical aphasia categories can't do for us, and why. *Brain Lang. 21:*1–8.

Wernicke, C. (1874). *Der Aphasische Symptomenkomplex.* Breslau: Cohn & Weigart. Reprinted in translation in *Boston Studies in Philosophy of Science 4:*34–97.

3

Phonologic Aspects of Language Disorders

Phonology is the subfield of linguistics concerned with the structure and systematic patterning of sounds in language (Akmajian et al., 1984). This chapter will focus on studies of acquired language disorders and on slip-of-the-tongue data (*spoonerisms*) in normal subjects, with reference to the experimental psychology literature where relevant.

The chapter begins with a review of disorders of phonological processing. Following this, a theoretical model employing the conceptual framework of parallel distributed processing (PDP) is introduced as a means of both explaining empirical observations in a cogent fashion and of potentially relating behavior to neural microstructure. The chapter concludes with a consideration of the anatomy of phonological processing. See Nadeau (2001) for more detailed review.

DISORDERS OF PHONOLOGICAL PROCESSING

PHONOLOGICAL SELECTION ERRORS

Phonological selection errors result in the production of incorrect phonemic sequences, easily recognizable when they constitute neologisms. Such errors provide the best evidence that the

brain does implicitly recognize phonemes as operational units, and that this sublexical knowledge is accessible from the neural representation of concepts and meaning. Several major types of single phoneme errors may be observed (Blumstein, 1973a):

Non-environmental:
Substitution:	/timz/"teams" →	/kimz/
Simplification:	/prIti/"pretty" →	/pIti/
Addition:	/papa/"papa" →	/papra/

Environmental:
Assimilation within a word:	"Crete" →	/trit/
Assimilation across word boundaries:	"roast beef" →	/rof bif/
Metathesis (exchange):	"degrees" →	/gedriz/

Environmental (*sequential*, *contextual*) errors may account for over 70% of errors in slip-of-the-tongue corpora and for 50%–70% of phonological errors in the language of patients with jargon aphasia (Lecours and Lhermitte, 1969; Schwartz et al., 1994). Substitution errors are more common than other non-environmental errors, and they tend to be relatively more common in aphasic language than in slip-of-the-tongue corpora (Poncet et al., 1972; Halpern et al., 1976; Niemi and Koivuselkä-

Sallinen, 1985; Caramazza et al., 1986; Valdois et al., 1988; Wilshire, 1998).

Several major studies of phonemic selection errors in aphasic patients have yielded a wealth of data on the phenomenological principles that govern such errors. The relative frequency of phoneme use is the same in aphasic as in normal language (Blumstein, 1973b). Errors may occur at any position within a word (Marquardt et al., 1979; Valdois et al., 1988). There is considerable variability in the phonemes most prone to selection error. However, patients tend to have the least difficulty with frequently used phonemes such as vowels and the consonants /t/, /n/ and /s/, and they tend to have the most difficulty with consonant clusters, fricatives (thin, shoe, then) and affricates (chin, just), phonemes that occur with the lowest frequency and require more muscles and closer control of movement than any other class (Shankweiler and Harris, 1966; Shankweiler et al., 1968; Johns and Darley, 1970; Blumstein, 1973a,b; Dubois et al., 1973; Trost and Canter, 1974; La Pointe and Johns, 1975; Halpern et al., 1976; Burns and Canter, 1977; Dunlop and Marquardt, 1977; Klich et al., 1979; Shewan, 1980; Canter et al., 1985). A similar phenomenon has been noted in slip-of-the-tongue collections (Motley and Baars, 1976; Ellis, 1980; Levitt and Healy, 1985).

Phoneme selection errors are influenced by lesion locus. Patients with Broca's aphasia tend to replace consonant clusters with a single consonant, whether the cluster is intrasyllabic or bridges two syllables, and they rarely create consonant clusters in lieu of a single consonant. In contrast, whereas patients with conduction aphasia alter consonants and consonant clusters just as often, they are more likely to replace a cluster with a different cluster, or to replace a single consonant with a cluster (Nespoulous et al., 1984).

Distinctive Features

Many observations regarding phonemic selection errors in aphasic patients are most usefully viewed in terms of distinctive features. Distinctive features are the specific states of roughly 18 dimensions of the orofacial–pharyngeal speech apparatus that, in particu-

lar combinations, operationally define all the phonemes. Some phonemic selection errors can equally well be viewed as distinctive feature selection errors (Lecours and Lhermitte, 1969). For example:

/bat/	→	/pat/	(deletion of voice)
/not/	→	/dot/	(deletion of nasality)
/fat/	→	/pat/	(deletion of continuance)

In these examples, it is impossible to determine whether it is a distinctive feature error or a phoneme selection error. However, in some rare cases, it is difficult to conceive that the error involves anything but a distinctive feature (Fromkin, 1971; Shattuck-Hufnagel and Klatt, 1979):

clear blue sky → glear plue sky
(an exchange of the voice feature between the initial phonemes of the first two words)

The following is equally suggestive:

Cedars of Lebanon → Cedars of Lemadon
(movement of the nasality feature from the first /n/ to the /b/)

In the substitution of one phoneme for another, the change tends to involve a minimum number of distinctive features, usually one or two, rarely more than three (Green, 1969; Lecours and Lhermitte, 1969; MacKay, 1970; Poncet et al., 1972; Blumstein, 1973b; La Pointe and Johns, 1975; Burns and Canter, 1977; Keller, 1978; Klich et al., 1979; Shinn and Blumstein, 1983; Niemi and Koivuselkä-Sallinen, 1985; Caramazza et al., 1986; Valdois et al., 1988). Blumstein (1973b) found that this principle applies equally to all types of perisylvian aphasia, and several investigators have noted it in slip-of-the-tongue errors (MacKay, 1970; van den Broecke and Goldstein, 1980; Stemberger, 1982; Poncet et al., 1972; Trost and Canter, 1974; Burns and Canter, 1977; MacNeilage, 1982; Nespoulous et al., 1984, 1987; Canter et al., 1985; Valdois et al., 1988). However, other studies of aphasic subjects have shown that distance 2 and 3 errors are relatively more common in conduction than in

Broca's aphasia, and Miller and Ellis (1987) made a parallel observation in a patient with jargon aphasia. Furthermore, in slip-of-the-tongue corpora, single, isolated phonemic errors are likely to differ from their target by only one or two distinctive features, but in cases in which phonemic errors are environmentally influenced (see below), this constraint does not seem to apply (Stemberger, 1985). These observations are consistent with the concept that in patients with Broca's aphasia, particularly those with phonetic disintegration (apraxia of speech), and in normal subjects who produce isolated phonemic paraphasias, selection errors are determined to a greater degree by the properties of the phoneme itself (and near misses tend to yield single distinctive feature slips). With more posterior aphasias, and with contextually induced slips in normal subjects, phonemic environment (i.e., the influences of preceding and following phonemes in the language stream) plays a greater role, and slips do not reflect the influence of distinctive feature distance.

SUPERORDINATE INFLUENCES ON PHONOLOGICAL SELECTION ERRORS

A number of observations indicate that even when the reliability of phonemic selection is reduced, there are still some persistent overarching influences that tend to rein in or modify phonemic selection errors.

Environmental Influences on Phonemic Selection Errors

Phonemic selection errors are frequently influenced by their phonemic environment (Blumstein, 1973a). Lecours and Lhermitte (1969) suggested that most phonemic additions, deletions, and substitutions in jargon aphasia can be viewed as sequential errors. These are errors in which a phoneme or phoneme cluster is altered such that, most often, it becomes closer to (in number of distinctive features) a preceding or following phoneme or phoneme cluster that resembles it in terms of distinctive features. The similarity between interacting phonemes observed by Lecours and Lhermitte has also been demon-

strated in normal subjects (Garrett, 1975; Ellis, 1980). In two French patients with jargon aphasia that Lecours and Lhermitte studied, nearly 80% of phonemic selection errors could be classified as sequential errors. The following are examples of transformations they observed (Lecours and Lhermitte, 1969):

Pair destruction:	/dɛsada/ →	/ɛsada/
	/koplɛks/ →	/koplɛs/
Pair creation:		
Anticipatory	/deabyla/ →	/debabyla/
Perseverative	/trist/ →	/tristr/
Metathesis		
Pre-positioning	/pulaje/ →	/apulje/
Post-positioning	/dekala/ →	/ekalad/

Sequential (contextual, environmental) phonemic errors are less common in aphasic language than in slip-of-the-tongue corpora (Wilshire, 1998). They are less common in Broca's aphasia and apraxia of speech than in conduction aphasia, and less common in conduction aphasia than in jargon aphasia (Poncet et al., 1972; Trost and Canter, 1974; La Pointe and Johns, 1975; Burns and Canter, 1977; Shewan, 1980; MacNeilage, 1982; Nespoulous et al., 1984, 1987; Canter et al., 1985; Miller and Ellis, 1987; Valdois et al., 1988). This suggests that as the production of language nears the output phase, the instantiation of phonemes as patterns of activity in articulatory motor representations matures and becomes less susceptible to the effects of perversions of knowledge of the phoneme sequences constituting words or phrases. In contrast, at earlier stages, at which word and even phrase level effects are prominent and environmentally linked phoneme errors are generated, these errors will tend to reflect the properties of the words and multiphoneme sublexical elements rather than the properties of the phoneme.

The occurrence of both anticipatory and perseverative errors reinforces the concept that as the brain processes phonemes, a number of them are maintained in a similar state of activity for some time, even when they occur sequentially in the output phoneme stream. Thus, a given phoneme may have as much opportunity to influence phonemes later in the stream (perseverative errors) as later phonemes have to influence it (anticipatory errors). The relative frequency of anticipatory and perseverative errors in different types of aphasia may be related in good part to some mix of speech rate effects and impairment of lexical–semantic access (Dell, 1986). Slow speech rates and better lexical–semantic access will tend to correct perseverative errors. Most sequential phoneme errors involve phonemes that are physically near each other (MacKay, 1970; Blumstein, 1973a; Niemi and Koivuselkä-Sallinen, 1985).

Phonemic Clumping

Phonemic substitutions, additions, deletions, or metatheses, whether in aphasic speech or slip-of-the-tongue errors, may involve phonemic aggregations or clumps of various sizes. These include joint phonemes (e.g., a consonant cluster), syllables, rhymes (e.g., "stop"), affixes, and stems (Lecours and Lhermitte, 1969; Fromkin, 1971; Blumstein, 1978; Buckingham et al., 1978; Shattuck-Hufnagel, 1979; Shewan, 1980; Stemberger, 1982; Dell, 1986). Phoneme and joint phoneme exchanges seldom involve words separated by more than one or two other words, whereas exchanges of larger entities may occur over longer distances (the "structural distance constraint"; (Garrett, 1975).

Malapropisms (in aphasic speech, often referred to as "formal," "form-related," or "verbal paraphasias") represent substitutions at the word level that are driven by similarity in phonology, number of syllables, stress pattern, and grammatic form, and are unconstrained or only partially constrained by meaning (unlike semantic paraphasias). They provide evidence that word representations exist, independent of meaning, as large phonemic clumps (Fay and Cutler, 1977; Blanken, 1990).

Functors or free grammatical morphemes (closed-class items such as articles, prepositions, and conjunctions) are rarely involved in phonemic paraphasic errors, which suggests that they exist as nearly indissoluble clumps of phonemes (Blumstein, 1973a; Garrett, 1975; Lecours, 1982; Stemberger, 1984; Kohn and Smith, 1990). There are exceptions, however: Kohn and Smith (1993) reported four patients

with jargon aphasia who made frequent phonemic paraphasias during repetition and reading of functors. Many have suggested that the relative preservation of functors is a word frequency effect, functors being the most commonly used words (Ellis et al., 1983; Stemberger and MacWhinney, 1986; Ellis and Young, 1988). Neologisms involving major lexical items also exhibit a strong word frequency effect (Strub and Gardner, 1974; Allport, 1984b; McCarthy and Warrington, 1984; Ellis, 1985; Bub et al., 1987; Miller and Ellis, 1987; Pate et al., 1987; Martin and Saffran, 1992).

The size of the units of substitution, addition, deletion, and metathesis is roughly correlated with the posterior extent of the lesion responsible for aphasia. Patients with Broca's aphasia (anterior lesions) are most likely to exhibit literal paraphasias best characterized as single phoneme or distinctive feature alterations. Patients with posterior lesions with Wernicke's or, even more so, jargon aphasia (Kertesz and Benson, 1970) are most likely to exhibit paraphasias best characterized as joint phoneme, syllable, or morpheme alterations. These observations suggest that the functional hierarchical organization of phonemic sequences is anatomically organized as well.

Other Constraints on Phonemic
Selection Errors

Sublexical substitutions obey phonetic rules (phonotactic constraints), indicating that rarely in either aphasic or slip-of-the-tongue errors is there evidence of a capability for producing phonemic sequences that are beyond the native speaker (Fromkin, 1971; MacKay, 1972; Blumstein, 1973a, 1978; Buckingham and Kertesz, 1974; Garrett, 1975; Butterworth, 1979; Buckingham, 1980; Niemi and Koivuselkä-Sallinen, 1985). For example:

plant the seed/z/ → plan the seat/s/
sphinx in the moonlight → minx in the spoonlight

Failure to modify these selection errors would have resulted in the impermissible sequences seat/z/ and "sphoonlight." Blumstein (1973a) found that only 2.6% of phonemic errors resulted in non-English sequences.

Lexical and Semantic Influence

As phonological processing proceeds over time, it continues to be influenced by lexical and semantic constraints, even in aphasia. There are three lines of evidence of lexical-semantic constraints on phonological processing.

First, phonemic selection errors are constrained by the lexical target and both normal subjects and aphasic patients make more phonological errors repeating nonwords than real words (Brener, 1940; Alajouanine and Lhermitte, 1973; Martin and Rigrodsky, 1974). Aphasic patients with relatively good access to lexical targets (e.g., patients with Broca's and conduction aphasia) demonstrate conduite d'approche (continuous improvement in their effort to zero in on the target through successive attempts), whereas those with poor lexical–semantic access (e.g., patients with Wernicke's aphasia) are much less likely to exhibit this phenomenon (Butterworth, 1979; Joanette et al., 1980; Miller and Ellis, 1987; Valdois et al., 1989; Gandour et al., 1994; but see also Goodglass et al., 1997). The phonological improvement noted during conduite d'approche is seen only with real words, and not with nonwords. Mistakes by patients who make errors only during nonword repetition tend to reflect lexicalization (Bub et al., 1987). Normal subjects are more likely to produce real word spoonerisms (e.g., "barn door" → "darn boor," than nonword spoonerisms (e.g., "dart board" → "bart doard") (Baars et al., 1975; Garrett, 1976; Dell and Reich, 1981). The likelihood of such real word spoonerisms can be enhanced by semantic priming. For example, Motley and Baars (1976) found that "get one" is more likely to slip to "wet gun" if preceded by "damp rifle."

Second, observations on abstruse neologisms (neologisms without evident relationship to a plausible target) suggest that lexical–semantic constraints reach deep into the phonological processor even as excessive noise within that processor interferes with the correct selection of phonemic sequences from concept representations. Neologisms in jargon aphasia have the same number of syllables as the target up to 80% of the time and they share a greater than chance number of phonemes (and particularly the initial phoneme) with the target, suggesting substantial sublexical access from se-

mantics (concept representations), even when the target is not sufficiently resolved to assure correct output (Ellis et al., 1983; Miller and Ellis, 1987; Valdois et al., 1989; Wilshire, 1998). These observations are remarkably similar to observations made on the tip-of-the-tongue phenomenon (see below). Butterworth (1979) found that 57% of neologisms in patients with jargon aphasia were phonologically linked to other neologisms. In patients with conduction aphasia, the successive approximations during conduite d'approche reflect a gamut of associations, rarely involving the whole word (malapropisms) (e.g., "dominoes" → "dynamos"), more commonly involving syllables, joint phonemes and phonemes (e.g., "pretzel" → "trep, tretz . . . fretful") (Kohn, 1984). Thus, neologisms in general reflect excessive noise and the presence of phonological factors influencing the selection of lexical and sublexical components, as opposed to purely lexical–semantic constraints. In jargon aphasia, there is less semantic influence, and the lexical target constantly shifts so that successive neologisms do not exhibit conduite d'approche. In conduction aphasia, relatively greater semantic influence preserves a lexical target most of the time, except in rare malapropisms, providing the basis for conduite d'approche.

Third, in experiments in which normal subjects are given the definition of low-frequency words and develop the *tip-of-the-tongue* (TOT) phenomenon (have a sense that they know the word but cannot actually produce it), there is evidence of sublexical access from concept representations despite unsuccessful lexical access. Despite anomia, subjects are able to guess the number of syllables in the target word with high accuracy, show knowledge of letters within the word—for example, guessing the first letter with 57% accuracy, and show knowledge of which syllable in the target is accented (Brown and McNeill, 1966; Yarmey, 1973; Koriat and Lieblich, 1974; Brown, 1991; Burke et al., 1991). In many cases, joint morphemes and syllables are retrieved (Rubin, 1975). Many of the products of naming attempts are phonologically related to the target and many are nonwords that obey the phonotactic rules of the native language and share an affix or root with the target (Kohn et al., 1987). Aphasic patients are also able to guess the first letter and the number of syllables with far greater than chance accuracy when they develop the TOT phenomenon; however, patients with conduction or Broca's aphasia are far better than are patients with Wernicke's or anomic aphasia (Barton, 1971; Goodglass et al., 1976; Laine and Martin, 1996). Even patients with anomic aphasia may be able to correctly identify the rhyming properties of the names of pictures they cannot actually name (Marin et al., 1976; Feinberg et al., 1986; Bub et al., 1988). These data suggest that neural activity representing meaning engages phonemes and sublexical clumps of phonemes even when the word representation in aggregate is not sufficiently engaged to elevate it above the threshold for production.

Summary

The data I have reviewed on phonological selection errors in normal and aphasic subjects provide evidence of several essential properties of the cerebral system instantiating phonological processing: (1) hierarchical structure; (2) simultaneous influence by lexical–semantic and phonological effects; (3) simultaneous processing of a chunk of the language stream, such that lexical and sublexical elements influence other elements that both precede and follow them; (4) anatomic distribution such that lesion locus has major effects on the pattern of breakdown observed; (5) substantial but not absolute similarity between the errors made by aphasic patients and errors made by normal subjects in slips of the tongue; and (6) stochastic function, such that lesions are associated with a reduced probability of correct phonological selection, with actual performance that is variable, and relative preservation of ability to distinguish correct from incorrect.

PHONOLOGICAL DECODING

Errors in acoustic processing exhibit some of the same features as errors in articulatory processing. "Slips of the ear" by normal subjects tend to involve errors of one distinctive feature (Bond and Garnes, 1980). Patients with aphasias of all types do better with discriminations involving two or more distinctive features relative to discriminations involving a single distinctive feature (Blumstein et al., 1977a; Miceli et al., 1978, 1980). Although most aphasic patients retain some ability to discriminate voice onset time (e.g., /t/ from /d/), some investigators have found patients with Wernicke's aphasia to be particularly impaired in their ability to use that discriminative ability to actually identify a phoneme (Blumstein et al., 1977b; Caramazza et al., 1983), whereas others have found impairment almost as severe in patients with Broca's or conduction aphasia (Gandour and Dardarananda, 1982). Difficulty in discriminating or labeling bears little relation to comprehension ability, which is probably defined to a far greater degree by lexical–semantic access, i.e., the integrity of the connections between acoustic representations and concept representations (Baker et al., 1981).

Lexical–semantic effects are evident in auditory perception. Aphasic patients make more errors with discriminations involving phonemes in nonwords than in real words (Blumstein et al., 1977a; see also Elman and McClelland, 1988). If patients with Broca's aphasia are faced with difficult phonetic discriminations involving ambiguous stimuli (e.g., indicate whether the first phoneme in "duke" is /d/ or /t/ when the actual /d/ sound is synthesized with voice onset time spanning the range between normal /d/ and /t/), they are unduly biased by lexical effects, compared to normal subjects (e.g., more likely to answer /d/ if the word is "duke" than if it is "doot"), consistent with impaired phonetic processing (Blumstein et al., 1994). However, patients with Wernicke's aphasia, like normal subjects, exhibit little or no lexical bias, which suggests either that they are able to rely on relatively intact phonetic discrimination capabilities in this task or are less capable of lexical bias. Normal subjects will exhibit lexical bias when additional semantic influences are brought to bear. When they hear synthetic words containing acoustically ambiguous phonemes, they will "hear" the form that is semantically congruent. For example, when /b-deIt/ is preceded by "there's the fishing gear and the . . .", they will hear "bait," whereas when it is preceded by "check the time and the . . .", they will hear "date" (Bond and Garnes, 1980).

CONDUCTION APHASIA

Conduction aphasia is characterized by impaired repetition, in most cases frequent phonemic paraphasias, occasional semantic and verbal paraphasias, and variable lexical access in spontaneous language and naming to confrontation, with relative sparing of comprehension and grammar (Benson et al., 1973; Dubois et al., 1973; Green and Howes, 1977; Kohn, 1984). Patients are not anosognosic and characteristically make extensive attempts to correct their errors. Conduction aphasia is essentially a disorder of phonological processing, and it is caused by a lesion at the core of the neural substrate for phonological processing. Because patients with conduction aphasia have relatively spared lexical access and normal articulation, however, they are able to produce voluminous output. For these reasons, conduction aphasia provides an ideal situation for the study of phonological processing, and studies of patients with conduction aphasia have contributed a great deal to our understanding of phonological processing.

Two different types of conduction aphasia have been defined: repetition conduction aphasia and reproduction conduction aphasia. *Repetition conduction aphasia* is characterized by relatively normal naming and spontaneous language, no phonemic paraphasias, even in repetition, usually poor phonetic discrimination, impaired auditory–verbal short-term memory, and severely impaired repetition. *Reproduction conduction aphasia* is characterized by impaired repetition, naming, and spontaneous language with the production of phonemic paraphasic errors in all three. Whether spontaneous language or repetition is more impaired depends on the distribution of the lesion. Auditory–verbal short-term memory may be nearly normal. Since many individual patients exhibit features of both, these two disorders are probably best viewed as defining the two ends of a spectrum.

Repetition Conduction Aphasia and Auditory–Verbal Short-Term Memory

Warrington and Shallice have suggested that the fundamental problem in repetition conduction aphasia is one of auditory–verbal short-term memory, based on observations that these patients have auditory digit spans of 1–3; they fail to exhibit a recency effect in digit recall (thought to depend on phonological short-term memory stores; Brooks and Watkins, 1990); they demonstrate a primacy effect, and perform better with familiar, meaningful, and more slowly presented stimuli (suggesting reliance on lexical–semantic short-term memory stores; Posner, 1964; Watkins and Watkins, 1977); and they perform poorly on the Brown-Petersen procedure. In contrast, patients with reproduction conduction aphasia often have relatively preserved digit spans (Damasio and Damasio, 1980). The auditory–verbal short-term memory hypothesis has been extensively debated (Warrington et al., 1971; Warrington and Shallice, 1972; Strub and Gardner, 1974; Saffran and Marin, 1975; Shallice and Warrington, 1977; Caramazza et al., 1981; Friedrich et al., 1984; Vallar and Baddeley, 1984; Shallice and Vallar, 1990). There are two possible ways in which the neural substrate for phonological processing could support short-term memory: *(1)* through the transient sustained activation of the acoustic and articulatory motor phonological networks (phonological working memory), and *(2)* through use of linked acoustic and articulatory motor networks for silent rehearsal (the phonological loop posited by Baddeley et al., 1998).

To the extent that auditory–verbal short-term memory deficits reflect impaired ability to silently rehearse, they are a result rather than a cause of the behavior observed. However, to the extent that auditory–verbal short-term memory deficits reflect damage to the neurologic substrate for phonological working memory (the phonological processor itself), it is reasonable to view them as indicative of a genuine deficit in immediate memory (Caramazza et al., 1981). Because damage to articulatory motor representations impairs both silent rehearsal and the substrate for phonological working memory, one would expect auditory–verbal short-term memory deficits in patients with Broca's aphasia or apraxia of speech, something that has been shown (Goodglass et al., 1970; Heilman et al., 1976; Cermak and Tarlow, 1978; Waters et al., 1992).

Reproduction Conduction Aphasia

Word Length Effects. Longer words pose greater problems for repetition because they increase the number of sublexical elements that are simultaneously being processed. This increases the opportunity for these elements to induce errors by interacting with each other and their various associated sublexical elements. Also, because the lesion reduces the reliability of bringing every one of multiple syllables above production threshold, this increases the opportunity for sublexical omissions (Alajouanine and Lhermitte, 1973; Dubois et al., 1973; Yamadori and Ikumura, 1975; McCarthy and Warrington, 1984; Caplan et al., 1986; Caramazza et al., 1986; Bub et al., 1987; Pate et al., 1987; Valdois et al., 1988; Kohn, 1989; Friedman and Kohn, 1990; Kohn and Smith, 1991, 1995; Gandour et al., 1994). Repetition of long words is less likely to result in verbal paraphasias, however, because a single phonemic error is less likely to generate patterns of activity corresponding to other real words.

Variable Lexical Bias Effects. Lexical bias varies with lesion locus. To the extent that concept representations or the pathways from them are damaged (manifested by anomia plus or minus phonemic paraphasias) and phonological representations are spared, repetition of nonwords will be spared, and lexical bias effects will be reduced. In addition, the lexical effect in repetition of real words may paradoxically have a corrupting influence, as the damaged pathway from concept representations to phonological representations serves as an additional potential source of phonemic paraphasias (Dubois et al., 1973; Caplan et al., 1986; Martin et al., 1999). To the extent that the phonological representations are damaged and pathways from concept representations are spared, lexical bias effects will be increased and repetition of nonwords will be impaired.

Lexical bias effects are more apparent during spontaneous language than during repetition. Not only do patients with conduction aphasia fair worse during repetition, but they also exhibit less successful conduite d'approche

during repetition (Joanette et al., 1980). Among fluent aphasic patients in general, semantic influences are most evident during naming and phonological influences are most evident during repetition (Dell et al., 1997).

Frequency and Imageability Effects. Normal subjects repeat high-frequency words better than low-frequency words (Watkins and Watkins, 1977). Naming errors in aphasia are more likely with low-frequency targets (Kay and Ellis, 1987). Neologistic errors and phonemic paraphasias in jargon and conduction aphasia are more common with low-frequency than high-frequency targets (Strub and Gardner, 1974; Allport, 1984b; McCarthy and Warrington, 1984; Bub et al., 1987; Miller and Ellis, 1987; Pate et al., 1987; Martin and Saffran, 1992), as are phonological slips in naturally occurring and experimentally induced slip-of-the-tongue errors (Stemberger, 1984; Stemberger and MacWhinney, 1986; Dell, 1988). In both aphasic and slip-of-the-tongue errors, less common phonemes and phoneme combinations tend to be replaced by more common phonemes and combinations.

A corollary to the effect of word frequency is the effect of imageability. Highly imageable words are likely to have extensive representations in sensory association cortices (most often visual) that in turn serve as an additional source of input to these words. Imageability effects on repetition have been reported (Allport, 1984a; Howard and Franklin, 1988; Martin and Saffran, 1992).

Word frequency and imageability effects are constrained by the same factors that govern lexical bias. Thus, frequency and imageability effects in repetition are maximal when concept representations and the pathways that link them to the phonological apparatus are intact and there is damage to phonological representations. If repetition can occur rapidly and accurately, however, then access to concept representations has minimal impact (still less if there is damage to links to concept representations), and frequency, imageability, and lexical bias effects are minimal (Martin and Saffran, 1997). Because imageability effects reflect only the impact of semantic influence, and not the effect of phonological knowledge, the discrepancy between imageability and frequency effects will be a measure of the relative contribution of the "pseudo-lexical" bias provided by phonological representations.

A MODEL TO ACCOUNT FOR PHONOLOGICAL PROCESSING DISORDERS

Linguistic theories have not yet provided a satisfactory account for the phonological processing disorders observed either in aphasic patients or in normal subjects demonstrating slips of the tongue. Three major reasons can be identified: *(1)* linguistic theories have been founded on the concept of serial processing, whereas abundant data suggest that language production incorporates parallel processing (Stemberger, 1985); *(2)* linguistic theories have difficulty capturing effects that are easily explained by bottom-up and top-down processing interactions, such as the occurrence of paraphasic errors that have both semantic and phonological similarity to the target (Dell and Reich, 1981; Harley, 1984; Dell et al., 1997); and *(3)* linguistic theories do not enable us to explain behavior in terms of the properties of neural network function, or to use what is known about neural network function as an aid to understanding the complexities of behavior.

Parallel distributed processing models, also called "connectionist models," offer an alternative approach. The PDP models are neural-like in that they incorporate large arrays of simple units that are heavily interconnected with each other, like neurons in the brain. A PDP model that fully emulates neural network principles constitutes a hypothesis not just about the organization of cognitive processes but also about neural organization. The processing sophistication of PDP models stems from the simultaneous interaction of large numbers of units (hundreds or even thousands). These models incorporate explicitly defined assumptions that are "wired" into them in the mathematical details of their computer implementation. They produce large numbers of predictions that can be (and have been) empirically tested through observations of normal subjects and patients. They exhibit properties of graceful degradation and probabilistic selection, that is, when damaged or fed noisy input, they do not produce novel or bizarre output unachievable by an intact network with good input; rather, they tend to produce output that is not so reliably correct but is rule-bound—quite reminiscent of many of the observations that have been made about phonological selection errors. This property obviates the need to postulate "error correction devices" in normal and aphasic subjects that filter out bizarre constructions (e.g., Garrett, 1975; Shattuck-Hufnagel, 1979; Buckingham, 1980). The latency of activity pattern shifts, related ultimately to the slowness of neural physiology, provides one potential basis for the sequential aspect of language in general and phonological processing in particular. The instantiation of short- and long-term memory in the same neural nets that are responsible for processing, in conjunction with processes underlying the engagement of working memory (Goldman-Rakic, 1990), also eliminates the need to posit buffers. Parallel distributed processing models are particularly appealing in the context of phonological processing because they involve simultaneous processing at a number of levels and locations, apparently mimicking what is going on in the brain. Finally, and perhaps most important of all, pure PDP models (models without incorporated digital devices) implicitly learn the rules governing the data they process in the course of their experience with that data (e.g., Plaut et al., 1996). Thus, in a pure PDP model of phonology, there is no need to build in specific structures to account for specific phonological phenomena. The structure of the model is defined entirely in terms of the domains of information accessible to it and the necessary relationship of these domains to each other. The absence of specific, ad hoc devices motivated by models (e.g., linguistic) designed to account for particular phonological phenomena in an orderly fashion is also crucial to the maintenance of neurological plausibility. In humans, as in PDP models, the phonological phenomena we observe reflect entirely the emergent behavior of the networks.

DISTRIBUTED REPRESENTATION MODELS OF PHONOLOGICAL PROCESSING

Perhaps surprisingly, PDP models can be related in a very direct way to information-processing models. However, in order to do this, it is necessary to inquire into the nature of the representations signified by the boxes and arrows of information-processing models. In what follows, I will take this approach to the Lichtheim model (Lichtheim, 1885) (Fig. 3–1). Figure 3–2 depicts a PDP version of Lichtheim's model.

In Figure 3–1, the boxes (sparely designated as *A*, *M*, and *Concepts*) represent very large numbers of units. Particular patterns of activity, called "distributed representations," involving subsets of these units define the represented entities. For example, the concept representation of "house" might correspond to activation of units representing features of houses such as visual attributes, construction materials, and contents (physical and human). The exact nature of the feature units that are activated in various aggregates to define articulatory motor representations and acoustic

representations is not important to our discussion, so long as they are discrete (rather than continuous and infinitely modifiable, like a motor program). For example, the feature units of articulatory motor representations might correspond to phonemic distinctive features. Thus, the model is explicitly phonological rather than phonetic. The model employs left–right position in acoustic and articulatory motor representations as a surrogate for temporal order in precisely the same way as the PDP reading model of Plaut et al. (1996). Thus, articulatory motor representations would feature positions for each output phoneme, ordered as they are in the phonological word form. Acoustic representations would involve an analogous representational scheme.

Each arrow in Lichtheim's model (Fig. 3–1) corresponds to the entire set of connections between every unit in one representational field and every unit in the connected field, e.g., between all the units in concept representations, all the hidden units between concept representations and articulatory motor representations, and all the units in articulatory motor representations (Fig. 3–2). Thus, each arrow in Lichtheim's model defines a *pattern associator network*—a network that translates distributed representations in one domain into distributed representations in a different domain. It is beyond the scope of this chapter to enter into a full discussion of hidden units, which individually do not exhibit patterns of activity that are easily defined in behavioral terms. Suffice it to say that hidden units enable the establishment of a functional linkage between forms that have an arbitrary relationship to each other (e.g., word meaning and word phonology). They also provide the basis for much of the computational power of PDP models. The knowledge represented in the model lies in the strengths of the connections between the units. One could set these connection strengths by hand. However, given models with connections numbering in the hundreds of thousands or millions, it makes much more sense to have models develop their own connection strengths through learning. In the most widely employed algorithm, back-propagation, a particular pattern of input, e.g., at acoustic representations, is allowed to generate a stable pattern of activation in a linked representational field of in-

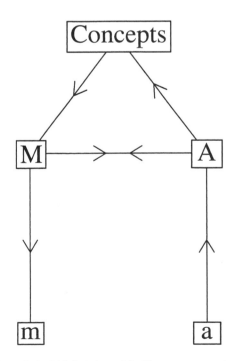

Figure 3–1. Lichtheim's model of language processing. *A* represents acoustic representations; *M*, motoric representations; *a*, acoustic impulses; and *m*, motor impulses (Lichtheim, 1885).

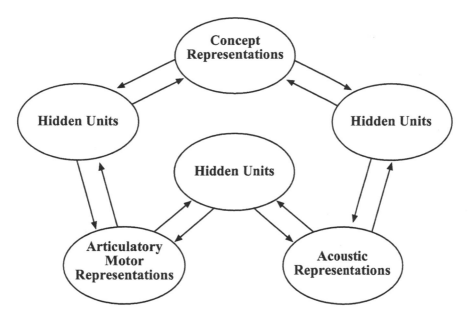

Figure 3–2. A parallel distributed processing (PDP) instantiation of Lichtheim's model.

terest, e.g., articulatory motor representations. The actual pattern of activity in articulatory motor representations is compared with the desired or target pattern of activity. To the extent that there is a discrepancy between actual output and target output, the connection strengths between acoustic representations and hidden units, and between hidden units and articulatory motor representations, are adjusted slightly (in proportion to their contribution to the error) such that the discrepancy is slightly reduced. With repeated cycling through the entire learning corpus, the model eventually develops the set of connection strengths that enables it to generate the correct pattern of activity within articulatory motor representations (within some defined error criterion) given a particular input to acoustic representations.

It is worth taking a moment to consider the issue of lexicons in this model. In the most general neural network conceptualization, a *lexicon* is defined by any pattern associator network in which one of the patterns instantiates declarative memory—that is, memory of discrete, consciously accessible "facts." Thus, the model in Figure 3–2 incorporates three pattern associator networks, but only two of them, the concept to articulatory motor representations pathway (the phonological output lexicon) and

the acoustic representations to concept representations pathway (the phonological input lexicon), instantiate lexicons because only these two incorporate the one type of representation that is declarative—concepts. Acoustic and articulatory motor representations derive meaning and conscious accessibility only by virtue of their links to concept representations. There are two lexicons in this system because the neural substrates, articulatory and acoustic, are fundamentally different. This conceptualization of a lexicon as a pattern of connectivity rather than a locus of discrete pieces of knowledge is at substantial odds with the intuitive way of thinking about lexicons that has been engendered by information-processing models. However, it is well accepted in the connectionist literature and is the only way of conceptualizing the instantiation of a lexicon in a machine, the brain, in which the knowledge is represented in the connections.

At this point it is worth inquiring more deeply into the nature of the processes subsumed in the links between representational fields and hidden unit fields. I will begin with a focus on the acoustic–to–articulatory motor pathway. Specifically, what is the nature of the knowledge represented in this pathway? A reading model developed by Plaut and colleagues (1996) provides crucial insight into this question (see also Seidenberg and McClelland, 1989). This model fundamentally recapitulates the acoustic–articulatory motor pathway of Figure 3–2, the major difference (inconsequential to this discussion) being that in place of acoustic representations, it incorporates orthographic representations. Specifically, it consists of three layers: *(1)* an input layer of 105 grapheme units divided into three groups, the first group consisting of all possibilities for the one or more consonants of the onset (e.g., "st̲op"); the second group, all the possible vowels in the nucleus (e.g., "sto̲p"); and the third group, all possibilities for the one or more consonants in the coda (e.g., "sto̲p̲"); *(2)* a hidden unit layer of 100 units; and *(3)* an output layer of 61 phoneme units divided into groups consisting of all the possibilities for onset, nucleus, and coda, respectively (as for the graphemes). Local representations are used for the graphemes and phonemes. There are one-way connections from each of the grapheme input units to each of the hidden units, and two-way connections between each of the hidden units and each of the phoneme output units. Every output unit is connected to every other output unit, giving the network attractor properties (a capability for settling precisely into one of the available output states, the time to settle corresponding to a response latency). The model was trained, using the back-propagation algorithm, by successively presenting, in pairs, the orthographic representation of 3000 English single-syllable words, and the desired phonological output. Ultimately, it learned to produce the correct pronunciation of all the words. One of the most striking things about the trained model is that it is able to produce correct pronunciations of plausible English nonwords (i.e., orthographic sequences it has never encountered before). How is this possible?

One might have inferred that the model simply learned the pronunciation of all the words by rote. If this were the case, however, the model would be incapable of applying what it has learned to novel words. In fact, what the model learned was the relationships between *sequences* of graphemes and *sequences* of phonemes that are characteristic of the English language. To the extent that there is a limited repertoire of such sequences, the model was

able to learn it and then apply that knowledge to novel forms that incorporated some of the sequential relationships in this repertoire. The information the model acquired through its long experience with English orthographic–phonological sequential relationships goes considerably beyond this, however. Certain sequences, those most commonly found in English single-syllable words, are more thoroughly etched in network connectivity. The model encounters difficulty (reflected in prolonged reading latency) only with low-frequency words, and only to the extent that it incorporates different, competing pronunciations of the same orthographic sequence. Thus, it is slow to read "pint" because in every case but "pint," the sequence "int" is pronounced /Int/ (e.g., "mint, tint, flint, lint"). It is also slow, though not quite so slow, to read words like "shown" because there are two equally frequent alternatives to the pronunciation of "own" ("gown, down, town" vs. "shown, blown, flown"). This behavior precisely recapitulates the behavior of normal human subjects given reading tasks.

To be more precise, the knowledge the model acquires reflects competing effects of type frequency and token frequency. If a single word is sufficiently common (high token frequency), the model acquires enough experience with it that competing orthographic–phonologic sequential relationships have a negligible impact on naming latency. However, if a word is relatively uncommon (e.g., "pint"), its naming latency will be significantly affected by the knowledge of other words that, though equally uncommon, together constitute a competing type (e.g., "mint, flint, tint, sprint").

The capacity of the model to read nonwords reflects its ability to capture patterns in the sequential relationships between orthographic and articulatory word forms and to apply this knowledge to novel word forms. Plaut et al. (1996), as well as Seidenberg and McClelland (1989), in their earlier work on this reading model, focused on differences in rhyme components of single-syllable words because these are the major determinants of whether a word is orthographically regular or irregular. However, as Seidenberg and McClelland point out, the network architecture in these models is capable of capturing any kind of regularity in the orthographic and phonological sequences it is exposed to, limited only by the extent of exposure. Such regularities would include joint phonemes (e.g., "str" of "stream," "street," "stray," and "strum"),[1] and, in a multisyllabic version, syllables and morphemes (particularly prefixes and very high–frequency words such as functors).

The acoustic–articulatory motor pathway in the model of Figure 3–2 would capture analogous patterns in the sequential relationships between acoustic and articulatory word forms (actually somewhat more redundantly, since in English, acoustic–articulatory correspondences are substantially more consistent than are orthographic-articulatory correspondences). These sequential relationship patterns potentially involve sequences of varying length, from phoneme pairs (joint phonemes) up to and including whole words and, possibly, multiple word compounds. These patterns represent the repository of knowledge about sublexical entities in general, as well as our knowledge of phonotactic constraints.

Whereas the acoustic–articulatory motor pathway of the model depicted in Figure 3–2 has the capability for representing sequence

knowledge and, hence, knowledge of sublexical entities, the linkage between concept representations and articulatory motor representations in this model provides relatively little basis for this type of knowledge. A unitary semantic representation, defined by a pattern of activity over concept features, elicits a unitary articulatory motor compound representation— in effect the reverse of the process by which an orthographic word image elicits a concept when one reads via the semantic route. Even though the ultimate output of the concept–articulatory motor pathway is a sequence of movements, the network architecture provides a poor substrate for capturing the regularities of phonologic sequences. Therefore, the fact that in the process of engaging articulatory motor representations from concept representations, normal subjects experience slips of the tongue and aphasic subjects produce phonemic paraphasias in naming and spontaneous language quite comparable to those produced during repetition tells us that this model cannot be correct. There must be a means by which concept representations access the sublexical, phoneme sequence knowledge within the acoustic–articulatory motor pathway. Thus we arrive at the model depicted in Figure 3–3.

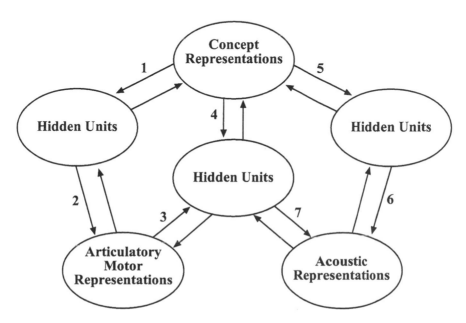

Figure 3–3. Parallel distributed processing instantiation of Lichtheim's model modified to account for the presence of literal paraphasic errors in the spontaneous language of patients with Wernicke's or conduction aphasia.

In the model in Figure 3–3, concept representations interface with the domain of sequence knowledge at the hidden units of the acoustic–articulatory motor pattern associator. Although this semantic input constrains the sequence knowledge in the latter, it tends to bind phonological sequences only to the extent that they form words, rather than to the extent that they instantiate phonotactic relationships. Thus, in all that follows, I will refer to this as *lexical–semantic input*, and reserve the term *sequence knowledge* for the phonotactic knowledge in the acoustic-to-articulatory motor pattern associator.

In the model of Figure 3–3, a direct, concept representations–to–articulatory motor representations pathway (pathway 1–2) has been left in place. The two pathways posited in this model offer a convenient explanation for certain phenomena (e.g., data on verb past tense formation (Ullman et al., 1997; Joanisse and Seidenberg, 1999), and the existence of pathway 1–2 finds direct support in observations of patients with repetition conduction aphasia and deep dysphasia who can repeat words and apparently do so using this pathway because they do not make phonemic paraphasias.

A RECONSIDERATION OF PHONOLOGY FROM A CONNECTIONIST PERSPECTIVE

This section briefly reviews the disorders of phonological processing discussed earlier in the chapter and shows how the PDP model of phonological processing just introduced can, at least in principle, provide a cogent explanation for most of these observations. Five fundamental attributes of the model, three of them characteristic of PDP models in general (graceful degradation, top-down/bottom-up processing interactions, and the representation of memory), and two of them specific to this particular model (the existence of two repositories of knowledge, lexical–semantic, and sequence, and of extensive connectivity between them) can account for most of the phonological phenomena described above.

Graceful Degradation

Graceful degradation refers to the fact that while network damage or noisy input enhances

the likelihood of errors, the errors themselves reflect the knowledge that was and, to some degree, still is represented in the network. Consequently, the errors do not suggest the acquisition of new knowledge and they respect the constraints that were built into the original network. Graceful degradation occurs because the knowledge, represented in the connection strengths, is distributed throughout the model. Thus, a lesion of part of the model leaves intact other portions of the model that support *all* of the knowledge it has acquired. At the same time, it is worth recalling that PDP networks are intrinsically probabilistic, and that different constraints are instantiated to varying degrees, reflecting the learning experience of the network. Graceful degradation means that damaged or noisy networks are intrinsically self-correcting, but absolutely correct output is rendered less certain in such networks and near misses are more likely. The corrective forces within the model vary with type of error, reflecting the heterogeneity of constraint instantiation, and the corrective forces vary somewhat from moment to moment, reflecting the probabilistic aspect of network operations.

Top-Down/Bottom-Up Processing Interactions

Top-down/bottom-up processing interactions stem from the flow of activation up and down, back and forth, throughout the model, no matter where input occurs (e.g., from the top, during naming or spontaneous language, or from the bottom, during repetition). This means that the output of the model is shaped both by the input and by the knowledge existent in connections throughout the model, knowledge whose reliability may have been (gracefully) degraded by lesions. Output is also shaped by the distribution of activation throughout the model (in effect, "noise") at the moment that input occurs, hence slip-of-the-tongue errors occur. Because of top-down/bottom-up processing, for example, input to acoustic representations in a repetition task will be influenced by the connectivity from concept representations, which will confer lexical frequency and imageability effects. Also, because of top-down/bottom-up effects, activation will flow up and down through representations of sequence knowledge, such that in a repetition task, the output will be influenced by words containing similar phonemes, joint phonemes, rhymes, syllables, and morphemes.

The Representation of Memory

In neural network models, long-term memories are represented in the strengths of the connections between units (as in the brain, where the units correspond to neurons), and short-term memory corresponds to the pattern of activation of all the units in the network at any given time. In these models, the neural substrates for memory and processing are one and the same—i.e., there are no physically separate memory stores. Functional imaging studies in humans also suggest that long-term memories are represented in the same cortices that process the substance of those memories, and single neuronal studies in monkeys indicate that the short-term or working memory of a cue corresponds either to sustained activity of neurons representing that cue (Ungerleider, 1995) or an alteration in their state such that they are more susceptible to depolarization by other inputs (Moran and Desimone, 1985). Thus, damage to a processor will inevitably be associated with concomitant impairment in both its short- and long-term mnestic capabilities (Martin et al., 1996; Martin and Saffran, 1997).

Impairment in phonological short-term memory is most likely to be evident in performance of non-rehearsal tasks such as the distraction condition of the Brown-Petersen consonant trigram test, on which patients with repetition conduction aphasia are impaired (Shallice and Warrington, 1977; Caramazza et al., 1981). The ability to use the phonological network for both recall and silent rehearsal is likely to be most important for verbatim repetition of sentences, recall of correct order in word lists, and comprehension of long or grammatically complex sentences. Patients with repetition conduction aphasia also show impairment on such tasks (Saffran and Marin, 1975; Shallice and Warrington, 1977; Vallar et al., 1990; Martin et al., 1994).

The long-term memory stored within the connections of the phonological processor corresponds to knowledge of phonological sequences that is commonly referred to, as in this chapter, as "phonological representations." The connections between the units of the phonological processor and concept representations, as we have discussed, instantiate the phonological lexicons and represent our lexical–semantic knowledge. The connectionist model proposed here, like the brain, would acquire long-term memory through experience with language. The extent of that experience provides the basis for several types of frequency effects. Phoneme sequences corresponding to commonly used words, e.g., "home," will receive particularly strong top-down support both because of the extensive representation of "home" and its manifest associations in association cortices throughout the brain, and because of particularly strong connectivity between the distributed concept representation of "home" and the phonological representation of home that has been acquired through highly repeated use. Sublexical phoneme sequences that are part of many words, e.g., "tion," will receive top-down reinforcement from phonological (sequence) representations because of the many words that contain them. All frequently used phonemic sequences, whether components of major lexical items such as "tion" or such things as free and bound grammatical morphemes (e.g., "the" and the past tense marker "ed," respectively), will also be instantiated in particularly strong connection strengths within the acoustic-articulatory motor pattern associator by virtue of their frequent use.

Two Repositories of Knowledge in the Phonological Processor

The model proposed reflects the now abundant evidence that two sources of knowledge are brought to bear on phonological processing: lexical–semantic and sequence. Connections between concept representations and the acoustic–articulatory motor pattern associator link particular phonological sequences to concepts, providing the basis for the input and output phonological lexicons. Connections within the acoustic–articulatory motor pattern associator provide the basis for knowledge of phonologic sequences in the abstract, devoid of meaning. This sequence knowledge provides the basis for a host of the phonological phenomena reviewed in this chapter. These include phonotactic constraints, clumping effects, and environmental constraints on phonemic selection. Because of phonotactic constraints, both normal and aphasic subjects could easily produce a phonological slip leading them to say "plame" in lieu of "blame." However, a slip from "blame" to "mlame" would be extremely unlikely because whereas both /pl/ and /bl/ are very strongly represented in neural connectivity within the acoustic–articulatory motor pattern associator, /ml/ has no representation at all, since there are no English words that begin with this sequence.

Sequence knowledge underlies the existence of phonological sequences that appear to resist decomposition, either in aphasia or slip-of-the-tongue errors. Rhymes and functors are most strongly represented in neural connectivity within the acoustic–articulatory motor pattern associator by virtue of their frequency of use, but so too, to some degree, are whole words, hence verbal paraphasias or malapropisms.

Environmental constraints on phonemic selection reflect the effect of top-down/bottom-up processing effects within the acoustic–articulatory motor pattern associator. A good example of what might be called a top-down/bottom-up/top-down effect is the tendency for repeated phonemes to induce misordering of phonemes around them (Wickelgren, 1969; MacKay, 1970). Dell (1986) elucidated the mechanism of this phenomenon in a spreading activation model of phonological processing (a connectionist model employing entirely local representations). In the model, as in normal subjects, a repeated phoneme such as /æ/ in the phrase "hat pad" could induce either an exchange, "pat had," an anticipation, "pat pad," or a perseveration, "hat had." The /æ/ gets double top-down activation, leading to particularly strong bottom-up activation of all syllables containing /æ/ throughout the time these syllables are being processed (only "hat" and "pad" were in the sequence vocabulary of Dell's model). These, in turn, provide top-down activation of all their constituent consonants, which then compete. In this example, at any one given time, all four component consonant phonemes, /h/, /t/, /p/, and /d/, are similarly activated and compete, leading to a significant probability that the wrong one will be selected at a particular instant.

Connectivity between Repositories of Lexical–Semantic and Sequence Knowledge

In the development of the connectionist model at the beginning of this section, much was made of the link between concept representations and the hidden units in the acoustic–articulatory motor pathway. This connectivity provides the explanation for the appearance of phonemic paraphasic errors in the naming and spontaneous language of patients with damage to the acoustic–articulatory motor processor and in normal subjects making slips of the tongue. However, this connectivity also provides the basis for a dynamic interaction between lexical–semantic and sequence knowledge that is actually observed in both aphasic and normal subjects. Malapropisms (formal verbal paraphasias) provide a particularly good illustration of this interaction. As a lexical item is activated (instantiated as a pattern of neural activity in the phonological apparatus), it activates all of its various sublexical components. These return activation to the lexical target, but also to phonologically similar targets, regardless of their degree of semantic unrelatedness. This pattern of top-down followed by bottom-up spread of activation can have perverse consequences. First, natural noise in the system can lead to selection of a lexical item phonologically similar to the lexical target because its activation level ends up being a little higher— a classic malapropism. Second, in the presence of a lesion of the phonological apparatus, the downward spread of activation from a lexical target may generate patterns of activity corresponding to a phonemic paraphasic error. This error in turn generates bottom-up spread of activation that enhances the likelihood that a phonologically similar word will receive higher activation than the target (Blanken, 1990). This process, the lexicalization of neologisms, adds one or more errors to the original phonological slip. Gagnon et al. (1995) have confirmed that formal paraphasias, on average, contain a greater number of phonological deviations from the target than do neologisms. Because formal paraphasias in aphasic language reflect an active, top-down mediated lexicalization process, they occur too often to be accounted for by the chance production of real words by single phonemic paraphasias, and they exhibit word frequency and grammatical class effects (greater than chance tendency to be nouns)— phenomena that would never be observed with single phonemic slips alone (Gagnon et al., 1997). A formal paraphasia loses its semantic relationship to the target because words with similar meaning do not generally sound alike.

Verbal paraphasias can arise in a completely different way, in which a phonological slip yields a real word by chance, without lexical or grammatic influence. For example, given the target "cat," a selection error late in phonological processing can result in "sat." However, verbal paraphasias commonly reflect what are referred to as "combination errors," in which phonological, semantic, and grammatic influences are evident. Combination errors may develop in two ways. First, a phonemic slip that initially eliminates semantic and grammatic resemblance to the target (e.g., "cat" → "sat") is followed by bottom-up/top-down processing that induces a second slip and generates a semantic, grammatic, and phonological associate of the target ("cat" → "sat" → "rat"), "rat" being the ultimate result because it received some direct activation as a semantic associate of "cat," and some bottom-up activation from sublexical elements of "sat." Second, the selection of a concept representation is associated with the activation of semantically related representations. All of these semantically related representations engage articulatory motor representations that then lead to bottom-up activation of phonologically related word forms. In the presence of natural or lesion-induced noise in the system that interferes with the engagement of the target word, an alternate that is both semantically and phonologically related, and thus receives activation from two sources, may be more likely to be selected than one that is only semantically related, only phonologically related, or unrelated (Dell and Reich, 1981; Harley, 1984, 1990; Martin et al., 1989; Brédart and Valentine, 1992; Laine and Martin, 1996; Dell et al., 1997; Goodglass et al., 1997).

These observations are paralleled by the findings of Motley and Baars (1976), alluded to earlier, that the likelihood of experimentally inducing a phonological slip is enhanced if the slip results in a real word (reflecting top-down influence of phoneme clumps corresponding to words), and it is further enhanced if that real word is related to a semantic priming stimulus (reflecting top-down influence from concept representations). Corresponding effects have been described in the formation of word blends (e.g., "solely/totally" → "sotally") (MacKay, 1973; Dell, 1980). Word blends are more likely to occur if the contributing words are both semantically and phonologically related, indicating the impact of both top-down and bottom-up effects in the production of these neologisms. These various observations provide very strong evidence of a highly dynamic top-down/bottom-up interactive process within the phonological processor, and a strong validation of PDP principles of parallel processing and both top-down and bottom-up spread of activation (Laine and Martin, 1996; Dell et al., 1997).

Conduction Aphasias

Finally, a brief explanation of the conduction aphasias in terms of the connectionist model introduced is in order. Repetition conduction aphasia can be attributed to *complete* destruction of pathway 7 and probably the hidden units of the acoustic–articulatory motor pathway and pathways 3 and 4 (the lesions are typically very large). As a result, naming and spontaneous language must take place via pathways 1 and 2, and repetition via pathways 6, 5, 1, and 2. Because these are essentially whole word pathways, substantially devoid of sequence knowledge, even if they are partially damaged, errors of phonemic sequence (phonemic paraphasias) will not occur. Furthermore, because acoustic and articulatory motor representations have been disconnected, the extent of the neural network capable of supporting phonological short-term memory is vastly reduced (now limited to acoustic representations), with the net result that these patients have severely impaired auditory–verbal short-term memory (and thus very short digit spans).

Nearly all the phenomena observed in reproduction conduction aphasia can be accounted for in terms of damage to the hidden units in the acoustic–articulatory motor pattern associator or their various connections to acoustic representations, articulatory representations, or concept representations. Consequently, these patients consistently demonstrate some disorder of sequence knowledge in some aspect of their language, resulting in production of phonemic paraphasic errors. To the extent that the acoustic–articulatory motor pattern associator is spared, repetition will be relatively preserved. To the extent that pathways 4 and 1–2 are spared, lexical access in naming and spontaneous language will be preserved and lexical effects will be evident during repetition as well.

ANATOMY OF PHONOLOGICAL PROCESSING

The conceptualization of the language processor developed in this chapter can be reconciled fairly easily with the traditional anatomic mapping of the Lichtheim model (Lichtheim, 1885), in which a center for auditory word images in area 22 is linked, presumably by the arcuate fasciculus, to the area of motor expression in posterior inferior frontal lobe (Broca's area) (Fig. 3–1).

ACOUSTIC–ARTICULATORY MOTOR PATTERN ASSOCIATOR

Whereas I have discussed a unitary processor that must implicitly incorporate a hierarchical structure, data from functional imaging studies (Démonet et al., 1992; Paulesu et al., 1993) and from intraoperative electrocortical stimulation studies (Ojemann, 1991) strongly suggest that there is a discontinuity in the perisylvian language cortex that supports phonological processing—that is, there is a posterior language region centered on area 22 and extending variably into area 40, and an anterior region centered on Broca's area and extending variably backwards into opercular areas 4 and 6. Parietal operculum between the central sulcus and area 40 appears less likely to be implicated directly in this process in most people. There is a caveat here, which is that data are emerging, particularly from Ojemann's electrocortical stimulation studies (Ojemann et al., 1989; Ojemann, 1991), but more recently from functional imaging studies (Binder et al., 1995; Cuenod et al., 1995), that support substantial individual variability in the location and extent of cortex devoted to language processing in general and to phonological processing in particular.

Disconnection theories of conduction aphasia originated with Carl Wernicke and have been a subject of continuous debate ever since (Palumbo et al., 1992). The long white matter links between Wernicke's and Broca's areas (e.g., the arcuate fasciculus) presumably evolved with the physical separation of these two cortices that developed during phylogenesis and ontogenesis. Thus, there is no particular reason to think that these long white matter tracts are either functionally more important or fundamentally different from white matter connections *within* Wernicke's and Broca's areas. If the arcuate fasciculus is part of the acoustic–articulatory motor pattern associator, it is not clear where within this hierarchical processor it is located, and the precise location may vary from subject to subject. It is also possible that this white matter pathway is not involved in phonological processing. Brown (1975) reported echolalia in a patient with an autopsy–documented lesion of the arcuate fasciculus, and Shuren et al. (1995) reported normal word and phrase repetition (nonword repetition was not tested) and mildly impaired digit span following a surgically produced arcuate lesion in a patient with a perisylvian glioma.

Reproduction conduction aphasia is produced by lesions in the supramarginal gyrus, posterior aspect of Wernicke's area, and the angular gyrus (Benson et al., 1973; Naeser and Hayward, 1978; Damasio and Damasio, 1980; Palumbo et al., 1992). This suggests that these regions comprise part of the acoustic–articulatory motor pattern associator. The insula is also commonly involved in patients with reproduction conduction aphasia, but it is unlikely that this phylogenetically ancient structure with predominantly orbitofrontal and limbic connectivity participates in language processes. However, white matter connections from the superior temporal gyrus to the frontal cortex do pass in the extreme capsule, immediately beneath the insula (Damasio and Damasio, 1980).

LINKS TO SEMANTIC REPRESENTATIONS

In a PDP framework, concepts are highly distributed over a network of subnetworks, each subnetwork instantiating features of a concept that fall within a particular domain. Thus, the concept "dog" corresponds to a pattern of neural activity in visual association cortices corresponding to visual attributes of dogs, a pattern in somatosensory association cortices corresponding to tactile aspects of dogs, a pattern in olfactory association cortex, a pattern in auditory association cortex, a pattern in limbic cortex (corresponding to emotional feelings regarding dogs in general or a particular dog), and a pattern in frontal cortex corresponding to predicative aspects of dogs (what they are likely to do). The fact that there is variability in the contribution of different feature domains to the meaning of particular entities provides the basis for category-specific naming deficits. Thus, the dominance of the visual representation in our conceptualization of dogs or other living things leads to a susceptibility of this knowledge to focal lesions of visual association cortex. This is essentially the explanation proposed by Warrington and Shallice years ago (Warrington and Shallice, 1984).

The links between the various networks supporting distributed concept representations and the various components of the acoustic–articulatory motor pattern associator appear to coalesce primarily in posterior perisylvian cortex (area 22) and immediately adjacent areas (areas 37 and 39) (Geschwind, 1965). In the view expanded in this chapter, the concept representations–hidden units–acoustic representations pathway instantiates the phonological input lexicon, and the concept representations–hidden units–articulatory motor representations pathways instantiate the phonologic output lexicon. In this way, lexicons are highly distributed and it is only the terminuses of the phonologic input and output lex-

icons that are actually located in dominant perisylvian cortices. This idea has been validated in an interesting way by a functional magnetic resonance imaging (fMRI) study. Binder et al. (1997) showed that during a tone sequence monitoring task, blood flow (a marker of synaptic activity) increased in the posterior two-thirds of the superior temporal gyri and the supramarginal gyri bilaterally. When this pattern of blood flow was contrasted (using a subtraction technique) with the pattern elicited by a semantic monitoring task (signal whether named animals were native to the United States and "used by humans"), increased blood flow was noted in posterior superior temporal sulcus, middle temporal gyrus, parts of the inferior temporal and fusiform gyri, angular gyrus, much of dorsolateral prefrontal cortex (including the frontal operculum), and the anterior and posterior cingulate gyri. Most notably, there was no increase in blood flow in Wernicke's area and supramarginal gyrus. Expectably, and entirely consistent with the model of distributed concept representations developed here, association cortices throughout the brain (the left cortices much more than the right) were differentially engaged by the semantic task. The semantic task also engaged Broca's area because it engaged the acoustic–articulatory motor pattern associator in a way that the tone-monitoring task could not. However, the acoustic representations and their various derivations in Wernicke's area and supramarginal gyrus were apparently engaged by both tasks equally. The lack of differential activation in these regions by the semantic task can partly be attributed to the limited ability of functional imaging studies to detect differential activation when both tasks engage a given region of cortex to some degree (Nadeau and Crosson, 1995). However, there is no avoiding the fact that in the study of Binder et al. (1997), the pure tone–monitoring task produced robust activation of area 22 and posterior area 40 (compared to rest). This seemingly paradoxical result becomes understandable when one appreciates that this cortex supports not the phonologic input lexicon but rather only the proximal, acoustic end of the phonologic input lexicon. This cortex can evidently be engaged by both pure tone and language sounds. However, because pure tones will not be translated by pattern associator networks into other language domains (semantic and articulatory motor), they do not elicit activity in the widely disseminated association cortices supporting the distal ends of the lexicons (distributed concept representations) or the distal end of the acoustic–articulatory motor pattern associator (Broca's area). Conversely, a lesion of Wernicke' area produces both anomia and phonologic paraphasias or neologistic jargon in output and impaired comprehension because it is usually damages the proximal portions of both the acoustic–articulatory motor pattern associator and the pattern associators supporting the input and output phonological lexicons. In this way, the somewhat unexpected results of this fMRI study are highly consistent with the concepts discussed in this chapter.

CONCLUSION

This brief review of disorders of phonological processing suggests that a PDP conceptualization of the phonological apparatus can account, in broad terms, for a large body of observational and experimental data, and at the same time be reconciled with what we know about the neuroanatomy involved. The specific structure of the model (Fig. 3–3) and, in particular, the posited links between concept representations and the hidden units of the acoustic–articulatory motor pattern associator bring two sources of knowledge to bear on phonological processing—sequence and lexical–semantic. This hypothesis of dual knowledge sources has great explanatory value, and it is hard to account for the full range of scientific observations without it. Other investigators (Dell, 1986) have implicitly posited dual knowledge sources in local representation-spreading activation models. Here, dual knowledge sources have been explicitly incorporated in a fully distributed representation model.

The model proposed here is merely a hypothesis about neural structure. It has not been subjected to simulations. Furthermore, the many studies reviewed here were motivated by a host of different models, most characterizable as serial and information-processing models. Inevitably, our conceptual biases color our perceptions. As has already occurred repeatedly in the brief history of PDP research, questions raised by PDP models, and particularly by PDP simulations, have led to re-examination of old and well-accepted ideas, often with startling results.

NOTE

1. The model of Plaut et al. (1996) coded such clusters as local representations, so it did not have the opportunity to learn these sequences.

REFERENCES

Akmajian, A., Demers, R. A., and Harnish, R. M. (1984). *Linguistics: An Introduction to Language and Communication*. Cambridge, MA: MIT Press.

Alajouanine, T., and Lhermitte, F. (1973). The phonemic and semantic components of jargon aphasia. In *Psycholinguistics and Aphasia*, H. Goodglass and S. Blumstein (eds.). Baltimore: Johns Hopkins University Press, pp. 318–329.

Allport, D. A. (1984a). Auditory–verbal short-term memory and conduction aphasia. In *Attention and Performance X. Control of Language Processes*, H. Bouma and D. G. Bouwhuis (eds.). London: Lawrence Erlbaum Associates, pp. 313–325.

Allport, D. A. (1984b). Speech production and comprehension: one lexicon or two? In *Cognition and Motor Processes*, W. Prinz and A. F. Sanders (eds.). Berlin/Heidelberg: Springer-Verlag, pp. 209–228.

Baars, B. J., Motley, M. T., and MacKay, D. G. (1975). Output editing for lexical status in artificially elicited slips of the tongue. *J. Verbal Learn. Verbal Behav. 14*:382–391.

Baddeley, A., Gathercole, S., and Papagno, C. (1998). The phonological loop as a language learning device. *Psychol. Rev. 105*:158–173.

Baker, E., Blumstein, S. E., and Goodglass, H. (1981). Interaction between phonological and semantic factors in auditory comprehension. *Neuropsychologia 19*:1–15.

Barton, M. I. (1971). Recall of generic properties of words in aphasic patients. *Cortex 7*:73–82.

Benson, D. F., Sheremata, W. A., Bouchard, R., Segarra, J. M., Price, N., Geschwind, N. (1973). Conduction aphasia. A clinicopathological study. *Arch. Neurol., 28*:339–346.

Binder, J. R., Frost, J. A., Hammeke, T. A., Cox, R. W., Rao, S. M., and Prieto, T. (1997). Human brain language areas identified by functional magnetic resonance imaging. *J. Neurosci.* 17:353–362.

Binder, J. R., Rao, S. M., Hammeke, T. A., Frost, J. A., Bandettini, P. A., Jesmanowicz, A. et al. (1995). Lateralized human brain language systems demonstrated by task subtraction functional magnetic resonance imaging. *Arch. Neurol.* 52:593–601.

Blanken, G. (1990). Formal paraphasias: a single case study. *Brain Lang* 38:534–554.

Blumstein, S. (1973a). *A Phonological Investigation of Aphasic Speech*. The Hague: Mouton.

Blumstein, S. (1973b). Some phonologic implications of aphasic speech. In *Psycholinguistics and Aphasia*, H. Goodglass and S. Blumstein (eds.). Baltimore: Johns Hopkins University Press, pp. 123–137.

Blumstein, S. E. (1978). Segment structure and the syllable in aphasia. In *Syllables and Segments*, A. Bell and J. B. Hooper (eds.). Amsterdam: North-Holland Publishing Company, pp. 189–200.

Blumstein, S. E., Baker, E., and Goodglass, H. (1977a). Phonological factors in auditory comprehension in aphasia. *Neuropsychologia* 15:19–30.

Blumstein, S. E., Burton, M., Baum, S., Waldstein, R., and Katz, D. (1994). The role of lexical status on the phonetic categorization of speech in aphasia. *Brain Lang.* 46:181–197.

Blumstein, S. E., Cooper, W. E., Zurif, E. B., and Caramazza, A. (1977b). The perception and production of voice-onset time in aphasia. *Neuropsychologia* 15:371–383.

Bond, Z.S., and Garnes, S. (1980). Misperceptions of fluent speech. In: *Perception and Production in Fluent Speech*, R. A. Cole (ed.) Hillsdale, NJ: Lawrence Erlbaum Associates, pp. 115–132.

Brédart, S., and Valentine, T. (1992). From Monroe to Moreau: an analysis of face naming errors. *Cognition* 45:187–223.

Brener, R. (1940). An experimental investigation of memory span. *J. Exp. Psychol.* 26:467–482.

Brooks, J. O., and Watkins, M. J. (1990). Further evidence of the intricacy of memory span. *J Exp. Psychol. Learn. Mem. Cogn.* 16:1134–1141.

Brown, A. S. (1991). A review of the tip-of-the-tongue experience. *Psychol. Bull.* 109:204–223.

Brown, J. W. (1975). The problem of repetition: a study of "conduction" aphasia and the "isolation" syndrome. *Cortex* 11:37–52.

Brown, R., and McNeill, D. (1966). The "tip of the tongue" phenomenon. *J. Verbal Learn. Verbal Behav.* 5:325–337.

Bub, D., Black, S., Howell, J., and Kertesz, A. (1987). Damage to input and output buffers—what's a lexicality effect doing in a place like that? In *Motor and Sensory Processes of Language*, E. Keller and M. Gopnik (eds.). Hillsdale, NJ: Lawrence Erlbaum Associates, pp. 83–110.

Bub, D. N., Black, S., Hamson, E., and Kertesz, A. (1988). Semantic encoding of pictures and words. Some neuropsychological observations. *Cogn. Neuropsychol.* 5:27–66.

Buckingham, H. W. (1980). On correlating aphasic errors with slips-of-the-tongue. *Appl. Psycholinguistics* 1:199–220.

Buckingham, H. W., Avakian-Whitaker, H., and Whitaker, H. A. (1978). Alliteration and assonance in neologistic jargon aphasia. *Cortex* 14:365–380.

Buckingham, H. W., and Kertesz, A. (1974). A linguistic analysis of fluent aphasia. *Brain Lang* 1:43–62.

Burke, D. M., MacKay, D.G., Worthley, J. S., and Wade, E. (1991). On the tip of the tongue: what causes word finding failures in young and older adults? *J. Mem. Lang.*, 30:542–579.

Burns, M. S., and Canter, G. J. (1977). Phonemic behavior of aphasic patients with posterior cerebral lesions. *Brain Lang.* 4:492–507.

Butterworth, B. (1979). Hesitation and the production of verbal paraphasias and neologisms in jargon aphasia. *Brain Lang.* 8:133–161.

Canter, G. J., Trost, J. E., and Burns, M. S. (1985). Contrasting speech patterns in apraxia of speech and phonemic paraphasia. *Brain Lang.* 24:204–222.

Caplan, D., Vanier, M., and Baker, C. (1986). A case study of reproduction conduction aphasia I: word production. *Cogn. Neuropsychol.* 3:99–128.

Caramazza, A., Basili, A. G., Koller, J. J., and Berndt, R. S. (1981). An investigation of repetition and language processing in a case of conduction aphasia. *Brain Lang.* 14:235–271.

Caramazza, A., Berndt, R. S., and Basili, A. G. (1983). The selective impairment of phonological processing: a case study. *Brain Lang.* 18:128–174.

Caramazza, A., Miceli, G., and Villa, G. (1986). The role of the (output) phonological buffer in reading, writing, and repetition. *Cogn. Neuropsychol.* 3:37–76.

Cermak, L. S., and Tarlow, S. (1978). Aphasic and amnesic patients' verbal vs nonverbal retentive capabilities. *Cortex* 14:32–40.

Cuenod, C. A., Bookheimer, S. Y., Hertz-Pannier, L., Zeffiro, T. A., Theodore, W. H., and Le Bihan, D. (1995). Functional MRI during word generation, using conventional equipment: a potential tool for language localization in the clinical environment. *Neurology* 45:1821–1827.

Damasio, H., and Damasio, A. R. (1980). The anatomical basis of conduction aphasia. *Brain* 103:337–350.

Dell, G. S. (1980). *Phonological and Lexical Encoding in Speech Production: An Analysis of Naturally Occurring and Experimentally Elicited Speech Errors.* Unpublished doctoral dissertation, University of Toronto.

Dell, G. S. (1986). A spreading-activation theory of retrieval in sentence production. *Psychol. Rev.* 93:283–321.

Dell, G. S. (1988). The retrieval of phonological forms in production: tests of predictions from a connectionist model. *J. Mem. Lang.* 27:124–142.

Dell, G. S., and Reich, P. A. (1981). Stages in sentence production: an analysis of speech error data. *J. Verbal Learn. Verbal Behav.* 20:611–629.

Dell, G. S., Schwartzm, M. F., Martin, N., Saffran, E. M., and Gagnon, D. A. (1997). Lexical access in normal and aphasic speakers. *Psychol. Rev.* 104:801–838.

Démonet, J.-F., Chollet, F., Ramsay, S., Cardebat, D., Nespoulous, J.-L., Wise, R., et al. (1992). The anatomy of phonological and semantic processing in normal subjects. *Brain* 115.1753 1768.

Dubois, J., Hécaen, H., Angelergues, R., Maufras de Chatelier, A., and Marcie, P. (1973). Neurolinguistic study of conduction aphasia. In *Psycholinguistics and Aphasia*, H. Goodglass and S. Blumstein (eds.). Baltimore: Johns Hopkins University Press, pp. 283–300.

Dunlop, J. M., and Marquardt, T. P. (1977). Linguistic and articulatory aspects of single word production in apraxia of speech. *Cortex* 13:17–29.

Ellis, A. W. (1980). Errors in speech and short-term memory: the effects of phonemic similarity and syllable position. *J Verbal Learn. Verbal Behav.* 19:624–634.

Ellis, A. W. (1985). The production of spoken words: a cognitive neuropsychological perspective. In *Progress in the Psychology of Language*, Vol. 2, A. W. Ellis, (ed.). Hillsdale, NJ: Lawrence Erlbaum Associates, pp. 107–145.

Ellis, A. W., Miller, D., and Sin, G. (1983). Wernicke's aphasia and normal language processing: a case study in cognitive neuropsychology. *Cognition* 15:111–144.

Ellis, A. W., and Young, A. W. (1988). *Human Cognitive Neuropsychology.* Hillsdale, NJ: Lawrence Erlbaum Associates.

Elman, J. L., and McClelland, J. L. (1988). Cognitive penetration of the mechanisms of perception: compensation for coarticulation of lexically restored phonemes. *J. Mem. Lang.* 27:143–165.

Fay, D., and Cutler, A. (1977). Malapropisms and the structure of the mental lexicon. *Linguist. Inquiry* 8:505–520.

Feinberg, T. E., Gonzalez Rothi, L. J., and Heilman, K. M. (1986). 'Inner speech' in conduction aphasia. *Arch. Neurol.* 43:591–593.

Friedman, R. B., and Kohn, S. E. (1990). Impaired activation of the phonological lexicon: effects upon oral reading. *Brain Lang.* 38:278–297.

Friedrich, F. J., Glenn, C. G., and Marin, O. S. M. (1984). Interruption of phonological coding in conduction aphasia. *Brain Lang.* 22:266–291.

Fromkin, V. A. (1971). The non-anomalous nature of anomalous utterances. *Language* 47:27–52.

Gagnon, D. A., Schwartz, M. F., Martin, N., Dell, G. S., and Saffran, E. M. (1995). The origins of form-related word and nonword errors in aphasic naming. *Brain Cogn.* 28:192.

Gagnon, D. A., Schwartz, M. F., Martin, N., Dell, G. S., and Saffran, E. M. (1997). The origin of formal paraphasias in aphasic's picture naming. *Brain Lang.* 59:450–472.

Gandour, J., Akamanon, C., Dechongkit, S., Khunadorn, F., and Boonklam, R. (1994). Sequences of phonemic approximations in a Thai conduction aphasic. *Brain Lang.* 46:69–95.

Gandour, J., and Dardarananda, R. (1982). Voice onset time in aphasia: Thai. I. Perception. *Brain Lang.* 17:24–33.

Garrett, M. F. (1975). The analysis of sentence production. In *The Psychology of Learning and Motivation*, G. H. Bower (ed.). New York: Academic Press, pp. 133–177.

Garrett, M. F. (1976). Syntactic processes in sentence production. In *New Approaches to Language Mechanisms*, R. J. Wales and E. Walker (eds.) Amsterdam: North-Holland Publishing, pp. 231–256.

Geschwind, N. (1965). Disconnexion syndromes in animals and man. *Brain* 88:237–294, 585–644.

Goldman-Rakic, P. S. (1990). Cellular and circuit basis of working memory in prefrontal cortex of nonhuman primates. *Prog. Brain Res.* 85:325–336.

Goodglass, H., Gleason, J. B., and Hyde, M. R. (1970). Some dimensions of auditory language comprehension in aphasia. *J Speech Hear. Res.* 13:595–606.

Goodglass, H., Kaplan, E., Weintraub, S., and Ackerman, N. (1976). The "tip of the tongue" phenomenon in aphasia. *Cortex* 12:145–153.

Goodglass, H., Wingfield, A., Hyde, M. R., Gleason, J. B., Bowles, N. L., and Gallagher, R. E. (1997). The importance of word initial phonology: error patterns in prolonged naming efforts by aphasic patients. *J Int. Neuropsychol. Soc.* 3:128–138.

Green, E. (1969). Phonological and grammatical aspects of jargon in an aphasic patient: a case study. *Lang. Speech* 12:103–118.

Green, E., and Howes, D. H. (1977). The nature of conduction aphasia: a study of anatomic and clinical features and of underlying mechanisms. In *Studies in Neurolinguistics*, Vol. 3, H. Whitaker and H. A. Whitaker (eds.). New York: Academic Press, pp. 123–156.

Halpern, H., Keith, R. L., and Darley, F. L. (1976). Phonemic behavior of aphasic subjects without dysarthria or apraxia of speech. *Cortex* 12:365–372.

Harley, T. A. (1984). A critique of top-down independent levels models of speech production: evidence from non–plan-internal speech errors. *Cogn. Sci.* 8:191–219.

Harley, T. A. (1990). Phonologic activation of semantic competitors during lexical access in speech production. *Lang. Cogn. Proc.* 8:291–309.

Heilman, K. M., Scholes, R., and Watson, R. T. (1976). Defects of immediate memory in Broca's and conduction aphasia. *Brain Lang.* 3:201–208.

Howard, D., and Franklin, S. (1988). *Missing the Meaning? A Cognitive Neuropsychological Study of the Processing of Words by an Aphasic Patient*. Cambridge, MA: MIT Press.

Joanette, Y., Keller, E., and Lecours, A. R. (1980). Sequences of phonemic approximations in aphasia. *Brain Lang.* 11:30–44.

Joanisse, M. F., and Seidenberg, M. S. (1999). Impairments in verb morphology after brain injury: a connectionist model. *Proc. Natl. Acad. Sci. U.S.A.* 96:7592–7597.

Johns, D. F., and Darley, F. L. (1970). Phonemic variability in apraxia of speech. *J. Speech Hear. Res.* 13:556–583.

Kay, J., and Ellis, A. W. (1987). A cognitive neuropsychological case study of anomia: implications for psychologic models of word retrieval. *Brain* 110:613–629.

Keller, E. (1978). Parameters for vowel substitutions in Broca's aphasia *Brain Lang.* 5:265–285.

Kertesz, A., and Benson, D. F. (1970). Neologistic jargon: a clinicopathological study. *Cortex* 6:362–386.

Klich, R. J., Ireland, J. V., and Weidner, W. E. (1979). Articulatory and phonological aspects of consonant substitutions in apraxia of speech. *Cortex* 15:451–470.

Kohn, S. E. (1984). The nature of the phonological disorder in conduction aphasia. *Brain Lang.* 23:97–115.

Kohn, S. E. (1989). The nature of the phonemic string deficit in conduction aphasia. *Aphasiology* 3:209–239.

Kohn, S. E., and Smith, K. L. (1990). Between-word speech errors in conduction aphasia. *Cogn. Neuropsychol.* 7:133–156.

Kohn, S. E., and Smith, K. L. (1991). The relationship between oral spelling and phonological breakdown in a conduction aphasic. *Cortex* 27:631–639.

Kohn, S. E., and Smith, K. L. (1993). Lexical–phonological processing of functors: evidence from fluent aphasia. *Cortex* 29:53–64.

Kohn, S. E., and Smith, K. L. (1995). Serial effects of phonemic planning during word production. *Aphasiology* 9:209–222.

Kohn, S. E., Wingfield, A., Menn, L., Goodglass, H., Gleason, J. B., and Hyde, M. (1987). Lexical retrieval: the tip-of-the-tongue phenomenon. *Appl. Psycholinguistics* 8:245–266.

Koriat, A., and Lieblich, I. (1974). What does a person in a "TOT" state know that a person in a "don't know" state doesn't know. *Mem. Cogn.* 2:647–655.

Laine, M., and Martin, N. (1996). Lexical retrieval deficit in picture naming: implications for word production models. *Brain Lang.* 53:283–314.

La Pointe, L. L., and Johns, D. F. (1975). Some phonemic characteristics in apraxia of speech. *J. Commun. Disord.* 8:259–269.

Lecours, A. R. (1982). On neologisms. In *Perspectives on Mental Representation*, J. Mehler, E. C. T. Walker, and M. Garrett (eds.). Hillsdale, NJ: Lawrence Erlbaum Associates, pp. 217–250.

Lecours, A. R., and Lhermitte, F. (1969). Phonemic paraphasias: linguistic structures and tentative hypotheses. *Cortex* 5:193–228.

Levitt, A. B., and Healy, A. F. (1985). The roles of phoneme frequency, similarity, and availability in the experimental elicitation of speech errors. *J Mem. Lang.* 24:717–733.

Lichtheim, L. (1885). On aphasia. *Brain* 7:433–484.

MacKay, D. G. (1970). Spoonerisms: the structure of errors in the serial order of speech. *Neuropsychologia* 8:323–350.

MacKay, D. G. (1972). The structure of words and syllables: evidence from errors in speech. *Cogn. Psychol.* 3:210–227.

MacKay, D. G. (1973). Complexity in output systems: evidence from behavioral hybrids. *Am. J. Psychol.* 86:785–806.

MacNeilage, P. (1982). Speech production mechanisms in aphasia. In *Speech Motor Control*, S. Grillner, B. Lindblom, J. Lubker, and A. Persson (eds.). London: Pergamon, pp. 43–60.

Marin, O. M., Saffran, E. M., and Schwartz, M. F. (1976). Dissociation of language in aphasia: implications for normal function. *Ann. NY Acad. Sci.* 280:868–884.

Marquardt, T. P., Reinhart, J. B., and Peterson, H. A. (1979). Markedness analysis of phonemic substitution errors in apraxia of speech. *J. Commun. Disord.* 12:481–494.

Martin, A. D., and Rigrodsky, S. (1974). An investigation of phonological impairment in aphasia, part 1. *Cortex* 10:317–346.

Martin, N., and Saffran, E. M. (1992). A computational account of deep dysphasia: evidence from a single case study. *Brain Lang.* 43:240–274.

Martin, N., and Saffran, E. M. (1997). Language and auditory-verbal short-term memory impairments: evidence for common underlying processes. *Cogn. Neuropsychol.* 14:641–682.

Martin, N., Saffran, E. M., and Dell, G. S. (1996). Recovery in deep dysphasia: evidence for a relation between auditory–verbal STM capacity and lexical errors in repetition. *Brain Lang.* 52:83–113.

Martin, N., Weisberg, R. W., and Saffran, E. M. (1989). Variables influencing the occurrence of naming errors: implications for a model of lexical retrieval. *J. Mem. Lang.* 28:462–485.

Martin, R. C., Lesch, M. F., and Bartha, M. C. (1999). Independence of input and output phonology in word processing and short-term memory. *J. Mem. Lang.* 41:3–29.

Martin, R. C., Shelton, J. R., and Yaffee, L. S. (1994). Language processing and working memory: neuropsychological evidence for separate phonological and semantic capacities. *J. Mem. Lang.* 33:83–111.

McCarthy, R., and Warrington, E. K. (1984). A two-route model of speech production. Evidence from aphasia. *Brain* 107:463–485.

Miceli, G., Caltagirone, C., Gainotti, C., and Payer-Rigo, P. (1978). Discrimination of voice versus place contrasts in aphasia. *Brain Lang.* 6:47–51.

Miceli, G., Gainotti, G., Caltagirone, C., and Masullo, C. (1980). Some aspects of phonological impairment in aphasia. *Brain Lang.* 11:159–169.

Miller, D., and Ellis, A. W. (1987). Speech and writing errors in "neologistic jargonaphasia": a lexical activation hypothesis. In *The Cognitive Neuropsychology of Language*, M. Coltheart, G. Sartori, and R. Job (eds.). Hillsdale, NJ: Lawrence Erlbaum Associates, pp. 253–271.

Moran, J., and Desimone, R. (1985). Selective attention gates visual processing in extrastriate cortex. *Science* 229:782–784.

Motley, M. T., and Baars, B. J. (1976). Semantic bias effects on the outcomes of verbal slips. *Cognition* 4:177–187.

Nadeau, S. E. (2001). Phonology: a review and proposals from a connectionist perspective.

Nadeau, S. E., and Crosson, B. (1995). A guide to the functional imaging of cognitive processes. *Neuropsychiatry Neuropsychol. Behav. Neurol.* 8:143–162.

Naeser, M. A., and Hayward, R. W. (1978). Lesion localization in aphasia with cranial computed tomography and the Boston Diagnostic Aphasia Exam. *Neurology* 28:545–551.

Nespoulous, J.-L., Joanette, Y., Béland, R., Caplan, D., and Lecours, A. R. (1984). Phonologic disturbances in aphasia: is there a "markedness effect" in aphasic phonetic errors? *Adv. Neurol.* 42:203–214.

Nespoulous, J.-L., Joanette, Y., Ska, B., Caplan, D., and Lecours, A. R. (1987). Production deficits in Broca's and conduction aphasia: repetition versus reading. In *Motor and Sensory Processes of Language*. E. Keller and M. Gopnik (eds.). Hillsdale, NJ: Lawrence Erlbaum Associates, pp. 53–81.

Niemi, J., and Koivuselkä-Sallinen, P. (1985). Phoneme errors in Broca's aphasia: three Finnish cases. *Brain Lang.* 26:28–48.

Ojemann, G. A. (1991). Cortical organization of language. *J. Neurosci.* 11:2281–2287.

Ojemann, G. A., Ojemann, J., Lettich, E., and Berger, M. (1989). Cortical language localization in left, dominant hemisphere. An electrical stimulation mapping investigation in 117 patients. *J. Neurosurg.* 71:316–326.

Palumbo, C. L., Alexander, M. P., and Naeser, M. A. (1992). CT scan lesion sites associated with conduction aphasia. In *Conduction Aphasia*, S. E. Kohn (ed.). Hillsdale, NJ: Lawrence Erlbaum Associates, pp. 51–75.

Pate, D. S., Saffran, E. M., and Martin, N. (1987). Specifying the nature of the production impairment in a conduction aphasic. *Lang. Cogn. Proc.* 2:43–84.

Paulesu, E., Frith, C. D., and Frackowiak, R. S. J. (1993). The neural correlates of the verbal component of working memory. *Nature* 362:342–345.

Plaut, D. C., McClelland, J. L., Seidenberg, M. S., and Patterson, K. (1996). Understanding normal and impaired word reading: computational principles in quasi-regular domains. *Psychol. Rev.* 103:56–115.

Poncet, M., Degos, C., DeLoche, G., and Lecours, A. R. (1972). Phonetic and phonemic transformations in aphasia. *Int. J. Ment. Health* 1:46–54.

Posner, M. I. (1964). Rate of presentation and order of recall in immediate memory. *Br. J. Psychol.* 55:303–306.

Rubin, D. C. (1975). Within word structure in the tip-of-the-tongue phenomenon. *J. Verbal Learn. Verbal Behav. 14*:392–397.

Saffran, E. M., and Marin, O. S. M. (1975). Immediate memory for word lists in a patient with deficient auditory short-term memory. *Brain Lang. 2*:420–433.

Schwartz, M. F., Saffran, E. M., Bloch, D. E., and Dell, G. S. (1994). Disordered speech production in aphasic and normal speakers. *Brain Lang. 47*:52–88.

Seidenberg, M. S., and McClelland, J. L. (1989). A distributed, developmental model of word recognition and naming. *Psychol. Rev. 96*:523–568.

Shallice, T., and Vallar, G. (1990). The impairment of auditory-verbal short-term storage. In *Neuropsychological Impairments of Short-term Memory*, G. Vallar and T. Shallice (eds.). Cambridge, UK: Cambridge University Press, pp. 11–53.

Shallice, T., and Warrington, E. K. (1977). Auditory–verbal short-term memory impairment and conduction aphasia. *Brain Lang. 4*:479–491.

Shankweiler, D., and Harris, K. S. (1966). An experimental approach to the problem of articulation in aphasia. *Cortex 2*:277–292.

Shankweiler, D., Harris, K. S., and Taylor, M. L. (1968). Electromyographic studies of articulation in aphasia. *Arch. Phys. Med. Rehabil. 49*: 1–8.

Shattuck-Hufnagel, S. (1979). Speech errors as evidence for a serial-ordering mechanism in sentence production. In *Sentence Processing: Psycholinguistic Studies*. W. E. Cooper and E. C. T. Walker (eds.). Hillsdale, NJ: Lawrence Erlbaum Associates, pp. 295–341.

Shattuck-Hufnagel, S., and Klatt, D. H. (1979). The limited use of distinctive features and markedness in speech production: evidence from speech error data. *J. Verbal Learn. Verbal Behav. 18*:41–55.

Shewan, C. M. (1980). Phonological processing in Broca's aphasics. *Brain Lang. 10*:71–88.

Shinn, P., and Blumstein, P. (1983). Phonetic disintegration in aphasia: acoustic analysis of spectral characteristics for place of articulation. *Brain Lang. 20*:90–114.

Shuren, J. E., Schefft, B. K., Yeh, H.-S., Privitera, M. D., Cahill, W. T., and Houston, W. (1995). Repetition and the arcuate fasciculus. *J. Neurol. 242*:596–598.

Stemberger, J. P. (1982). The nature of segments in the lexicon: evidence from speech errors. *Lingua 56*:235–259.

Stemberger, J. P. (1984). Structural errors in normal and agrammatic speech. *Cogn. Neuropsychol. 4*:281–313.

Stemberger, J. P. (1985). An interactive activation model of language production. In *Progress in the Psychology of Language*, Vol. 1. A. W. Ellis (ed.). Hillsdale, NJ: Lawrence Erlbaum Associates, pp. 143–186.

Stemberger, J. P., and MacWhinney, B. (1986). Frequency and the lexical storage of regularly inflected forms. *Mem. Cogn. 14*:17–26.

Strub, R. L., and Gardner, H. (1974). The repetition defect in conduction aphasia: mnestic or linguistic? *Brain Lang. 1*:241–255.

Trost, J. E., and Canter, G. J. (1974). Apraxia of speech in patients with Broca's aphasia: a study of phoneme production accuracy and error patterns. *Brain Lang. 1*:63–79.

Ullman, M. T., Corkin. S., Coppola, M., Hickok, G., Growdon, J. H., Koroshetz, W. J., et al. (1997). A neural dissociation within language: evidence that the mental dictionary in part of declarative memory, and that grammatical rules are processed by the procedural system. *J Cogn Neurosci. 9*:266–276.

Ungerleider, L. G. (1995). Functional brain imaging studies of cortical mechanisms of memory. *Science 270*:769–775.

Valdois, S., Joanette, Y., and Nespoulous, J.-L. (1989). Intrinsic organization of sequences of phonemic approximations: a preliminary study. *Aphasiology 3*:55–73.

Valdois, S., Joanette, Y., Nespoulous, J.-L., and Poncet, M. (1988). Afferent motor aphasia and conduction aphasia. In *Phonological Processes and Brain Mechanisms*, H. A. Whitaker (ed.). New York: Springer-Verlag, pp. 59–92.

Vallar, G., and Baddeley, A. D. (1984). Phonological short-term store, phonological processing and sentence comprehension: a neuropsychological case study. *Cogn. Neuropsychol. 1*:121–141.

Vallar, G., Basso, A., and Bottini, G. (1990). Phonologic processing and sentence comprehension: a neuropsychological case study. In *Neuropsychological Impairments of Short-term Memory*, G. Vallar and T. Shallice (eds.). New York: Cambridge University Press, pp. 448–476.

van den Broecke, M. P. R., and Goldstein, L. (1980). Consonant features in speech errors. In *Errors in Linguistic Performance. Slips of the Tongue, Ear, Pen, and Hand*. V. A. Fromkin (ed.). New York: Academic Press, pp. 47–65.

Warrington, E. K., Logue, V., and Pratt, R. T. C. (1971). The anatomical localization of selective impairment of auditory verbal short-term memory. *Neuropsychologia* 9:377–387.

Warrington, E. K., and Shallice, T. (1972). Neuropsychological evidence of visual storage in short-term memory tasks. *Q. J. Exp. Psychol.* 24:30–40.

Warrington, E. K., and Shallice, T. (1984). Category-specific semantic impairments. *Brain* 107:829–854.

Waters, G. S., Rochon, E., and Caplan, D. (1992). The role of high level speech planning in rehearsal—evidence from patients with apraxia of speech. *J. Mem. Lang.* 31:54–73.

Watkins, M. J., and Watkins, O. C. (1977). Serial recall and the modality effect: effects of word frequency. *J. Exp. Psychol. Hum. Learn. Mem.* 3:712–718.

Wickelgren, W. A. (1969). Context-sensitive coding, associative memory, and serial order in (speech) behavior. *Psychol. Rev.* 76:1–15.

Wilshire, C. E. (1998). Three "abnormal" features of aphasic phonologic errors. *Brain Lang.* 65:219–222.

Yamadori, A., and Ikumura, G. (1975). Central (or conduction) aphasia in a Japanese patient. *Cortex* 11:73–82.

Yarmey, A. D. (1973). I recognize your face but I can't remember your name: further evidence on the tip-of-the-tongue phenomenon. *Mem. Cogn.* 1:287–290.

4

Syntactic Aspects of Language Disorders

DAVID CAPLAN

SYNTACTIC STRUCTURES

Sentences convey relationships between the meanings of words, such as who is accomplishing an action or receiving it. These aspects of semantic meaning, collectively known as the *propositional content* of a sentence, vastly extend the power of language beyond what is available through single words and word formation processes to enable language to represent events and states of affairs. Propositions can be used for updating semantic memory, for reasoning, and for many other purposes. Thus, they constitute a vital link between language and other cognitive processes.

Syntactic structures, hierarchically organized sets of syntactic categories, provide the means through which the meanings of individual words are combined with one another to represent propositional meaning (Chomsky, 1965, 1981, 1986, 1995). In analyzing these structures, individual lexical items are marked for syntactic category (e.g., *cat* is a noun [N]; *read* is a verb [V]; *of* is a preposition [P]). These categories combine to create nonlexical nodes (or phrasal categories), such as noun phrase (NP), verb phrase (VP), sentence (S), etc. The way words are inserted into these higher-order phrasal categories determines a number of dif-

ferent aspects of sentence meaning. Consider, for instance, sentence 1:

1. The dog that scratched the cat killed the mouse.

In this sentence, there is a sequence of words, *the cat killed the mouse*, but *the cat* is not the subject of *killed*, and does not play a thematic role around *killed*, because of the position of these words in the syntactic structure of this sentence. *The cat* is the object of the verb *scratched* in the relative clause *that scratched the cat* and is the theme of *scratched*. *The dog* is the subject of the verb *killed* and is the agent of that verb. The syntactic structure of sentence 1 is shown in Figure 4–1, which demonstrates these relationships.

Researchers in modern linguistics try to represent the syntactic structure of sentences in such a way as to capture regularities in the relationship between sentence structure and propositional meaning. For instance, the mechanisms through which the subject of a sentence receives the role of agent in relation to a verb and the object of the verb receives the role of theme in sentence 1 apply generally to all sentences. These mechanisms postulate that each verb has a lexical entry that spec-

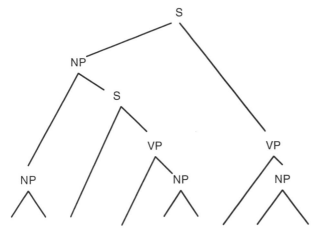

Figure 4–1. Structure of the sentence (S) *The dog that scratched the cat killed the mouse*, showing the hierarchical organization of syntactic categories that determine thematic roles. NP, noun phrase; VP, verb phrase.

ifies the nouns that can play thematic roles around it; these nouns are called the "arguments" of the verb. The *external* argument of the verb is assigned to the subject of the sentence; the *internal* argument (or arguments) is assigned to the object of the verb and other nouns. In this way, a verb such as *appreciate* can assign a thematic role other than agent to its subject: the external argument of *appreciate* is not an agent but an experiencer, and the subject of a sentence with the verb *appreciate* is the experiencer, not the agent, as in sentence 2:

2. The woman appreciated the concert.

The most interesting (and controversial) syntactic analyses are those in which these simple rules do not appear to hold. For instance, the generalization that the external argument of a verb is assigned to the subject of the sentence containing the verb is violated in passive voice sentences such as sentence 3:

3. The cat was scratched by the dog.

In this sentence, *the cat* is the subject of the sentence, but is the theme of *scratched*.

Chomsky (1957, 1965, 1981, 1986, 1995) developed models of syntactic structures that capture this phenomenon. These models postulate a so-called underlying syntactic structure at which thematic roles are directly related to

grammatical roles. This structure was known as "deep structure" in earlier models and is called "D-structure" in more recent work. In the D-structure of sentence 3, shown in Figure 4–2A, *the cat* is the object of *scratch*. To form the passive voice, *the cat* is moved by a syntactic rule from its position in D-structure to its final position in what is now called "S-structure" (formerly called "surface structure"), shown in Figure 4–2B. Chomsky's theory maintains that NPs leave "traces" when they move, which are assigned thematic roles. These thematic roles are transmitted to the NP whose movement left the trace and with which the trace is connected (*coindexed*). In sentence 3, theme is assigned to the trace of *the cat* and transmitted to *the cat*. The generalization that thematic roles are assigned to NPs in specific grammatical positions is thus maintained.

The reader may think that Chomsky has not achieved any overall simplification of syntactic representations, because he has had to introduce a new category, *trace*, to maintain the generalization about the assignment of thematic roles to subjects and objects. But this is not the case, because traces (or something like them) are necessary for structures other than passives. For instance, in the sentence *John seemed to his son to be flying*, the agent of *to be flying* is *John*. How did this happen? John is the subject of *seemed*, but *seemed* does not assign a thematic role to its subject: what "seemed" to John's son is not "John" but that

Figure 4–2. Formation of passive voice sentences, according to Chomsky. *a:* The underlying structure of the sentence (S) *The cat was scratched by the dog. e* is an empty noun phrase (NP) that is a placeholder for the subject of the sentence. *b:* The surface structure, showing the position of a trace. The trace is related to the subject. See text for additional details. PP, prepositional phrase; V, verb; VP, verb phrase.

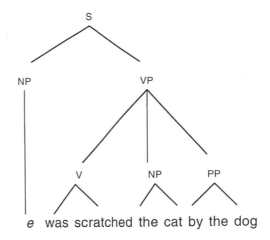

John is flying. A simple way to deal with *John seemed to his son to be flying* is to postulate a trace as subject of *to be flying*. This trace receives the thematic role assigned by *fly* and transmits it to *John*. This is similar to what happens in a passive voice sentence. Analyses like this indicate that languages need traces; therefore postulating them in passive sentences does not complicate the grammar beyond what is already necessary and does allow the generalization regarding assignment of thematic roles to be stated. I should emphasize, however, that many researchers do not agree with any of these analyses, and the postulation of empty categories (and many other aspects of Chomsky's theory) is highly controversial (see, e.g., Ellman, 1991).

Sentences convey many different semantic features, and each of these depends upon a dif-ferent relationship of nodes defined over a syntactic structure. One phenomenon that has been extensively studied is *co-reference*, the relationship of referentially dependent items such as pronouns (e.g., *him*) and reflexives (e.g., *himself*) to referring NPs. How syntactic structure affects the interpretation of reflexives and pronouns is illustrated in sentences 4 and 5. These sentences document an interesting fact that is true in all languages: if an NP is in a syntactic position where it can be the antecedent of a reflexive, then it cannot be the antecedent of a pronoun that occupies the same syntactic position as the reflexive. In sentence 4a, *herself* refers to *friend* and cannot refer to *Susan* or *Mary*. In sentence 4b, *her* cannot refer to *friend* but can refer to either *Susan* or *Mary*. Similarly, *herself* refers to *Mary* in sentence 5a, not *Susan* or *Helen*, and *her* cannot refer to *Mary* in sentence 5b but may refer to *Susan* or *Helen*.

4a. Susan said that a friend of Mary's washed herself.
4b. Susan said that a friend of Mary's washed her.
5a. Susan said that Mary's portrait of herself pleased Helen.
   b. Susan said that Mary's portrait of her pleased Helen.

Sentences 4 and 5 also illustrate which NP can function as the antecedent of a reflexive and be unable to be the antecedent of a pronoun. First, this NP must be within a particular syntactic domain. In the case of sentences 4a and 4b, this domain is the clause within

which the reflexive or pronoun occurs (*a friend of Mary's washed herself/her*); in sentences 5a and 5b, it is the complex NP within which the referentially dependent item occurs (*Mary's portrait of herself/her*). Second, an NP that must be the antecedent of a particular reflexive (or that cannot be the antecedent of a given pronoun) must stand in a particular structural relationship to the reflexive or pronoun. In sentences 4a and 4b, the head of the subject NP (*a friend*) stands in that relationship; in sentences 5a and 5b, the NP that occupies the determiner position in the complex NP (*Mary*) stands in that relationship. This relationship, known as *c-command* (Reinhardt, 1983), is illustrated in Figure 4–3. The point to appreciate here is that the structural relationship of c-

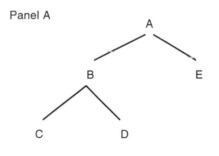

Panel A

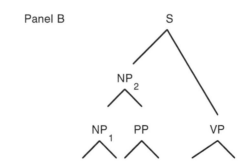

Panel B

Susan said that a friend of Mary's washed herself /her

Figure 4–3. Panel *A* is an abstract syntactic structure showing the syntactic relationship of c-command, which is relevant to the relationship of pronouns and reflexives to the nouns they refer to. A node c-commands another if (and only if) the branching node above the c-commanding node dominates the c-commanded node. C and D c-command each other, and B and E c-command each other. E also c-commands C and D, because the first branching node above E is A, which dominates C and D. However, neither C nor D c-command E, because C and D are both dominated by B, which does not dominate E. A reflexive can be co-indexed with a noun phrase (NP) that c-commands it. A pronoun cannot be co-indexed with such an NP. This is applied to sentence (S) 4 in panel *B*. Noun phrase 2 (NP_2) c-commands the reflexive/pronoun (*herself/her*), and can be co-indexed with the reflexive (*herself*) but not with the pronoun (*her*). *Mary* does not c-command the reflexive/pronoun, and can be co-indexed with the pronoun but not with the reflexive. PP, prepositional phrase; VP, verb phrase.

command, which is relevant to determining the antecedents of pronouns and reflexives, differs from the structural relationships of subject and object, which are relevant to thematic roles.

In summary, syntactic structures are hierarchically organized sets of syntactic categories, over which particular structural relations are defined that determine critical aspects of sentence meaning. These aspects of meaning (propositional content) are crucial to the communicative functions served by language.

CONSTRUCTING SYNTACTIC STRUCTURES IN COMPREHENSION

There is near universal agreement that syntactic structures are constructed from semantic and pragmatic representations as part of the production of spoken, written, and signed language, and from lexical, prosodic, and other perceptual cues in comprehension. There are different models to explain how this is accomplished, and these models can be divided into two main groups.

The first group consists of models in which syntactic structure is initially computed in relative (or total) isolation from other aspects of sentence structure, and integrated with other linguistic representations after it has been formed. For instance, these models maintain that when a sentence contains a syntactic ambiguity, the simplest syntactic structure is initially constructed, regardless of whether it makes sense in the context or not, and is revised if it is anomalous or contextually inappropriate. These models are often called "modular" because they postulate a "module" dedicated to syntactic processing.

In the second group of models, many different types of information interact at all stages of constructing syntactic structures. These different types of information include the likelihood that a word will occur after another word, the probability that subjects assign to the occurrence of events in the world, the discourse context, and others. These models view the assignment of syntactic structure as a part of a highly interactive process in which different types of information each constrain the possible meaning of a sentence.

Models of both types have been developed for sentence production as well as sentence comprehension, but because their empirical investigation is far more developed in the area of comprehension, we will focus on the kinds of evidence that support these models in comprehension. To do so, we need to take a closer look at how these models operate.

In *modular models*, rules are proposed for the creation of syntactic structures. What makes these models modular is the fact that these rules attach new words to existing syntactic structures solely on the basis of the syntactic category of a new word. The rules follow principles such as minimal attachment and right attachment. *Minimal attachment* requires the parser to create as few new syntactic nodes as possible when attaching a new word; *right attachment* requires it to continue adding words, if possible, to the node currently being developed. These principles, illustrated in Figure 4–4 can be conceived of as essentially constructing the simplest syntactic structure compatible with the lexical syntactic categories of the input on the initial pass through building a syntactic structure.

In *interactive models*, by contrast, a wide variety of types of information is used to create syntactic structures. Factors such as the plausibility of a noun playing a thematic role, the frequency with which particular words occur together in a language, and many other nonsyntactic factors all interact with each other as well as with the syntactic category of a word to "constrain" the possible syntactic structures and sentence-level semantic representations that could be assigned as each new word is recognized. Not only is the *process* of assigning syntactic structure different in these interactive, "constraint satisfaction" models of parsing and sentence interpretation, but the the syntactic structures themselves are different as well. Modular models tend to follow linguistic theories that postulate quite elaborate and abstract syntactic representations, such as those illustrated in Figures 4–3 and 4–4. Interactive models tend to postulate much less hierarchical and complex syntactic structures; some seem only to recognize the existence of sequences of lexical syntactic categories.

Panel A

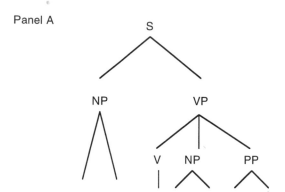

The policeman shot the robber with a gun

Panel B

The policeman shot the robber with a gun

Figure 4–4. Depiction of the structures associated with the parsing principles of minimal attachment and late closure. Two structures are associated with the ambiguous sentence *The policeman shot the robber with a gun.* Panel *A* shows the minimally attached structure, according to which the policeman used a gun to shoot the robber. The noun phrase (NP) in the verb phrase (VP) is simple and the prepositional phrase (PP) (*with the gun*) is attached with a minimum of nodes to the VP node being built. Panel *B* shows the structure associated with the sense of the sentence in which the policeman shot a robber who had a gun. The PP is attached in a way that requires additional structure (an extra NP) and it is not attached to the node under construction (the VP). This sense is available, but not preferred except under certain discourse conditions. V, verb.

The most intensively studied process that bears on the two types of models is the resolution of syntactic ambiguities. Sentence fragments such as the following are locally ambiguous:

6. The witness examined . . .

Sentence 6 can continue in a main verb (MV) reading, as in sentence 6a, or as a reduced relative (RR), in sentence 6b:

6a. The witness examined the evidence and implicated the defendant in the crime.
6b. The witness examined by the attorney implicated the defendant in the crime.

The sentence is disambiguated by the words following the verb. Psychologists have investigated the factors that make it easier for subjects to process one or the other of these disambiguating continuations. Two favorite experimental techniques that have been used are self-paced reading, in which subjects read sentences word by word or phrase by phrase, pushing a response key to call up successive words, and eye fixation duration measurements made while subjects read sentences such as sentences 6a and 6b. In both these techniques, the assumption is that, once allowance is made for the process of word recognition, words and phrases that are easier to integrate into the accruing representation of the sentence and discourse will be processed faster, leading to shorter reading times and eye fixation durations.

Using these techniques, psychologists confirmed the intuition that sentence 6b is initially difficult to structure. Eye fixation durations and self-paced reading times were found to be longer for the disambiguating phrase *by the attorney* in sentence 6b than the phrase *the evidence* in sentence 6a and longer than reading times for the same phrase in sentences with similar structures in which the verb clearly indicated that a RR structure is present, such as sentence 7:

7. The witness chosen by the attorney implicated the defendant in the crime.

This result was argued to be due to subjects taking the verb *examined* as a main verb, and having to revise this analysis to an RR structure when they encountered the phrase *by the attorney*. This process has been called being "led down the garden path," or being "garden pathed." In sentence 7, subjects cannot be garden pathed because *chosen* cannot be a main verb, hence the relative ease of integrating the phrase *by the attorney* into the structure that is being created.

Ferriera and Clifton (1986) then made an important and unexpected observation. They found that eye fixation durations were as long on the disambiguating phrase *by the attorney* in sentence 8, in which the RR structure was the only one that was semantically plausible, as they were in sentences such as sentence 6b:

8. The evidence examined by the attorney implicated the defendant in the crime.

The equal fixation times for this phrase in sentence 8 and 6b were taken as powerful evidence in favor of a modular model of syntactic processing, since the semantic implausibility of the first noun, *the evidence*, as the agent did not seem to stop subjects from being garden pathed. That is, these results were interpeted as evidence that subjects initially assign a main-verb reading to sentence 8, despite its semantic implausibility, presumably because the main-verb reading is easier to create, as predicted by principles of modular models such as minimal attachment.

Subsequent research has failed to replicate the results of Ferreira and Clifton. Trueswell et al. (1994), for instance, argued that, although Ferreira and Clifton used inanimate nouns as the initial nouns in sentences such as sentence 8, some of their sentences were plausible as main verb structures. Trueswell et al. replicated the Ferreira and Clifton experiment using new materials, and found that subjects had shorter eye fixation durations on the disambiguating phrase in sentences such as sentence 8 than in sentences such as 6b. Moreover, subtle semantic factors affected these fixation durations. Trueswell et al. found that the plausibility of the first noun of the sentence as the object of the verb (i.e., how likely it is that someone would examine either a witness or evidence) influenced fixation durations on the disambiguating phrase. The more plausible the first noun of the sentence was as the object of the verb, the shorter the eye fixations on the phrase indicating that the sentence was a RR clause, which suggests that subjects used plausibility information rapidly to aid in assigning sentence structure and meaning.

This result and several others in the recent literature have provided much evidence for a high degree of interaction between syntactic and nonsyntactic factors in the initial construction of sentence form. The debate continues, however. Advocates of modular models have argued that the interactive effects found in this literature arise after syntactic structures are initially created, and advocates of interactive models have responded by pointing out that there is no positive evidence for this postulated reanalysis.

In the discussion that follows, I shall use terminology employed more frequently by advocates of modular models, largely because studies of the neural basis for syntactic processing have mostly been undertaken within the linguistic and psycholinguistic frameworks associated with such models, not because these models are the only ones that can be used to describe aphasic disturbances of syntactic processing or the neural basis for this function. In fact, all of the claims made about aphasia and neural localization can be rephrased in terms of interactive models of syntactic processing.

THE FUNCTIONAL NEUROANATOMY OF SYNTACTIC PROCESSING

The neural basis for syntactic processing may differ in different tasks. In this review, I shall deal with studies of comprehension, because, as in the area of models of syntactic processing, it is the domain in which most studies have been done.

There is good evidence that syntactic processing in sentence comprehension involves the perisylvian association cortex—the pars triangularis and opercularis of the inferior frontal gyrus (Brodman's areas [BA] 45, 44: Broca's area), the angular gyrus (BA 39), the supramarginal gyrus (BA 40), and the superior temporal gyrus (BA 22: Wernicke's area)—in the dominant hemisphere. Patients with lesions in parts of this cortex have been described to have had long-lasting impairments of this function (Caramazza and Zurif, 1976). My colleagues and I have estimated that over 90% of patients with aphasic disorders who have lesions in this region have disturbances of syntactic comprehension (Caplan, 1987a). Disorders affecting syntactic comprehension after perisylvian lesions have been described in all languages studied, in patients of all ages, with written and spoken input, and after a variety of lesion types, indicating that this cortical region is involved in syntactic processing, independent of these factors (see Caplan, 1987b, for review). Functional neuroimaging studies by Stromswold et al. (1996), Caplan et al. (1998, 1999, 2000), Just et al. (1996), Dapretto and Bookheimer (1999), Stowe et al. (1998), and others have documented increases in regional cerebral blood flow (rCBF) using positron emission tomography (PET) or blood oxygenation level–dependent (BOLD) signal with functional magnetic resonance imaging (fMRI) in tasks in which subjects' processing of more and less syntactically complex sentences was compared. Event-related potentials (ERPs) whose sources are likely to be in this region (the left anterior negativity [LAN]) have been described in relation

to a variety of syntactic processes, including responses to category and agreement violations and comprehension of complex relative clauses, among others (Neville et al., 1991; Kluender and Kutas, 1993a, 1993b). These data lead to the conclusion that syntactic processing in comprehension is carried out in the dominant perisylvian cortex.

Regions outside the perisylvian association cortex might also support support syntactic processing. To date, there are no studies that document syntactic comprehension disorders following non-perisylvian association cortical lesions. However, evidence for the involvement of non-perisylvian regions in syntactic processing does come from functional neuroimaging and ERP studies.

Mazoyer et al. (1993) found increased rCBF in the anterior left temporal lobe when subjects heard French stories, French stories with all the content words replaced with nonwords, or French stories in which every content word was replaced with a semantically unrelated word from the same grammatical category, compared to when they listened to stories in a language they did not know (Tamil) or to lists of words. Bavelier et al. (1997) also found increased BOLD signal in anterior temporal, as well as perisylvian, cortex when subjects read sentences, compared to when they read word lists. These results are hard to interpret because there were many differences between the activation and baseline conditions in these studies, but both these studies have been taken as evidence that the anterior temporal cortex is involved in syntactic processing. More controlled activation studies of syntactic processing have also activated non-perisylvian regions. The cingulate gyrus and nearby regions of medial frontal lobe have shown increased blood flow when subjects processed syntactically more complex sentences (Caplan et al., 1998, 1999, 2000). In several studies (Caplan et al., 1998; Carpenter et al., 1999) activation has been found in superior parietal lobe on syntactic tasks. These activations have been attributed to non–domain-specific attentional processes (cingulate and midline frontal activation) and to visual–spatial processing (parietal activation), but they may reflect syntactic processing. The involvement of the superior parietal lobe in syntactic processing is supported by the existence of an ERP wave associated with syntactic anomalies and ambiguities—the P600, or syntactic positive shift (SPS), which is maximal over high parietal scalp electrodes. However, the brain origins of ERPs are hard to determine, so this electrophysiological result does not provide strong evidence for this localization.

The nondominant hemisphere may also be involved in syntactic comprehension. We found that 14 patients with nondominant hemisphere lesions showed effects of syntactic complexity on performance in a sentence enactment task, which were independent of sentence length (Caplan et al., 1996). Normal control subjects did not show these effects. We concluded that right hemisphere lesions affected syntactic comprehension. However, the control subjects performed at ceiling on the syntactically simple sentences, so the effect of the syntactic manipulation in that group may not have been apparent, and this conclusion needs to be reinvestigated. Just et al. (1996) reported activation results supporting a role for nondominant hemisphere homologues of Broca's and Wernicke's areas in syntactic comprehension; these areas increased their BOLD signal in response to processing syntactically complex sentences, though to a lesser extent than Broca's and Wernicke's areas themselves. A role for the nondominant hemisphere in this function is possible.

Finally, it has been suggested that subcortical structures involved in laying down procedural memories for motor functions, in particular, the basla ganglia, are involved in "rule-based" processing in language (Ullman et al., 1997a, 1997b). To date, data on the role of these structures in rule-based processes have come from studies of morphological processes, and the extent to which they may be involved in rule-based syntactic processing is unclear. These subcortical structures are nonetheless worth mentioning in this survey of possible neural loci of syntactic processing.

A major focus of investigation has been to examine how the perisylvian association cortex is organized to support syntactic comprehension. Different researchers endorse strongly localizationist models (Grodzinsky, 1990, 1995, 2000; Zurif et al. 1993; Swinney and Zurif, 1995), distributed net models (Mesulam, 1990; Damasio, 1992), and models that postulate individual variability in the neural substrate for this function (Caplan et al., 1985, 1996; Caplan 1987a, 1994). Localizationist models have focused on Broca's area as the locus of all or part of syntactic processing. Authors of distributed models have argued that the entire perisylvian association cortex constitutes a neural net in which this function takes place, although these theorists have also maintained that, within this net, Broca's area plays a more important role than other regions. Researchers who postulate individual variability maintain that different individuals use different parts of this cortex to process syntax, or different parts of syntax.

Data from deficit–lesion correlational studies bear on these models. These studies show that deficits in syntactic comprehension occur in all aphasic syndromes (Caplan et al., 1985, 1997; Berndt et al., 1996) and following lesions throughout the perisylvian cortex (Caplan et al., 1996). Conversely, patients of all types and with all lesion locations have been described with normal syntactic comprehension (Caplan et al., 1985; Caplan, 1987a). The fact that lesions throughout the perisylvian cortex are associated with syntactic processing deficits and that there is no clear relationship between these lesions or aphasic syndromes and these deficits is incompatible with localizationist models. The finding of spared comprehension after strokes in all parts of the perisylvian association cortex is also hard to reconcile with distributed models, since these models predict that there should be evidence of *some* syntactic impairment after *any* perisylvian lesion. It is possible, however, that seemingly unaffected patients have abnormalities of syntactic processing that would surface on more rigorous testing. It is also possible that patients who do not have syntactic comprehension disorders when tested months or years after a cerebral insult had such disorders initially. If all perisylvian lesions are initially associated with syntactic comprehension deficits and some of these deficits recover fully, the implication is that syntactic processing requires the entire perisylvian cortex in normal subjects and that it can be sustained by part of that cortex, or by other brain regions, in some individuals. Despite these considerations, the data from deficit–lesion correlations are most compatible with an individual variability model, and constitute the main reason for us postulating such a model (Caplan, 1987a, 1994; Caplan et al., 1985, 1996).

Advocates of localization have not accepted the conclusion that the data from deficit–lesion correlational analyses rule out localizationist models of syntactic processing. They have argued that a more detailed characterization of syntactic deficits leads to the conclusion that one syntactic process is localized in one cortical region. Specifically, Grodzinsky and colleagues have argued that Broca's aphasics, and not other aphasics, have impairments in the syntactic process of co-indexation of traces. Grodzinsky (2000) has also argued that this problem in co-indexing traces is the *only* syntactic processing problem that Broca's aphasics have. This hypothesis, known as the "trace deletion hypothesis," implies that traces are co indexed in Broca's area. There has been extensive discussion of the trace deletion hypothesis. In my view it is not supported by the evidence currently available from deficit–lesion correlations, but the reader is encouraged to consult the primary literature directly (see Grodzinsky, 2000, and commentaries on that article, as well as numerous articles in *Brain and Language* in 1995, 1999, and 2000).

Results from PET and, more recently, fMRI have become a major source of data regarding the location of the neural tissue involved in language processing. These technologies can be used to detect vascular responses to neural events associated with motor, sensory, and cognitive processes. Positron emission tomography and fMRI afford superior localization to deficit–lesion correlations because of the size of most lesions, and because the variability in many factors in most series of patients (age, education, neural structures affected, time since acute event, intervening therapy, etc.) makes it hard to attribute a particular deficit to a lesion in a particular structure independent of other factors. Use of PET and fMRI enables one to study a homogeneous group of subjects and to detect changes in vascular response associated with particular experimental manipulations.

Using PET, we found that rCBF increased in Broca's area in young adults when subjects made plausibility judgments about syntactically more complex sentences, compared to syntactically less complex sentences (Stromswold et al., 1996; Caplan et al., 1998, 1999). The syntactic differences were due to the structures of relative clauses (object *vs.* subject relativized stuctures). This brain region remained active in young adults when subjects made these judgments with concurrent articulation (Caplan et al., 2000), which impedes rehearsal. This indicates that the differences in rCBF were not due to increased rehearsal in the more complex condition but were due to more abstract aspects of sentence processing. Dapretto and Bookheimer (1999) have also found activation in Broca's area when subjects made judgments about the synonymity of two sentences in which the words in the sentences remained the same but the syntactic structure of the sentence changed from active to passive voice or vice versa.

However, not all studies show similar results. In our work, contrasting passive with active voice sentences in plausibility judgment tasks did not result in reliable increases in rCBF. In elderly subjects, the contrast involving relative clauses led to activation in the inferior parietal lobe. In many studies, blood flow was also increased in midline frontal structures and the cingulate gyrus. Just et al. (1996) reported an fMRI study in which subjects read and answered questions about conjoined, subject–subject and subject–object sentences. These authors reported an increase in rCBF in both Broca's area and in Wernicke's area of the left hemisphere, as well as smaller but reliable increases in rCBF in the homologous regions of the right hemisphere, when subjects were presented with the more complex subject–subject and subject–object sentences. Using event-related fMRI, we found that BOLD signal increased in the temporoparietal junction in young adults for plausible object- but not subject-relativized sentences at a time point that corresponds to their viewing the relative clause when sentences were presented word by word. The results across all experiments suggest that many regions show hemodynamic responses to processing more complex syntactic structures (including sentences in which the co-indexation of a trace is more difficult because of a greater separation between the trace and its antecedent NP).

Event-related potentials are of some help in localizing syntactic operations. These are electrophysiological responses to specific sensory, motor, and cognitive events that are discernable in the electroencephalographic (EEG) record by averaging over multiple trials, thereby increasing the signal-to-noise ratio for the part of the waveform related to a specific event. They are mostly used in normal subjects, although some ERP studies have investigated brain-damaged patients. Event-related potentials can be differentiated on the basis of their polarity, time course, and spatial localization, and researchers have developed models of the relationship between different aspects of ERPs and particular aspects of sentence processing.

Kutas and Hillyard (1983) first described a negative wave that arose when subjects were presented with sentences that contained errors in noun number, verb number, and verb tense. This wave, subsequently called the "left anterior negativity" (LAN), and a related earlier negative wave known as the "early left anterior negativity" (ELAN) have been described by a host of researchers in response to various syntactic violations (Neville et al., 1991; Kluender and Kutas, 1993a, 1993b; Munte et al., 1993; Rosler et al., 1993; Friederici et al., 1998) and are candidates for electrophysiological correlates of syntactic processing. It has been suggested that the LAN may arise from Broca's area, but this is uncertain because the location of the source of an ERP is difficult to determine. If it does, the data suggest that Broca's area participates in many syntactic operations.

Osterhout and Holcomb (1992) described a second wave that has been associated with syntactic processing—the P600, or syntactic positive shift (SPS) (Hagoort et al., 1993). The P600/SPS is a later, positive wave, arising about 500 msec or more after certain syntactic violations, with a centroposterior scalp distribution, that is often maximal over the right hemisphere electrodes. Osterhout and Holcomb found that this wave occurred after violations of subcategory restrictions on verbal complements, as in *The man persuaded to eat*, contrasted with *The*

man hoped to eat. Hagoort et al. (1993) found that it occurred after violations of subject–verb number agreement and violations of category sequences (which they called "phrase structure" violations). The P600/SPS has also been described and explored in numerous studies (Osterhout and Holcomb, 1992, 1993, 1995; Rosler et al., 1993; Osterhout and Mobley, 1995; McKinnon and Osterhout, 1996; Gunter et al., 1997). Its origin may be in the high parietal lobe but, as noted above, this is also unclear.

Overall, the data on the neural organization for syntactic processing in comprehension strongly implicate the dominant perisylvian association cortex in this process, but do not suggest further universal localization of aspects of this process to particular regions within this area. Much more work will undoubtedly be done on this topic, so this picture may well change in the future.

DISORDERS OF SYNTACTIC COMPREHENSION

Caramazza and Zurif (1976) first investigated the question of syntactic comprehension in aphasic patients. They tested Broca's, conduction, and Wernicke's aphasics on a sentence–picture matching test, using the four types of sentences illustrated in sentences 9–12:

9. The apple the boy is eating is red.
10. The boy the dog is patting is tall.
11. The girl the boy is chasing is tall.
12. The boy is eating a red apple.

The patients were scored on the number of errors they made in selecting the correct picture among a set of four. Broca's and conduction aphasics made almost no errors when pictures with incorrect adjectives or verbs were used as foils. Their errors were confined to pictures representing reversals of the thematic roles of the nouns in the sentences (so-called syntactic foils). Moreover, these patients only made errors on sentences such as sentences 10 and 11, in which the syntax of the sentences either indicated an improbable event in the real world or in which the thematic roles are reversible.

In the semantically irreversible sentences 9 and 12, these patients made no more errors than normal subjects. Caramazza and Zurif interpreted the results as indicating that some patients (those with Broca's and conduction aphasia) cannot construct syntactic structures.

However, to base this conclusion on these results is premature. One problem in interpretation involves the possibility of these results being based on how patients cope with the picture-matching task used in this research. Sentence–picture matching requires the use of nonsensical picture foils to depict "reversed" thematic roles in semantically irreversible sentences such as sentences 9 and 12 and the meaning of sentences such as sentence 10. The patients may have performed better on the irreversible sentences than on the reversible ones (sentences 9 and 12) and made errors on improbable sentences (sentence 10) by simply rejecting such pictures (Grodzinsky and Marek, 1988). The patients' selection of correct pictures over pictures in which lexical semantic foils appeared also does not prove that a patient can understand semantically irreversible sentences, only that she or he understands words. Proving that a patient assigns thematic roles in sentences without assigning syntactic structure is a nontrivial undertaking!

One study that provides an approach to this question is that of Schwartz et al. (1980), who reported that semantic features of single words played a disproportionately more important role in determining the sentence comprehension abilities of some aphasic patients than they did in normal subjects. In this study, five agrammatic patients did assign thematic roles, but relied heavily on the animacy of nouns in sentences to do so. Similar interactions between lexical semantic features of words and syntactic markers for thematic roles have been described in other studies of aphasic patients (Smith and Mimica, 1984; Smith and Bates, 1987; see Bates and Wulfeck, 1989, and Bates et al., 1991, for reviews). These studies thus show that nonsyntactic factors do appear to influence the assignment of sentential semantic meanings in aphasic patients to a greater degree than they do in normal subjects. They do not show that patients make no use of any syntactic information, however. On the contrary,

what has been found are complicated interactions between lexical semantic factors, such as the animacy of nouns, and simple aspects of sentence form, such as word order, subject–verb agreement, and case markings, that determine the assignment of thematic roles.

Regardless of whether disturbances of syntactic comprehension exist in isolation or are always accompanied by some form of impairment in nonsyntactic routes to sentence meaning, syntactic disturbances do exist, and their nature has been explored in several ways. In the following discussion I shall present a framework for viewing these impairments that arose from work undertaken by my colleagues and me, as it is a way to look at these disturbances that is comprehensive and flexible enough to provide niches for other types of studies.

Our research on syntactic comprehension disorders has led us to a framework in which we identified three components to a syntactic comprehension disorder: (1) a reduction in the processing resources used in this function; (2) specific impairments in the ability to assign or interpret particular aspects of syntactic structure; and (3) adaptations to the impaired construction and utilization of syntactic representations occasioned by components 1 and 2. Our research on syntactic comprehension deficits has provided evidence for all three aspects of these disorders. First I will review this research briefly, and then turn to studies by other researchers that amplify the picture in a variety of ways.

In our first studies of syntactic comprehension disorders, we explored the nature of disturbances in the process of syntactic comprehension along linguistic lines (Caplan et al., 1985; Caplan, 1987a). We used an object manipulation task, in which subjects manipulated toy animals to depict the thematic roles in sentences (who did what to whom). We studied nine syntactic structures in three studies of aphasic patients, testing over 150 patients in all. The results of the three studies were very similar. We found that mean group performance deteriorated on sentences that had more NPs, and more verbs and propositions, and in which NPs could not be linearly mapped onto the canonical order of thematic roles in English (agent, theme, goal). We also found that more impaired groups of patients performed increasingly poorly on sentences that were harder for the group overall. We suggested that this pattern could result from variable reductions in the availability of a processing resource used in syntactic comprehension.

We extended the analyses of patient groups to include a larger sentence set in the object manipulation task and the sentence–picture matching task. In the object manipulation study (Caplan et al., 1996), we analyzed the performance of 46 patients with left hemisphere strokes on 25 sentence types. These sentences were selected so that we might assess a subject's ability to process a wide range of syntactic structures. Six sentence types contained only "full" NPs, which are NPs such as *the dog* or *the cat* that refer directly to items in the real world. Six sentence types contained "referentially dependent" NPs—pronouns or reflexives (*himself* or *him*) that must be related to another NP to make reference to an item in the world. The remaining 13 sentence types contained what are known as "empty NPs" (Chomsky, 1986, 1995), or items such as the understood subject of *to jump* in the sentence *John promised Bill to jump* or the object of *scratched* in the sentence *The dog that the cat scratched chased the mouse* which are not physically signaled in the sentence but which are related to other NPs to determine thematic roles. Mean performance of the 46 patients deteriorated on sentences that required co-indexation of a pronoun or a reflexive, compared to their performance on sentences without such referentially dependent NPs, and it deteriorated even further on specific sentences in which there was an empty NP. In the sentence–picture matching task (Caplan et al., 1997), we tested two groups of aphasic patients with left hemisphere strokes (*N* = 52 and 17) on 10 examples of each of 10 sentence types. Performance was very similar to that on the object manipulation task. We also tested the group of 17 patients on both the object manipulation and sentence–picture matching tasks, and found that performance was highly correlated. These results replicate those of Caplan et al. (1985) and extend them to include analysis of a much larger set of sentences and a second test paradigm (sentence–picture matching). The results indicate that, in general, patients' performances are similar on different off-line tasks (though this is not always the case; see Cupples and Inglis, 1993).

All of these studies have shown that factors that add to the syntactic structural complexity of a sentence increase the error rate of aphasic patients, on average, in tasks that require patients to assign syntactic structure to determine sentence meaning. These studies are therefore consistent with the the view that patients have reduced processing capacity, or "working memory," in some sense of the term, that they can devote to the task of assigning syntactic structure and using it to determine sentence meaning. Normal language users run out of this resource when required to parse certain types of sentences, such as sentence 13, which is perfectly grammatical and means the same thing as *The woman hit the girl who kissed the boy who slipped*.

13. The boy who the girl who the woman hit kissed slipped.

Aphasic patients run out of this resource earlier and have trouble parsing sentences with less complex structures. One factor that determines the nature of a parsing disturbance in an individual patient is how much of this resource the patient retains.

A second finding in our studies is that individual patients can have selective impairments of syntactic comprehension. Published cases have had difficulty constructing hierarchical syntactic structures (Caplan and Futter, 1986); disturbances of co-indexation of empty NPs but not reflexives or pronouns (Caplan and Hildebrandt, 1988); dissociated disturbances of co-indexation of different empty NPs (Caplan and Hildebrandt, 1988, 1989); difficulty co-indexing empty NPs in structures that involve high memory demands (Hildebrandt et al., 1987); and dissociated disturbances of co-indexation of reflexives and pronouns (Caplan and Hildebrandt, 1988). The existence of double dissociations across these different types of structures makes it unlikely that all these deficits result from processing resource reductions, which would be expected to affect the more demanding of the two structures first.

Thus, these results provide support for the existence of different parsing operations by indicating that they are subject to selective impairments after brain damage.

These two types of impairments—a reduction in the processing resources available for parsing and sentence interpretation, and impairments of specific parsing and interpretive operations—constitute the two primary deficits that affect the parsing/interpretive process. By themselves, however, these deficits do not totally determine the interpretations that patients assign to sentences. These are determined by the operation of the residual parsing/interpretive system, coupled with the effects of adaptive interpretive mechanisms (*heuristics*) that apply when parsing fails.

Heuristics have been studied by analysing the systematic errors that patients make in syntactic comprehension tests. Our studies have reported error types for many sentence types in object manipulation tasks, in which subjects are free to assign any interpretation they wish to the sentence (Caplan et al, 1985, 1996; Caplan and Futter, 1986; Caplan and Hildebrandt, 1988a). Errors made by patients usually respect basic aspects of sentence structure and meaning, such as the number of thematic roles assigned by a verb, the number of propositions expressed in a sentence, and the distinction between referentially dependent NPs and referential expressions. We have found that what we have called "strictly linear interpretations," in which thematic roles are assigned to sequential NPs in canonical order (agent, theme, goal in English), are the most common error type, regardless of the syntactic structure of a sentence. In addition, patients appear to be sensitive to the relevance of some minor lexical items for thematic role assignment, such as the preposition *by* which signals the passive voice.

These heuristics would result from the operation of lexical identification processes, coupled with a memory system that maintains lexical items and their associated grammatical categories in linear sequences. In other languages, patients appear to make use of other readily available cues (declensional morphology, subject–verb agreement) in generating erroneous responses (Smith and Mimica, 1984;

see Bates and Wulfek, 1989, for review). The most significant feature of these heuristics is that they are closely related to normal syntactic operations. Patients' adaptations to parsing impairments make use of a subset of the items and operations found in normal parsing operations; they do not consist of behaviors based on other cognitive systems, such as spatial arrays or pragmatic factors. We conclude that patients retain elementary operations within the domain of parsing, and that their first attempts to deal with tasks that normally involve the parser make use of these retained abilities. These heuristics are exceptionally resistant to disturbance after brain damage. In the Caplan et al. (1985) study, only the most severely impaired subjects were unable to make use of at least some of them.

By specifying these three elements—the amount of processing resources, the nature of specific deficits in syntactic operations, and adaptive heuristics—a clinician or a researcher can completely describe an abnormality in syntactic processing. Of course, these elements of a deficit need to be described in relation to a model of normal syntactic and semantic structures and of normal parsing and sentence interpretation. Technically, these latter domains are not part of the theory of language deficits but of normal language, although they can, of course, be influenced by what is found to be the case in patients with impairments of syntactic (or other) processes.

The work reported above has a number of important limitations. We have not distinguished between disorders affecting the construction of syntactic structures and disorders affecting the use of those structures to determine sentence meaning. We have not provided evidence about unconscious operations that go on while subjects structure and interpret syntactic representations. Other researchers have studied these issues.

In 1983, Linebarger and colleagues surprised many researchers by showing that some patients (four agrammatic Broca's aphasics) retained the ability to indicate whether sentences were correct or syntactically ill-formed, despite performing at chance on tests of comprehension of reversible active, passive, and locative sentences. In their initial work, these authors did not carefully match sentences on which grammaticality judgment tasks were correctly made to sentences for which pictures could not be correctly selected, but in subsequent work they reported that these judgements can, at times, be made correctly for sentences that are not properly interpreted. For instance, Linebarger (1990) reported that some patients can correctly indicate that sentence 14 is ill-formed, but not match sentences like sentences 15 and 16 to pictures with thematic role reversal foils.

14. ° The woman was watched the man
15. The woman was watched by the man.
16. The woman was watched.

Linebarger and colleagues interpreted these results as indicating that these patients can assign syntactic structures, but not map them onto propositional semantic features. This interpretation suggests that the process of assigning the syntactic structure of a sentence is at least partially independent of the process of using that syntactic structure to interpret a sentence. In support of this analysis, Schwartz and colleagues (see Schwartz et al., 1985, 1987) cite the fact that their patients were able to judge the ill-formedness of sentences such as sentence 17, but not the anomalous nature of sentences such as sentence 18.

17. ° Who did the teacher smile?
18. ° It was the little boy that the puppy dropped.

In sentence 17, the ill-formedness is created by a syntactic violation—*smile* is an intransitive verb and cannot assign two thematic roles. In sentence 18, the anomaly is created by a violation of real-world probability—puppies are unlikely to drop boys. The fact that patients could detect the ill-formedness of sentence 17 suggests that they built the relevant syntactic structures. The fact that they did not detect the anomaly in sentence 18 suggests that they could not use more complex syntactic structures to assign thematic roles.

These studies suggest that a distinction needs to be made between disorders affecting the construction of syntactic form and those af-

fecting the use of syntactic form to determine aspects of sentence meaning. This in turn implies that these two processes are distinct, as captured in modular theories of sentence comprehension. In addition, one could ask whether disturbances of either of these functions, the construction of syntactic form and the use of syntactic form to determine aspects of sentence meaning, can be viewed within the framework outlined above, as reductions in processing resources, specific deficits in operations, and heuristic adaptations.

Another question that has been raised is whether the disturbances we have been describing reflect impairments of "on-line" or "off-line" processing. *On-line processing* is the unconscious, obligatory processing of a sentence as it is perceived. *Off-line processing* refers to the conscious, controlled processes that arise after a sentence has been understood. Most researchers assume that disorders of syntactic comprehension reflect abnormalities of on-line processing, but the evidence shows that the picture is more complicated than one might assume. Several studies have been interpreted by their authors as documenting comparable on-line and off-line syntactic processing in aphasics, but other studies have shown a dissociation between on-line and off-line tasks, with good-to-normal on-line and impaired off-line performances.

Swinney and colleagues (Zurif et al., 1993; Swinney and Zurif, 1995; Swinney et al., 1996) have presented evidence of comparable on-line and off-line syntactic processing in aphasics. These researchers tested eight Broca's aphasics and found that they performed below normal on sentence–picture matching for reversible passive sentences. They then tested them for on-line processing using a cross-modal lexical priming task. In this task, subjects heard a sentence and, at a point during the presentation of the sentence, saw a written stimulus that they had to classify as a word or a nonword as quickly as they could. Half of the visually presented real words were related to spoken words that had occurred previously in the sentence, and half were not related to any words in the sentence. Priming consists of faster reaction times (or, rarely, greater accuracy) in making decisions about visually presented words that are related to previously presented spoken words.

Swinney and colleagues tested priming for words that were related to the head noun of subject- and object-relativized clauses at the verb of the relative clause. This is demonstrated in sentences 19 and 20:

19. The nurse serving on the renal transplant unit [1] who administered [2] the injection replaced the vial.
20. The nurse serving on the renal transplant unit [1] who the injection dismayed [2] replaced the vial.

In these sentences, *nurse* is the head noun of the relative clause beginning with the word *who*. In sentence 19, *nurse* is the understood subject of the relative clause (the nurse gives the injection), and in sentence 20, *nurse* is the understood object of that clause (the nurse is dismayed). Normal subjects showed priming for words like *doctor* presented visually at point 2 but not at the control point 1 in auditorily presented sentences such as sentences 19 and 20. This indicates that, normally, the head noun is reactivated by the verb of the relative clause during on-line processing, when a thematic role is asigned to the head noun. The Broca's aphasics failed to show this effect. The authors attributed the Broca's aphasics' failure to show normal priming to an on-line delay in the reactivation of the head noun (in their terminology, based upon Chomsky's [1986, 1995] model of syntactic structure, the patients' disturbance was a disorder of co-indexation of traces due to slowed lexical activation). The authors argued that this disorder affected both on-line and off-line performance.

Other studies document abnormal off-line comprehension but appear to show good on-line syntactic processing in aphasic patients. Tyler (1985) studied one such patient, D.E., an agrammatic aphasic, whose off-line, end-of-sentence, anomaly judgments were much less accurate than those of normal subjects. D.E.'s on-line performances gave evidence of syntactic processing. In a word-monitoring task, he had longer latencies for word targets in syntactically correct, semantically anomalous prose than in normal prose, indicating a sensi-

tivity to sentential meaning, and even longer latencies in word salad, indicating a sensitivity to syntactic structure. His word-monitoring latencies also showed a normal tendency to have faster reaction times in the second and last thirds of normal prose but not in word salad, another indication of sensitivity to the accruing syntactic and sentential semantic representation. He showed normal effects of semantic and syntactic anomalies on monitoring times for the words following an anomalous word. These performances show on-line sensitivity to aspects of syntactic structure. A second study, by Swinney et al. (1996; Swinney and Zurif, 1995), also showed good on-line syntactic processing along with poor off-line comprehension in a group of aphasic patients. As noted above, Swinney and colleagues used cross-modal lexical priming to study Broca's aphasics. They also tested four fluent aphasics and found that the fluent aphasics performed poorly in a standard off-line sentence–picture matching task with reversible passive sentences. However, these patients showed cross-modal lexical priming for words related to the head noun of an object-relativized clause at the verb of the relative clause.

It is fairly easy to model what is going on when a patient does not show sensitivity to syntactic structure in on-line tasks and also makes errors on syntactically more complex sentences in off-line. Presumaby such a patient does not retain the unconscious processes that assign syntactic structure and use it to determine sentence meaning. It is another matter to understand what is going on when a patient performs normally in on-line tasks and makes errors on syntactically more complex sentences in off-line tasks. If a patient performs normally in on-line tasks, presumably the patient is assigning and interpreting syntactic structure normally at an unconscious level. It is not hard to understand how such a patient might fail to map this understanding onto actions, or a visual depiction of an event, or long-term memory, but it is not clear why a failure to use sentence meaning to accomplish tasks should occur only for syntactically more complex sentences, since accomplishing a task depends on the sentence's meaning (which has presumably been understood) not its form.

There are several possible ways out of this apparent dilemma. One is to inquire more carefully into what on-line tasks are sensitive to: might they be sensitive just to the assignment of syntactic structure and not to the determination of sentence-level meaning? If so, patients may assign syntactic structure in all sentences but only assign meaning in syntactically simple ones. Alternatively, off-line tasks such as sentence–picture matching and enactment might somehow be affected by the form of the sentence, not just its meaning. This could conceivably come about if subjects have an imperfect representation (or a short retention) of the entirety of the meaning of a sentence and have to refer back to the sentence and re-compute its meaning, which may be more difficult with more complex sentences. These studies of on-line processes thus raise important questions about the nature of the processing deficit in patients with syntactic comprehension disorders, to which we do not yet have answers.

We noted above that several researchers have suggested that one specific impairment in syntactic processing, the co-indexation of traces, is selectively affected in Broca's aphasia. I also indicated that I find the evidence for this suggestion weak, as it pertains to the relationship between lesions (and syndromes) and impairments in syntactic processing measured off-line. The reader will have appreciated that the research conducted by Swinney and colleagues suggests that this hypothesis may be true regarding on-line syntactic processing. Wernicke's aphasics showed cross-modal lexical priming for the antecedents of traces, as did normal subjects, but Broca's aphasics did not. However, not all studies have found this pattern of priming. Blumstein et al. (1998) repeated the Swinney study using purely auditory materials (the target word was presented in the voice of a speaker of the opposite sex from the speaker of the sentence). In eight Broca's aphasics they found priming for words semantically related to the antecedent of a trace, but no priming for words separated from a prime by an equal number of syllables in control sentences without traces. Balogh et al. (1998) argued that the Blumstein et al. results reflect end-of-sentence "wrap-up" reactivation of previously presented lexical items, not syn-

tactically based co-indexation of traces. However, this cannot be true of two sentence types in Blumstein et al.'s experiment 1 (their "wh-questions" and "relative clause as subject" materials), in which the trace was not at the end of the sentence and in which the Broca's aphasics showed priming effects. Five fluent (Wernicke's) aphasics did *not* show priming, which is also the opposite result from that reported by Swinney and colleagues. It does not appear that specific on-line deficits in syntactic processing are associated with specific syndromes or lesion sites within the perisylvian association cortex.

DISORDERS ASSOCIATED WITH IMPAIRMENTS OF SYNTACTIC COMPREHENSION

Studies of aphasic patients are relevant to the question of whether there is a single mechanism that computes syntactic structure in both input and output tasks. The discussion focuses on the fact that patients with expressive agrammatism often have syntactic comprehension disturbances (Heilman and Scholes, 1976; Schwartz et al., 1980; Caplan and Futter, 1986; Grodzinsky, 1986). Several authors have argued that the co-occurrence of deficits in sentence production and comprehension seen in these patients indicates that there are "central" or "overarching" syntactic operations, used in both comprehension and production tasks (Berndt and Caramazza, 1980; Zurif, 1984; Grodzinsky, 1986).

However, although deficits in syntactic comprehension frequently co-occur with expressive agrammatism, it does not appear that the two are due to a single functional impairment. Patients with agrammatism show a wide variety of performances in syntactic comprehension tasks. As noted above, several patients with expressive agrammatism have shown no disturbances of syntactic comprehension whatsoever (Miceli et al., 1983; Nespoulous et al., 1984; Kolk and van Grunsven, 1985) and some patients without agrammatism have syntactic comprehension disorders that are indistinguishable from those seen in agrammatic patients (Caramazza and Zurif, 1976; Caplan et al., 1985; Schwartz et al., 1987; Martin, 1987). To the extent that disturbances of syntactic comprehension and expressive agrammatism can be assessed in terms of degree of severity, there seems to be no correlation between the severity of a syntactic comprehension deficit and the severity of expressive agrammatism in an individual patient. These data constitute an argument against the view that there is only one impairment producing expressive agrammatism that necessarily entails a disturbance of syntactic comprehension. They are consistent with a model in which there are separate mechanisms for the construction of syntactic form in input and output side processing, and with the view that these mechanisms can be separately disturbed.

A second area of cognitive functioning that is often related to syntactic processing is short-term memory (STM), or working memory (WM). Research on memory has provided considerable evidence for a verbal STM system that is involved in memory tasks, such as free recall and serial probe recognition, in which subjects must retain small amounts of information over brief delays (Waugh and Norman, 1965). Some reserachers have suggested that the appropriate way to think of STM is as a system that maintains such information in the service of doing a task, hence as a "working memory" system. In one model (Baddeley, 1986), WM consists of a "central executive" (CE) that carries out computations on items held in part in the CE itself and in part in a "phonological store" (PS) that is refreshed by rehearsal in an "articulatory loop" (AL).

Since syntactic processing involves relating lexical items to each other over intervening material, it seems entirely natural to suppose that this system—the CE and possibly the PS and AL "slave systems" of a WM system—is needed for syntactic comprehension to proceed normally (Baddeley et al., 1987). However, a quite different point of view has been articulated by several researchers (Warrington and Shallice, 1969; Saffran and Marin 1975; McCarthy and Warrington, 1987, 1990; Caplan and Waters, 1990, 1999), who postulate no role for STM or WM, as conceived of above, in parsing. These

researchers have argued that the STM/WM system is involved in processes that arise after sentence meaning is assigned, such as mapping propositional content onto scenes, motor actions, and long-term memory.

Data from brain-damaged patients are relevant to these models. Researchers who maintain the view that STM/WM is used in comprehending more complex sentences have pointed to a variety of sentence comprehension disturbances found in patients with STM limitations (Vallar and Baddeley, 1984, 1987). Sentence length has been shown to affect certain comprehension tasks in some patients (Schwartz et al., 1987). However, in an extensive and detailed analysis of the comprehension abilities of all the STM patients in the recent neuropsychological literature, Caplan and Waters (1990) argued that the comprehension deficits found in these patients do not prove that STM limitations lead to syntactic comprehension deficits. In fact, case studies show that patients with STM impairments can have excellent syntactic comprehension abilities (McCarthy and Warrington, 1984; Butterworth et al., 1986). One such patient of ours, B.O., had a short-term memory span of two to three items but showed excellent comprehension of syntactically complex, semantically reversible sentences, even including those containing long-distance dependencies that spanned considerably more than three words (Waters et al., 1991). Thus data from B.O. and other STM patients provide strong evidence against any role of STM in parsing itself.

Cases such as B.O. also provide evidence against the role of the PS and AL in parsing. Patients with Alzheimer's disease show that the CE is also not needed for syntactic comprehension. Most patients with Alzheimer's disease have severe limitations of WM that are attributable to reduced CE capacity (Morris, 1984, 1986, 1987). Studies in our lab have found, however, that these patients have excellent syntactic comprehension abilities (Waters et al, 1995, 1998; Waters and Caplan, 1997).

The data from STM cases and patients with Alzheimer's diease are nonetheless compatible with the view that the WM system is involved in processes that arise after sentence meaning is determined on the basis of sentence structure. B.O. had problems understanding sentences that contained three or more noun phrases, especially if these were proper nouns. McCarthy and Warrington (1987, 1990) reported two STM patients who were unable to map commands onto actions when the task involved a pragmatically unpreferred arrangement of manipulanda. Vallar and Baddeley (1987) reported a STM patient who could not detect the discourse anomaly of referential dependencies. These data suggest that patients with compromised STM show deficits in a variety of situations in which the ability to review the initial analysis of a sentence could be useful (see Caplan and Waters, 1990, for discussion). Patients with Alzheimer's disease have trouble matching sentences with two propositions to a picture (Waters et al., 1995, 1998). This suggests that their CE problems interfere with postinterpretive processes.

The entire set of results indicates that there is a specialization within the verbal WM system for the assignment of the syntactic structure of a sentence and the use of that structure in the determination of sentence meaning. We have suggested that standard tests such as the reading span task (Daneman and Carpenter, 1980) are not measures of the WM or processing resource system discussed above, in which limitations lead to syntactic comprehension impairments (Caplan and Waters, 1999), but that standard WM tasks measure the capacity of a system involved in conscious, controlled, verbally mediated processes, which include the use of sentence meaning to accomplish many other functions.

CONSTRUCTING SYNTACTIC STRUCTURES IN SENTENCE PRODUCTION

In producing utterances, speakers (and writers) have to encode the concepts that they intend to convey. These concepts include items, actions, and features of those items and actions. These aspects of meaning are generally related to single words. The concepts also include the relationships between items, actions, and properties, and these features of meaning are encoded in the syntactic relationships between words. For instance, for many verbs, a noun can become the agent of a verb by making that noun the subject of the active form of that verb or by making it the object of the preposition *by* in a passive voice sentence. Aspects of meaning that arise at the level of discourse, whether an item is new in the discourse or is the focus of the discourse, also affect syntactic encoding. For instance, new information tends to come early in a sentence (van Dijk and Kintsch, 1983; Gross et al., 1989).

In this brief overview it is clear that the process of selecting (or constructing) a syntactic representation in the process of speech production is complex. It requires that syntactic structures be constructed to express both sentence-level semantic features (e.g., thematic roles) and discourse-level semantic features, and that semantic and syntactic features of lexical items, such as verbs, also affect the structures that are built. Models of normal sentence production have begun to suggest how syntactic structure is built.

Garrett (1975, 1976, 1978, 1980, 1982) studied a corpus of several thousand naturally occurring speech errors and suggested a model of the sentence production process based on the most frequent types of errors in speech production. Four error types considered to be especially revealing as to the nature of sentence production are the following:

1. Semantic substitutions, such as *boy* for *girl*, *black* for *white*, etc. These errors only occur with the content word vocabulary (nouns, verbs, adjectives) and certain prepositions.
2. Word exchanges, such as *he is planting the garden in the flowers* for *he is planting the flowers in the garden*. These exchanges affect words of similar categories (nouns exchange with nouns, adjectives with adjectives, verbs with verbs), and only affect the content word vocabulary. In addition, as would be expected with

these constraints, word exchanges do not affect words within a single phrase. For instance, exchanges of the form *this is a room lovely* for *this is a lovely room* do not occur.

3. Sound exchanges, such as *shinking sips* for *sinking ships*. Sound exchanges also affect the content word vocabulary, and usually affect adjacent words. They therefore are primarily phrase-internal and frequently affect words in different categories within the content word vocabulary, as in the example illustrated.

4. "Stranding" errors, as in *he is schooling to go*, for *he is going to school*, in which the suffix *ing* has been stranded in its original position and the verb stem to which it was originally attached has been moved elsewhere in the sentence. The elements that are stranded, that is, that are left in their syntactic positions, are affixes; it is the content words that are moved.

The stages of sentence planning identified in Garrett's model are illustrated in Figure 4–5. The first level is termed the *message level*. This is not a linguistic level, strictly speaking, but rather consists of the elaboration of the basic concepts that a speaker wishes to talk about. The first truly linguistic level is the *functional level*, at which lexical items are found for concepts. At this stage, the speaker has accessed the lexical semantic representation of a word but not its phonological representation. The functional level contains information about aspects of meaning that are related to sentences, such as thematic roles. As with lexical semantic information, this sentential semantic information is not related to the form of the sentence at this stage of processing. These "functional argument structures" do not, for instance, require that a sentence take a particular syntactic form, such as the active or the passive voice.

It is at the *positional level* that information about the form of words and sentences is specified. At the positional level, the syntactic form of a sentence is produced, and the phonological forms of words are inserted into their appropriate positions in the syntactic structure of

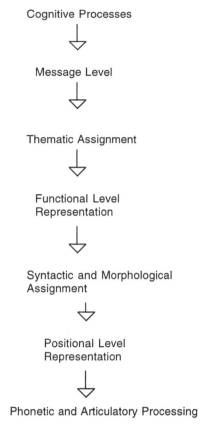

Cognitive Processes

↓

Message Level

↓

Thematic Assignment

↓

Functional Level
Representation

↓

Syntactic and Morphological
Assignment

↓

Positional Level
Representation

↓

Phonetic and Articulatory Processing

Figure 4–5. Schematic of Garrett's model of sentence production. For details, see text.

the sentence. An important feature of Garrett's model is that syntactic structures contain function words and bound morphemes at the point when they are accessed—that is, at the point when the positional level of representation is created. Following the creation of the positional level, the phonological form of words is specified in greater detail to yield a phonetic level of representation, which is ultimately transformed into a series of commands to the vocal apparatus.

The types of errors that Garrett has documented in normal speech can be attributed to disturbances arising at these different levels. Word exchanges and word substitutions arise at the functional level. Since the representations at the functional level only specify content words, these errors only apply to content words. Sound exchange errors arise during the insertion of content words into syntactic structures at the positional level. The fact that sound exchanges occur primarily between adjacent words suggests that the process of inserting the phonological form of content words into syntactic structures takes place on a phrase-by-phrase basis. Function words are not subject to sound exchanges because they are already present in the structures at the positional level. The stranding errors, in which function words and bound morphemes are stranded while the content words and stems are moved, also arise during the creation of the positional level, when content words are misordered. The fact that bound morphemes remain in place while stems move is one piece of evidence suggesting that the syntactic structures accessed during the creation of the positional level of representation already contain bound morphemes and function words in their final position.

Levelt, Bock, and colleagues (see Levelt, 1989, Chapter 7; Bock and Levelt, 1994) have expanded upon the process through which the functional and positional levels are created. In their model, which is based mostly upon experimental data, not speech errors, syntactic structures are highly dependent upon lexical items. For instance, to create a verb phrase, the speaker has to first access a verb: the building of a verb phrase comes along with activating the syntactic and semantic features of a verb. The model developed by Levelt, Bock, and colleagues differs in its details from that developed by Garrett. Both, however, share the feature that functional representations are constructed separately from some structural syntactic features of utterances.

In summary, the evidence from speech errors strongly supports a two-stage model of the generation of syntactic form. It also suggests that the insertion of nouns, verbs, and adjectives into syntactic structures takes place in a different fashion from that of function words and morphological affixes. In Garrett's model of sentence production, the second stage of generation of sentences, the creation of syntactic form, is closely tied in some way to accessing function words and morphological affixes. Levelt and Bock have developed models in which the creation of syntactic form is more closely tied to the structural implications of verbs and other content words.

DISORDERS OF SYNTACTIC PRODUCTION

DISTURBANCES OF PRODUCTION OF GRAMMATICAL VOCABULARY ELEMENTS

There are two aphasic disturbances that affect the production of function words—agrammatism and paragrammatism. We will describe each briefly.

In *agrammatism*, a component of the syndrome of Broca's aphasia, the most noticeable deficit is the widespread omission of function words and affixes and the greater retention of content words. This disparity is always seen in agrammatic patients' spontaneous speech and often occurs in their repetition and writing as well. The class of words affected in agrammatism has been described in two quite different frameworks. The first is a psychological framework; the second is linguistic. According to the psychological account, the words affected in agrammatism belong to the closed class of vocabulary elements. This set consists of all the vocabulary elements of English other than nouns, verbs, adjectives, and derived adverbs. An adult speaker does not learn new elements of this set, but still has the ability to learn new nouns, verbs, and adjectives. The linguistic approach to the characterization of agrammatism has been explored by several researchers. Kean (1977) proposed that the class of elements affected in this syndrome be defined in terms of aspects of their sound pattern—the retained words were ones that could be assigned stress in English. Other linguistic descriptions have also been suggested (Lapointe, 1983; Grodzinsky, 1984; Rizzi, 1985).

Many studies of agrammatic patients (Goodglass, 1973; Luria, 1973; Tissot et al., 1973; Miceli et al., 1983; 1989; Berndt, 1987; Parisi, 1987; Menn and Obler, 1990) have shown that patients with agrammatism can have different patterns of retention of the function word and bound morpheme vocabulary. For instance, one Italian patient showed preservation of free-standing function words but produced incorrect verbal inflections (Miceli et al., 1983). In contrast, one agrammatic English patient correctly inflected verbs (Goodglass, 1976). M.M., a French patient studied by Nespoulous and colleagues (1988) had trouble producing auxiliary verbs and certain pronouns in French (the "weak" forms of pronouns—*le*, *la*, *lui*—but not the "strong" forms—*il*, *elle*, *moi*, *toi*) but had considerably less trouble producing other function words. In a famous study, Goodglass and Berko (1960) studied the ability of 21 agrammatic aphasic patients to produce the suffix -*s*. They found that the possessive and third-person singular forms of -*s* were more frequently omitted than the plural, and that the third-person singular inflectional ending was omitted about as frequently as the possessive. These limited impairments indicate that there are many patterns of speech disturbance, all of which have traditionally been included in the category known as agrammatism.

A great deal of research has been directed at determining the factors involved in these patterns. One factor that influences variation in the manifestations of agrammatic speech is the patient's overall severity of impairment (Menn and Obler, 1990). Also, to some extent, the loss of affixes and function words mirrors their sequence of acquisition in reverse, although there are important exceptions to this effect (De Villers, 1974). Goodglass and Berko's (1960) patients had more trouble producing the nonsyllabic forms (e.g., bat*s*, cub*s*) of the suffix -*s* than in producing the syllabic form (e.g., church*es*). Kean (1977) pointed out that the differential susceptibility of syllabic and nonsyllabic affixes to omission can be explained in terms of the sonorance hierarchy: the syllabic form of -*s*, found in *churches*, is more sonorant than either of its nonsyllabic forms, /s/ and /z/.

Goodglass (1973) suggested that it is possible to integrate data from a number of experiments to define a class of words that are less "salient" and therefore more difficult for an agrammatic patient. Salience is the "psychological resultant of stress, of the informational significance, of the phonological prominence, and of the affective value of a word" (Goodglass, 1973; p. 204). Kean (1977) proposed that agrammatics are constrained to produce real words; this would explain the retention of affixes in languages in which roots without affixes are not well-formed words, such as Hebrew (Grodzinsky, 1984) and Italian (Miceli et al., 1983). Friedman and Grodzinsky (1999) have

argued that agrammatic patients omit affixes that are higher in a syntactic structure. Some variation in the production of function words and bound morphemes reflects control mechanisms. For instance, M.M. could read function words in isolation but not in sentences (Nespoulous et al., 1988).

The second major disturbance of function word production is *paragrammatism*, marked by substitutions of function words and morphological elements. Though separate disorders, agrammatism and paragrammatism often co-occur (Heeschen, 1985; de Bleser, 1987; Menn et al., 1990).

As with omissions in agrammatism, a wide variety of profiles of substitution of function words and bound morphemes is found in different patients. In some patients, the pattern of substitutions seems to be systematic. Lapointe (1983) suggested that infinitives and gerunds are the basic forms in the verbal system and that they are produced because they are the first to be accessed by patients with limited resources available for accessing verb forms. In other cases, substitutions are closely related to the inferred target (Miceli et al., 1990). In almost all cases, errors are "paradigm internal"; that is, they do not violate the word formation and even the syntactic processes of the language. Thus, in a language such as Italian that has several verb declensions marked by different thematic vowels, substitutions of verb affixes almost always respect the declension of the verb root. In Hebrew, substitutions of the vowels in words are always appropriate to the type of word being produced: shifts from one morphological paradigm to another and purely phonological errors do not occur with any frequency in paragrammatism. It thus appears that many constraints on word formation processes are respected in both paragrammatism and agrammatism.

There seem to be two broad sources of paragrammatism and agrammatism: an inability to access these lexical forms per se, and a disturbance of accessing them in sentence production. Some patients who omit function words and bound morphemes have disturbances affecting the production or processing of these items in isolation. Many patients with agrammatism have deep dyslexia and cannot read function words and bound morphemes aloud.

Others, such as patient F.S. (Miceli and Caramazza, 1988), have problems repeating some morphological forms. In cases such as this, several authors have suggested that the omission of function words and bound morphemes in sentence production is related to these processing disturbances at the single-word level.

In other patients, however, agrammatism occurs only in relation to sentence planning and production, without any disturbance of processing function words or bound morphemes in isolation. Caramazza and Hillis (1988) presented a patient of this sort, and, as noted above, M.M., also appears to have had trouble with auxiliary verbs and weak pronouns only when he had to produce sentences. This phenomenon was quite dramatic in M.M. Nespoulous tried an experiment in which he asked M.M. to read words written one to a page. M.M. did so perfectly, turning the pages over and reading each word, until he quite suddenly realized that the sequence of words formed a sentence. From that point on, he had difficulty with the items in these affected groups of words.

Overall, these studies illustrate the disturbances that patients can have affecting closed class vocabulary elements in sentence production tasks. Given the connection between production of function words and bound morphemes and the construction of syntactic form, we might expect that patients with agrammatism and paragrammatism have disturbances of this ability. We now turn to these disturbances.

DISTURBANCES OF GENERATING SYNTACTIC FORM

Disturbances in producing syntactic structures are extremely common in agrammatic patients. Goodglass et al. (1972) documented the syntactic constructions produced by one agrammatic patient and found virtually no syntactically well-formed utterances. All the agrammatic patients studied in a large contemporary cross-language study showed some impoverishment of syntactic structure in spontaneous speech (Menn and Obler, 1990). The failure to produce complex noun phrases and embedded verbs with normal frequency was the most striking feature of the syntactic simplification shown by these patients.

Studies of sentence repetition by agrammatic patients also document their syntactic planning limitations. Ostrin (1982) reported the performance of four agrammatic patients in repeating sentences with a variable number of noun phrases, prepositional phrases, and adjectives modifying nouns. She found that the patients had a strong tendency to repeat either a determiner and a noun (*the man*) or an adjective and a noun (*old man*), but not both (*the old man*). She interpreted this finding as showing that the presence of a determiner as a prenominal modifier was not independent of the presence of an adjective in the same position in these patients. Similarly, in sentences with both a noun phrase and a prepositional phrase in the verb phrase (*the woman is showing the dress to the man*), the patients showed a similar tendency to produce either the noun phrase or the prepositional phrase but not both. However, the patients' multiple attempts to repeat the target sentences often produced all the elements of the sentence, one on each attempt. These results indicated that the patients retained the entire semantic content of the presented sentence but could not produce all the elements they retained. Ostrin suggested that these patients had a reduced number of "planning frames" that they could use.

A second study of the repetition abilities of six agrammatic subjects introduces other considerations into the analysis of these patients' disorder. Ostrin and Schwartz (1986) had their patients repeat semantically reversible, semantically plausible, and semantically implausible sentences in the active and passive voice. They found that errors differed for plausible, reversible, and implausible sentences. Errors in plausible sentences were primarily lexical substitutions. Many errors in implausible sentences were an attempt to reverse the thematic roles in the sentence to render the resulting utterance plausible. The patients tended to retain the order of nouns and verbs in the presented sentence, and made many errors that the authors saw as efforts to produce passive forms ("mixed morphology errors" such as *The bicycle is riding by the boy* for *The bicycle is riding the boy*). The authors argued that the performances of their patients reflected a tendency to produce plausible sentences from an incomplete memory trace that contained the grammatical roles (subject, object) of the noun phrases in the presented sentence.

Despite these impairments in sentence production in agrammatic patients, it is not clear that these disturbances affecting syntactic forms are related to these patients' omission of function words and bound morphemes. First, there is no clear connection between the disturbances in production of function words and bound morphemes seen in individual patients and their syntactic abnormalities. Second, although many agrammatic patients show severe reductions in the production of syntactic structures, not all patients do. Miceli et al. (1983), Berndt (1987), and others have documented patients who omit disproportionally high numbers of function words and bound morphemes but who produce an apparently normal range of syntactic structures.

Turning to paragrammatic patients, several studies suggest that the syntactic production of these patients differs from that found in agrammatic patients. For instance, Butterworth and Howard (1987) described five paragrammatic patients who each produced many "long and complex sentences, with multiple interdependencies of constituents" (p. 23). Errors in paragrammatism include incorrect tag question formation, illegal noun phrases in relative clauses, and illegal use of pronouns to head relative clauses (Butterworth and Howard, 1987). A particular type of error that has often been commented on in paragrammatism is a "blend," in which the output seems to reflect two different ways of saying the same thing. These features of the speech of paragrammatic patients are not found in agrammatic patients, at least not with the same frequency as in paragrammatism, and they suggest that there are differences in the ability of these different patients to construct syntactic structures.

Very few studies of paragrammatic patients' performances on more constrained sentence production tasks have been undertaken. However, one well-known result based on a more constrained test, the anagram solution, also indicates differences in the ability of fluent paragrammatic and nonfluent agrammatic patients to construct syntactic structures. Von Stockardt (1972; von Stockhardt and Bader, 1976) found that paragrammatic patients solved anagram tasks according to syntactic constraints while agrammatic patients solved them using semantic constraints. Paragrammatic patients have not been tested as much as agrammatic patients on repetition, picture description, and story completion tasks, to ascertain whether they use both basic and more complex syntactic structures to convey specific propositional and discourse-level semantic features. The common belief is that they are much more capable of using a wide range of syntactic structures for these purposes than agrammatic patients, but make errors in their use.

Butterworth (1982, 1985; Butterworth and Howard, 1987) has argued that the syntactic and morphological errors in paragrammatism result from the failure of these patients to monitor and control their own output. If this is correct, the basic locus of the syntactic errors in paragrammatism may differ from those in agrammatism. Agrammatism would reflect a disturbance of one basic aspect of the sentence-building process, the construction of syntactic form, while paragrammatism would result from a disturbance of control mechanisms that monitor the speech planning process. This analysis assumes that normal subjects often generate erroneous utterances unconsciously, and that these errors are filtered out by control processes. Butterworth has argued that this is indeed the case.

Several studies indicate that aphasic patients' abilities to utilize syntactic devices to convey aspects of sentence meaning depends upon the devices commonly used in their language. Bates and colleagues have studied the abilities of patients to produce simple sentences in a language that makes extensive use of word order and little use of declensional or inflectional morphology (English), a language that makes extensive use of declensional morphology (German), a language that makes heavy use of inflectional agreement (Italian), and a language that uses both inflectional and declensional forms (Serbo-Croatian) (see Bates and Wulfeck, 1989, for a review of these studies). In each case, the patients tended to produce structures that incorporated the most commonly used syntactic markers in the language, and had difficulties producing sentences that required the use of less commonly used devices. This finding indicates that the "canonicity" of a structure or a grammatical device, or the degree to which it is used in a particular language, influences the ability of a patient to employ that device to express aspects of sentential meaning. These disturbances have been most clearly described in agrammatic patients, and it remains to be seen whether they affect patients with primarily paragrammatic output, as well as patients with other types of aphasic disturbances.

DISTURBANCES AFFECTING THE REALIZATION OF THEMATIC ROLES

Several researchers have suggested that there is a more profound disturbance of sentence production in certain patients. This disturbance has been said to affect the patient's ability to use the basic word order of English to convey propositional features such as thematic roles. Saffran et al. (1980) presented data regarding the order of nouns around verbs in sentences produced by five agrammatic patients describing simple pictures of actions. The authors noted a strong effect of animacy upon the position of the nouns around the verbs. They suggested that thematic roles were not mapped onto the canonical noun–verb–noun word order of English, and that animacy determined the position of nouns around verbs in these patients. They concluded that agrammatic patients have either lost the basic linguistic notions of thematic roles (agency, theme) or cannot use even the basic word order of the language to express this sentential semantic feature. They argued that this more profound deficit cannot be related to problems with the function word/inflection vocabulary. Therefore, agrammatic patients have more than one impairment affecting sentence planning and production. Although Caplan (1983) argued that the data in Saffran's et al.'s study did not support the authors' contention that animacy alone determined word order in the patients' responses, their report raises the question of whether the basic linguistic notions of thematic roles are always preserved in aphasia and whether patients always try to use some sort of structure to convey them. It is possible that some very severely affected patients lose these concepts or do not attempt to convey them. At the very least, it appears that some agrammatic patients tend to assign agency to animate items,

even where the task calls for the assignment of another thematic role to an animate noun. As discussed above, there are appear to be similar effects in comprehension.

The ability to produce utterances that convey thematic roles is closely linked to the ability to produce verbs. Many agrammatic patients have particular difficulties with the production of verbs. These difficulties do not entirely consist of trouble producing the correct inflectional and derivational forms of a verb in a given context. They also affect the ability to produce verbs themselves, resulting in omissions, paraphrases, and nominalizations of verbs.

Several studies have investigated this disturbance of verb production in agrammatic patients, with similar results. Miceli et al. (1984) compared 5 agrammatic, 5 anomic, and 10 normal subjects on tests requiring naming objects (the Boston Naming Test; Kaplan et al., 1976) or actions (the Action Naming Test; Obler and Albert, 1979). They found that the agrammatic patients were better at naming objects than actions, while the anomic patients and normal controls showed the opposite pattern. The agrammatic patients' difficulties in naming actions did not appear to arise at the level of achieving the concept of the action, since many erroneous responses were nouns, phrases, and nominalizations that were related to the intended verbs. Miceli and colleagues concluded that their agrammatic patients had a sort of anomia for verbs, a disturbance separate from the other aspects of their output.

Given the crucial role that verbs play in sentences, one would expect that a disturbance affecting the ability to use information regarding verbs would severely affect many other aspects of sentence production and comprehension. McCarthy and Warrington (1985) have argued that this is the case. Their patient, R.O.X., had a severe disturbance in naming actions and matching verbs to pictures. The authors argued that this disturbance was the result of a category-specific degradation of the meaning of verbs that also resulted in almost no production of verbs in speech and in difficulties in syntactic comprehension. However, the relationship between an inability to produce verbs and other abnormalities in the speech of agrammatic patients is not always so clear. In the

Miceli et al. study, patients' inabilities to produce verbs were only partially responsible for the shortened phrase length found in their speech, since the overall correlation between the noun/verb ratio and phrase length in the five agrammatic patients was not high. Berndt et al. (1997) also found that disturbances in verb production were variably related to disturbances in producing syntactic structures. It thus appears that some agrammatics have a disturbance affecting their ability to produce verbs, and that this disturbance can affect their ability to accomplish some sentence-processing tasks such as spontaneously producing a normal range of syntactic structures, but that some patients can build at least some phrasal structures despite poor verb production while others cannot produce normal phrase structure despite relatively good verb production.

SUMMARY

In this review, I have discussed the nature of syntactic representations and their role in expressing aspects of sentence (propositional) meaning, models of syntactic processing in sentence comprehension and production, the neural basis of syntactic processing in sentence comprehension, and disorders of syntactic comprehension and production. Many aspects of these disorders—their specificity for assignment vs. interpretation of syntactic structures, their occurrence during on-line processing— remain to be characterized in detail. Studies in the past 25 years have provided a basis upon which to develop more detailed models of these impairments.

ACKNOWLEDGMENTS

This work was supported in part by a grant from the National Institute of Deafness and Other Communication Disorders (DC00942).

REFERENCES

Baddeley, A. D. (1986). *Working Memory*. New York: Oxford University Press.

Baddeley, A. D., Vallar, G., and Wilson, B. (1987). Comprehension and the articulatory loop: some neuropsychological evidence. In *Attention and Performance XII*, M. Coltheart (ed.). Hillsdale, NJ: Lawrence Erlbaum Associates, pp. 509–530.

Balogh, J., Zurif, E. B., Prather, P., Swinney, D., and Finkel, L. (1998). Gap filling and end of sentence effects in real-time language processing: implications for modeling sentence comprehension in aphasia. *Brain Lang. 61:*169–182.

Bates, E., and Wulfeck, B. (1989). A cross-linguistic approach to language breakdown. *Aphasiology 3:*111–142.

Bates, E., Wulfeck, B., and McWhinney, B. (1991). Cross-linguistic research in aphasia: an overview. *Brain Lang. 41:*123–148.

Bavelier, D., Corina, D., and Jezzard, P. (1997). Sentence reading: a functional MRI study at 4 Telsa. *J. Cogn. Neurosci. 9:*664–686.

Berndt, R., and Caramazza, A. (1980). A redefinition of the syndrome of Broca's aphasia. *Appl. Psycholinguist. 1:*225–278.

Berndt, R., Mitchum, C., and Haendiges, A. (1996). Comprehension of reversible sentences in "agrammatism": a meta-analysis. *Cognition 58:* 289–308.

Berndt, R. S. (1987). Symptom co-occurrence and dissociation in the interpretatin of agrammatism. In *The Cognitive Neuropsychology of Language*, M. Coltheart, G. Sartori, and R. Job (eds.), London: Lawrence Erlbaum Associates, pp. 221–232.

Berndt, R. S., Haendiges, A. N., Mitchum, C. C., and Sandson, J. (1997). Verb retrieval in aphasia 2: relationship to sentence processing. *Brain Lang. 56:*107–110.

Blumstein, S., Byma, G., Hurowski, K., Huunhen, J., Brown, T., and Hutchison, S. (1998). On-line processing of filler-gap constructions in aphasia. *Brain Lang. 61:*149–169.

Bock, K., and Levelt, P. (1994). Language production: grammatical encoding. In *Handbook of Psycholinguistics*, M. Gernsbacher (ed.). New York: Academic Press, pp. 945–984.

Butterworth, B. (1982). Speech errors: old data in search of new theories. In *Slips of the Tongue in Language Production*, A. Cutler (ed.). The Hague: Mouton, pp. 73–108.

Butterworth, B., Campbell, R., and Howard, D. (1986). The uses of short-term memory: a case study. *Q. J. Exp. Psychol. 38:*705–737.

Butterworth, B., and Howard, D. (1987). Paragrammatisms. *Cognition 26:*1–38.

Butterworth, B. L. (1985). Jargon aphasia: processes and strategies. In *Current Perspectives in Dysphasia*. S. Newman & R. Epstein (eds.). Edinburgh: Churchill Livingstone.

Caplan, D. (1983). A note on the "word order problem" in agrammatism. *Brain Lang. 20*, 155–165.

Caplan, D. (1987a). Discrimination of normal and aphasic subjects on a test of syntactic comprehension. *Neuropsychologia 25*:173–184.

Caplan, D. (1987b): *Neurolinguistics and Linguistic Aphasiology*. Cambridge, UK: Cambridge University Press.

Caplan, D. (1994). Language and the brain. In *Handbook of Psycholinguistics*, M. Gernsbacher (ed.). New York: Academic Press, pp. 1023–1053.

Caplan, D., Alpert, N., and Waters, G. (1998). Effects of syntactic structure and propositional number on patterns of regional cerebral blood flow. *J. Cogn. Neurosci. 10*:541–552.

Caplan, D, Albert, N., and Waters, G. S. (1999). PET studies of sentence processing with auditory sentence presentation. *Neuroimage 9*:343–351.

Caplan, D., Baker, C., and Dehaut, F. (1985). Syntactic determinants of sentence comprehension in aphasia. *Cognition 21*:117–175.

Caplan, D., and Futter, C. (1986). Assignment of thematic roles to nouns in sentence comprehension by an agrammatic patient. *Brain Lang. 27*:117–134.

Caplan, D., and Hildebrandt, N. (1988). *Disorders of Syntactic Comprehension*. Cambridge, MA: M.I.T. Press (Bradford Books).

Caplan, D., and Hildebrandt, N. (1989). Disorders affecting comprehension of syntactic form: preliminary results and their implications for theories of syntax and parsing. *Can. J. Linguist. 33*: 477–505.

Caplan, D., Hildebrandt, N., and Makris, N. (1996). Location of lesions in stroke patients with deficits in syntactic processing in sentence comprehension. *Brain 119*:933–949.

Caplan, D., and Waters, G. S. (1990). Short-term memory and language comprehension: a critical review of the neuropsychological literature. In *Neuropsychological Impairments of Short-Term Memory*, G. Vallar & T. Shallice (eds.). Cambridge, UK: Cambridge University Press, (pp. 337–389).

Caplan, D., and Waters, G. S. (1999). Verbal working memory and sentence comprehension. *Behav. Brain Sci. 22*:77–94.

Caplan, D., Waters, G., and Hildebrandt, H. (1997). Determinants of sentence comprehension in aphasic patients in sentence-picture matching tasks. *J. Speech Hear. Res. 40*:542–555.

Caplan, D., Alpert, N., Waters, G. S., and Olivieri, A. (2000). Activation of Broca's area by syntactic processing under conditions of concurrent articulation. *Hum. Brain Mapping 9*:65–78.

Caramazza, A., and Hillis, A. (1988). The disruption of sentence production: A case of selected deficit to positional level processing. *Brain Lang. 35*:625–650.

Caramazza, A. and Zurif, E. B. (1976). Dissociation of algorithmic and heuristic processes in language comprehension: evidence from aphasia. *Brain Lang. 3*:572–582.

Carpenter, P. A., Just, M. A., Keller, T. A., Eddy, W. F., Thulborn, K. R. (1999). Time course of fMRI-activation in language and spatial networks during sentence comprehension, *NeuroImage 10*:216–224.

Chomsky, N. (1957). *Syntactic Structures*. The Hague: Mouton.

Chomsky, N. (1965). *Aspects of the Theory of Syntax*. Cambridge, MA: MIT Press.

Chomsky, N. (1981). *Lectures on Government and Binding*. Dordrecht: Foris.

Chomsky, N. (1986). *Knowledge of Language*. New York, Praeger.

Chomsky, N. (1995). *Barriers*. Cambridge, MA: MIT Press.

Cupples, L., and Inglis, A.L. (1993). When task demands induce "asyntactic" sentence comprehension: a study of sentence interpretation in aphasia. *Cogn. Neuropsychol. 10*:201–234.

Damasio, A. R. (1992). Aphasia. *N. Engl. J. Med. 326*:531–539.

Daneman, M., and Carpenter, P. (1980). Individual differences in working memory and reading. *J. Verbal Learn. Verbal Behav. 19*:450–466.

Dapretto, M., and Bookheimer, S. Y. (1999). Form and content: dissociating syntax and semantics in sentence comprehension. *Neuron. 24*:427–432.

de Bleser, R. (1987). From agrammatism to paragrammatisms: German aphasiological traditions and grammatical disturbances. *Cogn. Neuropsychol. 4*:187–256.

De Villiers, J.G. (1974). Quantitative aspects of agrammatism in aphasia. *Cortex 10*:36–54.

Ellman, J. L. (1991). Distributed representations, simple recurrent networks, and grammatical structure. *Machine Learn. 7*:195–225.

Ferreira, F., and Clifton, C. (1986). The Independence of syntactic processing. *Mem. Lang. 25*:348–368.

Friederici, A. D., Steinhauer, K., Mechlinger, A., and Meyer, M. (1998). Working memory constraints on syntactic ambiguity resolution as revealed by electrical brain responses. *Biol. Psychol. 47*:193–221.

Friedman, N., and Grodzinsky, Y. (1999). Tense and

agreement in agrammatic production: pruning the syntactic tree. *Brain Lang.* 56:397–425.

Garrett, M. F. (1975). The analysis of sentence production. In *Psychology of Learning and Motivation*, Vol. 9, G. Bower (Ed.). New York: Academic Press, pp. 137–177.

Garrett, M. F. (1976). Syntactic processes in sentence production. In *New Approaches to Language Mechanisms,* R. J. Wales, and E. Walker (Eds.). Amsterdam: North-Holland, pp. 231–255.

Garrett, M. F. (1978). Word and sentence perception. In *Handbook of Sensory Physiology, Vol. 8: Perception,* R. Held, H. W. Liebowitz, and H.-L. Teuber (eds.), Berlin: Springer-Verlag, pp. 611–623.

Garrett, M. F. (1980). Levels of processing in sentence production. In *Language Production: Vol. 1: Speech and Talk*, B. Butterworth (ed.). London: Academic Press, pp. 177–220.

Garrett, M. F. (1982). Production of speech: observations from normal and pathological language use. In *Normality and Pathology in Cognitive Functions,* A. W. Ellis (ed.). Ondon: Academic Press, pp. 19–75.

Goodglass, H. (1973). Studies on the grammar of aphasics. In *Psycholinguistics and Aphasia,* H. Goodglass, and S. Blumstein (eds.). Baltimore: John Hopkins University Press.

Goodglass, H. (1976). Agrammatism. In *Studies in Neurolinguistics, Vol. 1*, H. W. a. H. A. Whitaker (ed.). New York: Academic Press, pp. 237–260.

Goodglass, H., and Berko, J. (1960). Agrammatism and inflectional morphology in English. *J. Speech Hear. Res.* 3:257–267.

Goodglass, H., Gleason, J. B., Bernholtz, N., and Hyde, M. R. (1972). Some linguistic structures in the speech of a Broca's aphasic. *Cortex* 8:191–212.

Grodzinsky, Y. (1984). The syntacic characterization of agrammatism. *Cognition* 16:99–120.

Grodzinsky, Y. (1986). Language deficits and the theory of syntax. *Brain Lang.* 27:135–159.

Grodzinsky, Y. (1990). *Theoretical Perspectives on Language Deficits*. Cambridge, MA: MIT Press.

Grodzinsky, Y. (1995). A restrictive theory of agrammatic comprehension. *Brain Lang.* 50:27–51.

Grodzinsky, Y. (2000). The neurology of syntax: language use without Broca'a area. *Behav. Brain Sci.* 23:47–117.

Grodzinsky, Y., and Marek, A. (1988). Algorithmic and heuristic processes revisited. *Brain Lang.* 33:316–325.

Grosz, B. J., Pollack, M. E., and Sidner, C. L. (1989). Discourse. In *Foundations of Cognitive Science,*

M. Posner (ed.). Cambridge, MA: MIT Press, pp. 437–468.

Gunter, T. C., Stowe, L. A., and Gunter, G. (1997). When syntax meets semantics. *Psychophysiology* 34:660–676.

Hagoort, P., Brown, C., and Groothusen, J. (1993). The syntactic positive shift (SPS) as an ERP measure of syntactic processing. *Lang. Cogn. Proc.* 8(4):485–532.

Heilman, K. M., and Scholes, R. J. (1976). The nature of comprehension errors in Broca's, conduction, and Wernicke's aphasics. *Cortex* 12: 258–265.

Heeschen, C. (1985). Agrammatism vs. paragrammatism: a fictitious opposition. In *Agrammatism.* M.-L. Kean (ed.), London: Academic Press, pp. 207–248.

Hildebrandt, N., Caplan, D., and Evans, K. (1987). The man$_i$ left$_i$ without a trace: a case study of aphasic processing of empty categories. *Cogn. Neuropsychol.* 4:257–302.

Jackendoff, R. (1983) *Semantics and Cognition.* Cambridge, MA: The MIT Press.

Just, M. A., Carpenter, P. A., Keller, T. A., Eddy, W. F., and Thulborn, K. R. (1996). Brain activation modulated by sentence comprehension. *Science* 274:114–116.

Kaplan, E., Goodglass, H., and Weintraub, S. (1976). *The Boston Naming Test*. Boston: Veterans Administration.

Kean, M.-L. (1977). The linguistic interpretation of aphasic syndromes: agrammatism in Broca's aphasia, an example. *Cognition* 5:9–46.

Kluender, R., and Kutas, M. (1993a). Bridging the gap: evidence from ERPs on the processing of unbounded dependencies. *J. Cogn. Neurosci.* 5:196–214.

Kluender, R., and Kutas, M. (1993b). Subjacency as a processing phenomenon. *Lang. Cogn. Proc.* 8:573–633.

Kolk, H. H., and van Grunsven, J. J. F. (1985). Agrammatism as a variable phenomenon. *Cogn. Neuropsychol.* 2:347–384.

Kutas, M., and Hillyard, S. A. (1983). Event-related potentials to grammatical errors and semantic anomalies. *Mem. Cogn.* 11:539–550.

Lapointe, S. (1983). Some issues in the linguistic description of agrammatism. *Cognition* 14:1–39.

Levelt, W. J. M. (1989). *Speaking: From Intention to Articulation*. Cambridge, MA: MIT Press.

Linebarger, M. C. (1990). Neuropsychology of sentence parsing. In *Cognitive Neuropsychology and Neurolinguistics: Advances in Models of Cognitive Function and Impairment,* A. Caramazza (ed.). Hillsdale, NJ: Lawrence Erlbaum Associates, pp. 55–122.

Linebarger, M. C., Schwartz, M. F., and Saffran, E. M. (1983). Sensitivity to grammatical structure in so-called agrammatic aphasics. *Cognition* 13:361–392.

Luria, A. R. (1973). *The Working Brain*. New York: Basic Books.

Martin, R. C. (1987). Articulatory and phonological deficits in short-term memory and their relation to syntactic processing. *Brain Lang.* 32:159–192.

Mazoyer, B. M., Tzourio, N., Frak, V., Syrota, A., Murayama, N., Levrier, O., Salamon, G., Dehaene, S., Cohen, L., and Mehler, J. (1993). The cortical representation of speech. *J. Cogn. Neurosci.* 5:467–479.

McCarthy, R. A., and Warrington, E. K. (1984). A two-route model of speech production: evidence from aphasia. *Brain* 107:463–485.

McCarthy, R., and Warrington, E. M. (1985). Category specificity in an agrammatic patient: the relative impairment of verb retrieval and comprehension. *Neuropsychologia* 23:709–727.

McCarthy, R., and Warrington, E. K. (1987). Understanding: a function of short-term memory? *Brain* 110:1565–1578.

McCarthy, R., and Warrington, E. K. (1990). Neuropsychological studies of short-term memory. In *Neuropsychological Impairments of Short-Term Memory*, G. V. a. T. Shallice (ed.). Cambridge, UK: Cambridge University Press, pp. XX–XX.

McKinnon, R., and Osterhout, L. (1996). Constraints on movement phenomena in sentence processing: evidence from event-related brain potentials. *Lang. Cogn. Proc.* 11:495–523.

Menn, L., and Obler, L. K. (eds.) (1990). *Agrammatic Aphasia: A Cross-Language Narrative Sourcebook*. New York: John Benjamins.

Menn, L., Obler, L., and Goodglass, H. (eds.). (1990). *A Cross-Language Study of Agrammatism*. Philadelphia: John Benjamins.

Mesulam, M.-M. (1990). Large-scale neurocognitive networks and distributed processing for attention, language, and memory. *Ann. Neurol.* 28(5):597–613.

Miceli, G., and Caramazza, A. (1988). Dissociation of inflectional and derivational morphology. *Brain Lang.* 35:24–65.

Miceli, G., Guistolisi, L., and Caramazza, A. (1990). The interaction of lexical and non-lexical processing mechanisms: evidence from anomia. Baltimore: The Cognitive Laboratory, The Johns Hopkins University.

Miceli, G., Mazzucchi, A., Menn, L., and Goodglass, H. (1983). Contrasting cases of Italian agrammatic aphasia without comprehension disorder. *Brain Lang.* 19:65–97.

Miceli, G., Silveri, M. C., Romani, C., and Caramazza, A. (1989). Variation in the pattern of omissions and substitutions of grammatical morphemes in the spontaneous speech of so-called patients. *Brain Lang.* 36:447–492.

Miceli, G., Silveri, M., Villa, G., and Caramazza, A. (1984). On the basis for the agrammatic's difficulty in producing main verbs. *Cortex* 20:207–220.

Morris, R. G. (1984). Dementia and the functioning of the articulatory loop system. *Cogn. Neuropsychol.* 1:143–157.

Morris, R. G. (1986). Short-term forgetting in senile dementia of the Alzheimer's type. *Cogn. Neuropsychol.* 3:77–97.

Morris, R. G. (1987). Articulatory rehearsal in Alzheimer's type dementia. *Brain Lang.* 30:351–362.

Munte, T. F., Heinze, H. J., and Mangun, G. R. (1993). Dissociation of brain activity related to syntactic and semantic aspects of language. *J. Cogn. Neurosci.* 5:335–344.

Nespoulous, J.-L., Dordain, M., Perron, C., Ska, B., Bub, D., Caplan, D., Mehler, J., and Lecours, A.-D. (1988). Agrammatism in sentence production without comprehension deficits: reduced availability of syntactic structures and/or of grammatical morphemes? A case study. *Brain Lang.* 33:273–295.

Nespoulous, J. L., Joanette, Y., Beland, R., Caplan, D., and Lecours, A. R. (1984). Phonological disturbances in aphasia: is there a "markedness" effect in aphasic phonemic errors? In *Progress in Aphasiology: Advances in Neurology, Vol. 42*, F. C. Rose (ed.). New York: Raven Press, pp. XX–XX.

Neville, H., Nicol, J. L., Barss, A., Forster, K. I., and Garret, M. F. (1991). Syntactically based sentence processing classes: evidence from event-related brain potentials. *J. Cogn. Neurosci.* 2:151–165.

Obler, L. K., and Albert, M. L. (1979). *Action Naming Test*. Unpublished.

Osterhout, L., and Holcomb, P. (1992). Event-related brain potentials elicited by syntactic anomaly. *J. Mem. Lang.* 31:785–806.

Osterhout, L., and Holcomb, P. (1993). Event-related potentials and syntactic anomaly: evidence of anomaly detection during the perception of continuous speech. *Lang. Cogn. Proc.* 8:413–437.

Osterhout, L., and Holcomb, P. J. (1995). Event-related brain potentials and language comprehension. In *Electrophysiological Studies of Human Cognitive Function*, M. Rugg and M. Coles (eds.). Oxford, UK, Oxford University Press, pp. 171–215.

Osterhout, L., and Mobley, L. A. (1995). Event-related brain potentials elicited by failure to agree. *J. Mem. Lang.* 34:739–773.

Ostrin, R. (1982). Framing the production problem in agrammatism. Unpublished paper, Department of Psychology, University of Pennsylvania.

Ostrin, R., and Schwartz, M. F. (1986). Reconstructing from a degraded trace: a study of sentence repetition in agrammatism. *Brain Lang.* 28:328–345.

Parisi, D. (1987). Dual coding: theoretical issues and empirical evidence. In *Structure/Process Models of Complex Human Behavior*, J. M. Scandura, and C. J. Brainerd (eds.). Leiden, The Netherlands: Nordhoff, pp. XX–XX.

Reinhart, T. (1983). *Anaphora and Semantic Interpretation*. London: Croom Helm.

Rizzi, L. (1985). Two notes on the linguistic interpretation of Broca's aphasia. In *Agrammatism*. M.-L. Kean (ed.). London: Academic Press, pp. 153–164.

Rosler, F., Putz, P., Friederici, A., and Hahne, A. (1993). Event-related potentials while encountering semantic and syntactic constraint violations. *J. Cogn. Neurosci.* 5:345–362.

Saffran, E. M., Bogyo, L. C., Schwartz, M. F., and Marin, O. S. M. (1980). Does deep dyslexia reflect right-hemisphere reading? In *Deep Dyslexia*, K. E. P. a. J. C. M. M. Coltheart (ed.), London: Routledge, pp. 381–406.

Saffran, E. M., and Marin, O. S. M. (1975). Immediate memory for word lists and sentences in a patient with deficient auditory short-term memory. *Brain Lang.* 2:420–433.

Schwartz, M. F., Linebarger, M. C., and Saffran, E. M. (1985). The status of the syntactic deficit theory of agrammatism. In *Agrammatism*, M.-L. Kean (ed.). New York: Academic Press, pp. 83–124.

Schwartz, M. F., Linebarger, M. C., Saffran, E. M., and Pate, D. S. (1987). Syntactic transparency and sentence interpretation in aphasia. *Lang. Cogn. Proc.* 2:85–113.

Schwartz, M., Saffran, E., and Marin, O. (1980). The word order problem in agrammatism I: comprehension. *Brain Lang.* 10:249–262.

Smith, S., and Bates, E. (1987). Accessibility of case and gender contrasts for assignment of agent–object relations in Broca's aphasics and fluent anomics. *Brain Lang.* 30:8–32.

Smith, S., and Mimica, I. (1984). Agrammatism in a case-inflected language: comprehension of agent-object relations. *Brain Lang.* 13:274–290.

Stowe, L. A., Broere, C. A. J., Paans, A. M., Wijers, A. A., Mulder, G. Vaalbur, W., and Zwarts, F. (1998). Localizing components of a complex task: sentence processing and working memory. *Neuroreport* 9:2995–2999

Stromswold, K., Caplan, D., Alpert, N., and Rauch, S. (1996). Localization of syntactic comprehension by positron emission tomography. *Brain Lang.* 52:452–473.

Swinney, D. and Zurif, E. (1995). Syntactic processing in aphasia. *Brain Lang.* 50:225–239.

Swinney, D., Zurif, E., Prather, P., and Love, T. (1996). Neurological distribution of processing resources underlying language comprehension. *J. Cogn. Neurosci.* 8:174–184.

Tissot, R. J., Mounin, G., and Lhermitte, F. (1973). *L'agrammatisme*. Brussels: Dessart.

Trueswell, J. C., Tanenhaus, M. K., and Garnsey, S. M. (1994). Semantic influence on syntactic processing: use of thematic information in syntactic disambiguation. *J. Mem. Lang.* 33:285–318.

Tyler, L. (1985). Real-time comprehension processes in agrammatism: a case study. *Brain Lang.* 26:259–275.

Ullman, M. T., Bergida, R., and O'Craven, K. M. (1997a). Distinct fMRI activation patterns for regular and irregular past tense. *Neuroimage* 5:S549.

Ullman, M. T., Corkin, S., Coppola, M., Hickok, G., Growdon, J., Koroshetz, W., and Pinker, S. (1997b). A neural dissociation within language: evidence that the mental dictionary is part of declarative memory and grammatical rules are processed by the procedural system. *J. Cogn. Neurosci.* 9:289–299.

Vallar, G., and Baddeley, A. D. (1984). Phonological short-term store, phonological processing and sentence comprehension: a neuropsychological case study. *Cogn. Neuropsychol.* 1:121–141.

Vallar, G., and Baddeley, A. D. (1987). Phonological short-term store and sentence processing. *Cogn. Neuropsychol.* 4:417–438.

van Dijk, T.A., and Kintsch, W. (1983). *Strategies of Discourse Comprehension*. New York: Academic Press.

von Stockardt, T. R. (1972). Recognition of syntactic structure in aphasic patients. *Cortex* 8:322–334.

von Stockhardt, T. R., and Bader, L. (1976). Some

relations of grammar and lexicon in aphasia. *Cortex* 12:49–60.

Warrington, E. K., and Shallice, T. (1969). The selective impairment of auditory verbal short-term memory. *Brain* 92:885–896.

Waters, G., and Caplan, D. (1997). Working memory and on-line sentence comprehension in patients with Alzheimer's disease. *J. Psycholinguist. Res.* 26:377–400.

Waters, G. S., Caplan, D., and Hildebrandt, N. (1991). On the structure of the verbal short-term memory system and its functional role in language comprehension: evidence from neuropsychology. *Cogn. Neuropsychol.* 8:81–126.

Waters, G. S., Caplan, D., and Rochon, E. (1995). Processing capacity and sentence comprehension in patients with Alzheimer's disease. *Cogn. Neuropsychol.* 12:1–30.

Waters, G. S., Rochon, E., and Caplan, D. (1998). Task demands and sentence comprehension in patients with dementia of the Alzheimer's type. *Brain Lang.* 62:361–397.

Waugh, N. C., and Norman, D. A. (1965). Primary memory. *Psychol. Rev.* 72:89–104.

Zurif, E. B. (1984). Psycholinguistic interpretation of the aphasis. In *Biological Perspectives on Language*. A. R. L. a. A. S. D. Caplan (ed.). Cambridge, MA: MIT Press, pp. 158–171.

Zurif, E., Swinney, D., Prather, P., Solomon, J., and Bushell, C. (1993). An on-line analysis of syntactic processing in Broca's and Wernicke's aphasia. *Brain Lang.* 45:448–464.

5

Lexical–Semantic Aspects of Language Disorders

RITA SLOAN BERNDT

Words are the primary units of human communication. They are abstract symbols that can be expressed in a number of distinct forms to convey ideas and refer to the physical world. In modern society, adults are typically proficient users of words in two forms, spoken and written.[1] Estimates are that the average high school graduate knows the meanings of approximately 60,000 root words plus their morphological variants (Miller, 1991). Psycholinguistic studies of word processing, i.e., of the use of words in speaking, writing, reading, and listening, refer to the component of the language system dealing with words and their meanings as the "lexical–semantic system," to distinguish these elements from components dedicated to structural (syntactic) and phonological aspects of language. This chapter will follow that terminology, and will focus on the impairment of spoken and written words produced and/or understood outside the context of a sentence.

Almost by definition, all aphasic patients have some difficulty with words. These impairments can take a surprising number of different forms, ranging from almost total inability to produce comprehensible words to very selective difficulties with words of a particular type. The study of these varieties of impairment in individual aphasic patients, and comparison of impairments across patients, can provide important information about how the

normal lexical–semantic system is likely to be organized. Moreover, detailed study of such impairments can isolate the apparent source(s) of a patient's symptoms so that treatment may be focused on the appropriate level of processing (e.g., Conway et al., 1998).

This chapter will consider word-level deficits in patients with aphasia and, to a lesser extent, with progressive neurologic disorders. We will organize this discussion around issues that are critical to the development of a model of the lexical–semantic system to illustrate the importance of data from aphasia to cognitive theory, and to demonstrate the value of a model in motivating the systematic study of patients' symptoms. We will leave to other chapters in this volume the questions of how words are phonologically encoded, and how they are incorporated into sentences.

SYMPTOMS IMPLICATING LEXICAL-SEMANTIC ASPECTS OF LANGUAGE

All aphasia test batteries include subtests in which the aphasic person is required to produce, understand, read, or repeat isolated words.[2] The classical typologies of aphasia are based in part on the long-recognized fact that an individual patient's performance can vary markedly across these tasks, even when the same words are the targets. For example, a patient with poor comprehension and naming will typically be classed as a Wernicke's aphasic if the patient has difficulty repeating, and as a transcortical sensory aphasic if he or she does not; a patient with frequent phonemic paraphasias and poor repetition will most likely be labeled a Wernicke's aphasic if comprehension is poor, and a conduction aphasic if it is not. Here we are not concerned with accounting for these differences across syndromes in aphasia, but with understanding the elements that must be included in the hypothesized lexical–semantic system to allow this variety of symptoms to occur.

ISOLABILITY OF SYMPTOMS

As these clinical examples suggest, it is possible to find aphasic patients whose word-processing impairments are relatively isolated to a specific task, or to a single modality of input or output. The neurological literature of the nineteenth century is replete with examples of exquisitely selective deficits or sparings: difficulty naming objects when they are viewed but not when touched or described orally ("optic aphasia"; Freund, 1889); difficulty comprehending spoken words despite the ability to repeat and to read them aloud ("word meaning deafness"; Bramwell, 1897); severe difficulty reading aloud words that can be easily written ("pure alexia"; Dejerine, 1892). These and other interesting patterns were interpreted primarily in terms of neuroanatomical theories of brain–function relationships, although some functional model of language organization was often implied or explicated as well. More recently, these same symptom patterns have been interpreted with the goal of creating a cognitive, rather than a neuroanatomic, framework that can accommodate them. In the long run, of course, both are critical to understanding how the brain processes words.

CONTRASTING PATTERNS
AND THE IMPORTANCE OF
DOUBLE DISSOCIATIONS

One important problem in interpreting the occurrence of isolated symptoms concerns the possibility that the symptom reflects inherent differences in task "difficulty," a construct that is not easily measured or quantified. One might argue, for example, that spared repetition in the context of otherwise apparently abolished language abilities (e.g., Whitaker, 1976) simply reflects the relative ease of repetition ("even a parrot can do it!") compared to other language functions. On the other hand, one might just as easily argue that repetition is particularly vulnerable to injury because it is relatively unpracticed and has little functional value in human communication. The impact of these types of arguments can be blunted by the description of *double dissociations* of symptoms, i.e., of two different patients with contrasting performance patterns. A model that can explain the occurrence of patients whose repetition is selectively spared, and of patients whose repetition is selectively impaired, will need to provide an account of the cognitive demands of repetition compared to other language tasks.

The importance of the double dissociation in the interpretation of aphasic symptoms has been discussed in detail elsewhere (Shallice, 1988; McCarthy and Warrington, 1990). One important contribution of an emphasis on double dissociations is the identification of contrasting patterns that, though perhaps less striking than the classic cases mentioned above, have been important in illuminating the structure of the lexical–semantic system. Examples of these dissociations will be discussed below.

IDENTIFYING COMPONENTS OF
THE LEXICAL–SEMANTIC SYSTEM

Many of the assumptions currently made about the structure of the lexical–semantic system have been motivated by patterns of impairment and sparing in aphasia.

FORM VS. MEANING

There is evidence from a number of sources that the meanings of words are represented separately from their forms. It has long been noted that normal subjects in a "tip-of-the-tongue" state have detailed knowledge of a word's meaning, yet remain unable to produce its spoken form (Brown and McNeill, 1966).

This phenomenon is magnified in the symptom of anomia, in which a patient's attempts to name objects often provide compelling evidence of knowledge of meaning. In one study of a severely anomic patient (H.Y.), we elicited many accurate descriptions of objects that the patient could not name (Zingeser and Berndt, 1988). For example, H.Y.'s attempt to name a *camera* elicited "to take a picture"; his attempt to name *lamp* elicited "turns the lights on in the evening." These examples illustrate that H.Y.'s recognition of the picture and his understanding of the concept that was to be named by the elusive word were largely intact. But the lexical form associated with the object was rarely produced in picture-naming tasks.

A contrasting pattern of impaired meanings and relatively intact access to spoken word forms has been described in studies of patients with progressive dementing illnesses. In the variant known as "semantic dementia" (Hodges et al., 1992), semantic deterioration appears to progress more rapidly than does the ability to produce spoken word forms. For example, patient W.L.P. (Schwartz et al., 1980) showed a profound semantic impairment for words that she could read aloud and repeat without difficulty. Perhaps even more surprising is a pattern described in a patient with Alzheimer's disease who could name objects normally while performing significantly worse than controls on numerous tests of semantic knowledge for the same objects (Shuren et al., 1993).

These examples indicate that the lexical–semantic system must represent word meaning largely independently of word form; different types of brain damage can selectively affect either meaning or form, or (perhaps more frequently) can affect them both but to very different degrees.

THE ORGANIZATION OF THE SEMANTIC SYSTEM

The semantic component of the lexical–semantic system must contain a wide range of information of different types in order to encode the meanings of all of the concepts and categories that human speakers understand. How this information is organized within the cognitive system has been debated for many years; currently there are at least two basic views. One argument is that meanings are composed of networks of discrete semantic features (Bierwisch and Schreuder, 1992). A concept such as *dog* might be represented by features such as [living], [four legged], [domestic], etc. Another view holds that meaning is nondecompositional, i.e., that there is a single semantic concept associated with each known lexical concept (Roelofs, 1993). In this view, the meaning of *dog* is reperesented through its network of connections to other (superordinate, coordinate, and subordinate) lexical concepts such as *animal, cat, dachsund*, etc. Interpretations of neuropsychological data have generally adopted the decompositional (i.e., featural) model, assuming that a set of primitive features jointly determines a concept's meaning.

Another contentious issue about the organization of semantics is motivated by findings from patients with modality-specific semantic deficits. The most studied phenomenon among these is *optic aphasia*, in which the patient can name objects when they are described aloud or touched, but not when they are simply viewed (Freund, 1889; Beauvois, 1982).[3] Importantly, patients with optic aphasia are often reported to show some spared knowledge of viewed objects and may be able to gesture their use appropriately, indicating residual recognition. This type of pattern and analogous modality-specific naming impairments such as tactile aphasia (Beauvois et al., 1978) have led to the proposal that there are separate semantic systems linked to specific sensory modalities (Shallice, 1987, 1988). The idea is that such patients succeed in gaining access to a modality-specific semantic system (visual semantics in the case of optic aphasia), which allows them to gesture appropriate use of viewed objects and demonstrate other limited understanding. A separate verbal semantic system is also assumed to be intact, since objects can be named when encountered via non-affected sensory modalities. The problem, it is argued, lies in transmitting information from intact visual semantics to intact verbal semantics. This type of framework is depicted in Figure 5–1.

This "multiple semantics" hypothesis has been challenged by proponents of a model

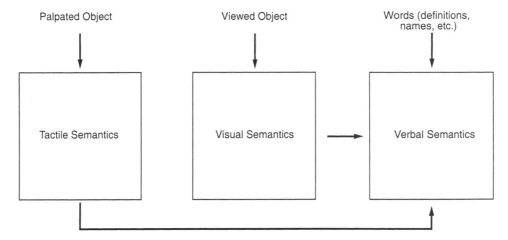

Figure 5–1. Schematic depiction of a "multiple semantics" model in which distinct semantic representations are associated with information obtained through each sensory modality.

such as that shown in Figure 5–2 with a single, amodal semantic system that can be accessed through all sensory modalities (Riddoch et al., 1988; Caramazza et al., 1990; Shelton and Caramazza, 1999). The primary arguments in favor of this position invoke natural differences in the relationships that hold between objects and their meanings on one hand, and words and their meanings on the other. Whereas words have a completely arbitrary relation to meaning, objects do not. For example, nothing about the spoken or written word form "scissors" gives a hint of its meaning, while the viewed object *scissors* (even if it is not identified) may be readily interpreted as something to be grasped with the hand and manipulated. Thus, if a single, amodal semantic system were

impaired, patients might still be able to gesture an object's use or give other minimal evidence of understanding of its function, but still fail to access the full semantic representation needed to generate its name.

Another approach to this issue has been offered by Coslett and Saffran (1989, 1992), who carried out detailed studies of two optic aphasic patients. These investigators argue that the demonstration of some residual recognition of visually presented objects (and words), despite inability to name such objects, reflects a rudimentary semantic system available in the right hemisphere that is disconnected from left hemisphere verbal capacities. The right hemisphere semantic system does not constitute a "visual semantics system" that supports all pro-

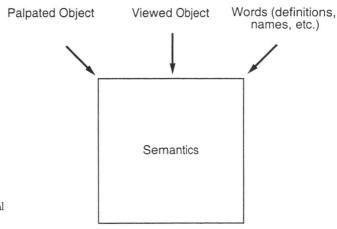

Figure 5–2. Schematic depiction of an amodal semantic system.

cessing of the meaning of viewed objects, but has limited ability to process objects and highly imageable written words (see also Coltheart, 1980).

Although we will adopt here the proposal of a single, amodal semantic system, we will revisit this issue below in the context of semantic category-specific effects.

ARE THERE SEPARATE LEXICONS FOR SPOKEN AND WRITTEN INPUT AND OUTPUT?

Another basic but controversial question concerning the structure of the lexical–semantic system involves the number of separate lexical components that must be postulated to accommodate a range of results from patients. Traditional linguistic models of the language system have assumed a single lexicon containing phonological entries abstract enough to support acoustic–phonetic input and articulatory–phonetic output (see Coleman, 1998, for a recent review of arguments). Linguistic conceptions of the lexicon do not generally touch upon written language, but when they do they are explicit in their argument that lexical knowledge is "medium neutral," accessible for use in spoken and written domains (Lyons, 1981). Such a framework is depicted in Figure 5–3.

In contrast, cognitive models, especially those incorporating data from neuropsychology, have assumed that there are separate lexicons for input and output, and separate phonological and orthographic lexical systems to support spoken and written words, respectively (Ellis and Young, 1996; Shelton and Caramazza, 1999). This framework is shown in Figure 5–4.

The single, amodal lexicon depicted in Figure 5–3 has difficulty accommodating a number of symptom dissociations found among aphasic patients. For example, patients with "word meaning deafness" (Bramwell, 1897; Franklin et al., 1994) cannot understand spoken words that they can repeat and, in some cases, spell to dictation (Hall and Riddoch, 1997). These patients can also understand written words, suggesting that word meanings can be accessed through the visual modality and are not themselves compromised. This pattern appears to require a very specific degradation of transmission between speech and the semantic system that will allow successful processing of spoken words for repetition and spelling. It is not clear how such fine distinctions could arise in a single lexicon model. Allport and Funnell (1981) discuss other evidence from patients weighing against the idea that all lexical processing gains access to an amodal store of lexical representations.

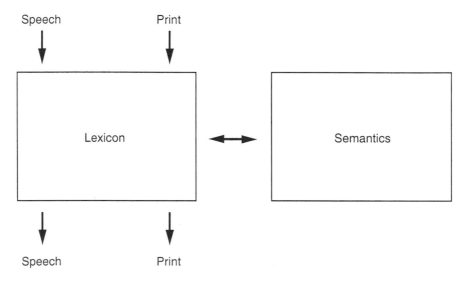

Figure 5–3. Schematic representation of a model with a single, amodal lexicon that supports spoken and written input and output.

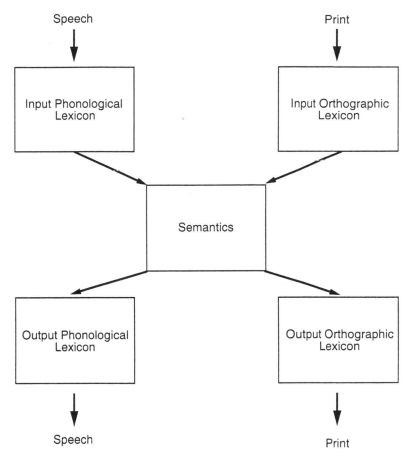

Figure 5–4. Schematic diagram of a model with separate lexical representations for spoken and written input and output.

If the single-lexicon approach cannot be supported, does that necessitate adoption of the four-lexicon model shown in Figure 5–4? There seem to be compelling reasons to require independent spoken (phonological) and written (orthographic) lexicons, and this distinction will be discussed further below. However, the additional separation of phonological and orthographic systems into stores dedicated to input and output processing is not so clearly mandated by the patient data. This is so because the mechanisms that mediate between lexical information and the outside world (i.e., the acoustic, articulatory, visual and motor components that stimulate receptive processes and execute expressive processes) have not been specified, and might themselves be selectively affected by brain injury. Thus, findings that appear to compel a separation of in-

put and output lexicons might be explainable as selective disruption of pathways into or out of a single phonological or orthograhic lexicon. It has proven to be extremely difficult to distinguish between these possibilities using data from normal subjects (e.g., Monsell, 1987).

The attempts to address this issue using neuropsychological data appear to support different conclusions for spoken and written words. The need for separate input and output lexicons for spoken words is supported by findings that the same words that appear to be no longer accessible for production remain easily accessible for comprehension. For example, Howard (1995) described an aphasic patient who showed a very consistent inability to produce specific lexical items across a variety of tasks, even when given phonemic cues. The same words, when spoken to the patient, were recognized and understood normally. The severity, specificity, and consistency of this patient's production impairment, within the context of normal word recognition and comprehension, is difficult to accommodate in a model with a single, amodal lexicon. Martin and colleagues (1999) reached a similar conclusion based on detailed analyses of the performance of an anomic patient on memory tasks requiring retention of input vs. output phonological codes.

In contrast to these findings for spoken words, similarly detailed studies across orthographic input and output tasks have thus far supported the existence of a single orthographic lexicon (Coltheart and Funnell, 1987; Behrmann and Bub, 1992; Greenwald and Berndt, 1999). A framework incorporating

these spoken and written differences might look something like that in Figure 5–5.

RELATIONSHIP BETWEEN SPOKEN AND WRITTEN WORD PROCESSING

The idea that there are separate input and output lexicons for speech, and a single lexicon for written words, may be unappealing because of its lack of symmetry. Nonetheless, it is possible that the differences in the manner in which spoken and written words are acquired during development are responsible for this asymmetry. That is, the understanding and production of spoken words are emergent abilities of the human cognitive system that may be tightly connected with the sensory (auditory) and mo-

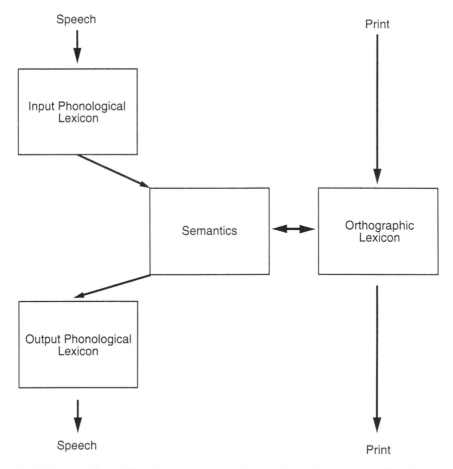

Figure 5–5. Diagram of a model with separate input and output lexicons for spoken words, and a single orthographic lexicon supporting reading and writing.

tor (speech) systems on which they rely. Written language is (for the most part) acquired through formal training that may blur distinctions between input and output. In fact, some techniques for the teaching of reading may mandate processing across modalities, as words are not only read aloud but spelled aloud and written as they are being learned. These speculations suggest that there may be reasons to expect that the lexical systems supporting spoken and written words may be differently organized.

An even stronger view about the differences between spoken and written words, which also has its roots in ontogenetic considerations, is that written word processing is in some sense parasitic on spoken word processing (Luria, 1966; Geschwind, 1969). This issue has been especially contentious in the cognitive literature as it relates to normal reading (Van Orden et al., 1988; Coltheart and Coltheart, 1997), but it is equally relevant to spelling (see Ellis, 1988, for review). The argument is that the recognition and production of written words *require* prior translation (to or from) phonological forms.

Recent neuropsychological evidence strongly suggests that there is no such requirement; rather, written words can be recognized and produced even when phonological systems are largely inoperative. The patients with word meaning deafness, described above, provide one source of evidence. These patients have no difficulty understanding words in written form, but cannot understand the same words in their spoken form. Thus, obligatory translation from orthographic to phonological form would result in degraded written word comprehension in these patients. Evidence from aphasia also supports independent orthographic and phonological representations for the production of words. For example, Shelton and Weinrich (1997) described a patient (E.A.) whose written picture naming was far superior to his spoken naming of the same pictures. Furthermore, E.A.'s ability to perform sublexical sound-to-print conversion was essentially abolished, suggesting that written picture naming was lexically mediated. These and other studies (Miceli et al., 1997; Rapp et al., 1997) support the view

that written word production and comprehension are not dependent on intact phonological representations but should be regarded as independent lexical components as depicted in Figures 5–4 and 5–5.

STIMULUS VARIABLES AFFECTING PATIENT PERFORMANCE

To this point, our discussion has focused on the effects of processing modality (auditory vs. visual) and type of task in highlighting the symptom dissociations that constrain construction of a model of the lexical–semantic system. Other types of performance dissociations appear to be related to characteristics inherent in the target words that must be produced or comprehended. The effects of these stimulus variables have frequently been interpreted as indicating a potential locus of patients' impairments within the lexical–semantic system.

FREQUENCY, IMAGEABILITY, AND AGE OF ACQUISITION

A long-standing clinical maxim is that aphasic word production is affected by word frequency (Howes, 1964). Frequency effects (found in both normal and aphasic subjects) are typically interpreted as reflecting heightened activation levels or lowered response thresholds for frequent word forms. Recent studies have emphasized the fact that lexical frequency is highly correlated with other variables such as subjective familiarity, age of acquisition, and length (Nickels and Howard, 1995). It is difficult to distinguish statistically the separate effects of these intercorrelated variables (Ellis et al., 1995/6); however, several recent studies have produced findings indicating that age of acquisition is a more reliable predictor than frequency of naming latencies in normal subjects (Morrison and Ellis, 1995) and of naming success in aphasic speakers (Feyereisen et al., 1988; Nickels and Howard, 1995). In a detailed study of a single anomic patient, Hirsh and Ellis (1994) demonstrated that production of words in spoken naming, written naming, and oral reading was affected by words' rated age of acquisition, but not by imageability or frequency when age of acquisition was controlled. The authors argue that the age at which words are acquired affects the stability (and vulnerability) of phonological word forms.

Since frequency and age of acquisition are highly correlated, it may seem unimportant to determine the relative contributions of each to normal or aphasic performance. However, resolution of this issue has important implications for models of lexical processing. Some models of how words are retrieved, for example, postulate a frequency-sensitive search process; others exhibit global frequency sensitivity because of the mechanisms hypothesized to underlie the dynamics of an interactive network (see Morrison and Ellis, 1995, for discussion). The age-of-acquisition findings suggest that words that are learned early have an advantage in normal processing over words that are learned late, and are less vulnerable to brain injury, even when they are not the words used more commonly later in life. This suggests that lexical retrieval mechanisms based on frequency of use, or recency of use, are likely to be incorrect.

The imageability of words' referents is another variable that may affect patient performance in tasks that do not require the testing of "picturable" words, such as oral reading (Coltheart, 1980), auditory comprehension (Franklin et al., 1994), writing to dictation and repetition (Howard and Franklin, 1988). The typical (and quite common) finding is that words with imageable referents (i.e., "concrete" words) are more likely to be correct than are words that refer to abstract concepts. Highly imageable words are also more likely to have been acquired early in development than less imageable words; this variable has not been systematically investigated in studies of imageability effects.

Unlike frequency, which has been assumed to exert its effects on lexical forms (especially forms in an output lexicon), imageability effects have been attributed to differences in words' semantic specifications. One hypothesis is that the semantic representations associated with more concrete referents necessarily include a wider range of semantic features that encode distinctions related to different sensory modalities. One effect of the learning of concrete concepts through multiple modalities might be that they are represented in both cerebral hemispheres, while more abstract concepts (which are learned primarily in verbal contexts) might be uniquely represented in the left hemisphere (Coltheart, 1980).

Another interpretation of the semantic differences between abstract and concrete concepts is that the latter are simply "richer" in terms of the information represented. This idea has been incorporated into computational models of lexical–semantic processing as a difference in the number of semantic features associated with words—i.e., more imageable (concrete) words are represented by more features (Plaut and Shallice, 1993). These accounts of imageability effects easily accommodate the typical finding that imageable words are more likely to be retained following brain damage, but they do not account for patients who show a reverse concreteness effect (Warrington, 1981; Breedin et al., 1994).

Although only a few such patients have been described, they form an important part of a double dissociation based on word imageability/concreteness. The patient studied by Breedin and colleagues (D.M., who suffered from semantic dementia) showed widespread semantic difficulties on clinical testing. He demonstrated significantly better understanding of abstract than concrete words across a range of tasks, including defining words, synonym judgments, and word–picture matching. Further testing suggested that D.M.'s impairment with concrete words was related to poor appreciation of visual–perceptual features. This problem was reflected in his word definitions, in which concrete objects were defined largely without reference to their appearance. For example, *carrot* was defined as "some kind of food you eat," and *ink* as "something that covers." In contrast, abstract words (which can be defined without the necessity of visual descriptors) elicited more identifiable definitions: *try*, "to endeavor to accomplish something"; *opinion*, "your concept or perspective."

Clearly, as Breedin and colleagues argue, the role of imageability/concreteness in word processing must be complex enough to allow different types of neural insult to lead to relatively selective disturbance of either concrete or abstract words; no unidimensional account based on number of semantic features can easily explain both patterns. It should also be noted that the reverse concreteness effect conflicts with results reviewed above, suggesting that the words most likely to be retained in conditions of brain damage are those learned early in life; here, less imageable words, which are generally learned later, are the words that are retained. This conflict may simply reflect the fact that concreteness effects, and age-of-acquisition effects, are operating at different levels of the lexical–semantic system (semantic representations and phonological output representations, respectively). Ultimately, however, a full account of the effects of these variables should incorporate an explanation of all of these phenomena.

SEMANTIC CATEGORY

Another variable that has been shown to affect patient performance is the semantic category of target words. Many aphasia batteries include tests that separately sample patients' knowledge of categories such as colors, letters, and body parts (e.g., Goodlass and Kaplan, 1983). As should be clear from the discussion thus far, before assuming that semantic category effects are real, it is critical to ensure that words from different categories are matched on other variables that are known to affect performance.

The most robust effect of semantic category to be reported to date involves the distinction between biological categories and human-made artifacts, usually referred to as the "animate/inanimate" contrast. In a review of this issue, Saffran and Schwartz (1994) listed 13 patients with relative impairment for living things, most of whom suffered from herpes simplex encephalitis affecting (often bilaterally) the temporal lobes. Several additional cases have now been reported. Fewer patients have been described who show a pattern of poorer performance on nonliving things, and their etiologies and correlated lesion sites are more variable (see Saffran and Schwartz, 1994).

The observance of this double dissociation is important because of the particular difficulty of matching the items tested in living/nonliving categories on all of the relevant variables. Funnell and Sheridan (1992) and Stewart and colleagues (1992) have argued that the early studies demonstrating a category-specific deficit for living things failed to match the categories adequately on variables such as familiarity and visual complexity. Such arguments may have some validity, but they do not apply to all relevant cases. For example, Hillis and Caramazza (1991) tested two patients on the same materials and found opposite patterns of selective disturbance for animate vs. inanimate objects. Clearly, *both* patterns could not arise because of failure to control confounding variables in a single set of stimuli.

Assuming, then, that category-specific deficits for living things vs. artifacts are real, what is the implication of this finding for models of lexical–semantic processing? One proposal is that the dissociation reflects differences in the types of features of objects that are most important in their semantic representations (Allport, 1985; Saffran and Schwartz, 1994). Exemplars of the category *living things* (animals, plants, etc.) are distinguished primarily by their perceptual properties (color, size, shape, etc.), while members of the category *artifact* are distinguished primarily by their function. As discussed above, it has been proposed that separate semantic systems are needed to encode semantic features that are tightly linked with specific sensory modalities. The relative impairment of such a sensory-specific semantic system (e.g., "visual semantics") could lead to category-specific effects.

The proposal that the living/nonliving dissociations reflect a distinction between perceptual and functional semantic features was supported by studies that manipulated the extent to which test questions were based on perceptual vs. functional information. For example, Silveri and Gainotti (1988) reported a patient with category-specific deficit for animals who was very poor (1/11 correct) at naming animals on the basis of a visual description (e.g., for *zebra:* a black and white striped wild horse). Performance improved markedly (8/14 correct) when the probe was a metaphorical expression (for *lion:* king of the jungle) or emphasized a distinctive sound and/or function (e.g., for *sheep:* the farm animal that bleats and supplies us with wool). Thus, this patient not only shows a category-specific impairment for living things but is particularly impaired for the visual–perceptual characteristics of living things.

The argument that category-specific deficits reflect a brain organization in which certain types of semantic features are tightly linked with specific sensory modalities has considerable appeal. As noted by Saffran and Schwartz (1994, p. 530), the implication of this view is that "information in semantic memory bears the stamp of the channels through which it was acquired"—i.e., semantic features may differ qualitatively on the basis of their links to different sensory modalities. Although it might be expected that such a sensory-based account of semantic deficits might lead to straightforward neuroanatomic correlations for semantic categories, this does not appear to be the case from current lesion data (Damasio, 1990).

A challenge to the sensory-specific semantics view has been mounted by Caramazza and Shelton, who favor a semantic system in which all information is represented in a single propositional format (Caramazza and Shelton, 1998; Shelton and Caramazza, 1999). Caramazza and Shelton report data from a patient (E.W.) with a category-specific impairment for animals who was equally impaired in demonstrating knowledge within that category for visual–perceptual properties ("has four legs?") and nonperceptual attributes ("lives on land?"). Furthermore, E.W. was unimpaired in making visual–perceptual judgments about inanimate objects. The authors argue that previous demonstrations of a link between animate category deficits and visual–perceptual features had inadequately matched the probe items for difficulty.

Caramazza and Shelton (1998) propose that the categories that have been distinguished in category-specific impairments (animals, plants, and inanimate things) constitute evolutionarily motivated conceptual–semantic domains with dedicated neural circuitry. Within the domains of animals and plants, which have obvious evolutionary significance, concepts will tend to have highly intercorrelated features (i.e., things that have eyes will tend to be self-locomoting, will ingest food, etc.) Such intercorrelations

among semantic features, it is argued, create a textured semantic network with considerable overlap among features within particular domains. Category-specific impairments arise when brain damage selectively affects specific areas of semantic space.

GRAMMATICAL CLASS

Another important performance dissociation found in aphasia that may be related to semantic category is grammatical class, i.e., the designation of how words are used within the context of a sentence. One of the most obvious contrasts found among aphasic patients involves the dissociation between noun production (good in Broca's aphasics and poor in severe anomic and Wernicke's aphasics) and the production of grammatical function words (poor in Broca's aphasics and good in anomic and Wernicke's aphasics). However, since nouns are generally more imageable than grammatical words, and grammatical words are more frequent than nouns, it is possible that this double dissociation can be reduced to a difference based on these other variables (see, e.g., Ellis et al., 1983, for one argument along these lines). Other explanations for content–function word dissociations implicate syntactic processes and are therefore outside the scope of this chapter (see Berndt, 2001, for discussion).

Another double dissociation based on grammatical class is that between nouns and verbs, which can be matched for other variables that might affect performance. Numerous cases have now been described of patients whose production of nouns is either much better or much worse than their production of frequency-matched verbs in picture naming (Miceli et al., 1984; Zingeser and Berndt, 1990; Berndt et al., 1997b). These results were initially linked to the clinical categories of Broca's aphasia (verbs impaired) and anomia (nouns impaired), which was consistent with neuroanatomic findings suggesting a frontal lobe locus for verb deficits and a temporal lobe locus for noun deficits (Damasio and Tranel, 1993). However, exceptions to the correlations with both clinical category and responsible lesion locus have been reported (Caramazza and Hillis, 1991; Berndt et al., 1997a).

Most of the follow-up studies on grammatical class effects have focused on relative impairment of verbs, but it is important that some patients show the opposite pattern of poorer performance with nouns. Thus, it cannot be argued that verbs are simply more difficult, and more vulnerable to brain injury, than nouns, perhaps because of their complex relationships to sentence processing. It is also true that most studies to date have shown selective verb impairments only in production tasks (but see Miceli et al., 1984; McCarthy and Warrington, 1985). Studies that have looked for but failed to find verb impairments in comprehension comparable to those found in production (Caramazza and Hillis, 1991; Berndt et al., 1997b) are always subject to the criticism that comprehension tasks (involving forced choice, etc.) may be inherently easier than production tasks.

The status of patients' comprehension of verbs is a critically important issue in evaluating the theoretical importance of modality-specific verb deficits in production. Caramazza and Hillis (1991) described two patients with problems producing verbs relative to nouns: one patient showed a verb-specific impairment only when speaking, and the other, only when writing. Because neither patient demonstrated an apparent problem understanding verbs, the authors argued that the locus of the patients' impairment must be in a component of the lexical–semantic system that is dedicated to one modality of output, i.e., to the phonological or the orthographic output lexicons within a four-lexicon model such as that shown in Figure 5–4 (Caramazza, 1997). This argument has generated considerable controversy, since grammatical class has typically been viewed as an element of an amodal component of lexical representations (Levelt, 1989; Bock and Levelt, 1994; see Garrett, 1992, for discussion).[4]

Further complicating interpretation of grammatical class effects in aphasia are results indicating that different underlying functional deficits might lead to selective problems with verbs. Breedin and Martin (1996) studied four aphasic patients who had more difficulty naming action than object pictures. The patients were tested with six tasks probing production and comprehension of different aspects of verbs, including elements of their meaning, of the thematic roles associated with different verbs, and of their subcategorization frames. The patients showed distinct impairments across the tasks, suggesting that different aspects of verb representations were affected in different patients. This result suggests that grammatical class impairments may arise for a number of different reasons, and that some of them may also affect comprehension and may be closely linked with the role of the word in sentence processing (see also Berndt et al., 1997a).

CURRENT ISSUES AND FUTURE DIRECTIONS

This review has described some of the components of the lexical–semantic system that appear to be required, based on neuropsychological data. The primary goal has been to use patient data to decide how hypothesized components of this system are organized and interrelated, and at the same time to use the model to interpret a variety of symptom patterns. We have not yet considered important issues regarding the dynamics of this skeletal system, i.e., the direction and chronology of information flow.

Much contemporary psycholinguistic research on this issue characterizes perturbations in information availability during lexical processing as reflections of differences in activation levels across networks of lexical or semantic units, usually referred to as "nodes" (Dell, 1986; Bock and Levelt, 1994). In some cases, such lexical networks have been implemented as computational models so that different processing dynamics can be tested in attempting to model experimental data. Performance patterns found in aphasic patients have been used to test aspects of such models, especially within the domain of word production.

For example, Dell and colleagues (1997) simulated picture-naming error patterns from 21 fluent aphasic patients using a two-step interactive model in which semantic features activate word nodes, which in turn activate the relevant phoneme nodes. Critically, the model allows feedback from later levels (e.g., activation of phoneme nodes) to influence earlier levels. The parameters of the model were chosen to fit patterns produced by normal speakers, then the model was "lesioned" by altering two parameters: global connection weight (which results in an overall decrease in flow of activation spreading through the network) and global decay rate (which increases the rate at which each unit in the network loses activation). Patients' error patterns were simulated by individually fitting these parameters to the data. These parameter values were then used to make predictions about other aspects of patients' errors, about recovery, and about their word repetition pattern. Manipulation of these two parameters successfully reproduced the major characteristics of the error patterns, and most predictions were upheld. However, there is continuing debate about the importance of performance patterns that were not successfully simulated (Foygel and Dell, 2000; Ruml and Caramazza, 2000).

The view that semantic and phonological information can mutually influence one another, which is instantiated in Dell's interactive activation model, is not shared by all modelers of lexical production. An opposing view is that word production proceeds strictly serially from semantics to phonology, without the possibility of phonological influences on semantic processing (e.g., Levelt, 1989). Using computational models in which the degree and type of interaction was systematically manipulated, Rapp and Goldrick (2000) evaluated the success of serial and interactive models in accounting for naming data from three aphasics patients. These studies led to the conclusion that, although some degree of interaction appears to be required to account for patients' error patterns, there are also clear limits on the types of interaction that might be allowed. For example, there was compelling evidence for the need for feedback from phoneme nodes to lexical nodes, but considerably less evidence for the need for feedback from word nodes to semantics.

These types of studies can be expected to play an increasingly important role in analyses of the implications of aphasic data. Moreover, the idea that word processing involves distributed networks of nodes specialized for different types of information is consonant with views of language–brain relationships that are emerging from functional neuroimaging studies (see Small and Burton, 2001, for review). In contrast to earlier views in which neural "centers" were dedicated to specific language operations (e.g., comprehension), functional imaging studies suggest that the performance of specific tasks can lead to widespread cortical activation. It has frequently been suggested that computational models of cognitive processes that employ interactive networks of nodes constitute "neurobiologically plausible" accounts of information representation, and efforts are now being made to combine functional brain imaging, computational modeling, and behavioral analyses (e.g., Horwitz et al. 1999). This review suggests that such studies need to incorporate detailed consideration of the patterns of word processing impairments that occur following brain damage.

ACKNOWLEDGMENTS

The preparation of this chapter was supported by grants R01-DC00262 and R01-DC00699 from the National Institute on Deafness and Other Communication Disorders to the University of Maryland School of Medicine.

NOTES

1. Another type of word form that has been subjected to experimental investigation is the gestural/spatial system of American Sign Language, which is affected by focal brain damage in native users of sign in much the same way as is spoken language in auditory–verbal language users (for a recent review, see Hickok and Bellugi, 2001). Other word forms (e.g., coded signal systems such as Morse code, tactile systems such as Braille, etc.) are also available to some word users.
2. Although such tasks can be very revealing, and in fact are the basis of the studies discussed here, it should be kept in mind that these uses of words are quite divorced from the normal use of words in sentences, in the service of communication.
3. Again it is important to note that a contrasting pattern has been found in some patients with Alzheimer's disease who are better able to name objects from visual presentation than from auditory definitions (Shuren et al., 1993; Lauro-Grotto et al., 1997). This finding indicates that no simple explanation based on the relative difficulty of object naming or the relative vulnerability of visual processes is a tenable explanation for optic aphasia.

4. The modality-neutral lexical representations postulated to encode grammatical class information in the cited papers are referred to as "lemmas". This element has not been incorporated into the models discussed here because its role is relevant primarily to sentence production.

REFERENCES

Allport, D. A. (1985). Distributed memory, modular subsystems and dysphasia. In *Current Perspectives in Dysphasia*, S. Newman and R. Epstein (eds.). London: Churchill Livingston, pp. 32–60.

Allport, D. A. and Funnell, E. (1981). Components of the mental lexicon. *Phil. Trans. R. Soc. Lond. Ser. B* 295:397–401.

Beauvois, M. F. (1982). Optic aphasia: a process of interaction between vision and language. *Phil. Trans. R. Soc. Lond. Ser. B* 298:35–47.

Beauvois, M. F., Saillant, B., Meininger, V., and Lhermitte, F. (1978). Bilateral tactile aphasia. A tacto-verbal dysfunction. *Brain* 101:381–401.

Behrmann, M., and Bub, D. (1992). Surface dyslexia and dysgraphia: dual routes, single lexicon. *Cogn. Neuropsychol.*, 9:209–251.

Berndt, R. S. (2001). More than just words: Sentence production in aphasia. In R.S. Berndt (Ed.) *Language and Aphasia*. Amsterdam: Elsevier, pp. 173–187.

Berndt, R. S., Haendiges, A. N., Mitchum, C. C., and Sandson, J. (1997a). Verb retrieval in aphasia. 2. Relationship to sentence processing. *Brain Lang.* 56:107–137.

Berndt, R. S., Mitchum, C. C., Haendiges, A. N., and Sandson, J. (1997b). Verb retrieval in aphasia. 1. Characterizing single word impairments. *Brain Lang.* 56:68–106.

Bierwisch, M., and Schreuder, R. (1992). From concepts to lexical items. *Cognition* 42:23–60.

Bock, K., and Levelt, W. (1994). Language production: grammatical encoding. In *Handbook of Psycholinguistics*, M. Gernsbacher (ed.). New York: Academic Press, pp. 945–984.

Bramwell, B. (1897). Illustrative cases of aphasia. *Lancet* 1:1256–1257 (reprinted 1984, *Cogn. Neuropsychol.* 1:245–258).

Breedin, S. D., and Martin, R. C. (1996). Patterns of verb impairment in aphasia: an analysis of four cases. *Cogn. Neuropsychol.* 13:51–91.

Breedin, S. D., Saffran, E. M., and Coslett, H. B. (1994). Reversal of the concreteness effect in a patient with semantic dementia. *Cogn. Neuropsychol.* 17:617–660.

Brown, R., and McNeill, D. (1966). The "tip-of-the-tongue phenomenon." *J. Verbal Learn. Verbal Behav.* 5:325–337.

Caramazza, A. (1997). How many levels of processing are there in lexical access? *Cogn. Neuropsychol.* 14:177–208.

Caramazza, A., and Hillis, A. E. (1991). Lexical organization of nouns and verbs in the brain. *Nature* 349:788–790.

Caramazza, A., Hillis, A. E., Rapp, B., and Romani, C. (1990). Multiple semantics or multiple confusions? *Cogn. Neuropsychol.* 7:161–190.

Caramazza, A. and Shelton, J. R. (1998). Domain-specific knowledge systems in the brain: the animate–inanimate distinction. *J. Cogn. Neurosci.* 10:1–34.

Coleman, J. (1998). Cognitive reality and the phonological lexicon: a review. *J. Neurolinguistics* 11:295–320.

Coltheart, M. (1980). Deep dyslexia: a right hemisphere hypothesis. In *Deep Dyslexia*, M. Coltheart, K. E. Patterson, and J. C. Marshall (eds.). London: Routledge & Kegan Paul, pp. 22–47.

Coltheart, M., and Coltheart, V. (1997). Reading comprehension is not exclusively reliant upon phonological representation. *Cogn. Neuropsychol.* 14:167–175.

Coltheart, M., and Funnell, E. (1987). Reading and writing: one lexicon or two? In *Language Perception and Production: Relationships between Listening, Speaking, Reading and Writing*, A. Allport, D. C. Mackay, W. Prinz, and E. Scheerer (eds.). London: Academic Press, pp. 313–339.

Conway, T. W., Heilman, P., Gonzalez Rothi, L. J., Alexander, A. W., Adair, J., Crosson, B. A. and Heilman, K. M. (1998). Treatment of a case of phonological alexia with agraphia using the ADD program. *J. Int. Neuropsychol. Soc.* 4:608–620.

Coslett, H. B., & Saffran, E. M. (1989) Preserved object recognition and reading comprehension in optic aphasia. *Brain* 112:1091–1110.

Coslett, H. B., and Saffran, E. M. (1992). Optic aphasia and the right hemisphere: a replication and extension. *Brain Lang.* 43:148–161.

Damasio, A. R. (1990). Category-related recognition defects as a clue to the neural substrates of knowledge. *Trends Neurosci.* 13:95–98.

Damasio, A. R., and Tranel, D. (1993). Nouns and verbs are retrieved with differently distributed neural systems. *Proc. Natl. Acad. Sci. U.S.A.* 90:4957–4960.

Dejerine, J. (1892). Contribution a l'etude anatomoclinique et clinique des differentes varietes de cecite verbale. *Memoire Soc. Biol.* 4:61–90.

Dell, G. S. (1986). A spreading activation theory of retrieval in sentence production. *Psychol. Rev.* 93:283–321.

Dell, G. S., Schwartz, M.F., Martin, N., Saffran, E. M., and Gagnon, D. A. (1997). Lexical access in aphasic and nonaphasic speakers. *Psychol. Bull.* 104:801–838.

Ellis, A. W. (1988). Modeling the writing process. In *Perspectives in Cognitive Neuropsychology*, C. Denes, C. Semenza, and F. P. Bisiacchi (eds.). London: Lawrence Erlbaum Associates.

Ellis, A. W., Lum, C., and Lambon Ralph, M. A. (1995/6). On the use of regression techniques for the analysis of single case aphasic data. *J. Neurolinguistics* 9:165–174.

Ellis, A. W., Miller, D., and Sin, G. (1983). Wernicke's aphasia and normal language processing: a case study in cognitive neuropsychology. *Cognition* 15:111–114.

Ellis, A. W., and Young, A. W. (1996). *Human Cognitive Neuropsychology. A Textbook with Readings*. Hove: Psychology Press.

Feyereisen, P., Van der Borght, F., and Seron, X. (1988). The operativity effect in naming. A reanalysis. *Neuropsychologia* 26:401–415.

Foygel, D. and Dell, G. S. (2000). Models of impaired lexical access in speech production. *J. Mem. Lang.* 43:182–216.

Franklin, S., Howard, D., and Patterson, K. (1994). Abstract word meaning deafness. *Cogn. Neuropsychol.* 11:1–34.

Freund, D. C. (1889). Uber optische Aphasie und Seelenblindheit. *Arch Psychiatrie Nervenkrankheim* 20:276, 297.

Funnell, E., and Sheridan, J. S. (1992). Categories of knowledge? Unfamiliar aspects of living and nonliving things. *Cogn. Neuropsychol.* 9:135–153.

Garrett, M. F. (1992). Disorders of lexical selection. *Cognition* 42:143–180.

Geschwind, N. (1969). Problems in the anatomical understanding of aphasia. In *Contributions of Clinical Neuropsychology*, A. L. Benton (ed.). Chicago: University of Chicago Press.

Goodglass, H., and Kaplan, E. (1983). *The Assessment of Aphasia and Related Disorders* (2nd edition). Philadelphia: Lea & Febiger

Greenwald, M. L., and Berndt, R. S. (1999). Impaired encoding of abstract letter order: severe alexia in a mildly aphasic patient. *Cogn. Neuropsychol.* 16:513–556.

Hall, D. A., and Riddoch, M. J. (1997). Word meaning deafness: spelling words that are not understood. *Cogn. Neuropsychol.* 14:1131–1164.

Hickok, G., and Bellugi, U. (2001). The signs of aphasia. In *Handbook of Neuropsychology: Vol. 2. Language and Aphasia*, 2nd ed., F. Boller and J. Grafman (series eds.) and R. S. Berndt (vol. ed.). Amsterdam: Elsevier, pp. 31–50.

Hillis, A. E., and Caramazza, A. (1991). Category-specific naming and comprehension impairment. A double dissociation. *Brain* 114:2081–2094.

Hirsh, K. W., and Ellis, A. W. (1994). Age of acquisition and lexical processing in aphasia: a case study. *Cogn. Neuropsychol.* 11:435–458.

Hodges, J. R., Patterson, K., Oxbury, S., and Funnell, E. (1992). Semantic dementia. Progressive fluent aphasia with temporal lobe atrophy. *Brain* 115:1783–1806.

Horwitz, B., Tagamets, M., and McIntosh A. (1999). Neural modeling, functional brain imaging and cognition. *Trends Cogn. Sci.* 3:91–98.

Howard, D. (1995). Lexical anomia: or the case of the missing entries. *Q. J. Exp. Psychol.* 48A:999–1023.

Howard, D., and Franklin, S. (1988). *Missing the Meaning?* Cambridge: The MIT Press.

Howes, D. (1964). Application of the word frequency concept in aphasia. In *Disorders of Language*, A. V. S. De Reuck, and M. O'Connor, (eds.). London: Churchill, pp. 47–75.

Lauro-Grotto, R., Piccini, C., and Shallice, T. (1997). Modality-specific operations in semantic dementia. *Cortex* 33:593–622.

Levelt, W. J. M. (1989). *Speaking: From Intention to Articulation*. Cambridge, MA: MIT Press.

Luria, A. R. (1966). *Higher Cortical Functions in Man*. New York: Basic Books.

Lyons, J. (1981). Language and speech. *Phil. Trans. R. Soc. Lond. Ser. B* 295:215–222.

Martin, R. C., Lesch, M. F., and Bartha, M. C. (1999). Independence of input and output phonology in word processing and short-term memory. *J. Mem. Lang.* 41:3–29.

McCarthy, R., and Warrington, E. K. (1985). Category-specificity in an agrammatic patient: the relative impairment of verb retrieval and comprehension. *Neuropsychologia* 23:709–727.

McCarthy, R. A., and Warrington, E. K. (1990). *Cognitive Neuropsychology*. San Diego: Academic Press.

Miceli, G., Benvegnu, B., Capasso, R., and Caramazza, A. (1997). The independence of phonological and orthographic lexical forms: evidence from aphasia. *Cogn. Neuropsychol.* 14:35–69.

Miceli, G., Silveri, M. C., Nocentini, U., and Caramazza, A. (1988). Patterns of dissociation in comprehension and production of nouns and verbs. *Aphasiology* 2:351–358.

Miceli, G., Silveri, M. C., Villa, G., and Caramazza, A. (1984). On the basis for the agrammatic's difficulty in producing main verbs. *Cortex* 20:207–220.

Miller, G. A. (1991). *The Science of Words.* New York: Scientific American Library.

Monsell, S. (1987). On the relation between lexical input and output pathways for speech. In *Language Perception and Production: Relationships Between Listening, Speaking, Reading, and Writing*, D. A. Allport, D. MacKay, W. Prinz, and E. Scheerer (eds.), London: Academic Press, pp. 273–316.

Morrison, C. M., and Ellis, A. W. (1995). Roles of word frequency and age of acquisition in word naming and lexical decision. *J. Exp. Psychol.* 21:116–133.

Nickels, L., and Howard, D. (1995). Aphasic naming: what matters? *Neuropsychologia* 33:1281–1303.

Plaut, D. C., and Shallice, T. (1993). Deep dyslexia: a case study of connectionist neuropsychology. *Cogn. Neuropsychol.* 10:377–500.

Rapp B., Benzing, L., and Caramazza, A. (1997). The autonomy of lexical orthography. *Cogn. Neuropsychol.* 14:71–104.

Rapp, B., and Goldrick, M. (2000). Discreteness and interactivity in spoken word production. *Psychol. Rev.* 107(3):460–499.

Riddoch, M. J., Humphreys, G. W., Coltheart, M., and Funnell, E. (1988). Semantic systems or system? Neuropsychological evidence re-examined. *Cogn. Neuropsychol.* 5:3–25.

Roelofs, A. (1993). Testing a non-decompositional theory of lemma retrieval in speaking: retrieval of verbs. *Cognition* 47:59–87.

Ruml, W., and Caramazza, A. (2000). An evaluation of a computational model of lexical access: comments on Dell et al. (1997). *Psychol. Rev.* 107(3): 609–634.

Saffran, E. M., and Schwartz, M. F. (1994). Of cabbages and things: semantic memory from a neuropsychological perspective—a tutorial review. In *Attention and Performance XV. Conscious and Neuroconscious Information Processing*, C. Umilta and M. Moscovitch, (eds.). Cambridge, MA: MIT Press, pp. 507–536.

Schwartz, M. F., Saffran, E. M., and Marin, O. S. M. (1980). Fractionating the reading process in dementia: evidence for word-specific print-to-sound associations. In *Deep Dyslexia*, M. Coltheart, K. E. Patterson, and J. C. Marshall (eds.),

London: Routledge and Kegan Paul, pp. 259–269.

Shallice, T. (1987). Impairments of semantic processing: multiple dissociations. In *The Cognitive Neuropsychology of Language*, M. Coltheart, G. Sartori, and R. Jobs (eds.). London: Lawrence Erlbaum Associates, pp. 111–127.

Shallice, T. (1988). *From Neuropsychology to Mental Structure.* Cambridge, UK: Cambridge University Press.

Shelton, J. R., and Caramazza, A. (1999). Deficits in lexical and semantic processing: implications for models of normal language. *Psychon. Bull. Rev.* 6:5–27.

Shelton, J. R., and Weinrich, M. (1997). Further evidence of a dissociation between output phonological and orthographic lexicons: a case study. *Cogn. Neuropsychol.* 14:105–129.

Shuren, J., Geldmacher, D., and Heilman, K. (1993). Nonoptic aphasia: aphasia with preserved confrontation naming in Alzheimer's disease. *Neurology* 43:1900–1907.

Silveri, M. C., and Gainotti, G. (1988). Interaction between vision and language in category specific impairment. *Cogn. Neuropsychol.* 5:677–709.

Small, S. L., and Burton, M. W. (2001). Functional neuroimaging of language. In *Handbook of Neuropsychology, Vol. 2, Language and Aphasia*, 2nd ed., F. Boller and J. Grafman (series eds.) and R. S. Berndt (volume ed.). Amsterdam: Elsevier, pp. 335–351.

Stewart, F., Parkin, A. J., and Hunkin, N. M. (1992). Naming impairments following recovery from herpes simplex encephalitis: category-specific? *Q. J. Exp. Psychol.* 4A.261–284.

Van Orden, G. C., Johnston, J. C., and Hale, B. L. (1988). Word identification in reading proceeds from spelling to sound to meaning. *J. Exp. Psychol.* 14:371–386.

Warrington, E. K. (1981). Concrete word dyslexia. *Br. J. Psychol.* 72:175–196.

Whitaker, H. (1976). A case of the isolation of the language function. In *Studies in Neurolinguistics, Vol. 2*, H. Whitaker and H. A. Whitaker (eds.). New York: Academic Press, pp. 1–58.

Zingeser, L. B. and Berndt, R. S. (1988). Grammatical class and context effects in a case of pure anomia: implications for models of language production. *Cogn. Neuropsychol.* 5:473–516.

Zingeser, L. B. and Berndt, R. S. (1990). Retrieval of nouns and verbs in agrammatism and anomia. *Brain Lang.* 39:14–32.

6

Acquired Dyslexia

H. BRANCH COSLETT

Unlike the ability to speak, which has presumably evolved over hundreds of thousands of years, the ability to read is a relatively recent development that is dependent upon both the capacity to process complex visual stimuli and the ability to engage phonologic, syntactic, and other language capacities. Perhaps as a consequence of the wide range of cognitive operations required, reading is compromised in many patients with cerebral lesions, particularly those involving the left hemisphere. The resultant reading impairments, or acquired dyslexias, take many different forms, reflecting the breakdown of specific aspects of the reading process. In this chapter, we briefly review the history of the study of acquired dyslexia and discuss a model of the processes involved in normal reading. Specific syndromes of acquired dyxlexia are discussed. We also briefly discuss connectionist accounts of reading and the anatomic basis of reading as revealed by recent functional imaging studies. Lastly, the clinical assessment of reading and attempts at reading remediation are briefly described.

HISTORICAL OVERVIEW

Investigations of acquired dyslexia commenced in the late nineteenth century, a time at which a number of now classical disorders were first described. Perhaps the most influential early contributions to the understanding of dyslexia were provided by Dejerine, who described two patients with quite different patterns of reading impairment. Dejerine's first patient (1891) manifested impaired reading and writing subsequent to an infarction involving the left parietal lobe. Dejerine termed this disorder "alexia with agraphia" and attributed the disturbance to a disruption of the "optical image for words," which he thought to be supported by the left angular gyrus. In an account that in some respects presages contemporary psychological accounts, Dejerine concluded that reading and writing required the activation of these "optical images" and that the loss of the images resulted in the inability to recognize or write even familiar words.

Dejerine's second patient (1892) was quite different. This patient exhibited a right homonymous hemianopia and was unable to read aloud or for comprehension, but could write. This disorder, designated "alexia without agraphia" (also known as "agnosic alexia" and "pure alexia"), was attributed by Dejerine to a "disconnection" between visual information presented to the right hemisphere and the left angular gyrus, which he assumed to be critical for the recognition of words.

After the seminal contributions of Dejerine, the study of acquired dyslexia languished for decades, during which the relatively few investigations that were reported focused primarily on the anatomic underpinnings of the disorders. Although a number of interesting observations were reported, they were often either ignored or their significance not appreciated. For example, Akelaitis (1944) reported that patients whose corpus callosum had been severed were unable to read aloud stimuli presented in the left visual field; this observation provided powerful support for Dejerine's interpretation of alexia without agraphia as a disconnection syndrome, but was reported only in passing in a series of contributions that failed to demonstrate a substantial role of the corpus callosum in behavior.

The study of acquired dyslexia was revitalized by the elegant and detailed analysis by Marshall and Newcombe (1966, 1973), which demonstrated that by virtue of a careful investigation of the pattern of reading deficits exhibited by dyslexic subjects, distinctly different and reproducible types of reading deficits could be elucidated. The insights provided by Marshall and Newcombe provided much of the basis for the "dual-route" model of word reading, to which we return below.

READING MECHANISMS AND THE CLASSIFICATION OF READING DISORDERS

Reading is a complicated process that involves many different procedures, including low-level visual processing, accessing meaning and phonology, and motor aspects of speech production. Figure 6–1 provides a graphic depiction of the relationship between these procedures. This "information-processing" model will serve as the basis for the discussion of the mechanisms involved in reading and the specific forms of acquired dyslexia to be presented below. Alternatives to the information-processing accounts will also be discussed.

Reading requires that the visual system efficiently process a complicated stimulus that, at least for alphabet-based languages, consists of smaller meaningful units, letters. Given the morphosyntactic constraints of languages as well as the relatively small number of letters in relation to the number of words, many words are visually quite similar, a fact that places a substantial burden on the visual system.

Under normal circumstances, however, written words are recognized so rapidly and accurately that one might suspect that the word is identified as a unit, much as we identify an object from its visual form. The evidence, however, does not support such a model. It appears that the letters must first be identified as alphabetic symbols. It has been shown that presenting words in a format that is not familiar to the reader—for example, by alternating the case of the letters (e.g., *wOrD*)—has minimal effects on reading speed (e.g., McClelland and Rumelhart, 1977). This finding suggests that the processing of written words includes a stage of letter identification, in which the graphic form (whether printed or written) is transformed into a string of alphabetic characters (*W-O-R-D*), sometimes referred to as "abstract letter identities." In addition, the positions of the letters must be maintained. How this is accomplished has yet to be determined. Possibilities include associating the letter in position 1 to the letter in position 2, and so on; binding each letter to a frame that specifies letter position; or labeling each letter with its position in the word. Finally, it should be noted that under normal circumstances letters are not processed in a strictly serial fashion but letter strings are processed in parallel (provided they are not too long). Disorders of reading resulting from impairment in the processing of the visual stimulus or the failure of this visual information to contact stored knowledge appropriate to a letter string, designated "peripheral dyslexias," are discussed below.

On dual-route models of reading, the identity of a letter string may be determined by a number of distinct procedures. The first is a "lexical" procedure by which the letter string is identified by means of matching the letter string to an entry in a stored catalog of familiar words, or *visual word form system*. As indicated in Figure 6–1 and discussed below, this procedure, which in some respects is similar to looking up a word in a dictionary, provides access to the meaning, phonologic form, and at

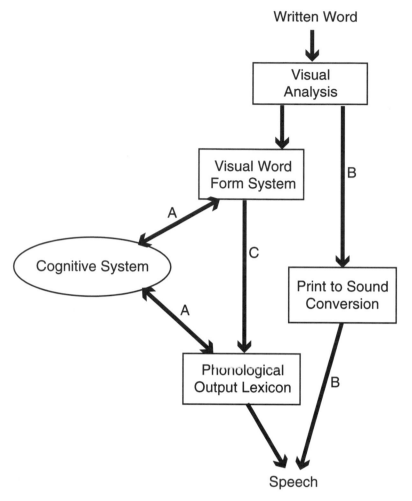

Figure 6–1. Information-processing model of reading depicting three distinct procedures for oral reading: the lexical pathway (A), the nonlexical grapheme-to-phoneme or print-to-sound pathway (B), and the direct pathway (C). See text for details.

least some of the syntactic properties of the word. Dual-route models of reading also assume that the letter string can be converted directly to a phonological form by means of the application of a set of learned correspondences between orthography and phonology. On this account, meaning may then be accessed from the phonologic form of the word.

Support for dual-route models of reading comes from a variety of sources. For present purposes, perhaps the most relevant evidence was provided by Marshall and Newcombe's ground-breaking description of "deep" and "surface" dyslexia (1966, 1973). These investigators described a patient (G.R.) who read ap-

proximately 50% of concrete nouns (e.g., *table, doughnut*) but was severely impaired in the reading of abstract nouns (e.g., *destiny, truth*) and all other parts of speech. The most striking aspect of G.R.'s performance, however, was his tendency to produce errors that appeared to be semantically related to the target word (e.g., *speak* read as "talk"). Marshall and Newcombe (1973) designated this disorder "deep dyslexia." These investigators also described two patients whose primary deficit appeared to be an inability to reliably apply "grapheme–phoneme" correspondences. Thus, J.C., for example, rarely applied the "rule of e" (which lengthens the preceding vowel in words such as *like*) and experienced great difficulties in deriving the appropriate phonology for consonant clusters and vowel digraphs. The disorder characterized by impaired application of print-to-sound correspondences was termed "surface dyslexia."

On the basis of these observations, Marshall and Newcombe (1973) argued that the meaning of written words could be accessed by two distinct procedures. The first was a direct procedure whereby familiar words activated the appropriate stored representation (or visual word form) which, in turn, activated meaning directly; reading in deep dyslexia, which was characterized by semantically based errors (of which the patient was often unaware), was assumed to involve this procedure. The second procedure was assumed to be a phonologically based process in which "grapheme-to-phoneme" or "print-to-sound" correspondences were employed to derive the appropriate phonology (or "sound out" the word); the reading of surface dyslexics was assumed to be mediated by this nonlexical procedure. Although a number of Marshall and Newcombe's specific hypotheses have subsequently been criticized, their argument that reading may be mediated by two distinct procedures has received considerable empirical support.

The information-processing model of reading depicted in Figure 6–1 provides three distinct procedures for oral reading. Two of these procedures correspond to those described by Marshall and Newcombe (1973). The first (labeled *A* in Figure 6–1) involves the activation of a stored entry in the visual word form system and the subsequent access to semantic information and ultimately activation of the stored sound of the word at the level of the phonologic output lexicon. The second (*B* in Figure 6–1) involves the nonlexical grapheme-to-phoneme or print-to-sound translation process; this procedure does not entail access to any stored information about words but rather is assumed to be mediated by access to a catalog of correspondences stipulating the pronunciation of phonemes. Many information-processing accounts of the language mechanisms subserving reading incorporate a third reading procedure. This mechanism (*C* in Fig. 6–1) is lexically based, in that it is as-

sumed to involve the activation of the visual word form system and the phonologic output lexicon. The procedure differs from the lexical procedure described above, however, in that there is no intervening activation of semantic information. This procedure has been called the "direct" reading mechanism or route. Support for the direct lexical mechanism comes from a number of sources including observations that some subjects read aloud words that they do not appear to comprehend (Schwartz et al., 1979; Coslett, 1991). For example, we reported a patient whose inability to read aloud nonwords (e.g., *flig*) suggested that she was unable to employ print-to-sound conversion procedures. Additionally, she exhibited semantic errors in writing and repetition and performed poorly on a synonymy judgement task with low-imageability words, suggesting that semantic representations were imprecise. Semantic errors and imageability effects were not observed in reading; additionally, she read aloud low-imageability words as well as many other words that she appeared to be unable to comprehend. Both observations suggest that her oral reading was not mediated by semantics. We argued that these data provided evidence for a reading mechanism that is independent of semantic representations and does not entail print-to-sound conversion—that is, a "direct" route from visual word forms to the phonological output representations.

PERIPHERAL DYSLEXIAS

A useful starting point in the discussion of the alexias is provided by the distinction made by Shallice and Warrington (1980) between "peripheral" and "central" dyslexias. *Peripheral dyslexias* are conditions characterized by a deficit in the processing of visual aspects of the stimulus that prevent the patient from reliably matching a familiar word to its stored visual form, or "visual word form" (Shallice and Warrington, 1980). In contrast, *central dyslexias* reflect impairment to the "deeper" or "higher" reading functions by which visual word forms mediate access to meaning, or speech production mechanisms. In this section we discuss the major types of peripheral dyslexia.

ALEXIA WITHOUT AGRAPHIA (PURE ALEXIA; LETTER-BY-LETTER READING)

This disorder is among the most common of the peripheral reading disturbances. It is associated with a left hemisphere lesion affecting left occipital cortex (responsible for the analysis of visual stimuli on the right side of space) and/or the structures (left lateral geniculate nucleus of the thalamus; white matter, including callosal fibers from the intact right visual cortex) that provide input to this region of the brain. It is likely that the lesion either blocks direct visual input to the mechanisms that process printed words in the left hemisphere or disrupts the visual word form system itself (Warrington and Shallice, 1980; Cohen et al., 2000). Some of these patients seem to be unable to read at all, while others do so slowly and laboriously by means of a process that involves serial letter identification (often termed "letter-by-letter" reading). At first, letter-by-letter readers often pronounce the letter names aloud; in some cases, they misidentify letters, usually on the basis of visual similarity, as in the case of $N \rightarrow M$ (see Patterson and Kay, 1982, for relevant data). Their reading is also abnormally slow.

It was long thought that patients with pure alexia were unable to read, except letter by letter. There is now evidence that some of them do retain the ability to recognize letter strings, although this does not guarantee that they will be able to read aloud. Several different paradigms have demonstrated the preservation of word recognition. Some patients demonstrate a word superiority effect (e.g., Bub et al., 1989; Reuter-Lorenz and Brunn, 1990; Friedman and Hadley, 1992; Bowers et al., 1996); this effect reflects superior letter recognition when the letter is part of a word (e.g., the R in WORD) to that when it occurs in a string of unrelated letters (e.g., WKRD). Second, some patients have been able to perform lexical decision tasks (determining whether a letter string constitutes a real word or not) and semantic categorization tasks (indicating whether or not a word belongs to a category, such as foods or animals) at above-chance levels when words are presented too rapidly to support letter-by-letter reading (e.g., Shallice and Saffran, 1986; Coslett and Saffran, 1989a). Brevity of

presentation is critical, in that longer exposure to the letter string seems to engage the letter-by-letter strategy, which appears to interfere with the ability to perform the covert reading task (Coslett and Saffran, 1989a; Coslett et al., 1993). In fact, the patient may show better performance on lexical decision at shorter (e.g., 250 msec) than at longer presentations (e.g., 2 seconds) that engage the letter-by-letter strategy but do not allow it to proceed to completion (Coslett and Saffran, 1989a). A compelling example comes from the patient reported by Shallice and Saffran (1986), who was given 2 seconds to scan the card containing the stimulus. The patient did not take advantage of the full inspection time when he was performing lexical decision and categorization tasks; instead, he glanced at the card briefly and looked away, perhaps to avoid letter-by-letter reading. The capacity for covert reading has also been demonstrated in two pure alexics who were completely unable to employ the letter-by-letter reading strategy (Coslett and Saffran, 1989b, 1992). These patients appeared to recognize words but were rarely able to report them, although they sometimes generated descriptions that were related to the word's meaning (for example, cookies → "candy, a cake"; Coslett and Saffran, 1992). In some cases, patients have shown some recovery of oral reading over time, although this capacity appears to be limited to concrete words (Coslett and Saffran, 1989a; Buxbaum and Coslett, 1996).

The mechanisms that underlie implicit or covert reading remain controversial. Dejerine (1892), who provided the first description of pure alexia, suggested that the analysis of visual input in these patients is performed by the right hemisphere, as a result of the damage to the visual cortex on the left. (It should be noted, however, that not all lesions to the left visual cortex give rise to alexia. A critical feature that supports continued left hemisphere processing is the preservation of callosal input from the visual processing on the right.) One possible account is that covert reading reflects printed word recognition on the part of the right hemisphere, which is unable either to articulate the word or (in most cases) to adequately communicate its identity to the language area of the left hemisphere (e.g., Coslett and Saffran, 1989a; Saffran and Coslett, 1998). On this account, letter-by-letter reading is carried out by the left hemisphere using letter information transferred serially and inefficiently from the right. Furthermore, the account assumes that when the letter-by-letter strategy is implemented, it may be difficult for the patient to attend to the products of word processing in the right hemisphere. Consequently, performance on lexical decision and categorization tasks declines (Coslett and Saffran, 1989a; Coslett et al., 1993). Additional evidence supporting the right hemisphere account of reading in pure alexia is presented below.

Alternative accounts of pure alexia have also been proposed. Behrmann and colleagues (Behrmann and Shallice, 1995; Behrmann et al., 1998), for example, have proposed that the disorder is attributable to impaired activation of orthographic representations. On this account, reading is assumed to reflect the "residual functioning of the same interactive system that supported normal reading premorbidly" (Behrmann et al., 1998, p. 7).

Other investigators have attributed pure dyslexia to a visual impairment that precludes activation of orthographic representations (Farah and Wallace, 1991). Chialant and Caramazza (1996), for example, reported a patient, M.J., who processed single, visually presented letters normally and performed well on a variety of tasks assessing the orthographic lexicon with auditorily presented stimuli. In contrast, M.J. exhibited significant impairments in the processing of letter strings. The investigators suggest that M.J. was unable to transfer information from the intact visual-processing system in the right hemisphere to the intact language-processing mechanisms of the left hemisphere. For additional information regarding these and additional accounts of pure alexia, the interested reader is referred to *Cognitive Neuropsychology* 15(1–2), 1998.

NEGLECT DYSLEXIA

Parietal lobe lesions can result in a deficit that involves neglect of stimuli on the side of space contralateral to the lesion, a disorder referred to as "hemispatial neglect." In most cases, this disturbance arises with damage to the right parietal lobe; therefore, attention to the left

side of space is most often affected. The severity of neglect is generally greater when there are stimuli on the right as well as on the left; attention is drawn to the right-sided stimuli, at the expense of those on the left, a phenomenon known as "extinction." Typical clinical manifestations include bumping into objects on the left, failure to dress the left side of the body, drawing objects that are incomplete on the left, and reading problems that involve neglect of the left portions of words, i.e., *neglect dyslexia*.

With respect to neglect dyslexia, it has been found that such patients are more likely to ignore letters in nonwords (e.g., the first two letters in *bruggle*) than letters in real words (compare with *snuggle*). This suggests that the problem does not reflect a total failure to process letter information but rather an attentional impairment that affects conscious recognition of the letters (e.g., Sieroff et al., 1988; Behrmann et al., 1990a,b; see also Caramazza and Hillis, 1990). Performance often improves when words are presented vertically or spelled aloud. In addition, there is evidence that semantic information can be processed in neglect dyslexia, and that the ability to read words aloud improves when oral reading follows a semantic task (Ladavas et al., 1997).

Cases of neglect dyslexia have also been reported in patients with left hemisphere lesions (Caramazza and Hillis, 1990; Greenwald and Berndt, 1999). In these patients, the deficiency involves the right sides of words. Here, visual neglect is usually confined to words, and is not ameliorated by presenting words vertically or spelling them aloud. This disorder has therefore been termed a "positional dyslexia," whereas the right hemisphere deficit has been termed a "spatial neglect dyslexia" (Ellis et al., 1993). Greenwald and Berndt (1999) have proposed that positional dyslexia arises in encoding the order of abstract letter identities prior to lexical access, that is, in an "ordinal graphemic code."

ATTENTIONAL DYSLEXIA

Attentional dyslexia is a disorder characterized by at least relatively preserved reading of single words but impaired reading of words in the context of other words or letters. This uncommon disorder was first described by Shallice and Warrington (1977), who reported two patients with brain tumors involving (at least) the left parietal lobe. Both patients exhibited relatively good performance with single letters or words but were significantly impaired in the recognition of the same stimuli when presented as part of an array. For example, both patients read single letters accurately but made significantly more errors naming letters when presented as part of 3 × 3 or 5 × 5 arrays. Similarly, both patients correctly read greater than 90% of single words but read only approximately 80% of words when presented in the context of three additional words. Although not fully investigated, it is worth noting that the patients were also impaired in recognizing line drawings and silhouettes when presented in an array.

Two additional observations from these patients warrant attention. First, Shallice and Warrington (1977) demonstrated that, for both patients, naming of single black letters was adversely affected by the simultaneous presentation of red flanking stimuli and flanking letters were more disruptive than numbers. For example, both subjects were more likely to correctly name the black (middle) letter when presented "37L82" as compared to "ajGyr". Second, the investigators examined the errors produced in the tasks in which patients were asked to report letters and words in rows of two to four items. They found different error patterns with letters and words. Whereas both patients tended to err in the letter report task by naming letters that appeared in a different location in the array, patients often named words that were not present in the array. Interestingly, many of these errors were interpretable as letter transpositions between words. This phenomenon was extensively investigated by Saffran and Coslett (1996; see also Shallice and McGill, 1977) and will be discussed in more detail below.

Citing the differential effects of letter vs. number flankers as well as the absence of findings suggesting a deficit in response selection, Shallice and Warrington (1977) attributed the disorder to a "failure of transmission of information from a non-semantic perceptual stage to a semantic processing stage" (p. 39; but see

Shallice, 1988). We will return to alternative accounts of these data below.

A second report of attentional dyslexia was provided by Warrington and colleagues (1993). These investigators reported a patient, B.A.L., who suffered a left frontoparietal intracerebral hemorrhage. B.A.L. was able to read single words but exhibited a substantial impairment in the reading of letters and words in an array. Like the patients reported by Shallice and Warrington (1977), B.A.L. exhibited no evidence of visual disorientation and was able to identify a target letter in an array of Xs or Os. He was impaired, however, in the naming of letters or words when these stimuli were flanked by other members of the same stimulus category. He differed from Shallice and Warrington's patients, however, in that naming of line drawings was not adversely affected by flanking line drawings.

Warrington et al. (1993) explored the effect of a number of additional manipulations. They found, for example, that the naming of individual letters was not significantly influenced by flanking words, nor was the naming of words impacted by flanking letters. Finally, the investigators demonstrated that the naming of individual letters was not significantly influenced by the case of the flanking letters (e.g., *ULH* vs. *uLh*).

In light of the stimulus class effects of flanking stimuli, Warrington et al. (1993) attributed the performance of B.A.L. as well as that of Shallice and Warrington's patients to an impairment in the "filter" mechanism controlling the transition from a parallel to a serial stage of lexical processing. These investigators differ from Shallice (1988) in that they consider the deficit to be post-lexical, arising "after letters and words are processed as units" (Warrington et al., 1993, p. 883).

Price and Humphreys (1993) reported a patient with alexia without agraphia and anomia, P.R., who also exhibited an impairment in the naming of stimuli in an array. P.R. named 94% of single letters and 93% of three-letter words but was able to name only 48% of letters within three-letter arrays. Similarly, she was able to name 75% of pictures presented individually but only 25% of the same pictures when the pictures were presented in an array of three.

Interestingly, she performed relatively well on tests requiring access to semantics from three-item picture arrays; for example, she scored 45/52 correct on the Pyramids and Palm Trees Test (Howard and Patterson, 1992). The investigators attributed her impairment in naming items in an array to a combination of a deficit in access from semantics to phonology and an impairment in the selective allocation of attention to elements in the array (see also Buxbaum and Coslett, 1996).

More recently, Saffran and Coslett (1996) reported a patient, N.Y., with biopsy-proven Alzheimer's disease that appeared to selectively involve posterior cortical regions (c.f., Saffran et al., 1990; Coslett et al., 1995), who exhibited attentional dyslexia. N.Y. scored within the normal range on verbal subtests of the (WAIS-R) but was unable to perform any of the performance subtests. He performed normally on the Boston Naming Test. N.Y. performed quite poorly on a variety of experimental tasks assessing visuospatial processing and visual attention. Despite his visuoperceptual deficits, however, N.Y.'s reading of single words was essentially normal. He read 96% of 200 words presented for 100 msec. (unmasked). Like previously reported patients with this disorder, N.Y. exhibited a substantial decline in performance when asked to read two words presented simultaneously. He read both words correctly on only 50% of 385 trials with a 250-msec stimulus exposure. Most errors were omissions of one word. Of greatest interest, however, was the fact that N.Y. produced a substantial number of "blend" errors in which letters from the two words were combined to generate a response that was not present in the display. For example, when shown *flip shot*, N.Y. responded "ship." Like the blend errors produced by normal subjects with brief stimulus presentation (Shallice and McGill, 1977), N.Y.'s blend errors were characterized by the preservation of letter position information; thus, in the preceding example, the letters in the blend response ("ship") retained the same serial position in the incorrect response. N.Y. produced significantly more blend errors than five controls whose overall level of performance had been matched to N.Y.'s by virtue of brief stimulus exposure (range: 83–17 msec).

A subsequent experiment demonstrated that for N.Y., but not controls, blend errors were encountered significantly less often when the target words differed in case (*desk FEAR*).

Like Shallice (1988; see also Mozer, 1991), we consider the central deficit in attentional dyslexia to be an impairment in the control of a filtering mechanism that normally serves to suppress input from unattended words or letters in the display. More specifically, we suggest that as a consequence of the patient's inability to effectively deploy the "spotlight" of attention to a particular region of interest (e.g., a single word or a single letter), multiple stimuli fall within the attentional spotlight. As on many accounts, visual attention serves to integrate visual feature information; impaired modulation of the spotlight of attention would be expected to generate word blends and other errors reflecting the incorrect concatenation of letters. We note that the frequency effects exhibited by N.Y. and other subjects with attentional dyslexia are also consistent with this account; partial letter information (e.g., *ta-*) is more likely to activate a high-frequency word (e.g., *table*) that it is a low-frequency word (e.g., *talon*).

We have previously argued that, at least for N.Y., loss of location information also contributed to N.Y.'s reading deficit. Several lines of evidence support such a conclusion. First, N.Y. was impaired relative to controls both with respect to accuracy and reaction time on a task in which he was required to indicate if a line was inside or outside a circle. Second, N.Y. exhibited a clear tendency to omit one member of a double-letter pair (e.g., *reed > red*). This phenomenon, which has been demonstrated in normal subjects (Mozer, 1991), has been attributed to the loss of location information that normally helps to differentiate two tokens of the same object (Mozer, 1989; cf., Kanwisher, 1991). Finally, we note in this context that the well-documented observation that the blend errors of normal subjects as well as of attentional dyslexics preserve letter position is not inconsistent with the claim that impaired location information contributes to attentional dyslexia. We suggest that migration or blend errors reflect a failure to link words or letters to a location in space, whereas the letter position constraint reflects the properties of the word-processing system. The latter, which is assumed to be at least relatively intact in patients with attentional dyslexia, specifies letter location with respect to the word form rather than space.

This account of attentional dyslexia is consistent with data from N.Y. as well as from the patients reported by Shallice and Warrington (1977) and Price and Humphreys (1993). It does not, however, provide a complete account of the impairment demonstrated by B.A.L. (Warrington et al., 1993), whose deficit was restricted to verbal materials and was not influenced by physical properties of the stimuli (e.g., color, case). Whether the difference in performance exhibited by these patients reflects different loci of impairment, as suggested by Warrington et al. (1993), or is attributable to differences between the patients with respect to severity or site of brain dysfunction is not clear.

OTHER PERIPHERAL DYSLEXIAS

Peripheral dyslexias may be observed in a variety of conditions involving visuoperceptual or attentional deficits. Patients with *simultanagnosia*, a disorder characterized by an inability to "see" more than one object in an array, are often able to read single words but are incapable of reading text (Coslett and Saffran, 1991; Baylis et al., 1994). Other patients with simultanagnosia exhibit substantial problems in reading even single words (Wolpert, 1924).

Patients with degenerative conditions involving the posterior cortical regions may also exhibit profound deficits in reading as part of their more general impairment in visuospatial processing. Several patterns of impairment may be observed in these patients. Patients such as N.Y. (Saffran and Coslett, 1996) may exhibit attentional dyslexia with letter migration and blend errors, whereas other patients exhibiting deficits that are in certain respects rather similar do not produce migration or blend errors in reading or illusory conjunctions in visual search tasks (Treisman and Souther, 1985). We have suggested that at least some patients with these disorders suffer from a pro-

gressive restriction in the domain to which they can allocate visual attention. As a consequence of this impairment, these patients may exhibit an effect of stimulus size such that they are able to read words in small print, but when shown the same word in large print, see only a single letter (Saffran et al., 1990; Coslett et al., 1995).

CENTRAL DYSLEXIAS

DEEP DYSLEXIA

Deep dyslexia, initially described by Marshall and Newcombe in 1973, is the most extensively investigated of the central dyslexias (see Coltheart et al., 1980) and, in many respects, the most compelling. Interest in deep dyslexia is due in large part to the hallmark of the syndrome, the production of semantic errors. Shown the word *castle*, a deep dyslexic may respond "knight"; shown the word *bird*, the patient may respond "canary." At least for some deep dyslexics, it is clear that these errors are not circumlocutions. Semantic errors may represent the most frequent error type in some deep dyslexics, whereas in other patients they comprise a small proportion of reading errors. Deep dyslexics also typically produce frequent "visual" errors (e.g., *skate* read as "scale") and morphological errors in which a prefix or suffix is added, deleted, or substituted (e.g., *scolded* read as "scolds"; *governor* read as "government").

Additional features of the syndrome include a greater success in reading words of high as compared to low imageability. Thus, words such as *table, chair, ceiling,* and *buttercup,* the referent of which is concrete or imageable, are read more successfully than words such as *fate, destiny, wish,* and *universal,* which denote abstract concepts.

Another characteristic feature of deep dyslexia is a part of speech effect such that nouns are typically read more reliably than modifiers (adjectives and adverbs), which are, in turn, read more accurately than verbs. Deep dyslexics manifest particular difficulty in the reading of functors (a class of words that includes pronouns, prepositions, conjunctions, and interrogatives including *that*, *which*, *they*, *because*, *under*, etc.) The striking nature of the part of speech effect may be illustrated by one patient (Saffran and Marin, 1977) who correctly read the word *chrysanthemum* but was unable to read the word *the*! Most errors to functors involve the substitution of a different functor (*that* read as "which") rather than the production of words of a different class such as nouns or verbs. As functors are in general less imageable than nouns, verbs, or adjectives, some investigators have claimed that the apparent effect of part of speech is in reality a manifestation of the pervasive imageability effect (Allport and Funnell, 1981). We (Coslett, 1991) have reported a patient, however, whose performance suggests that the part of speech effect is not simply a reflection of a more general deficit in the processing of low-imageability words.

Finally, all deep dyslexics exhibit a substantial impairment in the reading of nonwords. When confronted with letter strings such as *flig* or *churt*, deep dyslexics are typically unable to employ print-to-sound correspondences to derive phonology; nonwords frequently elicit "lexicalization" errors (e.g., *flig* read as "flag"), perhaps reflecting a reliance on lexical reading in the absence of access to reliable print-to-sound correspondences.

How can deep dyslexia be accommodated by the information-processing model of reading illustrated in Figure 6–1? Several alternative explanations have been proposed. Some investigators have argued that the reading of deep dyslexics is mediated by a damaged form of the left hemisphere–based system employed in normal reading (Morton and Patterson, 1980; Shallice, 1988; Glosser and Friedman, 1990). On such an account, multiple processing deficits must be hypothesized to accommodate the full range of symptoms characteristic of deep dyslexia. First, the strikingly impaired performance in reading nonwords and other tasks assessing phonologic function suggests that the print-to-sound conversion procedure is disrupted. Second, the presence of semantic errors and the effects of imageability (a variable thought to influence processing at the level of semantics) suggest that these patients

also suffer from a semantic impairment (but see Caramazza and Hills, 1990b). Lastly, the production of visual errors suggests that these patients suffer from an impairment in the visual word form system or in the processes mediating access of the stimulus to the visual word form system.

Other investigators (Coltheart, 1980, 2000; Saffran et al., 1980) have argued that deep dyslexics' reading is mediated by a system not normally used in reading—that is, the right hemisphere. We will return to the issue of reading with the right hemisphere below.

Although deep dyslexia has occasionally been associated with posterior lesions, the disorder is typically encountered in association with large perisylvian lesions extending into the frontal lobe (Coltheart et al., 1980, Appendix A). As might be expected given the lesion data, deep dyslexia is usually associated with global or Broca's aphasia but may rarely be encountered in patients with fluent aphasia.

PHONOLOGICAL DYSLEXIA: READING WITHOUT PRINT-TO-SOUND CORRESPONDENCES

First described in 1979 by Derouesne and Beauvois, phonologic dyslexia is perhaps the purest of the central dyslexias in that the syndrome appears to be attributable to a selective deficit procedure mediating the translation from print to sound. Thus, although in many respects less arresting than deep dyslexia, phonological dyslexia is of considerable theoretical interest (see Coltheart, 1996, for a recent discussion of this disorder).

Phonologic dyslexia is a relatively mild disorder in which reading of real words may be nearly intact or only mildly impaired. Patients with this disorder, for example, correctly read 85%–95% of real words (Funnell, 1983; Bub et al., 1987). Some patients with this disorder read all different types of words with equal facility (Bub et al., 1987) whereas other patients are relatively impaired in the reading of functors (or "little words") (Glosser and Friedman, 1990). Unlike patients with surface dyslexia, described below, the regularity of print-to-sound correspondences is not relevant to their performance; thus, phonologic dyslexics are as likely to correctly pronounce orthographically irregular words such as *colonel* as words with standard print-to-sound correspondences such as *administer*. Most errors in response to real words bear a visual similarity to the target word (e.g., *topple* read as "table").

The striking and theoretically relevant aspect of the performance of phonologic dyslexics is a substantial impairment in the oral reading of nonword letter strings. We have examined patients with this disorder, for example, who read greater than 90% of real words of all types yet correctly pronounced only approximately 10% of nonwords. Most errors involve the substitution of a visually similar real word (e.g., *phope* read as "phone") or the incorrect application of print-to-sound correspondences (e.g., *stime* read as "stim" [to rhyme with "him"]).

Within the context of the reading model depicted in Figure 6–1, the account for this disorder is relatively straightforward. Good performance with real words suggests that the processes involved in normal "lexical" reading—that is, visual analysis, the visual word form system, semantics, and the phonological output lexicon—are at least relatively preserved. The impairment in nonword reading suggests that the print-to-sound translation procedure is disrupted.

Recent explorations of the processes involved in nonword reading have identified a number of distinct procedures involved in this task (Coltheart, 1996). If these distinct procedures may be selectively lesioned by brain injury, one might expect to observe different subtypes of phonologic dyslexia. Although the details are beyond the scope of this chapter, it should be noted that Coltheart (1996) has reviewed evidence suggesting that such subtypes may be observed. Lastly, it should be noted that Farah et al. (1996) have suggested an alternative account of phonologic dyslexia. Noting that the vast majority of patients with phonologic dyslexia are impaired on a wide variety of non-reading tasks assessing phonology, these investigators have suggested that the disorder is attributable to a general phonologic deficit rather than to a specific impairment in reading mechanisms.

Phonologic dyslexia is, in certain respects, similar to deep dyslexia, the critical difference being that semantic errors are not observed in phonologic dyslexia. Citing the similarity of reading performance and the fact that deep dyslexics may evolve into phonologic dyslexics as they improve, Glosser and Friedman (1990) have argued that deep dyslexia and phonologic dyslexia are on a continuum of severity.

Phonologic dyslexia has been observed in association with lesions in a number of sites in the dominant perisylvian cortex, and, on occasion, with lesions of the right hemisphere (e.g., Patterson, 1982). Damage to the superior temporal lobe and angular and supramarginal gyri in particular is found in most but not all patients with this disorder. Although quantitative data are lacking, the lesions associated with phonological dyslexia appear, on average, to be smaller than those associated with deep dyslexia.

SURFACE DYSLEXIA: READING WITHOUT LEXICAL ACCESS

Surface dyslexia, first described by Marshall and Newcombe (1973), is a disorder characterized by the inability to read words with "irregular" or exceptional print-to-sound correspondences. Patients with surface dyslexia are thus unable to read aloud words such as *colonel, yacht, island, have,* and *borough,* the pronunciation of which cannot be derived by sounding-out strategies. In contrast, these patients read words containing regular correspondences (e.g., *state, hand, mosquito, abdominal*) as well as nonwords (e.g., *blape*) quite well.

As noted above, some accounts of normal reading postulate that familiar words are read aloud by matching the letter string to a stored representation of the word and retrieving the pronunciation by means of a mechanism linked to semantics or by means of a "direct" route. A critical point to note is that as reading involves stored associations of letter strings and sounds, the pronunciation of the word is not computed by rules but is retrieved, and therefore, whether the word contains regular or irregular correspondences does not appear to play a major role in performance.

The fact that the nature of the print-to-sound correspondences significantly influences performance in surface dyslexia demonstrates that the deficit in this syndrome is in the mechanisms mediating lexical reading—that is, in the semantically mediated and "direct" reading mechanisms. Similarly, the preserved ability to read words and nonwords demonstrates that the procedures by which words are "sounded out" are at least relatively preserved.

What, then, is the level at which the processing impairment gives rise to surface alexia? Scrutiny of the model depicted in Figure 6–1 suggests that the lexical mechanisms mediating reading may be disrupted at a number of different levels; thus, for example, surface dyslexia may be associated with disruption of the visual word form system, with a disruption of semantics (in conjunction with a deficit in the "direct" route; Schwartz et al., 1979) or with a lesion involving the phonologic output lexicon (Howard and Franklin, 1987). Using the traditional logic of neuropsychology, the putative locus of the processing disturbance is inferred on the basis of the overall pattern of deficits. Consider the patient described by Marshall and Newcombe (1973), who, in response to the word *listen*, said, "Liston" (a former heavyweight champion boxer), and added, "that's the boxer." The fact that the patient knew the word Liston suggests that the problem was not at the semantic level at which information about the meaning of the word would be stored.

Surface dyslexia is infrequently observed in patients with focal lesions. Rather, the disorder is more often encountered in patients with widespread or poorly localized lesions such as intracerebral hemorrhage (Margolin et al., 1985) or closed head injury. Surface dyslexia is most frequently encountered in patients with progressive, degenerative dementias such as Alzheimer's disease (Raymer and Berndt, 1996) or frontotemporal dementia (Shallice et al., 1983). In fact, surface dyslexia is characteristic of semantic dementia, a variant of frontotemporal dementia associated with left temporal atrophy (Hodges et al., 1992; Breedin et al., 1994).

The reader is referred to a volume edited by Patterson and colleagues (1985) for a more complete discussion of surface dyslexia.

READING AND THE RIGHT HEMISPHERE

One important and controversial issue regarding reading concerns the putative reading capacity of the right hemisphere. For many years, investigators argued that the right hemisphere was "word blind" (Dejerine, 1892; Geschwind, 1965). In recent years, however, several lines of evidence have suggested that the right hemisphere may possess the capacity to read. Indeed, as previously noted, a number of investigators have argued that the reading of deep (Coltheart, 1980, 2000; Saffran et al., 1980) and pure (Coslett and Saffran, 1989a; Bartolomeo et al., 1998) alexics is mediated at least in part by the right hemisphere.

One seemingly incontrovertible finding demonstrating that at least some right hemispheres possess the capacity to read comes from the performance of a patient who underwent a left hemispherectomy at age 15 for treatment of seizures caused by Rasmussen's encephalitis (Patterson et al., 1989b). After the hemispherectomy, the patient was able to read approximately 30% of single words and exhibited an effect of part of speech; she was unable to use a grapheme-to-phoneme conversion process. Thus, as noted by the authors, this patient's performance was similar in many respects to that of patients with deep dyslexia, a pattern of reading impairment that has been hypothesized to reflect the performance of the right hemisphere.

The performance of some split-brain patients is also consistent with the claim that the right hemisphere is literate. These patients may, for example, be able to match printed words presented to the right hemisphere with an appropriate object (Zaidel, 1978; Zaidel and Peters, 1983). Interestingly, the patients are apparently unable to derive sound from the words presented to the right hemisphere; thus, they are unable to determine if a word presented to the right hemisphere rhymes with an auditorally presented word.

The patient reported by Michel and colleagues (1996) is particularly interesting in this regard. This 23-year-old man with an acquired posterior callosal lesion (A.C.) exhibited markedly different patterns of performance with words and nonwords presented to the right and left visual fields. Not surprisingly, he performed well on all reading tasks with stimuli projected to the right visual field/left hemisphere. Performance with stimuli directed to the left visual field/right hemisphere, however, was severely impaired in terms of accuracy and speed. Additionally, with stimuli presented to the left visual field/right hemisphere, A.C. was impaired in the reading of function words, performed better with high- than with low-imageability words, and exhibited a substantial deficit in the reading of nonwords. This pattern of performance, which the authors attributed to semantic processing in the right hemisphere, is, of course, typical of the syndrome of deep dyslexia.

Another line of evidence supporting the claim that the right hemisphere is literate comes from the evaluation of the reading of patients with pure alexia and optic aphasia (Coslett and Saffran, 1989a, 1989b). We reported data, for example, from four patients with pure alexia who performed well above chance on a number of lexical decision and semantic categorization tasks with briefly presented words that they could not explicitly identify. Three of the patients who regained the ability to explicitly identify rapidly presented words exhibited a pattern of performance consistent with the right hemisphere reading hypothesis. These patients read nouns better than functors and words of high imageability (e.g., *chair*) better than words of low imageability (e.g., *destiny*). Additionally, both patients for whom data are available demonstrated a deficit in the reading of suffixed (e.g., "flowed") but not in pseudo-suffixed (e.g., "flower") words. These data are consistent with a version of the right hemisphere reading hypothesis, which postulates that the right hemisphere lexical–semantic system primarily represents high-imageability nouns. On this account, functors, affixed words, and low-imageability words are not adequately represented in the right hemisphere. An important additional finding is that magnetic stimulation applied to the skull, which disrupts electrical activity in the brain below, interfered with the reading performance of a partially recovered pure alexic when it affected the parieto-occipital area of the right hemisphere (Coslett and

Monsul, 1994). The same stimulation had no effect when it was applied to the homologous area on the left. Bartolomeo et al. (1998) reported data from a patient with pure alexia and letter-by-letter reading after a left occipitotemporal who retained the ability to read aloud some words; this capacity was abolished after she had a stroke involving the right occipitotemporal, which suggests that her residual reading was mediated by the right hemisphere. Finally, Bone et al. (2000) reported data from an investigation involving functional magnetic resonance imaging (fMRI) in two subjects with pure alexia. They found that reading letter by letter resulted in activation in the posterior portion of the left hemisphere, whereas processing of briefly presented letter strings activated the right parietotemporal region.

Although a consensus has not yet been achieved, there is mounting evidence that, at least for some people, the right hemisphere is not word-blind but may support the reading of some types of words. The full extent of this reading capacity and whether it is relevant to normal reading, however, remain unclear.

THE ANATOMIC BASIS OF NORMAL AND DISORDERED READING

A variety of experimental techniques, including positron emission tomography (PET) imaging, MRI, and evoked potentials, have been employed to investigate the anatomic basis of reading in normal subjects. Although differences in experimental technique and design have inevitably led to some variability in reported sites of activation, there appears to be at least relative agreement regarding the anatomic basis of several components of the reading system (see Fiez and Petersen, 1998).

As previously noted, most accounts of reading postulate that after initial visual processing, familiar words are recognized by comparison to a catalog of stored representations, which is often termed the "visual word form system." A variety of recent investigations involving visual lexical decision with fMRI (Madden et al., 1996; Rumsey et al., 1997), viewing of letter strings (Puce et al., 1996), and direct recording of cortical electrical activity (Nobre et al.,

1994) suggest that the visual word form system is supported by inferior occipital or inferior temporo-occipital cortex.

Additional evidence for this localization comes from an investigation of five normal subjects and two patients with posterior callosal lesions (Cohen et al., 2000). These investigators presented words and nonwords for lexical decision or oral reading to either the right or left visual fields. They found initial unilateral activation in what was thought to be V4 in the hemisphere to which the stimulus was projected. More importantly, however, for normal subjects, activation in the left fusiform gyrus (Talairach coordinates −42, −57, −6), which was independent of the hemisphere to which the stimulus was presented, was observed. The two patients with posterior callosal lesions were impaired in the processing of letter strings presented to the right but not the left hemisphere; fMRI in these subjects demonstrated that the region of the fusiform gyrus described above was activated in the callosal patients only by left hemisphere stimulus presentation. As noted by the investigators, these findings are consistent with the hypothesis that the hemialexia demonstrated by the callosal patients is attributable to a failure to access the visual word form system in the left fusiform gyrus.

Deriving meaning from visually presented words requires access to stored knowledge or semantics. While the architecture and anatomic bases of semantic knowledge remain controversial (Saffran and Schwartz, 1994; Damasio et al., 1996), investigations involving semantic access for written words implicate cortex at the junction of the superior and middle temporal gyrus (Brodman areas 22/21) (Pugh et al., 1997; Fiez and Petersen, 1998). A similar site of activation in the left temporal lobe (Talairach coordinates −58, −30, 0) was demonstrated by Vandenberghe et al. (1996).

CONNECTIONIST MODELS OF READING

Our discussion to this point has focused on an information-processing account of reading disorders. In recent years, fundamentally different types of reading models have been proposed. One account, originally developed by Seidenberg and McClelland (1989) and subsequently elaborated by Plaut and colleagues (Plaut et al., 1996; Plaut, 1997) belongs to the general class of parallel distributed processing, or connectionist, models. This model differs from information-processing accounts in that it does not incorporate word-specific representations (e.g., visual word forms, output phonologic representations). In this account, subjects learn how written words map onto spoken words through repeated exposure to familiar and unfamiliar words. Learning of word pronunciations is achieved by means of the development of a mapping between letters and sounds generated on the basis of experience with many different letter strings. The probabilistic mapping between letters and sounds is assumed to provide the means by which both familiar and unfamiliar words are pronounced. This model not only accommodates many of the classic findings in the literature on normal reading but has been "lesioned" in an attempt to reproduce the patterns of reading impairment characteristic of surface (Patterson et al., 1989a) and deep dyslexia (Plaut and Shallice, 1993).

An alternative computational account of reading has been developed by Coltheart and colleagues (Coltheart and Rastle, 1994; Rastle and Coltheart, 1999). Their "dual-route cascaded" model represents a computationally instantiated version of the dual-route theory, similar to that presented in Figure 6–1. This account incorporates a "lexical" route (similar to C in Figure 6–1) as well as a "nonlexical" route by which the pronunciation of graphemes is computed on the basis of position-specific correspondence rules. Like the parallel distributed processing model described above, the dual-route cascaded model accommodates a wide range of findings from the literature on normal reading. The debate regarding the relative merits of these and other (Van Orden et al., 1997) reading models continues.

ASSESSMENT OF READING

As previously noted, the specific types of dyslexia are distinguished on the basis of performance with different types of stimuli. For example, deep dyslexia is characterized by impaired performance on nonwords, an effect of part of speech such that nouns are read better than modifiers or functors, and an effect of imageability such that words denoting more abstract objects or concepts are read less well than words of high imageability. The assessment of patients with dyslexia should include stimuli varying along the dimensions discussed below.

The effect of imageability or concreteness should be assessed by presenting words of high (e.g., *desk*, *frog*, *mountain*) and low (e.g., *fate*, *universal*, *ambiguous*) imageability. Part of speech should be assessed by presenting nouns (e.g., *target*, *meatloaf*), modifiers (e.g., *beautiful*, *early*), verbs (e.g., *ambulate*, *thrive*), and functors (e.g., *because*, *their*). The effect of orthographic regularity should be assessed by presenting regular words that can be sounded out (e.g., *flame*, *target*) and irregular words that cannot be sounded out (e.g., *come*, *tomb*). The ability to sound out words is also assessed by presenting nonword letter strings that may ci ther sound like a real word (e.g., *kome*) or not (e.g., *blape*). As word frequency is typically an important determinant of performance, a wide range of word frequencies should also be employed. As word length frequently influences the performance of subjects with peripheral dyslexia, stimuli should include words of different letter (e.g., *top*, *chocolate*) and syllable (e.g., *mark*, *area*) length. Finally, to obtain a reliable assessment of performance, at least 10 words of each of the stimulus types noted above should be used. The compilation of the appropriate lists of stimuli may be time-consuming; consequently, many investigators employ published word lists, some of which are commercially available (Kay et al., 1993).

ACKNOWLEDGMENTS

This work was supported by the National Institute of Deafness and Other Communication Disorders (RO1 DC2754).

REFERENCES

Akelaitis AJ. (1944). A study of gnosis, praxis and language following section of the corpus Callosum and Anterior Commissure. *J Neurosurgery* 1:94–102.

Allport, D. A., and Funnell, E. (1981). Components of the mental lexicon. *Phil. Trans. R. Soc. Lond. Ser. B* 295:397–410.

Bartolomeo, P., Bachoud-Levi, A.-C., Degos, J.-D., and Boller, F. (1998). Disruption of residual reading capacity in a pure alexic patient after a mirror-image right-hemispheric lesion. *Neurology* 50:286–288.

Baylis, G. C., Driver, J., Baylis, L. L., and Rafal, R. D. (1994). Reading of letters and words in a patient with Balint's syndrome. *Neuropsychologia* 32:1273–1286.

Behrman, M., Moscovitch, M., Black, S. E., and Mozer, M. (1990a). Perceptual and conceptual mechanisms in neglect dyslexia. *Brain* 113:1163–1183.

Behrman, M., Moscovitch, M., and Mozer, M. C. (1990b). Directing attention to words and nonwords in normal subjects and in a computational model: implications for neglect dyslexia. *Cogn. Neuropsychol.* 8:213–248.

Behrmann, M., Plaut, D. C., and Nelson, J. (1998). A literature review and new data supporting an interactive account of letter-by-letter reading. *Cogn. Neuropsychol.* 15:7–52.

Behrmann, M., and Shallice, T. (1995). An ortho-graphic not spatial disorder. *Cogn. Neuropsychol.* 12:409–454.

Bone, R., Brenden, Maher, L., Mao, W., and Haist, F. (2000). Functional neuroimaging of implicit and explicit reading in patients with pure alexia [abstract]. *J Int. Neuropsychol. Soc.* 6:157.

Bowers, J. S., Bub, D. N., and Arguin, M. (1996). A characterization of the word superiority effect in a case of letter-by-letter surface alexia. *Cogn. Neuropsychol.* 13:415–442.

Breedin, S. D., Saffran, E. M., and Coslett, H. B. (1994). Reversal of the concreteness effect in a patient with semantic dementia. *Cogn. Neuropsychol.* 11:617–660.

Bub, D. N., Black, S., and Howell, J. (1989). Word recognition and orthographic context effects in a letter-by-letter reader. *Brain Lang.* 36:357–376.

Bub, D., Black, S. E., Howell, J., and Kertesz, A. (1987). Speech output processes and reading. In *Cognitive Neuropsychology of Language*, M. Coltheart, G. Sartori, and R. Job (eds.). Hillsdale, NJ: Lawrence Erlbaum Associates, pp. 79–109.

Buxbaum, L. J., and Coslett, H. B. (1996). Deep dyslexic phenomenon in pure alexia. *Brain Lang.* 54:136–167.

Caramazza, A., and Hills, A. (1990a). Levels of representation, coordinate frames and unilateral neglect. *Cogn. Neuropsychol.* 7:391–455.

Caramazza, A., and Hills, A. E. (1990b). Where do semantic errors come from? *Cortex* 26:95–122.

Chialant, D., and Caramazza, A. (1996). Perceptual and lexical factors in a case of letter-by-letter reading. *Cogn. Neuropsychol.* 15:167–202.

Cohen, L., Dehaene, S., Naccache L., Lehericy, S., Dehaene-Lambertz, G., Henaff, M.-A., and Michel, F. (2000). The visual word form area. *Brain* 123:291–307.

Coltheart, M. (1980). Deep dyslexia: a right hemisphere hypothesis. In *Deep Dyslexia*, M. Coltheart, K. Patterson, and J. C. Marshall (eds.). London: Routledge and Kegan Paul, pp. 326–379.

Coltheart, M. (1996). Phonological dyslexia: past and future issues. *Cogn. Neuropsychol.* 13:749–762.

Coltheart, M. (2000). Deep dyslexia is right-hemisphere reading. *Brain Lang.* 71:299–309.

Coltheart, M., Patterson, K., and Marshall, J. C. (eds.). (1980). *Deep Dyslexia*. London: Routledge and Kegan Paul.

Coltheart, M., and Rastle, K. (1994). Serial processing in reading aloud: evidence for dual-route models of reading. *J. Exp. Psychol. Hum. Percept. Perform.* 20:1197–1211.

Coslett, H. B. (1991). Read but not write 'idea': evidence for a third reading mechanism. *Brain Lang.* 40:425–443.

Coslett, H. B., and Monsul, N. (1994). Reading with the right hemisphere: evidence from transcranial magnetic stimulation. *Brain Lang.* 46:198–211.

Coslett, H. B., and Saffran, E. M. (1989a). Evidence for preserved reading in 'pure alexia'. *Brain* 112:327–359.

Coslett, H. B., and Saffran, E. M. (1989b). Preserved object identification and reading comprehension in optic aphasia. *Brain* 112:1091–1110.

Coslett, H. B., and Saffran, E. M. (1991). Simultanagnosia: to see but not two see. *Brain* 114:1523–1545.

Coslett, H. B., and Saffran, E. M. (1992). Optic aphasia and the right hemisphere: a replication and extension. *Brain Lang.* 43:148–161.

Coslett, H. B., and Saffran, E. M. (1998). Reading and the right hemisphere: evidence from acquired dyslexia. In *Right Hemisphere Language Comprehension*, M. Beeman and C. Chiarello (ed.). Mahway, NJ: Lawrence Erlbaum Associates, pp. 105–132.

Coslett, H. B., Saffran, E. M., Greenbaum, S., and Schwartz, H. (1993). Preserved reading in pure alexia: the effect of strategy. *Brain* 116:21–37.

Coslett, H. B., Stark, M., Rajaram, S., Saffran, E. M. (1995). Narrowing the spotlight: a visual attentional disorder in Alzheimer's disease. *Neurocase:* 1:305–318.

Damasio, H., Grabowski, T. J., Tranel, D., Hichwa, R. D., and Damasio, A. R. (1996). A neural basis for lexical retrieval. *Nature* 380:499–505.

Dejerine, J. (1891). Sur un cas de cécité verbale avec agraphie, suivi d'autopsie. *C. R. Séances Soc. Biol.* 3:197–201.

Dejerine, J. (1892). Contribution à l'étude anatomopathologique et clinique des différentes variétés de cécité verbale. *C. R. Séances Soc. Biol.* 4:61–90.

Derouesne, J., and Beauvois, M-F. (1979). Phonological processing in reading: data from dyslexia. *J. Neurol. Neurosurg. Psychiatry* 42:1125–1132.

Ellis, A. W., Young, A. W., and Flude, B. M. (1993). Neglect and visual language. In Unilateral Neglect: Clinical and Experimental Studies, I. H. Robinson and J. C. Marshall (eds.). Hove, UK: Lawrence Erlbaum Associates, pp. 233–256.

Farah, M. J., Stowe, R. M., and Levinson, K. L. (1996). Phonological dyslexia: loss of a reading-specific component of the cognitive architecture? *Cogn. Neuropsychol.* 13:849–868.

Farah, M. J., and Wallace, M. A. (1991). Pure alexia as a visual impairment: a reconsideration. *Cogn. Neuropsychol.* 8:313–334.

Fiez, J. A., and Petersen, S. E. (1998). Neuroimaging studies of word reading. *Proc. Natl. Acad. Sci. U.S.A.* 95:914–921.

Friedman, R. B., and Hadley, J. A. (1992). Letter-by-letter surface alexia. *Cogn. Neuropsychol.* 9:185–208.

Funnell, E. (1983). Phonological processes in reading: new evidence from acquired dyslexia. *Br. J. Psychol.* 74:159–180.

Geschwind, N. (1965). Disconnection syndromes in animals and man. *Brain* 88:237–294, 585–644.

Glosser, G., and Friedman, R. (1990). The continuum of deep/phonological dyslexia. *Cortex* 25:343–359.

Greenwald, M. L., and Berndt, R. S. (1999). Impaired encoding of abstract letter code order: severe alexia in a mildly aphasic patient. *Cogn. Neuropsychol.* 16:513–556.

Hodges, J. R., Patterson, K., Oxbury, S., and Funnell, E. (1992). Semantic dementia: progressive fluent aphasia with temporal lobe atrophy. *Brain* 115:1783–1806.

Howard, D,, and Franklin, S. (1987). Three ways for understanding written words, and their use in two contrasting cases of surface dyslexia (together with an odd routine for making 'orthographic' errors in oral word production). In *Language Perception and Production*, A. Allport, D.

Mackay, W. Prinz, and E. Scheerer (eds.). New York: Academic Press, pp. 340–366.

Howard, D., and Patterson, K. (1992). The Pyramid and Palm Trees Test. Suffolk, England: Thames Valley Test Company.

Kanwisher, N. (1991). Repetition blindness and illusory conjunctions: errors in binding visual types with visual tokens. *J. Exp. Psychol. Hum. Percept. Perform.* 17:404–421.

Kay, J., Lesser, R., and Coltheart, M. (1992). Psycholinguistic Assessment of Language Processing in Aphasia. Hove, UK: Psychology Press.

Ladavas, E., Shallice, T., and Zanella, M. T. (1997). Preserved semantic access in neglect dyslexia. *Neuropsychologia* 35:257–270.

Madden, D. J., Turkington, T. G., Coleman, R. E., Provenzale, J. M., Degrado, T. R., and Hoffman, J. M. (1996). Adult age differeences in regional cerebral blood flow during visual word identification: evidence from H215O PET. *Neuroimage* 31:127–142.

Margolin, D. I., Marcel, A. J., and Carlson, N. R. (1985). Common mechanisms in dysnomia and post-semantic surface dyslexia: process deficits and selective attention. In. *Surface Dyslexia*, K. E. Patterson, J. C. Marshall, and M. Coltheart (eds.). London: Lawrence Erlbaum Associates.

Marshall, J. C., and Newcombe, F. (1966). Syntactic and semantic errors in paralexia. *Neuropsychologia* 4:169–176.

Marshall, J. C., and Newcombe, F. (1973). Patterns of paralexia: a psycholinguistic approach. *J. Psycholinguist. Res.* 2:175–199.

McClelland, J. L., and Rumelhart, D. E. (1977). An interactive activation model of context effects in letter perception: part I. An account of basic findings. *Psychol. Rev.* 88:375–407.

Michel, F., Henaff, M.-A., and Intrilligator, J. (1996). Two different readers in the same brain after a posterior callosal lesion. *Neuroreport* 7:786–788.

Morton, J., and Patterson, K. E. (1980). A new attempt at an interpretation, or, an attempt at a new interpretation. In *Deep Dyslexia*, M. Coltheart, K. Patterson, and J. C. Marshall (eds.). London: Routledge and Kegan Paul, pp. 91–118.

Mozer, M. C. (1989). Types and tokens in visual letter perception. *J. Exp. Psychol. Hum. Percept. Perform.* 15:287–303.

Mozer, M. C. (1991). *The Perception of Multiple Objects.* Cambridge, MA: MIT Press.

Nobre, A. C., Allison, T., and McCarthy, G. (1994). Word recognition in the human inferior temporal lobe. *Nature* 372:260–263.

Patterson, K. (1982). The relation between reading and phonological coding: further neuropsychological observations. In *Normality and Pathology in Cognitive Functions*, A. W. Ellis (ed.). London: Academic Press, pp. 77–111.

Patterson, K., and Kay, J. (1982). Letter-by-letter reading: psychological descriptions of a neurological syndrome. *Q. J. Exp. Psychol.* 34A:411–441.

Patterson, K. E., Marshall, J. C., and Coltheart, M. (eds.) (1985). *Surface Dyslexia.* London: Routledge and Kegan Paul.

Patterson, K. E., Seidenberg, M. S., McClelland, J. L. (1989a). Connections and disconnections: acquired dyslexia in a computational model of reading processes. In *Parallel Distributed Processing: Implications for Psychology and Neurobiology*, R. G. M. Morris (ed.). Oxford: Oxford University Press, pp. 131–181.

Patterson, K. E., Vargha-Khadem, F., and Polkey, C. F. (1989b). Reading with one hemisphere. *Brain* 112:39–63.

Plaut, D. C. (1997). Structure and function in the lexical system: insights from distributed models of word reading and lexical decision. *Lang. Cogn. Proc.* 12:765–805.

Plaut, D. C., McClelland, J. L., Seidenberg, M. S., and Patterson, K. (1996). Understanding normal and impaired word reading: computational principles in quasi-regular domains. *Psychol. Rev.* 103:56–115.

Plaut, D. C., and Shallice, T. (1993). Deep dyslexia: a case study in connectionist neuropsychology. *Cogn. Neuropsychol.* 10:377–500.

Price, C. J., and Humphreys, G. W. (1993). Attentional dyslexia: the effects of co-occurring deficits. *Cogn. Neuropsychol.* 6:569–592.

Puce, A., Allison, T., Asgari, M., Gore, J. C., McCarthy, G. (1996). Differential sensitivity of human visual cortex to faces, letterstrings and textures: a functional magnetic resonance imaging study. *J. Neurosci.* 16:5205–5215.

Pugh, K. R., Shaywitz, B. A., Shaywitz, S. E., Shankweiler, D. P., Katz, L., Fletcher, J. M., Skudlarski, P., Fulbright, R. K., Constable, R. T., Bronen, R. A., Lacadie, C., and Gore, J. C. (1997). Predicting reading performance from neuroimaging profiles: the cerebral basis of phonological effects in printed word identification. *J. Exp. Psychol. Hum. Percept. Perform.* 23: 299–318.

Rastle, K., and Coltheart, M. (1999). Serial and strategic effects in reading aloud. *J. Exp. Psychol. Hum. Percept. Perform.* 25:482–503.

Raymer, A. M., and Berndt, R. S. (1996). Reading lexically without semantics: evidence from patients with probable Alzheimer's disease. *J. Int. Neuropyschol. Soc.* 2:340–349.

Reuter-Lorenz, P. A., and Brunn, J. L. (1990). A prelexical basis for letter-by-letter reading: a case study. *Cogn. Neuropsychol.* 7:1–20.

Rumsey, J. M., Horwitz, B., Donohue, B. C., Nace, K., Maisog, J. M., and Andreason, P. (1997). Phonological and orthographic components of word recognition. A PET-rCBF study. *Brain* 120:739–759.

Saffran, E. M., Bogyo, L. C., Schwartz, M. F., and Marin, O. S. M. (1980). Does deep dyslexia reflect right-hemisphere reading? In *Deep Dyslexia*, M. Coltheart, K. Patterson, and J. C. Marshall (eds.). London: Routledge and Kegan Paul, pp. 381–406.

Saffran, E. M., and Coslett, H. B. (1996). 'Attentional dyslexia' in Alzheimer's disease: a case study. *Cogn. Neuropsychol.* 13:205–228.

Saffran, E. M., and Coslett, H. B. (1998). Implicit vs. letter-by-letter reading in pure alexia: a tale of two systems. *Cogn. Neuropsychol.* 15:141–166.

Saffran, E. M., Fitzpatrick-DeSalme, E. J., and Coslett, H. B. (1990). Visual disturbances in dementia. In *Modular Deficits in Alzheimer-type Dementia*, M. F. Schwartz (ed.). Cambridge, MA: MIT Press, pp. 297–327.

Saffran, E. M., and Marin, O. S. M. (1977). Reading without phonology: evidence from aphasia. *Q. J. Exp. Psychol.* 29:515–525.

Saffran, E. M., and Schwartz, M. F. (1994). *Of Cabbages and Things: Semantic Memory from a Neuropsychological Perspective—A Tutorial Review. Attention and Performance XV.* C. Umilta and M. Moscovitch (eds.). Cambridge, MA: Bradford.

Schwartz, M. F., Saffran, E. M., and Marin, O. S. M. (1979). Dissociation of language function in dementia: a case study. *Brain Lang.* 7:277–306.

Seidenberg, M. S., and McClelland, J. L. (1989). A distributed, developmental model of word recognition and naming. *Psychol. Rev.* 96:523–568.

Sieroff, E., Pollatsek, A., and Posner, M. (1988). Recognition of visual letter strings following injury to the posterior visual spatial attention system. *Cogn. Neuropsychol.* 5:427–449.

Shallice, T. (1988). *From Neuropsychology to Mental Structure.* Cambridge, UK: Cambridge University Press.

Shallice, T., McGill, J. (1977). The origins of mixed errors. In *Attention and Performance VII*, J. Reguin (ed.). Hillsdale, NJ: Lawrence Erlbaum Associates, pp. 193–208.

Shallice, T., and Warrington E. K. (1977). The possible role of selective attention in acquired dyslexia. *Neuropsychologia* 15:31–41.

Shallice, T., and Saffran, E. M. (1986). Lexical processing in the absence of explicit word identification: evidence from a letter-by-letter reader. *Cogn. Neuropsychol.* 3:429–458.

Shallice, T., and Warrington, E. K. (1980). Single and multiple component central dyslexic syndromes. In *Deep Dyslexia*, M. Coltheart, K. Patterson, and J. C. Marshall (eds.). London: Routledge and Kegan Paul, pp. 326–353.

Shallice, T., Warrington, E. K., and McCarthy, R. (1983). Reading without semantics. *Q. J. Exp. Psychol.* 35A:111–138.

Sieroff, E., Pollatsek, A., and Posner, M. I. (1988). Recognition of visual letter strings following injury to the posterior visual spatial attention system. *Cogn. Neuropsychol.* 5:427–449.

Treisman, A., and Souther, J. (1985). Search asymmetry: a diagnostic for preattentive processing of separable features. *J. Exp. Psychol. Gen.* 114:285–310.

Vandenberghe, R., Price, C., Wise, R., Josephs, O., and Frackowiak, R. S. (1996). Functional anatomy of a common semantic system for words and pictures. *Nature* 383:254–256.

Van Orden, G. C., Jansen op de Haar, M. A., and Bosman, A. M. (1997). Complex dynamic systems also predict dissociations but they do not reduce to autonomous components. *Cogn. Neuropsychol.* 14:131–165.

Warrington, E., and Shallice, T. (1980). Word-form dyslexia. *Brain* 103:99–112.

Warrington, E. K., Cipolotti, L., and McNeil, J. (1993). Attentional dyslexia: a single case study. *Neuropsychologia* 31:871–886.

Wolpert, I. (1924). Die Simultanagnosie: Störung der Gesamtauffassung. *Z. Gesamte Neurol. Psychiatrie* 93:397–413.

Zaidel, E. (1978). Lexical organization in the right hemisphere. In *Cerebral Correlates of Conscious Experience*, P. Buser and A. Rougeul-Buser (eds.). New York: North Holland pp. 177–197.

Zaidel, E., and Peters, A. M. (1983). Phonological encoding and ideographic reading by the disconnected right hemisphere: two case studies. *Brain Lang.* 14:205–234.

7

Agraphia

DAVID P. ROELTGEN

For a century after Benedikt (1865) applied the term *agraphia* to disorders of writing, studies of agraphia focused on the relationship of agraphia to aphasia. Ogle (1867) found that although aphasia and agraphia usually occur together, they were occasionally separable. He concluded that there were distinct cerebral centers for writing and for speaking. Because agraphia and aphasia usually occur together, he concluded that the centers were anatomically close together. Ogle's classification of agraphia included amnemonic agraphia and atactic agraphia. Patients with amnemonic agraphia wrote well-formed, but incorrect letters. Patients with atactic agraphia made poorly formed letters but usually had an element of amnemonic agraphia as well. Ogle's two types of agraphia might be termed *linguistic* and *motor*.

In contrast to Ogle, Lichtheim (1885) proposed that disorders of writing usually were the same as disorders of speech. The exception was agraphia due to disruption of the "center from which the organs of writing are innervated," which was clinically similar to Ogle's atactic agraphia. Lichtheim proposed that agraphia and aphasia were similar because the acquisition of writing (and spelling) was superimposed on speech, and therefore utilized previously acquired speech centers. Head (1926) also

stressed this relationship. Goldstein (1948) also emphasized two types of agraphia: primary agraphia resulting from disruption of the motor act of writing, and secondary agraphia, resulting from disturbances of speech.

Nielson's classification (1946) reflected his view that writing is closely associated with speech but functionally and anatomically separable from it (a view similar to Ogle's). Nielson described three types of agraphia: apractic (apraxic), aphasic, and isolated. Apractic agraphia was characterized by poorly formed letters and was associated with various apraxias. Aphasic agraphia was associated with the various aphasias, and the patients' written errors reflected the aphasic disturbance. Agraphia without associated neuropsychological signs (isolated agraphia) resulted from a lesion of the frontal writing center (Exner's area). Nielson thought that isolated agraphias were rare. He theorized that Exner's area, the foot of the second frontal convolution, worked in close association with the angular gyrus and Wernicke's area to produce writing. He also proposed that the fibers carrying information from the angular gyrus to Exner's area passed close to Broca's speech area. Nielson suggested that these functional and anatomic connections accounted for the frequent association of agraphia and aphasia.

In addition to the dissociations between aphasia and agraphia and the contrast of motor agraphia and linguistic agraphia, as early as the 1880s, two different linguistic mechanisms were postulated for letter selection. Dejerine (1891) and Pitres (1894) postulated orthographic or visual word images. In contrast, Grashey (1885) and Wernicke postulated that writing utilized translation of sounded units (*phonemes*) into letters (*graphemes*).

Given this historical background, any assessment or classification of agraphia should probably address the following constructs: the relationship between agraphia and aphasia; the distinction between linguistic and motoric deficits underlying agraphias; and the distinction between deficits in orthographic word representations and in phoneme-to-grapheme conversion in linguistic agraphia.

TESTING FOR AGRAPHIA

In the evaluation of a patient with agraphia, both linguistic and motor components must be evaluated. The linguistic component includes the choice of the correct letters (spelling) and the choice of the correct word (meaning). The motor component includes those neuropsychological functions necessary for producing the correct letter form and the correct word form. In order to evaluate these features it is convenient to divide the tests into three types: spontaneous writing, writing to dictation, and copying.

To test *spontaneous writing*, the patient is asked to write sentences or words about a familiar topic. For maximum value the topic should be standard from patient to patient, and controlled. Therefore, we recommend having the patient write about a picture. The same picture can then be used with different patients and different times with the same patient to compare performance. Spontaneous writing allows an assessment of generative abilities, selection, and syntax, as well as the form of the patient's writing.

Writing to dictation, usually limited to single words or phrases, allows one to evaluate the effects of particular variables on writing, such as word length and frequency. The word type

can also be varied to test specific hypotheses based on models of agraphia, such as those presented later in this chapter. These models predict, for example, that certain patients may have more difficulty with a word depending on the class (noun, verb, adjective, adverb, or function word, i.e., conjunctions and prepositions), imageability (high or low), abstractness (high or low), regularity (regular or irregular), or lexicality (real or nonword). The mode of the patient's response may also be varied: the patient can be asked to spell orally, type, or spell using anagram letters (blocks with single letters written on them). This enables the examiner to distinguish motor or apraxic agraphias, in which typing and spelling are spared, from linguistic agraphias, in which letter choice is also impaired.

The third group of writing tests evaluates *copying*. Depending on the goals of the examination, the task may include copying simple nonsense figures (small configurations of strokes designed to imitate the strokes used in letters, but having no symbolic meaning), letters, words, sentences, or paragraphs. When one asks a patient to copy, it is important, but not always possible, to distinguish among three potential copy methods; slavish or "stroke-by-stroke" copying (drawing letters), "letter-by-letter" copying, and transcribing, in which the material is written fluently. It may be possible to distinguish these copying methods by (1) varying the length of material to be copied (increased length usually decreases slavish and letter-by-letter copying), (2) increasing the distance between the stimulus and the response (it is difficult to slavishly copy material from across the room), (3) having the patient copy nonsense figures (limiting the patient to slavish copying), and (4) performing delayed copying (showing the stimulus to the patient, removing the stimulus and then having the patient write it) (generally limiting the patient to transcribing).

After writing (or oral spelling) is produced, important information is frequently gleaned from the analysis of the product. Linguistic error analysis is important in assessing patients with linguistic agraphia. It is helpful to analyze performance related to specific word types (i.e., comparing frequency of correct performance on regular compared to irregular words) (see Lexical Agraphia, below). It may also be important to analyze syntax, content, and sentence length in spontaneous sentences or paragraphs (Rapcsak and Rubens, 1990), a level of analysis that has been ignored in most studies.

Analysis of handwriting form is necessary in assessing patients with motor agraphia. Such analysis in adults has not been systematic. However, there has been a systematic approach to the assessment of developmental dysgraphia in children (Denckla and Roeltgen, 1992, Roeltgen and Blaskey, 1992). In addition, we (Roeltgen et al., 1991; Denckla and Roeltgen, 1992) have developed a computerized system that effectively, efficiently, and accurately measures most of the structural components that are important in printed handwriting, *manuscript*.

In addition to these detailed tests of writing, it is important to evaluate patients for neurological or neuropsychological disorders that may interfere with writing, oral spelling, or copying. These include disorders of speech, reading, praxis, visuoperceptual, visuospatial, constructional abilities, attention, and elementary motor and sensory functions.

COMMON NEUROLOGICAL CLASSIFICATIONS OF AGRAPHIA

Classifications of agraphia by Leischner (1969), Hécaen and Albert (1978), Benson (1979), and Kaplan and Goodglass (1981), derived from clinical evaluations of agraphic patients, have generally distinguished five types of agraphia (Table 7–1): pure agraphia, aphasic agraphia, agraphia with alexia (also called "parietal agraphia") (Kaplan and Goodglass, 1981), apraxic agraphia, and spatial agraphia.

Table 7–1. Neurological Classification of the Agraphias

Pure agraphia
Aphasic agraphia
Agraphia with alexia (parietal agraphia)
Apraxic agraphia
Spatial agraphia

Pure agraphia is characterized by absence of any other language disturbance. Pure agraphia may result from a focal lesion or an acute confusional state. Patients with pure agraphia from focal lesions usually make well-formed graphemes (written letters) with spelling errors that vary in type, depending on the lesion location. Pure agraphia has been reported from focal lesions in the second frontal convolution (Exner's area) (Aimard et al., 1975; Hécaen and Albert, 1978; Marcie and Hécaen, 1979; Kaplan and Goodglass, 1981), the superior parietal lobule (Basso et al., 1978), the posterior perisylvian region (Auerbach and Alexander, 1981; Rosati and DeBastiani, 1981), the posterior parasagittal parieto-occipital region (Schomer et al. 1998), the region of the left caudate and internal capsule (Laine and Martilla, 1981), and other subcortical structures (Tanridag and Kirshner, 1985; Kertesz et al., 1990). Pure agraphia resulting from an acute confusional state (Chedru and Geschwind, 1972) is characterized by poorly formed graphemes, inability to write on a line, and writing over the model one is copying. When the letters are well formed, spelling errors may be recognized.

Aphasic agraphia has been described with Broca's aphasia, transcortical motor aphasia, conduction aphasia, Wernicke's aphasia, and transcortical sensory aphasia (Benson, 1979; Marcie and Hécaen, 1979; Kaplan and Goodglass, 1981; Grossfeld and Clark, 1983; Benson and Cummings, 1985). *Agraphia with alexia* has also been called "parietal agraphia" because these two symptoms, in the absence of significant aphasia, usually occur together in patients with parietal lesions (Kaplan and Goodglass, 1981). *Apraxic agraphia* is characterized by difficulty in forming graphemes when writing spontaneously and to dictation (Leischner, 1969; Hécaen and Albert, 1978; Marcie and Hécaen, 1979). Lesions in the nondominant parietal lobe may cause *spatial agraphia*, which is frequently associated with the neglect syndrome (Hécaen and Albert, 1978; Benson, 1979; Marcie and Hécaen, 1979).

Although we have attempted to classify agraphia into five well-defined groups, detailed analysis of agraphic patients reveals difficulty in classifying many of them (Roeltgen and Heilman, 1985). For example, some patients with Broca's aphasia have agraphias that more closely resemble the agraphias of patients with Wernicke's aphasia than the agraphias of patients with Broca's aphasia. Also, certain lesion sites may be associated with multiple agraphias. For example, parietal lesions may cause parietal agraphia (agraphia with alexia) but may also cause apraxic agraphia. In some reports, parietal and apraxic agraphia may represent the same abnormality seen from two different perspectives (Roeltgen and Heilman, 1985). One way that these difficulties may be resolved is by using an alternative approach to classifying the agraphias. Rather than base the classification on clinical descriptions of agraphic patients, the classification can be based on the neuropsychological mechanisms of writing that appear to be disturbed.

A NEUROPSYCHOLOGICAL MODEL OF WRITING

To develop a neuropsychologically based classification system, one must first appreciate what neuropsychological mechanisms may be involved in writing. It is best to begin with the two general categories of functions that Ogle (1867) first delineated: linguistic and motor components. To these must be added attentional functions and certain visual spatial skills.

In the last three decades, numerous information-processing or cognitive neuropsychological models have been proposed to explain the ability to write (and spell aloud) (Ellis, 1982; Margolin, 1984; Roeltgen, 1985; Roeltgen and Heilman, 1985; Patterson, 1986; Lesser, 1990; Rapcsak and Rubens, 1990; Roeltgen and Rapcsak, 1993). These models contain many similar components although the terms used to describe the components and the subtleties of functional capacity among them often differ. Unfortunately, only rarely has there been an attempt to correlate the cognitive components and the brain regions that might be associated with them (Roeltgen, 1985; Roeltgen and Heilman, 1985; Roeltgen and Rapcsak, 1993). The model of writing described here (Fig. 7–1), a modification of one

we have presented before (Roeltgen, 1985; Roeltgen and Heilman, 1985), defines many of the linguistic and motor components thought to be important for writing and oral spelling. It also addresses the mode of interaction between components and visual–spatial skills. Lastly, it suggests certain anatomic regions that may be associated with specific types of agraphia. Among the linguistic components, there are at least two parallel systems available for spelling and a mechanism by which semantics (meaning), interacts with these systems. This interaction enables one to spell or write with meaning. The motor components include mechanisms by which words can be spelled or written. It appears that the parallel spelling systems converge prior to motor output, as drawn in Figure 7–1. A detailed discussion of this model follows.

For convenience, this chapter will refer to the general output of both writing and oral spelling systems as "spelling." "Writing" will refer to written production (handwriting) and "oral spelling" will refer to oral production.

LINGUISTIC COMPONENTS

Lexical Agraphia

There are at least two general systems available to adults for spelling words: lexical and phonological (Beauvois and Deroucsnc, 1981; Ellis, 1982; Roeltgen et al., 1982a, 1983a; Hatfield and Patterson, 1983; Roeltgen and Heilman, 1984, 1985; Patterson 1986; Bub and Chertkow, 1988; Roeltgen and Rapcsak, 1993). The *lexical system* (Fig. 7–1, pathway 4–5–6), probably functionally the more important, has also been called "lexical–orthographic" (Margolin, 1984) or orthographic (Patterson, 1986; Rapcsak and Rubens, 1990). This system appears to utilize a whole-word retrieval process that may incorporate visual word images. It has been proposed that these visual word images arise from word engrams that are visual rather than phonological (Roeltgen et al., 1983a). In some patients the lexical system may also use whole-word processing that is not entirely based on visual word images but may include certain phonological components, word analogies, and mnemonic rules (Hatfield, 1985). The

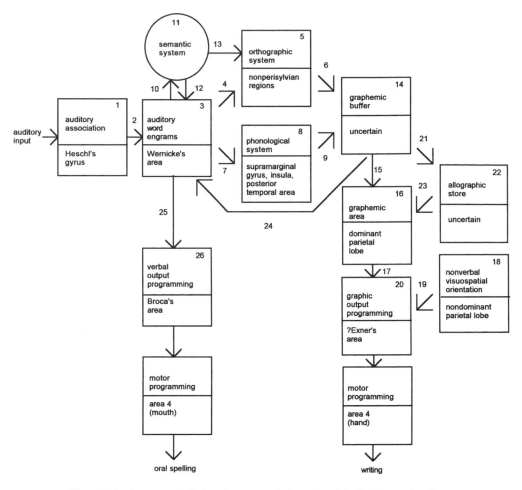

Figure 7–1. An anatomically based neuropsychological model of writing and spelling.

lexical strategy is necessary for spelling familiar orthographically irregular words (words that cannot be spelled utilizing direct sound-to-letter correspondence rules, e.g., "calm") and ambiguous words (words with sounds that may be represented by multiple letters or letter clusters e.g., "phone"). The lexical system can also be used for spelling familiar orthographically regular words (words with direct sound-to-letter correspondence, e.g., "animal") that the phonological system can also handle (see below).

Dysfunction of the lexical writing system is called "lexical agraphia" (Beauvois and Derouesne, 1981; Roeltgen and Heilman, 1984). It has also been called "phonological spelling" (Hatfield and Patterson, 1983). This disorder is characterized by impaired ability to spell ir-

regular and ambiguous words with a relatively preserved ability to spell regular words and nonwords. These patients usually make errors that are phonologically correct (e.g.,"gelosy" for "jealousy"). At least 20 patients with lexical agraphia have been reported (Beauvois and Derouesne, 1981; Hatfield and Patterson, 1983; Roeltgen and Heilman, 1984; Goodman-Shulman and Caramazza, 1987; Rapcsak et al., 1988, 1990; Croisile et al. 1989; Friedman and Alexander, 1989; Alexander et al., 1990; Roeltgen and Rapcsak, 1993).

Previously, Roeltgen and Heilman (1984) attempted to delineate the anatomy underlying lexical agraphia. They studied the computerized tomograms (CT) of four patients with lexical agraphia by plotting the lesions seen on CT on a lateral view of the left hemisphere. Overlap of these plots revealed that the junction of the posterior angular gyrus and the parieto-occipital lobule was lesioned in each patient. In addition, the lesion extended subcortically into the white matter in all patients. This suggested that this area is an important anatomic substrate for lexical agraphia.

Since then there have been reports of additional patients with lexical agraphia who have lesions at or around the dominant angular gyrus (Roeltgen, 1989; Alexander et al., 1990), while others have lesions outside that region. These have included the right parietal lobe (in a right-hander without aphasia or alexia) (Rothi et al., 1987), the left posterior temporal region (middle temporal gyrus) (Croisile et al., 1989), the left frontal region (Rapcsak et al., 1988), the left caudate (Roeltgen, 1989), and left thalamus (Roeltgen, 1989). Roeltgen and Rapcsak (1993) reviewed reports of previous patients with lexical agraphia and added seven new cases. They concluded that patients with lexical agraphia had lesions that usually spared the immediate perisylvian region, especially the anterior supramarginal gyrus and insula, areas thought to be important for the production of phonological agraphia (see below). They also noted a degree of linguistic heterogeneity that was consistent with the pathological heterogeneity. They concluded that the most striking cases of lexical agraphia appeared to have lesions of the angular gyrus but that the clinical and pathological heterogeneity were consistent with Hatfield's (1985) position that the lexical system might contain multiple cognitive components.

Phonological Agraphia

The alternative parallel spelling system is the *phonological system* (Fig. 7–1, pathway 7–8–9). Words and speech sounds must be phonologically decoded and then converted into letters. One way that this may occur is through what has been termed "sublexical sound-letter" or "phoneme–grapheme" conversion. For this method to occur, there are at least two necessary components: segmentation and sound–letter conversion. The former parses the phoneme or word–sound string into separate phonemes and the latter converts the single

phonemes into letters (graphemes). Alternatively, it has been suggested that the phonological system is lexically based and spells unknown words by an analogy method (Campbell, 1985). An analogy system chooses a spelling for a nonword by associating the phonology of the stimulus with similar-sounding real words and then chooses the best combination of sounds for the response. The phonological system is used for spelling unfamiliar orthographically regular words and pronounceable nonwords (e.g., "flig"). It is probable that this system is used to spell familiar regular words only when the lexical system is dysfunctional or when there is no available lexical item for the word that is to be spelled (an unfamiliar word).

Dysfunction of the phonological system causes phonological agraphia (Shallice, 1981; Roeltgen et al., 1983a). This disorder is characterized by impaired ability to spell nonwords and preserved ability to spell familiar words, both regular and irregular. Spelling errors by patients with phonological agraphia are usually not phonologically correct. They may have a high degree of visual resemblance to the stimulus, supporting a role of visual word images in the lexical system.

Roeltgen and colleagues (Roeltgen et al., 1983a; Roeltgen and Heilman, 1984) have investigated the anatomic basis of phonological agraphia using a method similar to the methods they used with lexical agraphia. The lesion site common to patients with phonological agraphia was the supramarginal gyrus or the insula medial to it. In addition, one patient with an isolated phonological agraphia (that is with no additional language deficits) had a small lesion confined to the insula or possibly extending to the surface of the supramarginal gyrus as revealed by CT scan (Roeltgen et al., 1982). They concluded that the lesions of the supramarginal gyrus or the insula medial to it (or both) are the critical anatomic loci for inducing phonological agraphia. Other patients with phonological agraphia had been reported to have lesions that included this area (Shallice, 1981; Bub and Kertesz, 1982; Nolan and Caramazza, 1982; Alexander et al., 1992). As in the case of lexical agraphia, subsequent studies of phonological agraphia have yielded patients with lesions that did not precisely correspond to the lesion locations of Roeltgen and colleagues' hypothesis. Baxter and Warrington (1986) described a patient with phonological agraphia who had a lesion that appeared to be slightly posterior to that proposed by Roeltgen and colleagues. Bolla-Wilson et al. (1985) described a left-handed patient with phonological agraphia who had a lesion in the right frontal parietal region (involving the supramarginal gyrus and insula). Also, Roeltgen (1989) described patients with still other lesion locations, including the caudate plus internal capsule and the thalamus plus posterior internal capsule. On the basis of these data, we have concluded that phonological agraphia is usually associated with lesions of the posterior perisylvian region and certain subcortical structures. In addition, there may be functional diversity similar to that proposed for lexical agraphia, and there are also individual variations in cerebral architecture and functional representation.

The presence of two parallel systems (phonological and lexical) for the production of correct spellings is one of the basic linguistic features of this model. Although it is applied here to English, similar models have been applied to Japanese writing. The presence of Kanji (morphograms) and Kana (phonograms) have enabled Japanese investigators to develop similar "dual-route" models (Iwata, 1984; Sakurai et al., 1997).

Deep Agraphia

Bub and Kertesz (1982), Roeltgen and colleagues (1983a), and Hatfield (1985) described patients who, like those with phonological agraphia, had trouble spelling nonwords, but also had more trouble spelling function words than nouns. They spelled nouns of high imageability (e.g., "arm") better than nouns of low imageability (e.g., "law"). They also made semantic paragraphic errors. These are spelling errors that consist of real words related in meaning to the target word, but with little phonological or visual resemblance to the target. For example, one patient wrote "flight" when the stimulus was "propeller" (Roeltgen et al., 1983a). Bub and Kertesz termed this disorder "deep agraphia."

All reported cases of deep agraphia, like those with phonological agraphia, have had lesions of the supramarginal gyrus or insula (Bub and Kertesz, 1982; Nolan and Caramazza, 1982; Roeltgen et al., 1983a), but their lesions have been large, extending well beyond the circumscribed area thought to be important for phonological agraphia. It is possible that deep agraphia reflects right hemisphere writing processes (Roeltgen and Heilman, 1982; Rapcsak et al., 1991). This hypothesis is similar to a proposed explanation for *deep dyslexia*, a reading disorder that is clinically similar to deep agraphia. Patients with deep dyslexia have trouble reading nonwords and make frequent semantic errors. Also, their reading ability is affected by word class and imageability (Coltheart, 1980, Saffran et al., 1980). The alternative hypothesis is that residual left hemisphere mechanisms are important for the residual abilities in patients with deep agraphia (Roeltgen and Heilman, 1982). A possible anatomic correlate of this hypothesis is that the left posterior angular gyrus has frequently been spared in patients with deep agraphia. Rapcsak and colleagues' patient is a clear exception to this. Their patient had complete loss of the left hemisphere, indicating with reasonable certainty that their patient used right hemispheric mechanisms.

Semantic Influence on Writing

The incorporation of meaning into writing is termed the "semantic influence on writing." The classical view of the interaction between semantics and language is that semantics interacts directly with oral language through auditory word images (Heilman et al., 1976, 1982; Fig. 7–1, pathway 12). Such an interaction enables a writer to incorporate meaning into words utilizing both the lexical strategy and the phonological strategy. With this arrangement the incorporation of meaning into spelling is indirect: it must come through auditory word images. There is evidence to suggest, however, that semantics may directly influence the lexical strategy (Brown and McNeill, 1966; Hier and Mohr, 1977; Morton, 1980; Shallice, 1981; Roeltgen et al., 1983a) (Fig. 7–1, pathway 13).

Recent evidence strongly supports the existence of this influence (Rapp et al., 1999).

Semantic Agraphia. A disruption of semantic ability (Fig. 7–1, component 11) or a disconnection of semantics from spelling (disruption of pathways 12 and 13, Fig. 7–1) has been termed "semantic agraphia" (Roeltgen et al., 1986). Patients with semantic agraphia lose their ability to spell and write with meaning. They may produce semantic jargon in sentence production (Rapcsak and Rubens, 1990). Also, they write and orally spell semantically incorrect but correctly spelled dictated homophones. For example, when asked to write "doe" as in "the doe ran through the forest," these patients may write "dough." They may write irregular words and nonwords correctly, demonstrating intact lexical and phonological systems (Fig. 7–1, pathways 4–5–6 and 7–8–9). The pathology of the reported patients with semantic agraphia is variable but frequently involves anatomic substrates important for accessing meaning in speech (Roeltgen and Rapcsak, 1993). Semantic agraphia is a common finding in early Alzheimer's disease (Niels and Roeltgen, 1995a).

Lexical Agraphia with Semantic Paragraphia. Many patients with lexical agraphia have difficulty utilizing semantic information when writing (Hatfield and Patterson, 1983; Roeltgen, personal observation). These patients, when asked to spell dictated homophones, frequently spell the semantically incorrect homophone (as do patients with semantic agraphia). They differ from some patients with semantic agraphia in that they are able to comprehend the meaning of the words when they read or hear them. Therefore, general semantic knowledge (Fig. 7–1, component 11) is preserved, but interacts poorly with spelling. This is presumably because there is a disturbance of the direct semantic influence on spelling (through the lexical system).

A Test of the Model

The model described here, as well as other similar models of spelling, has been developed from single case reports and small series of pa-

tients. To test this model, Roeltgen (1989, 1991) prospectively studied 43 consecutive right-handed patients with left hemisphere lesions and compared them with controls matched for handedness, age, and education. In this study, classification was based on strict definitions of the linguistic disorders described here. Phonological agraphia required preserved ability to write real words, whereas some previous studies (Roeltgen et al., 1983a; Roeltgen and Heilman, 1984) required only a relatively better ability to write real as opposed to nonsense words. Using stricter criteria, the model successfully classified 33 of the 43 patients. Eight had no agraphia, 5 had lexical agraphia, 4 had phonological agraphia, 10 had semantic agraphia, and 6 had global agraphia (severely impaired performance on all word types). Most patients with semantic agraphia also had an additional linguistic impairment involving the phonological or lexical systems, or the graphemic buffer (see below). Therefore, the number of patients classified as having a specific type of agraphia exceeds the number of patients studied.

The patients not classified into the above groups were classified into three additional groups. Three patients had impaired performance when spelling nonwords and moderately or severely impaired performance when spelling real words. However, they had no difference in performance when spelling regular or irregular words. Such patients would have previously been classified as having phonological agraphia. For the prospective study, they were classified as having phonological plus agraphia, indicating that, in addition to the impairment of the phonological system, they had a nonspecific impairment of spelling, such as would occur secondary to impairment of the graphemic buffer. Eight patients had a significant difference in performance when spelling regular as compared to irregular words (similar to lexical agraphia), but they also had impaired performance when spelling nonwords and overall poorer performance on spelling real words than the patients with either phonological or lexical agraphia. This group could represent lexical agraphia with a nonspecific impairment of spelling, such as would occur secondary to impairment of the graphemic buffer. This pattern of impaired performance is best termed "lexical plus agraphia." Eight patients had normal or nearly normal spelling performance when spelling nonwords but impaired performance when spelling real words, with an equal degree of impairment for both regular and irregular words. Although some of the patients in the last group may have had some impairment in the graphemic buffer, accounting for equal impairment on regular and irregular words, the good performance on nonwords makes that explanation unlikely. It is more likely that these patients, like patients with lexical agraphia, had impairment of the lexical system, but, unlike patients with lexical agraphia, they did not use the relatively preserved phonological system to compensate for difficulty spelling real words. This lack of compensation may be explained by the finding that patients with this type of agraphia were less likely to have chronic lesions than were patients with lexical agraphia. This pattern of performance may be termed "noncompensated lexical agraphia."

Attempts were made to correlate the type of agraphia with the locus of the cerebral lesion. Lesion locations of patients with lexical, phonological, and semantic agraphias were similar to those described previously. Patients with lexical agraphia had lesions sparing the mid-perisylvian region, specifically the insula, the anterior supramarginal, and the posterior superior temporal gyrus. In contrast, the patients with phonological agraphia had lesions involving these structures. The patients with semantic agraphia had various left hemispheric lesions.

Educational level significantly affected spelling performance after stroke. Better-educated subjects had better overall spelling ability after stroke and were less likely to have difficulty spelling nonwords.

In summary, the results from this prospective study supported the general framework of Roeltgen and Heilman's anatomically based information-processing model of spelling. However, analysis of the results also indicated that premorbid education level and chronicity of the lesion had an effect on the outcome. For example, it appears that for patients to develop lexical agraphia after stroke, they need chronic lesions in the non-perisylvian brain regions,

sparing the mid-insula, anterior supramarginal gyrus, and posterior superior temporal region, and usually 12 or more years of premorbid education.

The differences in results between previous studies and the prospective study also emphasize the different goals of these two types of analysis. Case studies and small group studies of the linguistic agraphias have helped delineate probable mechanisms of linguistic processing. The larger prospective study demonstrated the relative applicability of a model developed from such studies to a successive series of patients with left hemispheric strokes.

TRANSITION FROM LINGUISTIC INFORMATION TO MOTOR OUTPUT AND THE GRAPHEMIC BUFFER

Alternative spellings produced by the phonological and lexical systems must converge prior to motor output, since most patients with disorders of either spelling system produce substantially the same errors in oral spelling as those in writing.

Since the lexical and phonological systems need not produce the same spellings, there must be some way of choosing which spelling is to be produced. For example, in attempting to spell "comb," the lexical system, if familiar with the word, will produce "c-o-m-b." The phonological system, however, may produce "k-o-m" or "c-o-m," since the silent "b" does not conform to the rules of English orthography. Alternatively, "k-o-m-e" could be produced by analogy with "home." These alternative spellings will converge on the graphemic buffer (see below), which must transfer the correct spelling to the motor output systems. Because the lexical system produces only one response, which is dependent on prior experience, whereas the phonological system has the potential to produce multiple letter sequences for a single phonemic sequence, it is reasonable to assume that under normal circumstances the output of the lexical system is preferentially incorporated into written or oral spelling. Data from patients with semantic agraphia support this contention (Roeltgen et al., 1986). Patterns of response obtained from these patients suggest that the phonological system is probably only used for spelling non-words and unfamiliar regular words. Rarely, normal writers produce "slips of the pen" (spontaneous writing errors) that are phonologically correct (Hotopf, 1980). These errors (responses such as "k-o-m" for "comb") suggest that although most normal spelling (and writing) utilizes the lexical system, the phonological system continues to function in the background.

Graphemic Buffer

The output of the linguistic systems converge on what has been termed the "graphemic" or "orthographic buffer" (Fig. 7–1, component 14) (Margolin, 1984; Caramazza et al., 1987; Hillis and Caramazza, 1989; Lesser, 1990). This component of the model is thought to be a temporary working memory store of abstract letters. According to Caramazza and colleagues, disturbances of the graphemic buffer typically produce letter omissions, substitutions, insertions, and transpositions in nonwords and real words in oral and written spelling. Impairment occurs in spontaneous writing, writing to dictation, written naming, and delayed copying. Errors are not affected by linguistic factors (i.e., word class, regularity, and imageability) but are influenced by word length, with errors being more common in longer words (Cantagallo and Bonazzi, 1996). Errors also tend to be more prominent at the beginnings and ends of words. There is controversy as to whether there is an orthographic organization (allowing relative preservation of simple orthographic combinations) at the level of the orthographic buffer (Jonsdottir et al., 1996). Converging evidence is consistent with the conclusion that attentional mechanisms are very important for normal function of the graphemic buffer (Niels and Roeltgen, 1995b; Annoni et al., 1998). Although most patients with impairment of this type show similar disturbances in oral and written spelling, Lesser (1990) has described a dissociation, such that oral spelling was influenced by regularity and written spelling was not. She therefore suggested that there are separate graphemic buffers for oral and written spelling. A study of a Japanese dysgraphic has also suggested separate graphemic buffers. However, in that case, there were separate graphemic buffers for Kana and Kanji (Hashimoto et al., 1998). Dissociations between oral and written spelling may also be explained using the concept of a single graphemic buffer, but separate conversion systems from letters to shapes for writing and letters to sounds for oral spelling (Chialant, 2002).

Despite the fact that only a few reports have described patients with agraphia due to impairment of the graphemic buffer, the lesion loci have varied widely. These have included the left frontal parietal region (Hillis and Caramazza, 1989; Lesser, 1990), the left parietal region (Miceli et al., 1985; Posteraro et al., 1988; Annoni et al., 1998), and the right frontal parietal and basal ganglia region (Hillis and Caramazza, 1989). We (unpublished observation) and Laine (personal communication) have each observed patients with apparent agraphia due to impairment of the graphemic buffer. These patients had relatively discrete lesions of the left posterior dorsal lateral frontal lobe. Also, Niels and Roeltgen (1995b) described impairment of the graphemic buffer in early Alzheimer's disease. Because of the anatomic variability among the lesions in these patients, we feel no conclusive clinical–pathological correlation can be made.

MOTOR COMPONENTS

Motor output of spelled words may be either manual (written letters or graphemes) or oral (oral spelling). The dominant or nondominant hand may perform writing. Writing is not a unitary process, but includes motor and visuospatial skills, as well as knowledge of graphemes. Although there is some understanding of the neuropsychological bases of these skills, less is known about the components underlying oral spelling. Oral spelling and writing, however, do appear to be functionally dissociable.

Disorders of Writing with
Preserved Oral Spelling

Apraxic Agraphia. In order to write, motor functions are necessary. In addition to the pyramidal and extrapyramidal motor systems (which will not be discussed here), praxis is necessary for writing (see Chapter 11). Praxis includes the ability to properly hold a pen or pencil as well as the ability to perform the other learned movements necessary for forming written letters (graphemes). Apraxia usually results from lesions in the hemisphere opposite the preferred hand. In most right-handers this is also the hemisphere dominant for language, and consequently apraxia is often associated with aphasia. In aphasic apraxic patients, it may not be possible to separate clearly the aphasic from the apraxic elements of agraphia. Several patients have been described who have had language in the hemisphere ipsilateral to the preferred hand. When the hemisphere opposite the preferred hand was damaged, they developed ideomotor apraxia without aphasia (Heilman et al., 1973, 1974; Valenstein and Heilman, 1979). Patients with such disorders have illegible writing, both spontaneously and to dictation. Their oral spelling is preserved. Their writing typically improves with copying. They should be able to type or use anagram letters (Valenstein and Heilman, 1979). This syndrome may be termed "apraxic agraphia with ideomotor apraxia and without aphasia." Lesions in the parietal lobe opposite the hand dominant for writing may be the most common etiology for this disorder.

Apraxic Agraphia without Apraxia (Ideational Agraphia). The cognitive system necessary for performing handwriting, and thought to be important for knowledge of the features of letters, has been termed the "graphemic area" (Rothi and Heilman, 1981; Fig. 7–1, component 16). These space–time or visuokinesthetic–motor engrams for letters may be a subset of the engrams necessary to perform other skilled movements. Alternatively, letter engrams may be separate from other motor engrams. A syndrome of abnormal grapheme formation with normal praxis has been described and has been called "apraxic agraphia with normal praxis" (Roeltgen and Heilman, 1983). Patients produced poorly formed graphemes but have normal praxis, including the ability to imitate holding a pen or pencil. Apraxic agraphia with normal praxis is characterized by the pro-

duction of illegible graphemes in spontaneous writing and writing to dictation. Grapheme production improves with copying. Oral spelling and reading are intact. The initial patients described by Roeltgen and Heilman (1983) and Margolin and Binder (1984) also had disturbed visuospatial skills and therefore copying was moderately impaired. Baxter and Warrington (1986) have termed this disorder "ideational agraphia" and describe a patient with this disorder who had intact visuospatial skills. Their patient's writing improved substantially with copying. Croisile and co-workers (1990) have described a similar patient. This disorder may occur from a disruption of the graphemic area. Carey and Heilman (1988) described this form of agraphia in a patient with impaired letter imagery, despite normal reading, suggesting impaired letter engrams. In a study of a similar patient, analysis of errors suggested that this type of agraphia may also occur from a disconnection of the motor engrams from the motor output systems (Fig. 7–1, pathway 17). The patient studied by Otsuki and colleagues (1999) had a selective disorder of writing stroke sequences when writing. However, he was able to orally express the correct sequences.

The anatomic substrate for apraxic agraphia without apraxia appears to be the parietal lobe, perhaps the superior parietal lobule, either in the hemisphere contralateral to the hand used for writing (Margolin and Binder, 1984; Baxter and Warrington, 1986; Carey and Heilman, 1988; Otsuki et al., 1999) or in the ipsilateral hemisphere (Roeltgen and Heilman, 1983). However, there is at least one patient reported who had a dominant frontal lesion (Hodges, 1991).

Spatial Agraphia. Visuospatial skills are also necessary for the proper formation of letters and words. Spatial orientation must interact with graphic output in order that letter components (strokes) can be properly formed by the system of graphic output programming (Fig. 7–1, pathway 18–19–20). Disruption of this ability has been termed "visuospatial agraphia," "constructional agraphia," or "afferent dysgraphia" (Ellis et al., 1987). It is characterized by the following features: *(1)* reiteration of strokes, *(2)* inability to write on a straight horizontal line, and *(3)* insertion of blank spaces between graphemes. In patients with this disorder, the ability to copy is usually disturbed, but ability to spell orally and pronounce aurally perceived spelled words is preserved. This syndrome is usually due to nondominant parietal lobe lesions. It may also be seen with nondominant frontal lobe lesions (Ardila and Rosselli, 1993); however, these patients are typically not as severely impaired as are those with parietal lesions. It is also frequently associated with the syndrome of unilateral neglect, where the patient's writing may be confined to only one side of the paper, ipsilateral to the lesion (See Chapter 13). Ellis and colleagues (1987) have suggested that this may relate both to the left-sided neglect and to failure to utilize visual and kinesthetic feedback. Silveri and colleagues provided support for this latter hypothesis (1997) in a patient with spatial agraphia from a cerebellar lesion. Their patient performed much better with his eyes open than with his eyes closed.

Agraphia Due to Impaired Allographic Store. The allographic store (Fig. 7–1, component 22) is thought to be important for directing the handwriting systems in the production of correct case (upper and lower) and style (script [cursive] or manuscript [print]). Its existence was hypothesized by Ellis (1982) on the basis of analysis of slips of the pen. A few reports have described patients with acquired agraphia apparently due to impairment of the allographic store (Black et al., 1987; Yopp and Roeltgen, 1987; DeBastiani and Barry, 1989). These patients have better oral spelling than writing, normal praxis, normal visuospatial ability, and normal letter form. However, they make frequent case and style errors. These errors include difficulty producing a specific case or style or substitution of one particular case or style for another. Agraphia for words written in lower case with relatively preserved ability to write upper case and, in contrast, agraphia for upper case with preserved ability to write lower case supports the contention that graphic programs for different cases are dissociable (Kartsounis, 1992; Trojano and Chiacchio, 1994).

Unilateral (Callosal) Agraphia. In most agraphias the dominant and nondominant hands are equally affected, except when one hand is paretic. The spelling and grapheme systems of the left hemisphere have access via the neocommissures to the right hemisphere motor system responsible for controlling the nondominant hand. Disruption of this interhemispheric transfer results in unilateral agraphia (Liepman and Maas, 1907; Geschwind and Kaplan, 1962; Bogen, 1969; Levy et al., 1971; Rubens et al., 1977; Sugishita et al., 1980; Yamadori et al., 1980; Gersh and Damasio, 1981; Watson and Heilman, 1983; Tanaka et al., 1990). Most of these patients make unintelligible scrawls when they attempt to write with their left hands. Most improve with copying and are able to spell orally and read. Watson and Heilman (1983) described a patient with left unilateral agraphia who was able to type with her left hand. They termed this syndrome "unilateral apraxic agraphia," limited to the left hand. Their patient had a lesion affecting the body of the corpus callosum, sparing the genu and the splenium. Geschwind and Kaplan (1962) described a patient with an acquired callosal lesion and a unilateral left agraphia who was unable to type or use anagram letters with his left hand. This patient's lesion affected the entire anterior four-fifths of the corpus callosum. Watson and Heilman (1983) suggested that the difference between their patient and that of Geschwind and Kaplan (1962) was that the genu of the corpus callosum was spared in their patient. They hypothesized that the genu is important for the transmission of verbal–motor programs from the left to the right hemisphere and that the body of the corpus callosum is important for the transmission of visuokinesthetic (space–time) engrams. These engrams are thought to "command the motor system to adopt appropriate spatial positions of the relevant body parts over time" (Watson and Heilman, 1983). The disruption of transmission of these engrams was thought to account for the ideomotor apraxia observed in Watson and Heilman's patient (Fig. 7–2).

Some patients with left-sided unilateral agraphia do not have ideomotor apraxia (Sugishita et al., 1980; Yamadori et al., 1980; Gersh and Damasio, 1981). The agraphia of these pa-

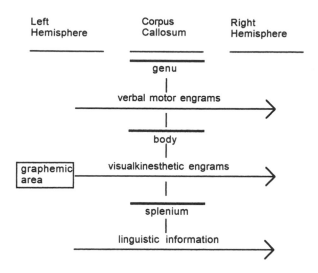

Figure 7–2. Transfer of information across the corpus callosum. Evidence suggests that there are at least three separable components necessary for writing and they cross at different levels of the callosum. Verbal motor programs cross in the genu, visuokinesthetic engrams cross in the body, and linguistic information crosses in the splenium.

tients consists of illegible scrawls as well as incorrect letters. The patient of Gersh and Damasio was also unable to write using anagram letters. This syndrome has been called "unilateral aphasic agraphia" (Watson and Heilman, 1983). The lesions in these patients were confined to the posterior portion of the corpus callosum. Gersh and Damasio suggested that the pathways for ideomotor praxis were more anterior in the callosum than those for writing. Watson and Heilman (1983) further suggested that although the body of the callosum was important for the transfer of visuokinesthetic engrams (ideomotor praxis for writing and other motor tasks), the posterior callosum (especially the splenium) was important for the transmission of linguistic information. This explanation, they felt, accounted for the apraxic agraphia in their patient and the aphasic agraphia in Gersh and Damasio's patient. These interhemispheric relationships are extremely complicated, as demonstrated by the results of a case study by Zesinger and colleagues (1994). Their patient had unilateral agraphia that included letter substitutions for upper-case letters and aborted letter formations for lower-case letters. These results suggest graphemic buffer dysfunction for upper case and graphemic area dysfunction for lower case. Therefore, the connection of the allographic store with the graphemic buffer (Fig 7–1, pathway 21) may be bidirectional.

Additionally, patients described by Sugishita and colleagues (1980) and Yamadori and colleagues (1980) showed a degree of dissociated linguistic agraphia with the left hand, in that they wrote Kanji characters better than Kana. Rothi et al. (1987) suggested that these results were consistent with the right hemisphere having a better ability to support both linguistic and motor mechanisms for the more ideographic Kanji characters than for the phonologic Kana.

Disorders of Oral Spelling

The mechanisms for oral spelling are not as well defined as those for writing. Two possible mechanisms exist. One mechanism would utilize the area of auditory word engrams (Wernicke's area) to guide the anterior perisylvian speech regions (e.g., Broca's area) to produce oral letters (Fig. 7–1, pathway 25–26). The other mechanism would utilize an independent area of oral motor engrams for letters to guide or program Broca's area. Evidence at this time supports the first mechanism. One patient with relatively spared writing but disturbed oral spelling has been well described (Kinsbourne and Warrington, 1965). This patient also had difficulty saying words spelled to him. This finding suggests that the system of auditory word images (Wernicke's area) is necessary for both perception of aurally perceived spelled words and the production of oral letters. Alternatively, there may be a close anatomic proximity between the area of auditory word images and the area of oral motor engrams for letters. If this hypothesis is correct, both systems were damaged in the patient of Kinsbourne and Warrington. Additionally, this hypothesis would predict that patients with destruction of auditory word images (Wernicke's aphasia) could have preserved oral spelling. Although patients with Wernicke's aphasia and preserved written spelling have been described (Hier and Mohr, 1977; Roeltgen et al., 1983a), no patients with preserved oral spelling have been described.

RELATIONSHIPS OF LINGUISTIC AND MOTOR AGRAPHIAS WITH OTHER NEUROPSYCHOLOGICAL DISORDERS

The association of the agraphias, as defined by the model discussed in this chapter, with other neuropsychological disorders, such as aphasia, alexia, the Gerstmann syndrome, and ideomotor apraxia, may reflect common neuropsychological and anatomic mechanisms, or the anatomic proximity of structures some serving different functions.

PHONOLOGICAL AGRAPHIA

Association with Aphasia

At least 21 patients with phonological agraphia have been described (Shallice, 1981; Bub and Kertesz, 1982; Roeltgen, 1983; Roeltgen et al., 1983a; Roeltgen and Heilman, 1984;, Baxter and Warrington, 1985; Bolla-Wilson et al., 1985; Hatfield, 1985; Goodman-Schulman and Caramazza, 1987). Nineteen of these patients had aphasia: there were seven Wernicke's, five Broca's, two conduction, two anomic, one global, one transcortical motor, and one transcortical sensory aphasia. Except for the transcortical aphasias, each of these aphasias is typically associated with perisylvian lesions (Benson, 1979). Phonological agraphia is also associated with perisylvian lesions. This shared anatomic relationship probably accounts for the association between phonological agraphia and the aphasias.

Phonological agraphia may be dissociated from aphasia, and in aphasic patients, writing may be dissociated from speech. Two patients with phonological agraphia (Roeltgen et al., 1983a) wrote better than they spoke. This type of dissociation has been previously described in aphasic patients (Weisenberg and McBride, 1964; Mohr et al., 1973; Hier and Mohr, 1977; Assal et al., 1981). Our evaluation suggested that this dissociation occurs because speech depends on left hemisphere phonological systems, whereas writing may be performed nonphonologically by a lexical system using structures outside the left perisylvian area.

Association with Alexia

Similarly, disorders of writing and disorders of reading are sometimes dissociable. Neuropsychological models have been proposed for reading that are similar to the model for writing discussed here (Shallice and Warrington, 1980; Beauvois and Derouesne, 1979). The reading models usually contain both a phonological system and a lexical system. Disruption of the phonological system, phonological alexia (dyslexia), is similar in many ways to phonological agraphia. In each of these disorders there is an inability to transcode nonwords. Also, each of these disorders may demonstrate the effects of imageability and word class with production of semantic paralexias and paragraphias resulting in the syndromes of deep dyslexia and deep dysgraphia. Most patients with phonological agraphia who have alexia have phonological alexia (Roeltgen, 1983). However, at least one patient had no alexia, and one patient had lexical (or surface) alexia (preserved ability to read nonwords along with impaired ability to read irregular words). These findings indicate that phonological agraphia and phonological alexia are dissociable. There are two possible explanations for this dissociation. First, phonological spelling and phonological reading may share neuropsychological mechanisms for conversion between phonemes and graphemes. A single lesion affecting this mechanism would disrupt both phonological spelling and reading, but lesions that disrupt information as it exits or enters the system would affect either reading or writing in isolation. Alternatively, each system may use different mechanisms, and the frequent association of phonological agraphia with alexia might relate to the anatomic proximity of these mechanisms. The anatomic substrate of phonological agraphia appears to be the supramarginal gyrus or insula, and the neighboring mid-perisylvian region has a role in the production of phonological alexia (Roeltgen, 1983).

Association with Gerstmann Syndrome and Apraxia

The proximity of the perisylvian lesions causing phonological agraphia to the angular gyrus and the dominant parietal lobe may also account for its association with the Gerstmann syndrome and ideomotor apraxia. The Gerstmann syndrome has been attributed to lesions in the angular gyrus (Nielson, 1938; Gerstmann, 1940; Roeltgen et al., 1983b), and ideomotor apraxia is frequently attributed to lesions in the dominant parietal lobe (Heilman, 1979). In our reported series of 14 patients with phonological agraphia (Roeltgen, 1983), 3 had other elements of the Gerstmann syndrome (right–left confusion, finger agnosia, or dyscalculia) in addition to agraphia. Also, seven of them had mild or severe ideomotor apraxia. It is probable that phonological agraphia is accompanied by the Gerstmann syndrome, ideomotor apraxia, or both when the extent of the lesion is sufficient to involve the anatomic substrates of the Gerstmann functions and praxis.

LEXICAL AGRAPHIA

Association with Aphasia

At least 19 patients with lexical agraphia have been described (Beauvois and Derouesne, 1981: Roeltgen and Heilman, 1983; Hatfield and Patterson, 1983; Goodman-Schulman and Caramazza, 1987; Rothi et al., 1987; Rapcsak et al., 1988; Croisile et al., 1989; Roeltgen and Rapcsak, 1993). For those patients for whom an aphasia diagnosis is known, the frequency of aphasia types differs from that found in phonological agraphia. Two patients had transcortical sensory aphasia, two had Wernicke's aphasia, seven had anomia, one had tactile aphasia, one had phonetic disintegration, and four had no aphasia. As is the case with phonological agraphia, the associations of lexical agraphia with aphasia appear to depend on the underlying pathological anatomy of the syndromes. Transcortical sensory aphasia may be caused by lesions of the posterior parietal region (Benson, 1979; Heilman et al., 1981; Roeltgen and Heilman, 1984), and Wernicke's aphasia is typically caused by lesions in the posterior superior temporal gyrus (Benson, 1979). Anomia may also be caused by lesions of the angular gyrus (Benson, 1979). Therefore, lexical agraphia, a disorder that frequently is caused by an angular gyrus lesion and other nonperisylvian structures, is associated with aphasias caused by lesions in and adjacent to the angular gyrus.

Association with Alexia

Of the reported patients with lexical agraphia, three had lexical (surface) alexia and had difficulty reading as well as spelling irregular words. Seven patients had phonological alexia and had relatively preserved ability to read irregular words but had difficulty reading nonwords and trouble spelling irregular words. One patient had a combination of lexical and phonological alexia, one was a letter-by-letter reader, and four had no alexia. Reading results from the other patients are uncertain. As with phonological agraphia, there are at least two explanations for the dissociation between lexical agraphia and lexical alexia. There may be two separate neural systems subserving spelling and reading individually. One, the other, or both could be disrupted, leading to the associations described. Alternately, there may be a single lexical system utilized for both spelling and reading. Disrupted flow of information out of this system would produce lexical agraphia and disrupted flow into it would produce lexical (surface) alexia. Dysfunction of the system itself would produce lexical agraphia and alexia. Having separate lexical systems for spelling and reading, similar to the possible separate phonological systems for spelling and reading proposed previously in this chapter, may appear to be redundant. However, Caramazza and Hillis (1991) have provided evidence to support the dissociation of lexical knowledge as it relates to speech and reading. Therefore, a similar dissociation between spelling and reading may also exist.

Association with Gerstmann Syndrome and Apraxia

Information about the occurrence of the Gerstmann syndrome and ideomotor apraxia in patients with lexical agraphia is available in only five and four patients, respectively. However, they occur sufficiently often (four of five and three of four) to conclude that these syndromes are probably frequently associated. Given the aforementioned anatomic pathology underlying the Gerstmann syndrome and ideomotor apraxia, it is not unexpected that lexical agraphia, a disorder commonly due to angular gyrus lesions, occurs with them.

SEMANTIC AGRAPHIA

At least 17 patients with semantic agraphia have been described. It has been associated with transcortical aphasia (motor, two patients; sensory, one patient; mixed one patient), anomia (seven patients), semantic jargon and global aphasia (one patient each), and no aphasia (three patients). The aphasia diagnosis in one patient was uncertain. The associations are not surprising, given the anatomic diversity of semantic agraphia. It is also not surprising that three patients developed what we termed "semantic alexia": fluent, preserved oral reading with absent comprehension (Roeltgen et al., 1986). This pattern of reading plus the semantic agraphia would appear to be secondary to a general disruption of semantics. The alexia in the remaining patients varies and includes phonological, mixed, global, and no alexia.

Other elements of the Gerstmann syndrome, as well as ideomotor apraxia, have been noted in the patients with semantic agraphia. However, because of the severe comprehension disturbance in many of these patients and the absence of data from others, it is difficult to interpret these results.

APRAXIC AGRAPHIA

Apraxic agraphia with ideomotor apraxia is typically associated with aphasia as well as alexia and other elements of the Gerstmann syndrome. However, other associations are variable because ideomotor apraxia, and therefore agraphia with ideomotor apraxia, may be due

to dominant parietal lesions or to lesions anterior to this region (Heilman et al., 1982). In those rare patients with crossed dominance (language in one hemisphere and motor in the other), apraxic agraphia with ideomotor apraxia may occur without aphasia (Heilman et al., 1973, 1974; Valenstein and Heilman, 1979).

Agraphia in patients without apraxia has been well described in only a limited number of patients (Roeltgen and Heilman, 1983; Margolin and Binder, 1984; Baxter and Warrington, 1986; Croisile et al., 1990). Therefore, it is difficult to draw any conclusions regarding the associations of this syndrome with disorders of other neuropsychological functions.

CONCLUSIONS

The neuropsychological approach to the agraphias offers a promising method of classifing these disorders. It complements, rather than supplants, the traditional classifications that rely on associated neurological findings, such as aphasia, alexia, or visuospatial disorders, rather than on the strict analysis of writing. Neuropsychological analysis may be of use not only in classifying agraphias but also in helping elucidate the underlying brain mechanisms. This approach may have heuristic value, including developing rational methods of therapy. An example of this last point is found in a review of a study by Schecter and colleagues (1985). They used phoneme analysis to treat patients with acquired agraphia and found that improvement correlated with phonemic analysis ability. There are few studies evaluating agraphia remediation. There are no studies that have used neuropsychological models, such as the one described here, to structure such remediation. The results from the study by Schecter and colleagues would suggest that remediation of agraphia should use such an approach.

REFERENCES

Aimard, G., Devick, Lebel, M., Trouillas, P., and Boisson, D. (1975). Agraphie pure (dynamique?) D'origine frontale. *Rev. Neurol. (Paris)* 7:505–512.

Alexander, M. P., Friedman, R., LoVerso (sic), F.,

and Fischer, R. (1990). Anatomic correlates of lexical agraphia. Presented at the Academy of Aphasia, Baltimore, MD.

Alexander, M. P., Friedman, R. B., Loverso, F., and Fischer, R. S. (1992). Lesion localization of phonological agraphia. *Brain Lang.* 43:83–95.

Annoni, J. M., Lemay, M. A., de Mattos Pimenta, M.A., and Lecours, A. R. (1998). The contribution of attentional mechanisms to an irregularity effect at the graphemic buffer level. *Brain Lang.* 63:64–78.

Ardila, A., and Rosselli, M. (1993). Spatial agraphia. *Brain Cogn.* 22:137–147.

Assal, G., Buttet, J., and Jolivet, R. (1981). Dissociations in aphasia: a case report. *Brain Lang.* 13:223–240.

Auerbach, S. H., and Alexander, M. P. (1981). Pure agraphia and unilateral optic ataxia associated with a left superior lobule lesion. *J. Neurol. Neurosurg. Psychiatry* 44:430–432.

Basso, A., Taborelli, A., and Vignollo, L. A. (1978) Dissociated disorders of speaking and writing in aphasia. *J. Neurol. Neurosurg. Psychiatry* 41:556–563.

Baxter, D. M., and Warrington, E. K. (1985). Category specific phonological dysgraphia. *Neuropsychologia* 23:653–666.

Baxter, D. M., and Warrington, E. K. (1986). Ideational agraphia: a single case study. *J. Neurol. Neurosurg. Psychiatry* 49:369–374.

Beauvois, M. F., and Derouesne, J. (1979). Phonological alexia: three dissociations. *J. Neurol. Neurosurg. Psychiatry* 42:1115–1124.

Beauvois, M. F., and Derouesne, J. (1981). Lexical or orthographic agraphia. *Brain* 104:2–49.

Benedikt, M. (1865). *Über Aphasie, Agraphie und verwandte pathologische Zustande.* Vienna: Wiener Medizische Presse, 6:897–899; 923–926.

Benson, D. F. (1979). *Aphasia, Alexia and Agraphia.* New York: Churchill Livingston.

Benson, D. F., and Cummings, J. L. (1985) Agraphia. In *Handbook of Clinical Neurology, Vol. 45, Clinical Neuropsychology,* J. A. M. Frederics (ed.). New York: Elsevier, pp. 457–472.

Black, S. E., Bass, K., Behrmann, M., and Hacker, P. (1987). Selective writing impairment: a single case study of a deficit in allographic conversion. *Neurology* 37:174.

Bogen, J. E. (1969). The other side of the brain. I. Dysgraphia and dyscopia following cerebral commissurotomy. *Bull. Los Angeles Neurol. Soc.* 34:3–105.

Bolla-Wilson, K., Speedie, J. J., and Robinson, R. G. (1985). Phonologic agraphia in a left-handed pa-

tient after a right-hemisphere lesion. *Neurology* 35:1778–1781.

Brown, R., and McNeill, D. (1966). The "tip of the tongue" phenomenon. *J. Verbal Learn. Verbal Behav.* 5:325–337.

Bub, D., and Chertkow, H. (1988). Agraphia. In *Handbook of Neuropsychology,* F. Boller and J. Grafman (eds.). Amsterdam: Elsevier, pp. 393–414.

Bub, D., and Kertesz, A. (1982). Deep agraphia. *Brain Lang.* 17:146–165.

Campbell, R. (1985). When children write nonwords to dictation. *J. Exp. Child Psychol.* 40:133–151.

Cantagallo, A., and Bonazzi, S. (1996). Acquired dysgraphia with selective damage to the graphemic buffer: a single case report. *Ital. J. Neurol. Sci.* 17:249–254.

Caramazza, A., and Hillis, A. E. (1991). Lexical organization of nouns and verbs in the brain. *Nature* 349:788–790.

Caramazza, A., Miceli, G., Vila, G., and Romani, C. (1987). The role of the graphemic buffer in spelling: evidence from a case of acquired dysgraphia. *Cognition* 26:59–85.

Carey, M. A., and Heilman, K. M. (1988). Letter imagery deficits in a case of pure apraxic agraphia. *Brain Lang.* 34:147–156.

Chedru, F., and Geschwind, N. (1972). Writing disturbances in acute confusional states. *Neuropsychologia* 10:343–354.

Chialant, D., Domoto-Reilly, K., Psoios, H., and Caramazza, A. (2002). Preserved orthographic length and transitional probabilities in written spelling and in a case of acquired dysgraphia. *Brain Lang.* 82:30–46.

Coltheart, M. (1980). Deep dyslexia: a review of the syndrome. In *Deep Dyslexia,* M. Coltheart, K. Patterson, and J. C. Marshall (eds.). London: Routledge and Kegan Paul, pp. 22–47.

Croisile, B., Laurent, B., Michel, D., and Trillet, M. (1990). Pure agraphia from a deep left hemisphere hematoma. *J. Neurol. Neurosurg. Psychiatry* 53:263–265.

Croisile, B., Trillet, M., Laurent, B., Latombe, D., and Schott, B. (1989). Agraphie lexicale par hematome temporo-parietal gauche. *Rev. Neurol. (Paris)* 145:287–292.

DeBastiani, K., and Barry, C. (1989). A cognitive analysis of an acquired dysgraphic patient with an "allographic" writing disorder. *Cogn. Neuropsychol.* 6:25–41.

Dejerine, J. (1891). Sur un cas de cecite verbale avec agraphie, suivi d'autopsie. *Mem. Soc. Biol.* 3:197–201.

Denckla, M. B., and Roeltgen, D. P. (1992). Disorders of motor function. In *Handbook of Neuropsychology. Section of Child Neuropsychology*, I. Rapin and S. Segalowitz (eds.). Amsterdam: Elsevier, pp. 455–476.

Ellis, A. W. (1982). Spelling and writing (and reading and speaking). In *Normality and Pathology in Cognitive Functions*, A. W. Ellis (ed.). London: Academic Press.

Ellis, A. W., Young, W. W., and Flude, B. M. (1987). "Afferent dysgraphia" in a patient and in normal subjects. *Cogn. Neuropsychol. 4:*465–487.

Friedman, R. B., and Alexander, M. P. (1989). Written spelling agraphia. *Brain Lang. 36:*5063–517.

Gersh, F., and Damasio, A. R. (1981). Praxis and writing of the left hand may be served by different callosal pathways. *Arch. Neurol. 38:*634–636.

Gerstmann, J. (1940). Syndrome of finger agnosia, disorientation for the right and left, agraphia and acalculia. *Arch. Neurol. Psychiatry 44:*398–408.

Geschwind, N., and Kaplan E. (1962). A human cerebral disconnection syndrome. *Neurology 12:*675–685.

Goldstein, K. (1948). *Language and Language Disturbances*. New York: Grune and Stratton.

Goodman-Schulman, R., and Caramazza, A. (1987). Patterns of dysgraphia and the nonlexical spelling process. *Cortex 23:*143–148.

Grashey, H. (1885). Uber aphasie und ihre Beziehungen zur Wahrnehmung. *Arch. Psychiatr. Nervenkr. 16:*654–688.

Grossfield, M. L., and Clark, L. W. (1983). Nature of spelling errors in transcortical sensory aphasia: a case study. *Brain Lang. 18:*47–56.

Hashimoto, R., Tanaka, R., and Yoshida, M. (1988). Selective Kana jargon agraphia following right hemispheric infarction. *Brain Lang. 63:*50–63.

Hatfield, F. M. (1985). Visual and phonological factors in acquired dysgraphia. *Neuropsychologia 23:*13–29.

Hatfield, F. M., and Patterson, K. E. (1983). Phonological spelling. *Q. J. Exp. Psychol. 35A:*451–468.

Head, H. (1926). *Aphasia and Kindred Disorders of Speech*. Cambridge, UK: Cambridge University Press.

Hécaen, H., and Albert, M. L. (1978) *Human Neuropsychology*. New York: John Wiley and Sons.

Heilman, K. M. (1979). Apraxia. In *Clinical Neuropsychology*, 1st ed., K. M. Heilman and E. Valenstein (eds.). New York: Oxford University Press, pp. 159–185.

Heilman, K. M., Coyle, J. M., Gonyea, E. F., and Geschwind, N. (1973). Apraxia and agraphia in a left hander. *Brain 96:*21–28.

Heilman, K. M., Gonyea, E. F., and Geschwind, N.

(1974). Apraxia and agraphia in a right hander. *Cortex 10:*284–288.

Heilman, K. M., Rothi, L., McFarling, D., and Rottman, A. L. (1981). Transcortical sensory aphasia with relatively spared spontaneous speech and naming. *Arch. Neurol. 38:*236–239.

Heilman, K. M., Rothi, L., and Valenstein, E. (1982). Two forms of ideomotor apraxia. *Neurology 32:*342–346.

Heilman, K. M., Tucker, D. M., Valenstein, E. (1976). A case of mixed transcortical aphasia with intact naming. *Brain 99:*415–426.

Hier, D. B., and Mohr, J. P. (1977). Incongruous oral and written naming. *Brain Lang. 4:*115–126.

Hillis, A. E., and Caramazza, A. (1989). The graphemic buffer and attentional mechanisms. *Brain Lang. 36:*208–235.

Hodges, J. R. (1991). Pure apraxic agraphia with recovery after drainage of a left frontal cyst. *Cortex 27:*469–473.

Hotopf, N. (1980). Slips of the pen. In *Cognitive Processes in Spelling*, U. Frith (ed.). London: Academic Press, pp. 287–307.

Iwata, M. (1984). Neuropsychological correlates of the Japanese writing system. *Trends Neurosciences 7:*290–293.

Jonsdottir, M. K., Shallice, T., and Wise, R. (1996). Phonological mediation and the graphemic buffer disorder in spelling: cross language differences. *Cognition 59:*169–197.

Kaplan, E., and Goodglass, H. (1981). Aphasia-related disorders. In *Acquired Aphasia*. M. T. Sarno (Ed.). New York: Academic Press.

Kartsounis, L. D. (1992). Selective lower-case letter ideational agraphia. *Cortex 28:*145–150.

Kertesz, A., Latham, N., and McCabe, P. (1990). Subcortical agraphia. *Neurology 40;S1:*172.

Kinsbourne, M., and Warrington, E. K. (1965). A case showing selectively impaired oral spelling. *J. Neurol. Neurosurg. Psychiatry 28:*563–566.

Laine, T. N., and Marttila, R. J. (1981). Pure agraphia: a case study. *Neuropsychologia 19:*311–316.

Leischner, A. (1969). The agraphias. In *Disorders of Speech, Perception and Symbolic Behavior*, P. J. Vinken and G. W. Bruyn (eds.). Amsterdam: North Holland, pp. 141–180.

Lesser, R. (1990). Superior oral to written spelling: evidence for separate buffers? *Cogn. Neuropsychol. 7:*347–366.

Levy, J., Nebes, R. D., and Sperry, R. W. (1971). Expressive language in the surgically separated minor hemisphere. *Cortex 7:*49–58.

Lichtheim, L. (1885). On aphasia. *Brain 7:*433–485.

Liepmann, H., and Maas, O. (1907). Ein Fall von

linksseitiger Agraphie und Apraxie bei rechtsseitiger Lahmumg. *J. Psychol. Neurol.* 10:214–227.

Marcie, P., and Hécaen, H. (1979). Agraphia. In *Clinical Neuropsychology*, 1st ed., K. M. Heilman and E. Valenstein (eds.). New York: Oxford University Press, pp. 92–127.

Margolin, D. I. (1984). The neuropsychology of writing and spelling: semantic phonological, motor, and perceptual processes. *Q. J. Exp. Psychol.* 36A:459–489.

Margolin, D. I., and Binder, L. (1984). Multiple component agraphia in a patient with atypical cerebral dominance: an error analysis. *Brain Lang.* 22:26–40.

Miceli, G., Silveri, M. C., and Caramazza, A. (1985). Cognitive analysis of a case of pure dysgraphia. *Brain Lang.* 25:187–212.

Mohr, J. P., Sidman, M., Stoddard, L. T., Leichester, J., and Rosenberger, P. B. (1973). Evaluation of the defect of total aphasia. *Neurology* 23:1302–1312.

Morton, J. (1980). The Logogen model and orthographic structure. In *Cognitive Processes in Spelling*, U. Frith (ed.). London: Academic Press, pp. 117–133.

Niels, J., and Roeltgen, D. P. (1995a). Decline in homophone spelling associated with loss of semantic influence on spelling in Alzheimer's disease. *Brain Lang.* 49:27–49.

Niels, J., and Roeltgen, D. P. (1995b). Spelling and attention in early Alzheimer's disease: evidence for impairment of the graphemic buffer. *Brain Lang.* 49:241–262.

Nielson, J. M. (1946). *Agnosia, Apraxia, Aphasia: Their Value in Cerebral Localization*. New York: Paul B. Hoeber.

Nielson, J. M. (1938). Gerstmann syndrome: finger agnosia, agraphia, confusion of right and left, acalculia. *Arch. Neurol. Psychiatry* 39:536–559.

Nolan, K. A., and Caramazza, A. (1982). Modality-independent impairments in word processing in a deep dyslexic patient. *Brain Lang.* 16:236–264.

Ogle, J. W. (1867). Aphasia and agraphia. *Rep. Med. Res. Counsel St. George's Hospital (Lond.)* 2:83–122.

Otsuki, M., Soma, Y., Aral, T., Otsuka, A., and Tsuji, S. (1999). Pure apraxic agraphia with abnormal writing stroke sequences: report of a Japanese patient with a left superior parietal hemorrhage. *J. Neurol. Neurosurg. Psychiatry* 66:233–237.

Patterson, K. (1986). Lexical but nonsemantic spelling? *Cogn. Neuropsychol.* 3:341–367.

Pitres, A. (1894). *Rapport sur la Question des Agraphies*. Bordeaux: Congres Francais de Medecine Interne.

Posteraro, L., Zinelli, P., and Mazzucci, A. (1988). Selective impairment of the graphemic buffer in acquired dysgraphia. *Brain Lang.* 35:274–286.

Rapcsak, S. Z., Arthur, S. A., and Rubens, A. B. (1988). Lexical agraphia from focal lesion of the left precentral gyrus. *Neurology* 38:1119–1123.

Rapcsak, S. Z., Beeson, P. M., and Rubens, A. B. (1991). Writing with the right hemisphere. *Brain Lang.* 41:510–530.

Rapcsak, S. Z., and Rubens, A. B. (1990). Disruption of semantic influence on writing following a left prefrontal lesion. *Brain Lang.* 38:334–344.

Rapcsak, S. Z., Rubens, A. B., and Laguna, J. F. (1990). From letters to words: procedures for word recognition in letter-by-letter reading. *Brain Lang.* 38:504–514.

Rapp, B., Boatman, D., and Gordon, B. (1999). The autonomy of lexical orthography: evidence from cortical stimulation. *Brain Lang.* 69:392–395.

Roeltgen, D. P. (1983). The neurolinguistics of writing: anatomic and neurologic correlates. Presented at the International Neuropsychological Society, Pittsburgh, PA.

Roeltgen, D. P. (1985). Agraphia. In *Clinical Neuropsychology*, 2nd ed., K. M. Heilman and E. Valenstein (eds.). New York: Oxford University Press, pp. 75–96.

Roeltgen, D. P. (1989). Prospective analysis of a model of writing, anatomic aspects. Presented at the Academy of Aphasia, Santa Fe, NM.

Roeltgen, D. P. (1991). Prospective analysis of writing and spelling. Part II. Results not related to localization. *J. Clin. Exp. Neuropsychol.* 13:48.

Roeltgen, D. P., and Blaskey, P. (1992). Processes, breakdowns and remediation in developmental disorders of written language. In *Cognitive Neuropsychology in Clinical Practice*, D. Margolin (ed.). New York: Oxford University Press, pp. 298–326.

Roeltgen, D. P., and Heilman, K. M. (1982). Global aphasia with spared lexical writing. Presented at the International Neuropsychological Society, Pittsburgh, PA.

Roeltgen, D. P., and Heilman, K. M. (1983). Apraxic agraphia in a patient with normal praxis. *Brain Lang.* 18:35–46.

Roeltgen, D. P., and Heilman, K. M. (1984). Lexical agraphia, further support for the two system hypothesis of linguistic agraphia. *Brain* 107:811–827.

Roeltgen, D. P., and Heilman, K. M. (1985). Review of agraphia and proposal for an anatomically based neuropsychological model of writing. *Appl. Psycholinguist.* 6:205–220.

Roeltgen, D. P., and Rapcsak, S. (1993). Acquired

disorders of writing and spelling. In *Linquistic Disorders and Pathologies*, G. Blanken (ed.). Berlin: Walter de Gruyter, pp. 262–278.

Roeltgen, D. P., Rothi, L. J. G., and Heilman, K. M. (1982). Isolated phonological agraphia from a focal lesion. Presented at the Academy of Aphasia, New Paltz, NY.

Roeltgen, D. P., Rothi, L. J. G., and Heilman, K. M. (1986). Linguistic semantic agraphia. *Brain Lang.* 27:257–280.

Roeltgen, D. P., Sevush, S., and Heilman, K. M. (1983a). Phonological agraphia: writing by the lexical–semantic route. *Neurology* 33:733–757.

Roeltgen, D. P., Sevush, S., and Heilman, K. M. (1983b). Pure Gerstmann syndrome from a focal lesion. *Arch. Neurol.* 40:46–47.

Roeltgen, D. P., Siegel, J., and Davis J. P. (1991). Influence of task demands on handwriting performance: a computer-assisted analysis. Poster presented at TENNET, Montreal.

Rosati, G., and de Bastiani, P. (1981). Pure agraphia: a discreet form of aphasia. *J. Neurol. Neurosurg. Psychiatry* 3:266–269.

Rothi, L. J. G., and Heilman, K. M. (1981). Alexia and agraphia with spared spelling and letter recognition abilities. *Brain Lang.* 12:1–13.

Rothi, L. J. G., Roeltgen, D. P., and Kooistra, C. A. (1987). Isolated lexical agraphia in a right-handed patient with a posterior lesion of the right cerebral hemisphere. *Brain Lang.* 301:181–190.

Rubens, A. B., Geschwind, N., Mahowald, M. W., and Mastri, A. (1977). Posttraumatic cerebral hemispheric disconnection syndrome. *Arch. Neurol.* 34:750–755.

Saffran, E. M., Bogeyo, L. C., Schwartz, M. F., and Martin, O. S. M. (1980). Does deep dyslexia reflect right-hemisphere reading? In *Deep Dyslexia*, M. Coltheart, K. E. Patterson, and J. C. Marshall (eds.). London: Routledge and Kegan Paul, pp. 381–406.

Sakurai, Y., Matsumura, K., Iwatsubo, T., and Momose, T. (1997). Frontal pure agraphia for Kanji or Kana: dissociation between morphology and phonology. *Neurology* 49:946–952.

Schecter, I., Bar-Isreal, J., Ben-Nun, Y., and Bergman, M. (1985). The phonemic analysis as a treatment method in dysgraphic aphasic patients. *Scand. J. Rehabil. Med. (Suppl.)* 12:80–83.

Schomer, D. L., Pegna, A., Matton, B., Sheck, M.,

Bidaut, L., Slossman, D., Roth, S., and Landis, T. (1998). Ictal agraphia, a patient study. *Neurology* 50:542–545.

Shallice, T. (1981). Phonological agraphia and the lexical route in writing. *Brain* 104:412–429.

Shallice, T., and Warrington, E. K. (1980). Single and multiple component central dyslexic syndromes. In *Deep Dyslexia*, M. Coltheart, K. E. Patterson, and J. C. Marshall (eds.). London: Routledge and Kegan Paul, pp. 119–145.

Silveri, M. C., Misciagna, S., Leggio, M. G., and Molinari, M. (1997). Spatial dysgraphia and cerebellar lesion: a case report. *Neurology* 48:1529–1532.

Sugishita, M., Toyokura, Y., Yoshioka, M., and Yamada, R. (1980). Unilateral agraphia after section of the posterior half of the truncus of the corpus callosum. *Brain Lang.* 9:212–223.

Tanaka, Y., Iwasa, H., and Obayashi, T. (1990) right hand agraphia and left hand apraxia following callosal damage in a right-hander. *Cortex* 26:665–671.

Tanridag, O., and Kirshner, H. S. (1985). Aphasia and agraphia in lesions of the posterior internal capsule and putamen. *Neurology* 35:1797–1801.

Trojano, L., and Chiacchio, L. (1994). Pure dysgraphia with relative sparing of lower-case writing. *Cortex* 30:499–501.

Valenstein, E., and Heilman, K. M. (1979). Apraxic agraphia with neglect-induced paragraphia. *Arch. Neurol.* 67:44–56.

Watson, R. T., and Heilman, K. M. (1983). Callosal apraxia. *Brain* 106:391–404.

Weisenberg, T., and McBride, K. E. (1964). Types of aphasia: the expressive. In *Aphasia, a Clinical and Psychological Study*, T. Weisenberg and K. E. McBride (eds.). New York: Hafner.

Wernicke, C. (1886). Nervenheilkunde. Die neueren Arbeiten uber Aphasie. *Fortschr. Med.* 4:463–482.

Yamadori, A., Osumi, Y., Ikeda, H., and Kanazawa, Y. (1980). Left unilateral agraphia and tactile anomia. Disturbances seen after occlusion of the anterior cerebral artery. *Arch. Neurol.* 37:88–91.

Yopp, K. S., and Roeltgen, D. P. (1987). Case of alexia and agraphia due to a disconnection of the visual input to and the motor output from an intact graphemic area. *J. Clin. Exp. Neuropsychol.* 9:42.

Zesinger, P., Pegna, A., and Rilleit, B. (1994). Unilateral dysgraphia of the dominant hand in a left-hander: a disruption of graphic motor pattern selection. *Cortex* 30:673–683.

8

Disorders of Visual–Spatial Perception and Cognition

MARTHA J. FARAH

Humans are visual creatures, and our brain organization reflects this. Vision is the main function of occipital cortex, and occupies much of parietal and temporal cortex as well. Even in the most anterior parts of the brain, as physically distant as possible from primary visual cortex, are areas dedicated to eye movement programming and visual working memory. One consequence of this organization is that lesions to many different parts of the brain can affect vision. The nature of the visual disturbance depends on the particular contribution that the damaged area would normally have made to vision.

This chapter will review disorders of visual processing in an order roughly corresponding to the stages of visual processing beginning with the earliest stages. For each disorder, its main behavioral features, associated lesion site, and implications for our understanding of normal vision will be discussed.

DISORDERS OF EARLY AND INTERMEDIATE VISION

VISUAL FIELD DEFECTS AND CORTICAL BLINDNESS

After the visual signal leaves the eye, where it receives some initial filtering, it projects to the thalamus, where it receives further processing, and then on to primary visual cortex, situated at the very back of the brain. Total destruction of primary visual cortex causes cortical blindness. Partial destruction causes partial blindness, and the location of the lesion within primary visual cortex corresponds to the location of the visual field defect, in a highly systematic way that reflects the retinotopic organization of primary visual cortex. With vascular lesions, it is common for some or all of the primary cortex in one hemisphere to be damaged, while the opposite hemisphere is unaffected. This results in blindness restricted to one-half of the visual field, or *hemianopia*. It sometimes called "homonymous hemianopia" to indicate that the blind regions are the same regardless of which eye is used to see.

In the days before computed tomographic (CT) scanning, the anatomy of primary visual cortex and the pathways from thalamus to visual cortex allowed lesions to be roughly localized from visual field defects. As shown in Figure 8–1, homonymous visual field defects imply that the lesion is posterior, because input from the two eyes merges anteriorly. Because the left optic radiation projecting to left visual cortex represents only the right visual field, and visa versa, visual field defects also reveal the side of the lesion. The altitude of the visual field defect is also informative, with lower-quadrant blindess suggesting a parietal

Figure 8–1. Correspondences between location of lesion within the visual system and pattern of visual field defects. (From Homans, J. (1945). *A Textbook of Surgery*. Springfield, IL: Charles C. Thomas.)

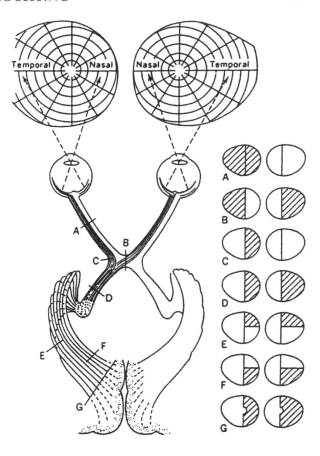

or superior occipital lesion because of the dorsal course of the pathways from thalamus to cortex, and upper-quadrant blindness suggesting a temporal or inferior occipital lesion because of the ventral course. An early and classic generalization about the anatomy of face recognition was based on this type of analysis. J.C. Meadows (1974) reviewed the visual field charts of a large number of cases of *prosopagnosia*, or face recognition impairment, and found a preponderance of left upper-quadrant defects, often with defects in the upper right as well. From this he was able to infer that the critical substrates for face recognition are in the right temporal cortex or bilateral temporal cortices in most people, a conclusion that has been confirmed with the advent of structural and functional brain imaging in recent years.

ACQUIRED COLOR BLINDNESS

Surrounding primary visual cortex is a set of cortical regions that receive their input principally from primary visual cortex. They maintain a retinotopic organization, although it is somewhat less precise than in primary visual cortex, and they carry out additional processing of the visual signal. The nature of this processing is not thoroughly understood, but at least one area, on the ventral surface of the brain, is known to play an important role in color perception.

The existence of a specialized cortical visual area for color was first suggested by patients with acquired cortical color blindness, also called acquired "cerebral achromotopsia" (see Zeki, 1990, for a review). Such patients report that the world seems drained of color, like a black-and-white movie. In other respects, their vision may be at least roughly normal. For example, they may have good acuity, motion and depth perception, and object recognition. It should be added that problems with face, object, and printed word recognition do sometimes accompany achromotopsia, but they are often transient and are likely to be caused by impairment to areas neighboring the color area. Cases in which the color vision impairment is truly selective imply that there is a brain region dedicated to color perception that is necessary for color perception and not for other aspects of vision.

The sudden loss of color vision has an impact on patients' lives in numerous ways. In one case, for example, a man was stopped by the police for running red lights. He could no longer select his own clothes each day, and required that food be placed in set positions so that he could discriminate mayonnaise and mustard from jam and ketchup. He found the changed appearance of food unappetizing, and began to eat only those foods that are naturally black and white: rice, olives, black coffee, and yogurt (Sacks and Wasserman, 1987).

In some cases, a unilateral lesion will result in color loss in just one hemifield, consistent with retinotopic mapping of the area responsible for color vision. A particularly selective and well-studied case of this was described by Damasio and colleagues (1980). Although acuity, depth perception, motion perception, and object recognition were normal in both hemifields, they differed strikingly for color perception: "He was unable to name any color in any portion of the left field of either eye, including bright reds, blues, greens and yellows. As soon as any portion of a colored object crossed the vertical meridian, he was able instantly to recognize and accurately name its color. When an object such as a red flashlight was held so that it bisected the vertical meridian, he reported that the hue of the right half appeared normal while the left half was gray." He was also unable to match colors in the left visual field.

The lesions in achromotopsia are usually on the inferior surface of the temporo-occipital region, in the lingual and fusiform gyri. In full achromotopsia they are bilateral, and in hemi-achromotopsia they are confined to the hemisphere contralateral to the color vision defect. This localization accords well with functional neuroimaging studies in which the substrates of color perception have been isolated by comparing cerebral activation patterns while subjects view colored displays to patterns resulting when gray-scale versions of the same displays are viewed (e.g., Zeki et al., 1991).

Achromotopsia should be distinguished from three other color-related disorders that sometimes follow brain damage in humans. *Color anomia* refers to an impairment in producing the names of colors. It is sometimes seen in isolation from anomia for other types of words (Goodglass et al., 1986) but it is not a disorder of color perception. There is no difficulty performing nonverbal tests of color perception and no subjective loss of color perception.

Color–object association is a task that has been used with a variety of different neuropsychological populations, from visually impaired to language impaired (DeRenzi and Spinnler, 1967). In a pure *disorder of color–object association*, the patient sees colors normally and knows how to use color names in the context of overlearned or abstract associations ("lemon yellow" or "green with envy"). But knowledge of the typical colors of objects in the absence of a verbal association is impaired. This could be one specific result of a more general impairment in visual image generation, to be discussed later in this chapter.

Color agnosia is a less clearly defined entity, said to involve a loss of knowledge about colors, and distinct from the other disorders reviewed here. Different authors seem to have different meanings in mind when they use this term (Farah, 2000). At least some of the data on color agnosia seem to require an explanation that is neither perceptual nor linguistic per se: Kinsbourne and Warrington (1964) showed that their patient could learn arbitrary associations between pairs of objects, noncolor names, and numbers, but could not learn associations between colors and noncolor names or numbers, nor between color names and other things. Furthermore, in these and other tasks, both the "colors" black, white and gray, and the names "black," "white," and "gray" were spared.

ACQUIRED MOTION BLINDNESS

There have been a small number of cases described of acquired cerebral motion blindness, or *cerebral akinotopsia* (see Zeki, 1993, for a review). By far the best-studied case is that of Zihl et al., (1983). This was case L.M., a 43-year-old woman who, following bilateral strokes in the posterior parietotemporal and occipital regions, was left with but one major impairment, namely the complete inability to perceive visual motion. Zihl et al. (1983) tested L.M.'s visual perception in a variety of simple experimental tasks and compared her performance with that of normal subjects. In her color and depth perception, object and word recognition, and a variety of other visual abilities tested by these authors, L.M. did not differ significantly from normal subjects. In addition, her ability to judge the motion of a tactile stimulus (wooden stick moved up or down her arm) and an auditory stimulus (tone-emitting loudspeaker moved through space) was also normal. In contrast, her perception of direction and speed of visual motion in horizontal and vertical directions within the picture plane and in depth was grossly impaired.

In her everyday life she was profoundly affected by her visual impairment. When pouring tea or coffee the fluid appeared to be frozen, like a glacier. Without being able to perceive movement, she could not stop pouring at the right time and frequently filled the cup to overflowing. Following conversations was difficult without being able to see the facial and mouth movements of each speaker, and gatherings of more than two other people left her feeling unwell and insecure. She complained that "people were suddenly here or there but I have not seen them moving." The patient could not cross the street because of her inability to judge the speed of a car. "When I see the car at first, it seems far away. But then, when I want to cross the road, suddenly the car is very near." She gradually learned to estimate the distance of moving vehicles by means of the sound becoming louder.

As with achromotopsia, the existence of akinotopsia implies a high degree of cerebral specialization, with one cortical area being necessary for motion perception and not necessary for other aspects of perception. Although L.M.'s lesions were fairly large and encompassed both parietal and temporal cortex, the critical lesion site has been inferred to be the posterior middle temporal gyrus. Functional neuroimaging studies of motion perception, comparing brain activation patterns to moving and static displays, show their maximum in this same region (Zeki et al., 1991).

DISORDERS OF HIGHER-LEVEL VISUAL–SPATIAL FUNCTION

AN ORGANIZING FRAMEWORK: THE TWO CORTICAL VISUAL SYSTEMS

Higher-level vision has two main goals; the identification of stimuli and their localization. Although a bit of an oversimplification, this dichotomy of function has provided a useful organizing framework for the neuropsychology of high-level vision. The two goals, sometimes abbreviated as "what" and "where," are achieved by relatively independent and anatomically separate systems, located in ventral and dorsal visual cortices, respectively, as shown in Figure 8–2. These have been termed "the two cor-

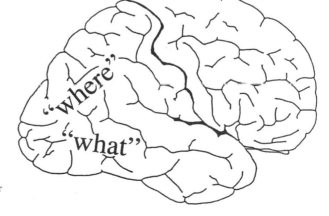

Figure 8–2. The two cortical visual systems. Dorsal visual areas are particularly important for spatial, or "where," processing, and ventral visual areas are particularly important for appearance, or "what," processing.

tical visual systems" (Ungerleider and Mishkin, 1982).

The earliest evidence for the existence of two cortical visual systems came from neurological case reports. Neurologists noted that some patients were selectively impaired at object recognition but retained good spatial abilities, and others were impaired at spatial vision but failed in object recognition (Potzl, 1928; Lange, 1936). Given the subjectively seamless experience of knowing what and where an object is when we look at it, these dissociations are striking. Dorsal simultanagnosic patients, with bilateral posterior parietal damage, may quickly and easily recognize an object (at least, once they have found it), but cannot point to it or describe its location relative to other objects in the scene (Holmes, 1918). Conversely, agnosic patients, with bilateral inferior occipitotemporal damage, may perform well on these simple localization tests as well as more complex tests of spatial cognition, while failing to recognize simple drawings of familiar objects, short printed words, or the faces of loved ones (Farah, 1990).

The same dissociation, in a weaker form, is found after unilateral right hemisphere brain damage. Newcombe and Russell (1969) tested World War II veterans with penetrating head wounds on two kinds of task. In the "closure" task, designed to tax visual recognition, patients had to judge the age and gender of faces rendered as fragmentary regions of light and shadow. In the maze task, designed to tax spatial processing, patients had to learn, by trial and error, the correct path through a matrix. Two subgroups of patients were defined, corresponding to the lowest 20% of scores on each of the two tests. The resulting subgroups were nonoverlapping, and indeed each group performed on a par with the remaining subjects on the other test, supporting the idea that "what" and "where" are processed independently. Furthermore, the men with poor closure performance all had posterior temporal lesions, whereas the men with poor maze performance all had posterior parietal lesions. Experimental studies of animals, using both lesions and single-unit recordings, add further support to the idea of a dorsal spatial visual system and a ventral pattern recognition system.

The clearest case of a visual disorder due to ventral system damage is *visual agnosia*, the impairment of visual recognition not due to more elementary visual problems or more general intellectual problems. Depending upon the precise location of damage, and whether it is confined to the left or right hemisphere or is bilateral, a patient may be agnosic for some kinds of object and not others. Face recognition may be primarily or perhaps even exclusively impaired (*prosopagnosia*), and the ability to recognize printed words may also be affected selectively (*pure alexia*). Visual agnosia, in its many forms, is the subject of Chapter 10 in this volume, and of a book by Farah (1990).

The most common form of visual disorder due to dorsal system damage is *hemispatial neglect*, a fascinating condition in which patients lose awareness of stimuli contralateral to a dorsal system lesion, but have no problem perceiving those same stimuli if moved to a non-neglected region of space. Neglect is also the subject of Chapter 13 in this volume. In addition to neglect, several other distinct problems with visual–spatial perception and cognition can follow lesions of the dorsal visual system. Four general types of visual–spatial disorders are reviewed here.

IMPAIRED PERCEPTION OF LOCATION

The ability to perceive the location of a single object can be impaired, resulting in a condition known as *visual disorientation*. Whether asked to point to or describe an object's location, the patient is grossly inaccurate. This is, not surprisingly, a disabling problem. The critical lesion site is the occipital–parietal junction, and in some cases a unilateral form of the disorder is observed after damage to either the left or right hemisphere alone (Riddoch, 1935).

IMPAIRED PERCEPTION OF LINE ORIENTATION

A subtler impairment of spatial perception, generally brought out by testing, is the impaired perception of line orientation. A widely used test of orientation perception is that of Benton et al. (1978), illustrated in Figure 8–3.

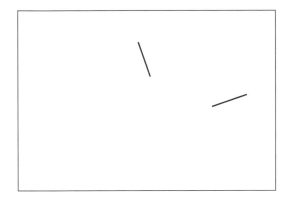

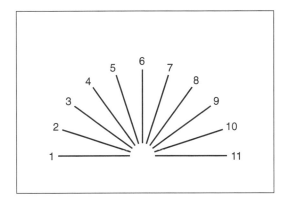

Figure 8–3. A typical item from the Benton, Varney, and Hamsher's (1978) test of orientation perception. The patient's task is to match the orientations of the test lines (*above*) with lines from the response set (*below*).

The spatial nature of the judgement and the minimal nature of the shape information involved suggests that this ability would depend strongly on parietal cortex and, indeed, that is the case. There is also a pronounced asymmetry in favor of greater right hemisphere involvement in this ability (De Renzi, 1982).

IMPAIRED VISUALLY GUIDED REACHING

Although it can be difficult to disentangle impairments of visual localization from impairments of visually guided reaching, a number of careful studies have done so (De Renzi, 1982). The latter impairment, also known as *optic ataxia*, is usually observed in unilateral form, but this generality covers a surprising array of variants. The left–right division may pertain to the hemispace, the reaching limb, or both, as when the left arm's reaches into the left hemi-

space are disproportionately less accurate than other limb–space combinations. In addition, some patients with unilateral lesions show a milder level of optic ataxia on the ispilesional side of space. Optic ataxia usually follows damage high in the parietal lobe, anterior to the regions most likely to cause visual disorientation. The precise scope of the impairment presumably depends on what parts of parietal gray and underlying white matter are damaged. Figure 8–4 shows how different combinations of hemispace and limb selectivity could result from interruption of the pathways from visual to motor cortex at different points.

IMPAIRED DRAWING AND BUILDING

This category has persisted in the clinical neuropsychology literature, under the label *constructional apraxia*, for many decades, probably because drawing and assembling objects are handy bedside tasks and are effective at revealing a range of spatial impairments. However, it is such a heterogeneous category that it is hardly a category at all. An enormous number of different underlying impairments can cause poor drawing or disorganized arrangements of puzzle parts, including motor and executive impairments as well as spatial impairments. Even for constructional apraxia following posterior lesions, there are pronounced differences between the effects of left and right hemisphere lesions, with the former generally resulting in spare, impoverished constructions and the latter resulting in abundantly detailed but disorganized constructions as illustrated in Figure 8–5 (McFie and Zangwill, 1960).

IMPAIRED TOPOGRAPHIC KNOWLEDGE

Patients can lose the ability to navigate their environment following damage to regions as diverse as posterior parietal cortex, and cingulate, parahippocampal, and lingual gyri. Their associated impairments are likewise variable. These two forms of variability can be understood in terms of differences in the underlying neurocognitive systems that are damaged in the different cases. A recent review by Aguirre and D'Esposito (1999) used cognitive theories of topographic orientation and information

Figure 8–4. Schematic diagram of different possible lesions interrupting visuomotor control, which would result in different patterns of limb and visual field differences in visually guided reaching. Lesions at points marked *1* and *4* would result in pure field selectivity and limb selectivity, respectively. Lesions at points marked *2* and *3* would result in both field and limb selectivity, contralateral and ispilateral, respectively. A lesion at *C* would result in a different pattern of field and limb selectivity, with contralateral combinations of limb and field, on either side, impaired (as in callosotomy patients). (From DeRenzi, E. (1982). *Disorders of Space Exploration and Cognition.* New York: John Wiley and Co.)

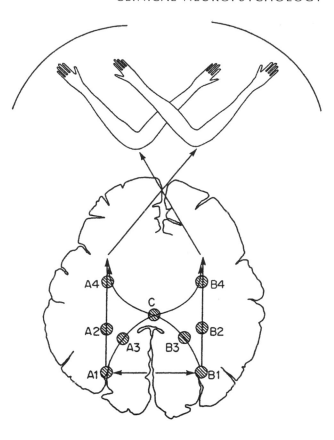

about lesion localization to arrive at a useful taxonomy of topographic disorders, which is summarized here. The different forms of topographic disorientation are informative about the organization of topographic knowledge in the normal brain. The patterns of preserved and impaired abilities described below suggest that spatial orientation in the environment involves both specialized topographic representations and more general spatial abilities, that spatial and landmark knowledge of the environment are subserved by different systems, and that the acquisition of topographic knowledge may be carried out by a specialized learning system.

Egocentric disorientation is the term used to describe patients whose topographic disorientation is secondary to visual disorientation. Not surprisingly, patients who cannot localize seen objects in space are severely handicapped in navigating both familiar and unfamiliar terrain. Of course, this form of topographic impairment is not specific to topographic knowledge. A representative case, described by Levine and col-

leagues (1985), was unable even to find his way around his own home, despite intact recognition of objects and landmarks. The critical lesion site, as noted earlier, is the posterior parietal and occipital juncture zone bilaterally.

Heading disorientation is a more specific impairment in spatial representation, consisting of the inability to perceive and remember the spatial relations among landmarks in the environment, and one's orientation relative to them. These patients, who are rare in the literature, do not have a more global form of visual disorientation, but are selectively impaired at way-finding, map use, and other tests of orientation in the environment. Three cases described by Takahashi et al. (1997) illustrate this disorder. The critical lesion site appears to be the posterior cingulate gyrus.

Landmark agnosia is an impairment of visual recognition that is selective or disproportionate for objects in the environment that normally serve as landmarks. These include buildings, monuments, squares, and so on. Patients with landmark agnosia, such as Pallis'

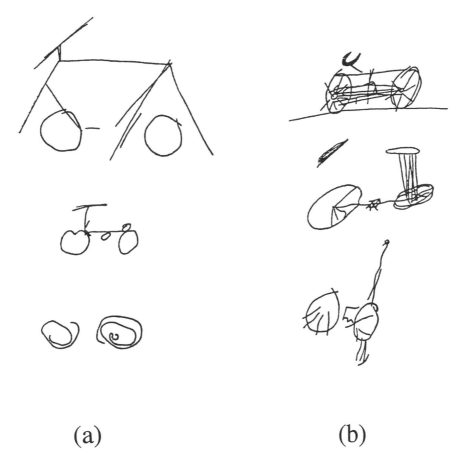

(a)   (b)

Figure 8–5. Examples of constructional apraxia in a bicycle drawing task following (a) left and (b) right hemisphere lesions. (From McFie, J., and Zangwill, O. L. (1960). Visual-constructive disabilities associated with lesions of the left cerebral hemisphere. *Brain 83*, 243–261.)

(1955) case, retain their spatial knowledge of the environment, as evidenced by good descriptions of routes, layouts, and maps. However, without the ability to discriminate one building from another, they cannot apply this knowledge. The typical lesions in landmark agnosia are similar to those of other visual agnosias, especially prosopagnosia, that is, the inferior surface of the occipitotemporal regions, either bilateral or right-sided.

Anterograde disorientation refers to a topographic impairment that encompasses both spatial and landmark knowledge, and is selective for the acquisition of this knowledge. Such patients show normal topographic abilities for environments that were familiar before their brain injury, but cannot learn to navigate new environments. Habib and Sirigu (1987) describe a typical case. The critical lesion site for

anterograde disorientation appears to be the right parahippocampal gyrus.

MENTAL IMAGERY

The most obvious function of the cortical visual system is the analysis of retinal inputs. Yet it is also used to represent visual and spatial information in the absence of triggering stimuli. When we imagine the appearance of an object or the layout of a scene from memory, we are using some of the same mechanisms in the occipital, temporal, and parietal lobes that are used when we recognize and localize physically present and visible stimuli.

Disorders of mental imagery can be grouped into three main categories: disorders of image representation, disorders of image generation, and disorders of image transformation. The first set includes imagery problems that appear secondary to loss of the underlying representations used in both imagery and perception. The second two include problems with imagery per se—either the ability to activate intact visual representations for the purpose of forming a mental image, or the ability to manipulate an image once formed.

DISORDERS OF IMAGE REPRESENTATION

If imagery and perception are both impaired after brain damage, this suggests that the functional locus of damage is the representations of visual appearance used by both. There are many reports of parallel impairments of imagery and perception, and these have attracted interest for what they can tell us about mental image representation. Specifically, they imply that mental imagery shares representations with the cortical visual system. A representative sample of these reports is presented here.

Color

Disorders of color imagery have often been noted, and the nature of the imagery impairment is generally similar to the perceptual impairment. For example, De Renzi and Spinnler (1967) investigated various color-related abilities in a large group of unilaterally brain-damaged patients and found an association between impairment on color vision tasks, such as the Ishihara test of color blindness, and on color imagery tasks, such as verbally reporting the colors of common objects from memory. Beauvois and Saillant (1985) studied the imagery abilities of a patient with a visual–verbal disconnection syndrome. The patient could perform purely visual color tasks (e.g., matching color samples) and purely verbal color tasks (e.g., answering questions such as "What color is associated with envy?") but could not perform tasks in which a visual representation of color had to be associated with a verbal label (e.g., color naming). When the patient's color imagery was tested purely visually, by selecting the color sample that represents the color of an object depicted in black and white, she did well. However, when the equivalent problems

were posed verbally (e.g., "What color is a peach?") she did poorly. In other words, mental images interacted with other visual and verbal task components as if they were visual representations. De Vreese (1991) reported two cases of color imagery impairment, one who had left occipital damage and displayed the same type of visual–verbal disconnection as the patient just described, and one who had bilateral occipital damage and parallel color perception and color imagery impairments.

Hemispatial Attention

In one of the best-known demonstrations of parallel impairments in imagery and perception, Bisiach and Luzzatti (1978) found that patients with hemispatial neglect for visual stimuli also neglected the contralesional sides of their mental images. Their two right parietal–damaged patients were asked to imagine a well-known square in Milan, shown in Figure 8–6. When they were asked to describe the scene from vantage point A on the map, they tended to name more landmarks on the east side of the square (marked with lower case a's in the figure)—that is, they named the landmarks on the right side of the imagined scene. When they were then asked to imagine the square from the opposite vantage point, marked B on the map, they reported many of the landmarks previously omitted (because these were now on the right side of the image) and omitted some of those previously reported.

"What" and "Where"

Levine and colleagues (1985) studied the roles of the two cortical visual systems in mental imagery. One patient had visual disorientation following bilateral parieto-occipital damage, and the other had visual agnosia following bilateral inferior temporal damage. We found that the preserved and impaired aspects of visual imagery paralleled the patients' visual abilities: the first case could neither localize visual stimuli in space nor accurately describe the locations of familiar objects or landmarks from memory. However, he was good at both perceiving object identity from appearance and describing object appearance from memory.

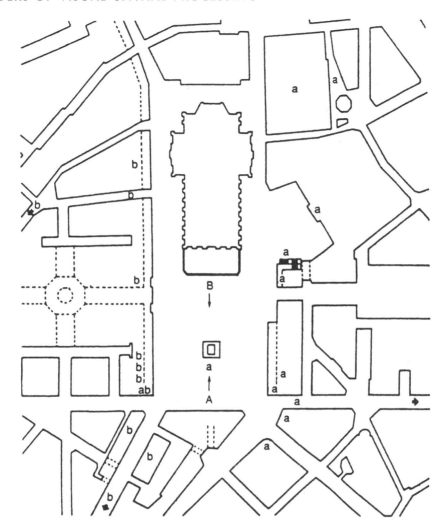

Figure 8–6. A map of the Piazza Del Duomo in Milan. When patients with left neglect were asked to imagine themselves standing at point A looking toward the cathedral, and to report what they saw in their "mind's eye," the locations they mentioned were those marked with a. When they repeated the procedure from the vantage point of B, they then mentioned the locations marked b. (From Farah, M. J. (1996). In *The Cognitive Neurosciences*, M. S. Gazzaniga (ed.). Cambridge, MA: MIT Press, p. 965.)

The second was impaired at perceiving object identity from appearance and describing object appearance from memory, but was good at localizing visual stimuli and at describing their locations from memory. In subsequent testing of the second patient, we found that he was impaired relative to control subjects on tasks that require imagining visual appearance (such as imagining animals and reporting whether they had long or short tails, imagining common objects and reporting their colors, and imagining triads of states within the U.S. and reporting which two are most similar in outline shape) but performed well on tasks that require imagining spatial properties (such as paths through a martix, mental rotation, and imagining triads of states and reporting which two are closest to one another; see Farah et al., 1988).

Visual Field

Shared representations for imagery and perception exist within occipital cortex as well. This was demonstrated by a patient with hemianopia for images and percepts following occipital resection. Our patient was an epileptic woman who was undergoing right occipital lobectomy. By testing her before and after her surgery, she could serve as her own control. If mental imagery consists of activating representations in the occipital lobe, then it should be impossible to form images in regions of the visual field that are blind because of occipital lobe destruction. This predicts that patients with homonymous hemianopia should have a smaller maximum image size, or visual angle of the mind's eye. By asking her to report the distance of imagined objects, such as a horse, breadbox, or ruler, when visualized as close as possible without "overflowing" her imaginal visual field, we could compute the visual angle of that field. We found that the size of her biggest possible image was reduced after surgery, as represented in Figure 8–7. Furthermore, by measuring maximal image size in the vertical and horizontal dimensions separately, we found that only the horizontal dimension of her imagery field was significantly reduced. These results provide strong evidence for the use of occipital visual representations during imagery.

Exceptions

Although patients with cortical visual damage usually manifest parallel impairments in their mental imagery, this is not always the case. For example, Bartolomeo and colleagues (1994) described preserved attention to the left sides of mental images in the presence of left visual neglect. Behrmann and colleagues (1992) and Servos and Goodale (1995) described severely agnosic patients who demonstrated good visual mental imagery abilities. On the face of things, these observations conflict with the hypothesis that imagery and visual perception share representations. Of course, earlier levels of representation in the central visual system may be less engaged by, and needed for, imagery than later levels, and it is possible that these cases of preserved imagery suffered damage to relatively earlier stages of processing. Even in the patient with the seemingly highest-level impairment, Behrmann et al.'s agnosic, there is evidence that the locus of damage is relatively early, in visual segmentation and grouping processes. A more detailed consideration of these discrepant findings and their implications is provided in Farah (2000).

To conclude, in most but not all cases of selective visual impairments following damage to the cortical visual system, patients manifest qualitatively similar impairments in mental imagery and perception. Central impairments of color perception tend to co-occur with impair-

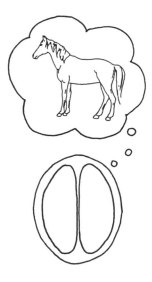

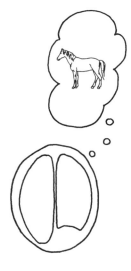

"I can get to within 15 feet of the horse in my imagination before it starts to overflow"

"The horse starts to overflow at an imagined distance of about 35 feet"

Figure 8–7. Depiction of the effects of unilateral occipital lobectomy on the visual angle of the mind's eye. (From Farah, M. J. (1996). In *The Cognitive Neurosciences*, M. S. Gazzaniga (ed.). Cambridge, MA: MIT Press, p. 968.)

ments of color imagery. Spatial attention impairments for the left side of the visual scene also affect the left side of mental images. Higher-order impairments of visual spatial orientation, sparing visual object recognition, and the converse, are associated with impairments of spatial imagery, sparing imagery for object appearance, and the converse. Finally, hemianopia resulting from surgical removal of one occipital lobe is associated with a corresponding loss of half the mind's eye's visual field. Taken together, these findings imply that at least some cortical visual representations perform "double duty," supporting both imagery and perception.

DISORDERS OF IMAGE GENERATION

If imagery consists of activating some of the same cortical visual areas used for perception, this raises the question of how these representations become activated in the absence of a stimulus. Whereas one cannot see a familiar object without recognizing it, one can think about familiar objects without inexorably calling to mind a visual mental image. This suggests that the activation of visual representations in imagery is a separate, voluntary process, needed for image generation but not for visual perception and object recognition.

Farah (1984) reviewed the neurological literature on imagery and identified a set of cases in which the underlying impairment seemed to be in image generation per se. In these cases perception was grossly intact, yet the patients complained of difficulty visualizing objects and scenes from memory. A few years later my colleagues and I encountered such a patient (Farah et al., 1988). The imagery impairment was demonstrated in a number of ways, including a sentence verification task developed by Eddy and Glass (1981). Half of the sentences required the use of visual imagery to verify a claim (e.g., "A grapefruit is larger than a canteloupe") and half did not (e.g., "The U.S. government functions under a two-party system"). Eddy and Glass had shown that normal subjects find the two sets of questions equally difficult (as did right hemisphere–damaged control subjects tested by Farah et al.), and that performance on the imagery questions was se-

lectively impaired by visual interference, thus validating them as imagery questions. R.M. showed a selective deficit for imagery on this validated task: he performed virtually perfectly on the nonimagery questions, and performed significantly worse on the imagery questions.

R.M. was also tested on imagery for the colors of objects, using black-and-white drawings of characteristically colored objects (e.g., a cactus, an ear of corn) for which we was to select the appropriate colored pencil. His imagery was further tested with drawing tasks. By these measures, too, his imagery was poor.

To infer a problem with image generation per se, as opposed to shared image–percept representations, R.M.'s object recognition and perceptual abilities were also tested. R.M. was not agnosic, and passed a stringent test of object recognition designed to assess long-term visual memory of the same items he was asked to image. In this test, R.M. was asked to select the correct drawing of an object from a pair. For example, a fish was either the correct shape or peanut-shaped. He performed this test perfectly. To assess color perception and long-term memory for object colors, different-colored versions of each drawing were presented and R.M. had to recognize which drawing was correctly colored. Although he did not perform perfectly on the color perception control condition, he did significantly better in this condition than in the imagery condition, with the same objects and colors.

The pattern of preserved and impaired abilities in R.M. is consistent with an impairment of mental image generation. In subsequent years, a small number of additional cases of selectively impaired imagery have been reported (e.g., Grossi et al., 1986; Riddoch, 1990; Goldenberg, 1992), as well as similar but weaker dissociations in subgroups of patients in group studies (Goldenberg, 1989; Bowers et al., 1991; Goldenberg and Artner, 1991; Stangalino et al., 1995).

What parts of the brain carry out image generation? This question has evoked controversy. Although mental imagery was for many years assumed to be a function of the right hemisphere, Ehrlichman and Barrett (1983) pointed out that there was no direct evidence for this assumption. Farah (1984) noted a trend in the cases she reviewed for left posterior damage. Farah et al. (1988) suggested that the left temporo-occipital area may be critical. This idea has met with a range of reactions.

Sergent (1990) argued against the hypothesis of left hemisphere specialization for image generation, concluding that "in spite of recent claims that the left hemisphere is specialized for the generation of visual mental images, an examination of the relevant data and experimental procedures provides little support for this view, and suggests that both hemispheres simultaneously and conjointly contribute to this process" (p. 98). Her conclusions followed persuasively from her reading of the literature, although one could take issue with this reading at a number of points. For example, our case study of patient R.M., whose performance on tests of image generation, object recognition, and color perception was described in the previous section, was discounted on the grounds that his object recognition and color perception were not tested.

Tippett (1992) arrived at a less extreme conclusion, declaring that "what is striking in this area is the pervasiveness of findings (especially with brain-damaged patients) that seem to implicate the left hemisphere in the image generation process" (p. 429) and concluded that "support is found for the involvement of the left hemisphere, although many researchers claim that the posterior regions of both hemispheres contribute to image generation" (p. 415).

A third view was expressed by Trojano and Grossi (1994), who reviewed the case report literature on mental imagery defects with and without accompanying visual recognition impairments. For the latter type of imagery defect, corresponding to the hypothesized image generation defect, they concluded that "mental imagery relies on dissociable processes which are localized in left hemisphere posterior areas" (p. 213). The recent focally damaged cases mentioned above (Grossi et al., 1986; Farah et al., 1988; Riddoch, 1991a; Goldenberg, 1992) have supported this suggestion, as have the group studies, to varying degrees (most clearly Goldenberg and Artner, 1991; Stangalino et al., 1995). The rarity of cases of image generation deficit suggests that this function may not be strongly lateralized in most

people; however, when impairments are observed after focal unilateral damage, the left or dominant hemisphere is implicated.

DISORDERS OF IMAGE TRANSFORMATION

The ability to visualize the spatial transformation of an object, whether currently in view or purely imaginary, allows one to simulate mentally the translation, enlargement, or rotation of the object. This ability is frequently called into play by our everyday spatial problem solving, for example, figuring out how to fit a big suitcase into a car trunk. Mental rotation is the most intensively studied mental image transformation, and virtually the only one studied in neurological patients.

As might be expected, given the fundamentally spatial character of mental rotation, the parietal lobes appear to be essential for this ability. Group studies of focally brain-damaged patients have invariably localized mental rotation to the parietal lobes, with some investigators supporting a predominantly right parietal locus (Ratcliff, 1979; Ditunno and Mann, 1990) and others suggesting left parietal superiority (Mehta and Newcombe, 1991). Consistent with these localizations, many functional neuroimaging studies have mapped the anatomy of mental rotation and almost invariably find bilateral parietal activation, greater on the right (e.g., see Corballis, 1997, for a review).

REFERENCES

Aguirre, G. K., and D'Esposito, M. (1999). Topographical disorientation: a synthesis and taxonomy. *Brain* 122:1613–1628.

Bartolomeo, P., D'Erme, P., and Gainotti, G. (1994). The relationship between visuospatial and representational neglect. *Neurology* 44:1710–1714.

Beauvois, M. F., and Saillant, B. (1985). Optic aphasia for colors and color agnosia: A distinction between visual and visuo-verbal impairments in the processing of color. *Cognitive Neuropsychology* 2:1–48.

Behrmann, M., Winocur, G., and Moscovitch, M. (1992). Dissociation between mental imagery and object recognition in a brain-damaged patient. *Nature* 359:636–637.

Benton, A. L., Varney, N. R., and Hamsher, K.

(1978). Visuospatial judgment: a clinical test. *Arch. Neurol.* 35:364–367.

Bisiach, E., and Luzzatti, C. (1978). Unilateral neglect of representational space. *Cortex* 14:129–133.

Bowers, D., Blonder, L. X., Feinberg, T., and Heilman, K. M. (1991). Differential impact of right and left hemisphere lesions on facial emotion and object imagery. *Brain* 114:2593–2609.

Corballis, M. C. (1997). Mental rotation and the right hemisphere. *Brain and Language* 57: 100–121.

Damasio, A. R., Yamada, T., Damasio, H., Corbett, J., and McKee, J. (1980). Central achromatopsia: behavioral, anatomic, and physiologic aspects. *Neurology* 30:1064–1071.

Davidoff, J., and Wilson, B. (1985). A case of visual agnosia showing a disorder of pre-semantic visual classification. *Cortex* 21:121–134.

De Renzi, E. (1982). *Disorders of Space Exploration and Cognition*. New York: John Wiley and Sons.

De Renzi, E., and Spinnler, H. (1967). Impaired performance on color tasks in patients with hemispheric lesions. *Cortex* 3:194–217.

De Vreese, L. P. (1991). Two systems for color naming defects. *Neuropsychologia* 29:1–18.

Ditunno, P. L., and Mann, V. A. (1990). Right hemisphere specialization for mental rotation in normals and brain damaged subjects. *Cortex* 26: 177–188.

Eddy, P., and Glass, A. (1981). Reading and listening to high and low imagery sentences. *J. Verbal Learn. Verbal Behav.* 20:333–345.

Ehrlichman, H., and Barrett, J. (1983). Right hemispheric specialization for mental imagery: a review of the evidence. *Brain Cogn.* 2:55–76.

Farah, M. J. (1984). The neurological basis of mental imagery: a componential analysis. *Cognition* 18:245–272.

Farah, M. J. (1990). *Visual Agnosia: Disorders of Object Recognition and What They Tell Us About Normal Vision*. Cambridge, MA: MIT Press/Bradford Books.

Farah, M. J. (2000). *The Cognitive Neuroscience of Vision*. Oxford: Blackwell Publishers.

Farah, M. J., Hammond, K. L., Levine, D. N., and Calvanio, R. (1988). Visual and spatial mental imagery: dissociable systems of representation. *Cogn. Psychol.* 20:439–462.

Goldenberg, G. (1989). The ability of patients with brain damage to generate mental visual images. *Brain* 112:305–325.

Goldenberg, G. (1992). Loss of visual imagery and loss of visual knowledge—a case study. *Neuropsychologia* 30:1081–1099.

Goldenberg, G., and Artner, C. (1991). Visual imagery and knowledge about the visual appearance of objects in patients with posterior cerebral artery lesions. *Brain Cogn.* 15:160–186.

Goodglass, H., Wingfield, A., Hyde, M. R., and Theurkauf, J. C. (1986). Category-specific dissociations in naming and recognition by aphasic patients. *Cortex* 22:87–102.

Grossi, D., Orsini, A., and Modafferi, A. (1986). Visuoimaginal constructional apraxia: On a case of selective deficit of imagery. *Brain Cogn.* 5:255–267.

Habib, M., and Sirigu, A. (1987). Pure topographical disorientation and anatomical basis. *Cortex* 23:73–85.

Holmes, G. (1918). Disturbances of visual orientation. *Br. J. Ophthalmol.* 2:449–468, 506–518.

Kinsbourne, M. and Warrington, E. K. (1964). Observations on colour agnosia. *J. Neurol. Neurosurg. Psychiatry* 27:296–299.

Lange, J. (1936). Agrosien und Apraxien. In *Handbuch der Neurologie*, O. Bunke and O. Foerster (eds.). Berlin: Springer-Verlag.

Levine, D. N., Warach, J., and Farah, M. J. (1985). Two visual systems in mental imagery: dissociation of "what" and "where" in imagery disorders due to bilateral posterior cerebral lesions. *Neurology* 35:1010–1018.

McFie, J., and Zangwill, O. L. (1960). Visual constructive disabilities associated with lesions of the left cerebral hemisphere. *Brain* 83:243–260.

Meadows, J. C. (1974). The anatomical basis of prosopagnosia. *J. Neurol. Neurosurg. Psychiatry* 37:489–501.

Mehta, Z., and Newcombe, F. (1991). A role for the left hemisphere in spatial processing. *Cortex* 27:153–167.

Newcombe, F., and Russell, W. (1969). Dissociated visual perceptual and spatial deficits in focal lesions of the right hemisphere. *J. Neurol. Neurosurg. Psychiatry* 32:73–81.

Pallis, C. A. (1955). Impaired identification of faces and places with agnosia for colors. *J. Neurol. Neurosurg. Psychiatry* 18:218–224.

Potzl, O. (1928). *Die Aphasielehre vom Standpunkte der Klinishcen Psychiatrie*. Leipzig: Franz Deudicte.

Ratcliff, G. (1979). Spatial thought, mental rotation and the right cerebral hemisphere. *Neuropsychologia* 17:49–54.

Riddoch, G. (1935). Visual disorientation in homonymous half-fields. *Brain* 58:376–382.

Riddoch, J. M. (1990). Loss of visual imagery: a generation deficit. *Cogn. Neuropsychol.* 7:249–273.

Sacks, O., and Wasserman, R. (1987). The case of the colorblind painter. *New York Review of Books* 25–34.

Sergent, J. (1990). The neuropsychology of visual image generation: data, method, and theory. *Brain Cogn.* 13:98–129.

Servos, P., and Goodale, M. A. (1995). Preserved visual imagery in visual form agnosia. *Neuropsychologia* 33:1383–1394.

Stangalino, C., Semenza, C., and Mondini, S. (1995). Generating visual mental images: deficit after brain damage. *Neuropsychologia* 33:1473–1483.

Takahashi, N., Kawamura, M. K. S., Kasahata, N., and Hirayama, K. (1997). Pure topographic disorientation due to right retrosplenial lesion. *Neurology* 49:464–469.

Tippett, L. J. (1992). The generation of visual images: a review of neuropsychological research and theory. *Psychol. Bull.* 112:415–432.

Trojano, L., and Grossi, D. (1994). A critical review of mental imagery defects. *Brain Cogn.* 24:213–243.

Tranel, D. (1997). Disorders of color processing (perception, imagery, recognition, and naming). In *Behavioral Neurology and Neuropsychology*, T. E. Feinberg and M. J. Farah (eds.). New York: McGraw Hill, pp. 257–265.

Ungerleider, L. G., and Mishkin, M. (1982). Two cortical visual systems. In *Analysis of Visual Behavior*, D. J. Ingle, M. A. Goodale, and R. J. W. Mansfield (eds.). Cambridge, MA: MIT Press, pp. 549–586.

Zeki, S. (1990). A century of cerebral achromatopsia. *Brain* 113:1721–1777.

Zeki, S. (1993). *A Vision of the Brain*. Oxford: Blackwell Scientific Publications.

Zeki, S., Watson, J. D. G., Lueck, C. J., Friston, K., Kennard, C., and Frackowiak, R. S. (1991). A direct demonstration of functional specialization in human visual cortex. *J. Neurosci.* 11:641–649.

Zihl, J., von Cramon, D., and Mai, N. (1983). Selective disturbance of movement vision after bilateral brain damage. *Brain* 106:313–340.

9

Acalculia and Disturbances of the Body Schema

NATALIE L. DENBURG AND DANIEL TRANEL

We review in this chapter the recent literature on acalculia and body schema disturbances. Neither of these conditions is common in clinical neuropsychology, although interestingly, both have attracted a considerable amount of research attention. Both conditions have been inconsistently defined, and not surprisingly, this has contributed to a tremendous confusion in the literature as to their specific neuropsychological and neuroanatomical correlates. Moreover, the disorders of acalculia, finger agnosia, and right–left disorientation have the (mis)fortune of being part of the tetrad of manifestations which comprise the Gerstmann syndrome (the other being agraphia), the reality and significance of which has been repeatedly and forcefully questioned (e.g., Benton, 1961, 1977, 1992; Critchley, 1966). Thus, a review of the literature on the topics of acalculia and body schema disturbances immediately encounters some major obstacles: neither condition has a consensual set of neuroanatomical correlates, which means the "localizing" value of these signs in clinical neuropsychology is fairly weak; moreover, both conditions are relatively infrequent, at least in terms of being the nuclear component of a neuropsychological presentation, and, thus, both are frequently ne-

glected in the clinical training of neuropsychologists, and both have suffered from a lack of availability of well-standardized and validated assessment procedures. Nonetheless, the conditions remain viable topics for clinical neuropsychology, and in fact, there have been a recent resurgence of interest in different aspects of mathematical (cf. Butterworth, 1999) and body schema processing (cf. Damasio, 1999).

Our review focuses on the recent literature, and in particular, on studies published in the past decade. As will be seen, the majority of investigations are case studies, covering a wide range of neurological conditions, including focal lesions, head injuries, cerebral tumors, degenerative diseases, and many others. We have chosen to be fairly inclusive in our review, in order to give a flavor for the wide variety of disturbances of math processing or body schema processing that can develop in connection with brain injury. One ramification of our inclusive approach, though, is that the reader will encounter a somewhat bewildering array of different lesion types, different lesion loci, and different profiles of neuropsychological dysfunction. We will attempt a synthesis of the main findings, with regard to each of the main topics.

ACALCULIA

Acalculia refers to an acquired neuropsychological condition in which patients with previously normal calculation abilities develop impairments in processing numbers as a consequence of acquired brain dysfunction. The prevailing conception is that acalculia is caused by a left parietal lobe lesion, and that it is frequently accompanied by aphasia. However, as the studies reviewed below indicate, it is evident that acalculia can result from damage to numerous brain regions, in either hemisphere. As alluded to earlier, these rather equivocal findings are likely attributable to a multitude of issues, including how the condition is defined, strategies employed in clinical and research studies, and the complex, multifaceted nature of the cerebral and cognitive processes involved in calculation. Furthermore, acalculia can arise in connection with a variety of neurological conditions which cause cerebral lesions, including stroke, tumor, traumatic brain injury, and degenerative conditions.

TERMINOLOGY

In 1919, Henschen coined the term "Akalkulia" to refer to an acquired calculation disturbance. Berger (1926) and later Grewel (1952) offered and further refined, respectively, the terms "primary" and "secondary" acalculia. *Primary* (also known as "pure") *acalculia* refers to acalculia that cannot be attributed to defects in other cognitive domains. In *secondary acalculia*, calculation disturbances are attributable, at least in part, to defects of attention, memory, or language. Hécaen et al., (1961) proposed a heuristically useful tripartite system for classifying patients with acalculia. Their classification involved the following:

1. *Acalculia with alexia and agraphia for numbers* may or may not be accompanied by aphasia. Here, calculation disturbances occur as a result of impaired reading or writing of numbers. This form of acalculia is thought to be caused primarily by left hemisphere (especially parietal) lesions. An example of this type of impairment is shown in Figure 9–1.

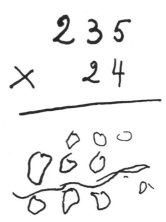

Figure 9–1. Example of agraphia for numbers. (From Hécaen et al., 1961. Reprinted with permission of the publisher.)

2. *Acalculia of the spatial type* refers to disordered spatial organization of numbers, related to visual neglect, misalignment of numbers, and number inversions. This form of acalculia is thought to be caused primarily by right hemisphere lesions. An example of this type of impairment is shown in Figure 9–2.

3. *Anarithmetria* is diagnosed when acalculia does not conform to either of the above two classifications. The term denotes a primary acalculia. This form of acalculia is thought to be caused primarily by left hemisphere lesions, but can occur, albeit with less frequency, following right hemisphere lesions.

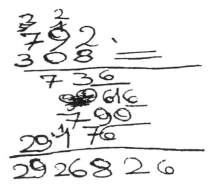

Figure 9–2. Example of disordered spatial alignment of numbers. (From Semenza et al., 1997. Reprinted with permission of the publisher.)

Taken together, the two classification systems outlined above have considerable overlap. That is, Hécaen et al.'s (1961) first two classifications fit nicely with Berger (1926) and Grewel's (1952) term "secondary acalculia." As stated previously, Hécaen et al.'s (1961) third classification is more or less synonymous with primary acalculia (Berger, 1926; Grewel, 1952).

To our knowledge, the last comprehensive review of acalculia appeared in the early 1990s, and we will concentrate on the literature published since that time. For reviews of the historical literature, the reader is referred to Boller and Grafman (1983), Grafman (1988), and Levin et al. (1993). In an attempt to synthesize the acalculia literature, we have organized our review according to a framework adapted from McCloskey and associates (McCloskey et al., 1985; McCloskey, 1992). We will outline a number of notable dissociations, which suggest that a significant degree of modularity exists for calculation in the human brain. We begin by reviewing case studies, and then turn our attention to group studies.

CASE STUDIES

Selective Impairment of Numeral Production

This refers to a dissociation between numeral comprehension (intact) and numeral production (impaired). Benson and Denckla (1969) illustrated two left hemisphere–damaged cases in which calculation disturbance appears attributable to paraphasic or paragraphic errors (i.e., substituting one number for another) and not defective computational processing, per se. That is, when presented with verbal or written calculation problems, the subjects committed errors (e.g., when asked to write "two hundred and twenty-one," case 1 produced "215"); however, when presented with the answers in a multiple-choice format, the subjects were able to discern the correct answer.

Selective Impairment of Syntactic Processing in Arabic Numeral Production

This refers to impairments in syntactic processing of numbers in the context of intact lexical processing. Singer and Low (1933) pre-

sented the unusual case of a patient who became acalculic following carbon monoxide poisoning. When verbal numbers (e.g., two hundred forty-two) were presented aurally and the patient was asked to write the Arabic equivalents, he produced responses in which the individual digits were correct but the order of magnitude was incorrect (e.g., "two hundred and forty-two" was written as "20042"). However, intact comprehension was assumed, given that the patient was accurate in his judgment of which of two spoken verbal numbers were larger. Macoir et al., (1999) observed a similar deficit in a patient with acalculia and language disturbances following a left inferior and posterior parietal cerebrovascular accident (CVA). The patient demonstrated a selective impairment in number transcoding (e.g., "nine thousand nine hundred and one" was written as "90901"), in the context of intact numerical comprehension abilities. A similar case was presented by Cipolotti and colleagues (1994).

Selective Impairment of Operation Symbol Comprehension

This refers to a selective deficit in the comprehension of written operation symbols. Ferro and Botelho (1980) presented two cases that illustrate this condition. A patient who suffered an intracerebral hematoma in the left temporo-occipital junction and a patient who suffered a left hemisphere stroke manifested a disturbance of processing arithmetical signs (e.g., they could not differentiate + from −) as their only symptom of acalculia. The authors termed this condition "asymbolic acalculia." Although both of these patients were also aphasic, their asymbolic acalculia could not be accounted for by their aphasia.

Selective Impairment of Calculation Ability

This refers to a dissociation between fact retrieval (intact) and calculation ability (impaired). Warrington (1982) presented the case of a severely acalculic patient who suffered a left parietal intracerebral hematoma. Although he demonstrated preserved counting and estimation of quantity and knowledge of number facts (e.g., he knew the boiling point of water), simple calculations were impaired. Similarly, Hittmair-Delazer and colleagues (1995) studied a patient who demonstrated severe problems with basic arithmetic following a bone marrow transplant with extensive irradiation and chemotherapy. Although the patient was unable to answer very simple arithmetic problems ("What is 2 + 3?"), he maintained intact processing of algebraic expressions and an understanding of complex arithmetic text problems. Semenza and colleagues (1997) followed a 17-year-old male who suffered from some prenatal or early developmental neurological insult that began to reveal itself at 6 months of age (asymmetry in posture and movement). Early computed tomography (CT) visualized hydrocephalus affecting right dorsolateral cortex as well as the right upper parietal lobe. These authors report a specific deficit for calculation ability, in the context of intact arithmetic factual knowledge (e.g., counting dots, transcoding from spoken to arabic numerals, magnitude estimation, recounting personal and nonpersonal number facts, such as dates).

Multiple Deficits in Calculation

Delazer and Benke (1997) assessed a patient with severe calculation problems (in addition to agraphia, finger agnosia, right–left disorientation, and apraxia) resulting from a left parietal lobe tumor. The patient maintained some "memorized fact knowledge" described as superficial (times tables, and some additions and subtractions), while she completely lost conceptual knowledge of arithmetic and performed very poorly on most calculation tasks. In terms of conceptual knowledge, the patient lost all ability to implement back-up strategies when faced with a calculation task for which she was unable to work out the answer. That is, when offered strategies such as using paper and pencil, a written number line, her fingers, or a pile of tokens, the patient was unable to implement these strategies effectively. Similarly, the patient demonstrated an inability to derive unknown facts from known ones; for example, two arithmetic problems were presented pairwise so that the answer for one problem could be inferred from the other (commutativity; "If 13 + 9 = 22, what is 9 + 13?"). The authors noted that the patient's ability to reason verbally, as measured by tasks of conceptualization and matrix reasoning, was preserved despite impaired conceptual knowledge of arithmetic.

Dissociation of Arithmetic Operations

This refers to the ability to execute particular, but not all, arithmetic operations. Benson and Weir (1972) presented the case of a patient with a generally isolated calculation disturbance resulting from left parietal lobe pathology. An intriguing dissociation was demonstrated in that the patient maintained the ability to complete addition and subtraction problems accurately, while displaying grave difficulty with multiplication and division problems. Grafman and colleagues (1989) studied the case of a patient with Alzheimer's disease who presented with primary calculation complaints. Two years of follow-up evaluations revealed an ensuing dissolution of his arithmetic abilities. This patient showed the functional dissociation of being able to add and subtract accurately, but not being able to multiply or divide. A similar case, albeit resulting from a left frontal infarction, demonstrated intact addition and subtraction in the context of impaired multiplication (Tohgi et al., 1995). Finally, Lampl and colleagues (1994) examined a patient with acalculia following a left parietotemporal hemorrhage. The patient retained the ability to subtract, without being able to perform any other arithmetic operations, which supports the idea that different processing systems may underlie each of the basic arithmetic operations.

Selective Impairment of Digit Naming

Digit naming can be impaired in patients who otherwise have no difficulty in mental arithmetic. Cipolotti and Butterworth (1995; see also Butterworth, 1999) described a patient with a progressive neurological degenerative condition of unknown etiology. Neuropsychological testing revealed multiple language deficits, including nonfluent, telegraphic speech and a deterioration of writing skills. On the calculation test, the patient manifested a severe and isolated difficulty in transcoding skills; that is, he demonstrated impairments in the reading of arabic numerals and written number names, the writing of arabic numerals from dictation, and the transcoding from written number names to arabic numerals (e.g., stimulus: "seven hundred thousand," response: "7,000,000"). In contrast, the patient was able to perform oral and written calculations, including number repetition, without error. The authors concluded that naming a digit can occur without necessarily accessing its semantic code.

Case Studies of Subcortical Lesions and Acalculia

Acalculia has been historically associated with lesions of the cortex, but a number of recent case studies demonstrate that subcortical impairments can also cause acalculia. Corbett and colleagues (1986) presented the case of a patient with acalculia following a subcortical infarct involving the head of the left caudate nucleus, the anterior superior putamen, and the anterior limb of the internal capsule extending superiorly into the periventricular white matter. Similarly, Whitaker et al. (1985) illustrated a severe acalculic presentation with normal language functions in a 79-year-old woman who suffered a deep left hemisphere infarction that involved the anterior and posterior lentiform nucleus.

Other Case Studies

Dehaene and Cohen (1997) reported two patients with "pure anarithmetria." Case 1 sustained a left subcortical lesion and case 2 sustained a right inferior parietal lesion. Both patients could read arabic numerals and write them to dictation, but they experienced a notable calculation deficit. In addition, case 1 demonstrated a selective deficit of rote verbal knowledge (e.g., arithmetic tables) despite intact semantic knowledge of numerical quantities. Case 2 showed the opposite pattern. This double dissociation suggests that distinct arithmetic cerebral pathways exist, with the left subcortical network being specialized for storage and retrieval of verbal arithmetic facts, while the bilateral inferior parietal network is dedicated to mental manipulation of numerical quantities. Acalculia arising from frontal lesions has also been reported (Lucchelli and De Renzi, 1993; Tohgi et al., 1995).

GROUP STUDIES

Group studies have been utilized primarily to study the relationship between hemispheric impairment and calculation abilities, and to further validate the findings from case studies. Many aspects of calculation involve verbal processing, hence, acalculia is commonly associated with aphasia. However, as suggested by Hécaen et al. (1961), acalculia can also be caused by right hemisphere lesions. According to Cohn (1961), right hemisphere–damaged individuals may demonstrate left visual field neglect and visuospatial defects, including difficulties in horizontal positioning, vertical columnar alignment, and transportation of numbers, that contribute to calculation disturbances.

Left Hemisphere Lesions

Delazer and associates (1999) studied the calculation abilities in 50 patients with focal left hemisphere lesions and in 15 control subjects. On the basis of aphasia testing, patients were placed in one of five groups: amnesic aphasics, Broca aphasics, global aphasics, Wernicke aphasics, and nonaphasics. Calculation error rates correlated with the severity of the language deficit: global aphasics displayed the most severe defects, while amnesic aphasics displayed the mildest impairments. In all patient groups, addition was the strongest operation while multiplication proved the most difficult. Additionally, Broca aphasics displayed a number of interesting findings, including particularly poor reading of Arabic numerals (relative to number words), a high incidence of syntactic errors, which was thought to reflect a more general impairment in syntactic skills, and disordered multiplication as compared to subtraction. These authors concluded that calculation abilities are mediated to a significant degree by linguistic functions.

Right Hemisphere Lesions

Ardila and Rosselli (1994) assessed the performance of 21 patients with right hemisphere damage. Of note, the average educational level of this sample was 7.01 years (range 5–15), which is very low given current education trends (U.S. Census, 1987). The patient group was further broken down by lesion site into prerolandic (6 patients) and retrorolandic (15 patients). For both groups, written calculation was considerably more difficult and error-prone than mental arithmetic. Spatial problems in the reading and writing of numbers were also observed. Error analysis suggested that acalculia was more frequently observed in the retrorolandic group.

Left and Right Hemisphere Lesions

One of the first large-scale studies to compare left and right hemisphere damaged patients on the same battery of calculation tasks was undertaken by Grafman et al. (1982). These investigators studied the presence of two of Hécaen et al.'s (1961) three acalculia classifications (i.e., anarithmetria and acalculia of the spatial type) in left and right hemisphere–damaged patients. Seventy-six patients with in-

tact ability to read and write numbers and 26 controls were administered a written calculation task and a brief neuropsychological battery. The patients were further divided into the following experimental groups: left anterior without visual field defect, left posterior with visual field defect, right anterior without visual field defect, and right posterior with visual field defect. The calculation task was scored both quantitatively and qualitatively; this latter scoring attribute involved application of Benton's Visual Retention Test scoring scheme (Sivan, 1992). Figure 9–3 displays the performance of patients and controls. As can be seen, patients with left hemisphere lesions committed the greatest number of errors; furthermore, the left posterior lesion group performed the most poorly relative to the other experimental groups for qualitative errors. The results were unchanged when these investigators employed age-, education-, and neuropsychological-group adjustments. Therefore, this study demonstrates that acalculia is particularly salient in left posterior lesions irrespective of language and visuospatial abilities.

Jackson and Warrington (1986) studied acalculia in 56 left hemisphere–damaged patients, 67 right hemisphere–damaged patients, and 100 control subjects. All subjects were admin-

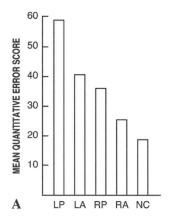
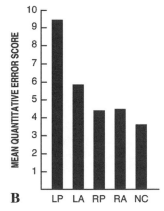
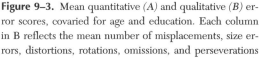

Figure 9–3. Mean quantitative (A) and qualitative (B) error scores, covaried for age and education. Each column in B reflects the mean number of misplacements, size errors, distortions, rotations, omissions, and perseverations for each group. LP, left posterior; LA, left anterior; RP, right posterior; RA, right anterior; NC, controls. (From Grafman et al., 1982. Reprinted with permission of the publisher.)

istered the Graded Difficulty Arithmetic Test (GDA; Jackson and Warrington, 1986), which is a speeded test of addition and subtraction abilities. The left hemisphere group was significantly impaired on the GDA relative to the right hemisphere group and controls. In contrast, the right hemisphere group's performance did not differ from that of the controls.

Dahmen and colleagues (1982) compared 20 Wernicke's aphasics, 20 Broca's aphasics, 20 patients with right retrorolandic lesions, and 40 normal controls on a calculation task that involved items differing in the degree of spatial and linguistic processing required for successful completion. Wernicke aphasics performed significantly poorer than the other subjects on calculation tasks with a spatial component (e.g., alignment of numbers). The investigators summarized their findings as being consistent with the lesion location in Wernicke's aphasia, involving the temporoparietal cortices, and suggested that spatial visualization plays an important role in the calculation disorders of Wernicke's aphasics.

Given the high comorbidity between language disorders and acalculia, Deloche and Seron (1982) investigated whether these two disorders are the result of damage to a cognitive component shared by the two systems, or from damage to two different components. Seven Broca aphasics and seven Wernicke aphasics were administered two tasks, involving the transcoding of written numerals (e.g., two hundred and forty-eight) into digit strings (248), and the error types of each aphasic group were compared. It was hypothesized that Broca aphasics would evidence faulty calculation as a result of grammatical errors, while Wernicke aphasics would demonstrate acalculia as a result of lexical and serial order errors. As hypothesized, the authors found distinct error patterns in the two groups of aphasics. It was concluded that the number-processing disorders in Broca and Wernicke aphasics were parallel to their language deficits, thus suggesting that the disorders result from damage to a shared cognitive component. In a follow-up study, Seron and Deloche (1983) reversed their task to the transcoding of digit strings (248) into written numerals (two hundred and forty-

eight), and found results comparable to the Deloche and Seron (1982) findings.

Rosselli and Ardila (1989) examined the calculation deficits of 41 left hemisphere– and 21 right hemisphere–damaged patients. Patients with left hemisphere lesions were further subdivided into seven subgroups: prefrontal, Broca aphasics, conduction aphasics, Wernicke aphasics, anomic aphasics, alexia without agraphia, and global aphasias. Right hemisphere patients were subdivided into anatomical groups of prerolandic and retrorolandic. As in other studies, the aphasic subgroups performed differentially on a calculation task, evincing discrete degrees and types of errors. More specifically, the patients with global aphasia displayed the greatest number of calculation disturbances. In contrast, prefrontal patients performed more strongly on the calculation task. Finally, Wernicke aphasics demonstrated relatively greater difficulty on tasks that necessitated spatial abilities.

Basso and colleagues (2000) compared the calculation performance of 50 left hemisphere–damaged patients, 26 right hemisphere–damaged patients, and 211 control subjects using the Assessment Battery for Calculation and Number Processing (Deloche et al., 1994), which consists of 13 tasks and numerous subtasks. On the basis of performance on language tests, the left hemisphere group was further divided into the following experimental groups: Broca aphasics (16), Wernicke aphasics (18), and nonaphasics (16). Using the number of tasks failed by normal controls as a marker, these authors were able to classify patients as "clinically acalculic" if they failed three or more tasks on the Calculation Battery. Eight Broca (50%) and 11 Wernicke (61%) aphasics fell in this acalculic classification. However, the authors underscored that a high percentage of aphasic patients were not clinically acalculic. Using this same criterion, only two of the nonaphasics (13%), three of the right hemisphere–damaged (12%), and four of the controls (2%) were deemed acalculic. The relationship between acalculia and spatial disorders was less clear-cut, with the exception of finding that the three right brain–damaged acalculic patients also had constructional apraxia.

EXPERIMENTAL INVESTIGATION OF NEURAL CORRELATES OF NUMBER PROCESSING

The findings described above highlight the widespread distribution of calculation processes in the brain. The case studies, in particular, additionally suggest that there are dissociable brain circuits for different aspects of number processing. However, the precise functional role of particular brain regions in calculation remains uncertain, and researchers have recently employed a number of other methods to corroborate and extend lesion studies conducted in acalculic patients. These methods include cortical and thalamic stimulation, electrophysiology event-related potentials [ERPs], metabolic studies, and functional neuroimaging (positron emission tomography [PET], functional magnetic resonance imaging [fMRI]).

Ojemann (1974) tested the effect of thalamic stimulation on calculation abilities. Specifically, 26 patients were asked to complete a simple mental arithmetic task of counting backwards by 3's while undergoing therapeutic stereotaxic thalamotomy. Acceleration in the rate of counting backwards and an increase in error rate were demonstrated in patients who underwent left thalamic stimulation. In contrast, right thalamic–stimulated patients displayed a slowed rate of counting, as well as an increase in error rate, and a longer latency to state the first serial subtraction. The findings suggest that both the right and left thalamus contribute to mental arithmetic.

Papanicolaou and colleagues (1983) administered arithmetic and visuospatial tasks to 14 normal participants, while recording ERPs at the temporal and parietal areas of both the left and right hemispheres. Left temporal lobe activation was observed during the arithmetic task. The visuospatial task activated left temporal, left parietal, and right parietal brain regions, with the greatest amount of activation occurring in the right hemisphere relative to the left.

Whalen and associates (1997) studied a young patient with a left parasagittal parietal region brain tumor and associated seizure disorder. At the age of 9, the patient underwent surgery to remove the tumor; however, recurrence was noted at the age of 16. Prior to a second neurosurgery, electrodes were placed in the patient's left hemisphere in an effort to localize the seizure focus and to map the cognitive functions that may be affected by the resection. In doing so, the researchers were able to examine the effects of mild stimulation of localized brain regions on sensory, motor, and cognitive tasks, including calculation. Neuropsychological examination revealed average intellect for both verbal and performance domains and normal academic achievement, in addition to intact language abilities. After determining that stimulation of particular sites did not affect the patient's attentional or expressive speech abilities, the results revealed that multiplication was significantly disrupted relative to addition. More specifically, stimulation at a left parietal site impaired performance on single-digit multiplication problems, likely also disrupting the retrieval of stored multiplication facts.

Using PET, Dehaene et al. (1996) examined the regional cerebral blood flow patterns underlying two simple mental calculation tasks—single-digit multiplication and number comparison (i.e., selection of which of two numbers is largest)—relative to a resting condition, in eight healthy participants. For the comparison task, there was an absence of activation of critical brain regions with the exception of those areas necessary for basic stimulus identification and response selection. However, a trend for bilateral inferior parietal region activity was noted. Regarding multiplication, the inferior parietal region was activated bilaterally, as were the left fusiform–lingual region and left lenticular nucleus, suggesting a role for these structures in multiplication. The authors underscore that no activation was found in the left and right angular gyri for either task. Finally, the rather distinct neuroanatomical activation involved in number comparison versus multiplication suggested that these two arithmetic functions may be subserved by distinct cerebral networks.

Burbaud et al. (1995) investigated the role of the right and left prefrontal cortices in calculation using fMRI techniques. Eight right-handed and eight left-handed subjects participated in the study and were asked to complete two numerical tasks (mental recitation of numbers and mental calculation). Recitation of numbers resulted in little cerebral activation. Mental calculation, by contrast, with its working memory demands, activated prefrontal brain regions. Furthermore, in right-handed subjects, activation was clearly lateralized to the left dorsolateral prefrontal cortex, whereas bilateral activation was found in left-handed subjects. In another fMRI study, Rueckert et al. (1996) measured activation in 12 right-handed subjects performing a mental calculation task involving subtraction by serial sevens. All subjects showed significant activation in left prefrontal cortex, left posterior parietal cortex (angular and/or supramarginal gyri), and bilateral motor/premotor cortex. There were additional areas of activation that varied from subject to subject (e.g., right prefrontal, left temporal lobe), suggesting a great deal of individual variability. Rueckert et al. (1996) concluded that their findings corroborated the important role of the posterior parietal area in calculation, while not supporting a differential role for the angular gyrus.

Chochon and colleagues (1999) attempted to distinguish between calculation tasks lateralized to the left parietal lobe from calculation tasks lateralized to the right parietal lobe. Eight healthy subjects underwent fMRI while completing tasks of digit naming, number comparison, subtraction, and multiplication. On the basis of the fMRI results, the four tasks could be ordered hierarchically with each higher task causing additional activation: naming < comparison < multiplication < subtraction. With the exception of digit naming, all of the tasks activated the parieto-occipital and cingulate regions. In terms of differential parietal lobe activity, number comparison relied more heavily on right parietal and prefrontal activation; the opposite pattern (i.e., left hemisphere activation) was suggested by the multiplication task. Finally, bilateral activation occurred during the subtraction task. These authors concluded that distinct parietal pathways exist for different arithmetic operations.

Using fMRI, Rickard et al. (2000) explored the patterns of neural activation for two relatively simple arithmetic tasks, multiplication verification and magnitude judgment, in eight right-handed healthy adult participants. The authors attempted to improve on prior functional imaging studies by utilizing simple arithmetic tasks rather than complex ones, given that complex tasks may engage ancillary cognitive processes that are not directly associated with arithmetic per se. For the multiplication verification task, bilateral activation in multiple brain regions was demonstrated, involving Brodmann's area 44 (left greater than right), dorsolateral prefrontal cortex (areas 9 and 10), inferior and superior parietal areas (left greater than right), and lingual and fusiform gyri. Regarding magnitude judgment, the results were even more variable, with the greatest and most consistent activation occurring in bilateral inferior parietal cortex. Interestingly, like Deheane et al. (1996), these investigators found no activation (and actually detected deactivation) in angular and supramarginal gyri, a finding that appears inconsistent with the neuropsychological literature. In sum, the functional imaging literature to date has provided a somewhat different set of findings regarding neural correlates of number processing, and this issue clearly warrants further investigation.

NEUROPSYCHOLOGICAL EVALUATION OF ACALCULIA

Paying bills, balancing a checkbook, addressing letters, counting out money for a purchase, and understanding the measurement aspects of a recipe are just a few examples of how meaningful calculation is to our daily life. Ideally, assessment of calculation skills should be varied, and should cover aural and written calculation, the comprehension and use of operations, and the spatial components of arithmetic.

Comprehensive Assessment

One especially comprehensive calculation test battery is that of Benton (1963), which comprises 12 tasks:

1. Appreciation of number values when presented verbally with a pair of numbers such as 28 and 31, where the task is to say which is greater

2. Appreciation of number values when presented visually, and the response is either oral or pointing to the larger of two numbers
3. Reading numbers aloud
4. Pointing to written numbers that are named by the examiner
5. Writing numbers to dictation
6. Writing numbers from copy
7. Counting out loud from 1 to 20, from 20 to 1, and from 1 to 20 by 2's
8. Estimating the number of items in a series of continuous dots and again in a discontinuous series of dots (e.g., four groups of five dots each arranged horizontally)
9. Oral arithmetic calculation in which simple examples are given using each of the four basic operations
10. Written arithmetic calculation in which the examples are similar to those given orally
11. Arithmetic reasoning ability via the Arithmetic Reasoning subtest of the Wechsler Adult Intelligence Scale (WAIS)
12. Immediate memory for calculation problems. This measure is a component of test 9 and serves as a control to ascertain whether a memory deficit is responsible for inability to perform calculation problems given orally.

Other comprehensive tests include the Verbal and Spatial Reasoning Test (VESPAR) (Langdon and Warrington, 1995), which measures arithmetic reasoning while minimizing attention and language contributions. An experimental battery discussed previously is the EC301 Assessment Battery for Calculation and Number Processing (Deloche et al., 1993, 1994). Subsequent research (Deloche et al., 1996) has demonstrated that the EC301 has strong ecological validity, as demonstrated by strong correlations with an activities in daily life (ADL) questionnaire that measured daily numerical activities (e.g., reading time on a digital clock). The Graded Difficulty Arithmetic test (Jackson and Warrington, 1986), alluded to earlier, contains 12 addition and 12 subtraction calculation problems. On the GDA, subjects

are presented the problems orally, in order of increasing difficulty, and a 10-second time limit is imposed for each calculation.

Diagnostic Assessment

There are numerous diagnostic tests of calculation available for purchase from commercial sources. Although widely utilized, these tests do not provide evaluation of all facets of calculation disturbances discussed in this chapter. On a positive note, all tests reviewed in this section, with the exception of WAIS-III Arithmetic, have available two parallel forms for uncomplicated repeat administration.

KeyMath Diagnostic Arithmetic Test–Revised (KeyMath-R). The KeyMath-R (Connolly, 1991) consists of 13 subtests that are further organized into three major areas: *(1)* Basic Concepts, which measures basic mathematical knowledge and contains three subtests (numeration, rational numbers, and geometry); *(2)* Operation, which measures computation and contains five subtests (addition, subtraction, multiplication, division, and mental computation); and *(3)* Applications, which measures mathematics encountered in everyday life and contains five subtests (measurement, time and money, estimation, interpreting data, and problem solving). The KeyMath-R normative data have an upper limit of 15 years, 5 months, but may prove useful with older individuals.

Peabody Individual Achievement Test–Revised (PIAT-R). The PIAT-R (Markwardt, 1989) Mathematics subtest consists of 100 multiple-choice items that range in difficulty from simple matching tasks to high school arithmetic. The examiner reads each item aloud while visually displaying the question and response options to the examinee. The PIAT normative data have an upper limit of 18 years, 11 months, but may prove useful with older individuals.

Wechsler Adult Intelligence Scale-III Arithmetic Subtest. The WAIS-III Arithmetic (Wechsler, 1991) is a widely utilized test of mental arithmetic. This subtest ranges from the counting of blocks to verbally presented mathematical problems involving fractions and proportions. A time limit is instituted for all problems, with bonus points given for quick, accurate responding. Use of pencil and paper to complete the problems is not allowed. The WAIS-III Arithmetic normative data are excellent, with norms through 89 years of age.

Wechsler Individual Achievement Test (WIAT). The WIAT (1992) contains two subtests that address calculation and, together, they can be combined to form a composite Mathematics score: *(1)* Mathematics Reasoning, which measures the ability to perform geometry, measurement, and statistics, in addition to problem-solving ability; and *(2)* Numerical Operations, which measures written calculation abilities for problems involving addition, subtraction, multiplication, and division. The WIAT normative data have an upper limit of 19 years, 11 months, but may prove useful with older individuals.

Wide Range Achievement Test, Third Edition (WRAT3) Arithmetic Subtest. The WRAT3 (Wilkinson, 1993) Arithmetic is a timed (15 minute) test of written calculation. Problems on the typical adult level involve simple and complex written calculation, in addition to questions that could be found in college-level mathematics courses. The WRAT3 normative data are excellent, with norms through 75 years of age.

The Woodcock-Johnson Tests of Achievement–Revised (WJ-R). The WJ-R Tests of Achievement (Woodcock and Mather, 1989) contain three calculation subtests: *(1)* Calculation, which measures the ability to perform written calculation problems ranging from simple addition to calculus-based problems; *(2)* Applied Problems, which measures the ability to solve practical problems, the complex problems necessitating written calculation; and *(3)* Quantitative Concepts, which measures knowledge of mathematical concepts and vocabulary. A Broad Mathematics Cluster score can be calculated following the administration of the Calculation and Applied Problems subtests; in addition, the Applied Problems subtest allows for a Mathematics Reasoning Cluster score. The

WJ-R normative data are excellent, with norms through 95 years of age.

Qualitative Assessment

Error analyses are often a very useful addition to traditional assessment. Grafman et al. (1982) utilized the Benton Visual Retention Test scoring criteria (Sivan, 1992) to examine calculation errors qualitatively. Specifically, they scored six types of errors: misplacement, size error, distortion, rotation, omission, and perseveration. Qualitative testing may be particularly important when addressing spatial forms of calculation disorders.

Other Issues in Assessment

It is critically important to gain a sense of the patient's premorbid calculation abilities to rule out developmental problems, relatively undeveloped math skills, or lack of opportunity to learn calculation skills. Furthermore, one must keep in mind the presence of gender-typical discrepancies in mathematical reasoning abilities, which favor males (Benbow and Stanley, 1983). Consideration of these concerns can be accomplished in a number of ways, including examination of academic records, knowledge of the patient's occupation and job responsibilities, or discussion with the patient and family members. Furthermore, given the high comorbidity between aphasia and acalculia, it is essential to evaluate the patient's language abilities thoroughly. Finally, calculation tasks should be administered as part of a full neuropsychological battery, as calculation disturbances may arise secondary to defects in attention, memory, or executive functions.

SUMMARY AND COMMENTS

It is evident from this brief review that acquired disturbances of mathematical ability can appear in many different forms, in the setting of many different types of neurological disease, and in connection with many different lesion sites. Nonetheless, the preponderance of the evidence indicates that left-sided lesions to the parietal region, especially in the inferior parietal lobule, are most consistently associated with acalculia, especially the primary type. It has even been suggested that the left parietal region constitutes the "mathematical brain" in humans (Butterworth, 1999). While acalculia has often been reported in patients who also manifest disturbances of language processing, this association is not a necessary one, as some cases have been described in whom acalculia occurred without an accompanying aphasia. The neuroanatomical separation of mathematical and language processing is supported further by cases of the reverse dissociation, i.e., impaired processing of linguistic information with preserved processing of numbers and mathematical calculations (e.g., Anderson et al., 1990). Finally, there is recent evidence from functional imaging (fMRI) that while "exact" types of mathematical knowledge (e.g., number facts, math tables) may depend on language and on inferior prefrontal structures that are also used for word association tasks, "approximate" arithmetic (e.g., quantity manipulation, approximation of magnitudes) may be language-independent and rely on bilateral areas of the parietal lobes that are also involved in visuospatial processing (Dehaene et al. 1999). In our view, the distinction between exact and approximate types of arithmetic reasoning has considerable appeal, and may prove very fruitful in future attempts to define the neural correlates of mathematical capacity.

Acalculia is a relatively rare disorder, but its study has provided several important insights into the neural basis of calculation. Studies based on the lesion method have furnished testable hypotheses, which are beginning to be pursued with group studies and functional imaging techniques. Furthermore, studies of normal individuals and acalculic brain-damaged patients have been essential to the development of theoretical models of number comprehension and production (e.g., Mc-Closkey et al., 1985; Ashcraft, 1987; Dehaene, 1992; McCloskey, 1992; Dehaene and Cohen, 1997; Butterworth, 1999). Such models will undoubtedly help in the creation of effective rehabilitation techniques for children with learning disorders and adults with acquired brain damage. Work along these lines is already underway (Sullivan et al., 1996; Guyard et al., 1997).

DISTURBANCES OF THE BODY SCHEMA

Body schema disturbances is a broad term that, in principle, can be applied to a wide variety of disorders of processing related to the representation and spatial location of the body, including conditions such as anosognosia, autoscopia, tactile extinction, and the phantom limb phenomenon (cf. Frederiks, 1985; Denes, 1989). Here, following the tradition of previous authors (e.g., Benton, 1985; Benton and Sivan, 1993), we focus on three specific manifestations of body schema disturbance: autotopagnosia, finger agnosia, and right–left disorientation. Two of these, right–left disorientation and finger agnosia, are part of the tetrad of signs included under the classic Gerstmann syndrome, and thus they are to some extent cognate to the condition of acalculia described earlier. And as we will highlight below, all of the body schema disturbances reviewed here tend to be related neuroanatomically to structures in the left parietal region, although the relationship is far less robust and reliable than many of the more well-studied neuropsychological syndromes (e.g., aphasia).

Several factors may explain the rather murky status of body schema disturbances in the neuropsychological literature. As Benton and Sivan (1993) noted, the term "body schema" has never received a standard, widely accepted definition, with different authors offering their own, often fairly idiosyncratic, explications. Also, the explanatory value of the concept of body schema has been repeatedly questioned (Benton, 1959; Poeck and Orgass, 1971; Denes, 1989). Some authors have argued that the term is useful in explaining the so-called phantom limb phenomenon, but newer studies have provided the basis for more parsimonious and compelling formulations of this condition (Ramachandran, 1998; Ramachandran and Rogers-Ramachandran, 2000). Perhaps of greatest importance, there has been a marked paucity of theoretical frameworks within which the concept of body schema could be properly situated and interpreted. The older literature, for example, appealed to simple distinctions such as unconscious versus conscious body representation knowledge (e.g., Head, 1920). This situation may finally be changing, though, as comprehensive, detailed theoretical accounts of the neurobiology of emotion, feeling, and consciousness have recently become available (e.g., Damasio, 1994, 1999). One can even be somewhat sanguine that in the context of such theoretical frameworks, it may be possible to conduct hypothesis-driven investigations of body schema disturbances that will lead to far more precision and clarity in this literature than has existed heretofore (Bechara et al., 1997; Adolphs et al., 1999, 2000; Damasio et al., 2000).

AUTOTOPAGNOSIA

Autotopagnosia (AT) can be defined as an inability to identify body parts, either on one's self, on the examiner, or on a human picture. The deficit may encompass both verbal (e.g., on verbal command, the patient is asked to point to a body part) and nonverbal (e.g., the patient is asked to imitate on his or her own body what body part the examiner is pointing to on him- or herself) modalities. In strict terms, AT should occur in relationship to both sides of the body (cf. Benton and Sivan, 1993), i.e., as a bilateral condition; however, some authors have allowed a broader conceptualization, in which unilateral manifestations (e.g., hemisomatoagnosia) are considered. Some rather surprising dissociations have been described, such as De Renzi and Scotti's (1970) account of a patient with AT who maintained the isolated ability to report when an examiner pointed incorrectly to a named body part. This rare disorder has been described both as the result of dementia (Pick, 1922) and focal left hemisphere damage (e.g., Selecki and Herron, 1965; Sauguet et al., 1971), usually involving the parietal lobe. It is usually accompanied by aphasia, reaching disorders, apraxia, neglect, or visuospatial disturbances, and, according to Benton and Sivan (1993), a "pure" case of AT has never been reported in the literature.

Many explanations for AT have been posited, perhaps nearly as many as there are cases reported in the literature. First, the patient's inability to point to body parts may be due to an underlying language disturbance (e.g., anomia). Related to aphasia, another explanation is that AT is attributable to a category-specific comprehension deficit in which the patient has difficulty understanding the names of body parts (Goodglass et al., 1966). Third, a parts–whole hypothesis has been raised, which suggests that the affected patient has an inability to separate a whole into its component parts (De Renzi and Faglioni, 1963; De Renzi and Scotti, 1970).

Semenza and Goodglass (1985) examined 32 brain-damaged patients and underscored the important role of language in body part identification. On the basis of clinical and neuroimaging data, the patients were divided into the following subgroups: global aphasics (2); Broca's aphasics (10); Wernicke's aphasics (10); anomics, left posterior lesion (2); conduction aphasics, left parietal lesion (3); mixed aphasics, left frontoparietal lesion (2); and bilateral posterior lesions (3). The investigators administered a comprehensive test battery involving body part identification in which certain tasks required verbal mediation and others were nonverbal or imitative (Semenza and Goodglass, 1985; this battery is described below in Neuropsychological Evaluation). Results revealed that the body part identification tasks that were administered verbally rather than nonverbally proved more difficult for all patients regardless of subgroup classification; however, this was not surprising, given that all patients had some degree of impairment in auditory comprehension. More impressive was the finding that the likelihood of success or failure in body part identification was a function of a single factor: lexical frequency. That is, accuracy of body part identification increased with frequency of use in the respective language ($r = 0.69$ for Italian-speaking patients and $r = 0.75$ for English-speaking patients).

Ogden (1985) reported the case of a patient with a left parietal lobe tumor that resulted in AT. The patient's AT could be attributed neither to language or mental status abnormalities nor to an inability to separate a whole into its component parts. Although this patient is one of the purest cases of AT to be reported to date, he demonstrated all aspects of the Gerstmann syndrome, in addition to ideomotor apraxia, dressing apraxia, and visuospatial deficits. Evaluation of the patient for AT was complex and thorough, and his deficits fell into the classic dissociation discussed by Denes (1989): Intact "what" tasks, which involve understanding, naming, and describing the functions of the body and body parts singled out by the examiner, in the context of impaired "where" tasks, which involve pointing to a specific body part on verbal command or imitation or describing the precise location of a specific body part in relation to other body parts. Similar findings were demonstrated for Semenza's (1988) examination of a patient with a left parieto-occipital tumor.

Sirigu and colleagues (1991) carried out a unique experiment to discern whether the ability to identify body parts could be dissociated from the ability to identify inanimate objects placed on the body. The investigators studied a patient with probable dementia of the Alzheimer's type who was roughly 3 years into the progression of the disease. As would be expected, she presented on neuropsychological testing with broad cognitive impairments, including the full tetrad of Gerstmann's syndrome, and dressing apraxia. Twenty-five body parts distributed over the entire body were chosen for study. In terms of body part identification in verbal and nonverbal conditions, the patient displayed difficulty localizing body parts on herself and on others, but was able to demonstrate naming and functional comprehension of body parts. Interestingly, when 10 inanimate objects were placed on her body at roughly the same locations as the body identification task (e.g., a figurine placed on the left knee), she successfully and reliably pointed to these objects and even recalled their position after their removal. The results of this study led the investigators to conclude that two systems of body knowledge exist, one for semantic and lexical information (intact in this patient) and the other for storing a body-specific visuospatial representation (impaired in this patient).

Denes and colleagues (2000) studied two AT patients who presented with somewhat complicated neurological pictures. Case 1 suffered a left posterior parietal lobe hemorrhage accompanied by significant calculation and writing disturbances, as well as mild language disturbances. Case 2, a left-handed woman,

suffered a vascular lesion of the right temporoparietal region and demonstrated aphasia and mild apraxia. Both patients were administered a comprehensive battery of body knowledge tasks, which involved body part naming on a human picture, self, and other, and body part localization. Both patients performed at ceiling in naming body parts. However, localization proved much more difficult, although their errors were meaningful and demonstrated some degree of body knowledge. For example, "vicinity" errors, in which the patient pointed to a body part close in location to the target, were common. These authors also found a lack of support for the proposal that AT is a function of an inability to separate a whole into its component parts. Rather, the investigators hypothesized that AT was attributable to an impairment in the ability to encode body position information for self and others. In a same–different matching task, patients decided whether two pictures of static body positions and two pictures of building block figures were the same or different. In contrast to controls who found the matching of body positions easier than the blocks, the patients demonstrated a comparable performance for the two tasks, suggesting a lack of the usual proclivity for body positions. The investigators concluded that lesions of the parietal lobe of the language-dominant hemisphere can impair the ability to locate body parts on verbal command and to detect changes in body position in a model.

Other Considerations

As the studies reviewed above illustrate, there is considerable confusion in the literature regarding the extent to which language disturbances play a role in AT. In our view, a strict definition of AT would exclude a role for language entirely; that is, AT should be considered a disturbance of the knowledge of body parts that cannot be attributed to or explained by an impairment of language, and especially, an impairment in retrieving and comprehending words for body parts. This formulation of AT is more in keeping with the notion that the core feature of the disorder is a disturbance of the body schema, and with the idea that AT can be classified as a disturbance of knowledge retrieval, i.e., an "agnosia." Our concerns here are not just specious; in fact, there are a number of studies which have demonstrated that the naming of body parts can be impaired quite independently of body part knowledge (De Renzi and Scotti, 1970; Ogden, 1985); moreover, it has been shown that the naming and comprehending of body parts can be impaired or preserved quite selectively in relationship to naming items from other conceptual categories (e.g., Goodglass et al., 1966; Yamadori and Albert, 1973; McKenna and Warrington, 1978; Suzuki et al., 1997).

Neuropsychological Evaluation of Autopagnosia

Virtually no systematic approaches to the neuropsychological assessment of AT exist. A review of common neuropsychological assessment and neurological exam texts revealed little attention to the topic. Research studies, however, have tended to use or adapt the approach set forth by Semenza and Goodglass (1985). Their battery includes 18 body parts (i.e., nose, knee, chest, eye, shoulder, ear, hip, wrist, toe, neck, elbow, hair, thigh, chin, ankle, cheek, thumb, and lips), and their localization is required in each of the following nine experimental conditions:

Verbal Tasks
1. On verbal command, the subject points to their own body parts.
2. On verbal command, the subject points to body parts on a full-size drawing of a human figure.
3. On verbal command, the subject points to a drawing of a single body part that has been presented in a multiple-choice paradigm. The four choices involve the target picture, a picture of a contiguous body part, a picture of a conceptually related body part, and a randomly chosen, unrelated body part.

Nonverbal Tasks
4. After being shown an isolated drawing of a single body part, the subject points to

the synonymous body part on their own body.
5. After being shown an isolated drawing of a single body part, the subject points to the synonymous body part on a full-size drawing of a human figure.
6. While the subject's eyes are closed, the examiner touches a part of the subject's body, then the subject must point to the synonymous body part on a full-size drawing of a human figure.
7. While the subject's eyes are closed, the examiner touches a part of the subject's body, then the subject must point to a drawing of a single body part, presented in a multiple-choice paradigm.
8. The examiner points to body parts on a full-size drawing of a human figure, and the subject must point to his or her own corresponding body parts.
9. Seated side by side, the examiner points to his or her own body parts and the subject must imitate on him- or herself.

A less complicated bedside approach was outlined by Frederiks (1985). Patients are asked to name or move body parts touched or named by the examiner, and this is conducted both with the patient's eyes open and with the eyes closed. As described previously, another task involves asking the patient to identify body parts on the examiner and on a picture. Finally, asking the patient to draw or assemble a face or human figure may demonstrate AT through the omission or distortion of body parts.

Error Analysis

Error analysis (after Denes, 1996) is used to test for three types of errors:

1. *Contiguity errors* refer to errors in which the patient touches the wrong body part, but it is located in close proximity to the target body part (e.g., touches shoulder rather than elbow).
2. *Semantic (also referred to as conceptual) errors* refer to errors in which the patient touches the wrong body part, but it is functionally related to the target body part (e.g., touches hand rather than foot).

3. *Random errors* refer to errors that cannot be classified into either of the other two error groupings. For example, this label is appropriate when the patient searches rather aimlessly (often in a fumbling, groping manner) for the body part.

It has been reported (Denes, 1989) that body parts devoid of definite boundaries, such as joints or cheeks, are more difficult for AT patients to localize than perceptually well-defined body parts, such as ear and nose.

Finally, as reflected in the research studies reviewed earlier, it is essential to test the patient's language, motor, and visuospatial abilities, which have the potential of contributing to or even explaining their AT. Such testing should ideally include naming of body parts displayed in isolation; describing the function of different body parts; naming parts/details and the whole of non-body pictures that are approximately as complex as the human body (e.g., maps and animals); and pointing to paraphernalia located on their body (e.g., watch, glasses, ring) to address the selectivity of the body part pointing deficit.

FINGER AGNOSIA

Finger agnosia (FA) can be defined as a finger localization deficit (Benton, 1959). Patients with FA demonstrate a loss of the ability to name fingers, show fingers on verbal command, or localize fingers following tactile stimulation. They are typically able to use their fingers for everyday life activities, often with an added degree of clumsiness. Of the body schema disturbances reviewed in this chapter, FA occurs with the greatest frequency (Frederiks, 1985) and is considered a hallmark feature of Gerstmann's syndrome. Finger agnosia is most commonly considered a bilateral condition in which both hands are affected. However, a unilateral version has been described, thought to be attributable to a sensory defect arising from brain damage contralateral to the affected hand (Head, 1920). (We would question the validity of applying the term "agnosia" to a condition that is primarily sensory based.) Finally, FA is most pronounced on examina-

tion of the middle three fingers (Frederiks, 1985).

Whether FA can occur as an isolated phenomenon continues to be an issue of great debate. Many believe it is truly a function of AT, aphasia, dementia, or visuospatial dysfunction (see Benton, 1992, for a review). Morris and colleagues (1984) demonstrated that through stimulation of perisylvian cortical areas, FA can be elicited while unaccompanied by other defects, and therefore suggest that, in principle, FA could exist in isolation. The most common neural correlate of FA is left parietal-occipital dysfunction. However, a sizeable minority of the literature reviewed below suggests that FA can occur with lesions on either side of the brain (e.g., Kinsbourne and Warrington, 1962).

Benton (1959) took the view that finger localization involves a language function or a symbolic process, and that FA is due to "an impairment of language function in which the patient has lost the ability to handle the symbols that related to the fingers (p. 159)." Benton's hypothesis was tested by Kinsbourne and Warrington (1962). They administered verbal and nonverbal tests of finger localization to 12 patients with elements of Gertsmann's syndrome (one-third of whom had bilateral lesions, one-third had left hemisphere lesions, and one-third had right hemisphere lesions) and 20 brain-damaged control patients without any Gerstmann symptoms. Results revealed that all patients with elements of the Gerstmann syndrome failed at least three of five finger localization tests administered, with much lower rates of failure observed among the brain-damaged control patients. Moreover, the performance of target patients was significantly worse on the nonverbal finger localization tests than on verbal tasks of finger localization. In contrast, brain-damaged controls performed equally well on both the verbal and nonverbal finger localization tasks. In summary, these authors concluded that their findings challenge Benton's view that language disturbance is essential to finger agnosia.

Ettlinger (1963) studied finger localization in 13 patients with known parietal lobe lesions (9 of the 13 had left parietal lesions; 2 had bilateral and 2 had right parietal lesions). All patients were administered 12 tasks of finger localization. Results revealed that correlations among tests were not high, and that failure on one finger localization task did not predict failure on others.

Matthews and colleagues (1966) assessed nonverbal finger localization in 237 subjects with mental retardation (mean full-scale IQ = 60.8 ± 13.3). These investigators found a stronger correlation between finger localization performance level and Wechsler-Bellevue (W-B) Performance IQ than that with W-B Verbal Scale IQ. Similarly, Poeck and Orgass (1969), in an unselected group of unilateral brain damaged patients, demonstrated that nonverbal testing of finger localization was most closely correlated with Wechsler Performance IQ, whereas verbal testing of finger localization correlated highly with Wechsler Verbal IQ.

Gainotti and colleagues (1972) studied finger localization in 162 unselected patients with unilateral brain damage (88 left and 74 right hemisphere brain damaged). The results demonstrated that the incidence of FA did not differ significantly in right and left brain–damaged patients when nonverbal procedures and larger samples are used. What did play a significant role in FA, however, was the presence of aphasia and/or general mental impairment: the poor performance of the right brain–damaged group was associated with general mental impairment, while the left brain–damaged group showed a relatively higher incidence of aphasia and sensory impairment.

Benke and colleagues (1988) studied FA in groups of right brain–damaged, left brain–damaged without aphasia, and aphasic patients. The investigators confirmed the high frequency of FA in aphasic patients, but also noted its occurrence in nonaphasic patients. In all the groups, the presence of FA was related to the severity of the defect in visuospatial, language-related cognitive functions, and mental imagery. The authors concluded that, rather than being the direct expression of a focal lesion, finger agnosia reflects impairment in higher-level cognitive systems.

Tucha and colleagues (1997) studied a patient with a tumor of the left angular gyrus. The patient presented with Gerstmann's syndrome. Neuropsychological evaluation was unremarkable except for acalculia, agraphia, and spelling impairments. Neurological testing revealed that she additionally manifested toe agnosia. These investigators suggest that patients should more regularly be evaluated for toe agnosia, and if occurrence is common, a new term, "digit agnosia," is recommended. However, Fein (1987) warns that normal adults misidentify toes with great regularity.

Neuropsychological Evaluation of Finger Agnosia

Benton (1959) and Benton et al. (1994) developed a 60-item test consisting of three parts (i.e., 10 items for each part below for each of the hands) to assess FA:

1. With the hand visible, localization of single fingers touched by the examiner
2. With the hand hidden from view, localization of single fingers touched by the examiner
3. With the hand hidden from view, localization of pairs of fingers simultaneously touched by the examiner.

Mode of response on the part of the examinee can take a number of forms, including naming, pointing on a drawing, or referring to the fingers with numbers.

RIGHT–LEFT DISORIENTATION

Right–left orientation refers to the ability to identify the right and left sides of one's own body, and to identify the right and left sides of a person seated opposite or in a photo or drawing. It additionally necessitates both spatial and symbolic elements for successful performance. Individuals with right–left disorientation (RLD) often demonstrate the sparing of other spatial concepts, such as up–down and front–back (Denes, 1989). As noted earlier, RLD is one of the Gerstmann signs, and it has been described most frequently in connection with at least some of the other components of Gerstmann syndrome. Right–left disorientation may develop consequent to broader disturbances of body schema or language processing, but it can exist as a fairly isolated symptom (Benton, 1958; Gold et al., 1995), which suggests that it is useful to retain RLD as a meaningful neuropsychological entity. As we have alluded, the most common neural correlate of RLD is left parietal dysfunction.

It is not rare to observe some degree of right–left confusion in healthy adults. Wolf (1973) examined the incidence of right–left confusion in a sample of physicians and their spouses. Results revealed that 17.5% of women and 8.8% of men sampled admitted to "frequent" right–left confusion. Harris and Gitterman (1978) assessed the frequency of right–left confusion in a sample of 364 university faculty members, and found greater error rates among females, especially left-handed females. No relationship between males and handedness emerged. These results are consistent with the premise that women generally have inferior spatial skills relative to men (De Renzi, 1982). In children, this ability appears to follow a developmental trajectory with own body right–left orientation developing before the ability to identify right from left on an opposing individual (Benton, 1959; Clark and Klonoff, 1990; Benton and Sivan, 1993). Assessment of RLD is evident on developmental tests of adaptive behavior, such as the Vineland Adaptive Behavior Scales (Sparrow et al., 1984). By the age of 12, however, most children show an adult level of success in right–left opposing orientation tasks (Clark and Klonoff, 1990).

Head (1926) and Bonhoeffer (1923) demonstrated that RLD was a consequence of left hemisphere lesions with associated aphasia, and specifically implicated the left retrorolandic area. McFie and Zangwill (1960) found RLD in 5 of 8 patients with left hemisphere lesions; in contrast, none of the 21 patients with right hemisphere lesions demonstrated the deficit. Successful right–left orientation necessitates numerous cognitive abilities, including mental rotation. Although RLD is classically thought of as being related to left hemisphere damage, work by Ratcliff (1979) suggests some right hemisphere contribution to right–left orientation. Ratcliff (1979) found

that patients with right parietal-temporal-occipital lesions were impaired at making right–left judgments about inverted (upside down) figures, but not with upright figures. Ratcliff (1979) summarized his findings as lending support to the notion that the right posterior cortex was specialized for mental rotation.

In one of the few group studies conducted to date, Saugert et al. (1971) examined 31 patients with right hemisphere lesions and 49 patients with left hemisphere lesions. The left hemisphere group was divided into 21 patients with "sensory" aphasia and 28 patients without aphasia. All patients completed, among other tasks, right–left orientation in four formats: (1) right–left orientation of one's own body; (2) confronting front view of examiner and model; (3) confronting back view of examiner; and (4) imitation of a three-step movement. For format 1, nonaphasic patients, regardless of side of lesion, performed relatively strongly; however, two-thirds of left hemisphere patients with aphasia performed defectively. For formats 2 and 3, 50% of left hemisphere patients with aphasia performed defectively, as did 13% of nonaphasic patients with right hemisphere lesions. Interestingly, all left hemisphere nonaphasics performed relatively strongly. For format 4, 48% of left hemisphere patients with aphasia performed defectively as did 32% of nonaphasic patients with right hemisphere lesions and 14% of left hemisphere nonaphasics. This study suggests that the relationship of RLD with side of lesion and the presence or absence of aphasia is not a simple one; rather, the performance of different unilateral lesion groups depends on what aspect of RLD is assessed. The study additionally suggests that right hemisphere damage contributes to RLD, especially during imitation tasks.

Fischer and colleagues (1990) examined whether patients with probable dementia of the Alzheimer's type (DAT) would show right–left disorientation, suggestive of left parietal dysfunction. Eighteen patients with DAT were matched on age, education, and dementia severity with 18 multi-infarct dementia (MID) patients. All participants were administered a shortened version of the Right–Left Orientation Test involving six questions addressing right–left orientation on their own body and six questions addressing right–left orientation on a confronting doll (Benton, 1959; Benton et al., 1994). Participants were also administered tests of language and visuospatial ability. The investigators found that DAT and MID groups did not differ on their own body right–left orientation. In contrast, the DAT group performed significantly poorer than the MID group on right–left orientation on a confronting doll, and this impairment was independent of language and visuospatial dysfunction. The authors suggest that their findings are consistent with the PET biparietal hypometabolism commonly seen in DAT patients.

Neuropsychological Evaluation of Right–Left Disorientation

Formal examination of RLD makes demands on numerous cognitive abilities, including auditory comprehension, verbal expression of the labels "left" and "right," short-term memory for the instructions, sensory discrimination, and mental rotation. Furthermore, the mode of response is varied, including naming, executing movements in response to verbal command, and imitation of movement (Benton and Sivan, 1993). Finally, identification of "right" and "left" may occur on one's own body, when confronting the examiner or picture, or during a combination of the two.

Benton and Sivan (1993) underscore the importance of taking a hierarchical approach to the assessment of RLD in which the execution of each lower level is a prerequisite for successful performance at higher levels. Table 9–1 demonstrates that the ability to execute double uncrossed commands (I-C) is a prerequisite for success on double crossed commands (I-D). Occasional exceptions to the rule do occur with failures on an easier item (I-D), while success occurs for an apparently more difficult item (III-B). According to Benton et al. (1994), successful completion of III-A and III-B requires a rotation of 180° in orientation.

Diagnostic Assessment

The following tests allow one to determine the presence or absence of a clinically significant RLD. If RLD is present, it is important to get a notion of whether the patient had an unusual premorbid weakness of these capacities. Furthermore, aphasic patients present a particularly challenging puzzle since their RLD may be driven by primary language factors such as comprehension deficits; anomia, which could cause confusion in the use of the "right" and "left" labels; and deficits in auditory retention.

Right-Left Orientation Test (RLOT). The RLOT (Benton, 1959; Benton et al., 1994) is a

Table 9–1. Components of Right–Left Orientation

I. Orientation toward one's own body
  A. Naming single lateral body parts touched by examiner
  B. Pointing to single lateral body parts on verbal command
  C. Executing double uncrossed movements on verbal command (e.g., touching left ear with left hand)
  D. Executing double crossed movements on verbal command (e.g., touching right ear with left hand)
II. Orientation toward one's own body without visual guidance (blindfolded or eyes closed)
  A. Naming single lateral body parts touched by examiner
  B. Pointing to single lateral body parts on verbal command
  C. Executing double uncrossed movements on verbal command (e.g., touching left ear with left hand)
  D. Executing double crossed movements on verbal command (e.g., touching right ear with left hand)
III. Orientation toward confronting examiner or picture
  A. Naming single lateral body parts touched by examiner
  B. Pointing to single lateral body parts on verbal command
  C. Imitating uncrossed movements of examiner (e.g., left hand on left ear)
  D. Imitating crossed movements of examiner (e.g., left hand on right ear)
IV. Combined orientation toward one's own body and confronting person
  A. Placing either left or right hand on specified part of confronting person on verbal command (e.g., placing right hand on confronting person's left ear)

Source: Benton and Sivan (1993).

20-item test of simple (e.g., "Show me your right hand") and complex (e.g., "Touch your right ear with your right hand") verbal commands to assess right–left orientation. The first 12 items involve discerning right from left on the subject's own body. The final eight questions necessitate right–left discrimination on the examiner or on a model that is at least 15 inches in height. Alternative forms of this test exist.

Standardized Road-Map Test of Direction Sense. This is a test of right–left orientation in extrapersonal space (Money, 1976). On an unmarked road map, the examiner draws a dotted pathway and the subject is asked to tell the direction (right or left) at each turn. Normative data above 18 years of age do not exist; however, for individuals above age 18, a cutoff value has been established to categorize the subject as intact or impaired.

Laterality Discrimination Test (LDT). The LDT (Culver, 1969) is a speeded task of laterality judgment and spatial perception. The stimuli consist of 32 line drawings of body parts (16 hands, 8 feet, 4 eyes, and 4 ears). Subjects are shown one card at a time, and are asked to judge whether the picture is a right or left body part.

As can be seen from the above diagnostic tests, there is a lack of nonverbal tests of right–left orientation available. However, most can be adapted for a nonverbal administration that involves pointing responses and imitation (Head, 1926). Inclusion of a few nonverbal tasks seems important, given the dissociation in performance on verbal and nonverbal right–left orientation that was revealed in a patient with a left anterior temporal lobe tumor (Dennis, 1976).

SUMMARY

Our review indicates that the neural basis of body schema representation remains poorly understood (for a review, see Berlucchi and Aglioti, 1997). The specific disorders of autotopagnosia, finger agnosia, and right–left dis-

orientation seem linked primarily to dysfuncion of the left parietal regions and, as suggested by other authors (e.g., Denes, 1989), seem to depend on an altered conceptual representation of the body and body parts; moreover, much of this alteration seems attributable in many cases to linguistic factors. Insofar as clinical practice is concerned, though, it seems that the utility of these constructs, and of the entire Gerstmann syndrome for that matter, remains viable, and we would encourage the continued use and teaching of these terms in clinical neuropsychology.

ACKNOWLEDGMENTS

This work was supported by Program Project Grant NINDS NS19632.

REFERENCES

Adolphs, R., Damasio, H., Tranel, D., Cooper, G., and Damasio, A. R. (2000). A role for somatosensory cortices in the visual recognition of emotion as revealed by three-dimensional lesion mapping. *J. Neurosci.* 20:2683–2690.

Adolphs, R., Russell, J. A., and Tranel, D. (1999). A role for the human amygdala in recognizing emotional arousal from unpleasant stimuli. *Psychol. Sci.* 10:167–171.

Anderson, S. W., Damasio, A. R., and Damasio, H. (1990). Troubled letters but not numbers. *Brain* 113:749–766.

Ashcraft, M. H. (1987). Children's knowledge of simple arithmetic: a developmental model and simulation. In *Formal Methods in Developmental Psychology: Progress in Cognitive Developmental Research*, J. Bisanz, C.J. Brainerd, and R. Kail (eds.). New York: Springer-Verlag.

Ardila, A., and Rosselli, M. (1994). Spatial acalculia. *Int. J. Neurosci.* 78:177–184.

Basso, A., Burgio, F., and Caporali, A. (2000). Acalculia, aphasia, and spatial disorders in left and right brain-damaged patients. *Cortex* 36:265–280.

Bechara, A., Damasio, H., Tranel, D., and Damasio, A. R. (1997). Deciding advantageously before knowing the advantageous strategy. *Science* 275:1293–1295.

Benbow, C. P., and Stanley, J. C. (1983). Sex differences in mathematical reasoning ability: more facts. *Science* 222:1029–1031.

Benke, T., Schelosky, L., and Gerstenbrand, F. (1988). A clinical investigation of finger agnosia. *J. Clin. Exp. Neuropsychol.* 10:335.

Benson, D. F., and Denckla, M. B. (1969). Verbal paraphasia as a source of calculation disturbance. *Arch. Neurol.* 21:96–102.

Benson, D. F., and Weir, W. F. (1972). Acalculia: acquired anarithmetia. *Cortex* 8:465–472.

Benton, A. L. (1958). Significance of systematic reversal in right-left discrimination. *Acta Psychiatr. Neurol. Scand.* 33:129–137.

Benton, A. L. (1959). *Right–Left Discrimination and Finger Localization: Development and Pathology*. New York: Hoeber-Harper.

Benton, A. L. (1961). The fiction of the "Gerstmann syndrome." *J. Neurol. Neurosurg. Psychiatry* 24:176–181.

Benton, A. L. (1963). *Assessment of Number Operations*. Iowa City: University of Iowa Hospital, Department of Neurology.

Benton, A. L. (1977). Reflections on the Gerstmann syndrome. *Brain Lang.* 4:45–62.

Benton, A. L. (1985). Body schema disturbances: finger agnosia and right–left disorientation. In *Clinical Neuropsychology*, K. M. Heilman and E. Valenstein (eds.). New York: Oxford University Press, pp. 115–129.

Benton, A. L. (1992). Gerstmann's syndrome. *Arch. Neurol.* 49:445–447.

Benton, A. L., and Sivan, A. B. (1993). Disturbances of the body schema. In *Clinical Neuropsychology*, K. M. Heilman and E. Valenstein (eds.), New York: Oxford University Press, pp. 123–140.

Benton, A. L., Sivan, A. B., Hamsher, K. S., Varney, N. S., and Spreen, O. (1994). *Contributions to Neuropsychological Assessment. A Clinical Manual*. New York: Oxford University Press.

Berger, H. (1926). Ueber Rechenstörungen bei Herderkrankungen des Grosshirns. *Arch. Psychiatrie Nervenkrankheiten* 78:238–263.

Berlucchi, G., and Aglioti, S. (1997). The body in the brain: neural bases of corporeal awareness. *Trends Neurosci.* 20:560–564.

Boller, F., and Grafman, J. (1983). Acalculia: historical development and current significance. *Brain Cogn.* 2:205–223.

Bonhoeffer, K. (1923). Zur Klinik und Lokalisation des Agrammatismus und der Rechts-Links-Desorientierung. *Monatsschr. Psychiatrie Neurol.* 54:11–42.

Burbaud, P., Degreze, P., Lafon, P., Franconi, J.-M., Bouligand, B., Bioulac, B., Caille, J.-M., and Allard, M. (1995). Lateralization of prefrontal activation during internal mental calculation: a functional magnetic resonance imaging study. *J. Neurophysiol.* 74:2194–2200.

Butterworth, B. (1999). *What Counts: How Every Brain is Hardwired for Math*. New York: The Free Press.

Chochon, F., Cohen, L., van de Moortele, P. F., and Dehaene, S. (1999). Differential contributions of the left and right inferior parietal lobules to number processing. *J. Cogn. Neurosci.* 11:617–630.

Cipolotti, L., and Butterworth, B. (1995). Toward a multiroute model of number processing: impaired number transcoding with preserved calculation skills. *J. Exp. Psychol.: Gen.* 124:375–390.

Cipolotti, L., Butterworth, B., and Warrington, E. K. (1994). From "one thousand nine hundred and forty-five" to 1,000,945. *Neuropsychologia* 32:503–509.

Clark, C. M., and Klonhoff, H. (1990). Right and left orientation in children aged 5 to 13 years. *J. Clin. Exp. Neuropsychol.* 12:459–466.

Cohn, R. (1961). Dyscalculia. *Arch. Neurol.* 4:301–307.

Connolly, A. J. (1991). *KeyMath Diagnostic Arithmetic Test-Revised*. Toronto: PsyCan Corporation.

Corbett, A. J., McCusker, E. A., and Davidson, O. R. (1986). Acalculia following a dominant-hemisphere subcortical infarct. *Arch. Neurol.* 43:964–966.

Critchley, M. (1966). The enigma of Gerstmann's syndrome. *Brain* 89:183–198.

Culver, C. M. (1969). Test of right–left discrimination. *Percept Mot Skills* 29:863–867.

Dahmen, W., Hartje, W., Büssing, A., and Sturm, W. (1982). Disorders of calculation in aphasic patients—spatial and verbal components. *Neuropsychologia* 20:145–153.

Damasio, A. R. (1994). *Descartes' Error: Emotion, Reason, and the Human Brain*. New York: Grosset/Putnam.

Damasio, A. R. (1999). *The Feeling of What Happens: Body and Emotion in the Making of Consciousness*. Orlando, FL: Harcourt/Brace.

Damasio, A. R., Grabowski, T. J., Bechara, A., Damasio, H., Ponto, L. L. B., Parvizi, J., and Hichwa, R. D. (2000). Subcortical and cortical brain activity during the feeling of self-generated emotions. *Nat. Neurosci.* 3:1049–1056.

Dehaene, S. (1992). Varieties of numerical abilities. *Cognition* 44:1–42.

Dehaene, S., and Cohen, L. (1997). Cerebral pathways for calculation: double dissociation between rote verbal and quantitative knowledge of arithmetic. *Cortex* 33:219–250.

Dehaene, S., Spelke, E., Pinel, P., Stanescu, R., and Tsivkin, S. (1999). Sources of mathematical thinking: behavioral and brain-imaging evidence. *Science* 284:970–974.

Dehaene, S., Tzourio, N., Frak, V., Raynaud, L., Cohen, L., Mehler, J., and Mazoyer, B. (1996). Cerebral activations during number multiplication and comparison: a PET study. *Neuropsychologia* 34:1097–1106.

Delazer, M., and Benke, T. (1997). Arithmetic facts without meaning. *Cortex* 33:697–710.

Delazer, M., Girelli, L., Semenza, C., and Denes, G. (1999). Numerical skills and aphasia. *J. Int. Neuropsychol. Soc.* 5:213–221.

Deloche, G., Dellatolas, G., Vendrell, J., and Bergego, C. (1996). Calculation and number processing: Neuropsychological assessment and daily life activities. *J. Int. Neuropsychol. Soc.* 2:177–180.

Deloche, G., and Seron, X. (1982). From three to 3: a differential analysis of skills in transcoding quantities between patients with Broca's and Wernicke's aphasia. *Brain* 105:719–733.

Deloche, G., Seron, X., Baeta, E., Basso, A., Salinas, D. C., Gaillard, F., Gondenberg, G., Stachowiak, F. J., Temple, C., Tzavaras, A., and Vendrell, J. (1993). Calculation and number processing: the EC301 Assessment Battery for brain-damaged adults. In *Developments in the Assessment and Rehabilitation of Brain Damaged Patients*, F. J. Stachowiak (ed.). Tübingen: Gunter Narr Verlag.

Deloche, G., Seron, X., Larroque, C., Magnien, C., Metz-Lutz, M. N., Noel, M. N., Riva, I., Schils, J. P., Dordain, M., Ferrand, I., Baeta, E., Basso, A., Cipolotti, L., Claros-Salinas, D., Howard, D., Gaillard, F., Goldenberg, G., Mazzucchi, A., Stachowiak, F., Tzavaras, A., Vendrell, J., Bergego, C., and Pradat-Diehl, P. (1994). Calculation and number processing: assessment battery; role of demographic factors. *J. Clin. Exp. Neuropsychol.* 16:195–208.

Denes, G. (1989). Disorders of body awareness and body knowledge. In *Handbook of Neuropsychology, Vol. 2*, F. Boller and J. Grafman (eds.). Amsterdam: Elsevier, pp. 207–228.

Denes, G. (1996). Autotopagnosia. In *The Blackwell Dictionary of Neuropsychology*, J. G. Beaumont, P. M. Kenealy, and M. J. C. Rogers (eds.). Cambridge, MA: Blackwell Publishers, pp. 137–142.

Denes, G., Cappelletti, J. Y., Zilli, T., Porta, F. D., and Gallana, A. (2000). A category-specific deficit of spatial representation: the case of autotopagnosia. *Neuropsychologia* 38:345–350.

Dennis, M. (1976). Dissociated naming and locating of body parts after left anterior temporal lobe resection: An experimental case study. *Brain and Language*, 3:147–163.

De Renzi, E. (1982). *Disorders of Space Exploration and Cognition*. New York: John Wiley and Sons.

De Renzi, E., and Faglioni, P. (1963). L'autotopagnosia. *Arch. Psicol. Neurol. Psychiatr.* 24:1–34.

De Renzi, E., and Scotti, G. (1970). Autotopagnosia: fiction or reality? *Arch. Neurol. (Chicago)* 23: 221–227.

Ettlinger, G. (1963). Defective identification of fingers. *Neuropsychologia* 1:39–45.

Fein, D. (1987). Systematic misidentification of toes in normal adults. *Neuropsychologia* 25:293–294.

Ferro, J. M., and Botelho, M. A. S. (1980). Alexia for arithmetical signs. A cause of disturbed calculation. *Cortex* 16:175–180.

Fischer, P., Marterer, A., and Danielczyk, W. (1990). Right–left disorientation in dementia of the Alzheimer type. *Neurology* 40:1619–1620.

Frederiks, J. A. M. (1985). Disorders of the body schema. In *Handbook of Clinical Neurology, Vol. 4*, F. J. Vinken and G. W. Bruyn (eds.). Amsterdam: North-Holland.

Gainotti, G., Cianchetti, C., and Tiacci, C. (1972). The influence of the hemispheric side of lesion on non verbal tasks of finger localization. *Cortex* 8:364–381.

Gerstmann, J. (1940). Syndrome of finger agnosia, disorientation for right and left, agraphia, and acalculia. *Arch. Neurol. Psychiatry* 44:398–408.

Gold, M., Adair, J. C., Jacobs, D. H., and Heilman, K. M. (1995). Right–left confusion in Gerstmann's syndrome: a model of body centered spatial orientation. *Cortex* 31:267–283.

Goodglass, H., Klein, B., Carey, P., and Jones, K. (1966). Specific semantic word categories in aphasia. *Cortex* 2:74–89.

Grafman, J. (1988). Acalculia. In *Handbook of Neuropsychology, Vol. 1*, F. Boller and J. Grafman (eds.). New York: Elsevier, pp. 415–431.

Grafman, J., Kampen, D., Rosenberg, J., Salazar, A. M., and Boller, F. (1989). The processing breakdown of number processing and calculation ability: a case study. *Cortex* 25:121–133.

Grafman, J., Passafiume, D., Faglioni, P., and Boller, F. (1982). Calculation disturbances in adults with focal hemispheric damage. *Cortex* 18:37–50.

Grewel, F. (1952). Acalculia. *Brain* 75:397–407.

Guyard, H., Masson, V., Quiniou, R., and Siou, E. (1997). Expert knowledge for acalculia assessment and rehabilitation. *Neuropsychol. Rehabil.* 7:419–439.

Harris, L. J., and Gitterman, S. R. (1978). University professors' self-descriptoins of left–right confusability: sex and handedness differences. *Percept. Mot. Skills 47*:819–823.

Head, H. (1920). *Studies in Neurology*. London: Oxford University Press.

Head, H. (1926). *Aphasia and Kindred Disorders of Speech*. Cambridge, UK: Cambridge University Press.

Hécaen, H., Angelergues, R., and Houillier, S. (1961). Les varietes cliniques des acalculies au cours des lesions retrorolandiques: approche statistique du probleme. *Rev. Neurol. 105*:85–103.

Henschen, S. E. (1919). Über Sprach-, Musik-, und Rechenmechanismen und ihre Lokalisation im Grosshirm. *Z. gesamte Neurol. Psychiatrie 52:* 273–298.

Hittmair-Delazer, M., Sailer, U., and Benke, T. (1995). Impaired arithmetic facts but intact conceptual knowledge—a single-case study of dyscalculia. *Cortex 31*:139–147.

Jackson, M., and Warrington, K. (1986). Arithmetic skills in patients with unilateral cerebral lesions. *Cortex 22*:611–620.

Kinsbourne, M., and Warrington, E. K. (1962). A study of finger agnosia. *Brain 85*:47–66.

Lampl, Y., Eshel, Y., Gilad, R., and Sarova-Pinhas, I. (1994). Selective acalcula with sparing of the subtraction process in a patient with left parietotemporal hemorrhage. *Neurology 44*:1759–1761.

Langdon, D. W., and Warrington, E. W. (1995). *The VESPAR: A Verbal and Spatial Reasoning Test*. Hove, England: Lawrence Erlbaum Associates.

Levin, II. S., Goldstein, F. C., and Spiers, P. A. (1993). Acalculia. In *Clinical Neuropsychology*, K. M. Heilman and E. Valenstein (eds.). New York: Oxford University Press, pp. 91–122.

Lucchelli, F., and De Renzi, E. (1993). Primary dyscalculia after a medial frontal lesion of the left hemisphere. *J. Neurol. Neurosurg. Psychiatry 56*:304–307.

Macoir, J. Audet, T., and Breton, M.-F. (1999). Code-dependent pathways for number transcoding: evidence from a case of selective impairment in written verbal numeral to arabic transcoding. *Cortex 35*:629–645.

Markwardt, F. C. (1989). *Peabody Individual Achievement Test-Revised*. Circle Pines, MN: American Guidance Service.

Matthews, C. G., Folk, E. D., and Zerfas, P. G. (1966). Lateralized finger localization deficits and differential Wechsler-Bellevue results in retardates. *Am. J. Ment. Defic. 70*:695–702.

McCloskey, M. (1992). Cognitive mechanism in nu-

merical processing: evidence from acquired dyscalculia. *Cognition 44*:107–157.

McCloskey, M., Caramazza, A., and Basili, A. (1985). Cognitive mechanisms in number processing and calculation: evidence from dyscalculia. *Brain Cogn. 4*:171–196.

McFie, J., and Zangwill, O. L. (1960). Visual-constructive disabilities associated with lesions of the left cerebral hemisphere. *Brain 83*:243–260.

McKenna, P., and Warrington, E. K. (1978). Category-specific naming preservation: a single case study. *J. Neurol. Neurosurg. Psychiatry 41*:571–574.

Money, J. A. (1976). *Standardized Road Map of Direction Sense*. San Rafael, CA: Academic Therapy Publications.

Morris, H. H., Lüders, H., Lesser, R. P., Dinner, D. S., and Hahn, J. (1984). Transient neuropsychological abnormalities (including Gertsmann's syndrome) during cortical stimulation. *Neurology 34*:877–883.

Ogden, J. A. (1985). Autotopagnosia. *Brain 108*: 1009–1022.

Ojemann, G. A. (1974). Mental arithmetic during human thalamic stimulation. *Neuropsychologia 12*:1–10.

Papanicolaou, A. C., Schmidt, A. L., Moore, B. D., and Eisenberg, H. M. (1983). Cerebral activation patterns in an arithmetic and a visuospatial processing task. *Int. J. Neurosci. 20*:283–288.

Pick, A. (1922). Storung der Orientierung am eigenen Korper. *Psychol. Forsch. 1*:303–318.

Poeck, K., and Orgass, B. (1969). An experimental investigation of finger agnosia. *Neurology 19*:801–807.

Poeck, K., and Orgass, B. (1971). The concept of the body schema: a critical review and some experimental results. *Cortex 7*:254–277.

Ramachandran, V. S. (1998). Consciousness and body image: lessons from phantom limbs, Capgras syndrome, and pain asymbolia. *Phil. Trans. R. Soc. Lond. Ser. B Biol. Sci. 353*:1851–1859.

Ramachandran, V. S., and Rogers-Ramachandran, D. (2000). Phantom limbs and neural plasticity. *Arch. Neurol. 57*:317–320.

Ratcliff, G. (1979). Spatial thought, mental rotation and the right cerebral hemisphere. *Neuropsychologia 17*:49–54.

Rickard, T. C., Romero, S. G., Basso, G., Wharton, C., Flitman, S., and Grafman, J. (2000). The calculating brain: an fMRI study. *Neuropsychologia 38*:325–335.

Rosselli, M., and Ardila, A. (1989). Calculation deficits in patients with right and left hemisphere damage. *Neuropsychologia 27*:607–617.

Rueckert, L., Lange, N., Partiot, A., Appollonio, I., Litvan, I., Le Bihan, D., and Grafman, J. (1996). Visualizing cortical activation during mental calculation with functional MRI. *Neuroimage* 3:97–103.

Sauguet, J., Benton, A. L., and Hécaen, H. (1971). Disturbances of the body schema in relation to language impairment and hemispheric locus of lesion. *J. Neurol. Neurosurg. Psychiatry* 34:496–501.

Selecki, B. R., and Herron, J. T. (1965). Disturbances of the verbal body image: a particular syndrome of sensory aphasia. *J. Nerv. Ment. Dis.* 141:42–52.

Semenza, C. (1988). Impairment in localization of body parts following brain damage. *Cortex* 24:443–449.

Semenza, C., and Goodglass, H. (1985). Localization of body parts in brain injured subjects. *Neuropsychologia* 23:161–175.

Semenza, C., Miceli, L., and Girelli, L. (1997). A deficit for arithmetical procedures: lack of knowledge or lack of monitoring? *Cortex* 33:483–498.

Seron, X., and Deloche, G. (1983). From 4 to four. A supplement to 'From three to 3.' *Brain* 106:735–744.

Singer, H. D., and Low, A. A. (1933). Acalculia (Henschen): a clinical study. *Arch. Neurol. Psychiatry* 29:467–498.

Sirigu, A., Grafman, J., Bressler, K., and Sunderland, T. (1991). Multiple representations contribute to body knowledge processing. *Brain* 114:629–642.

Sivan, A. B. (1992). *Benton Visual Retention Test* (5th Edition). San Antonio, TX: The Psychological Corporation.

Sparrow, S. S., Balla, D. A., and Cicchetti, D. V. (1984). *Vineland Adaptive Behavior Scales*. Circle Pines, MN: American Guidance Services.

Sullivan, K. S., Macaruso, P., and Sokol, S. M. (1996). Remediation of arabic numeral processing in a case of developmental dyscalculia. *Neuropsychol. Rehabil.* 6:27–53.

Suzuki, K., Yamadori, A., and Fujii, T. (1997). Category-specific comprehension deficit restricted to body parts. *Neurocase* 3:193–200.

Tohgi, H., Satoshi, K., Takahashi, S., Takahashi, H., Utsugisawa, K., Yonezawa, H., Hatano, K., and Sasaki, T. (1995). Agraphia and acalculia after a left prefrontal (F1, F2) infarction. *J. Neurol. Neurosurg. Psychiatry* 58:629–632.

Tucha, O., Steup, A., Smely, C., and Lange, K. W. (1997). Toe agnosia in Gerstmann syndrome. *J. Neurol. Neurosurg. Psychiatry* 63:399–403.

U.S. Bureau of the Census. (1987). Estimates of the population of the United States, by age, sex, and race: 1980–1986. *Current Population Reports* (Series P-25, No. 1000). Washingotn, DC: Author.

Warrington, E. K. (1982). The fractionation of arithmetical skills: a single case study. *Q. J. Exp. Psychol.* 34A:31–51.

Wechsler, D. (1991). *Wechsler Adult Intelligence Scale–III*. New York: The Psychological Corporation.

Wechsler Individual Achievement Test (WIAT). (1992). San Antonio: The Psychological Corporation.

Whalen, J., McCloskey, M., Lesser, R. P., and Gordon, B. (1997). Localizing arithmetic processes in the brain: evidence from a transient deficit during cortical stimulation. *J. Cogn. Neurosci.* 9:409–417.

Whitaker, H., Habiger, T., and Ivers, R. (1985). Acalculia from a lenticular-caudate infarction. *Neurology* 35(Suppl 1):161.

Wilkinson, G. S. (1993). *WRAT3 Administration Manual*. Wilmington, DE: Wide Range.

Wolf, S. M. (1973). Difficulties in right–left discrimination in a normal population. *Arch. Neurol.* 29:128–129.

Woodcock, R. W., and Mather, N. (1989). *Woodcock-Johnson Tests of Achievement*. Allen, TX: DLM Teaching Resources.

Yamadori, A., and Albert, M. L. (1973). Word category aphasia. *Cortex* 9:112–125.

10

Anosognosia

JOHN C. ADAIR, RONALD L. SCHWARTZ, AND ANNA M. BARRETT

Anosognosia refers to a state in which patients with brain injury deny their disabilities or lack awareness of their deficits. The relationship of anosognosia to other behavioral disorders is complex. Many authorities view the phenomenon as part of the spectrum of the neglect syndrome. Others emphasize the parallels between anosognosia and confabulatory behavior. Anosognosia also bears some resemblance to disorders of body schema such as asomatognosia or autotopagnosia.

Several descriptions of anosognosia were published before Babinski coined the term in 1914 (Babinski, 1914). As introduced, anosognosia referred only to lack of awareness or recognition of a specific neurologic disturbance (i.e., hemiparesis). Subsequently, the term has been applied more broadly to describe unawareness of any neurological or neuropsychological deficit (Fisher, 1989). A wide variety of clinical syndromes have been associated with anosognosia, including visual loss (hemianopia or cortical blindness), amnesia, dementia, aphasia, cortical deafness, movement disorders (hemiballismus, chorea, tardive dyskinesia), apraxia, and thought disorders associated with schizophrenia.

Understanding anosognosia may contribute to improvements in patient care for several rea-sons. First, current treatments for ischemic stroke depend critically on initiation within a short period after onset of injury. While specific data do not exist on this point, a lack of deficit awareness may be an important factor in determining why patients and their families delay seeking care after stroke (Grotta and Bratina, 1995). Second, patients who do not apprehend deficits may not understand the rationale for rehabilitation therapy. This may account for observations that patients with anosognosia recover incompletely and take longer to attain benefit from rehabilitation (Gialanella and Mattioli, 1992; Maeshima et al., 1997). Third, anosognosia may preclude patients from making appropriate concessions to residual disability. Patients lacking awareness of their deficit expose themselves to further harm, falling when they fail to use their assist device or colliding with hazards when they fail to remain vigilant for objects in a blind hemi-field (Cole, 1999).

This chapter describes anosognosia for several major neurological deficits, including hemiparesis, visual loss, and disorders of cognition such as dementia, memory loss, and aphasia. For each disorder, the text reviews the clinical characteristics and their anatomic correlates. The putative mechanisms of anosognosia are summarized and, despite the diversity of impairments, many share the same explanations.

ANOSOGNOSIA FOR HEMIPARESIS

CLINICAL CHARACTERISTICS

Anosognosia for hemiparesis (AHP) occurs most frequently after large brain injuries that render a patient severely disabled. Thus, the patient's inability to report their symptoms will dramatically strike even the most casual examiner. When asked about the nature of their visit to the hospital, such individuals may produce a broad range of responses that evade the issue of physical impairment (Bisiach and Geminiani, 1991; Feinberg, 1997). Often they will complain of other unrelated symptoms (e.g., indigestion). Some patients displace illness, stating that they merely accompanied a sick family member to the hospital. Others create delusional rationalizations for being at the hospital by claiming, for example, that they work on the nursing staff.

Denial of deficit may result from reduced deficit awareness, although individuals may display either denial or lack of insight separately. Those exhibiting denial might, for example, adamantly reject assertions that they are weak but act disabled, obeying ordered activity restrictions without objection. Those lacking insight freely admit that half of their body is paralyzed but betray profound lack of insight when attempting to ambulate on a weak leg or making abortive attempts to perform bimanual tasks. When asked specifically about the function of paretic extremities, patients with AHP may concede impairment but often underestimate its severity or appear unmoved by its consequences. *Anosodiaphoria* refers to this condition in which patients show "awareness" of their impairment but express indifference toward the implications of disability (Critchley, 1953). Such patients defy unambiguous determination of where deficit awareness ends and deficit underestimation begins. While many patients with AHP tenaciously disagree with examiners about weakness, others acknowledge differential strength but view it on their own terms. Cutting (1978) observed that, when

properly interrogated, most patients will admit they have some problem with the paretic limb, often phrasing symptoms in terms of "stiffness" or "heaviness." Patients may also rationalize impairment, blaming left-sided weakness on the fact that they are right-handed. Within the individual, depth of insight can vary over brief intervals, with patients acknowledging hemiparesis at one point of an interview only to recant their statements shortly thereafter (Ramachandran, 1995). Recent attempts to grade or quantify anosognosia for research and clinical purposes incorporate the concept that deficit awareness can be described in terms of a spectrum of severity (see below).

In addition to ignorance of their own bodily functions, patients with AHP may exhibit "productive" manifestations. These behaviors suggest that the brain injury can lead to alternative, confabulatory self-interpretations regarding an individual's somatic condition as well as their environment. Such phenomenon may be as ordinary as patients who, when asked to use the weak extremity, perform the task with the intact appendage and then, despite evidence to the contrary, assert with conviction that they followed the examiner's instructions. Other patients report peculiar and complex delusions regarding the affected body parts. While such individuals appear to concede some awareness of disturbed bodily function, they can elaborate on the affected extremity's function in an extraordinary manner. For example, some patients express intense hatred toward the limb, known as *misoplegia*, and threaten the limb for disobeying them (Critchley, 1974). Weinstein and Kahn (1955) reported patients who expressed resentment toward the disabled body part, calling it pejorative names (e.g., "lazy" or "dumb"). Other patients disown the limb, such as the patient of Gerstmann (1942) who claimed that the paretic arm and leg belonged to a sleeping child lying next to her. Patients may also personify the extremity, claiming that it is actually another individual. Examples include the patient of Bisiach et al. (1991) who stated flatly that his paretic arm was in fact his mother and the patient of Anton who believed that his daughter was lying next to him, rather than his lifeless extremity (Förstl et al., 1993). Productive manifestations associated with AHP may consist of peculiar verbal expressions called "paraphasic" substitutions by Weinstein and Kahn (1955). The patient's language distortions typically bear some relationship to their illness, such as calling a syringe a "used radio tube" or calling a bedpan a "piano stool." Patients may also refer to themselves in the second or third person and use excessive slang or malapropisms when speaking of their symptoms. Such patients appear to retain some awareness of deficit but, through the use of metaphor, acknowledge illness with some words but not others.

ASSESSMENT

The primary means of determining AHP remains a judgment by the clinician that the patient fails to acknowledge problems apparent to the examiner. This approach generates a crude determination of AHP as either present or absent. Lack of precision regarding what constitutes AHP has been cited as one of the main reasons for discrepant results between studies.

More recently, investigators have incorporated the concept of deficit awareness as falling along a continuum as suggested by Critchley (1953). Bisiach et al. (1986) ranked the severity of AHP on a four-point Likert scale. Different grades of awareness ranged from spontaneous reporting of deficit during routine interview to persistent denial of weakness even after explicit demonstration during the physical examination. More involved approaches include instruments such as the Denial of Illness Scale, which uses a semi-structured interview to rank a patient's responses to questions about their symptoms (Starkstein et al., 1993b). Others have indirectly measured anosognosia based on the discrepancy between the patient's rating of their own ability to perform activities (e.g., dressing) and the same rating made about the patient by collateral observers such as family members or nursing staff (Blonder and Ranseen, 1994).

ANATOMIC CORRELATES

The preponderance of clinical studies (Nathanson et al., 1952; Cutting, 1978; Starkstein et al.,

1992; Stone et al., 1993) indicate that AHP most frequently follows injury to the right or nondominant hemisphere. Selection bias might partly account for right–left asymmetry, however, since aphasia from dominant hemisphere injury tends to confound a patient's ability to acknowledge deficit awareness verbally. Indeed, many studies of AHP exclude such patients as "unassessable." Friedlander (1967) made an estimate of the frequency of AHP after left brain injury by assuming that AHP was as common among patients with and without severe aphasia. Inclusion of severely aphasic patients reduced but did not completely negate asymmetry that favored the right hemisphere, a finding reported by others (Cutting, 1978; Starkstein et al., 1992). Furthermore, Bisiach and colleagues (1991) emphasized that observers can reliably detect a patient's nonverbal expressions of AHP. For example, patients who admit that their left arm and leg are weak, only to abortively attempt ambulation or bimanual activity, provide such nonverbal confirmation of AHP.

A number of studies (Buchtel et al., 1992; Gilmore et al., 1992; Kaplan et al., 1993; Durkin et al., 1994; Breier et al., 1995; Carpenter et al., 1995; Dywan et al., 1995) examined AHP produced by hemispheric inactivation through intracarotid barbiturate infusion (Table 10–1). By testing patients shortly after recovery from anesthesia, aphasia should no longer bias assessment of deficit awareness. While the frequency of anosognosia differs from that in the clinical series mentioned above and varies considerably among studies, the conclusion remains that AHP occurs more frequently during right hemisphere inactivation.

Table 10–1. Incidence of Anosognosia for Hemiparesis during Wada Test

Study	Right Hemisphere (%)	Left Hemisphere (%)
Gilmore et al. (1992)	100	0
Buchtel et al. (1992)	92	57
Kaplan et al. (1993)	100	71
Durkin et al. (1994)	94	86
Dywan et al. (1995)	67	65
Breier et al. (1995)	89	49

Radiographic studies fail to define one particular neuroanatomic feature most characteristic of patients with AHP. On the basis of brain computerized tomographic (CT) scan data, Levine et al. (1991) reported that patients with AHP showed slightly larger lesions and marginally greater atrophy of the uninjured hemisphere. Besides involvement of the caudate nucleus in the anosognosic group, anatomic overlap among patients with preserved deficit awareness was extensive. In a similar study, Bisiach and colleagues (1986) mapped lesions from CT scans from a group of patients after right hemisphere stroke. Their conclusion that AHP was associated with damage to the inferoposterior parietal region was based on qualitative analysis of composite scans and they did not provide quantitative support for their assertion. They also found that thalamic injury was more common among the anosognosic group (3 of 4) than in those with insight into their deficit awareness (1 of 15). Starkstein and associates (1992) performed an analysis of CT scans from patients stratified according to severity of AHP. Patients with mild or severe AHP showed significantly higher frequencies of temporoparietal and thalamic lesions than those of patients with no or moderate anosognosia. The latter group of patients demonstrated a higher frequency of lesions involving the basal ganglia. After combining data across different levels of severity, Starkstein et al. observed a higher frequency of temporoparietal lesions, larger lesion area, and greater degrees of cerebral atrophy among patients with AHP. The association of AHP with larger lesion volume has also been reported with intracerbral hemorrhage (Maeshima et al., 1997).

Some authorities contend that AHP arises only with injury to association cortex and that patients remain aware of deficit after lesions confined to primary motor cortex or its projections. Since neural systems that support so-called intermediary processing, responsible for conscious awareness (Mesulam, 1998), reside within association areas, the argument has some theoretical foundation. However, several well-documented cases of AHP following injury to subcortical structures argue against this strict anatomical association. For example, cases of AHP after pontine infarction (Evya-

pan and Kumral, 1999) or hemorrhage (Bakchine et al., 1997) have been described. Likewise, several groups have reported AHP following hemorrhage within the caudate nucleus (Healton et al., 1982; Jacome, 1986). Lastly, in agreement with anatomic correlates defined by CT scans, several cases of AHP have been associated with focal thalamic injury (Zoll, 1969; Watson and Heilman, 1979; Graff-Radford et al., 1984; Liebson, 2000). The functional consequences of these subcortical injuries remain obscure since, in at least some cases, brainstem insult resulted in bilaterally reduced cerebral perfusion in the frontal region while the caudate lesions produced diffuse slowing of electrical activity throughout the affected hemisphere.

MECHANISMS UNDERLYING ANOSOGNOSIA FOR HEMIPARESIS

A unifying explanation of AHP in psychobiological terms remains elusive. The most enduring account of AHP views loss of insight as a psychological mechanism for moderating the impact of impairment on the patient's ego. This type of theory, termed "global" by some authors, posits that a single mechanism can account for anosognosia in all its diverse forms. Another such global hypothesis considers AHP as resulting from diffuse cognitive impairment. Other explanations invoke modular and dissociable processes that can be discretely disrupted. These hypotheses view AHP in terms of aberrant feedback to brain systems that "monitor" self status or, alternatively, disconnection of feedback from these systems. Lastly, AHP may result from defects in feedforward processes that attune the monitor in anticipation of incipient motor activity.

Psychologically Motivated Denial

Anosognosia has been explained by some authorities in terms of an unconscious defense mechanism that reduces distress engendered by loss of function. Most sources attribute the psychodynamic interpretation of anosognosia to the work of Weinstein and Kahn (1955). In fact, Sandifer (1946) identified motivational factors a decade earlier, viewing anosognosia as a means of avoiding the "catastrophic reaction," and Wortis and Dattner (1942) described personality features that they felt typified patients with denial of deficit.

In their book *Denial of Illness*, Weinstein and Kahn (1955) provided detailed observations on patients who lacked awareness for a broad range of deficits. Anosognosia always accompanied more generalized alteration in behavior including disorientation, "paraphasic" language errors, confabulations, mood disturbance, and reduplicative phenomena. However, in trying to understand how other equally impaired patients with similarly severe injuries retained awareness of their deficits, they speculated that "denial . . . was a continuation of a preexisting personality trend." In support of this claim, they studied two groups of patients who differed regarding whether or not they explicitly denied their deficits. After defining each patient's premorbid personality traits from close collateral sources, they found that patients with anosognosia had always regarded infirmity as a basis for shame and embarrassment and had actually denied the existence of other illness at earlier junctures. The group without denial of current symptoms varied considerably. While variability precluded generalizations about a typical personality type, the tendency to deny or ignore illness was not present.

Several clinical observations contradict the defense mechanism hypothesis of anosognosia. First, problems with deficit awareness are almost always maximal soon after injury with improvement in the ensuing days or weeks. This pattern is exactly opposite that predicted by a psychological coping strategy, which should evolve as orientation and level of alertness improve. Second, weakness developing slowly should engender the same threat to self-image as that associated with a deficit that develops rapidly. However, certain data indicate that AHP more frequently accompanies acute rather than slowly progressive weakness. Third, Bisiach and colleagues (1986) cited examples of individuals who deny hemiparesis but remain aware of speech impairment, and Berti et al. (1996) described a hemiparetic patient who acknowledged weakness in the arm but not in the leg. Any concession of dysfunction would presumably undermine the effectiveness of psychologically motivated denial. Fourth, assuming motivated denial requires high-level cognitive processes, then AHP would most often follow small, deep strokes since these would least impact cognitive function. However, as noted above, AHP most frequently accompanies large, cortically based injuries. Fifth, some deficits (e.g., hemianopia) cause relatively minor disability or disfigurement, thus posing little threat to the patient's self-perception of their own abilities. Since patients deny such deficits just as obstinately as those patients with anosognosia following more overt deficits, there is poor correlation between the need to preserve the ego from perception of deficiency and the severity of the injury. Lastly, while psychological defense might explain denial of deficit, such mechanisms poorly explain delusional phenomena such as misoplegia and personification.

Research pertaining to the relationship between affective disorders and AHP also provides persuasive evidence against the defense mechanism hypothesis. Starkstein and colleagues (1992) reasoned that if defense mechanisms served to protect patients from negative reactions to disability, then patients with anosognosia should demonstrate less anxiety and depression than those who retain deficit awareness. In their study of a large group of patients who had suffered left and right hemisphere stroke, they found no difference in the frequency of affective disorders between patients with and without anosognosia. Similar observations have been made by others (Blonder and Ranseen, 1994). Starkstein et al. (1990) reported two patients in whom depression followed right hemisphere stroke despite anosognosia. Treatment of affective disorders in such patients seems to have little effect on anosognosia. The data, supporting a double dissociation between adverse psychological outcomes and AHP, pose a formidable challenge to the defense mechanism hypothesis.

Studies of anosognosia during the Wada test mentioned above provide additional arguments against the defense mechanism hypothesis. First, as mentioned above, AHP follows barbiturate infusion into the right carotid artery more often than after left-sided injections. As noted by many authors (Friedland and Weinstein, 1977; Bisiach and Geminiani, 1991; Heilman, 1991), a psychological defense explanation provides no reason for observed left–right asymmetry. Second, the Wada technique permits inquiry about drug-induced weakness after symptoms have resolved. These patients without symptoms should have no motivation for denial. Third, the defense mechanism hypothesis predicts that left hemisphere–dominant individuals with AHP after left hemisphere anesthesia would also deny aphasia. However, Breier et al. (1995) described patients who denied hemiplegia while acknowledging speech disturbance and vice versa, a finding consistent with clinical experience after left brain injury.

Cognitive Impairment

Some authorities assert that AHP occurs when general mental impairments impede the processes of self-observation and inference necessary for accurate appraisal of bodily function (Hécaen and Albert, 1978; Levine, 1990). Support for this view comes from studies showing disorientation in 71% of patients with AHP compared to only 6% of patients who remain aware of deficits (Cutting, 1978). Other investigators have attempted to specify which cognitive disorders promote anosognosia. One investigation compared two groups of right brain–damaged patients that differed with respect to deficit awareness (Levine et al., 1991). While complete data were not available for every case, those with AHP showed "lack of mental clarity" and scored lower on nearly every measure of memory and intellect. Starkstein et al. (1993b) sought to define the cognitive correlates of AHP after right and left hemisphere injury. Patients with AHP performed significantly worse on a test of general cognition (Mini-Mental State Examination) as well as on tasks sensitive to frontal brain injury. In contrast, no significant between-group differences were found on tests of simple attention, verbal comprehension, constructional abilities, or memory.

Some of the arguments against the defense mechanism hypothesis also pertain to explanations of AHP in terms of general intellectual deterioration. For example, diffuse cognitive

problems cannot easily account for the ways that anosognosia can dissociate across modalities (Bisiach et al., 1986). Within an individual, reduced mental capacity would be predicted to preclude insight into all deficits to the same degree, a position conclusively refuted by the literature. The observation of AHP in Wada test subjects also argues against mental impairment as a cause of AHP (Buchtel et al., 1992; Gilmore et al., 1992; Kaplan et al., 1993; Durkin et al., 1994). Specifically, these subjects denied weakness even after resolution of barbiturate effects, a time when mental function was back to baseline levels.

Sensory Defects, Neglect, and Asomatognosia

One of the simplest accounts of AHP, termed the "feedback hypothesis," attributes lack of awareness to lack of sensory information. As noted by Heilman (1991), patients derive information about limb function through somatic sensations or visual inspection or both. The distribution of most lesions causing AHP also results in cortical deprivation of either visual or somatic afferent information about contralesional body parts. Hence, a number of authors emphasize the strong association between the presence of elemental sensory loss, particularly defective proprioception, and the presence of AHP (Anton, 1898; Weinstein and Kahn, 1950; Gerstmann 1942; Critchley, 1953; Zoll, 1969; Levine et al., 1991). Indeed, somatosensory evoked potential observations provide indirect support for the feedback hypothesis (Green and Hamilton, 1976). Other investigators failed to confirm abnormal evoked responses in patients with AHP, however (Maugiere et al., 1982). Regardless of electrophysiological data, the fundamental reason that AHP does not appear to be simply reducible to or equated with deafferentation remains clinical: patients with equally severe sensory loss can differ in their awareness of deficit.

Some authorities consider anosognosia as part of a larger disorder of processing information from contralesional space. For example, the neglect syndrome encompasses a set of disorders that preclude normal orientation toward or response to stimuli despite intact elementary sensorimotor function (see Chapter 13). The spatial distribution of neglect behaviors can independently involve extrapersonal space, the immediate extrapersonal environment, or personal space itself. The phenomenon of *personal neglect* (PN), otherwise known as *verbal asomatognosia*, refers to a condition in which patients lack regard for certain parts of their own body. Such individuals may fail to acknowledge the existence of the contralesional half of their body, dressing only the right arm and leg or grooming only half of their face and hair (Feinberg et al., 1990). Neglect might lead to AHP if it impedes self-assessment of limb function. For example, an individual with PN who lacks an adequate concept of half of their body might not make reliable judgments about the function of these parts.

A number of clinical studies provide evidence that anosognosia and neglect behavior are not synonymous conditions. Levine and colleagues (1991) divided right hemispheric stroke patients into two groups that differed only with regard to deficit awareness. Using tests of extrapersonal neglect, they found that all patients with AHP showed severe neglect compared to a minority of patients with transient or no AHP. Despite the strong correlation between neglect and AHP, they reported that patients retained "orientation" to the paretic extremities, suggesting that PN was not present. Other investigators have established a double dissociation between AHP and neglect. For example, Bisiach and colleagues (1986) systematically examined the relationship between different forms of neglect and deficit awareness in 97 right brain–damaged patients. While both personal and extrapersonal neglect frequently co-occurred with AHP, they observed cases of neglect without AHP as well as AHP without neglect. Cutting (1978) assessed neglect behaviors in 100 hemiplegic patients with AHP or "anosognosic phenomena" such as anosodiaphoria. Findings termed "visuospatial neglect" were found in 52% of patients with impaired awareness of deficit in contrast to 6% of those with retained awareness. Furthermore, while Cutting (1978) found PN only among patients with anosognosia or related phenomena, it was present in only a minority (32%) of this group. Starkstein et al. (1992) examined the relationship between different types of neglect and the level of severity of anosognosia. While neglect behaviors were

more common among patients with AHP, there was no relationship between neglect and the severity of AHP. In fact, other studies have reported an inverse relationship between neglect and anosognosia (Blonder and Ranseen, 1994), with neglect patients actually tending to overestimate the severity of their deficits.

To formally evaluate the association between AHP and PN, Adair et al. (1995) asked patients undergoing the Wada test to distinguish their own hands from those of the examiners. The weak extremity was positioned within ipsilesional visual space and unequivocal visual apprehension of the body part was documented. Only a small minority of patients with AHP failed to acknowledge ownership of affected extremities. The opposite dissociation was not observed, however, since no patient who retained awareness of deficit concurrently showed PN. In agreement with the earlier clinical series, the study illustrated how PN by itself is neither necessary nor sufficient to preclude insight into motor deficit.

Disconnection, Confabulation, and Illusory Limb Movement

Geschwind (1965) attributed anosognosia for left hemiparesis to disconnection of the left body's self-monitoring apparatus, presumably in the right hemisphere, from the language centers of the left hemisphere. Deprived of input, the left hemisphere produces "confabulatory" responses to inquiries regarding the function of the left half of their body. Appealing features of this hypothesis include providing a rationale for the delusional, productive aspects of AHP, as well as accounting for the asymmetric lateralization of lesions causing AHP. The disconnection hypothesis received indirect support from Feinberg and associates (1994), who studied two groups of patients with similar clinical and radiographic features after right brain injury. Asked to make forced-choice identification of objects presented briefly in the left visual hemifield, patients with AHP produced random (i.e., confabulatory) responses whereas the group without anosognosia more readily admitted that they did not perceive stimuli.

Several observations undermine disconnection as the sole explanation for AHP. Even if information about the paretic limb failed to access the language-dominant hemisphere, most patients should be able to convey deficit awareness nonverbally (Bisiach and Geminiani, 1991). In one study, patients were asked to communicate their insight through nonverbally selecting their preference from either physically feasible unimanual tasks associated with small rewards or physically impossible bimanual tasks associated with large rewards (Ramchandran, 1995). If AHP resulted from disconnection alone, the right hemisphere would presumably choose tasks that could be successfully completed. In nearly all trials, however, subjects with AHP selected bimanual tasks. Since subjects indicated their preference with their right hands, the left hemisphere may have still been "confabulating nonverbally." Hence, Adair and colleagues (1997) used the Wada test to more directly test the disconnection hypothesis. They speculated that providing the intact hemisphere with visual and kinesthetic information about the paretic limb should lead to deficit awareness if interhemispheric disconnection caused AHP. As mentioned above, positioning the weak left extremity in the right visual hemispace failed to alter AHP in most subjects, arguing against disconnection as a common etiologic factor.

A recent investigation failed to support a direct relationship between confabulation and AHP. During the Wada test, Lu et al. (1997) asked patients to make tactile discriminations of differently textured stimuli. After barbiturate injection, examiners apposed the fingertips of the paretic limb against one of several materials. The subject pointed with the intact extremity to the corresponding material from a board that contained all stimuli as well as a question mark to indicate identification failure. On some trials, no stimulus was delivered, thereby providing an opportunity for confabulation. The results indicated dissociations between confabulation and AHP. Some subjects were aware of weakness but confabulated on the task, whereas other individuals showed AHP but never made confabulatory responses.

In another study, Lu et al. (1997) assessed the patient's perception of illusory limb movements and their relationship to AHP. Preliminary results failed to establish a link between "phantom" percepts and AHP in patients undergoing the Wada test. Although several individuals reported illusory movements in the paretic extremity, some of these people retained awareness of deficit. In contrast, others who did not report illusory movement showed AHP.

The Feedforward Hypothesis

For an individual to detect their deficit, some hypothetical intentional mechanism within the brain presumably primes another hypothetical comparator mechanism regarding anticipated movement. When kinesthetic signals match expectations, the comparator detects no error. Hence, lack of deficit awareness might arise if the intentional system fails to alert the comparator, since lack of motion in the paralyzed limb will not signal mismatch. Accordingly, Heilman (1991) hypothesized that AHP may originate from defective processing within the intentional motor system.

Subjective reports of patient's experiences during recovery of awareness provide support for the feedforward hypothesis. Chatterjee and Mennemeier (1996) interviewed stroke patients about introspection into their illness within 2 weeks of brain injury. The individuals became aware of weakness only after attempts to move were prompted, either by another person or through their own volition. Similar findings have been obtained during Wada testing; some subjects discover their weakness during the procedure (Adair et al., 1997). Simple visual inspection, even with the limb clearly presented to the intact hemifield, failed to promote insight about the deficit. Those who acknowledged weakness did so only after commands to move the paralyzed limb, even if the attempt was not directly visualized. Likewise, a study of patients recovering from stroke within 24 hours examined awareness of the circumstances surrounding onset of deficit in addition to their introspections about awareness once the deficit was established (Grotta and Bratina, 1995). The majority of patients (80%) were aware of what they were doing at the time of stroke onset and were aware that some capacity relevant to their ability to continue this activity had changed. Nearly half of this group subsequently failed to recognize their deficit. One interpretation of their data, consistent with the feedforward hypothesis, is that patients involved in motor activity when injury occurs will show greater awareness of their deficit.

Limited experimental evidence also indicates dysfunction of intentional processes associated with AHP. In a pilot study, surface potentials were recorded from proximal muscles, which are normally activated bilaterally during maximal effort using only one limb (Gold et al., 1994). Normal controls and paretic patients without AHP activated truncal muscles bilaterally when asked to give maximal contractions with either the right or left hand. In contrast, a patient with AHP activated proximal muscles bilaterally only when giving maximal effort with the nonparetic hand; no muscle activity on either side accompanied attempted movements with the weak hand. Gold and associates (1994) interpreted these findings as indicating a loss of motor intention associated with AHP. In a similar manner, Hildebrandt and Zieger (1995) recorded motor responses from more distal parts of the plegic extremity in a patient with AHP after right hemisphere injury. Tasks that caused the largest response included recollection of past experiences of movement by the weak hand and tasks involving attempted bimanual manipulation of objects. Since these contexts may have invoked intact intentional processes of the left hemisphere to impel activity in the homolateral plegic extremity, the results do not contradict the feedforward hypothesis. In fact, commands to use the weak hand in isolation failed to invoke motor responses, consistent with the findings of Gold et al. (1994).

If attempts at movement represent a prerequisite to awareness, several predictions may be made. First, all injuries causing hemiplegia result in AHP, at least for a brief period of time until the attempt to move occurs and the resulting failure becomes detected. Indeed, some authorities assert that anosognosia to some degree accompanies all forms of brain injury (Fisher, 1989). Second, patients whose deficits develop during sleep, when intentional processes are presumably suspended, might be anticipated to show less awareness than those

whose deficits begin during wakefulness, particularly while engaged in some activity. Evidence on these points does not exist.

ANOSOGNOSIA FOR VISUAL DEFICITS

CLINICAL CHARACTERISTICS

Anosognosia for cortical blindness, known as *Anton's syndrome*, is relatively rare. Mentioned in the writings of Seneca 2000 years ago, von Monakow provided the first contemporary description of visual anosognosia in 1885. Severity of visual impairment typically includes at least an inability to discriminate shape and color; many patients cannot count fingers or even make light–dark discriminations. Patients act blind, failing to negotiate obstacles in their environment, and never establish eye contact with the examiner. Despite profound disability, patients deny visual symptoms and typically provide confident but incorrect responses when asked to make visual judgments. As with AHP, confronting patients with errors in judgment often leads to elaborate excuses for impaired performance (e.g., poor ambient light).

In contrast to the rarity of anosognosia for cortical blindness, between 55% and 88% of hemianopic patients fail to report their deficit (Warrington, 1962; Gassel and Williams, 1963; Bisiach et al., 1986; Celesia et al., 1997). Levine (1990) noted that patients with hemifield visual loss rarely complain of problems with vision. In fact, Bisiach and associates (1986) found that anosognosia for visual field defects occurred in 88% of their densely hemianopic patients, compared to the same degree of AHP in only 33% of their patients with severe motor weakness.

Deficits of higher-order visual processing can also be denied. For example, unawareness of dyslexia was originally reported by Bonhoeffer (1903) and more recently by Berti and colleagues (1996). A patient with prosopagnosia (difficulty in recognizing familiar people from their faces) who failed to recognize this deficit has also been described (Young et al., 1990). Subjects may also show anosognosia for color anomia after a brain lesion that disconnects the primary visual cortex from language areas (Geschwind and Fusillo, 1966). Lastly, while not specifically emphasized in the literature, loss of insight pervades other disorders of complex visual processing, such as visuospatial neglect and Balint syndrome.

Denial of cortical blindness may persist over time or evolve into partial deficit awareness. Anosognosia may abate completely if visual acuity sufficiently improves (Goldenberg, 1992). For hemianopia, there may exist a continuum of anosognosia, with some patients expressing incomplete awareness of their deficit (Critchley, 1949). For example, patients may acknowledge greater awareness of problems for stimuli from the temporal portion of the visual field, yet remain less aware of the nasal field defect (Teuber et al., 1960). Even patients who know they have homonymous visual loss may report that they forget its existence in ordinary visual-motor tasks (Cole, 1999).

ASSESSMENT

Few measures have been systematically developed to specifically gauge awareness of visual loss. For the cortically blind patient who produces fantastical responses to visual stimuli, such instruments may not add much beyond the examiner's narrative description. Bisiach and colleagues (1986) described a four-point Likert scale for grading awareness of hemianopia, ranging from spontaeous acknowledgment of deficit (score 0) to denial of deficit even after demonstration of defect by the examiner (score 3). More recently, other investigators (Celesia et al., 1997) have designed a scale based on a modification of Critchley's (1949) description of six levels of impaired awareness. Lastly, questionnaires of subjective disability exist for visual impairment (Kerkhoff et al., 1994). In principle, insight could be indexed by contrasting the responses of patients with those of collateral informants, though, to our knowledge, the application of such techniques has not yet been published.

ANATOMIC CORRELATES

While Anton's syndrome most frequently follows large, bilateral infarcts affecting the territory of the posterior cerebral arteries (Mohr

and Pessin, 1998), it may also result from brain tumors (Redlich and Dorsey, 1945) and intracerebral hemorrhages (Argenta and Morgan, 1998) involving the same region. Injury to the visual cortex and adjacent association areas is not necessary for anosognosia, however. Patients with a noncortical locus for blindness, including both ocular (Cohn, 1971) and prechiasmal optic nerve lesions (Redlich and Dorsey, 1945; Stengel and Steele, 1946), can also deny visual deficit. Visual anosognosia has even been reported among patients with apraxia of eyelid opening (Ellis and Small, 1994), a disorder with localization outside visual processing areas.

Using brain CT scans, Bisiach et al. (1986) generated composite images to compare patients with and without visual anosognosia. On average, patients who retained insight into visual loss harbored ventrally positioned occipital–temporal lesions. In contrast, brain damage in the group with visual anosognosia occupied more dorsal regions of the occipital–parietal junction.

As with AHP, the issue of laterality of injuries associated with unawareness of hemianopia remains somewhat unsettled. Some maintain that anosognosia for hemifield visual deficit, like AHP, occurs more frequently after right brain lesions (Koehler et al., 1986). Anosognosia for right homonymous field loss is not uncommon, however, and other studies indicate an approximately equivalent incidence of anosognosia after left brain injury (Milandre et al., 1994; Celesia et al., 1997). Subjects with anosognosia for blindness may have relatively larger brain lesions than those in subjects with anosognosia for hemianopia. It thus remains possible, as Celesia et al. (1997) speculate, that multiple or larger areas of cerebral dysfunction may predispose patients to experience visual anosognosia.

MECHANISMS UNDERLYING ANOSOGNOSIA FOR VISUAL LOSS

The theoretical accounts of anosognosia for blindness follow four main forms. First, as mentioned for AHP, visual anosognosia may result from reduced awareness due to generalized cognitive impairment. Second, a hypothetical brain monitor of visual input might be damaged. Alternatively, visual anosognosia may result from false feedback to an otherwise intact monitor. Lastly, anosognosia could result from disconnection of visual experience from the brain's language areas.

Global Cognitive Impairment

Patients with cortical blindness and Anton's syndrome may also suffer from other cognitive disturbances, especially memory loss (Mohr and Pessin, 1998). Besides the calcarine cortex, the posterior circulation supplies the medial temporal lobe as well as parts of the diencephalon, brain regions critical for memory and other cognitive processes. Confusional states have also been associated with injury to adjacent visual association areas such as the lingual and fusiform gyri (Medina et al., 1974; Devinsky et al., 1988). Therefore, several authorities have hypothesized that a generalized intellectual deficit interferes with awareness of blindness in these patients (Levine, 1990). In support of this claim, blind patients with anosognosia have been reported to be delirious, confused, amnestic, or inattentive (Redlich and Dorsey, 1945; Swartz and Brust, 1984; Verslegers et al., 1991; Ellis and Small, 1994). Failure to acknowledge blindness after lesions of the prechiasmal visual system may also be associated with diffuse cognitive impairment due to injury to adjacent frontal and diencephalic regions.

Several observations contradict the explanation of visual anosognosia based on cognitive impairment. First, patients have been reported who, despite alexia and amnesia, retained awareness of hemianopia. Conversely, many if not most individuals with anosognosia for hemianopia are not at all delirious, amnestic, or confused (Critchley, 1953; Warrington, 1962). Second, clearly documented cases of visual anosognosia for blindness without confusion have been described. For example, McDaniel and McDaniel (1991) reported denial for monocular visual loss in a patient with a normal level of consciousness and lack of "significant dementia." Mental processes were not completely normal in this patient, however, as they were remarkable primarily for executive dysfunction and verbal memory impairment.

Thus, the relationship between visual anosognosia and decrepit general cognition is ambiguous. At the least, such deficiencies appear neither necessary nor sufficient to preclude deficit awareness.

Sensory Defects/False Feedback

As in AHP, the inability to apprehend visual defects may relate to lack of access of sensory information to neural processes that monitor function within that modality. The relevant brain regions and basic functional properties for these processes remain vague and unspecified.

Evidence suggests that anosognosia for hemifield disturbances cannot be reduced to a manifestation of the neglect syndrome. While neglect and AHP occurred concurrently in 85% of patients in one study (Celesia et al., 1997), a double dissociation between these entities was found. Likewise, Bisiach and colleagues (1986) reported that cases without evidence of either personal or extrapersonal neglect could be identified even among patients with the most severe lack of insight into visual defects.

In the absence of input from geniculocalcarine pathways, visual input might originate in intact subcortical visual systems (Weiskrantz, 1986). In patients lacking so-called ventral stream afference, this auxiliary system can support activities such as target localization, a phenomenon referred to as *blindsight*. Other examples of visual parapathia might include patients with prosopagnosia who exhibit covert face recognition (Bauer, 1984; DeHaan et al., 1987) or patients with dyslexia who can extract meaning from words they can't read (Coslett and Saffran, 1989; Beversdorf and Heilman, 1998). While feedback into residual visual channels could in principle prevent the monitor's detection of deficit, they cannot by themselves explain anosognosia, since deficit awareness defines these parapathic states. In fact, the visual parapathias seem to represent something quite distinct from anosognosia for blindness, since patients lack awareness of residual capacity rather than deficit.

Alternatively, false feedback might originate from visual activities that are less dependent on sensory transduction. When patients retain some normal vision (e.g., hemianopia), the phenomenon of perceptual completion across the midline may explain why they disregard visual field defects (Warrington, 1962; Gassel and Williams, 1963; Celesia et al., 1997). Whether completion reflects residual sensory processing capacity in the damaged visual cortex is not clear. Some patients only complete whole stimuli, a finding referred to as "veridical completion," which suggests that the injured brain may support some level of visual perception (Torjussen, 1978). Other patients report whole percepts when presented with incomplete stimuli, a finding termed "confabulatory completion" (Feinberg and Roane, 1997). While not mutually exclusive, many investigators have commented on the inverse relationship between perceptual completion and awareness of visual dysfunction after brain injury. Indeed, the same phenomenon may account for the "normal unawareness" of the physiologic blind spot (Feinberg, 1997).

As noted above, patients with anosognosia for blindness maintain that they experience visual percepts (Anton, 1899; Levine, 1990; Goldenberg, 1995). In the context of cortical blindness, these "internal-origin" percepts have been considered visual confabulations (Feinberg et al., 1994) or hallucinations (Schultz and Melzack, 1991; Cole, 1999). While the basis for internal percepts remains poorly understood, they may represent disinhibited visual imagery or associations (Goldenberg, 1995; Goldenberg et al., 1995). Several authors (Gassel and Williams, 1963; Feinberg et al., 1994; Celesia et al., 1997) have postulated that confabulated percepts somehow prevent visual disturbance from reaching consciousness. Clinical and functional imaging studies support the notion that visual imagery and perception may compete for representation within the same neural networks. Indeed, studies in normal subjects show that visual imagery can interfere with visual perception (Segal and Fusella, 1970), suggesting capacity limitation within this representational medium. Heilman (1991) speculated that, under ordinary circumstances, "bottom-up" data from veridical transduction of visual stimuli have privileged access to these representations. In the absence of visual afference, patients may

perceive imagery as experience and the monitor may accept this input as confirmation of intact function. A sparse collection of clinical observations supports this interpretation. For example, Swartz and Brust (1984) described a blind alcoholic who claimed his vision was normal only during periods of visual hallucinosis. Free from constraints imposed by geniculocalcarine impulses, the patient's awareness of deficit may have been moderated by "parasitic" (i.e., internal) visual representations (Bisiach and Geminiani, 1991).

Other clinical data provide evidence against the false-feedback hypothesis as the sole explanation for visual anosognosia. First, there are reports of patients with awareness of a visual loss who concurrently report hallucinations (Cole, 1999). Indeed, some forms of "positive" visual phenomena (e.g., phosphenes) within the visual scotoma appear to enhance a patient's recognition of visual defects (Celesia et al., 1997). An objection might also be raised to the argument that such "top-down" processes can generate input to the monitor since the neural assemblies supporting visual imagery coincide with those supporting perception (Kosslyn et al., 1993). Goldenberg et al. (1995) reported, however, that a patient with anosognosia for cortical blindness experienced verbal, nonverbal auditory, and tactile information as visual percepts. Hence, synesthesia might explain why even patients lacking the neuronal apparatus necessary for visual imagery still report visual sensations. Regardless, the evidence indicates that it is unlikely that internal visual percepts invariably lead to anosognosia. Perhaps internal percepts produce anosognosia when accompanied by an as-yet unspecified cognitive disorder that disturbs the patient's ability to distinguish between internal- and external-origin material (Sergent, 1988; Levine, 1990).

Disconnection

Anton originally hypothesized that anosognosia may result from disconnection of damaged visual areas from parts of the brain responsible for conscious experience and verbal report (Heilman, 1991). Geschwind (1965) elaborated on the theory, asserting that, in the absence of generalized reduction in awareness, denial of blindness resulted from lesions that interrupted flow of information from primary visual areas to the rest of the brain. Heilman (1991) posited that disconnection from speech–language centers may be critical. Research in patients after cerebral commissurotomy supports this notion, as visual stimuli presented to the isolated right hemisphere in such patients can evoke confabulatory responses. While arguments against this explanation for AHP may also apply to visual anosognosia, no direct evidence exists to refute or confirm the disconnection hypothesis.

ANOSOGNOSIA FOR AMNESIA OR DEMENTIA

CLINICAL CHARACTERISTICS

Patients with amnesia typically retain general cognitive abilities but demonstrate a striking inability to remember past events or learn new information (see Chapter 18). In contrast, patients with dementia show impairment across multiple cognitive domains, usually including memory, that can impede functioning in social or occupational contexts (see Chapter 19). Both amnestic and demented patients often show lack of insight about their cognitive deficits.

Amnesia

Korsakoff's syndrome (KS) is a chronic amnesic state characterized by impaired recall of older information acquired over months or years (*retrograde amnesia*) and an impaired ability to learn new information (*anterograde amnesia*). The amnesic syndrome occurs with relative preservation of other cognitive functions. Patients with KS tend to be apathetic and unaware of their memory loss. Although patients with KS may admit a memory problem when interviewed, they lack insight into the severity of the deficit, with most patients showing little or no awareness of or concern about their memory deficits (Korsakoff, 1889; Talland, 1961). Squire and Zouzounis (1988) found that

patients with KS may be as severely impaired as other groups of amnesic patients yet report a less severe memory impairment on self-assessment ratings. Patients with KS may also confabulate elaborate explanations for their inability to recall information (Zangwill, 1966).

Although often associated, the relationship between confabulation and anosognosia for memory deficit remains controversial. Confabulation is considered a fundamental characteristic of KS (Victor et al., 1989) and, in general, patients are as unaware of the bizzare nature of their confabulations as they are of their memory impairment. Although confabulation may resolve as Korsakoff patients become more aware of their memory loss (Mercer et al, 1977; Stuss et al., 1978; Shapiro et al., 1981), the two phenomena are dissociable; anosognosia may persist despite the resolution of confabulations.

In contrast to KS, patients with other amnestic syndromes may demonstrate awareness of memory deficits. For example, transient global amnesia (TGA) results in profound but temporary anterograde amnesia, attributed to either ischemia (Ponsford and Donnan, 1980; Jensen and Olivarius, 1981) or epileptiform activity (Roman-Campos et al., 1980) affecting the medial temporal lobe. Patients with TGA show acute awareness of their memory problems and frequently ask repetitive questions in an attempt to orient themselves (Evans, 1966; Fisher, 1982; Kritchevsky, 1987). Patients with more enduring amnesia from temporal lobe lesions (e.g., encephalitis) may also show relatively preserved awareness of memory loss compared to patients with frontal or diencephalic injury (Rose and Symonds, 1960; Zangwill 1966; Kopelman et al., 1998). Similarly, rare cases of bilateral temporal lobectomy display severe anterograde amnesia but retain insight into their memory loss (Milner et al., 1968; Bennett-Levy et al., 1980).

Dementia

Patients with dementia may demonstrate lack of insight into or unawareness of their cognitive deficits as well as their functional impairment in activities of daily living. Fredericks (1985) termed this "anosognosia for dementia," a condition that hinders the management of demented patients and compromises the quality of life for patients and their caregivers.

Anosognosia for dementia may be present in 15%–24% of patients with Alzheimer's disease (AD), the most common cause of degenerative dementia (Reisberg et al., 1985; Lopez et al., 1993; Migliorelli et al., 1995). Some patients with AD often partially acknowledge their memory loss (McGlone et al., 1990; Michon et al., 1994) but claim that caregivers overstate the severity of impairment (Feher et al., 1991, Seltzer et al., 1995; Vasterling et al., 1995). Denial of dementia does not appear to correlate with other factors such as age at onset, duration of illness, or educational level (Feher et al., 1991, Mangone et al., 1991; Lopez et al., 1993; Sevush, 1999).

The relationship between deficit awareness and dementia severity in AD remains unsettled. Although awareness may be lacking from the earliest stages of AD (Joynt and Shoulson, 1985), patients tend to suffer further loss of insight as dementia severity increases (Neary et al., 1986; Schneck et al., 1992; McDaniel et al., 1995; Vasterling et al., 1995). However, many other investigators have failed to detect a consistent relationship between dementia severity and anosognosia for cognitive impairment (DeBettignies et al., 1990; Feher et al., 1991; Reed et al., 1993; Auchus et al., 1994; Michon et al., 1994; Weinstein et al., 1994; Kotler-Cope and Camp, 1995). The reason for discrepant results may relate to the fact that some studies made longitudinal conclusions on the basis of cross-sectional analyses. Alternatively, Zannetti et al. (1999) found that anosognosia for dementia proceeds through three phases corresponding to scores on the Mini-Mental Status Exam (MMSE). In the earliest stages (MMSE > 24), patients displayed relatively preserved insight. Patients in the middle stage (MMSE between 12 and 23) showed a linear decline in awareness while in the final stages (MMSE < 12), patients' insight remained stable at a very low level. This nonlinear loss of awareness may also explain why previous studies have failed to find a correlation between anosognosia and dementia severity.

Other diseases causing dementia may be associated with impaired insight into cognitive deficit. Gustafson and Nilson (1982) suggested that lack of insight may be an early sign of Pick's disease along with other indicators of frontal dysfunction, a claim supported by a number of studies. Likewise, patients with Huntington's disease, a degenerative condition with marked memory and executive impairments, lose insight into their cognitive problems, particularly in later stages (McGlynn and Kaszniak, 1991b). In contrast, Freedman et al. (1991) described a patient with posterior cortical atrophy with preserved insight until the later stages of the illness. Thus, anosognosia for cognitive impairment may help distinguish frontotemporal dementia and subcortical dementias from cortical degenerative disorders such as AD.

The published experience with vascular dementia (VD) and dementia in patients with Parkinson's disease (PD) indicates a more complicated relationship between executive deficits and anosognosia. Despite the salience of executive dysfunction in VD (Stuss and Cummings, 1990), AD patients tend to show greater anosognosia for both cognitive impairment (Wagner et al., 1997) and loss of independent living skills (DeBettignies et al., 1990) when compared to patients with VD. Other reports have failed to detect any difference between AD and VD with respect to deficit awareness (Verhey et al., 1995). In a similar fashion, the dementia that accompanies PD in 25%–40% of cases (Cummings et al., 1988) shows many features consistent with frontal lobe dysfunction (Taylor et al., 1986; Gotham et al., 1988; Sagar et al., 1991, Stam et al., 1993). Despite prominent executive dysfunction, however, Danielczyk (1983) described relatively preserved insight for cognitive funciton in PD patients. In fact, Starkstein et al. (1996b) encountered a greater degree of anosognosia in AD than in PD.

ASSESSMENT

Several techniques have been developed for assessing insight into cognitive disorders. As with AHP, some examiners simply employ a subjective clinical estimate of deficit awareness (McDaniel et al., 1995; Seltzer et al., 1995). Other investigators give questionnaires to both patients and their caregivers in order to rate memory loss and other cognitive symptoms (Feher et al., 1991; Mangone et al., 1991; Green et al., 1993; Correa et al., 1996). The difference between the patient's self-report and caregiver reports serves as an indirect indicator of the patient's anosognosia. As recently summarized by Sevush (1999), however, the primary weakness of such methods pertains to their disregard for factors unrelated to the patient's own awareness such as the accuracy of the informant. Caregiver's observations may be biased because of the stress of caring for a dementia patient (Seltzer et al., 1997) or their own health issues. Furthermore, even the introspections of normal elderly subjects regarding memory and functional capacity may be unreliable (Sunderland et al., 1986). Using a self-assessment questionnaire, McGlone and colleagues (1990) were not able to distinguish patients with early dementia from those with memory complaints from other causes (e.g., depression, anxiety). Given the lack of consistency in healthy and nondemented subjects, it seems unlikely that self-reported memory loss will be valid among patients with dementia.

Rather than relying on subjective reports, other investigators have combined a structured clinical interview with objective neuropsychological evaluations (Anderson and Tranel, 1989; Ott et al., 1996a; Wagner et al., 1997; Sevush, 1999). While more time intensive, these techniques avoid the systematic error introduced when difference scores become confounded with other related variables such as dementia severity.

ANATOMIC CORRELATES

Pathological examination of patients with KS indicates that injury to the dorsomedial nucleus of the thalamus may be the critical determinant for clinical manifestations (Victor et al., 1989). Anosognosia for amnesia may depend on secondary involvement of anatomically related frontal lobe structures. The dorsomedial nucleus has intricate connections to the prefrontal cortex (Goldman-Rakic, 1987; Pandya and Barnes, 1987) and damage to this structure may disrupt function in a thalamocortical circuit important for memory and awareness. In addition to in-

direct frontal injury, Korsakoff patients may also demonstrate frontal lobe atrophy (Shimamura et al., 1988). Detailed psychometric evaluation of patients with KS concurs with anatomic observations, often detecting impaired performance on tests sensitive to executive dysfunction (Squire, 1982; Schacter 1987).

Other patients with frontal lobe damage demonstrate unawareness of memory loss. For example, patients with rupture of the anterior communicating artery (ACoA) aneurysm may show a Korsakoff-like amnesia (Volpe and Hirst, 1983), including confabulation and denial of memory deficits. Vilkki (1985) examined the behavioral correlates of frontal lobe injury after rupture of ACoA aneurysms, finding that patients with frontal damage displayed anosognosia for amnesia while patients without frontal involvement retained awareness of memory loss. Regions vascularized by the ACoA contain other structures implicated in regulation of complex behavior, including the anterior hypothalamus, basal forebrain nuclei, corpus callosum, and anterior cingulate (Alexander and Freedman, 1984; Damasio et al., 1985; DeLuca, 1993). While the extent of injury in this group of patients varies widely (DeLuca and Diamond, 1995), the presence or absence of frontal brain dysfunction may determine their awareness of memory deficits.

Survivors of brain trauma, often the recipients of significant frontal lobe injury, also frequently fail to recognize their consequent memory disorders (Stuss and Benson, 1986). Jarho (1973) reported a Korsakoff-like syndrome in a small series of patients who had suffered penetrating brain injuries. Patients who lacked awareness of amnesia all suffered from frontal lobe damage; patients with traumatic injuries outside frontal regions were equally amnesic yet remained fully aware of their memory loss. Even patients with mild closed-head injuries may underestimate their memory problems (Rimel et al., 1981), showing a discrepancy between subjective ratings of their memory capacity and objective findings on psychometric assessment (Sunderland et al., 1983). Like KS patients, cases of traumatic injury frequently lack awareness of both memory loss and noncognitive behavioral changes (Boake et al., 1995).

Evidence from several sources suggests that, in AD patients, anosognosia for dementia may also relate to frontal brain dysfunction. For example, AD patients with anosognosia demonstrate behavioral disorders associated with frontal lobe impairment, such as disinhibition or elevated mood (Migliorelli et al., 1995). Impairment on psychometric measures of executive function also correlate highly with anosognosia in AD patients (Mangone et al., 1991; Michon et al., 1994; but see Auchus et al., 1994). Functional imaging studies further strengthen the link between anosognosia and frontal lobe dysfunction. Using single-photon emission computed tomography (SPECT) to measure regional cerebral blood flow (rCBF), Reed and associates (1993) compared AD patients with different degrees of insight, including 6 with complete deficit awareness, 10 with inconsistent or transient recognition of impairment, and 4 without deficit awareness. Patients with anosognosia showed a relative reduction of rCBF in the right dorsolateral frontal lobe. Starkstein et al. (1995) also used SPECT to measure rCBF in AD patients with and without anosognosia. The AD patients with anosognosia showed decreased rCBF in the right hemisphere, particularly in orbital and dorsolateral frontal cortex, compared to other AD patients. Another recent study in a larger group of AD patients (Ott et al., 1996b) also found that frontal hypoperfusion correlated with anosognosia, but only for the left hemisphere. In the right hemisphere, lack of insight correlated most with reduced rCBF in temporo-occipital cortex.

MECHANISMS UNDERLYING ANOSOGNOSIA FOR AMNESIA/DEMENTIA

Hypotheses about the mechanism of anosognosia for amnesia and dementia generally fall into one of the following categories. First, lack of deficit awareness may relate either to explicit memory loss alone or to confabulation. Patients simply cannot recall their cognitive problems, or confabulated memories convince patients that their memory function remains intact. Second, the neuropsychological theory claims that impaired self-monitoring processes resulting from frontal lobe and/or right hemisphere dys-

function produce anosognosia. Lastly, the defense mechanism hypothesis has also been proposed as the basis for anosognosia in the setting of amnesia and dementia.

Failure to Recall Deficits

This simple explanation for anosognosia derives from studies summarized above that show a correlation between dementia severity and lack of deficit awareness. The hypothesis founders on reports of profoundly amnestic patients who remain acutely aware of their problems. Some authors try to resolve the contradiction by proposing that amnesia alone may preclude initial insight, although some patients discover their deficit over time (Kopelman et al., 1998). However, "discovery" cannot readily explain patients with TGA who are aware of amnesia almost immediately. Although memory loss alone may not suffice to cause anosognosia, the amnesic syndrome may somehow help sustain unawareness.

Others speculate that confabulated "false" memories may deceive patients into believing that mental function is normal. This type of confabulation, often resulting from injury to basal forebrain nuclei (Fischer et al., 1995), will be discussed below.

A recent study suggested that anosognosia may be related to deficits in implicit, rather than explicit, memory. Starkstein and colleagues (1997b) gave tests of both explicit (i.e., declarative) and implicit (i.e., procedural) learning to a group of AD patients. All patients showed deficits in measures of explicit memory. In contrast, those with impaired deficit awareness performed significantly worse on measures of implicit memory.

Impaired Self-monitoring

Lack of insight into memory impairment may relate to a specific self-monitoring defect. Meta-memory, also known as *feeling-of-knowing*, refers to the ability to predict one's own performance on a memory test. Patients who lack the capacity to predict their own memory function may not detect abnormal memory performance as it occurs. Shimamura and Squire (1986) asked patients with KS to make predictions as to whether or not they could recognize information that they could not explicitly recall. Compared with other amnesic individuals, the Korsakoff group made impaired feeling-of-knowing judgements. Limited data from amnesia after diencephalic lesions suggest that the KS group's lack of self-awareness may result from frontal brain pathology. Kausall et al. (1981) described a patient who was amnesic from a discrete injury in the left dorsomedial thalamus but remained aware of his memory loss. In contrast to patients with KS, their patient demonstrated normal feeling-of-knowing predictions, providing support for the notion that self-monitoring problems correlate more with frontal lobe dysfunction than with diencephalic dysfunction (Shimamura and Squire, 1986).

Executive dysfunction, possibly including impaired meta-cognition, may also account for lack of awareness of dementia. As mentioned above, several studies document a correlation between impaired insight and impairment on psychometric tasks sensitive to frontal brain dysfunction (Mangone et al., 1991; Lopez et al., 1993; Michon et al., 1994). In one report (Weinstein et al., 1994), anosognosia in AD occurred significantly more often in patients whose initial manifestations indicated frontal brain involvement. The relationship between executive dysfunction and impaired meta-cognition in demented patients remains unclear, however, since available studies of metamemory in AD (Pappas et al., 1992; Lipinska and Backman, 1996) did not specifically assess its relationship to anosognosia.

As with KS patients, the phenomenon of confabulation may provide a link between anosognosia and frontal executive dysfunction (Stuss et al., 1978) in patients with dementia. Intrusions consist of confabulation-like responses on free-recall tasks in which patients give items that were not encountered during encoding. Dalla Barba et al. (1995) evaluated the relationship between anosognosia, intrusion errors, and performance on a test battery sensitive to frontal brain injuries. While they found an association between anosognosia for memory loss and intrusion errors; the only correlation with executive function was on the verbal fluency task. Intrusions were not associated with severity of memory impairment, only with lack of insight. Other studies in AD patients

showed that the production of confabulatory-type responses during psychometric testing correlated with an index of "frontal system functioning" (Kern et al., 1992). Unfortunately, analysis of deficit awareness was not included in the study design. Hence, while it is tempting to speculate that confabulations may preclude self-appraisal of cognitive potential, the causal relationship between confabulation and anosognosia remains undetermined.

Psychologically Motivated Denial

Anosognosia may be a defense mechanism that protects patients from realizing the extent of their cognitive deficits, thereby minimizing emotional distress (Reisberg et al, 1985; Weinstein et al., 1994). If this is true, then demented patients who lack deficit awareness should be less depressed. Evidence on this point is contradictory. Several investigations have reported modest correlations between awareness of memory loss and expressions of negative affect (Feher et al., 1991, 1993; Sevush and Leve, 1993; Seltzer et al., 1995). In contrast, many other researchers have failed to establish any relationship between depression and anosognosia for cognitive loss (DeBettignies et al., 1990; Reed et al., 1993; Cummings et al., 1995; Ott et al., 1996a; Zanetti et al, 1999).

One study (Starkstein et al., 1997a) distinguished between dysthymia and major depressive disorder. In patients with AD, dysthymia was common (34%) and often resolved over time. Major depression occurred less often (19%) and was more likely to persist. As dysthymia improved, the degree of anosognosia worsened, suggesting that initial dysphoria may have resulted from awareness of cognitive dysfunction. In contrast, major depression was not correlated with the severity of anosognosia. The authors tentatively concluded that different mechanisms produce unawareness, with psychological factors contributing to anosognosia in the dysthymic group and a neurological component (e.g., left fronto-temporo-parietal dysmetabolism) contributing to the unawareness in AD patients with depression.

Several observations argue against motivated denial as a cause of anosognosia for amnesia and dementia. If a psychological defense mechanism is primarily responsible for lack of insight, then denial should be greatest early in the course of disease as patients learn of their diagnosis. As mentioned above, however, awareness tends to fade with time as dementia severity escalates (McGlynn and Kasniak, 1991a). Reported dissociations between anosognosia for dementia and other deficits provide further evidence against this hypothesis. Wagner and Cushman (1994) found that patients with VD were aware of cognitive dysfunction much less often than patients with hemiparesis or aphasia. As in other types of anosognosia, the defense mechanism hypothesis predicts that patients should deny deficit without regard to modality. Lastly, although formal studies are lacking, anecdotal reports suggest that dementia patients with both depression and anosognosia fail to recover their awareness of cognitive impairment even after successful treatment for depression.

ANOSOGNOSIA FOR APHASIA

CLINICAL CHARACTERISTICS

Patients with anosognosia for aphasia do not attempt to correct errors in their speech and, when confronted with the error, deny its occurrence. Lack of insight most often accompanies *jargon aphasia* (Alajouanine, 1956), a fluent aphasia in which patients produce frequent semantic and phonemic paraphasias and neologisms (see Chapter 2). Patients typically remain unaware of the incomprehensibility of their speech and make no effort to correct their errors. Jargon aphasics make few of the hesitations, pauses, or self-corrections observed in other aphasic syndromes, a characteristic that may indicate failure of self-monitoring (see below). Jargon aphasia is commonly associated with Wernicke's aphasia but may also be seen in transcortical sensory aphasia or as part of the stereotyped perseverations associated with Broca's or global aphasia.

Global awareness of language impairment may be present despite unawareness for specific impairments caused by aphasia (Rubens and Garrett, 1991). Lecours and Joanette (1980) described an epileptic aphasic who pro-

duced jargon speech without comprehension. During seizures, his behavior reflected a general awareness of communication problems. Interictally, he could recount general impairment in speaking but could not convey awareness of the specific linguistic deficits, only that speech was not right. Butterworth (1979) found pauses in jargon speech just prior to production of neologisms and proposed that these hesitations reflect some degree of awareness for the lexical retrieval deficits. Other jargon aphasic patients retain the impulse to self-correct, indicating at least partial awareness of their language impairment (Wepman, 1958). Although jargon aphasics may retain at least some degree of insight (Cohn and Neumann, 1958), persistent logorrhea and lack of self-correction suggest that patients remain unaware that listeners do not understand them and that the patients themselves do not comprehend the feedback others give them about their deficit.

Anosognosia for language deficit is not limited to jargon aphasia. Patients with certain forms of Broca's aphasia demonstrate monophasic utterances, repeating stereotyped phrases continuously (Lebrun, 1987). These patients may be unaware of these repetitive utterances, even while displaying frustration regarding the difficulty of their volitional speech output. Several cases of optic aphasia have been described as lacking insight into their blatantly peculiar responses to naming tasks (Lhermitte and Beauvois, 1973). Lastly, Brown (1975) described anosognosia in a conduction aphasic whose efforts at self-correction increased as awareness of paraphasic errors returned.

ASSESSMENT

As Lebrun noted (1987), the judgment that a patient lacks insight into aphasia is largely based on circumstantial evidence because the language deficit precludes explicit verbal communication. A lack of attempt at error correction is interpreted by many clinicians as showing lack of insight into aphasia (Levelt, 1983; Marshall et al., 1985). However, as stressed by Maher et al. (1994), it may be overly simplistic to equate self-correction behavior with error awareness. One can infer at least some level of anosognosia when a patient manifests frustration and anger in response to the examiner's inability to comprehend their aphasic jargon (Alajouanine, 1956). The same judgment can safely be made about patients who offer confabulatory "definitions" when presented with nonword letter strings (Sandson et al., 1986).

Schlenck et al. (1987) described a technique for quantifying anosognosia through analysis of speech corrections. They referred to "repairs" as mistakes corrected immediately after production, while "prepairs" referred to "mistakes" presumably corrected prior to articulation, indirectly indicated by hesitation. This method can be applied to recordings of running discourse. Other investigators (Maher et al., 1994; Shuren et al., 1995) have described more time-intensive procedures in which patients respond with single words to target stimuli (e.g., confrontation naming) and are asked to indicate whether their response was correct after each presentation.

ANATOMIC CORRELATES

Kertesz (1979) concluded that lesions responsible for jargon aphasia involved the supramarginal gyrus and the posterior portion of the superior temporal gyrus. Semantic jargon may also be associated with transcortical sensory aphasia from more posteriorly situated lesions that involve the temporal–parietal–occipital junction. Semantic jargon in dementia (i.e., Alzheimer's disease) may also be seen in the context of transcortical sensory aphasia with relatively spared repetition but poor comprehension. The earliest cortical pathology in AD arises in the temporal–parietal association regions (Chui, 1989; Arnold et al., 1991) and functional neuroimaging studies show both hypoperfusion and hypometabolism in these same regions early in the course of AD (Foster et al., 1983; Friedland et al., 1984, 1985; Holman et al., 1992).

In a study comparing aphasia subtypes, Weinstein et al. (1966) reported that jargon aphasics typically exhibit evidence of bilateral brain damage. In contrast, other aphasic patients primarily showed signs of unilateral left hemisphere damage, leading the investigators to

posit that injury beyond the dominant hemisphere's language areas was necessary to produce anosognosia and jargon speech. Brown (1981) also reported a higher incidence of bilateral brain injury among patients without awareness of their aphasia. These findings are in accord with the observation that, for other focal neurological deficits, anosognosia most often follows lesions in the right hemisphere (see above). In contrast, Gainotti (1972) found anosognosia in 5 out of 16 Wernicke's aphasics with injury limited to the left hemisphere. Although bilateral brain injury may be conducive to anosognosia for aphasia, it appears neither necessary nor sufficient.

MECHANISMS UNDERLYING ANOSOGNOSIA FOR APHASIA

Although the neuropsychological basis of anosognosia for aphasia remains unknown, several hypotheses have been forwarded. Some theories emphasize problems within the complex process of self-monitoring of language. Alternative explanations include limited attentional capacity and psychologically motivated denial.

Disrupted Feedback or Self-monitoring

Aphasic patients may remain unaware of their language deficits because of a breakdown in the normal self-monitoring functions of speech. Self-monitoring ability likely entails access to lexical–semantic representations required for auditory comprehension (McGlynn and Schacter, 1989; Heilman, 1991; Rubens and Garrett, 1991). Since anosognosia for aphasia most commonly occurs in association with comprehension defects, lexical–semantic systems may be degraded. Alternatively, the lack of awareness may result from problems within more fundamental, nonlinguistic auditory processes (see below).

According to cognitive neuropsychological models (Ellis and Young, 1988), auditory comprehension depends on multiple dissociable processes including auditory analysis followed by activation of stored phonological forms (the lexicon) and their associated semantic representations. In principle, impairment at any of these stages could result in lack of error corrections. If disturbed auditory comprehension originates in faulty semantic processes with relative sparing of the lexicon, however, phonemic errors may be recognized and corrected despite poor comprehension. In general, spared auditory comprehension implies that the lexical–semantic system remains relatively intact and anosognosia must result from another mechanism.

Unawareness of aphasia may due to abnormal auditory feedback mechanisms. Self-monitoring may fail if intact cognitive systems receive corrupt input from the "early auditory analysis system" (Ellis and Young, 1988) that decodes speech sounds. When normal individuals receive delayed auditory feedback (DAF) of their own speech, their speech becomes distorted by phonemic substitutions, decreased rate of production, and increased voice amplitude (Fairbanks and Guttman, 1955; Timmons, 1983). Studies in aphasics have shown that fluent aphasics show minimal change in their speech patterns with DAF (Boller et al., 1978; Peuser and Temp, 1981), suggesting that impaired feedback may be responsible for their self-monitoring failure. However, since some of these patients also have impaired auditory comprehension, the lack of DAF response may relate to problems within the lexical–semantic system rather than the feedback loop. Accordingly, one study found normal DAF effects in jargon aphasics who made semantic paraphasic errors but absent DAF effect in those making phonemic paraphasic errors (Alajouanine and Lhermitte, 1964). More pertinent to abnormal DAF as the cause of anosognosia are reports of patients who lacked insight into their jargon aphasia yet showed a normal feedback response to DAF (Maher et al., 1994; Shuren et al., 1995). This observation directly refutes the notion that abnormal auditory feedback alone is a sufficient condition to prevent awareness of language disorders.

Although aphasic patients may be incapable of correcting errors, insight into their deficit should allow them to recognize abnormal utterances as incorrect. Marshall and Tompkins (1982) investigated verbal self-correction patterns in both fluent and nonfluent aphasics. The less impaired group with relatively preserved comprehension (Broca's and anomic aphasics) showed a higher proportion of successful self-correction compared to more severe dysfluent aphasics or those with significant comprehension impairment. Error detection occurred with equal frequency in Broca's and Wernicke's aphasia, however, showing that most aphasics have at least some degree of insight into their language disorder. Similar results have been reported in other studies contrasting these two types of aphasia (Schlenck et al., 1987). Likewise, Marshall et al. (1985) described an aphasic patient who was aware of her speech errors and could modify her verbal responses despite the loss of auditory comprehension. In contrast, several cases have been described where jargon aphasic patients remained unaware of aphasia despite relatively preserved auditory comprehension (Maher et al., 1994; Shuren et al., 1995). These double dissociations indicate that, although auditory comprehension may contribute to error detection and correction, self-monitoring depends on other language processes as well.

In theory, defective monitoring in jargon aphasia could result from defects within neural systems responsible for the representation of word sounds, known as the *lexicon*. Patients with anosognosia for recurrent monophasic utterances (Lebrun, 1986) may have deficiencies at this level since they are unable to detect that their speech repertoire consists of the same stereotyped sound. Studies indicate, however, that some aphasic patients may recognize speech errors produced by another person even while they remain oblivious to their own errors. Similar research demonstrates that these patients may not detect errors while speaking yet retain the ability to detect problems when their speech is played back to them on tape (Alajouanine, 1956; Alajouanine and Lhermitte, 1957; Kinsbourne and Warrington, 1963). If anosognosia resulted from a faulty lexicon alone, patients should not be better at detecting errors made by others or their own "off-line" mistakes.

Limited Attentional Capacity

Lebrun (1987) suggested that some aphasic patients with anosognosia may be unable to perform two simultaneous tasks. Reduced attentional capacity to concurrently speak and listen to one's own speech may result in unawareness of aphasia and explicit denial of deficit. Shuren et al. (1995) described a patient with jargon aphasia and established that their auditory analysis and lexical–semantic capacities were intact. In contrast, the patient had difficulty monitoring speech simultaneously produced by both him and the examiner. They posited that this reduced attentional capacity to attend to simultaneous language tasks may explain the patient's unawareness of specific language errors.

Other evidence supports the role of attentional factors in speech monitoring. Normal speakers are also frequently unaware of their language errors (Cutler, 1982). The speech of normal subjects may contain gross lexical or semantic substitutions; these are usually corrected when noted immediately, but may go unnoticed unless attention is directed to the error (Levelt, 1983). Likewise, aphasic patients self-correct errors on naming tasks more often than on other verbal output tasks such as picture description, presumably because the attentional demands of the tasks are different (Marshall and Tompkins, 1982). Normal speakers may self-correct lexical errors less often than phonemic errors (Nooteboom, 1980). To the extent that self-monitoring of language production relies on language comprehension, dual mechanisms (i.e., expressive and receptive) may interact to allow for conscious awareness of speech production errors in normal speakers (Rubens and Garrett, 1991).

Psychologically Motivated Denial

As with other forms of anosognosia, dynamic psychological factors have also been invoked to explain anosognosia for aphasia (Kinsbourne and Warrington, 1963). According to Weinstein et al. (1964), jargon aphasia provides an adaptive strategy for dealing with the psychic distress that accompanies loss of speech. Among 28 patients with left hemisphere lesions, one group of patients had severe AHP with minimal aphasia. Another group of aphasic patients did not display AHP and did not produce confabulations or jargon. Aphasic patients with anosognosia were unaware of both language and sensorimotor deficits and tended to produce jargon speech, leading Weinstein et al. (1964) to propose that jargon speech serves as an adaptive mechanism when aphasia and anosognosia occur simultaneously. The rapid flow of neologistic speech facilitated interpersonal interaction under the premise that dysfunctional communication was less threatening to the ego than no communication at all. Analogous to the defense mechanism hypothesis for AHP, there may also be a distinct premorbid personality profile for patients who develop jargon aphasia. Such characteristics include compulsiveness, excessive drive, excessive work orientation, and dread and denial of illness (Weinstein and Lyerly, 1976).

Some of the shortcomings of the defense mechanism hypothesis for AHP also apply to aphasic anosognosia. For example, it remains unclear why motivated denial would be associated with specific aphasic syndromes (e.g., jargon aphasia) when other forms of aphasia pose equivalent threats to one's self-perception of intact function. As mentioned above, some patients do not recognize their errors while speaking but detect errors when listening to taped recordings of their speech (Maher et al., 1994; Shuren et al., 1995). The defense mechanism hypothesis predicts that patients would not acknowledge such errors, assuming they recognized the voice as their own. Lastly, this hypothesis also fails to account for dissociations in which patients remain aware of disabling deficits such as a hemiparesis or hemianopia yet deny their aphasia (Breier et al., 1995).

RECOVERY AND TREATMENT

The course of anosognosia varies depending on the nature of the brain injury. For static pathologies such as ischemia or trauma, insight into hemiparesis increases with time since the injury. Longitudinal observations show that AHP resolves independently of other disorders including neglect and tends to remit long before the patient regains use of the extremity (Hier et al., 1983). From a group of over 50 stroke patients studied after transfer to a rehabilitation facility, Levine and colleagues

(1991) identified only 6 cases of persistent AHP. Some evidence suggests that resolution of AHP relates to the size of the brain injury, with lesions under 6% of hemispheric volume recovering significantly more rapidly than larger lesions. Less data exist regarding the natural history of anosognosia for visual loss or aphasia. The course of anosognosia into dementia is influenced by the cause of the symptoms. The studies summarized above primarily include patients with evolving defects due to degenerative conditions.

Certain maneuvers that ameliorate neglect behavior also improve awareness of deficit, at least for AHP. For example, in many patients with neglect of extrapersonal space, cold caloric stimulation of the right external auditory canal temporarily reduces bias on line bisection and omissions in target cancellation (see Chapter 13). Cappa et al. (1987) were the first to report that vestibular stimulation can also reduce personal neglect and increase awareness of hemiparesis. In contrast to performance on clinical tests of neglect, the influence on AHP outlasted the immediate stimulation period in this study. However, even patients who attained insight during stimulation would shortly relapse, indicating that memory of their transient experience could not override anosognosia (Ramchandran, 1995). In another report, caloric stimulation corrected both AHP and somatoparaphrenic delusions about the paretic extremity (Bisiach et al., 1991). A recent study may identify the limitations of caloric stimulation as it pertains to anosognosia. Vallar and colleagues (1995) gave caloric stimulation to a patient with right extrapersonal neglect and anosognosia for fluent aphasia. The intervention improved some of the patient's symptoms without altering the patient's awareness of disordered speech. Whether other pharmacological and behavioral interventions used in the treatment of neglect also modify anosognosia remains unknown.

The literature about therapeutically modifying insight into visual loss or aphasia remains even more sparse. Lebrun (1987) asserts that patients must first be "rendered conscious" of their errors for effective speech therapy to proceed, and suggests that, in some cases, audio-

and videotape recordings of their performance may prove useful. As the data summarized above indicate, not all patients will respond to such interventions.

REFERENCES

Adair,. J. C., Na, D. L., Schwartz, R. L., Fennell, E. M., Gilmore, R. L., and Heilman, K. M. (1995). Anosognosia for hemiplegia: test of the personal neglect hypothesis. *Neurology 45*:2195–2199.

Adair, J. C., Schwartz, R. L., Na, D. L., Fennell, E. B., Gilmore, R. L., and Heilman, K. M. (1997). Anosognosia: examining the disconnection hypothesis. *J. Neurol. Neurosurg. Psychiatry 63*:798–800.

Alajouanine, T. (1956). Verbal realization in aphasia. *Brain 79*:1–28.

Alajouanine, T., and Lhermitte, F. (1957). Des anosognosie electives. *Encephale 46*:505–519.

Alajouanine, T., and Lhermitte, F. (1964). The phonemic and semantic components of jargon aphasia. In *Psycholinguistic Aspects of Aphasia*, H. Goodglass and S. Blumstein (eds.). Baltimore: Johns Hopkins University Press, pp. 218–329.

Alexander, M. P., and Freedman, M. (1984). Amnesia after anterior communicating artery aneurysm rupture. *Neurology 34*:752–757.

Anderson, S. W., and Tranel, D. (1989). Awareness of disease states following cerebral infarction, dementia, and head trauma: standardized assessment. *Clin. Neuropsychol. 3*:327–339.

Anton, G. (1898). Herderkrankungen des Gehirnes, welche vom Patienten selbst nicht wahrgenommen werden. *Wien. Klin. Wochenschr. 11*:227–229.

Anton, G. (1899). Über die Selbstwahrnehmung der Herderkrankungen des Gehirns durch den Kranken bei Rindenblindheit und Rindentaubheit. *Arch. Psychiatrie Nervenkr. 32*:86–127.

Argenta, P. A., and Morgan, M. A. (1998). Cortical blindness and Anton syndrome in a patient with obstetric hemorrhage. *Obstet. Gynecol. 91*:810–812.

Arnold, S. E., Hyman, B. T., Flory, J., Damasio, A. R., and Van Hoesen, G. W. (1991). The topographical distribution of neurofibrillary tangles and neuritic plaques in the cerebral cortex of patients with Alzheimer's disease. *Cereb. Cortex 1*:103–116.

Auchus, A. P., Goldstein, F. L., Green, J., and Green, R. C. (1994). Unawareness of cognitive impairments in Alzheimer's disease. *Neuropsychiatry Neuropsychol. Behav. Neurol.* 7:25–29.

Babinski, J. (1914). Contribution a l'etude dies troubles mentaux dans l'hemiplegie organique cerebrale (anosognosie). *Rev. Neurol. (Paris)* 27:845–847.

Bakchine, S., Crassard, I., and Seilhan, D. (1997). Anosognosia for hemiplegia after a brainstem haematoma: a pathological case. *J. Neurol. Neurosurg. Psychiatry* 63:686–687.

Bauer, R. M. (1984). Autonomic recognition of names and faces in prosopagnosia: a neuropsychological application of the guilty knowledge test. *Neuropsychologia* 22:457–469.

Bennet-Levy, J., Polkey, C. E., and Powell, G. E. (1980). Self-report of memory skills after temporal lobectomy: the effect of clinical variables. *Cortex* 16:543–557.

Berti, A., Ladavas, E., and Corte, M. D. (1996). Anosognosia for hemiplegia, neglect dyslexia, and drawing neglect: clinical findings and theoretical considerations. *J. Int. Neuropsychol. Soc.* 2:426–440.

Beversdorf, D. Q., and Heilman, K. M. (1998). Progressive ventral posterior cortical degeneration presenting as alexia for music and words. *Neurology* 50:657–659.

Bisiach, E., and Geminiani, G. (1991). Anosognosia related to hemiplegia and hemianopia. In *Awareness of Deficit After Brain Injury*, G. P. Prigatano and D. L. Schacter (eds.). New York: Oxford University Press, pp. 17–39.

Bisiach, E., Rusconi, M. L., and Vallar, G. (1991). Remission of somatoparaphrenic delusion through vestibular stimulation. *Neuropsychologia* 29:1029–1031.

Bisiach, E., Vallar, G., Perani, D., Papagno, C., and Berti, A. (1986). Unawareness of disease following lesions of the right hemisphere: anosognosia for hemiplegia and anosognosia for hemianopia. *Neuropsychologia* 24:471–482.

Blonder, L. X., and Ranseen, J. D. (1994). Awareness of deficit following right hemisphere stroke. *Neuropsychiatry Neuropsychol. Behav. Neurol.* 7:260–266.

Boake, C., Freeland, J. C., Ringholz, G. M., Nance, M. L., and Edwards, K. E. (1995). Awareness of memory loss after severe closed-head injury. *Brain Inj.* 9:273–283.

Boller, F., Vrtunski, P. B., Kim, Y., and Mack, J. L. (1978). Delayed auditory feedback and aphasia. *Cortex* 14:212–226.

Bonhoeffer, K. (1903). Casuistische Beiträge zur Aphasielehre. *Arch. Psychiatrie* 37:564–597.

Breier, J. I., Adair, J. C., Gold, M., Fennell, E. B.,

Gilmore, R. L., and Heilman, K. M. (1995). Dissociation of anosognosia for hemiplegia and aphasia during left-hemisphere anesthesia. *Neurology* 45:65–67.

Brown, J. (1981). Introduction. In *Jargon Aphasia*, J. Brown (ed.). Orlando, FL: Academic Press.

Brown, J. W. (1975). The problem of repetition: a study of "conduction" aphasia and the "isolation syndrome". *Cortex* 11:37–52.

Brown, R. G., and Marsden, C. D. (1984). How common is dementia in Parkinson's disease? *Lancet ii*:1262–1265.

Buchtel, H., Henry, T., and Abou-Khalil, B. (1992). Memory for neurological deficits during the intracarotid amytal procedure: a hemispheric difference. *J. Clin. Exp. Neuropsychol.* 14:96–97.

Butterworth, B. (1979). Hesitation and the production of verbal paraphasias and neologisms in jargon aphasia. *Brain Lang.* 8:133–161.

Calvanio, R., Levine, D., and Petrone, P. (1993). Elements of cognitive rehabilitation after right hemisphere stroke. *Neurol. Clin.* 11:25–57.

Cappa, S., Sterzi, R., Vallar, G., and Bisiach, E. (1987). Remission of hemineglect and anosognosia during vestibular stimulation. *Neuropsychologia* 25:775–782.

Carpenter, K., Berti, A., Oxbury, S., Molyneaux, A. J., Bisiach, E., Oxbury, J. M. (1995). Awareness of and memory for arm weakness during intracarotid sodium amytal testing. *Brain* 118:243–251.

Celesia, G. G., Brigell, M. G., Vaphanides, M. S. (1997). Hemianopic anosognosia. *Neurology* 49:88–97.

Chatterjee, A., and Mennemeier, M. (1996). Anosognosia for hemiplegia: patient retrospections. *Cogn. Neuropsychiatry* 1:221–237.

Chui, H. C. (1989). Dementia: a review emphasizing clinicopathologic correlation and brain-behavior relationships. *Arch. Neurol.* 46:806–814.

Cohn, R. (1971). Phantom vision. *Arch. Neurol.* 25:468–471.

Cohn, R., and Neumann, M. A. (1958). Jargon aphasia. *J. Nerv. Ment. Dis.* 127:381–399.

Cole, M. (1999). When the left brain is not right the right brain may be left: report of personal experience of occipital hemianopia. *J. Neurol. Neurosurg. Psychiatry* 67:169–173.

Correa, D. D., Graves, R. E., and Costa, L. (1996). Awareness of memory deficit in Alzheimer's disease patients and memory-impaired older adults. *Aging Neuropsychol. Cogn.* 3:215–228.

Coslett, H. B., and Saffran, E. M. (1989). Evidence for preserved reading in pure alexia. *Brain* 112:327–359.

Critchley, M. (1949). The problem of awareness or nonawareness of hemianopic field defects. *Trans. Opthalmol. Soc. UK* 69:95–109.

Critchley, M. (1953). *The Parietal Lobes.* London: Edward Arnold.

Critchley, M. (1974). Misoplegia or hatred of hemiplegia. *Mt. Sinai J. Med.* 41:82–87.

Cummings, J. L., Darkins, A., Mendez, M., Hill, M. A., and Benson, D. F. (1988). Alzheimer's disease and Parkinson's disease: comparison of speech and language alterations. *Neurology* 38:680–684.

Cummings, J. L., Ross, W., Absher, J., Gornbein, J., and Hadjiaghai, L. (1995). Depressive symptoms in Alzheimer disease: assessments and determinants. *Alzheimer Dis. Assoc. Disord.* 9:87–93.

Cutting, J. (1978). Study of anosognosia. *J. Neurol. Neurosurg. Psychiatry* 41:548–555.

Cutler, A. (1982). The reliability of speech error data. In *Slips of the Tongue*, A. Cutler (ed.). The Hague: Mouton.

Dalla Barba, G., Parlato, V., Iavarone, A., and Boller, F. (1995). Anosognosia, intrusions, and 'frontal' functions in Alzheimer's disease and depression. *Neuropsychologia* 33:247–259.

Damasio, A. R., Graff-Radford, N. R., Eslinger, P. J., Damasio, H., and Kassell, N. (1985). Amnesia following basal forebrain lesions. *Arch. Neurol.* 42:263–271.

Danielczyk, W. (1983). Various mental behavioral disorders in Parkinson's disease, primary degenerative senile dementia, and multiple infarction dementia. *J. Neural Transm.* 56:161–176.

DeBettignies, B. H., Mahurin, R. K., and Pirozzolo, F. J. (1990). Insight for impairment in independent living skills in Alzheimer's disease and multi-infarct dementia. *J. Clin. Exp. Neuropsychol.* 12:355–363.

DeHaan, E. H. F., Young, A. W., and Newcombe, F. (1987). Face recognition without awareness. *Cogn. Neuropsychol.* 4:385–415.

Deluca, J. (1993). Predicting neurobehavioral patterns following anterior communicating artery aneurysm. *Cortex* 29:639–647.

Deluca, J., and Diamond, B. J. (1995). Aneurysm of the anterior communicating artery: a review of neuroanatomical and neuropsychological sequelae. *J. Clin. Exp. Neuropsychol.* 17:100–121.

Devinsky, O., Bear, D., and Volpe, B. T. (1988). Confusional states following posterior cerebral artery infarctions. *Arch. Neurol.* 45:160–163.

Durkin, M. W., Meador, K. J., Nichols, M. E., Lee, G. P., and Loring, D. W. (1994). Anosognosia and the intracarotid amobarbital procedure (Wada Test). *Neurology* 44:978–979.

Dywan, D. A., McGlone, J., and Fox, A. (1995). Do intracarotid barbiturate injections offer a way to investigate hemispheric models of anosognosia? *J. Clin. Exp. Neuropsychol.* 17:431–438.

Ellis, A. W., and Young, A. W. (1988). *Human Cognitive Neuropsychology.* Hillsdale, NY: Lawrence Erlbaum Associates.

Ellis, S. J., and Small, M. (1994). Denial of eye closure in acute stroke. *Stroke* 25:1958–1962.

Evans, J. H. (1966). Transient loss of memory, an organic mental syndrome. *Brain* 89:539–548.

Evyapan, D., and Kumral, E. (1999). Pontine anosognosia for hemiplegia. *Neurology* 53:647–649.

Fairbanks, G., and Guttman, N. (1955). Effects of delayed auditory feedback upon articulation. *J. Speech Hear. Res.* 1:12–22.

Feher, E. P., Larrabee, G. J., Sudilovsky, A., and Crook, T. H. (1993). Memory self-report in Alzheimer's disease and in age-associated memory impairment. *J. Geriatr. Psychiatry Neurol.* 6:58–65.

Feher, E. P., Mahurin, R. K., Inbody, S. B., Crook, T., and Pirozzolo, F. P. (1991). Anosognosia in Alzheimer's disease. *Neuropsychiatry Neuropsychol. Behav. Neurol.* 4:136–146.

Feinberg, T. E. (1997). Anosognosia and confabulation. In *Behavioral Neurology and Neuropsychology*, T. E. Feinberg and M. J. Farah (eds.). New York: McGraw-Hill, pp. 369–390.

Feinberg, T. E., Haber, L. D., and Leeds, N. E. (1990). Verbal asomatognosia. *Neurology* 40:1391–1394.

Feinberg, T. E., and Roane, D. M. (1997). Anosognosia, completion and confabulation: the neutral-personal dichotomy. *Neurocase* 3:73–85.

Feinberg, T. E., Roane, D. M., Kwan, P. C., Schindler, R. J., and Haber, L. D. (1994). Anosognosia and visuoverbal confabulation. *Arch. Neurol.* 51:468–473.

Fischer, R. S., Alexander, M. P., D'Esposito, M., and Otto, R. (1995) Neuropsychological and neuroanatomical correlates of confabulation. *J. Clin. Exp. Neuropsychol.* 17:20–28.

Fisher, C. M. (1989). Neurologic fragments II. Remarks on anosognosia, confabulation, memory and other topics; and an appendix on self-observation. *Neurology* 39:127–132.

Fisher, C. M. (1982). Transient global amnesia: precipitating activities and other observations. *Arch. Neurol.* 39:605–608.

Förstl, H., Owen, A. M., and David, A. S. (1993). Gabriel Anton and "Anton's symptom": on focal diseases of the brain which are not perceived by the patient. *Neuropsychiatry Neuropsychol. Behav. Neurol.* 1:1–8.

Foster, N. L., Chase, T. N., Fedio, P., Patronas, N. J., Brooks, R. A., and DiChiro, G. (1983). Alzheimer's disease: focal cortical changes shown by positron emission tomography. *Neurology 33:* 961–965.

Frederiks, J. A. M. (1985). The neurology of aging and dementia. In *Handbook of Clinical Neurology, Vol. 2*, J. A. M. Frederiks (ed.). Amsterdam: Elsevier, pp. 199–219.

Freedman, L., Selchen, D. H., Black, S. E., Kaplan, R., Garnett, E. S., and Nahmias, C. (1991). Posterior cortical dementia with alexia: neurobehavioral, MRI, and PET findings. *J. Neurol. Neurosurg. Psychiatry 54:*443–448.

Friedland, R. P., and Bodis-Wollner, I. (1977). Absence of somatosensory evoked potentials in patients with anosognosia [letter]. *Neurology 27:* 695–696.

Friedland, R. P., Brun, A., and Budinger, T. F. (1985). Pathological and positron emission tomographic correlates in Alzheimer's disease. *Lancet 1(8422):*228.

Friedland, R. P., Budinger, T. F., Brandt-Zawadzki, M., and Jagust, W. J. (1984). The diagnosis of

Alzheimer-type dementia: a preliminary comparison of positron emission tomography and proton magnetic resonance. *JAMA 252:*2750–2752.

Friedland, R. P., and Weinstein, E. A. (1977). Hemiinattention and hemisphere specialization: introduction and historical review. *Adv. Neurol.* 18:1–31.

Friedlander, W. J. (1967). Anosognosia and perception. *Am. J. Phys. Med. 46:*1394–1408.

Gainotti, G. (1972). Emotional behavior and hemispheric side of lesion. *Cortex 8:*41–55.

Gassel, M., and Williams, D. (1963). Visual function in patients with homonymous hemianopia. III. The completion phenomenon: insight and attitude to the defect; and visual function efficiency. *Brain 86:*229–260.

Gerstmann, J. (1942) Problems of imperception of disease and of impaired body territories with organic lesions. *Arch. Neurol. Psychiatry 48:*890–913.

Geschwind, N. (1965). Disconnexion syndromes in animals and man. *Brain 88:*237–294.

Geschwind, N., and Fusillo, M. (1966). Color-naming defects in association with alexia. *Arch. Neurol.* 15:137.

Gialanella, B., and Mattioli, F. (1992). Anosognosia and extrapersonal neglect as predictors of functional recovery following right hemisphere stroke. *Neuropsychol. Rehabil.* 2:169–178.

Gilmore, R. L., Heilman, K. M., Schmidt, R. P., Fennell, E. M., and Quisling, R. (1992). Anosog-

nosia during Wada testing. *Neurology 42:*925–927.

Gold, M., Adair, J. C., Jacobs, D. H., Heilman, K. M. (1994). Anosognosia for hemiplegia: an electrophysiological investigation of the feedforward hypothesis. *Neurology 44:*1804–1808.

Goldenberg, G. (1992). Loss of visual imagery and loss of visual knowledge—a case study. *Neuropsychologia 30:*1081–1099.

Goldenberg, G. (1995). Dissociations entre l'imagerie et la perception visuelle lors de lesions des aires visuelles. *Rev. Neuropsychol.* 5:489–502.

Goldman-Rakic, P. S. (1987). Circuitry of primate prefrontal cortex and regulation of behaviors by representational memory. In *Handbook of Physiology: Nervous System V: Higher Functions of the Brain*, F. Plum (ed.). Bethesda, MD: American Physiological Society, pp. 373–417.

Gotham, A. M., Brown, R. G., and Marsden, C. D. (1988). 'Frontal' cognitive function in patients with Parkinson's disease 'on' and 'off' levodopa. *Brain 111:*299–321.

Graff-Radford, N. R., Eslinger, P. J., Damasio, A. R., and Yamada, T. (1984). Nonhemorrhagic infarction of the thalamus: behavioral, anatomic, and physiologic correlates. *Neurology 34:*14–23.

Green, J., Goldstein, F. C., Sirockman, B. E., and Green, R. C. (1993). Variable awareness of deficits in Alzheimer's disease. *Neuropsychiatry Neuropsychol. Behav. Neurol.* 6:159–165.

Green, J. B., and Hamilton, W. J. (1976). Anosognosia for hemiplegia: somatosensory evoked potential studies. *Neurology 26:*1141–1144.

Grotta, J., and Bratina, P. (1995). Subjective experiences of 24 patients dramatically recovering from stroke. *Stroke 26:*1285–1288.

Gustafson, I., and Nilsson, L. (1982). Differential diagnosis of presenile dementia on clinical grounds. *Acta Psychiatr. Scand.* 65:194–207.

Healton, E. B., Navarro, C., Bressman, S., and Brust, J. C. M. (1982). Subcortical neglect. *Neurology 32:*776–778.

Hécaen, H, and Albert, M. (1978). Disorders of somesthesia and somatognosis. In: *Human Neuropsychology*. New York: John Wiley & Sons.

Hedreen, J. C., Peyser, C. E., Folstein, S. E., and Ross, C. A. (1991). Neural loss in layers V and VI of cerebral cortex in Huntington's disease. *Neurosci. Lett.* 133:257–261.

Heilman, K. M. (1991). Anosognosia. Possible neuropsychological mechanisms. In *Awareness of Deficit After Brain Injury*, G. P. Prigatano and D. L. Schacter (Eds.). New York: Oxford University Press, pp. 53–62.

Hier, D. B., Mondlock, J., and Caplan, L. R. (1983). Recovery of behavioral abnormalities after right hemisphere stroke. *Neurology* 33:345–350.

Hildebrandt, H., and Zieger, A. (1995). Unconscious activation of motor responses in a hemiplegic patient with anosognosia and neglect. *Eur. Arch. Psychiatry Clin. Neurosci.* 246:53–59.

Holman, B. L., Johnson, K. A., Gerada, B., Carvalho, P. A., and Satlin, A. (1992). The scintigraphic appearance of Alzheimer's disease: a prospective study using technetium-99m-HMPAO SPECT. *J. Nucl. Med.* 33:181–185.

Jacome, D. E. (1986). Case report: subcortical prosopagnosia and anosognosia. *Am. J. Med. Sci.* 292:386–388.

Jarho, L. (1973). Korsakoff-like amnesic syndrome in penetrating brain injury. *Acta Neurol. Scand.* 55:49–67.

Jensen, T. S., and Olivarius, B. (1981). Transient global amnesia—its clinical and pathophysiological basis and prognosis. *Acta Neurol. Scand.* 63:220–230.

Joynt, R. J., and Shoulson, I. (1985). Dementia. In *Clinical Neuropsycholgy, 2nd edition*, K. M. Heilman and E. Valenstein (eds.). New York: Oxford Univeristy Press, pp. 453–479.

Kaplan, R. F., Meadows, M. E., Cohen, R. A., Bromfield, E. B., and Ehrenberg, B. L. (1993). Awareness of deficit after the sodium amobarbital (Wada) test. *J. Clin. Exp. Neuropsychol.* 15:383.

Kausall, P. I., Zetin, M., and Squire, L. R. (1981). A psychosocial study of chronic circumscribed amnesia. *J. Nerv. Ment. Dis.* 169:383–389.

Kerkhoff, G., MunBinger, U., and Meier, E. K. (1994). Neurovisual rehabilitation in cerebral blindness. *Arch. Neurol.* 51:474–481.

Kern, R. S., Van Gorp, W. G., Cummings, J. L., Brown, W. S., and Osato, S. S. (1992). Confabulation in Alzheimer's disease. *Brain Cogn.* 19:172–182.

Kertesz, A. (1979). *Aphasia and associated disorders*. New York:Grune and Stratton.

Kinsbourne, M., and Warrington, E. K. (1963). Jargon aphasia. *Neuropsychologia* 1:27–37.

Koehler, P. J., Endtz, l. J., TeVelde, J., and Hekster, R. E. (1986). Aware or non-aware. On the significance of the lesion responsible for homonymous hemianopia. *J. Neurol. Sci.* 75:255–262.

Kopelman, M. D., Stanhope, N., and Guinan, E. (1998). Subjective memory evaluations in patients with focal frontal, diencephalic, and temporal lobe lesion. *Cortex* 34:191–207.

Korsakoff, S. S. (1889). Etude medico-psychologique sur une forme des maladies de la memoire. *Rev. Philos.* 5: 501–30.

Kosslyn, S. M., Alpert, N. M., Thompson, W. L., Maljkovic, V., Weise, S. B., Chabris, C. F., Hamilton, S. E., Rausch, S. L., and Buonanno, F. S. (1993). Visual mental imagery activates topographically organized visual cortex: PET investigations. *J. Cogn. Neurosci.* 5:263–287.

Kotler-Cope, S., and Camp, C. J. (1995). Anosognosia in Alzheimer disease. *Alzheimer Dis. Assoc. Disord.* 9:52–56.

Kritchevsky, M. (1987). Transient global amnesia: when memory temporarily disappears. *Postgrad. Med.* 82:95–100.

Lebrun, Y. (1986). Aphasia with recurrent utterance: a review. *Br. J. Dis. Comm.* 21:3–10.

Lebrun, Y. (1987). Anosognosia in aphasics. *Cortex* 23:251–263.

Lecours, A. R., and Joanette, Y. (1980). Linguistic and other psychological aspects of paroxysmal aphasia. *Brain Lang.* 10:1–23.

Levelt, W. J. M. (1983). Monitoring and self-repair in speech. *Cognition* 14:41–104.

Levine, D. N. (1990). Unawareness of visual and sensorimotor defects: a hypothesis. *Brain Cogn.* 13:233–281.

Levine, D. N., Calvanio, R., Rinn, W. E. (1991). The pathogenesis of anosognosia for hemiplegia. *Neurology* 41:1770–1781.

Lhermitte, F., and Beauvois, M. A. (1973). A visual–speech disconnexion syndrome. *Brain* 96:695–714.

Liebson, E. (2000). Anosognosia and mania associated with right thalamic hemorrhage. *J. Neurol. Neurosurg. Psychiatry* 68:107–108.

Lipinska, B., and Backman, L. (1996). Feeling-of-knowing in fact retrieval: further evidence for preseveration in early Alzheimer's disease. *J. Int. Neuropsychol. Soc.* 2:350–358.

Lopez, O. L., Becker, J. T., Somsak, D., Dew, M. A., and DeKosky, S. T. (1993). Awareness of cognitive deficits in probable Alzheimer's disease. *Eur. Neurol.* 34:277–282.

Lu, L. H., Barrett, A. M., Schwartz, R. L., Cibula, J. E., et al. (1997). Anosognosia and confabulation during the Wada test. *Neurology* 49:1316–1322.

Maeshima, S., Dohi, N., Funahashi, K., Nakai, K., Itakura, T., and Komai, N. (1997). Rehabilitation of patients with anosognosia for hemiplegia due to intracerebral haemorrhage. *Brain Inj.* 11:691–697.

Maher, L. M., Gonzalez Rothi, L. J., and Heilman, K. M. (1994). Lack of error awareness in an aphasic patient with relatively preserved auditory comprehension. *Brain Lang.* 46:402–418.

Mangone, C. A., Hier, D. B., Gorelick, P. B.,

Ganellen, R. J., Langenberg, P., Boarman, R., and Dollear, W. C. (1991). Impaired insight in Alzheimer's disease. *J. Geriatr. Psychiatry Neurol.* 4:189–93.

Marshall, R. C., Rappaport, B. Z., and Garcia-Bunuel, L. (1985). Self-monitoring behavior in a case of severe auditory agnosia with aphasia. *Brain Lang.* 24:297–313.

Marshall, R. C., and Tompkins, C. A. (1982). Verbal self-correction behaviors of fluent and non-fluent aphasic subjects. *Brain Lang.* 15:292–306.

Mauguiere, F., Brechard, S., Pernier, J., Courjon, J., and Schott, B. (1982). Anosognosia with hemiplegia: auditory evoked potential studies. In *Clinical Applications of Evoked Potentials in Neurology*, J. Courjon, F. Maugiere, and M. Revol (eds.). New York: Raven Press, pp. 271–278.

McDaniel, K. D., Edland, S. D., Heyman, A., and the CERAD clinical investigators. (1995). Relationship between level of insight and severity of dementia in Alzheimer disease. *Alzheimer Dis. Assoc. Disord.* 9:101–104.

McDaniel, K. D., and McDaniel, L. D. (1991). Anton's syndrome in a patient with posttraumatic optic neuropathy and bifrontal contusions. *Arch. Neurol.* 48:101–105.

McGlone, J., Gupta, S., Humphrey, D., Oppenheimer, S., Mirsen, T., and Evans, D. R. (1990). Screening for early dementia using memory complaints from patients and relatives. *Arch. Neurol.* 47:1189–1193.

McGlynn, S. M., and Kaszniak, A. W. (1991a). Unawareness of deficits in dementia and schizophrenia. In *Awareness of Deficit After Brain Injury: Clinical and Theoretical Issues*, G. P. Prigatano and D. L. Schacter (eds.). New York: Oxford University Press, pp. 84–110.

McGlynn, S. M., and Kaszniak, A. W. (1991b). When metacognition fails: impaired awareness of deficit in Alzheimer's disease. *J. Cogn. Neurosci.* 3:183–189.

McGlynn, S. M., and Schacter, D. L. (1989). Unawareness of deficits in neuropsychological syndromes. *J. Clin. Exp. Neuropsychol.* 11:143–205.

Medina, J. L., Rubino, F. A., and Ross, E. (1974). Agitated delirium caused by infarctions of the hippocampal formation and fusiform and lingual gyri: a case report. *Neurology* 24:1181–1183.

Mercer, B., Wapner, W., Gardner, H., and Benson, D. F. (1977). A study of confabulation. *Arch. Neurol.* 34:429–433.

Mesulam, M. M. (1998). From sensation to cognition. *Brain* 121:1013–1052.

Michon, A., Deweer, B., Pilon, B., Agid, Y., and Dubois, B. (1994). Relation of anosognosia to frontal lobe dysfunction in Alzheimer's disease. *J. Neurol. Neurosurg. Psychiatry* 57:805–809.

Migliorelli, R., Tecson, A., Sabe, L., Petracca, G., Petracca, M., Leiguarda, R., and Starkstein, S. E. (1995). Anosognosia in Alzheimer's disease: a study of associated factors. *J. Neuropsychiatry Clin. Neurosci.* 7:338–344.

Milandre, L., Brosset, C., Botti, G., and Khalil, R. (1994). Étude de 82 infarctus du territoire des artères cérébrales postérieures. *Rev. Neurol. (Paris)* 150:133.

Milner, B., Corkin, S., and Teuber, H. L. (1968). Further analysis of the hippocampal amnesic syndrome: 14-year follow-up study of H.M. *Neuropsychologia* 6:215–234.

Mohr, J. P., and Pessin, M. (1998). Posterior cerebral artery disease. In *Stroke: Pathophysiology, Diagnosis and Management, third edition,* H. J. M. Barnett, J. P. Mohr, B. M. Stein, and F. M. Yatsu (eds.). New York: Churchill Livingstone, pp. 581–502.

Nathanson, M., Bergman, P. S., and Gordon, G. G. (1952). Denial of illness: its occurrence in one hundred consecutive cases of hemiplegia. *Arch. Neurol. Psychiatry* 68:380–397.

Neary, D., Snowden, J. S., Bowen, D. M., Sims, N. R., Mann, D. M. A., Benton, J. S., Northen, B., Yates, P. O., and Davison, A. N. (1986). Neuropsychological syndromes in presenile dementia due to cerebral atrophy. *J. Neurol. Neurosurg. Psychiatry* 49:163–74.

Neundorfer, M. M. (1997). Awareness of variability in awareness. *Alzheimer Dis. Assoc. Disord.* 11:125–131.

Nooteboom, S. (1980). Speaking and unspeaking: detection and correction of phonological and lexical errors in spontaneous speech. In *Errors in Linguistic Performance: Slips of the Tongue, Ear, Pen and Hand*, V. A. Fromkin (ed.). New York: Academic Press, pp. 87–95.

Ott, B. R., Lafleche, G., Whelihan, W. M., Buongiorno, G. W., Albert, M. S., and Fogel, B. S. (1996a). Impaired awareness of deficits in Alzheimer's disease. *Alzheimer Dis. Assoc. Disord.* 2:68–76.

Ott, B. R., Noto, R. B., and Fogel, B. S. (1996b). Apathy and loss of insight in Alzheimer's disease: a SPECT imaging study. *J. Neuropsychiatry Clin. Neurosci.* 8:41–46.

Pandya, D. N., and Barnes, C. L. (1987). Architecture and connections of the frontal lobe. In *The Frontal Lobes Revisited*, E. Perecman (ed.). New York: IRBN Press, pp. 41–72.

Pappas, B. A., Sunderland, T., Weingartner, H. M.,

Vitiello, B., Martinson, H., and Putnam, K. (1992). Alzheimer's disease and feeling-of-knowing for knowledge and episodic memory. *J. Gerontol. 47*:P159–P164.

Peuser, B., and Temp, K. (1981). The evolution of jargon aphasia. In *Jargon Aphasia*, J. Brown (ed.). Orlando, Academic Press.

Ponsford, J. L., and Donnan, G. A. (1980). Transient global amnesia—a hippocampal phenomenon? *J. Neurol. Neurosurg. Psychiatry 43*:285–287.

Ramachandran, V. S. (1995). Anosognosia in parietal lobe syndrome. *Conscious. Cogn. 4*:22–51.

Redlich, F. C., and Dorsey, J. F. (1945). Denial of blindness by patients with cerebral disease. *Arch. Neurol. Psychiatry 53*:407–417.

Reed, B. R., Jagust, W. J., and Coulter, L. (1993). Anosognosia in Alzheimer's disease: relationships to depression, cognitive function, and cerebral perfusion. *J. Clin. Exp. Neuropsychol. 15*: 231–244.

Reisberg, B., Gordon, B., and McCarthy, M. (1985). Insight and denial accompanying progressive cognitive decline in normal aging and Alzheimer's disease. In *Geriatric Psychiatry: Ethical and Legal Issues*, B. Stanley (ed.). Washington, DC: American Psychiatric Press, pp. 19–39.

Rimel, R. W., Giordani, B., Barth, J. T., Boll, T. J., and Jane, J. A. (1981). Disability caused by minor head injury. *Neurosurgery 9*:221–228.

Roman-Campos, G., Poser, C. M., and Wood, F. B. (1980). Persistent retrograde memory deficit after transient global amnesia. *Cortex 16*:509–518.

Rose, F. C., and Symonds, C. P. (1960). Persistent memory defect following encephalitis. *Brain 83*:195–212.

Rubens, A. B., and Garrett, M. F. (1991). Anosognosia of linguistic deficits in patients with neurological deficits. In *Awareness of Deficit After Brain Injury: Clinical and Theoretical Issues*, G. P. Prigatano and D. L. Schacter (eds.). New York: Oxford University Press, pp. 40–52.

Sagar, H. J., Sullivan, E. V., Cooper, J. A., and Jordan, H. (1991). Normal release from proactive interference in untreated patients with Parkinson's disease. *Neuropsychologia 29*:1033–1044.

Sandifer, P. H. (1946). Anosognosia and disorders of body scheme. *Brain 39*:122–137.

Sandson, J., Albert, M. L., and Alexander, M. P. (1986). Confabulation in aphasia. *Cortex 22*:621–626.

Schacter, D. L. (1987). Memory, amnesia, and frontal lobe dysfunction. *Psychobiology 15*:21–36.

Schacter, D. L. (1990). Toward a cognitive neuropsychology of awareness: implicit knowledge and anosognosia. *J. Clin. Exp. Neuropsychol. 12*:155–178.

Schacter, D. L. (1991). Unawareness of deficit and unawareness of knowledge in patients with memory disorders. In *Awareness of Deficit After Brain Injury: Clinical and Theoretical Issues*, G. P. Prigatano and D. L. Schacter (eds.). New York: Oxford University Press, pp. 127–151.

Schlenck, K. J., Huber, W., and Willmes, K. (1987). Prepairs and repairs: different monitoring functions in aphasic language production. *Brain Lang. 30*:224–226.

Schneck, M. K., Reisberg, B., and Ferris, S. H. (1992). An overview of current concepts of Alzheimer's disease. *Am. J. Psychiatry 139*:165–173.

Schultz, G., and Melzack, R. (1991). The Charles Bonnet syndrome: 'phantom visual images'. *Perception 20*:809–825.

Segal, S. J., and Fusella, V. (1970). Influence of imaged pictures and sounds on detection of visual and auditory signals. *J. Exp. Psychol. 83*:458–464.

Seltzer, B., Vasterling, J. J., Hale, M. A., and Khurana, R. (1995). Unawareness of memory deficits in Alzheimer's disease: relation to mood and other disease variables. *Neuropsychiatry Neuropsychol. Behav. Neurol. 8*:176–181.

Seltzer, B., Vasterling, J. J., Yoder, J., and Thompson, K. A. (1997). Awareness of deficit in Alzheimer's disease: relation to caregiver burden. *Gerontologist 37*:20–24.

Sergent, J. (1988). An investigation into perceptual completion in blind areas of the visual field. *Brain 111*:347–373.

Sevush, S. (1999). Relationship between denial of memory deficit and dementia severity in Alzheimer disease. *Neuropsychiatry Neuropsychol. Behav. Neurol. 12*:88–94.

Sevush, S., and Leve, N. (1993). Denial of memory deficit in Alzheimer's disease. *Am. J. Psychiatry 150*:748–751.

Shapiro, B. E., Alexander, M. P., Gardner, H., and Mercer, B. (1981). Mechanisms of confabulation. *Neurology 31*:1070–1076.

Shimamura, A., Jernigan, T. L., and Squire, L. (1988). Korsakoff's syndrome: radiological (CT) findings and neuropsychological correlates. *J. Neurosci. 8*:4400–4410.

Shimamura, A. P., and Squire, L. R. (1986). Memory and meta-memory: a study of feeling-of-known phenomenon in amnestic patients. *J. Exp. Psychol. Learn. Mem. 12*:452–460.

Shuren, J. E., Smith Hammond, C., Maher, L. M., Rothi, L. J. G., and Heilman, K. M. (1995). Attention and anosognosia: the case of a jargon aphasic patient with unawareness of language deficit. *Neurology* 45:376–378.

Squire, L. R. (1982). Comparisons between forms of amnesia: some deficits are unique to Korsakoff's syndrome. *J. Exp. Psychol. Learn. Mem.* 8:560–571.

Squire, L. R., and Zousounis, L. A. (1988). Self-rating of memory dysfunction: different findings in depression and amnesia. *J. Clin. Exp. Neuropsychol.* 10:727–738.

Stam, C. J., Visser, S. L., Op de Coul, A. A. W., DeSonneville, L. M. J., Schellens, R. L. L. A., Brunia, C. H. M., de Smet, J. S., and Gielen, G. (1993). Disturbed frontal regulation of attention in Parkinson's disease. *Brain* 116:1139–1158.

Starkstein, S. E., Chemerinski, E., Sabe, L., Kuzis, G., Petracca, G., Teson, A., and Leiguarda, R. (1997a). Prospective longitudinal study of depression and anosognosia in Alzheimer's disease. *Br. J. Psychiatry* 171:47–52.

Starkstein, S. E., Fedoroff, J. P., Price, T. R., Leiguarda, R., and Robinson, R. G. (1992). Anosognosia in patients with cerebrovascular lesions: a study of causative factors. *Stroke* 23:1446–1453.

Starkstein, S. E., Fedoroff, J. P., Price, T. R., Leiguarda, R., and Robinson, R. G. (1993a). Neuropsychological deficits in patients with anosognosia. *Neuropsychiatry Neuropsychol. Behav. Neurol* 6:43–48.

Starkstein, S. E., Fedoroff, J. P., Price, T. R., and Robinson, R. G. (1993b). Denial of illness scale: a reliability and validity study. *Neuropsychiatry Neuropsychol. Behav. Neurol.* 6:93–97.

Starkstein, S. E., Berthier, M. L., Fedoroff, P., Price, T. R., Robinson, R. G. (1990). Anosognosia and major depression in 2 patients with cerebrovascular lesions. *Neurology* 40:1380–1382.

Starkstein, S. E., Sabe, L., Cuerva, A. G., Kuzis, G., and Leiguarda, R. (1997b). Anosognosia and procedural learning in Alzheimer's disease. *Neuropsychiatry Neuropsychol. Behav. Neurol.* 10:96–101.

Starkstein, S. E., Sabe, L., Petracca, G., Chemerinski, E., Kuzis, G., Merello, M., and Leiguarda, R. (1996c). Neuropsychological and psychiatric differences between Alzheimer's disease and Parkinson's disease with dementia. *J. Neurol. Neurosurg. Psychiatry* 61:381–387.

Starkstein, S. E., Sabe, L., Vazquez, S., Teson, A., Petracca, G., Chemerinski, E., DiLorenzo, G., and Leiguarda, R. (1996b). Neuropsychological, psychiatric, and cerebral blood flow findings in vascular dementia and Alzheimer's disease. *Stroke* 27:408–414.

Starkstein S.E., Vazquez S., Migliorelli R., Vazquez S., Teson A., Sabe L., and Leiguarda R. (1995). A single-photon emission computed tomographic study of anosognosia in Alzheimer's disease. Arch. Neurol. 52: 415–420.

Stelmach, G. E., Worringham, C. J., and Strand, E. A. (1986). Movement preparation in Parkinson's disease. *Brain* 109:1179–1194.

Stengel, E., and Steele, G. D. F. (1946). Unawareness of physical disability (anosognosia). *J. Ment. Sci.* 92:379–388.

Stone, S. P., Halligan, P. W., and Greenwood, R. J. (1993). The incidence of neglect phenomena and related disorders in patients with an acute right or left hemisphere stroke. *Age Ageing* 22:46–52.

Stuss, D. T. (1991). Disturbance of self-awareness after frontal system damage. In *Awareness of Deficit After Brain Injury: Clinical and Theoretical Issues*, G. P. Prigatano and D. L. Schacter (eds.). New York: Oxford University Press, pp. 63–83.

Stuss, D. T. (1993). Assessment of neuropsychological dysfunction in frontal lobe degeneration. *Dementia* 4:220–225.

Stuss, D. T., Alexander, M. P., Lieberman, A., and Levine, H. (1978). An extraordinary form of confabulation. *Neurology* 28:1166–1172.

Stuss, D. T., and Benson, D. F. (1986). *The Frontal Lobes.* New York: Raven Press.

Stuss, D. T., and Cummings, J. L. (1990). Subcortical vascular dementias. In *Subcortical Dementia*, J. L. Cummings (ed.). New York: Oxford University Press, pp. 145–163.

Sunderland, A., Harris, J. E., and Baddeley, A. D. (1983). Do laboratory tests predict everyday memory? A neuropsychological study. *J Verbal Learn. Verbal Behav.* 22:341–357.

Sunderland, A., Watts, K., Baddeley, A. D., and Harris, J. E. (1986). Subjective memory assessment and test performance in elderly adults. *J. Gerontol.* 41:376–384.

Swartz, B. E., and Brust, J. C. M. (1984). Anton's syndrome accompanying withdrawal hallucinosis in a blind alcoholic. *Neurology* 34:696–673.

Talland, G. A. (1961). Confabulation in the Wernicke-Korsakoff syndrome. *J. Nerv. Ment. Dis.* 132:361–381.

Taylor, A. E., Saint-Cyr, J. A., and Lang, A. E. (1986). Frontal lobe dysfunction in Parkinson's disease: the cortical focus of neostriatal outflow. *Brain* 109:845–883.

Teuber, H. L., Battersby, W. S., and Bender, M. S. (1960). *Visual Field Defects After Penetrating Missile Wounds of the Brain.* Cambrigde, MA: Harvard University Press, p. 87.

Timmons, B. A. (1983). Speech disfluencies under normal and delayed auditory feedback conditions. *Percept. Mot. Skills* 56:575–579.

Torjussen, T. (1978). Residual function in cortically blind hemifields. *Neuropsychologia* 16:15–21.

Vallar, G., Papagno, C., Rusconi, M. L., and Bisiach, E. (1995). Vestibular stimulation, spatial hemineglect and dysphasia. Selective effects? *Cortex* 31:589–593.

Vasterling, J. J., Seltzer, B., Foss, J. W., and Vanderbrook, V. (1995). Unawareness of deficit in Alzheimer's disease: domain-specific differences and disease correlates. *Neuropsychiatry Neuropsychol. Behav. Neurol.* 8:26–32.

Vasterling, J. J., Seltzer, B., and Watrous, W. E. (1997). Longitudinal assessment of deficit unawareness in Alzheimer's disease. *Neuropsychiatry Neuropsychol. Behav. Neurol.* 10:197–202.

Verhey, F. R. J., Ponds, R. W. H. M., Rozendaal, N., and Jolles, J. (1995). Depression, insight, and personality changes in Alzheimer's disease and vascular dementia. *J. Geriatr. Psychiatry Neurol.* 8:23–27.

Verslegers, W., De Deyn, P. P., Saerens, J., Marien, P., Appel, B., Pickut, B. A., and Lowenthal, A. (1991). Slow progressive bilateral posterior artery infarction presenting as agitated delirium, complicated with Anton's syndrome. *Eur. Neurol.* 31:216–219.

Victor, M., Adams, R. D., and Collins, G. H. (1989). *The Wernicke-Korsakoff Syndrome, second edition.* Philadelphia: F. A. Davis.

Vilkki, J. (1985). Amnesic syndromes after rupture of anterior communicating artery aneurysms. *Cortex* 21:431–444.

Volpe, B. T., and Hirst, W. (1983). Amnesia following the rupture and repair of an anterior communicating artery aneurysm. *J. Neurol. Neurosurg. Psychiatry* 46:704–709.

Von Monakow, C. (1885). Experimentelle und pathologisch-anatomische Untersuchungen über die Beziehungen der sogenannten Sehsphäre zu den infracorticalen Opticuscentren und zum N. opticus. *Arch. Psychiatrie Nervenkr.* 16:151–199, 317–352.

Wagner, M. T., and Cushman, L. A. (1994). Neuroanatomic and neuropsychological predictors of unawareness of cognitive deficit in the vascular population. *Arch. Clin. Neuropsychol.* 9:57–69.

Wagner, M. T., Spangenberg, K. B., Bachman, D. L., and O'Connell, P. (1997). Unawareness of cognitive deficit in Alzheimer disease and related dementias. *Alzheimer Dis. Assoc. Disord.* 11:125–131.

Warrington, E. K. (1962). The completion of visual forms across hemianopic field defects. *J. Neurol. Neurosurg. Psychiatry* 25:208–217.

Watson, R. T., and Heilman, K. M. (1979). Thalamic neglect. *Neurology* 29:690–694.

Weinstein, E. A., Cole, M., Mitchell, M. S., and Lyerly, O. G. (1964). Anosognosia and aphasia. *Arch. Neurol.* 10:376–386.

Weinstein, E. A., Friedland, R. P., and Wagner, E. E. (1994). Denial/awareness of impairment and symbolic behavior in Alzheimer's disease. *Neuropsychiatry Neuropsychol. Behav. Neurol.* 7:176–184.

Weinstein, E. A., and Kahn, R. L. (1950). The syndrome of anosognosia. *Arch. Neurol. Psychiatry* 64:772–791.

Weinstein, E. A., and Kahn, R. L. (1953). Personality factors in denial of illness. *AMA Arch. Neurol. Psychiatry* 69:355–367.

Weinstein, E. A., and Kahn, R. L. (1955). *Denial of Illness: Symbolic and Physiological Aspects.* Springfield, IL: Charles C. Thomas.

Weinstein, E. A., and Lyerly, O. G. (1976). Personality factors in jargon aphasia. *Cortex* 12:122–33.

Weinstein, E. A., Lyerly, O. G., Cole, M., and Ozer, M. S. (1966). Meaning in jargon aphasia. *Cortex* 2:165–187.

Weiskrantz, L. (1986). *Blindsight: A Case Study and Implications.* New York: Oxford University Press.

Wepman, J. M. (1958). The relationship between self-correction and recovery from aphasia. *J. Speech Hear. Disord.* 23:302–305.

Wortis, H., and Dattner, B. (1942). Analysis of a somatic delusion: a case report. *Psychsom. Med.* 4:319–323.

Young, A. W., deHaan, E. H., and Newcombe, F. (1990). Unawareness of impaired face recognition. *Brain Cogn.* 14:1–18.

Zanetti, O., Vallotti, B., Frisoni, G. B., Geroldi, C., Bianchetti, A., Pasqualetti, P., and Trabucchi, M. (1999). Insight in dementia: when does it occur? Evidence for a nonlinear relationship between insight and cognitive status. *J. Gerontol.* 54B: P100–P106.

Zangwill, O. L. (1966). The amnesic syndrome. In *Amnesia,* C. W. M. Whitty and O. L. Zangwill (eds.). London: Butterworth, pp. 104–117.

Zoll, J. G. (1969). Transient anosognosia associated with thalamotomy: is it caused by proprioceptive loss? *Confin. Neurol.* 31:48–55.

11

Apraxia

KENNETH M. HEILMAN AND LESLIE J. GONZALEZ ROTHI

The motor systems are capable of directing muscles to make an almost infinite number of movements. In order to perform purposeful skilled movements, the brain must acquire the knowledge to program motor systems appropriately. *Apraxia* is a cognitive motor disorder that entails the loss or impairment of the ability to program motor systems to perform purposeful skilled movements. Because apraxia is a cognitive motor disorder, abnormal movements should not be called apraxic if they can be attributed to weakness, dystonia, tremor, chorea, athetosis, ballismus, seizures, myoclonus, ataxia, defects of sensory feedback, or if they result from non-motor cognitive disorders such as poor comprehension, agnosia, or inattention. Although apraxia is in part defined by exclusion, a variety of errors may characterize the apraxic patient's performance and these errors help define the variety of apraxias seen in the clinic. This chapter will be limited to descriptions of apraxias that are associated with forelimb and buccofacial movements. The forms of limb apraxia we will discuss include limb-kinetic, ideomotor, disassociation, conduction, ideational, and conceptual apraxias. We will also briefly discuss buccofacial apraxia. On the basis of these clinical descriptions, we will develop a model of how the brain mediates learned skilled movements. We will not discuss certain disorders that have been called apraxic, because they do not meet our definition of apraxia. Apraxia of eye opening and apraxia of gait are not cognitive motor disorders. Constructional apraxia and dressing apraxia are usually not movement program disorders, but are caused primarily by visuospatial disorders such as neglect.

EXAMINATION AND TESTING

GENERAL NEUROLOGICAL EXAMINATION

Since apraxia is in part defined by excluding the contribution of other disorders that may obscure apraxic errors, a thorough neurological examination is required. Diseases that affect either the basal ganglia or the cerebellum typically do not cause weakness or sensory change but can be associated with nonapraxic disorders of movement. Disorders of the basal ganglia and cerebellum are also manifested by changes in posture and tone and by tremors, dysmetria, or stereotypic movements that are evident on neurological examination. If motor, sensory, basal ganglia, or cerebellar signs are limited to one side, the normal side can still be tested for apraxia. If the abnormality is mild enough to permit use of the affected extremity, it should also be tested. In this case, the examiner should make allowance for the underlying disorder in judging whether apraxia is present.

Many apraxic patients are also aphasic, and aphasic disorders may be confused with apraxic disorders. For example, patients who do not understand commands may be thought to be apraxic when they fail to make an appropriate movement in response to a command. Conversely, apraxic patients with aphasia are occasionally mistakenly thought to have a comprehension disorder when their failure to accurately follow a command results from the inability to produce the correct movement. It is therefore important to test comprehension in other ways, such as with yes/no questions, pointing to objects on command, or by having the patient describe the movement they were asked to perform. Patients who fail to make correct movements but who demonstrate that they have comprehended of the command may be apraxic. Patients who fail to demonstrate comprehension, however, may still be apraxic, since aphasia and apraxia frequently coexist.

Apraxic patients may use body parts as objects or make spatial and temporal errors, but often these movements can be recognized as having the correct intent, providing evidence that the command has been understood. Such movement errors should therefore not be attributed to aphasia, even if the patient has a mild deficit in language comprehension.

TESTING FOR APRAXIA

Patients rarely complain of apraxia and often appear unaware of their defect. This unawareness may be a form of anosognosia (Rothi et al., 1990). Also, apraxic deficits, when recognized, are often explained away. For example, patients with right hemiparesis often think their left hand is clumsy because they are not accustomed to using it. When patients with Alzheimer's disease develop apraxia, it is often attributed to memory loss or to general intellectual decline. Furthermore, apraxia is usually mildest when a patient uses actual tools or objects and is most severe with pantomime. Since patients at home are rarely called upon to use

pantomime, they and their families are often not aware of this disorder. Therefore, in diagnosing apraxia, one cannot rely on history but must test patients.

The following are some suggested procedures for apraxia testing. Classification of apraxia is based on relative performance across these tasks and on the type of errors that the patients makes. The different forms of apraxia will be discussed in subsequent sections of this chapter.

The examiner should test both hands when possible. If one hand is severely paretic, the nonparetic hand should be tested. In addition to observing a patient's performance, the clinician should ascertain if a patient is disturbed by his or her errors or if the patient can even recognize that he or she has made errors. When testing aphasic patients, there is always the concern that the failure to perform correctly is related to a language comprehension error rather than to an apraxic error. Gesturing to command is most likely to be confounded by impaired language comprehension. However, while apraxic patients make errors, the intent of the gesture is often obvious. Comprehension of movement commands may also be tested by asking patients to describe what they were asked to do or by having patients point to the object (from an array of objects) that they would use to perform a specific action.

Gesture to command. This procedure should involve pantomiming both tool use (transitive movement), such as "Show me how you would use a pair of scissors," and emblems (intransitive movement), which are arbitrarily coded nonverbal communications, such as waving good-bye. Some of the gestures we use are listed in Table 11–1.

Frequently, when patients pantomime, they use a body part as the tool. They may perform in this manner either because they do not understand that they are supposed to pantomime (i.e., they are using the body part as a symbol of the tool) or because they cannot perform the task even though they understand it. If a patient uses a body part as the object, this performance should be corrected: "Do not use your finger as a key. Make believe you are re-

Table 11–1. Tests for Apraxia

Intransitive Limb Gestures	*Intransitive Buccofacial Gestures*
1. Wave good-bye	1. Stick out tongue
2. Hitchhike	2. Blow a kiss
3. Salute	
4. Beckon "come here"	*Transitive Buccofacial Gestures*
5. Stop	1. Blow out a match
6. Go	2. Suck on a straw
Transitive Limb Gestures	*Serial Acts*
1. Open a door with a key	1. Show how you would make a sandwich.
2. Flip a coin	2. Show how you would write and mail a letter.
3. Open a catsup bottle	
4. Use a screwdriver	
5. Use a hammer	
6. Use scissors	

ally holding a key." If verbal instructions do not help, the examiner should demonstrate the correct pantomime. If the patient still uses body part as tool, the patient is making an apraxic error.

Gesture to imitation. Some apraxic patients who cannot gesture to command can imitate gesture. Although some examiners only test imitation if the patient fails to perform the command correctly, there are patients who cannot imitate gestures, but who will perform correctly to command. Therefore, we advocate that imitation be tested in all patients. We also suggest that transitive as well as intransitive movements be tested and that meaningful and meaningless pantomimes also be tested.

Gesture (pantomime) in response to seeing a tool. This test may be especially useful when a patient has a language comprehension deficit and it is unclear if the failure to correctly gesture to command results from a language or apraxic disorder.

Gesture (pantomime) in response to seeing object upon which a tool works. This test may also be helpful when there is a comprehension disorder. Because seeing a tool may provide cues, this test may be more sensitive. This test is performed by showing the patient an object that receives the action of a tool (e.g., a nail partially driven into block of wood) and having the patient pantomime, using the tool.

Actual tool use. This task is performed by handing the tool to the patient (e.g., hammer) and may be performed with or without the object (e.g., nail) upon which the tool works.

Imitation of examiner using the tool. In this task, the patient is asked to imitate the examiner's pantomine of the use of tools or implements.

Discrimination between correct and incorrect movements pantomimed by the examiner. To determine if a patient can discriminate between correctly and incorrectly performed pantomime, the examiner performs pantomimes that randomly are either correct or incorrect and asks the patient if the gesture is well performed.

Pantomime and gesture comprehension. While the examiner makes a specific gesture, he or she can ask the patient to identify the action, e.g., "What tool am I using?".

Serial acts. To learn if a patient can perform a series of acts, in order, that leads to a goal, the examiner asks the patient to perform a multi-step task. (e.g., "How would you make a sandwich?") (see Table 11–1).

Action–tool associations. In this test the examiner displays an array of tools (e.g., hammer, screwdriver, knife, plier) and then pantomimes a target action (e.g., cutting) and asks the patient to point to the tool in the array that is associated with this action.

Tool–object associations. In this test the examiner displays an object (e.g., partially driven nail) and asks the subject to select from an array of tools the tool used to accomplish this action.

Conceptual knowledge. If the subject performs well on the tool–object association test, the tool is taken away and the patient is asked to select an alternative tool that could accomplish the same goal. For example, if the object is to remove a nail from a piece of wood, and the patient selects a hammer, the hammer is removed, and the patient can select another appropriate tool, such as a pair of pliers.

VARIETIES OF LIMB APRAXIA

Because of the diverse nature of the apraxic disorders, each will be discussed separately. Limb-kinetic, ideomotor, and ideational apraxia are terms used by Liepmann (1920). We also describe three forms of apraxia not discussed by Liepmann: disassociation, conduction, and conceptual apraxia.

LIMB-KINETIC APRAXIA

Clinical

Patients with limb-kinetic apraxia are incapable of making fine, precise movements with the limb contralateral to a central nervous system lesion. The disorder is more obvious when testing distal independent movements (finger movements) than when testing proximal movements, and is especially evident when the patient makes rapid finger movements such as tapping. The movement abnormality can be seen when the patient pantomimes, imitates, or uses objects. In the clinic, we ask patients to pick up a dime from a flat surface. Patients with limb-kinetic apraxia may not be able to perform the necessary pinching movement with their thumb and index finger and instead will slip the dime off the table and grasp the

coin between their fingers and their palm. We also ask patients to rotate a quarter between their thumb, index, and middle finger as rapidly as possible. We note if there are any between-hand asymmetries in this task.

Pathophysiology

The neuroanatomic correlates of limb-kinetic apraxia are unclear. Limb-kinetic apraxia is often unilateral (contralateral to the lesioned hemisphere). However, we recently demonstrated that in right-handers limb-kinetic apraxia of the ipsilateral (left) hand is more likely to result from left hemisphere than right hemisphere dysfunction (Heilman et al., 2000). Liepmann (1920) postulated that lesions in the sensory motor cortex may induce this disorder. It has been demonstrated that pyramidal lesions in monkeys can cause clumsiness and a loss of movement fractionation that is not completely accounted for by weakness or by change in tone or posture (Lawrence and Kuypers, 1968). This suggests that the clumsiness seen in patients with limb-kinetic apraxia may be induced by pyramidal or corticospinal tract lesions. The role of the premotor regions in the pathogenesis of limb-kinetic apraxia is also unclear. However, according to Freund and Hummelsheim (1985), manual dexterity and the capacity for relatively independent distal movements are unaffected in patients with lesions of convexity premotor cortex. Unfortunately, many patients with lesions of premotor and motor cortex have tone and posture changes that make testing for limb-kinetic apraxia difficult.

IDEOMOTOR APRAXIA

Clinical

Unlike patients with limb-kinetic apraxia, patients with ideomotor apraxia may have normal deftness (dexterity), especially when their ipsilesional arm is tested. Pieczuro and Vignolo (1967) tested the manual dexterity of 35 patients with lesions of the right hemisphere and 70 patients with lesions of the left hemisphere. The severity of the ideomotor apraxia was independent of manual dexterity. In addition, patients with ideomotor apraxia have greatest difficulty when asked to pretend they are making transitive movements (using a tool or instrument) (Goodglass and Kaplan, 1963). Although they may improve their performance by imitating, gesture to imitation is frequently still defective. Similarly, improvement may be noted when the actual object is used, but performance often remains defective (Poizner et al., 1989).

Patients with ideomotor apraxia make several types of errors. *Perseverative errors* entail execution of previously performed pantomimes when new pantomimes are requested. *Sequencing errors* involve reversal of the order of movements in a sequence of movements. For example, in pantomiming the use of a key, one needs to extend the arm at the elbow and then rotate the forearm; the patient who makes sequencing errors may reverse this order (rotate first, and then extend). Patients with idiomotor apraxia may use *body part as object* despite repeated reminders to act as if they were actually holding and using the object (Raymer et al., 1997). *Spatial errors* are most characteristic of ideomotor apraxia. There are three forms of spatial errors: errors of posture, spatial orientation, and spatial movement (Rothi et al., 1988b; Poizner et al., 1990). *Postural errors* entail the failure to position the hand to hold the imagined utensil or tool correctly. Body part as object errors are a special kind of postural error. Postural errors are seen primarily with pantomime and imitation and are not usually seen with actual object use, since the actual object constrains hand position. *Spatial orientation errors* denote hand movements that do not direct the imagined tool toward an imagined object. For example, when asked to pantomime the use of scissors, apraxic patients may move the scissors laterally instead of forward, or when asked to cut a slice of bread with a knife, they may fail to keep the imaginary knife in a constant sagittal plane. Haaland et al. (1999) demonstrated that aiming movement became worse when patients closed their eyes. *Spatial movement errors* denote movements at incorrect joints. For example, when asked to pantomime the use of a screwdriver,

the normal subject will fix the wrist and shoulder and twist the forearm, so that the imaginary screwdriver rotates on its axis. The apraxic patient may fix the wrist and forearm and rotate the shoulder, so that the screwdriver moves incorrectly in an arc. Movement errors can also occur when there is loss of coordination of movements at different joints. For example, normally when cutting a loaf of bread with a knife, the shoulder is flexed in order to bring the arm forward as the elbow is extended, and the shoulder is extended (to bring the arm back) as the elbow is flexed. With each successive cutting movement, the elbow is flexed less so that the knife moves downward. Patients with ideomotor apraxia primarily use one movement, usually the more proximal movement (shoulder), or may fail to coordinate the two movements (Poizner et al., 1990).

Patients with apraxia also make *timing errors* (Poizner et al., 1990). There may be a delay in the initiation of movement or occasional pauses, especially when the spatial trajectory must be changed. Patients may also fail to coordinate the speed of movement with its spatial components. For example, when cutting bread with an imaginary knife, one normally slows the movement when one is about to reverse the direction of the cut; once the direction has been changed, the speed of movement increases. Patients with ideomotor apraxia do not demonstrate this pattern of movement.

Pathophysiology

Callosal Lesions—Lateralized Movement Formula. Liepmann and Maas (1907) studied a patient with right hemiplegia who performed poorly when attempting to carry out verbal commands with his left hand. On postmortem examination he was found to have a lesion in the left basis pontis, which accounted for his right hemiplegia, and a lesion of the anterior four-fifths of the corpus callosum, which Liepmann and Maas thought accounted for his left-hand apraxia. Although it could be postulated that the callosal lesion resulted in apraxia because it disconnected the language areas in the left hemisphere (Wernicke, 1874) from areas of the right hemisphere that control fine movements of the left hand, Liepmann and Maas did not believe that a language–motor disconnection could fully explain their patient's movement deficits, because their patient also failed on nonverbal tasks. He could not correctly imitate skilled movements or manipulate actual tools. These deficits could not be accounted for by a primary sensorimotor disorder, because primary visual, visual association, primary somesthetic, somesthetic association, and premotor and motor areas in the right hemisphere were all intact. Liepmann and Maas concluded that the left hemisphere must contain "movement formulas" that control purposeful skilled movements. Their patient's apraxia resulted from the inability of right hemisphere sensorimotor areas to access left hemisphere movement formulas.

Liepmann (1920) proposed that these "movement formulas" contain the "time–space–form picture of the movement" (see Kimura, 1979). To perform a skilled learned act, one must place particular body parts in certain spatial positions in a specific order at specific times. The spatial positions assumed by the relevant body parts depend not only on the nature of the act but also on the position and size of an external object with which the body parts must interact. Skilled acts also require orderly changes in the spatial positions of the body parts over time. These movement formulas command the motor systems to adopt the appropriate spatial positions of the relevant body parts over time.

According to Liepmann's postulate, a callosal lesion in a right-handed patient who has both motor language engrams in the left hemisphere would not interfere with the ability of the patient to carry out commands, imitate, and use actual tools correctly with the right hand, but would result in the patient having difficulty with all these tasks when using the left hand. These predictions were not completely supported by subsequent cases. Geschwind and Kaplan (1962) described a patient with a left hemisphere glioblastoma and a postoperative left anterior cerebral artery infarction that had caused destruction of the anterior four-fifths of the corpus callosum. Their patient could not follow commands with his left hand but, unlike Liepman and Maas' patient, he could correctly

imitate and he could use actual tools. He was agraphic with the left hand and could not type or use anagram letters with the left hand but performed flawlessly with the right hand. He followed commands with his right hand but not with his left. A language–motor disconnection could explain both the left-hand aphasic agraphia and the left-hand apraxia. Similarly, surgical lesions of the corpus callosum (Gazzaniga et al., 1967) were not associated with the type of apraxia proposed by Liepmann and Maas (1907). Subsequently, however, Watson and Heilman (1983) and Graff-Radford et al. (1987) reported patients with acute naturally occurring callosal lesions who, unlike the patient of Geschwind and Kaplan (1962), had severe apraxia with imitation and object usage, thereby providing support for Liepmann's callosal motor disconnection hypothesis.

Why are some patients with callosal lesions apraxic with imitation and object use, while others are not? Patients with surgical callosal lesions have had prior seizures and brain injury that may have induced brain reorganization; however, Geschwind and Kaplan's patient did not have long-standing injury, suggesting that the absence of left-hand ideomotor apraxia cannot be entirely explained by brain reorganization. Extracallosal damage cannot explain the difference, since Geschwind and Kaplan's patient had considerable extracallosal damage, but he could imitate and use tools, whereas the computer tomographic (CT) scan of Watson and Heilman's patient (1983) did not show any extracallosal damage. Variability in brain organization may explain the difference. In right handers, right-hemisphere lesions almost never produce apraxia; however, left hemisphere lesions in areas known to induce both aphasia and apraxia more often induce aphasia. In one study, only 57% (20 of 35) of aphasic patients were also apraxic (Heilman, 1975), suggesting that movement formula or space–time movement representations are bilaterally represented in a considerable minority of right-handers (Heilman, 1979). It should therefore not be surprising that callosal damage does not induce apraxia in all patients. The patients of Watson and Heilman and Graff-Radford et al. probably had language and movement representations restricted to the left hemisphere, which might represent the more common pattern. The patients reported by Gazzaniga et al. (1967) and Geschwind and Kaplan (1962) were left hemisphere dominant for language but probably had bilateral movement representations. Geschwind (1965) remarked that the independence of the right hemisphere in nonlanguage skilled motor function manifested by his patient may have been exceptional.

The nature of the apraxic deficit seen with callosal lesions depends on the pattern of language and motor dominance in the individual patient. For example, we have seen two left-handed patients who were apraxic but not aphasic following right hemisphere lesions (Heilman et al., 1973; Valenstein and Heilman, 1979). Movement representations in these two patients were stored in the right hemisphere while language was mediated by the left hemisphere. We can speculate that if, prior to their right hemisphere lesion, these patients had a lesion of their corpus callosum, the right hand, deprived of the movement representations, would perform poorly to command, to imitation, and with the use of the actual object. The left hand, deprived of language, should perform poorly to gestural command but perform well with imitation and with an actual object. This pattern of deficits has not yet been reported.

Left Hemisphere Lesions (Intrahemispheric)

Defective symbolization. In right-handed patients, almost all cases of apraxia are associated with left hemisphere lesions (Goodglass and Kaplan, 1963; Hécaen and Ajuriaguerra, 1964; Geschwind, 1965; Hécaen and Sanguet, 1971). In right-handers, the left hemisphere is also dominant for language. Apraxia therefore is commonly associated with aphasia. This has led to the suggestion that apraxia and aphasia may both be manifestations of a primary defect in symbolization: aphasia is a disturbance of verbal symbolization, while apraxia is a defect of nonverbal symbolization (e.g., emblem and pantomime) (Goldstein, 1948). The observation that patients with apraxia perform poorly to command and imitation but improve with the use of the actual object (Goodglass and Kaplan, 1963) lends support to Goldstein's pos-

tulate. In addition, Dee et al. (1970) and Kertesz and Hooper (1982) found a close relationship between language impairment and apraxia.

However, several studies lend support to Liepmann's hypothesis that the left hemisphere controls skilled movements and that destruction of the movement representations or separation of these representations from the motor areas controlling the extremity causes abnormalities of skilled movement. Goodglass and Kaplan (1963) tested apraxic and nonapraxic aphasic subjects with the Wechsler Adult Intelligence Scale and used the performance-scaled score as a measure of intellectual ability. They also tested their subjects' ability to gesture and perform simple and complex pantomimes. Although apraxic aphasics performed less well on these motor skills than did their intellectual counterparts in the control groups, no clear relationship emerged between the severity of aphasia and the degree of gestural deficiency. Apraxic aphasic patients were also less able to imitate than were nonapraxic aphasic controls. Although Goodglass and Kaplan believed that their results supported Liepmann's hypothesis, they noted that their apraxic subjects did not have any difficulty in handling tools. Liepmann, however, thought apraxic patients were clumsy with tools, and Poizner et al. (1989) observed and quantified motor and spatial errors of apraxic patients' use of actual objects. Kimura and Archibald (1974) studied the ability of left hemisphere–impaired aphasics and right hemisphere–impaired controls to imitate unfamiliar, meaningless motor sequences. The performance of aphasic apraxic patients with left hemisphere impairment was poorer than that of the controls, again supporting Liepmann's hypothesis. The strongest support for the postulate that apraxia is a disorder of skilled movement rather than a symbolic defect comes from Liepmann's own observations that only 14 of 20 apraxic patients were aphasic. Goodglass and Kaplan (1963) and Heilman et al. (1973, 1974) have also described similar patients. In addition, aphasic patients are often not apraxic (Heilman, 1975). In summary, because there is a poor correlation between the severity of symbolic disorders (aphasia) and disorders of skilled movements

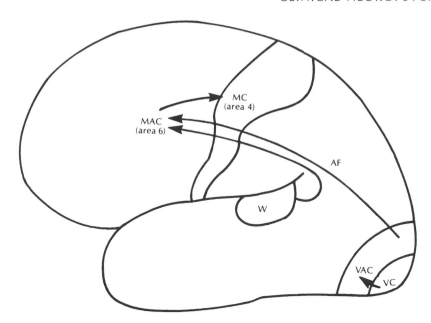

Figure 11–1. Geschwind's schema. Lateral view of the left side of the brain. AF, arcuate fasciculus; MAC, motor association cortex; MC, motor cortex; VAC, visual associa- tion cortex; VC, visual cortex. The arrows indicate major connections of the areas shown.

and because even nonsymbolic movements are poorly performed by apraxic patients, there is little evidence to support the hypothesis that apraxia is a disorder of symbolic behavior.

Disconnection hypothesis of apraxia. Geschwind (1965) proposed that language elic- its motor behavior by using a neural substrate similar to that proposed by Wernicke (1874) to explain language processing (see Fig. 11–1). Auditory stimuli travel along auditory pathways and reach Heschl's gyrus (primary auditory cortex). From Heschl's gyrus, the auditory message is relayed to the posterior superior portion of the temporal lobe (auditory associ- ation cortex). In the left hemisphere, this is called "Wernicke's area," and is important in language comprehension. Wernicke's area is connected to premotor areas (motor associa- tion cortex) by the arcuate fasciculus, and the motor association area on the left is connected to the left primary motor area. When someone is told to carry out a command with the right hand, this pathway is used. To carry out a ver- bal command with the left hand, information

must be carried to the right premotor cortex. Since it is rare to find fibers that run obliquely in the corpus callosum, fibers either cross from Wernicke's area to the contralateral auditory association area or cross from the premotor area on the left to the premotor area on the right. The information is then conveyed to mo- tor areas on the right side. Geschwind (1965) postulated that the connections between the premotor cortical areas are the active pathways. Support for the hypothesis that the active path- way for praxis crosses the callosum anteriorly comes from the observation that a selective an- terior callosal section induced an ideomotor apraxia of the left hand (personal observation by K.M.H.).

Geschwind believed that disruption of cor- tical-cortical pathways explained most apraxic disturbances. As we have already discussed, ac- cording to Geschwind, callosal lesions produce unilateral ideomotor apraxia by disconnecting the left premotor region from the right. Le- sions that destroy the left convexity premotor cortex also cause ideomotor apraxia, because the cell bodies of neurons that cross the corpus callosum are destroyed. Therefore, a lesion in the left convexity premotor cortex would cause a defect similar to that induced by a lesion in the body of the corpus callosum (sympathetic dyspraxia). Lesions of the left convexity premotor cortex are often associated with right hemiplegia, so the right limb frequently cannot be tested. If these patients were not hemiparetic, however, they would probably be apraxic on the right.

According to Geschwind's schema (1965), lesions of the arcuate fasciculus should disconnect the posterior language areas, important for language comprehension, from the convexity premotor cortex, important for implementing programs. Therefore, patients with parietal (or arcuate fasciculus) lesions that spare convexity premotor cortex should be able to comprehend commands but not perform skilled movements in response to command. More posterior lesions, affecting Herschl's gyrus, Wernicke's area, or the connections between them, cause abnormalities in language comprehension, but not apraxia. These patients fail to carry out commands because they cannot understand the command, not because they have difficulty performing skilled movements.

One problem in Geschwind's interpretation is that patients with arcuate fasciculus lesions should theoretically be able to correctly imitate using their left hand, but often they cannot. Geschwind attempted to explain this discrepancy by noting that the arcuate fasciculus also contains fibers passing from visual association cortex to premotor cortex. He proposed that the arcuate fasciculus of the left hemisphere is dominant for visuomotor connections; but there is no evidence to support this hypothesis. Even if one assumes that the left arcuate fasciculus is dominant for visuomotor connections and interruption of this dominant pathway explains why patients cannot imitate, it could not explain why these patients are clumsy when they use actual tools. One would have to assume that the arcuate fasciculus also carries somesthetic-motor impulses and that the left arcuate fasciculus is also dominant for this function.

Representational hypothesis. After one learns a skilled motor behavior, future behav-

iors that require that same skill are expedited. In addition, even in the absence of specific instruction or cues, one can pantomime learned skilled behaviors. These observations suggest that the nervous system stores knowledge of motor skills. When this knowledge must be called into use, it is retrieved from storage and implemented rather than constructed de novo. A hypothesis that may explain why patients with parietal lesions cannot properly pantomime, imitate the use of, or use an object postulates that movement formulas or learned time–space movement representations are stored in the dominant parietal cortex (Heilman, 1979; Kimura, 1979). These representations help program the premotor cortex, which in turn implements the required movements by selectively activating the motor cortex. This innervates the specific muscle motor neuron pools needed to carry out the skilled act (Fig. 11–2). We call these movement formula or time–space motor representations "praxicons."

Theoretically, it should be possible to distinguish between dysfunction caused by destruction of parietal areas where praxicons are stored and apraxia resulting from disconnection of this parietal area from motor areas that implement these representations. Although patients with either disorder should experience difficulty in performing a skilled act in response to command, imitation of, or use of an object, patients whose representations for skilled acts are retained but whose premotor areas are disconnected (or whose premotor cortex is destroyed) should be able to differentiate a correctly performed skilled act from an incorrectly performed one because they still have these praxic representations (praxicons) and, therefore, have the information characterizing distinctive features of learned skilled movements. Patients with parietal lesions that have destroyed these representations (praxicons) should not be able to perform this analysis.

To test the postulate that praxicons are stored in the dominant parietal lobe and that destruction of these representations induces a discrimination deficit, we (Heilman et al., 1982; Rothi et al., 1985) gave a gestural recognition and discrimination task to apraxic and nonapraxic patients with anterior lesions or nonfluent aphasia and to patients with poste-

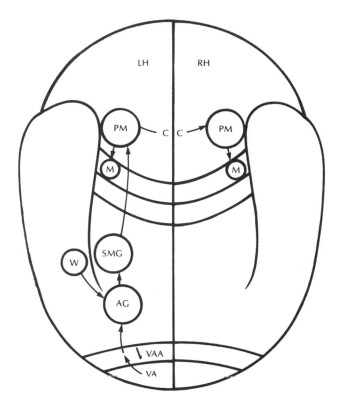

Figure 11–2. Authors' schema. View from top of brain. AG, angular gyrus; CC, corpus callosum; LH, left hemisphere; M, motor cortex; PM, premotor area (motor association cortex); RH, right hemisphere; SMG, supramarginal gyrus; VA, primary visual area; VAA, visual association area; W, Wernicke's area. The arrows show major connections of the areas shown.

rior lesions or fluent aphasia. In the discrimination task, the subject was to select a correctly performed act from a poorly performed act (e.g., using a body part as an object). In the comprehension task, the subject was asked to select the requested (target) act from foils consisting of movements that were correctly executed but not the correct movement. Thus, if the target movement was "open a door with a key," the foil might be using scissors or a screwdriver. On both the discrimination and comprehension tasks, the posterior/fluent patients performed worse than the other subjects. On the basis of these observations, we believe that there are at least two forms of ideomotor apraxia. One is induced by a loss of praxicons stored in the supramarginal or angular gyrus. These patients perform poorly to command, are unable to comprehend gestures, and are also unable to discriminate poorly performed from well-performed acts. The other results from lesions anterior to the angular or supramarginal gyrus that either disconnect praxicons from the premotor and motor areas important

in implementing skilled movements or destroy premotor areas. Support for this hypothesis comes from functional imaging studies of normal subjects in whom pantomiming tool use activated the left parietal cortex (Moll et al., 1998).

If ideomotor apraxia results from destruction of movement representations or praxicons, patients with this disorder should have difficulty acquiring new motor skills and retaining new gestures in memory. In regard to the former, Heilman et al. (1975) studied nine right-handed hemiparetic patients with apraxia and aphasia and eight right-handed hemiparetic controls with aphasia but without apraxia. These subjects were given six trials on a rotary pursuit apparatus (five acquisition trials and one retention trial). All subjects used their left, nonparetic hand. The performance of the control group on the sixth trial was significantly better than on the first trial; however, there was no significant difference between the first and sixth trials in the apraxic group, which suggests that these patients had a defect in motor learning. The defect appeared to be caused by a combined impairment of acquisition and retention. Wyke (1971), who studied patients with either right or left hemisphere lesions, gave her subjects a motor acquisition task that required bimanual coordination. Although patients with left hemisphere disease demonstrated acquisition, it was below the level of skill demonstrated by patients with right hemisphere disease. Since Wyke did not separate her left hemisphere group into apraxic and nonapraxic patients, one could not be certain whether apraxic patients would have demonstrated poorer learning than nonapraxic left hemisphere–damaged patients. Rothi and Heilman (1985) used a modified Buschke (1973) paradigm to study apraxic subjects' ability to learn a list of gestures. We noted significantly more consolidation errors in the apraxic than control groups, a finding that suggests apraxic patients have a memory consolidation deficit. Pistarini and co-workers (1991) also studied gesture and skill learning in patients with ideomotor apraxia and found that these patients were impaired. Lastly, if patients with apraxia have a loss of movement representations (praxicons), they should also demonstrate imagery deficits. Ochipa et al. (1997) demonstrated that ideomotor apraxia may be associated with movement imagery deficits.

Innervatory patterns. Praxicons stored in the inferior parietal lobe are in a three-dimensional supramodal code that has to be translated into a motor plan before the target movement can take place. Although Geschwind (1965) thought that lesions in convexity premotor cortex might induce apraxia, the role of the convexity premotor cortex in praxis is unclear. Many complex movements require the simultaneous movement of multiple joints. Barrett et al. (1998) suggested that convexity premotor cortex may be important in binding these movement programs. The convexity premotor cortex may also be important in adapting the motor program to environmental perturbations.

The premotor cortex in the medial frontal lobe is called the supplementary motor area (SMA). Whereas stimulation of the primary

motor cortex (Brodmann's area 4) induces simple single movements, SMA stimulation induces complex movements of the fingers, arms, and hands (Penfield and Welch, 1951). The SMA receives projections from parietal neurons and projects to convexity premotor cortex and to primary motor neurons. The SMA neurons discharge before neurons in the primary motor cortex (Brinkman and Porter, 1979). Studies of cerebral blood flow, an indicator of cerebral metabolism, reveal that a single repetitive movement increases activation of the contralateral motor cortex. However, complex movements increase flow in contralateral motor cortex and bilaterally in the SMA. When subjects think about making complex movements but do not move, blood flow is increased to the SMA but not to primary motor cortex (Orgogozo and Larsen, 1979).

Watson et al. (1986) reported several patients with left-sided medial frontal lesions that included the SMA who had bilateral ideomotor apraxia. However, unlike patients with parietal lesions, these patients could both comprehend and discriminate pantomimes. Because the SMA has connections with the primary motor cortex and the parietal lobe, is activated before motor cortex, becomes activated with complex learned movements, and when ablated induces apraxia, we believe the SMA is the site where praxic representations are translated into motor programs or innervatory patterns that activate motor cortex.

Basal ganglia. Whereas lesions and dysfunction of the basal ganglia are thought to induce alterations of muscle tone, abnormal movement, decreased spontaneous movements, and slowing of movements, the role of basal ganglia dysfunction in apraxia remains unclear. There have been several reports of patients who demonstrated ideomotor apraxia from lesions that involved the basal ganglia and/or thalamus (Basso et al., 1980; Agostini et al., 1983). Rothi et al. (1988a) described two patients with left-sided lenticular infarctions that did not involve cerebral cortex or associative pathways. Both patients had spatial movement errors that were similar to errors seen in patients with cortical lesions. However, both patients also showed frequent perseverative errors.

Alexander et al. (1986) described five discrete cortical striatal–pallidal–thalamic-cortical circuits. We have already provided evidence that lesions of left SMA are associated with apraxia. The SMA is a part of the motor circuit that projects to the putamen. The putamen projects to the globus pallidus and the globus pallidus projects to the ventrolateral nucleus of the thalamus. Finally, the ventrolateral nucleus projects back to the SMA. This discrete "motor loop" may control the flow of information into the SMA. Therefore, lesions of the loop may cause SMA dysfunction and SMA dysfunction may lead to apraxia.

Support for the observation that the basal ganglia are important in praxis also comes from reports of patients with degenerative basal ganglia diseases. For example, Shelton and Knopman (1991) reported that apraxia was associated with Huntington's disease and Leiguarda et al. (1997) reported that 27% of patients with Parkinson's disease have ideomotor apraxia. Ideomotor apraxia has also been reported in the Parkinson-plus syndromes of progressive supranuclear palsy (PSP) (Leiguarda et al., 1997) and corticobasal degeneration (Jacobs et al., 1999; Merians et al., 1999). In addition, patients with basal ganglia disease such as Parkinson's disease may be impaired at learning new skills. However, even nondemented patients with basal ganglia disease may have cortical dysfunction. Pramstaller and Marsden (1996) performed a detailed review and meta-analysis of the relationships between basal ganglia injury and apraxia and concluded that diseases confined to the basal ganglia "rarely, if ever, cause apraxia."

CONDUCTION APRAXIA

Clinical

Although most patients with ideomotor apraxia imitate transitive gestures better than they can pantomime transitive gestures to command, Ochipa et al. (1990) described a patient whose imitation of learned transitive and symbolic movements was worse than his pantomime of these same movements to command. This patient had no difficulty comprehending the examiners' pantomimes and gestures.

Pathophysiology

Unfortunately, the praxis model we have developed thus far (Fig. 11–3) cannot account for these findings. Such findings suggest that there are two independent sets of movement representations or praxicons—one for processing gestural input (input praxicon) and one for processing movement output (output praxicon) (Rothi et al., 1991) (see Fig. 11–4). A preserved ability to comprehend gesture in conjunction with impaired imitation would suggest that the input praxicon remains intact and that the impairment occurs after the input praxicon. The observation that the patient was better able to pantomime to command than imitate would suggest that verbal language is capable of activating the output praxicon (bypassing processing by the input praxicon) (see Fig. 11–4) and that this patient's deficit was a dissociation between the input and output praxicon. Unfortunately, the localization of lesions that cause conduction apraxia is unknown.

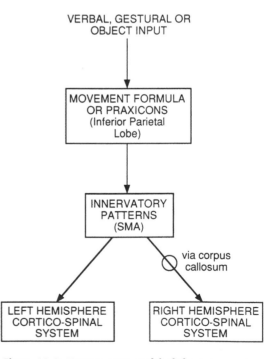

VERBAL, GESTURAL OR OBJECT INPUT

↓

MOVEMENT FORMULA OR PRAXICONS (Inferior Parietal Lobe)

↓

INNERVATORY PATTERNS (SMA)

via corpus callosum

LEFT HEMISPHERE CORTICO-SPINAL SYSTEM   RIGHT HEMISPHERE CORTICO-SPINAL SYSTEM

Figure 11–3. Diagrammatic model of ideomotor praxis system. SMA, supplementary motor area.

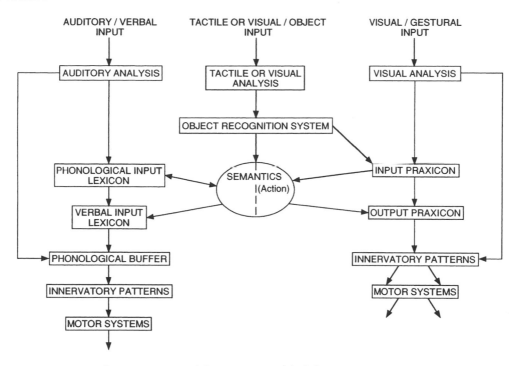

Figure 11–4. Revised diagrammatic model of ideomotor praxis system.

DISCONNECTION AND DISASSOCIATION APRAXIAS

Verbal–Motor Disassociation Apraxia

Clinical. Heilman (1973) described three patients who, when asked to gesture, hesitated to make any movements and often appeared as if they did not understand the command. They could, however, demonstrate both verbally and by picking out the correct act from several performed by the examiner that they understood the command. Unlike patients with ideomotor apraxia, these patients were able to imitate and use actual tools flawlessly. Because imitation and actual object use was performed well, it would seem that their representations of motor skills (praxicons) were intact. What seemed to be defective in these patients was the ability to elicit the correct motor sequences in response to language.

Pathophysiology. Although we hypothesized that the lesions were in, or deep to, the parietal region (angular gyrus), we never learned

the exact locations of the left hemisphere lesions that induce this apraxia.

The patients with callosal lesions described by Geschwind and Kaplan (1962) and Gazzaniga et al. (1967) could not perform with their left hand in response to command, but they could imitate and use tools. Performance with the left hand of these patients with callosal disconnection was similar to the performance with both hands of patients with the left hemisphere lesions described above (Heilman, 1973). If normal performance on imitation and use-of-object tasks suggests that movement representations (praxicons) are intact and connected to premotor and primary motor areas, then patients with callosal lesions and patients with angular gyrus or subcortical lesions deep in the parietal lobe must have a dissociation between language areas and the area where motor representations (praxicons) are stored. In patients with callosal lesions, these movement representations are presumed to be in both hemispheres, whereas comprehension of commands is being mediated by the left hemisphere. In patients with left hemisphere lesions, both speech comprehension and the learned motor skills are being mediated by the left hemisphere, and the lesion disassociates language areas from praxicons such that language is not able to activate the appropriate praxicon (see Fig. 11–4). An alternative hypothesis is that in patients with left hemisphere lesions, the right hemisphere is mediating language comprehension, the left hemisphere contains the praxic representations, and the lesions disconnect the language areas from these representations.

Visuomotor and Tactile–Motor Disassociation Apraxia

Clinical. De Renzi et al. (1982) replicated Heilman's (1973) observations of a verbal–motor dissociation apraxia and also described a patient who performed in the opposite manner. The patient failed to correctly perform gestures with visual stimuli but performed well to verbal command. Although most patients perform skilled actions better with tactile stimuli than to command, the authors described two patients who performed better with visual and verbal stimuli than with tactile stimuli.

Pathophysiology. The mechanism proposed by De Renzi et al. to explain these modality-specific apraxias was similar to that proposed by Heilman (1973); namely, there is a disconnection between modality-specific pathways and the center where movements are programmed.

PANTOMIME AGNOSIA

Clinical

Agnosia is a failure of recognition that cannot be attributed to deafferentation or a naming disorder. Disorders of discrimination and recognition associated with ideomotor apraxia from posterior lesions (described above) may not be considered to be a form of agnosia because of the associated production deficits. Rothi et al. (1986) reported two patients who could not comprehend or discriminate visually presented gestures, but who performed gestures normally. These patients could, however,

recognize tools. These patients could be considered to have pantomime agnosia without object agnosia. Both patients could imitate better than they could comprehend or discriminate gestures. Because they could imitate, their inability to discriminate or comprehend gestures could not be accounted for by a defect in vision or perception. The patients had left-sided temporo-occipital lesions that may have disconnected visual input from the input praxicon. Schwartz et al. (1998) and Larrabee et al. (1985) reported patients who had the opposite dissociation. They could not recognize tools but could recognize pantomimes.

Pathophysiology

Studies of patients with object agnosia suggest that these patients have injury to their ventral temporal-occipital "what" system. Whereas Rothi et al. (1986) thought that the ventral "what" visual stream is also important for gesture comprehension, the loss of the ability to name tools with a preserved ability to comprehend gestures reported by Schwartz et al. (1998) in a patient with a ventral lesion suggests that it may be the dorsal "where" visual stream that is important for gesture recognition.

In regard to the neuropsychological mechanism, patients with Wernicke's aphasia and pure word deafness can neither comprehend spoken language nor repeat. Whereas the former is thought to be related to destruction of the lexicon (representations of learned word sounds), the latter disorder is thought to be related to an inability of auditory input to gain access to the phonological lexicon. However, patients with transcortical sensory aphasia can repeat (i.e., imitate) in spite of being unable to comprehend, demonstrating that comprehension and imitation are dissociable. This comprehension–imitation disassociation suggests that these two processes are at least in part divergent and are mediated by different parts of the brain. Lichtheim (1885) suggested that while repetition is mediated by a phonological–lexical system that is still functional in transcortical sensory aphasia, comprehension unlike repitition requires semantic processing. Thus, in transcortical sensory aphasia the systems that mediate semantic processing of language are impaired, or auditory input cannot gain access to these semantic systems (Heilman et al., 1976). The neuropsychological mechanisms underlying impaired gesture comprehension with spared imitation reported by Rothi et al. could be similar. These patients can gain access to the input praxicon but the activated praxic representations could not access semantics (see Fig. 11–4).

Several authors have suggested that speech repetition (i.e., imitation) may be performed by using either stored word representations (lexical) or a nonlexical route (McCarthy and Warrington, 1984; Coslett et al., 1987). Just as we can repeat words we have not heard, we can also mimic movements we have never seen or previously engaged in. Perhaps imitation, like repetition, can take place without having to access stores of previously learned skilled movement, the praxicon (see Fig. 11–4). Support for this alternative imitation system comes from the observation of a patient whose deficit was limited to the imitation of nonfamiliar limb movement (Mehler, 1987). Because there are no memory stores for unfamiliar movements, the praxicon could not be accessed and the patient had to rely on a nonrepresentational route that was impaired. Perhaps the patients with ideomotor apraxia who improve with imitation can use this nonrepresentational route, whereas those who do not improve may have an additional deficit in this nonrepresentational route.

IDEATIONAL APRAXIA

Clinical

There has been much confusion about the term *ideational apraxia*. The disassociation apraxias discussed above were unfortunately originally called "ideational apraxia" (Heilman, 1973). The inability to carry out a series of acts, an ideational plan, has also been called "ideational apraxia" (Marcuse, 1904; Pick, 1905). These patients have difficulty sequencing acts in the proper order. For example, instead of cleaning the pipe, putting tobacco in, lighting it, and smoking it, the patient with ideational apraxia may first put tobacco in the pipe and then clean it. As noted by Pick (1905), most of the patients

with this type of ideational apraxia have had dementing illnesses or confusional states.

Most patients with ideomotor apraxia improve with actual object use; however, De Renzi et al. (1968) reported patients who made gross errors with the use of actual tools. De Renzi et al. considered the inability to use actual tools a sign of ideational apraxia. While the inability to use actual tools may be induced by a conceptual disorder, Zangwell (1960) noted that failure to use actual tools may be related to a severe production disorder, ideomotor apraxia. However, as we will discuss in the next section, the nature of the error may reveal if the patient is suffering from a production or conceptual disorder. To avoid confusion between those patients who cannot sequence acts and are said to have ideational apraxia and those who have a conceptual disorder, we term this latter disorder *conceptual apraxia*.

Pathophysiology

Most patients with ideational apraxia are suffering with some form of dementia. Both lesion (Mateer, 1999) and functional imaging studies (Wildgruber et al., 1999) suggest that the frontal lobes are critical for sequencing. Vascular or arteriosclerotic dementia is more often associated with frontal dysfunction that is early Alzheimer's disease and vascular dementia is more often associated with sequencing deficits (Starkstein et al., 1996); however, no studies have attempted to determine which forms of dementia are most frequently associated with ideational apraxia or if ideational apraxia can be observed with isolated lesions.

CONCEPTUAL APRAXIA

Clinical

Whereas patients with ideomotor apraxia make production errors (e.g., spatial and temporal errors) when pantomiming, imitating, or even using actual tools, patients with conceptual apraxia may make content errors resulting from an inability to select the actions associated with the use of specific tools, utensils, or objects (tool–object action knowledge). Therefore, patients with this type of conceptual error make content errors (De Renzi and Lucchelli, 1988; Ochipa et al., 1989). For example, when asked to pantomime how to use a screwdriver, the patient may pantomime a hammering movement or use the screwdriver as if it were a hammer. Patients with ideomotor apraxia may make arcs rather than twisting on fixed axis, but do demonstrate the knowledge of the screw-turning action of screwdrivers. Making content errors (i.e., using a tool as if it were another tool) can also result from object agnosia. However, Ochipa et al. (1989) reported a patient who could name tools but used them inappropriately (e.g., used a tube of toothpaste as a toothbrush and a toothbrush as a fork). Because this patient could name the tool he was not agnosic. However, because he could not associate the correct action with the tool he was considered to have a conceptual apraxia.

Patients with conceptual apraxia may be unable to recall which tool is associated with an object (tool–object association knowledge). For example, when shown a nail that has been partially nailed into a piece of wood, they may be unable to select a hammer from an array of tools. Instead, they may select a screwdriver. This conceptual defect may also be in the verbal domain: patients may be unable to name or point to a tool when its function is discussed, even though they can name the actual tool and point to it when named by the examiner. They may also be unable to describe verbally the function of a particular tool.

Patients with conceptual apraxia may also be unaware of the mechanical advantage afforded by tools (mechanical knowledge). Therefore, when they are presented with a partially driven-in nail and are expected to complete the task without an available hammer, these patients may not select an alternate tool that is hard, rigid, and heavy, such as a wrench or pliers. Instead, they may select an alternate that is flexible and lightweight, such as a hand-saw. Lastly, patients with conceptual apraxia may also be unable to construct tools (tool fabrication).

Because patients with Alzheimer's disease may have impaired semantic memory even early in the course of the disease, Ochipa et al. (1992) studied patients with degenerative dementia of the Alzheimer type for these four components of conceptual apraxia. They found that patients with Alzheimer's disease often have conceptual apraxia. When compared to controls, they were impaired on all four levels discussed above. It was also learned that some elements of conceptual apraxia may even be seen in patients who do not have either ideomotor apraxia or semantic language impairment.

Heilman et al. (1997) also demonstrated that conceptual apraxia may be associated with focal cerebral diseases such as cerebral infarction. In right-handers, it was primarily injury to the left hemisphere that induced conceptual apraxia. Further evidence that these representations are lateralized comes from the observation of a patient who had a callosal disconnection and demonstrated conceptual apraxia of the nonpreferred (left) hand (Watson and Heilman, 1983). However, the subject investigated by Ochipa et al. (1989) was left-handed and rendered conceptually apraxic by a lesion in the right hemisphere, suggesting that both production and conceptual knowledge have lateralized representations and that such representations are usually contralateral to the preferred hand.

Pathophysiology

The lesion associated with conceptual apraxia when testing tool use (tool–object action and tool–object association knowledge) has been localized to the posterior regions of the left hemisphere by Liepmann (1920), who thought that this knowledge was stored in the caudal parietal lobe. De Renzi and Lucchelli (1988) thought that the critical area was in the temporoparietal junction. Although Heilman et al. (1997) found that in right-handers conceptual apraxia was associated with left hemisphere lesions, they did not find a critical hemispheric locus.

Ideomotor and conceptual apraxia often co-occur, but the finding that there are patients with ideomotor apraxia who do not demonstrate conceptual apraxia and patients with conceptual apraxia who do not demonstrate ideomotor apraxia provides evidence for the postulate that the conceptual and production systems are independent (Rapcsak et al., 1995; Heilman et al., 1997). However, to perform skilled acts to command or when presented visually with tools or objects, these conceptual and production systems must interact. The recognition and naming of gestures also require that these systems interact. This is diagrammatically depicted in Figure 11–4 (Rothi et al., 1991).

BUCCOFACIAL APRAXIA (ORAL APRAXIA)

Clinical

Hughlings Jackson (cited by Taylor, 1932) was the first to describe buccofacial or oral apraxia (nonprotrusion of the tongue). Patients with oral apraxia have difficulty performing learned skilled movements with the face, lips, tongue, cheeks, larynx, and pharynx on command. For example, when they are asked to pretend to blow out a match, suck on a straw, lick a sucker, or blow a kiss, they will make incorrect movements. Poeck and Kerschensteiner (1975) found several types of errors. Verbal descriptions may be substituted for the movement: the oral apraxic asked to pantomime blowing out a match may respond by saying "blow." Other error types include movement substitutions and perseverations. Raade et al. (1991) noted that patients with buccofacial apraxia make content, spatial, and temporal errors. Mateer and Kimura (1977) demonstrated that imitation of meaningless movements was also impaired, providing evidence that oral apraxia is not a form of asymbolia. Although many of these patients do not improve with imitation, they consistently improve dramatically when seeing or using an actual object (e.g., a lighted match). Raade et al. (personal communication) also demonstrated that some patients with buccofacial apraxia have impaired comprehension of buccofacial gestures.

Pathophysiology

In order to learn if impairment of the same system could account for both buccofacial and limb ideomotor apraxia, Raade et al. (1991) studied the co-occurrence of these apraxias, the type of errors made by apraxic patients, and lesion sites. Forty percent of their subjects had only one type of apraxia. Basso et al. (1980) re-ported dissociations in 23% of their subjects, and De Renzi et al. (1968), in 28% of theirs. Raade et al. (1991) also found different error types. Whereas patients with limb apraxia made more errors with transitive than with intransitive movements, Raade and colleagues found no difference in errors between transitive and intransitive movements in patients with buccofacial apraxia. Lastly, lesion sites were found to be different.

Tognola and Vignolo (1980) studied patients who were unable to imitate oral gestures. The critical areas for lesions included the frontal and central opercula, anterior insula, and a small area of the first temporal gyrus (adjacent to the frontal and central opercula). Tognola and Vignolo (1980) and Kolb and Milner (1981) found that parietal lesions were not associated with oral apraxia, but they did not test performance to command. Benson et al. (1973), however, described patients with parietal lesions who exhibited oral apraxia to command.

Some authors have classified the phonological selection and sequencing deficit of nonfluent aphasia as "apraxia of speech" (Johns and Darley, 1970; Deal and Darley, 1972). Although Pieczuro and Vignolo (1967) noted that 90% of patients with Broca's aphasia have oral apraxia, it would seem unlikely that buccofacial apraxia causes this phonological disturbance because there are patients with nonfluent aphasia who do not have oral apraxia. It can be argued, however, that oral and verbal apraxias are points along a continuum, sharing a common underlying mechanism. It could be hypothesized that speech requires finer coordination than does response to a command such as "blow out a match"; therefore, the effortful, phonologically inaccurate speech of the nonfluent aphasic may still be caused by an apraxic disturbance affecting speech more than oral, nonverbal movement. Oral apraxia and the speech production deficits associated with Broca's aphasia often coexist, but they can also be completely dissociated (Heilman et al., 1974), suggesting that, at least in part, the anatomic system that mediates facial praxis is not the same as those that mediate the movements used in speech. Furthermore, because patients may have conduction aphasia with or without oral apraxia (Benson et al., 1973), oral apraxia may coexist with fluent speech. If one attributes the nonfluent disorders of speech in patients with Broca's aphasia to a generalized oral motor programming deficit, one cannot explain how oral apraxia may be associated with the fluent speech seen in conduction aphasia. In addition, we have examined a patient with aphemia (nonfluent speech with intact writing skills) who did not have oral apraxia. If the speech deficits exhibited by left hemisphere–impaired patients is induced by a motor defect, this motor programming defect is strongly linked to the language and phonological systems and is not a generalized oral motor programming deficit.

DISEASES THAT MAY INDUCE APRAXIA

Any disease that destroys or injures portions of the cerebral cortex or portions of the thalamus (Nadeau et al., 1994) may induce apraxia, including stroke (infarctions and hemorrhages), trauma, and tumors. Apraxia may also be associated with degenerative diseases. For example, ideomotor, ideational, and conceptual apraxias are often seen in patients with Alzheimer's disease (Ochipa et al., 1989; Rapcsak et al., 1989). In corticobasal degeneration, ideomotor and limb kinetic apraxia may be one of the first symptoms or signs. Usually the ideomotor apraxia is of the innervatory-executive type (Jacobs et al., 1999) Often this apraxia is asymmetrical or even unilateral. Although Leiguarda et al. (1997) reported that apraxia may be associated with Parkinson's disease, other laboratories have been unable to replicate this finding. Apraxia has also been reported to be associated with Huntington's disease (Shelton and Knopman, 1991) Finally, apraxia may also be sign and symptom of a developmental disorder.

RECOVERY FROM APRAXIA AND TREATMENT

After a stroke, spontaneous recovery from apraxia may occur over a period of 6 months.

However, some degree of apraxia may persist (Sunderland, 2000) and may cause disability, as it can interfere with activities of daily living (Bjorneby and Reinvang, 1985). Basso et al. (1987) demonstrated that patients with apraxia from anterior lesions recover better than those with posterior lesions. In addition, the presence of a right hemisphere lesion did not appear to retard recovery, suggesting that recovery was mediated by uninjured portions of the left hemisphere. The portions of the brain that are responsible for recovery are unknown. There are several possible scenarios. Damaged areas may recover. Undamaged portions of the hemisphere dominant for praxis may take over function for the damaged areas. Possibly, the nondominant hemisphere may also have a residual ability to compensated for the damaged hemisphere.

Stroke patients are often anosognosic for their apraxic disability (Rothi et al., 1990) or attribute their disabilities to right hemiparesis and inexperience using their left arm. Therefore, these patients often do not request therapy. In addition, no information is presently available on methods for, or efficacy of, treatment of apraxia. However, information from animal recovery models (Rothi and Horner, 1983) suggests that therapy should be aimed initially at restitution of function: the underlying disorder should be treated so that maximum function can be achieved within the limits set by the recovery process. Then other therapeutic measures can be attempted to foster substitutive strategies. Compensatory strategies can help these apraxic patients develop the skills needed to perform activities of daily living (van Heugten et al., 1998). Apraxic patients should be taught alternative strategies for performing tasks that pose difficulty for them.

REFERENCES

Agostoni, E., Coletti, A., Orlando, G., and Fredici, G. (1983). Apraxia in deep cerebral lesions. *J. Neurol. Neurosurg. Psychiatry* 46:804–808.

Alexander, G. E., DeLong, M. R., and Strick, P. L. (1986). Parallel organization of functionally segregated circuits linking basal ganglia and cortex. *Annu. Rev. Neurosci.* 9:357–381.

Barrett, A.M., Schwartz, R.L., Raymer, A.L., Crucian, G.P., Rothi, L.J.G., Heilman, K.M. (1998). Dyssynchronous apraxia: Failure to combine simultaneous preprogramed movements. *Cogn. Neuropsychol.* 15:685–703.

Basso, A., Capitani, E., Della-Sala, S., Laiacona, M., and Spinnler, H. (1987). Recovery from ideomotor apraxia. A study on acute stroke patients. *Brain* 110(Pt 3):747–760.

Basso, A., Luzzatti, C., and Spinnler, H. (1980). Is ideomotor apraxia the outcome of damage to well-defined regions of the left hemisphere? Neuropsychological study of CT correlation. *J. Neurol. Neurosurg. Psychiatry* 43:118–126.

Benson, F., Shermata, W., Bouchard, R., Segarra, J., Prie, D., and Geschwind, N. (1973). Conduction aphasia. A clinicopathological study. *Arch. Neurol.* 28:339–346.

Bjorneby, E. R., and Reinvang, I. R. (1985). Acquiring and maintaining self-care skills after stroke. The predictive value of apraxia. *Scand. J. Rehabil. Med.* 17:75–80.

Brinkman, C., and Porter, R. (1979). Supplementary motor area in the monkey: activity of neurons during performance of a learned motor task. *J. Neurophysiol.* 42:681–709.

Buschke, H. (1973). Selective reminding for analysis of memory and learning. *J. Verbal Learn. Verbal Behav.* 12:543–550.

Coslett, H. B., Roeltgen, D. P., Rothi, L. G., and Heilman, K. M. (1987). Transcortical sensory aphasia: evidence for subtypes. *Brain Lang.* 32:362–378.

Deal, J. L., and Darley, F. L. (1972). The influence of linguistic and situational variables on phonemic accuracy in apraxia of speech. *J. Speech Hear. Res.* 15:639–653.

Dee, H. L., Benton, A., and Van Allen, M. W. (1970). Apraxia in relation to hemisphere locus lesion, and aphasia. *Trans. Am. Neurol. Assoc.* 95:147–150.

De Renzi, E., Faglioni, P., and Sorgato, P. (1982). Modality-specific and supramodal mechanisms of apraxia. *Brain* 105:301–312.

De Renzi, E., and Lucchelli, F. (1988) Ideational apraxia. *Brain* 113:1173–1188.

De Renzi, E., Pieczuro, A., and Vignolo, L. (1968). Ideational apraxia: a quantitative study. *Neuropsychologia* 6:41–52.

Freund, H., and Hummelsheim, H. (1985). Lesions of premotor cortex in man. *Brain* 108:697–733.

Gazzaniga, M., Bogen, J., and Sperry, R. (1967). Dyspraxia following diversion of the cerebral commissures. *Arch. Neurol.* 16:606–612.

Geschwind, N. (1965). Disconnection syndromes in animals and man. *Brain* 88:237–294, 585–644.

Geschwind, N., and Kaplan, E. (1962). A human cerebral disconnection syndrome. *Neurology* 12:65–685.

Goldstein, K. (1948). *Language and Language Disturbances*. New York: Grune and Stratton.

Goodglass, H., and Kaplan, E. (1963). Disturbance of gesture and pantomime in aphasia. *Brain* 86:703–720.

Graff-Radford, N. R., Welsh, K., and Godersky, J. (1987). Callosal apraxia. *Neurology* 37:100–105.

Haaland, K.Y., Harrington, D.L., and Knight, R.T. (1999). Spatial deficits in ideomotor limb apraxia. A kinematic analysis of aiming movements. *Brain* 122(Pt 6):1169–1182.

Hécaen, H., and de Ajuriaguerra, J. (1964). *Left Handedness*. New York: Grune and Stratton.

Hécaen, H., and Sanguet, J. (1971). Cerebral dominance in left-handed subjects. *Cortex* 7:19–48.

Heilman, K. M. (1973). Ideational apraxia—a redefinition. *Brain* 96:861–864.

Heilman, K. M. (1975). A tapping test in apraxia. *Cortex* 11:259–263.

Heilman, K. M. (1979). Apraxia. In *Clinical Neuropsychology*, K. M. Heilman and E. Valenstein (eds.). New York: Oxford University Press, pp. 159–185.

Heilman, K. M., Coyle, J. M., Gonyea, E. F., and Geschwind, N. (1973). Apraxia and agraphia in a left-hander. *Brain* 96:21–28.

Heilman, K. M., Gonyea, E. F., and Geschwind, N. (1974). Apraxia and agraphia in a right-hander. *Cortex* 10:284–288.

Heilman, K. M., Maher, L. M., Greenwald, M. L., and Rothi, L. J. (1997). Conceptual apraxia from lateralized lesions. *Neurology* 49:457–464.

Heilman, K. M., Meador, K. J., and Loring, D. W. (2000). Hemispheric asymmetries of limb-kinetic apraxia: a loss of deftness. *Neurolgy* 55:523–526.

Heilman, K. M., Rothi, L. J., and Valenstein, E. (1982). Two forms of ideomotor apraxia. *Neurology* 32:342–346.

Heilman, K. M., Schwartz, H. D., and Geschwind, N. (1975). Defective motor learning in ideomotor apraxia. *Neurology* 25:1018–1020.

Heilman, K. M., Tucker, D. M., and Valenstein, E. (1976). A case of mixed transcortical aphasia with intact naming. *Brain* 99:415–426.

Jacobs, D. H., Adair, J. C., Macauley, B., Gold, M., Gonzalez-Rothi, L. J., and Heilman, K. M. (1999). Apraxia in corticobasal degeneration. *Brain Cogn.* 40(20):336–354.

Johns, D. F., and Darley, F. L. (1970). Phonemic

variability in apraxia of speech. *J. Speech Hear. Res.* 13:556–583.

Kertesz, A., and Hooper, P. (1982). Praxis and language: the extent and variety of apraxia in aphasia. *Neuropsychologia* 20:275–286.

Kimura, D. (1979). Neuromotor mechanisms in the evolution of human communication. In *Neurobiology of Social Communication in Primates: An Evolutionary Perspective*, H. D. Steklis and M. J. Raleigh (eds.). New York: Academic Press

Kimura, D., and Archibald, Y. (1974). Motor function of the left hemisphere. *Brain* 97:337–350.

Kleist, K. (1934). *Gehirnpathologie.* Leipzig: Barth.

Kolb, B., and Milner, B. (1981). Performance of complex arm and facial movements after focal brain lesions. *Neuropsychologia* 19:491–503.

Larrabee, G. J., Levin, H. S., Huff, F. J., Kay, M. C., Guinto, F. C. Jr. Visual agnosia contrasted with visual-verbal disconnection. *Neopsychologia* 23:1–12.

Lawrence, D. G., and Kuypers, H. G. J. M. (1968). The functional organization of the motor system in the monkey. *Brain* 91:1–36.

Leiguarda, R. C., Pramstaller, P. P., Merello, M., Starkstein, S., Lees, A. J., and Marsden, C. D. (1997). Apraxia in Parkinson's disease, progressive supranuclear palsy, multiple system atrophy and neuroleptic-induced parkinsonism. *Brain* 120(Pt 1):75–90.

Lichtheim, L. (1885). On aphasia. *Brain* 7:733–784.

Liepmann, H. (1920). Apraxia. *Ergebn. Ges. Med.* 1:516–543.

Liepmann, H., and Mass, O. (1907). Fall von linksseitiger Agraphie und Apraxie bei rechsseitiger Lahmung. *Z. Psychol. Neurol.* 10:214–227.

Marcuse, H. (1904). Apraktiscke Symptome beim linem Fall von seniler Demenz. *Zentralbl. Nervheilkd. Psychiatrie.* 27:737–751.

Mateer, C.A. (1999). Executive function disorders: rehabilitation challenges and strategies. *Semin. Clin. Neuropsychiatry* 4:50–59.

Mateer, K., and Kimura, D. (1977). Impairment of nonverbal movements in aphasia. *Brain Lang.* 4:262–276.

McCarthy, R., and Warrington, E. K. (1984). A two route model of speech production: evidence from aphasia. *Brain* 107:463–485.

Mehler, M. F. (1987). Visuo-imitative apraxia. *Neurology* 37:129.

Merians, A. S., Clark, M., Poizner, H., Jacobs, D. H., Adair, J. C., Macauley, B., Gonzalez Rothi, L. J., and Heilman, K. M. (1999). Apraxia differs in corticobasal degeneration and left-parietal stroke: a case study. *Brain Cogn.* 40: 314–335.

Moll, J., De-Oliveira-Souza, R., De-Souza-Lima, F., and Andreiuolo, P. A. (1998). Activation of left intraparietal sulcus using fMRI conceptual praxis paradigm. *Arq. Neuropsiquiatr.* 56:808–811.

Nadeau, S. E., Roeltgen, D. P., Sevush, S., Ballinger, W. E., and Watson, R. T. (1994). Apraxia due to a pathologically documented thalamic infarction. *Neurology* 44:2133–2137.

Ochipa, C., Rapcsak, S. Z., Maher, L. M., Rothi, L. J., Bowers, D., and Heilman, K. M. (1997). Selective deficit of praxis imagery in ideomotor apraxia. *Neurology* 49:474–480.

Ochipa, C., Rothi, L. J. G., and Heilman, K. M. (1989). Ideational apraxia: a deficit in tool selection and use. *Ann. Neurol.* 25:190–193.

Ochipa, C., Rothi, L. J. G., and Heilman, K. M. (1990). Conduction apraxia. *J. Clin. Exp. Neuropsychol.* 12:89.

Ochipa, C., Rothi, L. J. G., and Heilman, K. M. (1992). Conceptual apraxia in Alzheimer's disease. *Brain* 115:1061–1071.

Orgogozo, J. M., and Larsen, B. (1979). Activation of the supplementary motor area during voluntary movement in man suggests it works as a supramotor area. *Science* 206:847–850.

Penfield, W., and Welch, K. (1951). The supplementary motor area of the cerebral cortex. *Arch. Neurol. Psychiatry* 66:289–317.

Pick, A. (1905). *Studien uber Motorische Apraxia und ihre Nahestenhende Erscheinungen.* Leipzig: Deuticke.

Pieczuro, A., and Vignolo, L. A. (1967). Studio sperimentale sull'aprassia ideomotoria. *Sisterma Nerv.* 19:131–143.

Pistarini, C., Majani, G., Callegari, S., and Viola, L. (1991). Multiple learning tasks in patients with ideomotor apraxia. *Riv. Neurol.* 61:57–61.

Poeck, K., and Kerschensteiner, M. (1975). Analysis of the sequential motor events in oral apraxia. In *Otfried Foerster Symposium*, K. Zulch, O. Kreutzfeld, and G. Galbraith (eds.). Berlin: Springer, pp. 98–109.

Poizner, H., Mack, L., Verfaellie, M., Rothi, L. J. G., and Heilman, K. M. (1990). Three-dimensional computer graphic analysis of apraxia. *Brain* 113:85–101.

Poizner, H., Soechting, J. F., Bracewell, M., Rothi, L. J. G., and Heilman, K. M. (1989). Disruption of hand and joint kinematics in limb apraxia. *Soc. Neurosc. Abstr.* 15:196.2.

Pramsmtaller, P. P., and Marsden, C. D. (1996). The basal ganglia and apraxia. *Brain* 119(Pt 1): 319–340.

Raade, A. S., Rothi, L. J. G., and Heilman, K. M.

(1991). The relationship between buccofacial and limb apraxia. *Brain Cogn. 16:*130–146.

Rapcsak, S. Z., Croswell, S. C., and Rubens, A. B. (1989). Apraxia in Alzheimer's disease. *Neurology 39:*664–668.

Rapcsak, S. Z., Ochipa, C., Anderson, K. C., and Poizner, H. (1995). Progressive ideomotor apraxia: evidence for a selective impairment of the action production system. *Brain Cogn. 27:*213–236.

Raymer, A. M., Maher, L. M., Foundas, A. L., Heilman, K. M., and Rothi, L. J. (1997). The significance of body part as tool errors in limb apraxia. *Brain Cogn. 34:*287–292.

Rothi, L. J. G., and Heilman, K. M. (1985). Ideomotor apraxia: gestural learning and memory. In *Neuropsychological Studies in Apraxia and Related Disorders*, E. A. Roy (ed.). New York: Oxford University Press, pp. 65–74.

Rothi, L. J. G., Heilman, K. M., and Watson, R. T. (1985). Pantomime comprehension and ideomotor apraxia. *J. Neurol. Neurosurg. Psychiatry 48:*207–210.

Rothi, L. J. G., and Horner, J. (1983). Restitution and substitution: two theories of recovery with application to neurobehavioral treatment. *J. Clin. Neuropsychol. 5:*73–82.

Rothi, L. J. G., Kooistra, C., Heilman, K. M., and Mack, L. (1988a). Subcortical ideomotor apraxia. *J. Clin. Exp. Neuropsychol. 10:*48.

Rothi, L. J. G., Mack, L., and Heilman, K. M. (1986). Pantomime agnosia. *J. Neurol. Neurosurg. Psychiatry 49:*451–454.

Rothi, L. J. G., Mack, L., and Heilman, K. M. (1990). Unawareness of apraxic errors. *Neurology 40(Suppl. 1):*202.

Rothi, L. J. G., Mack, L., Verfaellie, M., Brown, P., and Heilman, K. M. (1988b). Ideomotor apraxia: error pattern analysis. *Aphasiology 2:*381–387.

Rothi, L. J. G., Ochipa, C., and Heilman, K. M. (1991). A cognitive neuropsychological model of limb praxis. *Cogn. Neuropsychol. 8:*443–458.

Schwartz, R. L., Barrett, A. M., Crucian, G. P., and Heilman, K. M. (1998). Dissociation of gesture and object recognition. *Neurology 50:*1186–1188.

Shelton, P. A., and Knopman, D. S. (1991). Ideomotor apraxia in Huntington's disease. *Arch. Neurol. 48:*35–41.

Starkstein, S. E., Sabe, L., Vazquez, S., Teson, A., Petracca, G., Chemerinski, E., Di-Lorenzo, G., and Leiguarda, R. (1996). Neuropsychological, psychiatric, and cerebral blood flow findings in vascular dementia and Alzheimer's disease. *Stroke 27:*408–414.

Sunderland, A. (2000). Recovery of ipsilateral dexterity after stroke. *Stroke 31:*430–433.

Taylor, J. (1932). *Selected Writings*. London: Hodder and Stoughton.

Tognola, G., and Vignolo, L. A. (1980). Brain lesions associated with oral apraxia in stroke patients: a cliniconeuroradiological investigation with the CT scan. *Neurophysiologica 18:*257–272.

Valenstein, E., and Heilman, K. M. (1979). Apraxic agraphia with neglect induced paragraphia. *Arch. Neurol. 36:*506–508.

Van-Heugten, C. M., Dekker, J., Deelman, B. G., Van-Dijk, A. J., Stehmann-Saris, J. C., and Kinebanian, A. (1998). Outcome of strategy training in stroke patients with apraxia: a phase II study. *Clin. Rehabil. 12:*294–303.

Watson, R. T., Fleet, W. S., Rothi, L. J. G., and Heilman, K. M. (1986). Apraxia and the supplementary motor area. *Arch. Neurol. 43:*787–792.

Watson, R. T., and Heilman, K. M. (1983). Callosal apraxia. *Brain 106:*391–403.

Wernicke, E. (1874). *Der Aphasische Symptomenkomplex*. Breslau: Cohn and Weigart.

Wildgruber, D., Kischka, U., Ackermann, H., Klose, U., and Grodd, W. (1999). Dynamic pattern of brain activation during sequencing of word strings evaluated by fMRI. *Brain Res. Cogn. Brain Res. 7:*285–294.

Wyke, M. (1971). The effects of brain lesions on the learning performance of a bimanual coordination task. *Cortex 7:*59–71.

Zangwell, O. L. (1960) L'apraxie ideatorie. *Nerve Neurol. 106:*595–603.

12

Agnosia

RUSSELL M. BAUER AND JASON A. DEMERY

Agnosia is a relatively rare neuropsychological symptom defined in the classical literature as a failure of recognition that cannot be attributed to elementary sensory defects, mental deterioration, attentional disturbances, aphasic misnaming, or unfamiliarity with external stimuli (Frederiks, 1969). Agnosia is most often modality-specific; the patient who fails to recognize material presented through a particular sensory channel (e.g., vision) is successful when allowed to perceive it in another channel (e.g., touch, hearing). Visual, auditory, and tactile agnosias have received the most attention, and will be reviewed here.

One of the most fundamental and difficult questions about agnosia concerns whether it is best thought of as a perceptual or memory impairment. In his classic definition, Teuber (1968) stated that "two limiting sets of conditions: failure of processing and failure of naming . . . bracket . . . the alleged disorder of recognition per se, which would appear in its purest form as a normal percept that has somehow been stripped of its meaning." Teuber's definition is significant since it "locates" the agnosias at the intersection of perception and memory, and in fact, seems to imply that "pure" agnosia is a disorder of memory access. In contrast, others have asserted that such a defect does not exist and that all so-called agnosics are either per-

ceptually impaired, or demented, or both (Bay, 1953; Bender and Feldman, 1972). Proponents on either side of this debate assume that perception and memory are dissociable. As we shall discuss, this assumption derives from serial information-processing models of the perceptual process, and alternative models that do not require such a separation are now available (Mc-Clelland and Rumelhart, 1986; Rumelhart and McClelland, 1986).

An early observation of agnosia-like phenomena was provided by Munk (1881), who observed that dogs with bilateral occipital lobe excisions neatly avoided obstacles placed in their paths, but failed to react appropriately to objects that previously had frightened or attracted them. Similar observations have been made by Horel and Keating (1969, 1972) in the macaque with lesions of the occipital lobe and its temporal projections. Munk felt that his dogs' behavior resulted from a loss of memory images of previous visual experience and termed the condition "Seelenblindheit" (mind blindness). Nine years later, Lissauer (1890) provided the first detailed report of a recognition disturbance in humans, and his views on different varieties of the disturbance have had important historical impact on theory and practice. The term "agnosia" was introduced by Freud (1891), eventually replacing "mind blindness" and other terms such as "asymbolia" (Finkelnburg, 1870) and "imperception" (Jackson, 1876). As with most neurobehavioral syndromes, significant debate has existed regarding the functional mechanisms responsible for agnosic phenomena. However, unlike most other neuropsychological phenomena, a major point of debate has centered on whether agnosia existed at all. Over the years, interpretation of agnosic syndromes has varied according to the zeitgeist prevailing at the time. In the early 20th century, when Gestalt psychology guided perceptual theory, published cases of agnosia were conceptualized with Gestalt concepts in mind (see Goldstein and Gelb, 1918; Goldstein, 1943, vs. Poppelreuter, 1923; Brain, 1941). With the reemergence of "disconnection theory" (Geschwind, 1965), cases of agnosia during the 1960s and 1970s were largely viewed as examples of sensory–verbal or sensory–limbic disconnections. In the past decade, with significant advancements in computational neuroscience and an increased componential understanding of visual cognition, clinical data have been reinterpreted in the language of cognitive neuropsychology. The history of agnosia contains several striking examples of the interplay between cognitive theory and clinical practice, and represents a good example of how scientific advancement is not always linear or cumulative. There has been a recent revolution in the field of agnosia as we have moved primarily from an almost exclusive emphasis on disconnection concepts to a more cognitive neuropsychological perspective. Because models of normal perception have always driven conceptualizations of agnosia, a brief review of four broad models will be provided before discussing the major agnosic syndromes.

MODELS OF RECOGNITION

STAGE MODELS

The earliest neuropsychological ideas of the process of object recognition were embodied in "stage models," which held that the cortex first built up a percept from elementary sensory impressions. Recognition was achieved in a subsequent stage in which the resulting per-

cept was "matched" to stored information about the object. Lissauer (1890) argued that recognition proceeds in two stages: apperception and association. By *apperception*, he meant the conscious perception of a sensory impression; the construction of separate visual attributes into a whole. By *association*, he meant the imparting of meaning to the content of perception by matching and linking it to a previous experience. A central idea in Lissauer's work is that object or face recognition depends not just on the integrity of early perceptual processes but also on a later, culminating "gnostic" stage in which the visual impressions are combined in such a way as to access an internal representation. Only after such a stage has been reached will conscious recognition occur. The distinction between apperception and association has had significant implications for clinical testing, since Lissauer felt that patients with a visual defect at the apperceptive level would be unable to match or copy a misidentified object or picture, while patients with an associative deficit will be able to copy because they perceive normally.

Although Lissauer's model has been historically important, recent analyses of normal and disordered perception have raised serious questions about its ability to accommodate the clinical data. The apperceptive stage is itself further divisible into a number of constituent visual abilities that can be selectively impaired with appropriately placed lesions (see Humphreys and Riddoch, 1987; Farah, 1990; Kaas, 1995). Also, it is becoming increasingly clear that perception is not entirely normal in the vast majority of so-called associative agnosics (Levine, 1978; Bauer and Trobe, 1984; Humphreys and Riddoch, 1987; Levine and Calvanio, 1989). Despite these problems, the apperceptive–associative distinction remains a useful descriptive framework, and will be used to organize the presentation of clinical material in this chapter.

DISCONNECTION MODELS

In 1965, Geschwind, in his classic paper on disconnection theory, defined agnosia in a different way. In Geschwind's view, agnosia resulted from a disconnection between visual and verbal processes. He cited anatomic evidence from the syndrome of visual object agnosia, which, in his view, was most often seen in the context of left mesial occipital lobe damage. According to Geschwind, this lesion not only induced a right homonymous hemianopia but also prevented information perceived by the intact right hemisphere from reaching the naming area because of impingement of crossing fibers. In advancing this hypothesis, Geschwind (1965) described several examples of patients who, after failing to identify objects on formal testing, later used or interacted normally with the object. In bringing attention to these phenomena, Geschwind (1965) provided clear evidence that recognition is not a unitary phenomenon. He wrote:

A fundamental difficulty has been in the acceptance of a special class of defects of 'recognition', lying somewhere between defects of 'perception' and 'naming'. What indeed are the criteria for recognition and is it a single function? I believe that there is no single faculty of recognition, but that the term covers the totality of all the associations aroused by any object. Phrased another way, we "manifest" recognition by responding appropriately; to the extent that any appropriate response occurs, we have shown 'recognition'. But this view abolishes the notion of a unitary step of 'recognition'; instead, there are multiple parallel processes of appropriate response to a stimulus. To describe the behavior correctly we must describe the pattern of loss and preservation of responses to each particular type of stimulus. (p. 587)

Although this idea is critical to an understanding of agnosia, it is now clear that disconnection theory cannot, by itself, account for the fact that most agnosics show abnormal verbal *and nonverbal* processing of viewed objects. Despite this, the major historical impact of this idea was to point out the fact that recognition behavior measures the output of many separate components. Thus, an answer to the basic question, "did the patient recognize?", depends on what response is required of the patient in a given task situation.

COMPUTATIONAL MODELS

The models proposed by Lissauer and Geschwind attempt to explain agnosic symptoms in terms that were consistent with available the-oretical constructs. An alternative approach is to begin by accounting for normal perceptual phenomena and to then determine whether such an account can explain recognition failures observed in the clinic. This approach begins by specifying the tasks that sensory–perceptual systems must perform to achieve the kind of powerful and flexible recognition abilities we as humans possess. We are able to recognize everyday objects and faces with remarkable ease across wide ranges in viewing distance, orientation, and illumination. We are able to "infer" depth, volume, and structure from relatively impoverished two-dimensional stimuli such as photographs and line drawings. We can determine with immediate certainty whether a pictured and real object are the same or different, or whether they would be used together. Thus, from perceptual analysis, we can derive an enormous amount of structural and semantic information about the world around us.

What is required to perform all these remarkable functions? In an attempt to answer this question, Marr (1982) started with the assumption that the brain must store some form of codified, symbolic description (a "representation") of known objects or faces that is sufficiently flexible to accommodate the perceptual variations inherent in everyday recognition tasks. His analysis led him to postulate three types of representations, which he referred to as *(1)* the primal sketch, *(2)* the viewer-centered, or $2^1/_2$-D, sketch, and *(3)* the object-centered, or 3-D, sketch. The *primal sketch* represents intensity (brightness) changes across the field of vision, resulting in a way of specifying the two-dimensional geometry (shape) of the image. The $2^1/_2$-D *sketch* represents the spatial locations of visible surfaces from the point of view of the observer. The essential feature of this type of representation is that it is computed on the basis of the spatial relationship between viewer and object. Because of this, the resulting representation is dependent on the point of view, and thus it is known as a "viewer-centered" or "viewpoint-dependent" description. The *3-D sketch* specifies the configuration of surfaces, features, and shapes within an object in an object-centered coordinate frame. An object-centered coordinate frame (in which shapes and features are represented in terms of their location *on the object*) yields a description that is not dependent upon the observer's point of view since, for example, simple rotation would not alter the spatial relationships among features of the object. Because of this, the 3-D representation has also been referred to as an "object-centered" or "viewpoint-independent" description. Presumably, achieving this kind of description is essential to flexible object recognition, although it is obvious that specific objects could sometimes be recognized using only a $2^1/_2$-D sketch (see below).

Marr's theoretical position is important for two reasons. First, it provides an priori conceptual approach to the study of object recognition disturbances. Indeed, we will see that Marr's ideas about multiple object representations provide a useful framework within which to understand the various ways that recognition can become disordered. Marr's ideas have led to the development of new, more refined, clinical assessment tools, and have clarified some of the intractable problems in this area. Second, it serves as a potent reminder that the various tests used to tap the apperceptive and associative stages of object recognition impose different demands on the recognition apparatus.

A contemporary computational model set in neural terminology has been proposed by Damasio (1989). Like its ancestors in the parallel-distributed processing framework (McClelland and Rumelhart, 1986; Rumelhart and McClelland, 1986; Goldman-Rakic, 1988). Damasio's model suggests that perception involves the evocation of a neural activity pattern in primary and first-order association cortex that corresponds to the various perceptual features extracted from viewed objects. Downstream, these features are combined in "local convergence zones," which serve to bind together the pattern of features into an "entity" (e.g, object). Damasio specifically rejects the view that recognition involves the activation of a packaged, locally stored memory representation of the stimulus. Instead, recognition occurs when the neural pattern defining a specific entity is reactivated in a time-locked fashion (in response to stimulation). The most important feature of Damasio's model is that *no fundamental distinction between perception and memory is made*; that is, information about

previously encountered items is stored in a pattern of neural activity, not in a localized representation. In this sense, recognition is indeed "re-cognition." Because the memory–perception distinction is abolished, this kind of model avoids many of the problems encountered in answering the question, "is agnosia a perceptual or memory deficit"? Damasio's model predicts that there can be no disorder of object recognition without attendant perceptual dysfunction. As we shall see, this seems entirely consistent with the behavior of most associative agnosics.

COGNITIVE NEUROPSYCHOLOGICAL MODELS

A fourth class of models has recently emerged in the tradition of the cognitive modular, or "box model," approach. These models attempt to outline, in cognitive terms, the functional components involved in object recognition. Such models have received significant attention only in the context of visual recognition. One representative model of object recognition, proposed by Ellis and Young (1988), is depicted in Figure 12–1. In this model, the initial, viewer-centered, and object-centered representations correspond to Marr's three levels of object description. According to Ellis and Young, the process of recognition begins by comparing viewer-centered and object-centered representations to stored structural descriptions of known objects (so-called object recognition units [ORUs]). The ORU acts as an interface between visual representations (which describe what an object looks like) and semantic information (which describes the object's functional properties and attributes). According to the model, when information in viewer- and object-centered representations adequately matches structural information in some ORU, the ORU becomes activated. This, in turn, gives rise to a sense of familiarity and unlocks semantic information about the object. Since the ORU receives independent input from viewer- and object-centered representations, it can be activated by either independently if a sufficient match is obtained. Name retrieval occurs in the final stage of the model. Its position at the bottom of the model assumes that the semantic system does not contain a

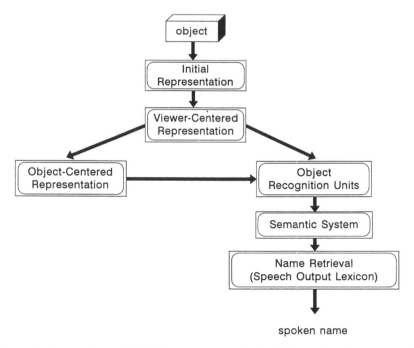

Figure 12–1. A working model of object recognition. (Adapted from Ellis and Young, 1988.)

record of the object's name, but can retrieve the name from a separate store or lexicon. There is no direct link between ORU and speech output lexicon; all retrieval of object names occurs via the semantic representation. Deficits prior to the level of the ORU roughly correspond to Lissauer's apperceptive agnosics; defects subsequent to this point are more or less associative.

CRITERIA OF RECOGNITION

In the literature, three general classes of responses have been used to provide evidence that an object has been recognized. First, the patient's ability to *overtly identify the stimulus* can be assessed. Responses in this category include confrontation naming, pointing, and demonstrating the use of the object in its presence. The second class involves *responses that indicate semantic knowledge about the object.* Tasks eliciting responses of this type include sorting and grouping objects on the basis of functional characteristics. It is obviously important to know whether a patient who has failed a recognition test can group the unrecognized object with other objects with which it

is semantically similar. If the patient can do this, some degree of meaningful information is being extracted from the stimulus. Third, the presence or absence of *discriminative responses adequate to the stimulus* (e.g., correct object use in the absence of direct naming or recognition, physiological or behavioral discrimination, and similar effectx) can be assessed. These three response classes measure different levels of performance in tasks of object recognition, and may be dissociated in specific instances. For example, a patient may "recognize" an object (by emitting a discriminative response to it or by sorting it with other like objects), without being able to identify it.

CLINICAL PHENOMENA

VISUAL AGNOSIA

Patients with visual agnosia cannot identify visually presented material even though language, memory, and general intellectual functions are preserved at sufficient levels so that their impairment cannot account singly or in combination for the failure to recognize. In the classic cases, the recognition defect is modality-specific. Identification is immediate and certain when the patient is presented the stimulus in other sensory modalities.

When the patient fails to name but can indicate visual recognition by verbal description or gesture, the failure is usually considered to be anomic in nature. Unlike the agnosic, the anomic generally does not improve when the material is presented through another sensory modality (Spreen et al., 1966; Goodglass et al., 1968), and is less apt to perform normally when asked to produce lists of words in specific categories, to complete open-ended sentences, or to respond to definitions. The conversational speech of the anomic may alert the examiner to the possibility of difficulty on visual confrontation naming because it contains word-finding pauses, circumlocutions, semantic paraphasias, and a general lack of substantives (see Chapter 2). We will later consider a syndrome called "optic aphasia," in which the naming disturbance is disproportionately severe for visually presented objects, and will consider whether this syndrome is agnosic or anomic.

Visual agnosia has been classified in a number of different ways. The most widely known classification is Lissauer's (1890) apperceptive–associative distinction discussed earlier, which, from a clinical perspective, is based primarily on the severity of perceptual impairment. Visual agnosia has also been classified according to the specific category of visual material that cannot be recognized. Impairments in the recognition of faces (prosopagnosia), colors (color agnosia), objects (object agnosia), and an agnosic inability to read (agnosic alexia) have been described in isolation and in various combinations (Farah, 1991). The co-occurrence of associative visual object agnosia with alexia, color agnosia, and prosopagnosia is common, though not obligatory.

Some types of agnosia (e.g., visual object agnosia) involve a defect that prevents the recognition not only of the specific identity of an object but also of the general semantic class to which it belongs. Other forms of agnosia (e.g., prosopagnosia) are characterized by an ability to recognize the general nature of the object (e.g., a face), but a profound inability to appreciate its individual identity within that class. It remains to be determined whether the distinction between agnosia for object classes and

agnosia for specific identities reflects a feature of brain organization or whether it represents the fact that visual and semantic information play different roles in the recognition of specific classes of objects (see below). It is possible that specific identity discriminations (e.g., "that's my wallet"), are more visually or semantically demanding than more general ones (e.g., "a wallet") and that certain classes of objects (e.g. faces) place special demands on sensory–perceptual systems (Damasio et al., 1982; Warrington and Shallice, 1984). Alternatively, it is possible that certain classes of objects demand qualitatively different types of processing that differ in kind, rather than degree, from processes involved in recognizing other objects (Farah et al., 1998). We will consider these issues later when we describe some strikingly specific agnosias.

Apperceptive Visual Agnosia

The term *apperceptive agnosia* has been applied to a broad spectrum of patients who have in common some measurable impairment at the perceptual level, but whose elementary sensory functions appear to be relatively intact. Farah (1990) points out that the term has been applied to a heterogeneous range of disabilities from patients whose visual impairments prevent them from negotiating their surroundings (Luria et al., 1963) to those without in vivo impairments in object recognition who fail specialized perceptual tests that require patients to match stimuli across different views (Warrington and Taylor, 1973). Most cases have been associated with pathological processes such as carbon monoxide poisoning (Von Hagen, 1941; Adler, 1944; Benson and Greenberg, 1969; Mendez, 1988; Milner and Heywood, 1989; Milner et al., 1991; Sparr et al., 1991), mercury intoxication (Landis et al., 1981), cardiac arrest (Brown [case Il], 1972), bilateral cerebrovascular accident (CVA) (Stauffenberg, 1914), basilar artery occulusion (Caplan, 1980), or bilateral posterior cortical atrophy (Benson et al., 1988; Mendez et al., 1990). The behavior of these patients suggests severe visual difficulties. Many are recovering from a state of cortical blindness. Because of their helplessness in the visual environment, many are considered blind until they report that they can indeed see, but not clearly or until they are observed avoiding obstacles in their environment. Standard testing then reveals normal or near-normal acuity in the spared visual field. Preservation of sufficient field and acuity to allow for recognition distinguishes the apperceptive agnosic from the patient with Anton's syndrome (Anton, 1899), denial of cortical blindness.

Apperceptive agnosics fail recognition tasks because of defects in perceptual processing. They cannot draw misidentified items or match them to sample. They are generally unable to point to objects named by the examiner. The impairment most often involves elements of the visual environment that require shape and pattern perception (faces, objects, letters). The recognition of even the simplest of line drawings may be impossible. However, bright and highly saturated colors may be better recognized. Some patients can trace the outlines of letters, objects, or drawings (Goldstein and Gelb, 1918; Landis et al., 1982), but often retrace them over and over because they lose the starting point. Many patients behave as if they are unaware or unconcerned about their deficit until they are given a visual recognition task. They will then acknowledge that they do not see clearly. Others are aware of their difficulty but try to conceal it.

Many patients complain that their visual environment changes or disappears as they try to scrutinize it. Recognition may improve when visual stimuli are moved or, in the case of reading, if letters are traced (Botez, 1975). This condition, known as visual static agnosia, has been thought to reflect residual capacity of the subcortical (tectopulvinar) visual system (Denny-Brown and Fischer, 1976; Zihl and Von Cramon, 1979; Celesia et al., 1980). Patients may claim they need new glasses, or may complain about poor lighting or the fact that they have not had much prior experience with the particular kind of visual material that they are being asked to identify. One of our patients, a retired architect, condescendingly remarked about the poor quality of our line-drawn stimuli. It has always been difficult to characterize the visual performance of these patients because of large inter- and intraindividual variability, and in fact there may be multiple forms

of deficit (Shelton et al., 1994). Cognizant of this variability, Farah (1990) attempted to bring order out of chaos by subdividing apperceptive agnosics into the following four behaviorally meaningful categories.

Narrow Apperceptive Agnosia. Representative cases in this category include patients reported by Adler (1944), Alexander and Albert (1983), Benson and Greenberg (1969), Campion and Latto (1985), Goldstein and Gelb (1918), Landis et al., (1982), and Milner et al. (1991). These patients all have seemingly adequate elementary visual function (acuity, visual fields, luminance detection, color vision, and depth and movement perception) but display a striking inability to recognize, match, copy, or discriminate simple visual forms. Benson and Greenberg's patient is a case in point.

The patient was a 25-year-old victim of accidental carbon monoxide poisoning. For several months he was thought to be blind and yet was seen one day navigating the corridor in his wheelchair. He could name colors and could often follow moving visual stimuli, yet could not identify by vision alone objects placed before him. He could occasionally identify the letters *x* and *o* if allowed to see them drawn or if they were moved slowly before his eyes. Visual acuity was at least 20/100, measured by his ability to indicate the orientation of the letter *E*, detect the movement of small objects at standard distances, and reach for fine threads on a piece of paper. Optokinetic nystagmus was elicited bilaterally with fine 1/8 inch marks on a tape. Visual fields were normal to 3 mm–wide objects with minimal inferior constriction bilaterally to 3 mm red and green objects. There was an impersistence of gaze with quasi-random searching movements, particularly when inspecting an object. His recognition deficit included objects, photographs, body parts, letters, and numbers, but not colors. He could tell which of two objects was larger and could detect very small movements of small targets. He easily identified and named objects when he could touch them or hear the sounds they made. He guessed at the names of objects, utilizing color, size, and reflectance cues. He was totally unable to match or copy material that he could not identify. However, he was taught to apply a name to each object in a small group of objects that were presented to him one at a time on a piece of white paper. For instance, after he was repeatedly shown the back of a red-and-white playing card and informed of its identity, he was able on later exposures to identify it. He was thus able to use color and size cues to learn and remember the names of various objects in a closed set. However, when these objects were placed out of context, he was no longer able to name them. His recent and remote memory, spontaneous speech, comprehension of spoken language, and repetition were intact. On psychophysical testing he was able to distinguish small differences in the luminance (0.1 log unit) and wavelength (7–10 μm) of a test aperture subtending a visual angle of approximately 2°, but was unable to distinguish between two objects of the same luminance, wavelength, and area when the only difference between them was shape. The deficit in this patient, therefore, was a low specificity for the attribute of shape while the specificity for the awareness of other stimulus attributes was retained (Efron, 1968). Benson and Greenberg (1969) referred to the patient's defect as a "visual form agnosia."

Many of these patients develop compensatory strategies, such as tracing of the outline of stimuli or executing small head movements as they explore their visual environment, perhaps as an attempt to use movement cues to aid form detection. The patient reported by Landis et al., (1982) developed an apperceptive visual agnosia secondary to mercury intoxication, and presented with a clinical picture similar to that of the famous patient Schn. (Goldstein and Gelb, 1918). The patient developed a strategy whereby he would trace letters, parts of letters, or words with the left hand alone or with both hands. He could trace simple geometric figures if the point of departure for tracing was unimportant. With more complex figures, unimportant lines misled him. He developed a sophisticated system of codes that aided in the identification of individual letters. Goldstein and Gelb's (1918) patient Schn. also developed a tracing strategy by using both his head and hand. Both patients' recognition abilities deteriorated instantly if they were prevented from using kinesthetic feedback.

Dorsal Simultanagnosia. The term "simultanagnosia" was introduced by Wolpert (1924) to refer to a condition in which the patient is unable to appreciate the meaning of a whole picture or scene even though the individual parts are well recognized. Luria (1959) used the term literally to indicate the inability to see or attend to more than one object at a time. Luria's use of the term has more generality since it is debatable, even in mildly impaired cases, whether the parts are recognized normally. Representative cases have been reported by Hécaen and de Ajuriaguerra (1954); Holmes (1918), Holmes and Horrax (1919), Luria (1959), Luria et al., (1963), and Tyler (1968). Most of these patients sustained bilateral parieto-occipital damage, although cases with superior occipital (Rizzo and Hurtig, 1987) or inferior parietal damage (Kase et al., 1977, case 1) have been reported. Simultanagnosia can also be present in the context of generalized or localized degenerative disease (Graff-Radford et al., 1993; Ardila et al., 1997; Beversdorf and Heilman, 1998; Mendez and Cherrier, 1998; Mendez, 2000).

As a result of their visual defect, these patients are impaired in counting tasks (Holmes, 1918) and on tasks that require the naming of a number of objects presented together (Luria et al., 1963). The disorder may also be evident in a dramatic inability to interpret the overall meaning of a line drawing or picture, with performance on such tasks often being a haphazard, inferred reconstruction of fragmented picture elements. On the basis of the study of such patients, Luria (Luria, 1959; Luria et al., 1963) concluded that simultanagnosia represents a complex perceptuomotor breakdown of the active, serial, feature-by-feature analysis necessary for processing elements of a visual scene or pattern. In the most severe cases, prominent features available in the stimulus array may themselves be fragmented and distorted.

Luria equates simultanagnosia with a perceptual defect often found as part of Balint's syndrome (Balint, 1909; Husain and Stein, 1988), which consists of (1) psychic paralysis of fixation with an inability to voluntarily look into the peripheral field (Tyler, 1968; Karpov et al., 1979), (2) optic ataxia, manifested by clumsiness or inability to manually respond to visual stimuli, with mislocation in space when pointing to visual targets (Holmes, 1918; Boller et al., 1975; Haaxma and Kuypers, 1975; Levine et al., 1978; Damasio and Benton, 1979), and (3) a disturbance of visual attention mainly affecting the periphery of the visual field and resulting in a dynamic concentric narrowing of the effective field (Hécaen and Ajuriaguerra, 1954; Levine and Calvanio, 1978; DeRenzi, 1982). Balint's syndrome is almost invariably associated with large biparietal lesions (but see Watson and Rapcsak, 1987), and is especially severe when frontal lobe lesions are also found (Hécaen and Ajuriaguerra, 1954). Frontal lobe involvement may lead to particularly severe psychic paralysis and optic ataxia, presumably because of disruption in visual–motor mechanisms and because of the role played by frontal eye fields and surrounding prefrontal cortex in the control of saccadic eye movements and visual attention (Lynch and McClaren, 1989).

Visual fields may be normal by standard perimetric testing but shrink to "shaft vision" when the patient concentrates on the visual environment. Performance may be worse in one hemifield, more often on the left. A striking example of narrowing of the "effective visual field" is given by Hécaen and Ajuriaguerra (1954; case 1). While their patient's attention was focused on the tip of a cigarette held between his lips, he failed to see a match flame offered him and held a few inches away. A good example of this deficit is presented by Tyler (1968), whose patient suddenly developed visual difficulties after segmental basal artery occlusion:

Visual acuity was 20/30 with glasses. Visual fields were at first considered normal, but careful retesting showed that while the left field was normal to movement of large objects, these objects faded from awareness in one or two seconds. With continued testing within that field, awareness of even the movement of large objects was lost. In the right visual field, the central two degrees around fixation were always normal, the surrounding outer 20 degrees fatigued rapidly, and beyond 20 degrees, movement was recognized but objects faded rapidly. The patient could see only one object or part of one object at a time with her central two to four degrees of vision. She scanned normally when looking at predictable objects such as a circle or a square but frequently lost her place when viewing objects and pictures. Slight movement of the page made her lose her place. She reported seeing bits and fragments. For instance, when shown a picture of a flag, she said, "I see a lot of lines, now I see some stars." When shown a dollar bill, she saw a picture of George Washington. Moments later when shown a cup, she said, "A cup with a picture of Washington on it." Eye movement studies revealed a normal number of visual fixations per unit of time and a normal pattern of fixation for small saccades or so-called visual steps. However, there were very few, if any, so-called long saccades or leaps that relate one part of the picture to another.

The three subjects described by Rizzo and Hurtig (1987) reported intermittent disappearance of a light target during electrooculogram (EOG)-verified fixation. Rizzo and Hurtig argue that a disorder of attentional mechanisms that permit sustained awareness of visual targets is involved. Verfaellie et al. (1990), using Posner's attentional cueing task, found that their Balint's patient had difficulty shifting attention to the left or right visual field, and benefited only from cues directing attention to the upper visual field. This patient also demonstrated a loss of spontaneous blinking, which may normally participate in a complex system mediating saccadic eye movement, sensory relay, and attentional deployment (Watson and Rapcsak, 1987).

Ventral Simultanagnosia. A second group of simultanagnosics appears to have lesions restricted to the left occipitotemporal junction. The primary feature that distinguishes these patients from dorsal simultanagnosics is that they succeed on dot-counting tasks and seem less impaired in negotiating their natural environment. Whether the disorder is one of degree or kind is debatable, though the anatomic pathology of this group is clearly distinct from that seen in dorsal simultanagnosia. The patients of Kinsbourne and Warrington (1962), Levine and Calvanio (1978), and Warrington and Rabin (1971), all presenting as letter-by-letter readers, are representative cases.

Kinsbourne and Warrington (1962) described a defect in "simultaneous form perception" which they believed accounted for the reading disturbance in these patients (see Levine and

Calvanio, 1978; Warrington and Shallice, 1980). Levine and Calvanio (1978) found that patients with simultanagnosia would report only one or two letters when presented with three letters simultaneously. If told in advance which letter to name, they successfully reported any single letter; if told after the exposure which letter to name, they performed poorly. The authors interpreted the defect as impairment in the perceptual analysis of compound visual arrays. Patients with this form of simultanagnosia thus do not perceive more than one object at a time. Their problem is compounded by an inability to relate small portions of what they see to the remainder of the stimulus by scanning.

Perceptual Categorization Deficit. Included in this category are patients who do not have deficits in the real-life recognition of objects but whose defect must be elicited experimentally. These patients, most of whom have unilateral posterior right hemisphere lesions, have difficulties matching two- or three-dimensional objects across different views. Such cases have been reported by De Renzi et al. (1969), Warrington and Taylor (1973), and Warrington and James (1988). Because they may recognize real-life objects, these patients are usually not considered agnosic but are included in Farah's (1990) classification system, because they appear to have a special kind of perceptual defect. Although Warrington's studies had localized the defect to the posterior right hemisphere, patients with unilateral left hemisphere lesions may also have the defect (Mulder et al., 1995). In Marr's (1982) terms, these patients fail to achieve a viewpoint-independent description of objects, and thus are impaired whenever an object identification or matching task requires them to match stimuli across views or to recognize a stimulus presented from a highly unconventional or noncanonical viewpoint.

Most of the controversy regarding the existence of agnosia has involved the apperceptive types. Given Teuber's classic definition of agnosia as a "normal percept stripped of its meaning," it is reasonable to question whether these patients qualify as agnosic. According to Bay (1953), there exists neither a specific gnostic function nor a specific disorder of gnosis, agnosia. For Bay, apparent cases of agnosia are

actually disorders of primary sensory function due to lesions of the primary sensory fields or their connections, and the occasional presence of a generalized dementing process further complicates the interpretation of faulty primary sensory data. Bay reported abnormalities in sensation time (the minimal exposure time sufficient for recognition of portions of the visual field) and local adaptation time (the elapsed time for a visual stimulus to fade from portions of the field) in patients with otherwise normal visual acuity and field. In these patients, visual stimuli tend to drop out of awareness because of abnormal fatiguability, particularly at the periphery (so-called Funktionswandel). Bay applied his tests to a patient with visual agnosia and, finding an abnormality of Funktionswandel, attributed the recognition deficit to primary visual sensory impairment.

Similarly, Bender and Feldman (1972) claimed that visual agnosia represented nothing more than a complex interaction between primary visual sensory abnormalities, various degrees of inattention, ocular fixation disturbance, and dementia. In their view, previously reported cases of visual agnosia were insufficiently examined. In a retrospective review of agnosia cases, they found that perceptuomotor defects and dementia were found in all instances, leading them to conclude that "visual agnosia is a result of a disorder of the total cerebral activity which renders performance of vision and/or other sensory functions inadequate." This kind of argument, of course, begs the question of just how adequate vision has to be to for object recognition to occur.

Despite their persistence, these criticisms are weakened by the fact that severe sensory abnormalities in the context of visual field defects, perceptual derangement, and dementia, do not necessarily lead to defects in object recognition (Ettlinger, 1956). The converse also seems true; one of Ettlinger's patients, a prosopagnosic, performed at a higher level on visuosensory tests than did most of the nonagnosic patients. Studies by Levine and Calvanio (1978) suggest that patients with agnosia do not differ from normals in sensation time or susceptibility to "backward masking." It is evident, therefore, that visual sensory abnormalities as measured by tests of sensation time and local adaptation time are not, even in the presence of dementia, sufficient in themselves to produce an agnosia-like recognition defect. It is true, however, that many patients with visual agnosia have elements of this type of disturbance and many also have abnormalities in visual attention, search, and exploration. Recent work suggests that there may be heterogeneous deficits within the general category of apperceptive agnosia. Studies in which stimulus manipulations seek to mimic apperceptive agnosia in normal subjects point to the special importance of perceptual grouping processes in producing the defect (Vecera and Gilds, 1998). In some cases, a combination of impaired feature recognition and limited cognitive resources available for processing demanding visual material may be present (Grossman et al., 1997). It seems likely that such defects represent a continuum on which impairment is a necessary, but not sufficient, characteristic of agnosia.

Although each of the four types of apperceptive agnosia has a relatively consistent lesion profile, it is impossible with our present level of knowledge to fully specify the functional anatomy underlying the various forms of visual apperceptive agnosia. It is clear that there is no singular entity called "apperceptive visual agnosia." Behaviorally, these patients differ along attentional, perceptual, oculomotor, and mnemonic dimensions; the relative contribution of each of these factors remains to be fully elucidated. However, it seems reasonable on clinical and experimental grounds to conclude that complex visual abilities are made up of dissociable ("modular") information-processing streams, including form discrimination, color perception, luminance, size, movement, and spatial localization and integration (Sprague et al., 1977; Perenin and Jeannerod, 1978; Berkley and Sprague, 1979; Maunsell and Newsome, 1987; DeYoe and Van Essen, 1988) and that the variability among apperceptive agnosics reflects the fact that these streams can be impaired singly or in combination at the individual case level.

Associative Visual Agnosia

The major distinguishing feature of associative visual agnosia is the presence of a modality-specific object identification defect in the context of a preserved ability to copy and/or match stimuli presented in the affected modality. Preserved copying or matching has often been taken as evidence of "normal" perception, an assumption that has been called into question by recent evidence (see below). Although, as we shall see, perception is not entirely normal in these patients, the degree of perceptual disturbance in this class of patients is different in degree and kind from that seen in apperceptive agnosia. A number of well-documented cases meeting the above criteria have appeared in the literature, leaving no doubt about the existence of this form of agnosia (Rubens and Benson, 1971; Taylor and Warrington, 1971; Lhermitte et al., 1973; Benson et al., 1974; Hécaen et al., 1974; Newcombe and Ratcliff, 1974; Albert et al., 1975a, 1979; Mack and Boller, 1977; Pillon et al., 1987a; Davidoff and Wilson, 1985; McCarthy and Warrington, 1986; McCarthy and Warrington, 1986; Riddoch and Humphreys, 1987a; Feinberg et al., 1994).

Pointing to objects named by the examiner, while characteristically impaired, may be better than identifying objects verbally or by gesture. This may reflect the fact that pointing takes place in the context of a closed set, while naming an object involves an almost infinite list of potential names. It is also possible that pointing to a named object is an easier task because it does not involve speaking and therefore reduces the chances that an incorrect verbal response will adversely affect nonverbal aspects of stimulus recognition. In many patients, picture identification is more impaired than is the identification of real objects and identification of line drawings is more impaired than either of these. A disturbance in the identification of line drawings or pictures may be the only residual defect after the acute disturbance has cleared. This dissociation is not seen in the naming performance of aphasics (Corlew and Nation, 1975; Hatfield and Howard, 1977), and may serve as a marker for the presence of agnosia in naming tasks.

Impairment of recognition of faces (prosopagnosia), color (so-called color agnosia), and of written material (alexia) are frequently but not invariably found with associative object agnosia (Farah, 1991). Object agnosia itself is more rare than these other conditions, each of which may occur in isolation or in various combinations. The patients of Hécaen and Ajuriaguerra (1956) and Lhermitte and Beauvois (1973) had no impairment in facial recognition, and reading was spared in the patients of Davidenkov (1956), Newcombe and Ratcliff (1974), Mack and Boller (1977), and Albert et al. (1975a). Levine's patient and case 1 of Newcombe and Ratcliff had no color agnosia or alexia. Alexia is commonly found alone or with color agnosia (see Geschwind and Fusillo, 1966); prosopagnosia is sometimes an isolated recognition disturbance (De Renzi, 1986a; Pallis, 1955), but is often associated with achromatopsia (Critchley, 1965). Much debate has centered around the coexistence of these various signs. Some authors believe that symptom co-occurrence is a simple "neighborhood sign," while others believe it reflects the fact that certain classes of objects (e.g., objects and faces) overlap in their visual processing demands. Tactile and auditory recognition are typically intact, although two patients of Newcombe and Ratcliff (1974) and the patients of Taylor and Warrington (1971) and Feinberg et al. (1986) were unable to identify objects by touch or vision.

The associative agnosic not only cannot name seen objects but also typically fails when asked to demonstrate semantic knowledge about the stimulus or its functional properties. The failure to sort objects and pictures into categories (e.g., articles of clothing, tools, etc.) or to match two different representations of the same object (a small line drawing of a wrist watch with a real watch) are typical examples. Some agnosics can classify objects according to their basic level (Rosch et. al., 1976) category (e.g., prosopagnosics always identify faces as faces) but are unable to identify the object at a more specific, individual level ("John's face" or "my wallet"). Others can identify neither the general class nor the individual-within-class. Such differences may signal important differences among agnosic syndromes or may more simply reflect the fact that different recognition tasks demand different levels of specificity. For example, "a key" is often an adequate answer in an object recognition paradigm, while

face recognition tasks require the subject to ascertain individual identity.

The role played by perceptual factors in associative agnosia has recently received attention. On the one hand, these patients are capable of remarkable visual achievements given the severity of their object recognition disturbances. The patients of Rubens and Benson, Taylor and Warrington, and Newcombe and Ratcliff (case 1) matched to sample and produced strikingly accurate drawings of pictures and objects they could not identify (Fig. 12–2). The patients of Rubens and Benson, and Taylor and Warrington were able to find hidden figures in figure-ground tests. Case 1 of Newcombe and Ratcliff showed no deficits on psychophysical tests of visual function.

On the other hand, two lines of evidence have made it clear that perceptual abilities are not normal in the vast majority of these patients and that such abnormalities may play a causative role in at least some aspects of the recognition disorder. First, although these patients may be capable of earning normal scores on tests of copying and matching, qualitative data suggest remarkably consistent evidence of slow, feature-by-feature, or "slavish" drawing and a reliance on local detail at the expense of the more global aspects of the stimulus (Levine, 1978; Humphreys and Riddoch, 1987; Levine and Calvanio, 1989; Farah, 1990; Suzuki et al., 1997). For example, Humphreys and Riddoch (1987) provide an exquisitely detailed report of a patient, H.J.A., who took hours to complete remarkably accurate drawings of objects he could not identify. Our own experience with the prosopagnosic patient L.F. revealed that performance on difficult facial matching tests (e.g., Benton Test of Facial Recognition), though quantitatively normal, proceeded in a feature-by-feature manner, resulting in extremely prolonged response times. Second, systematic variation of perceptual variables can significantly affect the recognizability of stimuli (Levine and Calvanio, 1978, 1989; Riddoch and Humphreys, 1987a). Stimulus complexity (e.g., presence of color, morphological similarity between items) appears to exert a strong effect on the frequency of semantic and morphological errors on object-naming tasks. Both the presence of fine-grained visual

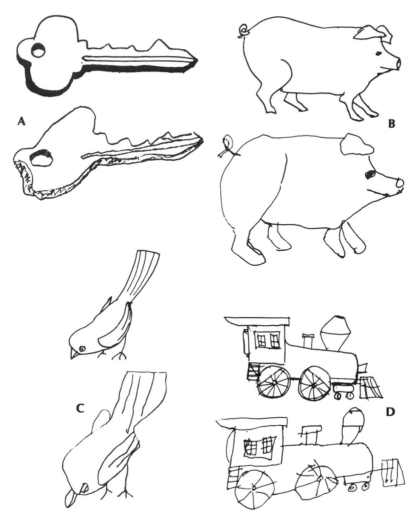

Figure 12–2. Copies of line drawings by a patient with associative visual agnosia. After copies were made, the patient still misidentified drawings as follows: *A:* "I still don't know." *B:* "Could be a dog or any other animal." *C:* "Could be a beach stump." *D:* "A wagon or a car of some kind. The larger vehicle is being pulled by the smaller one." (From Rubens and Benson, 1971.)

information as well as the presence in the stimulus of "compound" (multiple) information appear to contribute to ease of identification (see Levine and Calvanio, 1978). A frequently reported finding is that associative agnosics appear deficient in "gestalt perception," although they may perceive local details relatively normally. Partially covering an item or placing it in an unusual context hinders identification. Levine and Calvanio (1989) reported that their associative agnosic, L.H., was severely impaired on tasks of "visual closure"—the ability to perceive shape and identity of an object that has been degraded by visual noise (see also Farah, 1990). H.J.A., the patient reported by Humphreys and Riddoch (1987), performed poorly on a feature integration task requiring him to detect an upside down *T* among a group of upright *T*s. Unlike normals, H.J.A. did not show faster detection when the stimuli were arranged in a discrete circular configuration (as opposed to random presentation), suggesting a defect in integrating local feature details into an overall gestalt. These findings illustrate why there is growing discontent with the apperceptive–associative distinction, at least in its "strong" form. They also illustrate why parallel-distributed models of object recognition that posit no fundamental distinction between perception and memory/association (Goldman-Rakic, 1988; Damasio, 1989) deserve increased attention by neuropsychologists and behavioral neurologists interested in agnosic phenomena.

The cases of Kertesz (1979) and Wapner et al. (1978) further complicate the apperceptive–associative distinction. Kertesz's patient presents a challenge, as she had elements of Balint's syndrome, visual static agnosia (Botez and Serbanescu, 1967; Botez, 1975), alexia without agraphia, prosopagnosia, and amnestic syndrome. The patient performed poorly on copying tasks (her reproductions were poorly executed and contained only fragmented elements of the associated target stimuli), but matched real objects; line drawings, colors, letters, and geometric figures better than she named or pointed to them. Verbal responses were marked by perseverations and form confusions. The patient had 20/20 acuity (open E method), and a spiraling visual field defect. A computed tomography (CT) scan revealed right frontal and deep left occipital lobe lesions.

Wapner and colleagues (1978) presented a case report of visual agnosia in an artist whose drawing skills were specifically assessed. Their patient suffered a cerebral infarction with resulting variable right hemianopia, visual recognition defect, and amnesia. A brain scan revealed bilateral medial occipital infarctions. Visual acuity was 20/70. The patient showed poor visual recognition of objects and drawings in the context of moderately impaired design copying. Interestingly, the patient showed a striking dissociation in qualitative drawing performance between objects he could and could not recognize. With unrecognized objects, his drawings revealed piecemeal, slavish reproduction of recognized elements. Describing his drawing of a telephone dial, he said, "a circle, another circle, a square . . . things keep coming out . . . and this is as though it hooks into something." In contrast, when drawing an object he could identify, the patient relied on preserved structural knowledge of the essential components of the object, producing a sketch that was faithful to the specific target as well as to the general class of objects to which the target belonged. He remarked, "can't help but

use your natural knowledge in drawing the thing." These two cases are important for two reasons. First, they both showed dissociations among various tests classically used to tap the apperceptive level. Second, their combined defects at the levels of perception and recognition underscore the fact that agnosia is the final outcome of many different defects, and again illustrate that the apperceptive–associative distinction should be viewed as an heuristic and perhaps nothing more.

In addition to the contribution of perceptual factors, there is evidence that the initial verbalized response to visual presentation can adversely affect recognition ability in at least some of these patients. Identification errors are usually morphological confusions or perseverations, though semantic errors are not uncommon. The tendency to perseverate previous naming errors and the disruptive influence of visual naming on tactile identification are examples of this. One might expect that visual agnosic patients with normal blindfolded tactile naming would perform at least as well when they simultaneously inspect and handle an object. However, the otherwise superior tactile identification of the patients of Ettlinger and Wyke (1961) and Rubens et al. (1978; cited in Rubens, 1979) fell to the much lower level of visual identification alone when the patients were allowed to simultaneously view and handle the objects. Ettlinger and Wyke's patient, when given two exposures of each of 21 items, made 26 errors with vision alone, only 9 errors with touch alone, but 16 errors with vision and touch.

Prevention of the contaminating effect of verbal responses is not always easy. Many patients insist on speaking despite strict instructions to remain silent. Case 1 of Oxbury et al. (1969) was specifically instructed to demonstrate in silence the use of objects shown to her, but continued to name them aloud and then to produce an incorrect gesture that corresponded to her verbal misidentification. This same patient, when asked to match a line drawing to one of three real objects, would misname the drawing and then search in vain for an object corresponding to her incorrect name. It has been claimed that perseverations represent verbal reports of a lingering visual sensory experience of previously viewed material (Critchley, 1964; Cummings et al., 1982). However, when patients are asked to draw an object on which such perseverative errors occur, they draw the item they are viewing, not the item whose name has been perseverated (Rubens and Benson, 1971; Lhermitte and Beauvois, 1973; Rubens et al., 1978, cited in Rubens, 1979). Successfully copying a misidentified picture generally does not facilitate identification of that picture. This suggests that the motor system generally does not have the ability to cue the visual identification process in most patients, although requiring the patient to write the name (Lhermitte and Beauvois, 1973) or to supply a description (Newcombe and Ratcliff, 1974) of an object instead of naming it aloud normalized recognition in one case and enhanced it in the other.

The most common visual field defect in associative agnosia is a dense, right homonymous hemianopia. In the patient of Albert and colleagues (1975a), the right visual field defect was confined to the upper quadrant. Two left-handed patients with left homonymous hemianopia have been reported (Newcombe and Ratcliff, 1974 [case 2]; Levine, 1978). Interestingly, reading was spared in all three of these patients. Normal visual fields have also been reported (Davidenkov, 1956; Taylor and Warrington, 1971; Newcombe and Ratcliff, 1974 [case I]).

The marked variability in performance of patients in the natural setting as opposed to the test setting was noted by Geschwind (1965), who viewed misidentifications as confabulated responses elaborated by the intact speech area pathologically disconnected from intact visual sensory area. Failure to supply the correct gesture results from concomitant disconnection between motor and sensory areas. The common association of visual object agnosia with right homonymous hemianopia, alexia, and color agnosia, a triad occurring in the context of damage to mesial left occipital lobe and nearby posterior callosal fibers, supports the visual–verbal disconnection hypothesis. Authors arguing against the disconnection hypothesis cite (1) the occasional finding of normal visual fields or left homonymous hemianopia (Cambier et al., 1980); (2) the occasional absence of color agnosia and alexia in the same patient (Newcombe and Ratcliff, 1974 [case 1]; Levine, 1978); and (3) the question of why a left occipital-splenial lesion produces the syndrome of alexia without agraphia commonly but that of object agnosia only rarely. The pathology in some cases is inconsistent with a visual–verbal disconnection view. For example, Levine's (1978) patient had a unilateral right occipital lobe resection and was, in fact, able to verbally code some visually presented stimuli with remarkable accuracy (e.g., "something with 'U' in it," when looking at a padlock). In a series of recent cases of associative visual agnosia, consistent damage to the dominant parahippocampal, fusiform, and lingual gyri, but inconsistent damage to the callosal splenium was found (Feinberg et al., 1994).

Strictly speaking, the imperfect correlation between color agnosia, alexia, and visual object agnosia does not, by itself, invalidate the visual–verbal disconnection hypothesis. It remains possible that there may be highly specific forms of visual–verbal disconnection, and that unilateral or bilateral intrahemisphere disconnection and/or selective destruction of independent pathways mediating various elements of visual recognition plays a role (see Ratcliff and Ross, 1981). There is, for example, evidence for the specificity of neural pathways for color (Zeki, 1973, 1977; Meadows, 1974a). This kind of specificity is also implicit in the classical work of Hubel and Wiesel (1977). However, more damaging for the visual–verbal disconnection view is the fact that many associative agnosics fail on tasks that require nonverbal tasks, such as functional classification or gesturing.

Neuropathological data in associative agnosia present a confusing picture. Some authors (Warrington, 1985) suggest that diffuse damage may be involved, but that a lateralized left hemisphere lesion may be sufficient. Alexander and Albert (1983) argue for a bilateral occipitotemporal localization (see also Benson et al., 1974). Geschwind's (1965) visual–verbal disconnection model is based on a unilateral left mesial occipital localization, and other left-sided cases include the patients of Warrington and McCarthy (1987) and Feinberg et al. (1986, 1994). Levine's (1978) patient shows that associative agnosia can result from a unilateral right occipital lesion. Farah (1990) suggests that this heterogeneity might account for different perceptual impairments in patients with associative agnosia. For example, in the context of the debate regarding the relative significance of cortical and white matter lesions (Albert et al., 1979; Ross, 1980b), it seems possible, even likely, that there are multiple forms of associative visual agnosia representing impairment at different levels of processing (Damasio and Damasio, 1982). Patients such as those of Taylor and Warrington (1971) and Newcombe and Ratcliff (1974 [cases 1 and 2]) with diffuse bilateral disease processes, tactile agnosia, and normal visual fields probably form a separate group from those with right homonymous hemianopia associated with infarction in the territory of the left posterior cerebral artery.

Optic Aphasia

The term "optic aphasia" was introduced by Freund (1889) to describe the deficit of one of his patients with a right homonymous hemianopia and aphasia due to a left parieto-occipital tumor; the patient's naming ability was impaired primarily for visually presented objects. The case report is of little value because of its incompleteness, but Freund's speculations are pertinent. He hypothesized that a left speech area–right occipital disconnection was the basis for the visual naming deficit in the intact visual field. In current usage, *optic aphasia* refers to the condition in which patients are unable to name visually presented objects but are able to show that they recognize the object by indicating its use, by pointing to it when it is named, or by otherwise demonstrating knowledge of object meaning. Tactile and auditory naming are preserved. Representative cases have been reported by Lhermitte and Beauvois (1973), Riddoch and Humphreys (1987b), Larrabee et al. (1985), and Coslett and Saffran (1989b). Whether optic aphasia and associative agnosia differ in degree or kind remains a matter of controversy (De Renzi and Saetti, 1997; Chanoine et al., 1998), though the recent trend is to consider it a separate entity.

The patient of Lhermitte and Beauvois (1973) represents a good example of the syndrome of optic aphasia. Their patient suffered a left posterior cerebral artery territory infarction and presented with right homonymous hemianopia, moderately severe amnesia, and alexia. The most striking feature of his presentation was an inability to name visually presented objects. Naming errors consisted of perseverations of previously presented objects, semantic errors (in which an object was given the name of a semantically related object), and, less frequently, visual errors. At the same time, he could demonstrate that he knew what the object was by demonstrating how it would be used. Drawing of viewed objects was normal even when the object was misnamed. He showed normal tactile naming in both right and left hands and could name environmental sounds with little difficulty. Also, when given the name of an object he was viewing, he could provide an accurate definition of the object and its functional properties. Although he was aware of his visual field defect and his reading disturbance, he was not aware of his difficulty in visual naming.

What makes optic aphasia so important is that it challenges the widely held view that object naming is based on a common set of semantic representations of known objects that can be accessed from any sensory modality. The problem is this: why should a patient who shows intact verbal semantics (as evidenced, for example, by his good performance on the definitions task) and intact visual semantics (as evidenced by his accurate miming of object use) be able to name only those objects that are held in the hand? There have been several different answers to this question. Beauvois (1982) suggested that, in J.F., visual and verbal semantics became disconnected from each other, and that only tactile input had preserved access to verbal semantics. This view is based on the more general idea of multiple, modality-specific semantic systems, segregated according to the modality in which constituent information is represented (Warrington, 1985; Shallice, 1988).

Riddoch and Humphreys (1987b) suggest a different answer, based on their analysis of another case of optic aphasia. Riddoch and Humphreys presented an object decision task in which the patient had to decide whether a series of individual line drawings represented real objects or not. Their patient performed normally on this task, which suggests that he had preserved knowledge of object structure. However, the patient was impaired in grouping semantically related objects (e.g., hammer and nail), and could not draw named objects from memory. Thus, in either direction, the patient could not link semantic and visual information. On the basis of these results, Riddoch and Humphreys describe optic aphasia as a modality-specific semantic access problem. They further postulate that the knowledge of how to use objects is linked to structural rather than to semantic properties, and suggest that the patient may be able to demonstrate object use by a direct connection between visual object recognition units and motor action systems.

A third answer was provided by Coslett and Saffran (1989b), who suggested that at least some patients with optic aphasia are able to access semantic information contained in the right hemisphere but are unable to access the semantic system and speech production mechanisms within the left hemisphere. Like Warrington (1985) and Shallice (1988), these authors posit multiple semantic systems, but argue that these systems are differentiated not by the modality of input but by their anatomic locus in the right or left hemisphere. The patient described by Coslett and Saffran was a 67-year-old man with a large left occipital lobe infarct and a lacunar infarct in the right internal capsule. The patient was unable to name visually presented objects but was able to name them to palpation and visual description and could point to them when they were named. This latter ability is not easily accommodated by a model that dissociates all visual and verbal input. The patient could correctly categorize unnamed pictures and words and could group unrecognized objects according to their functional similarity and semantic association. This provides good evidence that the patient was able to access detailed semantic information from visually presented objects, which Coslett and Saffran argue reflects an intact right hemisphere semantic system.

While the mechanisms discussed above all invoke deficits of semantic access, Shuren et al. (1993) suggested that the critical deficit in optic aphasia may be lexical access. They reported three patients who named visually presented stimuli normally, but could not name the same objects when given a definition, nor could they demonstrate or describe the use of the objects. They called this disorder "non-optic aphasia" and suggested that while percepts could access an intact lexicon, the semantic representations were degraded. In contrast, patients with optic aphasia may be able to access semantics, but not the lexicon.

Although optic aphasia appears to be qualitatively different from associative agnosia, the possibility remains that, at least in some patients, the distinction may be a matter of degree (De Renzi and Saetti, 1997; Chanoine et al., 1998). Clinical lore suggests that patients may evolve into optic aphasia during recovery from classical associative visual agnosia. The fact that some patients can be made to oscillate between optic aphasia and visual agnosia by varying the instructions given them on a particular task blurs, at least in some cases, the distinction between a naming disorder and a disturbance of recognition.

Color Agnosia

Patients with color agnosia are, by classic definition, unable to name colors shown to them or to point to a color named by the examiner, yet perform normally on nonverbal tasks of color perception. One of the earliest cases was reported by Wilbrand (1887), who referred to the defect as "amnestic color blindness." Wilbrand observed that his patient could not find the appropriate word for a color displayed, that he frequently perseverated names across trials, and that naming the color of a familiar object out of sight was impaired. Wilbrand invoked an "amnestic" disorder because the patient often indicated that he had forgotten the name of the colors he was shown.

The term *color agnosia* presents something of a conceptual dilemma. Unlike objects, colors cannot be heard or palpated and cannot be shown in use; they can only be known through vision or visual representation (imagery). It is difficult to imagine a clinical tool to assess color recognition in other modalities and thus it is hard to establish the modality specificity of the deficit, although conceptual color tasks (e.g., "what color is associated with feelings of envy"?) have utility in assessing semantic aspects of color processing. Still, acquired anomalies of color vision and color performance do occur as a result of lesions to the posterior cortex (De Renzi and Spinnler, 1967). Four syndromes of color disturbance have been described: *(1) central achromatopsia/dyschromatopsia* (MacKay and Dunlop, 1899; Green and Lessell, 1977; Meadows, 1974a; Pearlman et al., 1979; Damasio et al., 1980; Young and Fishman, 1980), *(2)* color anomia, which is found in association with pure alexia and right homonymous hemianopia and is attributable to visual–verbal disconnection (Geschwind and Fusillo, 1966; Oxbury et al., 1969 [case I]; Meadows, 1974a; Beauvois and Saillant, 1985); *(3)* specific color aphasia, in which the patient

has linguistic defects but the impairment in utilizing color names is disproportionately severe (Kinsbourne and Warrington, 1964; Oxbury et al., 1969 [case 2]); and *(4)* color-naming and color association defects concomitant with aphasia (De Renzi et al., 1972, 1973; Wyke and Holgate, 1973; Cohen and Kelter, 1979). We will review the first three of these defects below. A summary of performance defects in patients with these various syndromes is presented in Table 12–1 (Bowers, 1981).

Central Achromatopsia/Dyschromatopsia. Central achromatopsia refers to a loss of color vision due to central nervous system (CNS) disease. The causative lesions can be in the optic nerve, chiasm, or in one or both of the cerebral hemispheres (Green and Lessell, 1977). The disorder can be hemianopic (Albert et al., 1975b), or can exist throughout the visual

Table 12–1. Summary of Color Performance Defects in Patients with Various Syndromes

Tasks		Achromatopsia	Color Anomia A (visual-verbal d/c)	Color Anomia B (specific color aphasia)	Aphasic Patients
Visual-visual	Ishihara	±*	+	+	+
	Hue discrimination	−	+	+	+
	Color matching	±°	+	+	+
	Coloring pictures	±	+[†]	−	−
	Color absurdities	±	+[†]	+	±[‡]
	Color sorting	±	+	−	−
Verbal-verbal	Color naming				
	Blood is _____	+	+	−	−
	What color is grass?	+	+	−	−
	Color fluency	+	+	NT	−
	Naming items of specific colors	+	+	−	NT
Visual-verbal	Color naming	±°	−	−	−
	Color pointing	±°	−	−	−
	Color-object naming	±°	−	−	−
	Color-object pointing	±°	−	−	−

The symbol + refers to intact performance and − refers to impaired performance.

*Performance depends upon severity of achromatopsia. In mild cases, only hue discrimination is impaired.

[†]Performance on these tasks is unimpaired as long as patient does not attempt to verbalize answers. If patient does attempt to do so, then verbalizations can interfere with performance.

[‡]Global and Wernike's aphasics are impaired; all other aphascis are OK.

fields. Although typically nonselective, achromatopsia may be partial, affecting one color more than others. Critchley (1965) described a patient with "xanthopsia" who suddenly felt as if all objects around him were covered with gold paint.

Patients with achromatopsia notice their loss of color vision, and describe their visual world as "black and white," "all grey," "washed out," or "dirty." Damasio et al. (1980) reported that one of their patients had every drapery in her house laundered because she thought they needed cleaning. Such patients perform poorly on tasks of color perception (Ishihara plates, Munsell Farnsworth 100-Hue Test, hue discrimination, color matching), but do well on verbal–verbal tasks (e.g., "What color is blood?"; "Name three blue things"). Performance on visual–verbal tasks (naming, pointing, color-object naming and pointing) varies with the severity of the disorder.

There is agreement in the literature that achromatopsia results from unilateral or bilateral lesions in the inferior ventromedial sector of the occipital lobe, involving the lingual and fusiform gyri (Meadows, 1974b; Green and Lessell, 1977; Damasio et al., 1980). Superior field defects are the rule. Prosopagnosia and topographical memory loss are found in the bilateral but not the unilateral cases (Damasio et al., 1980). Two patients (Green and Lessell, 1977 [case 4]; Pearlman et al., 1979) each had two separate unilateral posterior cerebral artery infarctions and did not become achromatopsic until their second strokes. At least one case of reversible achromatopsia and prosopagnosia associated with migraine has been reported (Lawden and Cleland, 1993). Visual evoked responses to alternating green and red checkerboard patterns may be abnormal (Damasio et al., 1980), although chromatic contrast sensitivity has been reportedly normal (Heywood et al., 1998; Hurlbert et al., 1998).

The physiologic work of Zeki (1973, 1977) has revealed that in rhesus monkey there are specialized areas (V-4 complex and an additional region in the superior temporal sulcus) containing "color-coded" cells that selectively respond to specific wavelengths of light. Heywood and colleagues (1995) have shown that lesions anterior to V4, but completely sparing it, can lead to achromatopsia in monkeys. Damasio et al. (1980) speculate that the lingual and fusiform gyri in humans may be the homologues of area V-4. The exact location is not currently known, though recent functional imaging evidence points to the fusiform gyrus (Sakai et al., 1995). What does seem clear from clinical data is that one single area in each hemisphere (eccentrically located in the lower visual association cortex) controls color processing for the entire hemifield (Damasio et al., 1980).

Color Anomia. The patient with color anomia succeeds on visual–visual and verbal–verbal tasks, but is unable to name colors, a visual–verbal task. The disorder is usually associated with the syndrome of alexia without agraphia (Stengel, 1948; Geschwind and Fusillo, 1966; Carlesimo et al., 1998), and frequently exists in the context of right homonymous hemianopia. The underlying neuroanatomic mechanism is a visual–verbal disconnection resulting from infarction in the left posterior cerebral artery (PCA) distribution. The patients of Geschwind and Fusillo (1966) and Oxbury et al. (1969 [case I]) are classic examples of this syndrome.

These patients may show impairment on some tasks related to color perception, such as coloring pictures or detecting errors in wrongly colored stimuli. This impairment is exacerbated if patients attempt to "verbalize" their answers (Bowers, 1981). Damasio and colleagues (1979) suggest that the type of stimuli, the demands of the task, and the patient's problem-solving approach can strongly influence the extent of visual–verbal dissociation. In their analysis, visual–verbal dissociation is maximized when, at the perceptual level, stimuli are purely visual (such as color), structurally less "rich," or low in association value. At the verbal end, visual–verbal dissociation is maximized when a specific name, rather than the name of a broad category, is involved (Boller and Spinnler, 1967). If the patient's verbalizations about the stimulus are incorrect, they may interfere with attempts to assign it the correct color.

Specific Color Aphasia. Patients with this syndrome are distinguished from color anomics by their poor performance on verbal–verbal tasks. The patients of Oxbury et al. (1969 [case 2] and Kinsbourne and Warrington (1964) are among the best documented cases of this variety. Aphasic symptoms are usually present, but the difficulty with color names and other color-associative skills is disproportionately severe. The patient of Oxbury et al. had head trauma (and probable bilateral lesions) with complete right homonymous hemianopia and mild right hemiparesis. Kinsbourne and Warrington's patient had a left posterior parietal subdural hematoma. These patients can generally sort colors categorically and according to hue, and can appropriately match colors. These deficits are similar to those reported in aphasic patients by De Renzi et al. (1972).

Prosopagnosia

The term "prosopagnosia" was formally introduced by Bodamer (1947) to describe an acquired inability to recognize previously familiar faces. Patients with this disorder often present with a dramatic and recognizable disability that comes to the attention of the clinician by personal encounter or by the report of distressed family members who are concerned about the patient's inability to recognize them. Typically, an inability to recognize newly encountered individuals (e.g., health-care workers and hospital personnel) is also present. The inability to recognize family members, friends, and hospital staff may lead to the mistaken conclusion that the patient is suffering from a severe memory defect or a generalized dementia. The disorder should be distinguished from Capgras syndrome, a psychiatric disturbance in which the patient believes that familiar persons have been replaced by imposters (Synodinou et al., 1978; Alexander et al., 1979; Shraberg and Weitzel, 1979). When formally tested, patients with prosopagnosia may score normally on face discrimination and matching tasks (Warrington and James, 1967; Benton and Van Allen, 1972). They almost invariably recognize faces as faces, and can often succeed at perceptually demanding tasks of age, gender, and expression discrimination (Tzavaras et al., 1970; Benton and Van Allen, 1972). Their primary defect is in identifying and recognizing whose face they are viewing. Such patients may be unable to recognize their own face in a mirror, though they often correctly infer that it must be themselves. The defect prevents the identification of famous personalities, family members, and other familiar persons, and often severely limits the ability to acquire familiarity with faces first encountered after illness onset (Beyn and Knyazeva, 1962).

Prosopagnosia typically presents as an acquired disorder, although convincing cases in which the problem in recognition exists on a developmental basis have been reported (De Haan et al., 1991; De Haan and Campbell, 1991; Kracke, 1994; Ariel and Sadeh, 1996; Duchaine, 2000). The patient typically reports, and demonstrates in everyday behavior, an inability to recognize the identity of individuals by their facial features. However, the patient is easily capable of recognizing others by voice or some other nonfacial cue. Prosopagnosia typically presents as a disabling condition, but affected patients are often able to compensate remarkably after an initial period of adjustment. For example, such patients often become able use extrafacial cues, including clothing, characteristic gait, length of hair, height, or distinguishing birthmark, to achieve recognition, though significant individual differences exist. In many cases, patients realize that they have a defect and are distressed by it, although there are cases in which the patient is unaware of the problem (Young et al., 1990). The variability in clinical presentation suggests that the clinician should always carefully evaluate the scope of the deficit as well as deficit awareness. Clinical examination often reveals additional neuropsychological deficits including central achromatopsia, constructional disability, topographical memory loss, and dressing apraxia, and the patient may or may not show more generalized signs of object agnosia (Hécaen and Angelergues, 1962). As with many cases of recognition disturbance, there is evidence that prosopagnosia may take apperceptive and associative forms (Gloning, et al., 1970; Levine, 1978; Bauer and Trobe, 1984; De Renzi et al.,

1991). Thus every patient with prosopagnosia should be examined with basic tests of facial discrimination, facial learning, and perceptual function to determine whether the recognition defect results from impairments in basic perceptual processes or at the stage in which perceptual inputs are compared with stored information about faces.

Although patients with prosopagnosia deny any familiarity with the faces they view, and fail miserably on tests of facial identification, many are able to demonstrate some degree of recognition ability if such ability is measured indirectly. This has been referred to as "covert recognition," and includes a number of distinct behavioral phenomena. For example, prosopagnosics can autonomically discriminate facial identity (Bauer, 1984) and facial familiarity (Tranel and Damasio, 1985) despite a total inability to recognize faces overtly. They can show cross-domain semantic priming using faces and names (Young et al., 1988). They show normal interference in name classification ("Is Brad Pitt a politician or an actor?") when a face from a different semantic category is presented (De Haan et al., 1987b, 1992). All of these data suggest that prosopagnosics can extract information from faces that is not reflected in their verbal report.

Lesions causing prosopagnosia are typically bilateral and involve the cortex and white matter in the mesial occipitotemporal region. Although it is widely accepted that most cases of prosopagnosia involve bilateral lesions, there are several recent cases suggesting that prosopagnosia can occur with unilateral lesions to the language-nondominant (right) hemisphere. There are now several well-documented cases of prosopagnosia with CT evidence of damage restricted to the right hemisphere (De Renzi, 1986b; Benton, 1990; Michel et al., 1989; Landis et al., 1986; Tohgi et al., 1994; Evans et al., 1995). The anatomic facts suggest that impairment in the right occipitotemporal junction is necessary, and at times sufficient, to produce prosopagnosia, although the typical lesion profile is bilateral in nature (Meadows, 1974b; Cohn et al., 1977; Whitley and Warrington, 1977; Damasio et al., 1982; Ettlin et al., 1992; Bauer, 1993). Some authors have argued that true prosopagnosia requires bilateral lesions, though atypical cases may appear with unilateral (right hemisphere) damage, much like the occasional case of "crossed aphasia" (Aptman et al., 1977). Some authors have distinguished among different types of prosopagnosia, each with its particular lesion profile. Damasio et al. (1990) described three subtypes: an associative type characterized by bilateral damage in Brodmann areas 18, 19, and 37; an amnestic–associative type resulting from damage to the hippocampus and surrounding cortex, and an apperceptive type resulting from extensive right hemisphere damage involving Brodmann areas 18, 19, 37, and 39. Likewise, De Renzi et al. (1991) distinguish between apperceptive and associative prosopagnosia.

Superior field defects (either altitudinal hemianopia or superior quadrantanopia) are most common, suggesting that causative lesions tend to occur inferiorly in the occipitotemporal region (Meadows, 1974b). Some authors believe that unilateral right hemisphere damage restricted to the inferior occipitotemporal does not produce full-blown prosopagnosia; for this to occur, more extensive superior damage, often extending into the parietal lobe, must be present (Damasio et al., 1990).

The occipitotemporal projection system (OTPS) is a series of short U-fibers tht course beneath the cortical mantle to connect adjacent regions in striate, prestriate, and inferior temporal cortex (Tusa and Ungerleider, 1985). This system, which serves as the functional interface between visual association cortex and temporal lobe, has been particularly implicated in prosopagnosia (Benson et al., 1974; Meadows, 1974b; Bauer, 1982). The regions in temporal lobe served by the OTPS subsequently project to the Iimbic system. Accordingly, prosopagnosia has been interpreted as a visual–limbic disconnection syndrome (Benson et al., 1974; Bauer, 1982). Evidence that prosopagnosics suffer from reductions in emotional responsivity to visual stimuli seem to support this idea (Bauer, 1982; Habib, 1986). However, the situation seems more complex, because OTPS lesions anterior to the occipitotemporal area (which, if complete, also produce visual–limbic disconnection) do not typically result in prosopagnosia (Meadows, 1974b). Intrinsic damage to the occipitotemporal area thus seems important. It is possible that intrinsic damage to the occipitotemporal region destroys or disconnects from visual input the association cortex in which visual representations of faces (or at least the "hardware" for activating such representations) reside (Damasio et al., 1982; Perrett et al., 1987; Perrett et al., 1982). Second, occipitotemporal lesions involving the OTPS are usually posterior enough to directly affect portions of inferotemporal cortex, a region that seems particularly critical in recognizing, categorizing, and discriminating visual forms (Iversen and Weiskrantz, 1964, 1967; Kuypers et al., 1965; Gross et al., 1972). This may contribute to the "underspecification" of visual detail, which recent authors (Levine, 1978; Shuttleworth et al., 1982) have considered important in the production of the defect.

Prosopagnosia has stimulated remarkable interest because it apparently represents a category-specific defect and thus may shed light on the manner in which perceptual representations are stored and organized in the brain. The pattern of spared and impaired abilities in these patients has led to the construction of models of the face recognition process. One critical question that still awaits final resolution is whether face recognition is special in any particular way, or whether it is simply distinct because of its complexity (Valentine, 1988; Nachson, 1995; Farah, 1996; Farah et al., 1998; Kreiman et al., 2000).

In the past decade, cognitive models of the face recognition process have been constructed as a way of understanding the various steps involved in extracting identity information from people's faces. One such model, similar to that proposed by Marr, and adapted from Ellis and Young (1988), is depicted in Figure 12–1. According to the model, faces are first subjected to complex visual analysis of the facial structure, including both featural and configural elements. Collectively, this step is referred to as "structural encoding," and includes the construction of two kinds of structural representations. The first, the "view-centered description," represents the image of the face from the viewer's perspective. Many such descriptions of each face are possible, depending upon point of view, momentary facial expression, lighting, and other factors. The second is a "viewpoint -independent description," which is a general structural description of the face that is not dependent upon either viewpoint or expression. The viewpoint-independent description allows us to recognize that two pictures of faces, seen from different points of view, may belong to the same person. While the "structural encoding" step is a critical first step in analyzing facial identity, other kinds of non–identity-based visual processing are going on simultaneously. The face may be analyzed for its emotional expression ("expression analysis") or might be visually inspected in such a way as to allow lip-reading ("facial speech analysis"). These two processes are depicted as outside the "structural encoding" box to emphasize that they are not involved in identity processing. In fact, many severely impaired prosopagnosics perform normally on emotion recognition or lip-reading tasks (Campbell et al., 1986; Tranel et al., 1988). Once a structural representation of the face is constructed, other forms of "directed visual processing" (e.g., gender, age discrimination, same–different judgments) are possible. Associative prosopagnosics rarely fail at this type of processing, while those with an apperceptive defect may have difficulty in performing complex facial discriminations.

An important component of the model is the "face recognition unit" (FRU), which receives input from structural encoding, and contains the visual structural descriptions that allow a particular known face to be discriminated from other familiar and unfamiliar faces. According to the model, each familiar face has its own FRU. Activation of the FRU leads to a sense of familiarity, but not to individual identification, since the FRU contains structural, but not semantic information. Activation of the FRU normally leads to the activation of a "person identity node" (PIN) that contains semantic information about the owner of the face. After activation of the FRU and PIN, a name might be assigned to the individual face. According to the model, naming occurs only after an appropriate PIN is activated.

This kind of model has been useful in organizing a large body of empirical findings on face recognition in normal subjects and is a useful heuristic in understanding patterns of impairment in face processing that occur after brain injury. As applied to prosopagnosia, the model is useful in describing the various stages at which a face recognition defect can occur. Some patients have difficulty at the structural encoding level, and thus have difficulty with a broad range of face discrimination and perception tasks. Others have defects much later in the processing chain. In some patients, the face recognition units themselves appear to be damaged, while in others, access to otherwise intact FRUs, or from the FRU to the PIN, appears to be impaired. Evidence of intact FRUs comes from case studies in which patients more easily learn correct face–name matches than incorrect ones (Bruyer, 1991; De Haan et al., 1991), and in studies demonstrating intact access to person information in semantic priming paradigms (Young et al., 1988).

Recent computational studies have attempted to use computer simulations to evaluate the degree to which impairments at particular stages of a cognitive model could account for the pattern of spared and impaired face identification abilities in at least some prosopagnosics. Using an interactive activation model patterned after similar models in word recognition, Burton et al. (1990) attempted to simulate the behavior of their prosopagnosic patient, P.H. This patient failed at all conventional tests of facial identification, but showed intact semantic priming of familiarity decisions with both faces and names. That is, when Prince Charles' face was presented as a prime, he was more likely to regard Princess Diana's face as familiar then when an unrelated face preceded Diana's face. Thus, despite a complete failure of overt recognition, P.H. showed that he could access some semantic information from viewed faces. Burton et al. attempted to simulate this finding by "lesioning" their interactive activation model. The basic architecture of the model, patterned after the Bruce and Young (1986) face recognition model, contained a number of distinct pools of units corresponding to names, faces (FRUs), persons (PINs), and semantic information. In their simulation, input was applied to an individual name or FRU, and activation of associated units was measured. The normal behavior of the model

accurately simulated cross-domain (face–name) and within-domain (name–name) semantic priming. For example, when input was applied to the Prince Charles PIN, increased activation (priming) occurred at the Diana FRU. On the basis of their behavioral data, Burton et al. hypothesized that P.H.'s lesion damaged the links between FRUs and PINs. In the normal simulation described above, all connections were equally weighted. To simulate damaged links between the FRUs and the PINs, the weights assigned to these links were halved and model was run again. Results from the simulations showed (1) normal name–name priming (expected in prosopagnosia, since the disorder does not affect the patient's ability to recognize names) and (2) intact cross-domain (face–name) priming for names despite the fact that activation at the FRU never reached recognition threshold. Thus, this computational model successfully simulated both normal and disordered face recognition performance.

Other researchers have utilized computational approaches to address the issue of whether the pattern of spared and impaired recognition abilities in prosopagnosia implies impaired access to an intact face recognition processor (Farah et al., 1993). Although the dominant view of covert recognition in prosopagnosia is that it represents a failure of the face processor to access conscious awareness, these researchers argued that the covert recognition phenomenon reflected damage to the face processor itself. They argued that the damaged neural network would manifest residual knowledge in the kinds of tasks used to measure covert recognition. They constructed a three-layer model consisting of face, name, and semantic (occupational) information for 16 units. The model contained face input and name units on the first level, face- and name-hidden units on the second level, and semantic units on the third level. Using a contrastive Hebbian learning algorithm, the network was first trained to associate an individual's face, name, and semantics whenever one of these was presented. The network was then lesioned by removing between 2 and 14 units from the 16-item face input pool and from the 16-item face hidden unit pool. In four simulations measuring face–name learning, speed of visual perception, semantic priming, and face recognition, they found that their lesioned model displayed behavior remarkably similar to that reported in experimental studies of prosopagnosics, showing covert without overt recognition.

Computational approaches are valuable because they provide dynamic, hypothesis-driven tests of models derived from clinical cases. Their success does not, of course, imply that the actual neural activity underlying face recognition is being accurately modeled. However, this overall approach does yield suggestive data regarding the structure of the neural architecture underlying face recognition abilities.

Recent neuromaging and electrophysiological investigations with humans and primates have also yielded important information about the neural basis of face recognition. A long tradition of electrophysiological work in the macaque has revealed populations of cells that respond selectively to faces, in some cases to particular faces (Bruce et al., 1981; Perrett et al., 1982; Baylis et al., 1985; Desimone, 1991). These findings have led to speculation that the temporal cortex contains the hardware that supports face-specific "modules" or at least dedicated face-specific perceptual mechanisms. While this view seems widely accepted, it has been observed that lesions to these regions do not clearly produce a serious impairment in face recognition ability (Baylis et al., 1985). Nevertheless, findings from electrophysiological and functional neuroimaging studies have continued to inform and constrain cognitive models of the face recognition process.

Some electrophysiological data from humans have yielded similar results. Studies with implanted electrodes have revealed patches of cells in extrastriate visual cortex that selectively respond to faces. Interestingly, evidence suggests that these cells are intermixed with others that are not face responsive, rather than forming a localized "face region" (Allison et al., 1994). In a study of facial repetition effects, scalp potential and current density maps revealed maximum activity in the inferotemporal and fusiform gyri (from 50 to at least 250 msec), mainly on the right, for both faces and shapes, and in the hippocampus and adjacent areas (around 300 msec), specifically for faces (George et al., 1997).

There have been few electrophysiological investigations with prosopagnosic patients. In a recent study, unfamiliar faces, inverted faces, and houses were shown to a prosopagnosic and controls. The controls showed consistent early negativity (N170) at the lateral temporal electrode sites, but the prosopagnosic did not (Eimer and McCarthy, 1999). This pattern was seen only for the faces. These data were interpreted as evidence of a deficit in structural encoding of faces in the prosopagnosic patient.

Recent neuroimaging studies have generally tended to confirm suspicions about functional location of face processing learned from patient studies, though it is apparent that many studies have found lateralized (left or right) rather than bilateral activations. Andreasen et al. (1996) measured cerebral blood flow with positron emission tomography (PET) while subjects performed one of three face processing tasks: classifying faces by gender, recognizing new faces, and recognizing familiar faces. Results showed activation of the left lingual and fusiform gyri during recognition of familiar, but not new, faces. A more recent study found greater activation in the right lingual and fusiform gyri when performing a familiar face recognition task than when performing a gender classification task (Kim et al., 1999). McIntosh and colleagues (1994) performed a network analysis of regions activated during face matching and dot–location matching and found greatest activity in right occipitotemporal regions for faces and in occipitoparietal regions for dot location. The functional network in the left hemisphere did not differ for the two tasks. One exception to the preponderance of unilateral activations (Sergent et al., 1992) reported that face–gender categorization resulted in activation changes in the right extrastriate cortex, and a face–identity condition produced additional activation of the fusiform gyrus and anterior temporal cortex of both hemispheres, and of the right parahippocampal gyrus and adjacent areas. Areas within the fusiform gyrus appear to be consistently active in many functional imaging studies of face recognition ability (Kanwisher et al., 1996, 1998).

The studies reviewed above could be taken to mean that tasks requiring the identification of familiar faces typically involve activation of occpititotemporal regions and associated structures that are normally involved in initial perceptual processing and encoding. Evidence that the situation is, in fact, far more complex is provided by a recent PET study (Haxby et al., 1996) that evaluated neural substrates of encoding and retrieval of new faces. A region in the right hippocampus and adjacent cortex was activated during memory encoding but not during recognition. The most striking finding in neocortex was the lateralization of prefrontal participation. Encoding activated left prefrontal cortex, whereas recognition activated right prefrontal cortex. These results suggest that face recognition is not mediated simply by recapitulation of operations performed at the time of encoding but, rather, involves regions that are anatomically distant from initial processing zones.

The nature of the cognitive defect(s) underlying prosopagnosia has been a matter of significant debate since the disorder was first formally described. While it is obvious that no single impairment can explain all the varieties of prosopagnosia, it has been tempting to search for a core deficit in cases in which elementary visual perception appears adequate to the task of face recognition.

Some consider prosopagnosia to be one of a number of category-specific agnosias. Although in prosopagnosia the defect in identifying individuals on the basis of their facial features is disproportionately impaired (compared, for example, to the identification of objects), the balance of available data suggests that, in most cases, impairment in recognizing other classes of objects co-exists with the face agnosia. Doubt is cast on a purely category-specific view by reports of prosopagnosics who concurrently lost the ability to recognize specific chairs (Faust, 1955) or automobiles (Lhermitte and Pillon, 1975). Bornstein and colleagues have reported two prosopagnosics, one a birdwatcher, the other a farmer, who concurrently lost the ability to recognize individual birds or cows, respectively (Bornstein and Kidron, 1959; Bornstein, 1963; Bornstein et al., 1969). Additional issues regarding the concept of category specificity are discussed below.

Another view is that prosopagnosia represents a limited form of amnesia. This hypothesis is supported by findings that patients with prosopagnosia cannot learn and remember new faces, because the causative lesions partially or completely disconnect vision from limbic structures important to initial encoding and storage of information (Ross, 1980a; Bauer, 1982). The basic idea is that the structural representations of faces that result from visual inspection cannot be matched to stored representations built up from past experience. However, doubt is cast on this view by the fact that many patients with complete visual–limbic disconnection (particularly those with anterior temporal lesions) or diencephalic pathology (e.g., alcoholic Korsakoff's syndrome) are not prosopagnosic, if one adopts the reasonable definition that a selective face recognition defect in the retrograde compartment must be present. In amnesic states, the impairment in both anterograde and retrograde memory is almost never absolute; such patients have a clinically significant defect in learning new information and in retrieving from the remote store, yet some new learning and remote recall is invariably possible and is accompanied by at least some degree of judged confidence or familiarity. In most forms of acquired amnesia, there is a relative preservation of remote memory, whereas in prosopagnosia, the recognition of remotely learned faces (friends, family members) is particularly impaired (Meadows, 1974b). In prosopagnosia, the impairment in face recognition is characteristically abolute and inspection of faces yields no subjective familiarity with the viewed person. Finally, most prosopagnosics, unlike amnesics, have significant perceptual dysfunction, including impairment in gestalt processing, and apparent defects in analyzing low spatial frequency components of faces (Sergent and Villemure, 1989).

One prominent view is that the underlying defect prevents the identification of individual items within a class of objects that are visually similar (Damasio et al., 1982). According to this view, recognition proceeds normally at the superordinate level (i.e., the patient concludes correctly that she is looking at a face) but breaks down at subordinate levels. Several relevant factors, including the similarity in physical structure among facial exemplars, the number of faces one must recognize, and familiarity with specific exemplars, can influence recognition in such a way as to make it appear category-specific (Damasio et al., 1990).

One study (Farah et al., 1995a) questioned this view by showing that a prosopagnosic patient had more difficulty recognizing faces than that in recognizing objects, even when the two tasks were equated for difficulty. This finding is relevant to the question of whether faces are special or unique as an object category, and the related issue of whether the brain has evolved a special-purpose module for face recognition. Evidence for a special-purpose face processor comes from the single-unit studies described above and from behavioral research showing unique perceptual effects found only with faces. The best example of the latter type of evidence is the "face inversion effect" (Yin, 1969; Valentine, 1988a). Compared to upright faces, recognizing and discriminating upside-down faces is much harder for normal subjects, and appears to proceed using different visual processes. This vastly inferior performance with inverted faces has been taken to suggest the presence of specialized recognition processes (or at least the development of special expertise) for upright faces. It has been reported that prosopagnosics may not show a normal face inversion effect, and, in fact, may show better performance with upside-down faces (i.e., an "inversion superiority effect"; Farah et al., 1995b). While this finding has been taken as support for the existence of a specialized face processor, a subsequent report (de Gelder et al., 1998) found an inversion superiority effect for faces and shoes in a prosopagnosic patient. Thus, the debate about whether face recognition is unique has not yet been fully resolved, though a likely answer to this important question is that face recognition involves some unique abilities that do not completely overlap with other visual recognition abilities (Yin, 1970).

Category-Specific Recognition Defects

Before leaving the topic of visual agnosia, it is important to mention several recent cases in which visual recognition disorders appear to be limited to a specific semantic category or class

of objects (Warrington and Shallice, 1984; Warrington and McCarthy, 1987; Farah et al., 1989; Damasio et al., 1990; Farah, 1991). As indicated earlier, questions regarding category specificity arise in the context of evaluating the significance of other selective forms of agnosia such as prosopagnosia. Although some prosopagnosics have a relatively pure face recognition defect (De Renzi, 1986a), others have difficulty in recognizing objects in other semantic classes, such as animals (Bornstein and Kidron, 1959; Damasio et al., 1982), plants (Shuttleworth et al., 1982), or foods (Damasio et al. 1982; Michel et al., 1986). When these problems have been considered together, it has been suggested that a supercategorical defect in recognizing living things might be involved (see Farah et al., 1991), reflecting primary neural organization along an animate–inanimate dimension (Caramazza and Shelton, 1998). However, it is unclear how other category-specific deficits involving, for example, musical instruments (Gainotti and Silveri, 1996), medical implements (Crosson et al., 1997), or cars (Forde et al., 1997) can be accommodated in this framework (Dixon, 2000; Dixon et al., 2000).

Two general explanations for such category specificity have been offered. One is that these disorders represent localized impairment in a semantic system that is organized according to conceptual categories. Another view suggests that living things are more visually complex (Gloning et al., 1970), are more visually similar to each other (Forde et al., 1997), or require for identification more specific names than do nonliving things (see Farah et al., 1991). The former explanation suggests that a selective disruption in the recognition of living things reveals something basic about the structure of semantic memory; the latter implies that such selective disruption results from task, processing, or response factors that have been confounded in the usual clinical tasks of object recognition (Dixon, 2000).

With these alternative explanations in mind, Farah et al. (1991) devised a series of object naming tasks that took account of visual complexity, interitem similarity, and response specificity (e.g., "table" vs. "picnic table") and gave them to two patients who became agnosic after sustaining severe closed head injury. They found that, despite efforts to control for these variables, living things remained selectively impaired relative to nonliving things. Their data do not allow them to specifically discern the locus of impairment (i.e., whether it is in a categorically organized semantic system or within a modularly organized visual system specialized for the recognition of living things), but they concluded that some level of visual or semantic representations specific to living things appeared to be involved.

The patient P.S.D. reported by Damasio et al. (1990) showed a similar, though apparently more complicated dissociation. This patient was able to visually recognize man-made tools, though his recognition of most "natural" stimuli was less than 30% accurate. At the same time, he showed normal recognition of some natural stimuli (e.g., body parts) and poor recognition of some man-made stimuli (e.g., musical instruments).

Recently, computational models have been applied to the problem of category specificity in visual recognition and naming (Farah and McClelland, 1991; Small et al., 1995; Devlin et al., 1998). In these accounts, stimuli are represented by sets of perceptual features that are then lesioned in an attempt to produce results analogous to human neurological syndromes. Although a detailed review of these models is beyond the scope of this chapter, the basic result that emerges from these simulations is that damage to feature-based computational models can accurately simulate category-specific naming and recognition deficits without having to postulate hierarchical or categorical organization within the semantic system itself.

AUDITORY AGNOSIA

The term *auditory agnosia* refers to the impaired capacity to recognize sounds in the presence of otherwise adequate hearing as measured by standard audiometry. The term has been used in a broad sense to refer to impaired capacity to recognize both speech and nonspeech sounds, and in a more narrow sense to refer to a selective deficit in the recognition of nonverbal sounds only. If one uses the broader definition, then the disorder is further subdi-

vided into auditory sound agnosia, auditory verbal agnosia, and a mixed group with deficits in both speech and nonspeech sounds. We prefer the more narrow definition, and will discuss pure word deafness (a selective impairment in speech-sound recognition) and auditory agnosia (selective impairment in recognizing nonspeech sounds) separately. The term *cortical deafness* generally has been applied to those patients whose daily activities and auditory behavior indicate an extreme lack of awareness of auditory stimuli of any kind, and whose audiometric pure tone thresholds are markedly abnormal. *Receptive* (sensory) *amusia* refers to loss of the ability to appreciate various characteristics of heard music. *Phonagnosia* refers to the loss of the ability to recognize familiar persons by voice.

Cortical Auditory Disorder and Cortical Deafness

In the large majority of cases, impairment of nonverbal sound recognition is accompanied by some degree of impairment in the recognition of speech sounds. The relative severity of these impairments may reflect premorbid lateralization of linguistic and nonlinguistic processes in the individual patient, and may depend upon which hemisphere is more seriously, or primarily, damaged (Ulrich, 1978). Terminologic confusion has arisen with regard to these "mixed" forms, with such terms as "cortical auditory disorder" (Kanshepolsky et al., 1973; Miceli, 1982), "auditory agnosia" (Oppenheimer and Newcombe, 1978; Rosati et al., 1982), "auditory agnosia and word deafness" (Goldstein et al., 1975), and "congenital aphasia" (Landau and Kleffner, 1957; Landau et al., 1960) all being used to describe similar phenomena. We will refer to these mixed forms as "cortical auditory disorders," and will discuss them together with cortical deafness. Cortical auditory disorders frequently evolve from a state of cortical deafness and, as we shall see, it is often difficult to define a clear separation between the two.

Patients with these disorders have difficulty recognizing auditory stimuli of many kinds, verbal and nonverbal (Vignolo, 1969; Lhermitte et al., 1971). Aphasic signs, if present, are mild, and do not prevent the patient from recognizing with incoming information provided audition is not required. Difficulties in temporal auditory analysis and localization of sounds in space are common. These disorders are rare, and their underlying neuroanatomic basis is poorly understood (Rosati et al., 1982). Some case reports have questioned the distinctive nature of "true" cortical deafness (Vignolo, 1969; Lhermitte et al., 1971; Kanshepolsky et al., 1973).

Distinguishing between cortical deafness and auditory agnosia continues to be problematic. It has been suggested that a diagnosis of cortical deafness requires a demonstration that brainstem auditory evoked responses are normal, but cortical evoked potentials are not (Coslett et al., 1984). One distinction which is frequently cited is that cortically deaf patients feel deaf and seem to be so, whereas auditory agnosics insist that they are not deaf (Michel et al., 1980). This turns out to be a poor criterion. Although it was originally believed that bilateral cortical lesions involving the primary auditory cortex resulted in total hearing loss, evidence from animal experiments (Neff, 1961; Massopoust and Wolin, 1967), cortical mapping of the auditory area (Celesia, 1976), and clinicopathological studies in humans (Wohlfart et al., 1952; Mahoudeau et al., 1956) indicate that complete destruction of primary auditory cortex does not lead to substantial permanent loss of audiometric sensitivity. It is more likely, however, for an asymptomatic patient with old unilateral temporal lobe pathology to suddenly become totally deaf with the occurrence of a second contralateral lesion in the auditory region.

A neuroanatomic distinction between cortical deafness and auditory cortical disorders has been tentatively offered by Michel et al. (1980). Recognizing the hazards of such a dichotomy, they distinguish between lesions of auditory koniocortex (41–52 of Brodmann) and lesions of pro- and para-konio cortex (22, 52 of Brodmann), respectively. While this distinction may prove useful, naturally occurring lesions do not typically obey architectonic boundaries (Michel et al., 1980).

In their article on cortical deafness, Michel et al. (1980) considered the possibility that the two syndromes could be differentiated on the basis of auditory evoked potentials (AEPs). Several studies (e.g., Jerger et al., 1969; Michel et al., 1980) have found either totally absent cortical AEPs or absent late components of AEP in patients with cortical auditory disorders. However, AEPs have been found to be present in other cases (Albert et al., 1972 [pure word deafness]; Assal and Despland, 1973 [auditory agnosia]), and in at least one case of cortical deafness (Adams et al., 1977), normal late AEPs were found. While results to date are conflicting, this remains a promising area of research. Such variability may be due in part to differing pathologies and recording methods. Michel et al. (1980) offer methodological suggestions designed to increase comparability among patients.

Cortical deafness is most commonly seen in bilateral cerebrovascular disease in which the course is commonly biphasic with a transient deficit (often aphasia and hemiparesis) related to unilateral damage followed by a second deficit associated with sudden transient total deafness (Jerger et al., 1969, 1972; Adams et al., 1977; Earnest et al., 1977; Leicester, 1980). A biphasic course is also typical of cases of auditory cortical disorder.

In cortical deafness, bilateral destruction of the auditory radiations or the primary auditory cortex has been a constant finding (Leicester, 1980). The anatomic basis of auditory cortical disorder is more variable. Although lesions can be quite extensive (see Oppenheimer and Newcombe, 1978), the superior temporal gyrus (i.e., efferent connections of Heschl's gyrus) is frequently involved. Several recent cases (Motomura et al., 1986; Kazui et al., 1990; Nishioka et al., 1993) suggest that generalized auditory agnosia can result from relatively circumscribed bilateral subcortical lesions that impinge upon the auditory radiations.

Pure Word Deafness (Auditory Agnosia for Speech, Auditory Verbal Agnosia)

Patients with pure word deafness are unable to comprehend spoken language although they can read, write, and speak in a relatively normal manner (Buchman et al., 1986; Ackermann and Mathiak, 1999). By definition, comprehension of nonverbal sounds is relatively spared. The syndrome is "pure" in the sense that it is relatively free of aphasic symptoms found with other disorders affecting language comprehension such as Wernicke's and transcortical sensory aphasia. The disorder was first described by Kussmaul (1877). Lichteim (1885) defined the disorder as "the inability to understand spoken words as an isolated deficit unaccompanied by disturbance of spontaneous speech or by severe disturbance in writing or understanding of the printed word." He used the term "subcortical sensory aphasia," and postulated a subcortical interruption of fibers from both ascending auditory projections to the left auditory word center. With few exceptions, pure word deafness has been associated with bilateral, symmetric cortical–subcortical lesions involving the anterior part of the superior temporal gyri with some sparing of Heschl's gyrus, particularly on the left. Some patients have unilateral lesions located subcortically in the dominant temporal lobe, presumably destroying the ipsilateral auditory radiation as well as callosal fibers from the contralateral auditory region (e.g., Liepmann and Storch, 1902; Schuster and Taterka, 1926; Kanter et al., 1986). Cases of word deafness after right hemisphere lesions (Roberts et al., 1987; Kitayama, Yamazaki et al., 1990; Bhaskaran et al., 1998) are quite rare and may be related to alterations in cerebral dominance. The neuroanatomic substrate is generally conceived, from a functional point of view, as a bilateral disconnection of Wernicke's area from auditory input (Geschwind, 1965; Hécaen and Albert, 1978). The low incidence of pure word deafness is explained by the fact that it takes an unusually placed, circumscribed lesion of the superior temporal gyrus to involve Heschl's gyrus or its connections and still selectively spare Wernicke's area.

Cerebrovascular disease is by far the most common cause of pure word deafness, though a recent case suggested neurodegenerative pathology (Otsuki et al., 1998). Developmental auditory verbal agnosia coincident with seizures or retardation is also a recognized syndrome in child neurology (Gascon et al., 1973; Rapin et al., 1977; Cooper and Ferry, 1978; Lamberts, 1980). The adult patient, when first seen, may be recovering from cortical deafness (Mendez and Geehan, 1988) or from a full-blown Wernicke's aphasia, though occasionally pure word deafness may actually give way to a Wernicke's aphasia (Ziegler, 1952; Klein and Harper, 1956; Gazzaniga et al., 1973; Albert and Bear, 1974). As the paraphasias and reading disturbances disappear, the patient still does not comprehend spoken language but can communicate by writing. Deafness can be ruled out by normal pure-tone thresholds on audiometry. At this stage, the patient may experience auditory hallucinations or exhibit transient euphoric (Shoumaker et al., 1977) or paranoid (Reinhold, 1950) ideation. The inability to repeat speech stimuli that are not comprehended distinguishes pure word deafness, generally viewed as a disturbance at the perceptual–discriminative level (Jerger et al., 1969; Kanshepolsky et al., 1973), from transcortical sensory aphasia in which word sounds are perceived normally, but in which sound is estranged from meaning. The absence of florid paraphasia and of reading and writing disruption distinguishes the disorder from Wernicke's aphasia. This having been said, it should be recognized that aphasic and agnosic symptoms may occasionally be difficult to separate in the individual case.

Many patients complain of dramatic, sometimes aversive, changes in their subjective experience of speech (dysacusis; see Mendez and Geehan, 1988). The patient with pure word deafness may complain that speech is muffled or sounds like a foreign language. Hemphill and Stengel's patient (1940) stated that "voices come but no words." The patient of Klein and Harper (1956) described speech as "an undifferentiated continuous humming noise without any rhythm" and "like foreigners speaking in the distance." Albert and Bear's (1974) patient said "words come too quickly," and, "they sound like a foreign language." The speech of these patients may contain occasional word-finding pauses and paraphasias and is often slightly louder than normal. Performance on speech perception tests is very inconsistent and highly dependent upon context (Caplan, 1978) and the linguistic structure of the material (Auerbach et al., 1982). Patients do much better when they are aware of the category under discussion, or when they can lip-read. Comprehension often drops suddenly when the topic is changed. Words embedded in sentences are more easily identified than are isolated words. Slowing the presentation rate of words in sentences sometimes facilitates comprehension.

Most studies of patients with pure word deafness have emphasized the role of auditory–perceptual processing in the genesis of the disorder (Jerger et al., 1969; Kansepolsky et al., 1973; Albert and Bear, 1976; Auerbach et al., 1982; Mendez and Geehan, 1988). Temporal resolution (Albert and Bear, 1974), and phonemic discrimination (Chocholle et al., 1975; Denes and Semenza, 1975; Saffran et al., 1976; Nakakoshi et al., 2001) have also received attention. In an exceptionally detailed case report and literature review, Auerbach et al. (1982) suggest that the disorder may take two forms: (1) a prephonemic temporal auditory acuity disturbance associated with bilateral temporal lesions, or (2) a disorder of phonemic discrimination attributable to left temporal lesions.

Albert and Bear (1974) suggested that the problem in pure word deafness is one of temporal resolution of auditory stimuli rather than specific phonetic impairment. Their patient demonstrated abnormally long click-fusion thresholds (time taken to perceive two clicks as one), and improved in auditory comprehension when speech was presented at slower rates. This may lessen the impact of abnormally slow temporal auditory analysis or may allow the patient to reconstruct the message strategically (Neisser, 1967). Saffran and colleagues (1976) showed, however, that informing their patient of the nature of the topic under discussion (indicating the category of words to be presented or giving the patient a multiple-choice array just before presentation of words) significantly facilitated comprehension. Words embedded in a sentence were better recognized, particularly when they occurred in the latter part of the sentence. Whereas a temporal auditory acuity disorder was likely present in Albert and Bear's (1974) patient, the patient of Saffran et al. (1976) displayed linguistic discrimination deficits that appeared to be independent of a disorder in temporal auditory acuity.

Several studies have reported brainstem and cortical auditory evoked responses in patients with pure word deafness (see Michel et al., 1980, for review). Brainstem evoked potentials are almost universally reported as normal, suggesting normal processing up to the level of the auditory radiations (Albert and Bear, 1974; Stockard and Rossiter, 1977; Auerbach et al., 1982). Results from studies of cortical AEPs are more variable, probably consistent with variable pathology (Auerbach et al., 1982). For example, the patient of Jerger et al. (1969) had no appreciable AEP, yet heard sounds. The patient of Auerbach et al. (1982) showed normal P1, N1, and P2 to right ear stimulation, but minimal response over either hemisphere to left ear stimulation. A recent study measuring auditory evoked magnetic fields (Makino et al., 1998) revealed no N100 m detected in the left temporal lobe with right ear stimulation in two patients with putaminal hemorrhages—one bilateral, the other only on the left. However, in both cases, normal N100 m was obtained in the right hemisphere with left ear stimulation. The location of the equivalent current dipole (ECD) of the intact N100 m in the right hemisphere was superimposed on the Heschl gyrus on brain magnetic resonance imaging (MRI). These results are consistent with the disconnection view of pure word deafness.

On tests of phonemic discrimination, patients with bilateral lesions tend to show distinctive deficits for the feature of place of articulation (Naeser, 1974; Chocholle et al., 1975; Auerbach et al., 1982). Those with unilateral left hemisphere disease showed either impaired discrimination for voicing (Saffran et al., 1976) or no distinctive pattern (Denes and Semeneza, 1975).

On dichotic listening, some patients show extreme suppression of right ear perception (Albert and Bear, 1974; Saffran et al., 1976), which suggests the inaccessibility of the left hemisphere phonetic decoding areas (Wernicke's area) to auditory material that has already been acoustically processed by the right hemisphere. However, the patient of Auerbach et al. (1982) showed marked left ear extinction, which the authors attribute to spared auditory processing in the left temporal lobe.

Patients with pure word deafness perform relatively well with environmental sounds, although the appreciation of music is sometimes disturbed (Buchman et al., 1986). Some patients may recognize foreign languages by their distinctive prosodic characteristics, and others can recognize *who* is speaking, but not what is said; this suggests preserved ability to comprehend paralinguistic aspects of speech. Coslett and colleagues (1984) described a word-deaf patient who showed a remarkable dissociation between the comprehension of neutral and affectively intoned sentences. He was asked to point to pictures of males and females depicting various emotional expressions. When verbal instructions were given in a neutral voice, he performed poorly. When instructions were given with affective intonations appropriate to the target face, he performed significantly better and at a level commensurate to his performance with written instructions. This patient had bilateral destruction of primary auditory cortex with some sparing of auditory association cortex, which suggests at least some direct contribution of the auditory radiations directly to the latter without initial decoding in Heschl's gyrus (Coslett et al., 1984). These authors speculate that one reason why patients with pure word deafness improve their auditory comprehension with lipreading is that face-to-face contact allows them to take advantage of visual cues (gesture and facial expression) that are processed by different brain systems. An alternative explanation is that lipreading provides information about place of articulation, a linguistic feature that is markedly impaired at least in the bilateral cases (Auerbach et al., 1982). In either instance, the finding of preserved comprehension of paralinguistic aspects of speech further reinforces the notion that comprehension of speech and nonspeech sounds may represent dissociable abilities.

There is evidence that unilateral left-sided lesions, particularly those producing Wernicke's aphasia with impaired auditory comprehension, are also associated with impaired ability to match nonverbal sounds with pictures (Vignolo, 1969). However, resulting errors are almost exclusively semantic, not acoustic, and thus do not suggest that unilateral left hemispheric temporal lobe damage produces a perceptual–discriminative sound recognition disturbance. For this reason, the finding of impaired ability to discriminate nonverbal speech

sounds in a patient with pure word deafness suggests bilateral disease, even in the absence of other neurological evidence of bilaterality. Since many of these patients have, by history, successive strokes, the primary and secondary side of damage may be important in producing a picture dominated either by pure word deafness or by auditory sound agnosia (Ulrich, 1978).

Although distinctions have been made between basic defects in auditory perception and defects in linguistic processing, few studies of pure word deafness have analyzed the defect in terms of the apperceptive–associative distinction so prominent in discussing visual agnosia (Polster and Rose, 1998). It has been suggested that word deafness may represent the apperceptive counterpart of a very rare and ill-defined disorder called "pure word meaning deafness," in which the patient can hear and repeat words, but does not know their meaning (Corballis, 1994; Franklin et al., 1996).

Auditory Sound Agnosia (Auditory Agnosia for Nonspeech Sounds)

Auditory agnosia for nonspeech sounds is by far more rare than pure word deafness. This may be because such patients are less likely to seek medical advice than those with a disorder of speech comprehension, and also because nonspecific auditory complaints may be discounted when pure tone audiometric and speech discrimination thresholds are normal. This is unfortunate, since normal or near-normal audiometric evaluation does not rule out the possible role played by primary auditory perceptual defects (Goldstein, 1974; Buchtel and Stewart, 1989).

Vignolo (1969) argued that there may be two forms of auditory sound agnosia: *(1)* a perceptual-discriminative type associated mainly with right hemisphere lesions involving Brodmann's areas 41, 42, and 52, and *(2)* an associative-semantic type associated with lesions of the left hemisphere involving Brodmann's areas 37 and 20, and closely linked to Wernicke's aphasia. This anatomic distinction is by no means settled. The former group makes predominantly acoustic (e.g., "man whistling" for birdsong) errors on picture–

sound matching tasks, while the latter group makes predominantly semantic (e.g., "train" for automobile engine) errors. This division follows the original classification of Kliest (1928), who distinguished between the ability to perceive isolated sounds or noises and the inability to understand the meaning of sounds. It also resembles the apperceptive–associative dichotomy made by Lissauer (1890). In the verbal sphere, the analogous distinction is between pure word deafness (perceptual-discriminative) and transcortical sensory aphasia (semantic-associative).

Few stable cases of "pure" auditory sound agnosia have been reported in the literature (Nielsen and Sult, 1939; Wortis and Pfeffer, 1948; Spreen et al., 1965; Albert et al., 1972; Fujii et al., 1990; Schnider et al., 1994). Sometimes a patient evolves into auditory sound agnosia from a more generalized agnosia for both verbal and nonverbal sounds (Motomura et al., 1986), and occasionally a patient evolves from an auditory sound agnosia into an auditory recognition defect that encompasses speech sounds and other auditory stimuli (Kaga, 1999). The patient of Spreen et al. was a 65-year-old right-handed male whose major complaint when seen 3 years after a left hemiparetic episode of "nerves" and headache. Audiometric testing demonstrated moderate bilateral high-frequency loss and speech reception thresholds of 12 dB for both ears. There was no aphasia. The outstanding abnormality was the inability to recognize common sounds; understanding of language was fully retained and there were no other agnosic defects. Sound localization was normal. Scores on the pitch subtest of the Seashore Tests of Musical Talent were at chance level. The patient claimed no experience or talent with music and refused to cooperate with further testing of musical ability. The patient could match previously heard but misidentified sounds with one of four tape-recorded choices, suggesting an associative defect. Postmortem examination revealed a sharply demarcated old infarct of the right hemisphere involving the superior temporal and angular gyri, as well as a large portion of the inferior parietal, inferior and middle frontal, and long and short gyri of the insula. This case represents one of the few examples of auditory sound agnosia with unilateral pathology. The lesion is too large to allow for precise anatomicoclinical correlation. Other cases with unilateral pathology include those reported by Fujii et al. (small posterior right temporal hemorrhagic lesion that involved the middle and superior temporal gyri), Nielsen and Sult (right thalamus and parietal lobe), and Wortis and Pfeffer (large lesion of the right temporoparietal–occipital junction). The case reported by Fujii et al. (1990) is informative because he was completely free of aphasic symptoms and his lesion was relatively small. In this patient, pure tone audiometry was within normal limits in spite of a 30 dB high-frequency hearing loss in the left ear. He showed marked suppression of the left ear during dichotic listening tests involving digits and words. Brainstem auditory evoked responses (BAERs) were normal and sound localization was intact. The patient was selectively impaired in identification of nonspeech sounds, and his errors consisted primarily of acoustic confusions ("sound of railroad crossing" for telephone ring). His agnosia cleared by the 16th post-stroke day.

Albert et al. (1972) described a patient with auditory sound agnosia with minimal dysphasia. Clinical evidence suggested bilateral involvement. The patient was able to attach meaning to word-sounds, but not to nonverbal sounds. Albert et al. also demonstrated marked extinction of the left ear to dichotic listening; impaired perception of pitch, loudness, rhythm, and time; and abnormally delayed and attenuated cortical AEPs, worse on the right. They concluded that the sound agnosia in their patient resulted from "an inability to establish the correspondence between the perceived sound and its sensory or motor associations" (associative defect), and suggested that the dissociation between verbal and nonverbal sound recognition in their patient reflected different processing mechanisms for linguistic and nonlinguistic aspects of acoustic input.

Sensory (Receptive) Amusia

Musical ability is a complex domain of functions in which selective impairments can occur after brain damage. Several distinct disorders have been identified, including vocal amusia, loss of skilled instrumental ability (instrumental amusia; McFarland and Fortin, 1982), loss of the ability to read write music (musical alexia and agraphia; Brust, 1980; Midorikawa and Kawamura, 2000), impaired recognition of music (receptive amusia; Procopis, 1983; Piccirilli et al., 2000; Schuppert et al., 2000), and disorders of rhythm (Berman, 1981). Analysis of the patient with reported musical impairments should take into account the multicomponential nature of musical abilities.

The subject of amusia has been reviewed in detail by Wertheim (1969), Critchley and Henson (1977), and Gates and Bradshaw (1977). *Sensory (receptive) amusia* refers to an inability to appreciate various characteristics of heard music. It occurs to some extent in all cases of auditory sound agnosia, and in most cases of aphasia and pure word deafness, but can occur independently of these other deficits (Piccirilli et al., 2000). As is the case with auditory sound agnosia, the loss of musical perceptual ability may be underreported because a specific musical disorder rarely interferes with everyday life. A major obstacle to systematic study of acquired amusia is the extreme variability of pre-illness musical abilities, interests, and skills. It was Wertheim's (1969) opinion that receptive amusia corresponds more frequently with a lesion of the left hemisphere, while expressive musical disabilities are more apt to be associated with right hemisphere dysfunction. Recent evidence indicates that cerebral organization of musical ability is dependent on degree of experience, skill, and musical sophistication. Musically skilled and trained individuals may be more likely to perceive music analytically and to rely more heavily on the dominant hemisphere. Dichotic listening studies show that the right hemisphere plays a more important role than the left in the processing of musical and nonlinguistic sound patterns (Blumstein and Cooper, 1974; Gordon, 1974). However, the left hemisphere appears to be of major importance in the processing of sequential (temporally organized) material of any kind, including musical series. According to Gordon (1974), melody recognition becomes less of a right-hemisphere task as time and rhythm factors become more important for dis-

tinguishing tone patterns (see also Mavlov, 1980), although it has been argued that rhythm and interval processing may be vulnerable to right hemisphere damage (Schuppert et al., 2000). Such complexities contribute to a lack of definition of the entity of receptive amusia and the difficulty of localizing the deficit to a particular brain region. Further complicating the picture is the fact that pitch, harmony, timbre, intensity, and rhythm may be affected to different degrees and in various combinations in the individual patient. Furthermore, there is evidence that aspects of musical denotation (the-so-called real-world events referred to by lyrics) and musical connotation (the formal expressive patterns indicated by pitch, timbre, and intensity) are selectively vulnerable to focal brain lesions (Gardner et al., 1977). For instance, on tests of musical denotation, right hemisphere–damaged patients perform well on items where acquaintence with lyrics is required; in contrast, aphasics with anterior lesions perform better than both right hemisphere–damaged patients and aphasics with posterior lesions on items where knowledge of lyrics is unnecessary. (Incidentally, Benton [1980] reports that aphasics with posterior lesions and comprehension disturbance are also most impaired among aphasics on tests of face recognition, another ostensibly "configurational" task). On tests of musical connotation, right hemisphere–damaged patients do better in matching sound patterns to temporally sequenced designs than to simultaneous gestalten. Aphasics with posterior lesions perform relatively well on tests of musical connotation. Comprehensive tests of musical ability that separate these many subskills are now available (Schuppert et al., 2000).

Peretz and colleagues (1994) applied comprehensive nonverbal auditory testing to two patients with bilateral lesions of auditory cortex. In their patients, the perception of speech and environmental sounds was spared, but the perception of tunes, prosody, and voice was impaired. On the basis of these behavioral dissociations, they argue that music processing is distinct from processing of speech or environmental sounds (Piccirilli et al., 2000). Their data led them to argue for a task- and process-specific approach to the analysis of cases of auditory agnosia. They suggest that nominally auditory tasks be broken down into their functional subcomponents and that more extensive component-based analysis of auditory processing deficits is warranted. For example, they distinguish between processes involved in the recognition of specific voices or musical instruments (which are timbre-dependent), and processes involved in recognition of tunes (which are pitch-dependent). The notion that nominally distinct classes of auditory material (e.g., melodies, prosody, and voice) share common processes may be critically important in developing a functional taxonomy of auditory recognition disorders in general, and of amusia in particular (Schuppert et al., 2000).

This suggestion points out certain significant deficiencies in the evaluation of amusic patients. Although theories linking brain function to music perception have long been available (Hécaen, 1962; Bever and Chiarello, 1974), such theories do not often contain sufficient process specificity to guide the clinical evaluation of amusic patients. Thus, for example, relatively little is known about the musical features that will be most informative in constructing a neuropsychological model of music perception. Another obstacle to systematic study of acquired amusia is the variability of pre-illness musical abilities, interests, and experience (see Wertheim [1969] for a system of classifying musical ability level). The cerebral organization of musical perception has been suggested to be dependent upon on the degree of these pre-illness characteristics (Bever and Chiarello, 1974).

Paralinguistic Agnosias: Auditory Affective Agnosia and Phonagnosia

Heilman and colleagues (1975) showed that patients with right temporoparietal lesions and the neglect syndrome were impaired in the comprehension of affectively intoned speech, but showed normal comprehension of speech content. Patients with left temporoparietal lesions and fluent aphasia comprehended both affective (paralinguistic) and content (linguistic) aspects of speech normally. Whether this defect represents a true agnosia remains to be determined, since auditory sensory–perceptual

skills were not assessed. It is possible that auditory affective agnosia is a variant of auditory sound agnosia; i.e., that it represents a category-specific auditory agnosia.

Studies by Van Lancker and associates (Van Lancker and Kreiman, 1988; Van Lancker et al., 1988, 1989) have revealed another type of paralinguistic deficit after right hemisphere disease. In their studies, patients with unilateral right hemisphere disease showed deficits in discriminating and recognizing familiar voices, while patients with left hemisphere disease were impaired only on a task that required discrimination between two famous (but not personally familiar) voices. The CT evidence suggested that right parietal damage was significantly correlated with voice recognition impairment, while temporal lobe damage in either hemisphere led to deficits in voice discrimination. The authors refer to this deficit as "phonagnosia," but, like auditory affective agnosia, it remains to be seen whether it is truly agnosic in nature. A recent functional imaging study revealed that a distributed cortical network may be involved in the processing of familiar visual and vocal stimuli (Shah et al., 2001). In this fMRI study, subjects viewed familiar and unfamiliar faces and listened to personally familiar and unfamiliar voices. Changes in neural activity associated with stimulus modality irrespective of familiarity were observed in regions known to be important for face recognition (fusiform gyrus bilaterally) and voice recognition (superior temporal gyrus bilaterally), while familiarity of faces and voices (relative to unfamiliar faces and voices) was associated with increased neural activity in the posterior cingulate cortex, including the retrosplenial cortex. Although the status of these defects vis-à-vis the concept of agnosia is uncertain, the discovery of seemingly specific impairments in the comprehension of affectively intoned speech and speaker identity is important, as paralinguistic abilities may be spared in cases of pure word deafness (Coslett et al., 1984). As indicated above, patients with pure word deafness frequently report that they are able to recognize the speaker of the message and, less frequently, the language in which it is transmitted. These findings lend further support to the idea that linguistic and nonlinguistic processing of auditory signals are based on different neuropsychological mechanisms and in fact may be preferentially processed by different hemispheres. Further research is needed to provide more precise neuroanatomic correlates of auditory affective agnosia and phonagnosia.

SOMATOSENSORY AGNOSIA

Compared to visual agnosia, somatosensory (tactile) agnosias have received less attention and are poorly understood. However, it is likely that loss of higher-order tactual recognition in the absence of elementary somatosensory loss is probably at least as common as visual or auditory agnosia. Several distinct disorders have been identified, and many classifications of somatosensory agnosia have been offered. A reasonable descriptive framework was proposed by Delay (1935), who identified *(1)* impaired recognition of the size and shape of objects ("amorphognosia"), *(2)* impaired discrimination of the distinctive qualities of objects such as density, weight, texture, and thermal properties ("ahylognosia"), and *(3)* impaired recognition of the identity of objects in the absence of amorphognosia and ahylognosia ("tactile asymboly"). Delay's scheme is similar to that of Wernicke (1895), who distinguished between primary agnosia and secondary agnosia, or *asymboly*. For Wernicke, primary agnosia involved a loss of primary identification because of a destruction of "tactile images." In contrast, secondary agnosia resulted from the inability of intact tactile images to be associated with other sensory representations, resulting in a loss of appreciation of the object's significance.

The systematic study of tactile recognition disturbances has been beset by terminologic confusion. The terms *tactile agnosia* and *astereognosis* have been used interchangeably by some authors, while others draw a sharp distinction between them. *Astereognosis* has been used to denote *(1)* loss of the ability to distinguish three-dimensional forms (Hoffman, 1884; cited by Gans, 1916), *(2)* the inability to make shape or size discriminations (Roland, 1976), and *(3)* the inability to identify objects by touch (Delay, 1935). This is confusing, since Hoffman and Roland use the term to describe

discrimination defects, while Delay and others use the term to denote defects of object *identification*. It is clear that defects in two-point discrimination, point localization, and position sense can impair tactile form perception, and thus object identification without producing concomitant defects in sensitivity to light touch, temperature, or pain (Gans, 1916; Campora, 1925; Corkin, 1978). However, significant defects in discriminative ability need not accompany disorders of tactual identification (Corkin, 1978). Thus, clinical data suggest that tactile discrimination and identification are dissociable. Unfortunately, the vast majority of the physiological and anatomic data on somatosensory agnosia have come from animal research using almost exclusively discrimination, rather than identification, paradigms.

With these considerations in mind, we will use the term *cortical tactile disorders* to refer to a diverse spectrum of defects in somatosensory discrimination or recognition of distinct object qualities. We will reserve the term *tactile agnosia* for those rare cases in which there is an inability to identify the nature of tactually presented objects despite adequate sensory, attentional, intellectual, and linguistic capacities. Although debatable, we will discuss *astereognosis* as an apperceptive form of tactile agnosia, recognizing that it represents a failure of complex perceptual processing that has, as an outcome, an impairment in tactile object recognition ability.

Before discussing disorders of tactile recognition, some comments about the functional anatomy of the somatosensory systems are necessary. An exhaustive review of this vast literature will not be undertaken here; the interested reader is referred to excellent reviews by Hécaen and Albert (1978), Corkin (1978), Mountcastle and Powell (1959a, 1959b), and Werner and Whitsel (1973).

Two relatively distinct somatosensory systems have been identified. One is the spinothalamic system: cutaneous nerve endings → spinothalamic tract → reticular formation → intrinsic thalamic nuclei → superior bank of Sylvian fissure (SII) (Hécaen and Albert, 1978; Brodal, 1981). This system is primarily responsible for the less precise aspects of somesthetic perception, and seems especially important in nocioception and perception of thermal properties. The other system is centered on the medial lemniscus: cutaneous and subcutaneous receptors → medial lemniscal tract → ventroposterolateral thalamic nuclei → postcentral gyrus (SI). The postcentral gyrus corresponds to Brodmann areas 3, 1, and 2. This system appears responsible for more precise discriminative aspects of touch, and carries information regarding form, position, and temporal change (Mountcastle, 1961). The two cortical somatosensory receiving areas (SI, SII) contain complex representations (homunculi) of body parts, with SI arranged somatotopically, and SII less so. The postcentral gyrus (SI) receives innervation from contralateral body parts, while SII receives bilateral input. It should be noted that other areas of cortex, including supplementary motor area and superior parietal lobe (areas 5, 7), also receive direct input from somatosensory thalamus (Brodal, 1981).

In the sections on visual agnosia, we noted that certain visual tasks place strong motor-exploratory demands on the visual system. This motor theme is also a striking characteristic of the somatosensory system. In a report of the results of cortical stimulation during craniotomy, Penfield (1958) found significant overlap between sensory and motor regions, in that 25% of stimulation points giving rise to somatosensory experiences were located in the precentral region. Woolsey (1952) found similar results in his electrophysiological studies of the alert monkey. Because of these and related findings, it has become common to speak of the sensorimotor cortex. Anatomic interconnections of SI and SII attest to the sensorimotor nature of these regions. Both SI and SII have reciprocal connections with thalamic nuclei, supplementary motor cortex, area 4, and with each other (Hécaen and Albert, 1978; Brodal, 1981). In addition, SI projects heavily to area 5 (superior parietal lobule) (Jones and Powell, 1969a, 1969b; Corkin, 1978), which is important for motor pursuit of motivationally relevant targets in extrapersonal space (Mountcastle et al., 1975).

Thus, the functional interconnections of cortical somatosensory areas involve regions that, from numerous other studies, have been found to subserve motor, proprioceptive, and spatial functions. The existence of such a complex system in the human brain is important for intentional, spatially guided motor movements that bring us into contact with tactile stimuli. Reciprocal connections between somatosensory, motor, proprioceptive, and spatial components of the system provide the mechanisms through which regulation of the perceptual act can be achieved. The complex functional organization of the somatosensory systems underscores the idea that perception is an active process and involves more than the mere passive processing of environmental input.

Although patients with lesions of the afferent somatosensory pathways frequently cannot identify tactually presented objects, this is due to a severe sensory loss, sometimes referred to as "steroanaesthesia." Lesions of the primary visual and auditory areas produce specific disorders of sensation that can vary in severity depending on the extent and location of the lesion. Total ablation of primary visual and auditory areas results in cortical blindness or deafness, respectively. In contrast, disorders of sensation for touch, temperature, pain, and vibration are rare following cortical lesions (Hécaen and Albert, 1978). Redundancy in representation seems to be an especially important characteristic of somatosensory systems. Paul et al. (1972) explored units in anatomic subdivisions of SI, and found multiple representations of the monkey's hand, one in each subdivision (see also Mountcastle and Powell, 1959a, 1959b; Powell and Montcastle, 1959). Randolph and Semmes (1974) selectively ablated each of the SI subregions (3b, 2, 1). Area 3b excisions resulted in impairment of all aspects of tactile discrimination learning. Lesions of area 1 produced loss of hard–soft and rough–smooth (texture) discrimination, but spared complex–concave and square–diamond (shape) discriminations. The opposite pattern was seen with area 2 lesions. Thus, the hand appears to be represented and re-represented within specific subdivisions of somatosensory cortex according to sensory "submodality."

The notion of sensory submodality dates back at least to von Frey (1895), who divided the tactile sense into light touch, pressure, temperature, and pain sensitivity. Head (1918) divided sensory functions into three categories: (1) recognition of spatial relations (passive movement, two-point discrimination, and point localization), (2) relative sensitivity to touch, temperature, and pain, and (3) recognition of similarity and difference (size, shape, weight, and texture). Submodalities may be selectively impaired, while others are spared, by circumscribed cortical lesions. Head's (1918) framework, for example, suggests that discriminatory defects are accompanied by defects in the discrimination of texture and weight, but not by impaired perception of spatial relations, touch, temperature, or pain (see Corkin, 1978). On the basis of studies of recovery from peripheral nerve injuries, Head and colleagues (1905), distinguished between "protopathic" and "epicritic" sensation. The epicritic system subserves local point sensibility, while the protopathic system is more diffuse. The protopathic–epicritic distinction has been widely accepted by anatomists and physiologists (Rose and Woolsey, 1949; Mountcastle, 1961), but unlike Head, these authors have emphasized the anatomic implications of this distinction at the cortical and thalamic levels, rather than at the peripheral level (Hécaen and Albert, 1978, p. 279 ff). As implied previously, the epicritic aspects of touch are more directly subserved by the medial lemniscal–SI system, while the protopathic dimension relates more closely to the functions of the bilaterally represented SII, although there is considerable functional overlap between the two systems.

Cortical Tactile Disorders

The brief review of the somatosensory systems has been designed to emphasize the complexity of this sensory modality and to enable the reader to anticipate the enormous variability in presentation among patients suffering from tactile recognition and identification disorders. Historically, there have been two views regarding the nature and functional localization of disorders of tactile sensation. The first, more traditional, view is that sensory defects are associated with the contralateral primary somatosensory projection area in the postcentral gyrus (Head, 1920). The other perspective is that more diffuse aspects of cortex (e.g., posterior parietal lobe) are involved in somatosensory perception (Semmes et al., 1960). In a series of studies, Corkin and colleagues (Corkin, 1964; Corkin et al., 1970, 1973) administered quantitative tasks of pressure sensitivity, two-point discrimination, point localization, position sense, and tactual object recognition to patients who had been operated on for relief of focal epileptic seizures. Lesions in the contralateral post-central gyrus produced the most severe disorders of cortical tactile sensation. Also, clear demonstration was made of the existence of bilateral sensory defects associated with a unilateral cortical lesion, as had been previously reported by Semmes et al. (1960) and Oppenheim (1906).

Corkin found that the most severe defects occurred in patients whose lesions encroached on the hand area. This is consistent with the findings of Roland (1976) in his studies of tactual shape and size discrimination impairment with focal cortical lesions. Corkin et al. (1970) also found that disorders of tactual object recognition were restricted to the contralateral hand in patients with lesions that involved the hand area in SI. Importantly, defects of tactile object recognition were always associated with significant defects in pressure sensitivity, two-point discrimination, and other elementary sensory functions. Patients with parietal lobe lesions sparing SI did not show object identification disturbances.

Twenty of 50 patients with parietal lobe involvement showed additional sensory defects ipsilateral to the damaged hemisphere (Corkin et al., 1970). This effect was found with equal frequency after left and right hemisphere excisions, in contrast to previous studies that had found the incidence of ipsilateral sensory impairment to be much more frequent following left hemisphere damage (Semmes et al., 1960). Differences in the extent of lesions in the samples used by Corkin et al. (circumscribed cortical excisions) and Semmes et al. (penetrating missile wounds) may account for some of these discrepancies. An important anatomic fact is that, in patients with bilateral sensory defects of the hand, the postcentral hand area needs not be involved (Corkin et al., 1973). The area of damage implicated in these patients was tentatively offered as SII. In summarizing these data, Corkin (1978) suggested that unilateral SI hand area lesions produce severe contralateral sensory defects, while unilateral SII lesions may produce milder defects that affect both hands.

There is growing evidence of hemispheric specialization for certain higher somesthetic functions. Data on this issue can be found in cerebral laterality studies, examinations of patients following brain bisection, and in studies of performance on complex somatosensory tasks after unilateral hemispheric lesions (Milner and Taylor, 1972; Corkin, 1978; Hécaen and Albert, 1978). While laterality studies have failed to show hemispheric specialization for elementary somesthetic functions such as pressure sensitivity (Fennell et al., 1967), vibration sensitivity (Seiler and Ricker, 1971; cited in Corkin, 1978), two-point discrimination (McCall and Cunningham, 1971), or point localization (Semmes et al., 1960; Weinstein, 1968), results of complex sensory tasks requiring spatial exploration of figures or fine temporal analysis reveal evidence of hemispheric specialization. The left hand–right hemisphere combination appears especially proficient at tasks in which a spatial factor is important, such as in ciphering braille (Rudel et al., 1974) or perceiving the spatial orientation of tactually presented rods (Benton et al., 1973). Results from studies of split-brain patients (reviewed in detail by Corkin, 1978) are consistent with these conclusions; the left hand–right hemisphere combination is better able to perform complex, spatially patterned discriminations, although the right hand–left hemisphere can succeed if familiar stimuli are presented, if a small array of objects is involved, or in other situations in which linguistic processing can be effectively used (Milner and Taylor, 1972).

Thus, patients with right hemisphere disease do worse than left hemisphere–damaged patients on tasks requiring the perception of complexly organized spatial stimuli, although any patient with elementary somatosensory dysfunction, regardless of hand, can be expected to do poorly with that hand (Corkin, 1978). Semmes (1965) has identified a group of patients without primary sensory tactile impairment who fail tests of object–shape discrimination. These patients were unimpaired

in roughness, texture, and size discrimination, but showed profound impairments on tests of spatial orientation and route finding. These patients suffered from lesions of the superior parietal lobe. Semmes concluded that there is a "non-tactual" factor in these discriminative defects that transcended sensory modality. According to her view, what is spatial for vision is represented in touch by the temporal exploration of object qualities. Teuber (1965a, 1965b) interpreted the difficulty as a special form of spatial disorientation, rather than one of "agnosia for shape."

To summarize, no hemispheric specialization appears to exist for elementary somatosensory function, although there is growing evidence that the right hemisphere is more strongly involved in processing the highly spatial character of some tactile discrimination and identification tasks. Postcentral gyrus lesions frequently result in severe and long-lasting defects in using the contralateral hand, while lesions of SII result in less severe, bilateral defects. A general conclusion from this extensive and complex literature is that the central regions (so-called sensorimotor cortex) are more directly involved in elementary somatosensory function, while complex somatosensory tasks possessing strong spatial or motor exploratory components involve additional structures posterior or anterior to the sensorimotor region (Corkin, 1978). This distinction makes it possible to see a higher somatosensory disorder in the absence of elementary sensory loss. Whether this higher disorder deserves to be called an "agnosia" is a subject to which we now turn.

Tactile Agnosia

The patient with tactile agnosia cannot appreciate the nature or significance of objects placed in the hand despite elementary somatosensory function, intellectual ability, attentional capacity, and linguistic skill adequate to the task of object identification. The terms *astereognosis* and *pure astereognosis* have been sometimes used synonymously with tactile agnosia, and sometimes used to describe basic defects in the appreciation of size, shape, and texture. Delay (1935) asserted that astereognosis was a complex disorder comprised of amorphognosis, ahylognosis, *and* tactile agnosia. In our view, astereognosis, as it has been described in the literature, essentially refers to "apperceptive tactile agnosia." We will use the term in this fashion, and will reserve the term *tactile agnosia* for cases in which a deficit of tactile object recognition exists without concomitant sensory–perceptual defects.

Clinical case reports of pure astereognosis are rare (Raymond and Egger, 1906; Bonhoeffer, 1918; Campora, 1925; Hécaen and David, 1945; Newcombe and Ratcliff, 1974). Frequently, obvious sensory defects do appear at some point in the clinical course of these patients, though not necessarily coincident with the identification disturbance. The astereognosic patient frequently has defects limited to one hand, usually the left, although patients with defects limited to the right hand have been reported (Hécaen and David, 1945). In some cases, the asymbolic hand can eventually achieve recognition of the object, but only after protracted linguistic analysis of the separate features.

Many astereognosic patients do not normally palpate the object when it is placed in the hand for identification (Oppenheim, 1906; 1911). This suggests a defect in the mechanism through which tactile impressions are collected to form an integrated percept of the whole object, or a defect in stored structural tactile representations. Motor and sensory information is highly integrated in the act of palpating an object; motor commands are issued that direct the hand in ongoing exploration. In a series of experiments using regional cerebral blood flow (rCBF) during astereognostic testing in humans, Roland and Larsen (1976), have shown that local rCBF increases occur most strongly in the contralateral sensorimotor hand area and the premotor region. Although sensorimotor integration and proprioception are crucial components in tactile identification, it should be noted that the motor component probably has a complex role and is not obligatory in any simple sense. This conclusion is warranted by two clinical facts: *(1)* motor paralysis does not necessarily cause tactile identification disturbances (Caselli, 1991b), and *(2)* objects can often be identified if they are passively moved across the subject's hand, independent of active manipulation. Still, the fact that true astereognosics do not palpate objects suggests that elementary sensory function is not actively brought to bear, nor is it adequately integrated with motor information, in the perceptual processing of the stimulus.

Evidence for an associative defect exists when elementary somatosensory defects are either absent or too mild to account for a tactile object recognition disturbance and when the patient can draw or match tactually presented stimuli. For example, the patient of Hécaen and David (1945) who could not name an object placed in the hand could draw an accurate picture of the object and could then name the picture. The patients of Newcombe and Ratcliff (1974) could tactually match to sample, even though they had a disturbance in recognition of the nature of objects.

As in other forms of agnosia, there has been significant debate regarding the existence of true tactile agnosia. Three general disclaimers have been proposed. The first is the familiar argument that all disturbances of tactile object identification can be traced to defects of elementary somatosensory dysfunction. The second states that the defect is not an agnosia, but instead represents a modality-specific anomia. Third, there are those who do not deny the existence of higher defects of tactile identification in the context of normal elementary somatosensory function, but say that the defect of function in astereognosis is spatial and supramodal, involving both tactile and visual disturbances. Because one of the hallmarks of the agnosia concept is its modality specificity, this third view rejects the notion that tactile object identification disturbances are agnosic in nature. Each of these views is capable of handling some, but not all, of the data. We will briefly examine the status of each of these arguments below.

The possible role of subtle somatosensory defects in producing disorders of tactile identification has been raised by several authors (Head and Holmes, 1911; Bay, 1944; Corkin et al., 1970). Bay (1944) stated that most putative cases of tactile agnosia had been inadequately tested for elementary somatosensory dysfunction, and specifically implicated labile thresholds and defects in performing complex sensory discriminations. Head and Holmes (1911) also stressed the importance of inconstant thresholds, and found that rapid local fatigue and abnormal persistence of sensations frequently accompanied defects of tactile object identification. Semmes (1953) mentioned the possible contributory role of tactile extinction revealed by the method of double simultaneous stimulation, and stated that "if one stimulus extinguishes or obscures the perception of another, or displaces the subjective position, the resultant impression might be sufficiently different from normal perception to make recognition impossible" (p. 144). In a recent study, somatosensory evoked potentials were measured as an index of early sensory–perceptual function and were found to be abnormal in every case of putative tactile agnosia (Mauguiere and Isnard, 1995).

Most studies fail to evaluate elementary sensory function to effectively refute the sensory argument. One exception is a careful study by Caselli (1991b) that examined tactile object recognition (TOR) disturbances in 84 patients with a variety of peripheral and CNS diseases. Using an extensive battery of tests of somatosensory function and two tests of TOR, Caselli found a number of patients who, despite normal or only mildly compromised somatosensory function, had disproportionate TOR impairment. According to Caselli, this type of impairment can result from unilateral damage (in either hemisphere) involving parietotemporal cortices, possibly affecting SII. Hécaen (1972) paid careful attention to somatosensory function in examining his agnosic patient, finding neither lability of threshold nor sensory perseveration. Although only one hand was agnosic, tactile discrimination, touch, and thickness discrimination were equal in both hands. There did appear to be a subtle defect in shape discrimination in the affected hand, as the patient could not accurately judge a series of objects on a continuum from ovoid to sphere, but, like many of Caselli's patients, this defect seemed insufficient in severity to account for the TOR disturbance. Delay (1935) found no differences between the hands for pain, temperature, pressure, kinesthesis, or vibration sense, although tactile localization and position sense were poorer in the affected hand (see Hécaen and Albert, 1978). Nakamura et al. (1998) found a bilateral impairment in rec-

ognizing palpated objects despite normal hylogonosis and morphognosis. This case had bilateral subcortical angular gyrus lesions, leading the authors to speculate that there was a bilateral disconnection of the somatosensory regions from semantic memory (Endo et al., 1992; Nakamura et al., 1998). Thus, there are cases in which defects in elementary somatosensory function cannot fully account for the observed defects in object identification.

Although the existence of tactile agnosia seems now established, the possibility that a modality-specific anomia might account for some instances of TOR impairment is raised by the remarkable patient of Geschwind and Kaplan (1962). This patient underwent surgical extirpation of a left hemisphere glioblastoma and postoperatively developed a left anterior cerebral artery infarction involving the anterior four-fifths of the corpus callosum. He was unable to name or to supply verbal descriptions of items placed in his left hand but could draw misidentified objects with the left hand and could tactually choose a previously presented object from a larger group.

It is important to emphasize the differences between Geschwind and Kaplan's patient and other patients with deficient tactile object identification. First, because their patient could demonstrate recognition nonverbally, the defect was not a tactile agnosia in the true sense, but instead represented a disconnection of right hemisphere (left hand) tactual input from the speech area in the left hemisphere. Second, their patient, who had bilateral lesions, demonstrated an object naming defect confined to the left hand (see also Geschwind and Kaplan, 1962; Gazzaniga et al., 1963; Gazzaniga and Sperry, 1967; Lhermitte et al., 1976; McKeever et al., 1981; Watson and Heilman, 1983; Boldrini et al., 1992). This defect is in contrast to bilateral impairments in TOR after a unilateral lesion insufficient in size or location to cause a complete tactile–verbal disconnection syndrome (e.g., Oppenheim, 1906; Goldstein, 1916; Lhermitte and Ajuriaguerra, 1938). It also contrasts with the defect of the patient reported by Beauvois et al. (1978), who, after surgical removal of a large left parietooccipital tumor, developed a modality-specific inability to name or verbally describe objects placed in either hand. When blindfolded, the patient could demonstrate the use of tactually presented objects. Naming errors were frequently semantic confusions. The authors interpreted the deficit as a "bilateral tactile aphasia," and suggested that it represents the tactile analogue of "optic aphasia" (Lhermitte and Beauvois, 1973). The third difference is that Geschwind and Kaplan's patient showed normal tactual exploration of objects, while patients with apperceptive tactile agnosia (astereognosis) show deficient palpation of objects, characterized either by a reluctance to manipulate the object or by a stereotypic pattern of manipulation that is independent of specific object qualities.

Supramodal Spatial Defects

Some patients with tactile recognition disorders also have profound defects in spatial localization, route-finding, and other visuospatial tasks (Semmes, 1965; Corkin, 1978). In concluding her review of somatosensory function, Corkin (1978) stated that it is "possible to observe an impairment of high tactile functions in an individual whose elementary sensory status is preserved. It is inappropriate, however, to call this impairment an agnosia, because the higher-order deficits seen are not specific to somesthesis" (p. 145). Recent evidence suggests that tactile recognition may be dependent on spatial and visual processing, perhaps representing the assembly of an object's structural description (Platz, 1996; Saetti 1999; Zangaladze et al., 1999). This is a persuasive and important argument, but should not be taken to mean that tactile agnosia as a modality-specific entity does not exist in some patients. It is possible, for example, to suffer from an isolated deficit in tactile shape perception without the contribution of apparent spatial disability (Reed et al., 1996). It is likely that, in many cases, large lesions involving parietal cortex and underlying white matter affect neural systems involved in supramodal spatial ability in addition to specifically involving the second somatosensory system. What may result from this kind of lesion is a sort of mixed defect in which somatosensory and spatial factors combine in unspecified amounts. The fact that such a complex disorder exists does not negate the possibility that, with more restricted lesions, a purer, modality-specific defect corresponding to tactile agnosia will result.

Although the anatomic and clinical evidence is far from clear, it seems reasonable to distinguish four defects of somatosensory recognition: cortical tactile disorders, astereognosis, tactile agnosia, and disorders of tactile naming secondary to tactile–verbal disconnection. Cortical tactile disorders involve defects in basic and and intermediate somatosensory function, the end result of which will be pervasive somatosensory impairment in addition to defects in TOR. We believe that astereognosis is a more specific defect, that it deserves a designation as an apperceptive tactile agnosia (but see Tranel, 1991), and that it is primarily caused by a lesion in the functional system subserved by the middle third of the postcentral gyrus (the hand area) and its cortical and subcortical connections. Tactile agnosia, in contrast, seems to result from parietotemporal lesions that primarily involve SII (Caselli, 1991a) and involve connections between somatosensory regions and semantic memory stores (Endo et al., 1992).

Understanding complex somatosensory function in the individual patient requires a systematic neuropsychological evaluation of the task of tactual object identification as well as an evaluation of elementary and intermediate somatosensory function (Caselli, 1991a). When an object is palpated, sensory and proprioceptive cues received by postcentral gyrus interact with the premotor region to direct a series of coordinated movements necessary to construct a tactile image of the object. Most TOR tasks contain components that could be described as sensory, spatial, proprioceptive, constructive, and motor. The functional interconnections between SI, premotor region, and more posterior portions of the parietal cortex highlight the challenges in functionally separating these task dimensions in tasks of TOR.

AGNOSIA AND CONSCIOUS AWARENESS

Despite a profound disability in direct identification of objects or faces, many agnosics are able to demonstrate some knowledge about the stimulus if appropriate tests of recognition are used. Generally speaking, such tests have the common characteristic of not requiring the patient to make direct conscious reference to stimulus identity. Instead, the task is structured such that knowledge is demonstrated in an indirect or implicit way.

Dissociations of this type have received substantial discussion in the memory and attentional literatures (see Chapters 13, 18, and 19). For example, it has been shown that severely amnesic patients are able to acquire new motor or perceptual skills and can demonstrate intact perceptual and conceptual priming of previously presented information (Roediger et al., 1994; Verfaellie and Keane, 1997). Similarly, patients with hemispatial neglect are capable of perceiving unattended information and, in some cases, engaging in high-level semantic processing of neglected stimuli despite being unaware of their perceptions (McGlinchey Berroth, et al., 1993; Farah and Feinberg, 1997). Other findings include lexical access without awareness in acquired alexia (Landis et al., 1980; Shallice and Saffran, 1986; Coslett and Safran, 1989a), preserved visual identification capacity in hemianopic fields ("blindsight"; Weiskrantz, et al., 1974, Weiskrantz, 1986), and preserved semantic priming in Wernicke's aphasia (Milberg and Blumstein, 1981; Blumstein et al., 1982). In all of these examples, evidence exists that the cognitive system thought to be impaired in these patients is capable of substantial processing. However, the results of such processing cannot, or do not, reach the level of conscious awareness.

The best evidence for covert recognition in agnosia has come from studies of patients with prosopagnosia. Bruyer et al. (1983) provided the first behavioral evidence of covert recognition when they showed that their prosopagnosic was more easily able to match unrecognized faces with their real names than with arbitrary names. De Haan et al. (1987a) found that their prosopagnosic, like normal controls, performed same–different judgments more rapidly when the task involved famous faces than when unknown faces were presented. In these two examples, performance benefited from familiarity, even though the patients never recognized specific faces as familiar.

In an elegant series of studies, De Haan et al. (1987a, 1987b) used the face–name interference (FNI) task to explore preserved semantic processing of faces in prosopagnosia. In FNI, subjects are asked to make a semantic classification judgment (e.g., "Is this an actor or politician?") when presented printed names. Presented along with the name, but irrelevant for the name classification task, is a face that is (a) the same person as the printed name, (b) from the same semantic category as the printed name, or (c) from a different category. In normal subjects, name classification is slowed by the presence of a face from a different category, presumably based on a Stroop-like phenomenon. Prosopagnosics also show this effect, even though they fail to recognize a single face (De Haan et al., 1987a, 1987b, 1992). This suggests that, at some level, they can extract semantic information from faces and can thus become distracted by it when they perform the name classification task.

Covert recognition in prosopagnosia has also been demonstrated using psychophysiological (Bauer, 1984; Tranel and Damasio, 1985, 1988; Bauer and Verfaellie, 1986), electrophysiological (Debruille et al., 1989; Renault et al., 1989), and oculomotor (Rizzo et al., 1987) measures. Bauer (1984) showed that electrodermal responses to correct face–name matches were greater than those to incorrect matches, while Tranel and Damasio (1985) showed a similar effect for face familiarity. Bauer and Verfaellie (1986) replicated this effect with a second prosopagnosic, but failed to show covert learning of new faces.

Renault et al. (1989) recorded evoked potentials while their prosopagnosic performed familiarity judgments to a series of faces in which the proportion of familiar and unfamiliar faces was varied. They found that, despite poor explicit recognition, P300 amplitude varied inversely with stimulus probability (e.g., was higher on series containing few familiar faces) and latency varied positively with face familiarity.

Rizzo et al. (1987) evaluated exploratory eye movements in two prosopagnosic patients while they viewed famous and unfamiliar faces. Like normals, these patients examined the whole face when encountering unfamiliar faces, but concentrated on internal features when viewing famous faces. Thus, the manner of visual exploration reveals that, at some level, facial familiarity is detected by the visual system, though it is not reflected in the patient's verbal report.

Similar techniques have been applied to the question of whether prosopagnosics can learn new faces. Sergent and Poncet (1990) asked their prosopagnosic to inspect a series of famous and novel faces in preparation for a subsequent recognition task. Afterward, some of these faces (old) were combined with series of new faces, and subjects were asked to perform an old–new discrimination. Although the patient was generally unable to discriminate between old and new faces, face familiarity led to increased accuracy in episodic recognition. Remarkably, the patient was able to directly recognize faces on some trials.

Greve and Bauer (1990) used a variant of Zajonc's "mere exposure" paradigm to demonstrate covert learning of faces in their prosopagnosic. The patient was shown a series of faces that were each later paired with a novel distractor for forced-choice recognition and preference judgments. In forced-choice recognition, the patient was asked to indicate which of the two faces had been previously presented. In the preference-judgment task, the patient was asked which of the two faces he liked better. He performed at chance in forced-choice recognition, but liked significantly more of the target faces than predicted by chance. Thus, both of these studies suggest that prosopagnosics can learn some aspects of new faces, provided that such learning is assessed indirectly.

In a few patients, psychophysiological (Bauer, 1986) and behavioral (Newcombe et al., 1989) measures have failed to reveal evidence of covert recognition (see Bruyer, 1991 for review). These patients had significant apperceptive defects, which suggest impairment prior to the level of the face-recognition unit. Thus covert recognition may be a characteristic of associative prosopagnosia.

These findings, and those in the literature on amnesia, alexia, aphasia, neglect, and blindsight, suggest that a substantial amount of perceptual and semantic processing must be intact in these patients prior to or independent of the

process that generates contextual or autobiographical recognition (Damasio, 1989; Schacter, 1989). Second, they imply that autobiographical recognition or appreciation of the nature of a stimulus involves mechanisms that are different from or additional to the mechanisms that process stimulus attributes.

One important issue concerns the implication that such findings have for the functional architecture of object recognition. One of the dominant viewpoints is that such findings imply a dissociation between stimulus processing and consciousness. Schacter (1989) offers a general account of such dissociations by proposing that implicit and explicit domains reflect parallel, nonoverlapping outputs of early, "modular" cortices dedicated to processing specific types of information. In this view, one set of outputs links the outputs from sensory cortex with motor, verbal, and visceroautonomic response systems that are themselves capable of reading out cortical activity without conscious or executive control. Another independent set of outputs links modular cortices with a conscious awareness system that is responsible, in the case of object recognition, for explicit stimulus identification. According to this model, covert recognition in agnosia would result when functional interaction between modular cortices is selectively interrupted or disconnected while modular outputs to motor, verbal, and autonomic response systems remain intact. This impairment of functional interaction between modular cortices and the awareness system would lead to the kind of deficit one sees in agnosia: a domain-specific impairment in conscious identification without a global impairment in conscious awareness.

An alternative model, not requiring a disconnection mechanism, posits that dissociations between implicit and explicit forms of object/face identification are the natural result of a damaged object recognition processor (Farah et al., 1993). This general approach was outlined above in the section on prosopagnosia, and is useful because (1) it begins to specify the nature of information processing taking place at different levels of the nervous system, and (2) it supplements lesion work in a way that informs and constrains the analysis of individual cases.

EXAMINATION OF THE PATIENT WITH AGNOSIA

Two basic principles should guide the examination of the agnosic patient. First, care should be taken to rule out the possibility that the recognition disorder is attributable to sensory–perceptual dysfunction, inattention, aphasia, generalized memory loss, or dementia. Second, an extensive analysis of the scope and limits of the patient's defect is required to characterize its functional locus.

RULING OUT ALTERNATIVE EXPLANATIONS

At the outset, it is important to remember that agnosic recognition failures are classically modality-specific. Patients who exhibit multimodal defects are more likely to be suffering from amnesic syndrome, language disturbance, dementia, or, in rarer cases, generalized impairments in semantic access. The nonaphasic agnosic patient will not usually manifest word-finding difficulty in spontaneous speech, and will generally succeed in generating lists of words in specific categories, in completing open-ended sentences, and in supplying words that correspond with definitions. Except in the rare case of optic aphasia, the agnosic will not be able to identify the misnamed objects by means of circumlocution, or by indicating function. It is thus important to determine whether the patient is able to demonstrate the use of objects not in his or her presence and to follow commands not requiring objects (e.g., salute, wave good-bye, make a fist, etc.). Failures of this type in the presence of otherwise intact auditory comprehension indicate apraxia; subsequent failure to demonstrate the use of objects presented on visual confrontation may therefore be apraxic, not agnosic.

In pointing and naming tasks, it is important to be certain that the patient is visually fixating on the objects to be identified and that pointing errors are not due to mislocation in space. Recognition should be examined both in the context of normal surroundings and in the formal test setting, taking care to ensure that the patient is familiar with target objects.

As a start, comprehensive neurologic and neuropsychological assessment of intellectual skill, memory function, language, constructional/perceptual ability, attention, problem-solving, and personality/emotional factors should be undertaken to rule out bracketing conditions.

CHARACTERIZING THE NATURE OF THE DEFECT

In the visual sphere, the recognition of objects, colors, words, geometric forms, faces, and emblems and signs should be evaluated. In the event of failure to recognize, the patient should be allowed to match misidentified items to sample and to produce drawings of objects not identified. Quantitative achievement and *qualitative performance* on these tasks should be carefully noted, keeping in mind that quantitatively correct matching and accurate drawing do not necessarily suggest intact perceptual processing. Poor drawing does not necessarily implicate an apperceptive defect, since visuomotor or constructional defects may also be present. For this reason, it is important to use tasks in addition to drawing to document intact perception, if possible. Cross-modal matching and matching objects across different views should be evaluated. Line drawings to be copied should contain sufficient internal detail so that slavish tracing of an outline can, if present, be elicited.

Other perceptual functions, such as figure–ground perception (hidden figures), closure and synthetic ability, topographical orientation, route-finding, and visual counting (counting dots on a white paper, picking up pennies spread over a tabletop) should also be evaluated. Visual memory for designs, objects, faces, and colors should be assessed by delayed recall (drawing from memory) and multiple-choice recognition tasks. The ability to categorize, sort misidentified objects, and pair similar objects that are not morphologically identical should be tested.

The patient should be asked to identify pictures of well-known people and to identify hospital staff by face. If recognition does not occur, the patient should be asked to determine whether the face is of a male or female or whether the face is of a human or animal. In the acutely hospitalized patient, ability to recognize visiting family can be assessed by dressing the family member in a white coat or other appropriate hospital garb to minimize the use of extrafacial cues by the patient. If face recognition impairment exists, it is important to demonstrate intact semantic (nonvisual) knowledge about persons that cannot be recognized visually. Failure to name a particular face should, therefore, be further examined by asking the subject to provide information (e.g., "Who is Tiger Woods?") about unrecognized personalities. Discrimination of faces across different viewpoints should be evaluated with matching tasks (e.g., Benton Facial Recognition Test).

Color perception should be tested with pseudoisochromatic plates and with the Munsell-Farnsworth 100 Hue Test ("visual" color tasks). The patient should be asked to respond to verbal tasks such as, "What is the color of a banana?", to list as many colors as possible in a minute, or to name as many items as possible of a certain color. Other visual tasks, including coloring line drawings with crayons, should be given. Finally, visual–verbal color tasks such as naming colors pointed out by the examiner or pointing to named colors should be routinely presented.

The possibility of confabulation interfering with identification performance should be kept in mind. Therefore, test performance when patients are allowed to verbalize should be compared with performance when they are prohibited from verbalizing by asking them to count backwards or by having them place their tongue between their teeth. Comparing naming in the tactile modality alone with simul-taneous visual and tactile presentation is also important.

Careful visual fields and visual acuity measures are crucial. In testing patients who cannot read, it may be necessary to construct tests of acuity that use nonverbal targets, such as the orientation of lines of various lengths and distances from the viewer, or the detection of two points at variable distances from each other and from the patient. If equipment is available, detailed psychophysical tests should be employed, including absolute threshold determination, local adaptation time, flicker fusion, contrast and spatial frequency sensitivity, movement aftereffect, and the brief presentation of single and multiple items. In patients with associated alexia without agraphia, tachistoscopic presentation of words and letters, as well as a neurobehaviorally oriented reading battery should be given. Depth perception using Julesz figures should be tested. Luminance discrimination should also be assessed. The use of an eye movement monitor may be useful in describing visual scanning behavior. In settings where such sophisticated equipment is not available, careful observational analysis of visual exploratory behavior, manifested in eye movements, head turning, and step-by-step feature comparisons, should nonetheless be conducted.

In the auditory sphere, standard audiometric testing using speech reception and pure-tone audiometry should be conducted. The ability to localize sounds in space should also be examined by using both absolute and relative localization tasks. It should be remembered that patients with acquired auditory sound agnosia do not ordinarily complain about their problems. Recognition of nonverbal sounds should be tested preferably with the use of a series of tape-recorded environmental sounds that are sufficiently familiar to unimpaired subjects to yield nearly perfect recognition. The Seashore Tests of Musical Talent may be used with the understanding that in the absence of history of proven musical ability and interest, results may be difficult to interpret.

In the tactile sphere, each hand should be assessed separately in the performance of basic somatosensory function (touch, pain, temperature, vibration, kinesthesia, proprioception, two-point discrimination, double simultaneous stimulation), as well as discrimination of weight, texture, shape, and substance. In assessing TOR, verbal, pointing, and matching tasks should be used. Cross-modal matching (tactual–verbal, tactual–visual) are alsoimportant in evaluating the scope of the recognition defect. It is important to allow the patient to draw misidentified objects or to after-select them from a group tactually. Tactual exploratory behavior (palpating of objects) should also be carefully observed.

CONCLUSION

During the past decade, significant advances have been made toward an understanding of the complex components of recognition processes. It is now clear that recognition is not a unitary, or even a two-step, process. Much of the historic debate about the existence of agnosia can be attributed to the fact that our models of recognition have generated some incorrect assumptions about what should happen when the recognition system becomes damaged. The best example is the debate over whether agnosia is a perceptual or memory access problem. Historically, the major problem with this question has been our assumption that it is the correct question to ask in the first place. We now know better, and, as a result, significant advances have been made in the last decade. The concept of recognition encompasses a broad range of behaviors, including attention, feature extraction, exploratory behavior, pattern and form perception, temporal resolution, and memory. New data on sensory and perceptual systems have revealed the exquisite complexity of the cortical and subcortical systems that support sensory and perceptual activities. Because of these advances, we have transcended the notion of a two-stage recognition process consisting of apperception and association. Instead, recognition of sensory stimuli is now understood as a complex outcome of parallel processing occurring simultaneously at cortical and subcortical levels.

These complexities make it extremely unlikely that a core defect responsible for all agnosic phenomena exists. It now seems more fruitful to specify the conditions under which stimuli can and cannot be recognized and to more precisely specify the input, processing, and output requirements of specific tasks of identification and recognition. By doing this, and by correlating the emerging clinical findings with available neuropathological data, a meaningful understanding of the spectrum of agnosic deficits and of normal recognition abilities is rapidly emerging.

REFERENCES

Ackermann, H., and Mathiak, K. (1999). *Fortschr. Neurol. Psychiatrie, 67:*509–523.

Adams, A. E., Rosenberger, K., Winter, H., and Zollner, C. (1977). A case of cortical deafness. *Arch. Psychiatrie Nervenkr. 224:*213–220.

Adler, A. (1944). Disintegration and restoration of optic recognition in visual agnosia. *Arch. Neurol. Psychiatry 51:*243–259.

Albert, M. L., and Bear, D. (1974). Time to understand: a case study of word deafness with reference to the role of time in auditory comprehension. *Brain 97:*373–384.

Albert, M. L., Reches, A., and Silverberg, R. (1975a). Associative visual agnosia without alexia. *Neurology 25:*322–326.

Albert, M. L., Reches, A., and Silverberg, R. (1975b). Hemianopic colour blindness. *J. Neurol. Neurosurg. Psychiatry 38:*546–549.

Albert, M. L., Soffer, D., Silverberg, R., and Reches, A. (1979). The anatomic basis of visual agnosia. *Neurology 29:*876–879.

Albert, M. L., Sparks, R., von Stockert, T., and Sax, D. (1972). A case study of auditory agnosia: linguistic and nonlinguistic processing. *Cortex 8:*427–433.

Alexander, M. P., and Albert, M. L. (1983). The anatomical basis of visual agnosia. In *Localization in Neuropsychology*, A. Kertesz (ed.). New York: Academic Press, pp. 393–415.

Alexander, M. P., Stuss, D. T., and Benson, D. F. (1979). Capgras syndrome: a reduplicative phenomenon. *Neurology 29:*334–339.

Allison, T., Ginter, H., McCarthy, G., Nobre, A. C., Puce, A., Luby, M., and Spencer, D. D. (1994). Face recognition in human extrastriate cortex. *J. Neurophysiol. 71:*821–825.

Andreasen, N. C., O'Leary, D. S., Arndt, S., Cizadlo, T., Hurtig, R., Rezai, K., Watkins, G. L., Ponto, L. B., and Hichwa, R. D. (1996). Neural substrates of facial recognition. *J. Neuropsychiatry Clin. Neurosci. 8:*139–146.

Anton, G. (1899). Ueber die Selbstwahrnehmungen der Herderkrankungen des Gehirns durch den Kranken bei Rindenblindheit und Rindentaubheit. *Arch. Psychiatrie 32:*86–127.

Aptman, M., Levin, H., and Senelick, R. C. (1977). Alexia without agraphia in a left-handed patient with prosopagnosia. *Neurology 27:*533–536.

Ardila, A., Rosselli, M., Arvizu, L., and Kuljis, R. O. (1997). Alexia and agraphia in posterior cortical atrophy. *Neuropsychiatry Neuropsychol. Behav. Neurol. 10:*52–59.

Ariel, R., and Sadeh, M. (1996). Congenital visual agnosia and prosopagnosia in a child: a case report. *Cortex 32:*221–240.

Assal, G., and Despland, P. A. (1973). Presentation d'un cas d'agnosie auditive. *Otoneuroophtalmologie 45:*353–355.

Auerbach, S. H., Allard, T., Naeser, M., et al. (1982). Pure word deafness: analysis of a case with bilateral lesions and a defect at the prephonemic level. *Brain 105:*271–300.

Balint, R. (1909). Seelenlahmung des "Schauens", optische Ataxie, raumliche Störung der Aufmerksamkeit. *Montasschr. Psychiatrie Neurol. 25*:57–71.

Bauer, R. M. (1982). Visual hypoemotionality as a symptom of visual-limbic disconnection in man. *Arch. Neurology 39*:702–708.

Bauer, R. M. (1984). Autonomic recognition of names and faces in prosopagnosia: a neuropsychological application of the Guilty Knowledge Test. *Neuropsychologia 22*:457–469.

Bauer, R. M. (1986). The cognitive psychophysiology of prosopagnosia. In *Aspects of Face Processing*, H. Ellis, M. Jeeves, F. Newcombe, and A. Young (eds.). Dordrecht, UK: Martinus Nijhoff, pp. 253–267.

Bauer, R. M. (1993). Agnosia. In *Clinical Neuropsychology, 3rd ed.*, K. M. Heilman and E. Valenstein (eds.). New York: Oxford University Press, pp. 215–278.

Bauer, R. M., and Trobe, J. (1984). Visual memory and perceptual impairments in prosopagnosia. *J. Clin. Neuroophthalmol. 4*:39–45.

Bauer, R. M., and Verfaellie, M. (1986). Electrodermal discrimination of familiar but not unfamiliar faces in prosopagnosia. *Brain Cognition 8*:240–252.

Bay, E. (1944). Zum Problem der taktilen Agnosie. *D. Z. Nervenkr. 156*:1–3, 64–96.

Bay, E. (1953). Disturbances of visual perception and their examination. *Brain 76*:515–550.

Baylis, G. C., Rolls, E. T., and Leonard, C. M. (1985). Selectivity between faces in the responses of a population of neurons in the cortex in the superior temporal sulcus of the monkey. *Brain Res. 342*:91–102.

Beauvois, M. F. (1982). Optic aphasia: a process of interaction between vision and language. *Phil. Trans. R. Soc. Lond. Ser. B Biol. 298*:35–47.

Beauvois, M. F., and Saillant, B. (1985). Optic aphasia for colors and color agnosia: a distinction between visual and visuo-verbal impairments in the processing of colors. *Cogn. Neuropsychol. 2*:1–48.

Beauvois, M. F., Saillant, B., Meininger, V., and Lhermitte, F. (1978). Bilateral tactile aphasia: a tacto-verbal dysfunction. *Brain 101*:381–401.

Bender, M. D., and Feldman, M. (1972). The so-called visual agnosias. *Brain 95*:173–186.

Benson, D. F., Davis, R. J., and Snyder, B. D. (1988). Posterior cortical atrophy. *Arch. Neurol. 45*:789–793.

Benson, D. F., and Greenberg, J. P. (1969). Visual form agnosia. *Arch. Neurol. 20*:82–89.

Benson, D. F., Segarra, J., and Albert, M. L. (1974). Visual agnosia-prosopagnosia. *Arch. Neurol. 30*:307–310.

Benton, A. (1990). Facial recognition. *Cortex 26*:491–499.

Benton, A. L. (1980). The neuropsychology of face recognition. *Am. Psychol. 35*:176–186.

Benton, A. L., Levin, A., and Varney, N. (1973). Tactile perception of direction in normal subjects. *Neurology 23*:1248–1250.

Benton, A. L., and Van Allen, M. W. (1972). Prosopagnosia and facial discrimination. *J. Neurol. Sci. 15*:167–172.

Berkley, M. A., and Sprague, J. M. (1979). Striate cortex and visual acuity functions in the cat. *J. Comp. Neurol. 187*:679–702.

Berman, I. W. (1981). Musical functioning, speech lateralization and the amusias. *S. Afr. Med. J. 59*:78–81.

Bever, T. G., and Chiarello, R. J. (1974). Cerebral dominance in musicians and nonmusicians. *Science 185*:137–139.

Beversdorf, D. Q., and Heilman, K. M. (1998). Progressive ventral posterior cortical degeneration presenting as alexia for music and words. *Neurology 50*:657–659.

Beyn, E. S., and Knyazeva, G. R. (1962). The problem of prosopagnosia. *J. Neurol. Neurosurg. Psychiatry 25*:154–158.

Bhaskaran, R., Prakash, M., Kumar, P. N., and Srikumar, B. (1998). Crossed aphasia leading to pure word deafness. *J. Assoc. Physicians India 46*:824–826.

Blumstein, S., and Cooper, W. (1974). Hemispheric processing of intonation contours. *Cortex 10*:146–158.

Blumstein, S. E., Milberg, W., and Shrier, R. (1982). Semantic processing in aphasia: evidence from an auditory lexical decision task. *Brain Lang. 17*:301–315.

Bodamer, J. (1947). Prosopagnosie. *Arch. Psychiatrie Nervenkr. 179*:6–54.

Boldrini, P., Zanella, R., Cantagallo, A., and Basaglia, N. (1992). Partial hemispheric disconnection syndrome of traumatic origin. *Cortex 28*:135–143.

Boller, F., Cole, M., Kim, Y., et al. (1975). Optic ataxia: clinical-radiological correlations with the EMI scan. *J. Neurol. Neurosurg. Psychiatry 38*:954–958.

Boller, F., and Spinnler, H. (1967). Visual memory for colors in patients with unilateral brain damage. *Cortex 3*:395–405.

Bonhoeffer, K. (1918). Partielle reine Tastlahmung. *Mtschr. Psychiatrie Neurol. 43*:141–145.

Bornstein, B. (1963). Prosopagnosia. In *Problems of*

Dynamic Neurology, L. Halpern (ed.). New York: Grune and Stratton.

Bornstein, B., and Kidron, D. P. (1959). Prosopagnosia. *J. Neurol. Neurosurg. Psychiatry* 22:124–131.

Bornstein, B., Sroka, H., and Munitz, H. (1969). Prosopagnosia with animal face agnosia. *Cortex* 5:164–169.

Botez, M. I. (1975). Two visual systems in clinical neurology: readaptive role of the primitive system in visual agnosic patients. *Eur. Neurol.* 13:101–122.

Botez, M. I., and Serbanescu, T. (1967). Course and outcome of visual static agnosia. *J. Neurol. Sci.* 4:289–297.

Bowers, D. (1981). Acquired color disturbances due to cerebral lesions. Presented at the Seventh Annual Course in Behavioral Neurology and Neuropsychology, Florida Society of Neurology, St. Petersburg Beach, Florida, December, 1981.

Brain, W. R. (1941). Visual object agnosia with special reference to the gestalt theory. *Brain* 64:43–62.

Brodal, A. (1981). *Neurological Anatomy in Relation to Clinical Medicine*, 3rd ed. New York: Oxford University Press.

Brown, J. W. (1972). *Aphasia, Apraxia, and Agnosia—Clinical and Theoretical Aspects*. Springfield, IL: Charles C. Thomas.

Bruce, C. J., Desimone, R., and Gross, C. G. (1981). Visual properties of neurons in a polysensory area in superior temporal sulcus of the macaque. *J. Neurosci.* 4:2051–2062.

Bruce, V. and Young, A. (1986). Understanding face recognition. *Brit. J. Psychology* 77:305–327.

Brust, J. C. (1980). Music and language: musical alexia and agraphia. *Brain* 103:367–392.

Bruyer, R. (1991). Covert face recognition in prosopagnosia: a review. *Brain Cogn.* 15:223–235.

Bruyer, R., Laterre, C., Seron, X., Feyereisen, P., Strypstein, E., Pierrard, E., and Rectem, D. (1983). A case of prosopagnosia with some preserved covert rememberance of familiar faces. *Brain Cogn.* 2:257–284.

Buchman, A. S., Garron, D. C., Trost-Cardamone, J. E., Wichter, M. D., and Schwartz, M. (1986). Word deafness: one hundred years later. *J. Neurol. Neurosurg. Psychiatry* 49:489–499.

Buchtel, H. A., and Stewart, J. D. (1989). Auditory agnosia: apperceptive or associative disorder? *Brain Lang.* 37:12–25.

Burton, A. M., Bruce, V., and Johnston, R. A. (1990). Understanding face recognition with an interactive activation model. *Br. J. Psychol.* 81:361–380.

Cambier, J., Masson, M., Elghozi, D., et al. (1980). Agnosie visuelle sans hemianopsie droite chez un sujet droitier. *Rev. Neurol. (Paris)* 136:727–740.

Campbell, R., Landis, T., and Regard, M. (1986). Face recognition and lipreading. A neurological dissociation. *Brain* 109(Pt 3):509–521.

Campion, J. and Latto, R. (1985). Apperceptive agnosia due to carbon monoxide poisoning: an interpretation based on critical band masking from disseminated lesions. *Behav. Brain Res.* 15:227–240.

Campora, G. (1925). Astereognosis: its causes and mechanism. *Brain* 18:65–71.

Caplan, L. R. (1978). Variability of perceptual function: the sensory cortex as a categorizer and deducer. *Brain Lang.* 6:1–13.

Caplan, L. R. (1980). "Top of the basilar" syndrome. *Neurology* 30:72–79.

Caramazza, A., and Shelton, J. R. (1998). Domain-specific knowledge systems in the brain the animate-inanimate distinction. *J. Cogn. Neurosci.* 10:1–34.

Carlesimo, G. A., Casadio, P., Sabbadini, M., and Caltagirone, C. (1998). Associative visual agnosia resulting from a disconnection between intact visual memory and semantic systems. *Cortex* 34:563–576.

Caselli, R. J. (1991a). Rediscovering tactile agnosia. *Mayo Clin. Proc.* 66:129–142.

Caselli, R. J. (1991b). Bilateral impairment of somesthetically mediated object recognition in humans. *Mayo Clin. Proc.* 66, 357–364.

Celesia, G. G. (1976). Organization of auditory cortical areas in man. *Brain* 99:403–414.

Celesia, G. G., Archer, C. R., Kuroiwa, Y., and Goldfader, P. R. (1980). Visual function of the extrageniculo-calcarine system in man. *Arch. Neurol.* 37:704–706.

Chanoine, V., Ferreira, C. T., Demonet, J. F., Nespoulous, J. L., and Poncet, M. (1998). Optic aphasia with pure alexia: a mild form of visual associative agnosia? A case study. *Cortex* 34:437–448.

Chocholle, R., Chedru, F., Bolte, M. C. et al. (1975). Étude psychoacoustique dun cas de surdite corticlae. *Neuropsychologia* 13:163–172.

Cohen, R., and Kelter, S. (1979). Cognitive impairment of aphasics in color to picture matching tasks. *Cortex* 15:235–245.

Cohn, R., Neumann, M. A., and Wood, D. H. (1977). Prosopagnosia: a clinico-pathological study. *Ann. Neurol.* 1:177–182.

Cooper, J. A., and Ferry, P. C. (1978). Acquired auditory verbal agnosia and seizures in childhood. *J. Speech Hear. Disord.* 43:176–184.

Corballis, M. C. (1994). Neuropsychology of perceptual functions. In *Neuropsychology*, D. W. Zaidel (ed.). San Diego: Academic Press, pp. 83–104.

Corkin, S. (1964). Somesthetic function after focal cerebral damage in man. Unpublished doctoral dissertation, McGill University.

Corkin, S. (1978). The role of different cerebral structures in somesthetic perception. In *Handbook of Perception, (Vol. VI B.)* C. E. Carterette and M. P. Friedman (eds.). New York: Academic Press, pp. 105–155.

Corkin, S., Milner, B., and Rasmussen, T. (1970). Somatosensory thresholds: contrasting effects of postcentral-gyrus and posterior parietal-lobe excision. *Arch. Neurol.* 23:41–58.

Corkin, S., Milner, B., and Taylor, L. (1973). Bilateral sensory loss after unilateral cerebral lesions in man. Presented at the joint meeting of the American Neurological Association and the Canadian Congress of Neurological Sciences, Montreal.

Corlew, M. M., and Nation, J. E. (1975). Characteristics of visual stimuli and naming performance in aphasic adults. *Cortex* 11:186–191.

Coslett, H. B., Brashear, H. R., and Heilman, K. M. (1984). Pure word deafness after bilateral primary auditory cortex infarcts. *Neurology* 34:347–352.

Coslett, H. B., and Saffran, E. (1989a). Evidence for preserved reading in "pure alexia". *Brain* 112:327–360.

Coslett, H. B., and Saffran, E. (1989b). Preserved object recognition and reading comprehension in optic aphasia. *Brain* 112:1091–1110.

Critchley, M. N. (1964). The problem of visual agnosia. *J. Neurol. Sci.* 1:274–290.

Critchley, M. N. (1965). Acquired anomalies of colour perception of central origin. *Brain* 88:711–724.

Critchley, M. M., and Henson, R. A. (1977). *Music and the Brain: Studies in the Neurology of Music.* Springfield, IL: Charles C. Thomas.

Crosson, B., Moberg, P. J., Boone, J. R., Rothi, L. J., and Raymer, A. (1997). Category-specific naming deficit for medical terms after dominant thalamic/capsular hemorrhage. Brain Lang. 60:407–442.

Cummings, J. L., Syndulko, K., Goldberg, Z., and Treiman, D. M. (1982). Palinopsia reconsidered. *Neurology* 32:331–341.

Damasio, A. R. (1989). Time-locked multiregional coactivation: a systems-level proposal for the neural substrates of recall and recognition. *Cognition* 33:25–62.

Damasio, A. R. (1990). Category-related recognition defects as a clue to the neural substrates of knowledge. *Trends Neurosci.* 13:95–98.

Damasio, A. R., and Benton, A. L. (1979). Impairment of hand movements under visual guidance. *Neurology* 29:170–174.

Damasio, A. R., and Damasio, H. (1982). Cerebral localization of complex visual manifestations: clinical and physiological significance [Abstract]. *Neurology* 32(Suppl.):A96.

Damasio, A. R., Damasio, H., and Van Hoesen, G. W. (1982). Prosopagnosia: anatomic basis and behavioral mechanisms. *Neurology* 32:331–341.

Damasio, H., McKee, H., and Damasio, A. R. (1979). Determinants of performance in color anomia. *Brain Lang.* 7:74–85.

Damasio, A. R., Tranel, D., and Damasio, H. (1990). Face agnosia and the neural substrates of memory. *Ann. Rev. Neurosci.* 13:89–109.

Damasio, A. R., Yamada, T., Damasio, H., et al. (1980). Central achromatopsia: Behavioral, anatomic, and physiologic aspects. *Neurology* 30:1064–1071.

Davidenkov, S. (1956). Impairments of higher nervous activity: lecture 8, visual agnosias. In *Clinical Lectures on Nervous Diseases*. Leningrad: State Publishing House of Medical Literature.

Davidoff, J., and Wilson, B. (1985). A case of visual agnosia showing a disorder of presemantic visual classification. *Cortex* 21:121–134.

Debruille, B., Breton, F., Robaey, P., Signoret, J. L., and Renault, B. (1989). Potentiels evoques cerebraux et reconnaisance consciente et non consciente des visages: application a l'etude de prosopagnosie. *Neurophsiol. Clin.* 19:393–405.

de Gelder, B., Bachoud Levi, A. C., and Degos, J. D. (1998). Inversion superiority in visual agnosia may be common to a variety of orientation polarised objects besides faces. *Vision Res.* 38:2855–2861.

De Haan, E. H., Bauer, R. M., and Greve, K. W. (1992). Behavioural and physiological evidence for covert face recognition in a prosopagnosic patient. *Cortex* 28:77–95.

De Haan, E. H., and Campbell, R. (1991). A fifteen year follow-up of a case of developmental prosopagnosia. *Cortex* 27(4):489–509.

De Haan, E. H. F., Young, A., and Newcombe, F. (1987a). Face recognition without awareness. *Cogn. Neuropsychol.* 4:385–415.

De Haan, E. H. F., Young, A., and Newcombe, F. (1987b). Faces interfere with name classification in a prosopagnosic patient. *Cortex* 23:309–316.

De Haan, E. H., Young, A. W., and Newcombe, F. (1991). Covert and overt recognition in prosopagnosia. *Brain,* 114(Pt 6):2575–2591.

Delay, J. (1935). *Les Astereognosies. Pathologie due Toucher. Clinique, Physiologie, Topographie.* Paris: Masson.

Denes, G., and Semenza, C. (1975). Auditory modality-specific anomia: evidence from a case of pure word deafness. *Cortex 11*:401–411.

Denny-Brown, D., and Fischer, E. G. (1976). Physiological aspects of visual perception II: the subcortical visual direction of behavior. *Arch. Neurol. 33*:228–242.

De Renzi, E. (1982). *Disorders of Space Exploration and Cognition.* New York: John Wiley and Sons.

DeRenzi, E. (1986a). Current issues in prosopagnosia. In *Aspects of Face Processing*, H. D. Ellis, M. A. Jeeves, F. Newcombe, and A. Young (eds.). Dordrecht: Martinus Nijhoff, pp. 243–252.

De Renzi, E. (1986b). Prosopagnosia in two patients with CT scan evidence of damage confined to the right hemisphere. *Neuropsychologia 24*:385–389.

De Renzi, E., Faglioni, P., Grossi, D., and Nichelli, P. (1991). Apperceptive and associative forms of prosopagnosia. *Cortex 27*:213–221.

De Renzi, E., Faglioni, P., Scotti, G., and Spinnler, H. (1972). Impairment in associating colour to form, concomitant with aphasia. *Brain 95*:293–304.

De Renzi, E., Faglioni, P., Scotti, G., and Spinnler, H. (1973). Impairment of color sorting: an experimental study with the Holmgren Skein Test. *Cortex 9*:147–163.

De Renzi, E., and Saetti, M. C. (1997). Associative agnosia and optic aphasia: qualitative or quantitative difference? *Cortex 33*:115–130.

De Renzi, E., Scotti, G., and Spinnler, H. (1969). Perceptual and associative disorders of visual recognition. *Neurology 19*:634–642.

De Renzi, E., and Spinnler, H. (1967). Impaired performance on color tasks in patients with hemispheric damage. *Cortex 3*:194–217.

Desimone, R. (1991). Face-selective cells in the temporal cortex of monkeys. *J. Cogn. Neurosci. 3*:1–8.

Devlin, J. T., Gonnerman, L. M., Andersen, E. S., and Seidenberg, M. S. (1998). Category-specific semantic deficits in focal and widespread brain damage: a computational account. *J. Cogn. Neurosci. 10*:77–94.

DeYoe, E. A., and Van Essen, D. C. (1988). Concurrent processing streams in monkey visual cortex. *Trends Neurosci. 11*:219–226.

Dixon, M. J. (2000). A new paradigm for investigating category-specific agnosia in the new millennium. *Brain Cogn. 42*:142–145.

Dixon, M. J., Piskopos, M., and Schweizer, T. A. (2000). Musical instrument naming impairments: the crucial exception to the living/nonliving dichotomy in category-specific agnosia. *Brain Cogn. 43*:158–164.

Duchaine, B. C. (2000). Developmental prosopagnosia with normal configural processing. *Neuroreport 11*:79–83.

Earnest, M. P., Monroe, P. A., and Yarnell, P. A. (1977). Cortical deafness: demonstration of the pathologic anatomy by CT scan. *Neurology 27*:1175–1175.

Efron, R. (1968). What is perception? In *Boston Studies in the Philosophy of Science, Vol. 4.* New York: Humanities Press.

Eimer, M., and McCarthy, R. A. (1999). Prosopagnosia and structural encoding of faces: evidence from event-related potentials. *Neuroreport 10*:255–259.

Ellis, A. W. and Young, A. W. (1988). *Human Cognitive Neuropsychology.* Hillsdale NJ: Lawrence Erlbaum.

Endo, K., Miyasaka, M., Makishita, H., Yanagisawa, N., and Sugishita, M. (1992). Tactile agnosia and tactile aphasia: symptomatological and anatomical differences. *Cortex 28*:445–469.

Ettlin, T. M., Beckson, M., Benson, D. F., Langfitt, J. T., Amos, E. C., and Pineda, G. S. (1992). Prosopagnosia: a bihemispheric disorder. *Cortex 28*:129–134.

Ettlinger, G. (1956). Sensory deficits in visual agnosia. *J. Neurol. Neurosurg. Psychiatry 19*:297–307.

Ettlinger, G., Warrington, E. K., and Zangwill, O. L. (1957). A further study of visual spatial agnosia. *Brain 80*:335–361.

Ettlinger, G., and Wyke M. (1961). Defects in identifying objects visually in a patient with cerebrovascular disease. *J. Neurol. Neurosurg. Psychiatry 24*:254–259.

Evans, J. J., Heggs, A. J., Antoun, N., and Hodges, J. R. (1995). Progressive prosopagnosia associated with selective right temporal lobe atrophy. A new syndrome? *Brain 118(Pt 1)*:1–13.

Farah, M. J. (1990). *Visual Agnosia: Disorders of Object Vision and What they Tell Us About Normal Vision.* Cambridge, MA: MIT Press/Bradford Books.

Farah, M. J. (1991). Patterns of co-occurrence among the associative agnosias: implications for visual object representation. *Cogn. Neuropsychol. 8*:1–19.

Farah, M. J. (1996). Is face recognition 'special'? Evidence from neuropsychology. *Behav. Brain Res. 76*:181–189.

Farah, M. J., and Feinberg, T. E. (1997). Consciousness of perception after brain damage. *Semin. Neurol.* 17:145–152.

Farah, M. J., Hammond, K. M., Mehta, Z., and Ratcliff, G. (1989). Category-specificity and modality-specificity in semantic memory. *Neuropsychologia* 27:193–200.

Farah, M. J., Levinson, K. L., and Klein, K. L. (1995a). Face perception and within-category discrimination in prosopagnosia. *Neuropsychologia,* 33:661–674.

Farah, M. J., and McClelland, J. L. (1991). A computational model of semantic memory impairment: modality specificity and emergent category specificity. *J. Exp. Psychol. Gen.* 120:339–357.

Farah, M. J., McMullen, P. A., and Meyer, M. M. (1991). Can recognition of living things be selectively impaired? *Neuropsychologia* 29:185–193.

Farah, M. J., O'Reilly, R. C., and Vecera, S. P. (1993). Dissociated overt and covert recognition as an emergent property of a lesioned neural network. *Psychol. Rev.* 100:571–588.

Farah, M. J., Wilson, K. D., Drain, H. M., and Tanaka, J. R. (1995b). The inverted face inversion effect in prosopagnosia: evidence for mandatory, face-specific perceptual mechanisms. *Vision Res.* 35:2089–2093.

Farah, M. J., Wilson, K. D., Drain, M., and Tanaka, J. N. (1998). What is "special" about face perception? *Psychol. Rev.* 105:482–498.

Faust, C. (1955). *Die zerebralen Herderscheinungen bei Hinterhauptsverletzungen und ihre Beurteilung.* Stuttgart: Thieme Verlag.

Feinberg, T. E., Gonzalez-Rothi, L. J., and Heilman, K. M. (1986). Multimodal agnosia after unilateral left hemisphere lesion. *Neurology* 36:864–867.

Feinberg, T. E., Schindler, R. J., Ochoa, E., Kwan, P. C., and Farah, M. J. (1994). Associative visual agnosia and alexia without prosopagnosia. *Cortex* 30:395–411.

Fennell, E., Satz, P., and Wise, R. (1967). Laterality differences in the perception of pressure. *J. Neurol. Neurosurg. Psychiatry* 30:337–340.

Finkelnburg, F. C. (1870]. Niederrheinische Gesellschaft in Bonn. Medicinische Section. *Berl. Klin. Wochenschr.* 7:449–450, 460–461.

Forde, E. M. E., Francis, D., Riddoch, M. J., Rumiati, R. L., and Humphreys, G. W. (1997). On the links between visual knowledge and naming: a single case study of a patient with a category-specific impairment for living things. *Cogn. Neuropsychol.* 14:403–458.

Franklin, S., Turner, J., Ralph, M., Morris, J., and Bailey, P. L. (1996). A distinctive case of word-meaning deafness. *Cogn. Neuropsychol.* 13: 1139–1162.

Frederiks, J. A. M. (1969). The agnosias. In *Handbook of Clinical Neurology, Vol. 4,* P. J. Vinken and G. W. Bruyn (eds.). Amsterdam: North Holland.

Freud, S. (1891). *Zur Auffasun der Aphasien. Eine Kritische Studie.* Vienna: Franz Deuticke.

Freund, D.C. (1889). Ueber optische Aphasie und Seelenblindheit. *Arch Psychiatrie Nervenkr.* 20:276–297, 371–416.

Fujii, T., Fukatsu, R., Watabe, S., Ohnuma, A., Teramura, K., Kimura, I., Saso, S., and Kogure, K. (1990). Auditory sound agnosia without aphasia following a right temporal lobe lesion. *Cortex* 26:263–268.

Gainotti, G., and Silveri, M. C. (1996). Cognitive and anatomic locus of lesion in a patient with a category-specific semantic impairment for living beings. *Cogn. Neuropsychol.* 13:352–389.

Gans, A. (1916). Uber Tastblindheit und uber Storungen der raumlichen Wahrnmungen der Sensibilitat. *Z. Gesamte Neurol. Psychiatrie 31:* 303–428.

Gardner, H., Silverman, H., Denes, G., et al. (1977). Sensitivity to musical denotation and connotation in organic patients. *Cortex* 13:242–256.

Gascon, G., Victor, D., Lombroso, C., and Goodglass, D. (1973). Language disorder, convulsive disorder, and electroencephalographic abnormalities. *Arch. Neurol.* 28:156–162.

Gates, A., and Bradshaw, J. L. (1977). The role of the cerebral hemispheres in music. Brain Lang. 4:403–431.

Gazzaniga, M. S., Bogen, J. E. and Sperry, R. W. (1963). Laterality effects in somesthesis following cerebral commisurotomy in man. *Neuropsychologia* 1:209–215.

Gazzaniga, M., Glass, A. V., and Sarno, M. T. (1973). Pure word deafness and hemi-spheric dynamics: a case history. *Cortex* 9:136–143.

Gazzaniga, M. S., and Sperry, R. W. (1967). Language after section of the cerebral commisures. *Brain* 90:131–148.

George, N., Jemel, B., Fiori, N., and Renault, B. (1997). Face and shape repetition effects in humans: a spatio-temporal ERP study. *Neuroreport* 8:1417–1423.

Geschwind, N. (1965). Disconnexion syndromes in animals and man. *Brain* 88:237–294; 585–644.

Geschwind, N., and Fusillo, M. (1966). Color-naming defects in association with alexia. *Arch. Neurol.* 15:137–146.

Geschwind, N., and Kaplan, E. F. (1962). A human disconnection syndrome. *Neurology* 12:675–685.

Gloning, I., Gloning, K., Jellinger, K., and Quatember, R. (1970). A case of prosopagnosia" with necropsy findings. *Neurospychologia* 8:199–204.

Goldman-Rakic, P. S. (1988). Topography of cognition: parallel distributed networks in primate association cortex. *Ann. Rev. Neurosci.* 11:137–156.

Goldstein, K. (1916). Uber kortikale Sensibilitsstorungen. *Neurol. Zentralbl.* 19:825–827.

Goldstein, K. (1943). Some remarks on Russell Brain's article concerning visual object-agnosia. *J. Nerv. Ment. Dis.* 98:148–153.

Goldstein, K., and Gelb, A. (1918). Psychologische Analysen hirnpathologischer Falle auf Grund von Untersuchungen Hirnverletzter. *Z. Gesamte Neurol. Psychiatrie* 41:1–142.

Goldstein, M. N. (1974). Auditory agnosia for speech ("pure word deafness"): a historical review with current implications. *Brain Lang.* 1:195–204.

Goldstein, M. N., Brown, M., and Holander, J. (1975). Auditory agnosia and word deafness: analysis of a case with three-year follow up. *Brain Lang.* 2:324–332.

Goodglass, H., Barton, M. I., and Kaplan, E. F. (1968). Sensory modality and object-naming in aphasia. *J. Speech Hear. Res.* 11:488–496.

Gordon, H. W. (1974). Auditory specialization of the right and left hemispheres. In *Hemispheric Disconnection and Cerebral Function*, M. Kinsbourne and W. L. Smith (eds.). Springfield, IL: Charles C. Thomas.

Graff-Radford, N. R., Bolling, J. P., Earnest, F. T., Shuster, E. A., Caselli, R. J., and Brazis, P. W. (1993). Simultanagnosia as the initial sign of degenerative dementia. *Mayo Clin. Proc.* 68:955–964.

Green, G. L., and Lessell, S. (1977). Acquired cerebral dyschromatopsia. *Arch. Ophthalmol.* 95:121–128.

Greve, K. W. and Bauer, R. M. (1990). Implicit learning of new faces in prosopagnosia: an application of the mere-exposure paradigm. *Neuropsychologia* 28:1035–1041.

Gross, C. G., Rocha-Miranda, C. E., and Bender, D. B. (1972). Visual properties of neurons in inferotemporal cortex of the macaque. *J. Neurophysiol.* 35:96–111.

Grossman, M., Galetta, S., and D'Esposito, M. (1997). Object recognition difficulty in visual apperceptive agnosia. *Brain Cogn.* 33:306–342.

Haaxma, R., and Kuypers, H. G. J. M. (1975). In-trahemispheric cortical connections and visual guidance of band and finger movements in the rhesus monkey. *Brain* 98:239–260.

Habib, M. (1986). Visual hypoemotionality and prosopagnosia associated with right temporal lobe isolation. *Neuropsychologia* 24:577–582.

Hatfield, F. M., and Howard, D. (1977). Object naming in aphasia—the lack of effect of context or realism. *Neuropsychologia* 15:717–727.

Haxby, J. V., Ungerleider, L. G., Horwitz, B., Maisog, J. M., Rapoport, S. I., and Grady, C. L. (1996). Face encoding and recognition in the human brain. *Proc. Natl. Acad. Sci. U.S.A.* 93:922–927.

Head, H. (1918). Sensation and the cerebral cortex. *Brain* 41:57–253.

Head, H. (1920). Studies in Neurology, vol. 2. London: Oxford University Press.

Head, H., and Holmes, G. (1911). Sensory disturbances from cerebral lesions. *Brain* 34:102–254.

Head, H., Rivers, W. H. R., and Sherren, J. (1905). The afferent system from a new aspect. *Brain* 28:99.

Hécaen, H. (1962). Clinical symptomatology in right and left hemispheric lesions. *Interhemispheric Relations and Cerebral Dominance*, In V. B. Mountcastle (ed.). Baltimore, MD: Johns Hopkins University Press.

Hécaen, H. (1972). *Introduction à la Neuropsychologie*. Paris: Larousse.

Hécaen, H., and Albert, M. L. (1978). *Human Neuropsychology*. New York: John Wiley and Sons.

Hécaen, H., and Angelergues, R. (1962). Agnosia for faces (prosopagnosia). *Arch. Neurol.* 7:92–100.

Hécaen, H., and David, M. (1945). Syndrome parietale traumatique: asymbolie tactile et hemiasomatognosie paroxystique et douloureuse. *Rev. Neurol.* 77:113–123.

Hécaen, H., and de Ajuriaguerra, J. (1954). Balint's syndrome (psychic paralysis of visual fixation) and its minor forms. *Brain* 77:373–400.

Hécaen, H., and de Ajuriaguerra, J. (1956). Agnosie visuelle pour les objets inanimes par lesion unilaterale gauche. *Rev. Neurol. (Paris)* 94:222–233.

Hécaen, H., Goldblum, M. C., Masure, M. C., and Ramier, A. M. (1974). Une nouvelle observation dagnosie dobjet. Deficit de lassociation ou de la categorisation, specifique de Ia modalite visuell? *Neuropsychologia* 12:447–464.

Heilman, K. M., Scholes, R., and Watson, R. T. (1975). Auditory affective agnosia. Disturbed comprehension of affective speech. *J. Neurol. Neurosurg. Psychiatry* 38:69–72.

Hemphill, R. C., and Stengel, E. (1940). A study of pure word deafness. *J. Neurol. Psychiatry* 3:251–262.

Heywood, C. A., Gaffan, D., and Cowey, A. (1995). Cerebral achromatopsia in monkeys. *Eur. J. Neurosci.* 7:1064–1073.

Heywood, C. A., Kentridge, R. W., and Cowey, A. (1998). Form and motion from colour in cerebral achromatopsia. *Exp. Brain Res.* 123:145–153.

Holmes, G. (1918). Disturbances of visual orientation. *Br. J. Ophthalmol.* 2:449–468.

Holmes, G., and Horrax, G. (1919). Disturbances of spatial orientation and visual attention with loss of stereoscopic vision. *Arch. Neurol. Psychiatry* 1:385–407.

Horel, J. A., and Keating, E. G. (1969). Partial Kluver-Bucy syndrome produced by cortical disconnection. *Brain Res.* 16:281–284.

Horel, J. A., and Keating, E. G. (1972). Recovery from a partial Kluver-Bucy syndrome induced by disconnection. *J. Comp. Physiol. Psychol.* 79:105–114.

Hubel, D. H., and Weisel, T. N. (1977). Functional architecture of macaque monkey visual cortex. *Proc. R. Soc. Lond. Biol.* 198:1–59.

Humphreys, G. W., and Riddoch, M. J. (1987). *To See But Not To See: A Case Study of Visual Agnosia.* London: Lawrence Erlbaum Associates.

Hurlbert, A. C., Bramwell, D. I., Heywood, C., and Cowey, A. (1998). Discrimination of cone contrast changes as evidence for colour constancy in cerebral achromatopsia. *Exp. Brain Res.* 123:136–144.

Husain, M., and Stein, J. (1988). Rezso Balint and his most celebrated case. *Arch. Neurol.* 45:89–93.

Iversen, S. D., and Weiskrantz, L. (1964). Temporal lobe lesions and memory in the monkey. *Nature* 201:740–742.

Iversen, S. D., and Weiskrantz, L. (1967). Perception of redundant cues by monkeys with inferotemporal lesions. *Nature* 214:241–243.

Jackson, J. H. (1876). Case of large cerebral tumour without optic neuritis and with left hemiplegia and imperception. *R. Lond Ophthalmol. Hosp. Rep.* 8:434. Reprinted in *Selected Writings of John Hughlings Jackson, Vol. 2.* (1932), I. Taylor (ed.). London: Hodder and Stoughton.

Jerger, J., Lovering, L., and Wertz, M. (1972). Auditory disorder following bilateral temporal lobe insult: report of a case. *J. Speech Hear. Disord.* 37:523–535.

Jerger, J., Weikers, N., Sharbrough, F., and Jerger, S. (1969). Bilateral lesions of the temporal lobe. A case study. *Acta Otolaryngol. Suppl.* 258:1–51.

Jones, E. G., and Powell, T. P. S. (1969a). Connections of the somatic sensory cortex of the rhesus monkey. I. Ipsilateral cortical connections. *Brain* 92:477–502.

Jones, E. G., and Powell, T. P. S. (1969b). Connections of the somatic sensory cortex of the rhesus monkey. II. Contralateral connections. *Brain* 92:717–730.

Kaas, J. H. (1995). Human visual cortex. Progress and puzzles. *Curr. Biol.* 5:1126–1128.

Kaga, M. (1999). Language disorders in Landau-Kleffner syndrome. *J. Child Neurol.* 14:118–122.

Kanshepolsky, J., Kelley, J., and Waggener, J. (1973). A cortical auditory disorder. *Neurology* 23:699–705.

Kanter, S. L., Day, A. L., Heilman, K. M., and Gonzalez-Rothi, L. J. (1986). Pure word deafness: a possible explanation of transient deterioration after extracranial–intracranial bypass grafting. *Neurosurgery* 18:186–189.

Kanwisher, N., Chun, M. M., McDermott, J., and Ledden, P. J. (1996). Functional imagining of human visual recognition. *Cogn. Brain Res.* 5:55–67.

Kanwisher, N., Tong, F., and Nakayama, K. (1998). The effect of face inversion on the human fusiform face area. *Cognition* 68:B1–B11.

Karpov, B. A., Meerson, Y. A., and Tonkonogii, I. M. (1979). On some peculiatities of the visuomotor system in visual agnosia. *Neuropsychologia* 17:231–294.

Kase, C. S., Tronscoso, J. F., Court, J. E., Tapia, F. J. and Mohr, J. P. (1977). Global spatial disorientation. *J. Neurol. Sci.* 34:267–278.

Kazui, S., Naritomi, H., Sawada, T., and Inque, N. (1990). Subcortical auditory agnosia. *Brain Lang.* 38:476–487.

Kertesz, A. (1979). Visual agnosia: the dual deficit of perception and recognition. *Cortex* 15:403–419.

Kim, J. J., Andreasen, N. C., O'Leary, D. S., Wiser, A. K., Ponto, L. L., Watkins, G. L., and Hichwa, R. D. (1999). Direct comparison of the neural substrates of recognition memory for words and faces. *Brain* 122(Pt 6):1069–1083.

Kinsbourne, M., and Warrington, E. K. (1962). A disorder of simultaneous form perception. *Brain* 85:461–486.

Kinsbourne, M., and Warrington, E. K. (1964). Observations on color agnosia. *J. Neurol. Neurosurg. Psychiatry* 27:296–299.

Kitayama, I., Yamazaki, K., Shibahara, K., and Nomura, J. (1990). Pure word deafness with possible transfer of language dominance. *Jpn. J. Psychiatry Neurol.* 44:577–584.

Klein, R., and Harper, J. (1956). The problem of agnosia in the light of a case of pure word deafness. *J. Ment. Sci.* 102:112–120.

Kliest, K. (1928). Gehirnpathologische und lokalisatorische Ergebnisse uber Hörstorungen, Geruschtaubheiten und Amusien. *Monatsschr. Psychiatrie Neurol.* 68:853–860.

Kracke, I. (1994). Developmental prosopagnosia in Asperger syndrome: presentation and discussion of an individual case. *Dev. Med. Child Neurol.* 36:873–886.

Kreiman, G., Koch, C., and Fried, I. (2000). Category-specific visual responses of single neurons in the human medial temporal lobc. *Nat. Neurosci.* 3:946–953.

Kussmaul, A. (1877). Disturbances of speech. In *Cyclopedia of the Practice of Medicine*, H. von Ziemssien (ed.). New York: William Wood and Co.

Kuypers, H. G. J. M., Szwarcbart, M. K., Mishkin, M., and Rosvold, H. E. (1965). Occipitotemporal corticocortical connections in the rhesus monkey. *Exp. Neurol.* 11:245–262.

Lamberts, F. (1980). Developmental auditory agnosia in the severely retarded: a further investigation. *Brain Lang.* 11:106–118.

Landau, W. U., Goldstein, R., and Kleffner, F. R. (1960). Congenital aphasia: a clinicopathologic study. *Neurology* 10:915–921.

Landau, W. U., and Kleffner, F. R. (1957). Syndrome of acquired aphasia with convulsive disorder in children. *Neurology* 7:523–530.

Landis, T., Cummings, J. L., Christen, L., Bogen, J. E., and Imhof, H. G. (1986). Are unilateral right posterior cerebral lesions sufficient to cause prosopagnosia? Clinical and radiological findings in six additional patients. *Cortex* 22:243–252.

Landis, T., Graves, R., Benson, D. F., and Hebben, N. (1982). Visual recognition through kinaesthetic mediation. *Psychol. Med.* 12:515–531.

Landis, T., Regard, M., and Serrant, A. (1980). Iconic reading in a case of alexia without agraphia caused by a brain tumor: a tachistoscopic study. *Brain Lang.* 11:45–53.

Larrabee, G. J., Levin, H. S., Huff, F. J., Kay, M. C., and Guinto, F. C. (1985). Visual agnosia contrasted with visual–verbal disconnection. *Neuropsychologia* 23:1–12.

Lawden, M. C., and Cleland, P. G. (1993). Achromatopsia in the aura of migraine. *J. Neurol. Neurosurg. Psychiatry* 56:708–709.

Leicester, J. (1980). Central deafness and subcortical motor aphasia. *Brain Lang.* 10:224–242.

Levine, D. N. (1978). Prosopagnosia and visual object agnosia: a behavioral study. *Brain Lang.* 5:341–365.

Levine, D. N., and Calvanio, R. (1978). A study of the visual defect in verbal alexia-simultanagnosia. *Brain* 101:65–81.

Levine, D. N., and Calvanio, R. (1989). Prosopagnosia: a defect in visual configural processing. *Brain Cogn.* 10:149–170.

Levine, D. N., Kaufman, K. J., and Mohr, J. P. (1978). Inaccurate reaching associated with a superior parietal Iobe tumor. *Neurology* 28:556–561.

Lhermitte, F., and Beauvois, M. F. (1973). A visual–speech disconnection syndrome. *Brain* 96:695–714.

Lhermitte, F., Chain, F. Chcdru, J., and Pcnct, C. (1976). A study of visual processes in a case of interhemispheric disconnexion. *J. Neurol. Sci.* 25:317–330.

Lhermitte, F., Chain, F. Escourolle, R., et al. (1971). Étude des troubles perceptifs auditifs dans les lesions temporales bilaterales. *Rev. Neurol. (Paris)* 128:329–351.

Lhermitte, F., Chedru, J., and Chain, F. (1973). A propos d'une cas d'agnosie visuelle. *Rev. Neurol. (Paris)* 128:301–322.

Lhermitte, J., and de Ajuriaguerra, I. (1938). Asymbolie tactile et hallucinations du toucher. Étude anatomoclinique. *Rev. Neurol. (Paris)* 70:492–495.

Lhermitte, F., and Pillon, B. (1975). La prosopagnosie: role de l'hemisphere droit dans la perception visuelle. *Rev. Neurol. (Paris)* 131:791–812.

Lichteim, L. (1885). On aphasia. *Brain* 7:433–484.

Liepmann, H., and Storch, E. (1902). Der mikroskopische Gehirnbefund bei dem Fall Gorstelle. *Monatsschr. Psychiatrie Neurol.* 11:115–120.

Lissauer, H. (1890). Ein Fall von Seelenblindheit nebst einem Beitrage zur Theorie derselben. *Arch. Psychiatrie* 21:222–270.

Luria, A. R. (1959). Disorders of "simultaneous perception" in a case of bilateral occipitoparietal brain injury. *Brain* 83:437–449.

Luria, A. R., Pravdina-Vinarskaya, E. N., and Yarbus, A. L. (1963). Disorders of ocular movement in a case of simultanagnosia. *Brain* 86:219–228.

Lynch, J. C., and McClaren, J. W. (1989). Deficits of visual attention and saccadic eye movements after lesions of parietooccipital cortex in monkeys. *J. Neurophysiol.* 61:74–90.

Mack, J. L., and Boller, F. (1977). Associative visual agnosia and its related deficits: the role of the minor hemisphere in assigning meaning to visual perceptions. *Neuropsychologia* 15:345–349.

MacKay, G., and Dunlop, J. C. (1899). The cerebral lesions in a case of complete acquired colourblindness. *Scott. Med. Surg. J.* 5:503–512.

Mahoudeau, D., Lemoyne, J., Dubrisay, J., and Caraes, J. (1956). Sur un cas dagnosie auditive. *Rev. Neurol. (Paris)* 95:57.

Makino, M., Takanashi, Y., Iwamoto, K., Yoshikawa, K., Ohshima, H., Nakajima, K., Hayashi, K., Hayashi, R., and Endo, K. (1998). Auditory evoked magnetic fields in patients of pure word deafness [in Japanese]. *No To Shinkei* 50:51–55.

Marr, D. (1982). *Vision: A Computational Investigation into the Human Representation and Processing of Visual Information*. New York: W. H. Freeman.

Massopoust, L. C., and Wolin, L. R. (1967). Changes in auditory frequency discrimination thresholds after temporal cortex ablation. *Exp. Neurol.* 19:245–251.

Mauguiere, F., and Isnard, J. (1995). Tactile agnosia and dysfunction of the primary somatosensory area. Data of the study by somatosensory evoked potentials in patients with deficits of tactile object recognition [in French]. *Rev. Neurol. (Paris),* 151:518–527.

Maunsell, J. H. R., and Newsome, W. T. (1987). Visual processing in monkey extrastriate cortex. *Ann. Rev. Neurosci.* 10:363–401.

Mavlov, L. (1980). Amusia due to rhythm agnosia in a musician with left hemisphere damage: a non-auditory supramodal defect. *Cortex* 16:331–338.

McCall, G. N., and Cunningham, N. M. (1971). Two-point discrimination: asymmetry in spatial discrimination on the two sides of the tongue, a preliminary report. *Percept. Mot. Skills* 32:368–370.

McCarthy, R. A. and Warrington, E. K. (1986). Visual associative agnosia: a clinico-anatomical study of a single case. *J. Neurol. Neurosurg. Psychiatry* 49:1233–1240.

McClelland, J. L., and Rumelhart, D. E. (1986). *Parallel Distributed Processing: Explorations in the Microstructure of Cognition II. Psychological and Biological Models*. Cambridge, MA: MIT Press.

McFarland, H. R., and Fortin, D. (1982). Amusia due to right temporoparietal infarct. *Arch. Neurol.* 39:725–727.

McGlinchey Berroth, R., Milberg, W. P., Verfaellie, M., Alexander, M., and et al. (1993). Semantic processing in the neglected visual field: evidence from a lexical decision task. *Cogn. Neuropsychol.* 10:79–108.

McIntosh, A. R., Grady, C. L., Ungerleider, L. G., Haxby, J. V., Rapoport, S. I., and Horwitz, B. (1994). Network analysis of cortical visual pathways mapped with PET. *J. Neurosci.* 14:655–666.

McKeever, W. F., Larrabee, G. J., Sullivan, K. F., Johnson, H. J., Ferguson, S., Rayport, M., et al. (1981). Unimanual tactile anomia consequent to corpus callosotomy: reduction of anomic deficit under hypnosis. *Neuropsychologia* 19:179–190.

Meadows, J. C. (1974a). Disturbed perception of colours associated with localized cerebral lesions. *Brain* 97:615–632.

Meadows, J. C. (1974b). The anatomical basis of prosopagnosia. *J. Neurol. Neurosurg. Psychiatry* 37:489–501.

Mendez, M. F. (1988). Visuoperceptual function in visual agnosia. *Neurology* 38:1754–1759.

Mendez, M. F. (2000). Corticobasal ganglionic degeneration with Balint's syndrome. *J. Neuropsychiatry Clin. Neurosci.* 12:273–275.

Mendez, M. F., and Cherrier, M. M. (1998). The evolution of alexia and simultanagnosia in posterior cortical atrophy. *Neuropsychiatry Neuropsychol. Behav. Neurol.* 11:76–82.

Mendez, M. F., and Geehan, G. R., Jr. (1988). Cortical auditory disorders: clinical and psychoacoustic features. *J. Neurol. Neurosurg. Psychiatry* 51:1–9.

Mendez, M. F., Mendez, M. A., Martin, R., Smyth, K. A., and Whitehouse, P. J. (1990). Complex visual disturbances in Alzheimer's disease. *Neurology* 40:439–443.

Miceli, G. (1982). The processing of speech sounds in a patient with cortical auditory disorder. *Neuropsychologia* 20:5–20.

Michel, F., Perenin, M. T., and Sieroff, E. (1986). Prosopagnosie sans hemianopsie apres lesion unilateralie occipito-temporale droite. *Rev. Neurol. (Paris)* 142:545–549.

Michel, J., Peronnet, F., and Schott, B. (1980). A case of cortical deafness: clinical and electrophysiological data. *Brain Lang.* 10:367–377.

Michel, F., Poncet, M., and Signoret, J. L. (1989). Are the lesions responsible for prosopagnosia always bilateral? [in French]. *Rev. Neurol. (Paris)* 145:764–770.

Midorikawa, A., and Kawamura, M. (2000). A case of musical agraphia. *Neuroreport* 11:3053–3057.

Milberg, W., and Blumstein, S. E. (1981). Lexical decision and aphasia: evidence for semantic processing. *Brain Lang.* 14:371–385.

Milner, A. D., and Heywood, C. A. (1989). A disorder of lightness discrimination in a case of visual form agnosia. *Cortex* 25:489–494.

Milner, A. D., Perrett, D. I., Johnston, R. S., Benson, P. J., Jordan, T. R., Heeley, D. W., Betucci, D., Mortara, F., Mutini, R., Terazzi, D., and Davidson, D. L. W. (1991). Perception and action in "visual form agnosia." *Brain* 114:405–428.

Milner, B., and Taylor, L. B. (1972). Right-hemisphere superiority in tactile pattern recognition after cerebral commisurotomy: evidence for nonverbal memory. *Neuropsychologia* 10:1–15.

Motomura, N., Yamadori, A., Mori, E., and Tamaru, F. (1986). Auditory agnosia: analysis of a case with bilateral subcortical lesions. *Brain* 109: 379–391.

Mountcastle, V. B. (1961). Some functional properties of the somatic afferent system. In *Sensory Communication*, W. A. Rosenblith (ed.). Cambridge, MA: MIT Press, pp. 403–436.

Mountcastle, V. B., Lynch, J. C., Georgopoulos, A., Sakata, H., and Acuna, C. (1975). Posterior parietal association cortex of the monkey: command functions for operations within extrapersonal space. *J. Neurophysiol.* 38:871–908.

Mountcastle, V .B., and Powell, T. P. S. (1959a). Central nervous mechanisms subserving position sense and kinesthesis. *Bull. Johns Hopkins Hosp.* 105:173–200.

Mountcastle, V. B., and Powell, T. P. S. (1959b). Neural mechanisms subserving cutaneous sensibility, with special reference to the role of afferent inhibition in sensory perception and discrimination. *Bull. Johns Hopkins Hosp.* 105: 201–232.

Mulder, J. L., Bouma, A., and Ansink, B. J. (1995). The role of visual discrimination disorders and neglect in perceptual categorization deficits in right and left hemisphere damaged patients. *Cortex* 31:487–501.

Munk, H. (1881). *Ueber die Functionen der Grosshirnrinde. Gesammelte Mittheilungen aus den Jahren 1877–80.* Berlin: Hirschwald.

Nachson, I. (1995). On the modularity of face recognition: the riddle of domain specificity. *J. Clin. Exp. Neuropsychol.* 17:256–275.

Naeser, M. (1974). The relationship between phoneme discrimination, phoneme/picture perception, and language comprehension in aphasia. Presented at the Twelfth Annual Meeting of the Academy of Aphasia, Warrenton, Virginia, October 1974.

Nakakoshi, S., Kashino, M., Mizobuchi, A., Fukada, Y., and Katori, H. (2001). Disorder in sequential speech perception: a case study on pure word deafness. *Brain Lang.* 76:119–129.

Nakamura, J., Endo, K., Sumida, T., and Hasegawa, T. (1998). Bilateral tactile agnosia: a case report. *Cortex* 34:375–388.

Neff, W. D. (1961). Neruonal mechanisms of auditory discrimination. In *Sensory Communication*, N. A. Rosenblith (ed.). Cambridge, MA: MIT Press.

Neisser, U. (1967). *Cognitive Psychology.* New York: Appleton-Century-Crofts.

Neisser, U. (1976). *Cognition and Reality.* San Francisco: W. H. Freeman.

Newcombe, F., and Ratcliff, G. (1974). Agnosia: a disorder of object recognition. In *Les Syndromes de Disconnexion Calleuse chez L'homme.* F. Michel and B. Schott (eds.). Lyon: Colloque International de Lyon.

Newcombe, F., Young, A. W., and DeHaan, E. H. F. (1989). Prosopagnosia and object agnosia without covert recognition. *Neuropsychologia* 27: 179–191.

Nielsen, J. M., and Sult, C. W., Jr. (1939). Agnosia and the body scheme. *Bull. Los Angeles Neurol. Soc.* 4:69–81.

Nishioka, H., Takeda, Y., Koba, T., Yano, J., Ohiwa, Y., Haraoka, J., and Ito, H. (1993). A case of cortical deafness with bilateral putaminal hemorrhage [in Japanese]. *No Shinkei Geka* 21:269–272.

Oppenheim, H. (1906). Uber einen bemerkenswerten Fall von Tumor cerebri. *Berl. Klin. Wochenschr.* 43:1001–1004.

Oppenheim, H. (1911). *Textbook of Nervous Diseases for Physicians and Students.* Edinburgh: Darien Press.

Oppenheimer, D. R., and Newcombe, F. (1978). Clinical and anatomic findings in a case of auditory agnosia. *Arch. Neurol.* 35:712–719.

Otsuki, M., Soma, Y., Sato, M., Homma, A., and Tsuji, S. (1998). Slowly progressive pure word deafness. *Eur. Neurol.* 39:135–140.

Oxbury, J., Oxbury, S., and Humphrey, N. (1969). Varieties of color anomia. *Brain* 92:847–860.

Pallis, C. A. (1955). Impaired identification of faces and places with agnosia for colors. *J. Neurol. Neurosurg. Psychiatry* 18:218–224.

Paul, R. L., Merzenich, M., and Goodman, H. (1972). Representation of slowly and rapidly adapting cutaneous mechanorceptors of the hand in Brodmanns areas 3 and 1 of *Macaca mulatta. Brain Res.* 36:229–249.

Pearlman, A. L., Birch, J., and Meadows, J. C. (1979). Cerebral color blindness: an acquired defect in hue discrimination. *Ann. Neurol.* 5:253–261.

Penfield, W. (1958). *The Excitable Cortex in Conscious Man.* Springfield, IL: Charles C. Thomas.

Perenin, M. T., and Jeannerod, M. (1978). Visual function within the hemianopic field following early cerebral hemidecortication in man. I. Spatial localization. *Neuropsychologia* 16:1–13.

Peretz, I., Kolinsky, R., Tramo, M., Labrecque, R., Hublet, C., Demeurisse, G., and Belleville, S.

(1994). Functional dissociations following bilateral lesions of auditory cortex. *Brain 117(Pt 6)*:1283–1301.

Perrett, D., Rolls, E. T., and Caan, W. (1982). Visual neurons responsive to faces in the monkey temporal cortex. *Exp. Brain Res. 47*:329–342.

Perrett, D., Mistlin, A. J., and Chitty, A. J. (1987). Visual cells responsive to faces. *Trends Neurosci. 10*:358–364.

Piccirilli, M., Sciarma, T., and Luzzi, S. (2000). Modularity of music: evidence from a case of pure amusia. *J. Neurol. Neurosurg. Psychiatry 69*: 541–545.

Pillon, B., Signoret, J. L., and Lhermitte, F. (1981). Agnosie visuelle associative. Role del hemisphere gauche dans la perception visuelle. *Rev. Neurol. (Paris) 137*:831–842.

Platz, T. (1996). Tactile agnosia. Casuistic evidence and theoretical remarks on modality-specific meaning representations and sensorimotor integration. *Brain 119(Pt 5)*:1565–1574.

Polster, M. R., and Rose, S. B. (1998). Disorders of auditory processing: evidence for modularity in audition. *Cortex 34*:47–65.

Poppelreuter, W. (1923). Zur Psychologie und Pathologie der optischen Wahrnehmung. *Arch. Gesamte Neurol. Psychiatrie 83*:26–152.

Powell, T. P. S., and Mountcastle, V. B. (1959). Some aspects of the functional organization of the cortex of the postcentral gyrus of the monkey: a correlation of findings obtained in a single unit analysis with cyto-architecture. *Bull. Johns Hopkins Hosp. 105*:123–162.

Procopis, P. G. (1983). A case of receptive amusia with prominent timbre perception defect. *J. Neurol. Neurosurg. Psychiatry 46*:464.

Randolph, M., and Semmes, J. (1974). Behavioral consequences of selective subtotal ablations in the postcentral gyrus of *Macaca mulatta*. *Brain Res. 70*:55–70.

Rapin, I., Mattis, S., Rowan, A. J., and Golden, G. G. (1977). Verbal auditory agnosia in children. *Dev. Med. Child Neurol. 19*:192–207.

Ratcliff, G., and Ross, J. E. (1981). Visual perception and perceptual disorder. *Br. Med. Bull. 37*:181–186.

Raymond, F., and Egger, M. (1906). Un cas d'aphasie tactile. *Rev. Neurol. (Paris) 14*:371–375.

Reed, C. L., Caselli, R. J., and Farah, M. J. (1996). Tactile agnosia. Underlying impairment and implications for normal tactile object recognition. *Brain 119*:875–888.

Reinhold, M. (1950). A case of auditory agnosia. *Brain 73*:203–223.

Renault, B., Signoret, J. L., Debruille, B., Breton, F., and Bolgert, F. (1989). Brain potentials reveal covert facial recognition in prosopagnosia. *Neuropsychologia 27*:905–912.

Riddoch, M. J., and Humphreys, G. W. (1987a). A case of integrative visual agnosia. *Brain 110*: 1431–1462.

Riddoch, M. J., and Humphreys, G. W. (1987b). Visual object processing in optic aphasia: a case of semantic access agnosia. *Cogn. Neuropsychol. 4*:131–185.

Rizzo, M., and Hurtig, R. (1987). Looking but not seeing: attention, perception, and eye movements in simultanagnosia. *Neurology 37*:1642–1648.

Rizzo, M., Hurtig, R., and Damasio, A. R. (1987). The role of scanpaths in facial recognition and learning. *Ann. Neurol. 22*:41–45.

Roberts, M., Sandercock, P., and Ghadiali, E. (1987). Pure word deafness and unilateral right temporo-parietal lesions: a case report. *J. Neurol. Neurosurg. Psychiatry 50*:1708–1709.

Roediger, H. L., III, Guynn, M. J., and Jones, T. C. (1994). Implicit memory: a tutorial review. In *International Perspectives on Psychological Science, Vol. 2: The State of the Art*. G. d'Ydewalle and P. Eelen (eds.). Hove, UK: Lawrence Erlbaum Associates, pp. 67–94.

Roland, P. E. (1976). Astereognosis. *Arch. Neurol. 33*:543–550.

Roland, P. E., and Larsen, B. (1976). Focal increase of cerebral blood flow during stereognostic testing in man. *Arch. Neurol. 33*:551–558.

Rosati, G., DeBastiani, P., Paolino, E., et al. (1982). Clinical and audiological findings in a case of auditory agnosia. *J. Neurol. 227*:21–27.

Rosch, E., Mervis, C. B., Gray, W., Johnson, D., and Boyes-Braem, P. (1976). Basic objects in natural categories. *Cogn. Psychol. 8*:382–439.

Rose, J. E., and Woolsey, C. N. (1949). Organization of the mammalian thalamus and its relationship to the cerebral cortex. *Electroencephalogr. Clin. Neurophysiol. 1*:391–400.

Ross, E. D. (1980a). Sensory-specific and fractional disorders of recent memory in man. I. Isolated loss of visual recent memory. *Arch. Neurol. 37*: 193–200.

Ross, E. D. (1980b). The anatomic basis of visual agnosia [letter]. *Neurology 30*:109–110.

Rubens, A. B. (1979). Agnosia. In *Clinical Neuropsychology*. K. M. Heilman and E. Valenstein (eds.). New York: Oxford University Press

Rubens, A. B., and Benson, D. F. (1971). Associative visual agnosia. *Arch. Neurol. 24*:304–316.

Rudel, R. G., Denckla, M. B., and Spalten, E. (1974). The functional asymmetry of Braille letter learning in normal, sighted children. *Neurology 24:*733–738.

Rumelhart, D. E., and McClelland, J. L. (1986). *Parallel Distributed Processing: Explorations in the Microstructure of Cognition I. Foundations.* Cambridge, MA: MIT Press.

Saetti, M. C., De Renzi, E., and Comper, M. (1999). Tactile morphagnosia secondary to spatial deficits. *Neuropsychologia 37:*1087–1100.

Saffran, E. B., Marin, 0. S. M., and Yeni-Komshian, G. H. (1976). An analysis of speech perception in word deafness. *Brain Lang. 3:*255–256.

Sakai, K., Watanabe, E., Onodera, Y., Uchida, I., Kato, H., Yamamoto, E., Koizumi, H., and Miyashita, Y. (1995). Functional mapping of the human colour centre with echo-planar magnetic resonance imaging. *Proc. R. Soc. Lond. Ser. B Basic Biol. Sci. 261(1360):*89–98.

Schacter, D. L. (1989). On the relation between memory and consciousness: dissociable interactions and conscious experience. In *Varieties of Memory and Consciousness: Essays in Honour of Endel Tulving:* H. L. Roediger and F. I. M. Craik (eds.). Hillsdale, NJ: Lawrence Erlbaum Associates, pp. 355–389.

Schnider, A., Benson, D. F., Alexander, D. N., and Schnider-Klaus, A. (1994). Non-verbal environmental sound recognition after unilateral hemispheric stroke. *Brain 117:*281–287.

Schuppert, M., Munte, T. F., Wieringa, B. M., and Altenmuller, E. (2000). Receptive amusia: evidence for cross-hemispheric neural networks underlying music processing strategies. *Brain 12:*546–559.

Schuster, P., and Taterka, H. (1926). Beitrag zur Anatomie und Klinik der reinen Worttaubheit. *Z. Gesamte Neurol. Psychiatrie 105:*494.

Seiler, J., and Ricker, K. (1971). Das Vibrationsempfinden. Eine apparative Schwellenbestimmung. *Z. Neurol. 200:*70–79.

Semmes, J. (1953). Agnosia in animal and man. *Psychol. Rev. 60:*140–147.

Semmes, J. (1965). A non-tactual factor in astereognosis. *Neuropsychologia 3:*295–314.

Semmes, J., Weinstein, S., Ghent, L., and Teuber, H.-L. (1960). *Somatosensory Changes After Penetrating Brain Wounds in Man.* Cambridge, MA: Harvard University Press.

Sergent, J., Ohta, S., and MacDonald, B. (1992). Functional neuroanatomy of face and object processing. A positron emission tomography study. *Brain 115:*15–36.

Sergent, J., and Poncet, M. (1990). From covert to overt recognition of faces in a prosopagnosic patient. *Brain 113:*989–1004.

Sergent, J., and Villemure, G. (1989). Prosopagnosia in a right hemispherectomized patient. *Brain 112:*975–995.

Shah, N. J., Marshall, J. C., Zafiris, O., Schwab, A., Zilles, K., Markowitsch, H. J., and Fink, G. R. (2001). The neural correlates of person familiarity: a functional magnetic resonance imaging study with clinical implications. *Brain 124:*804–815.

Shallice, T. (1988). *From Neuropsychology to Mental Structure.* Cambridge, UK: Cambridge University Press.

Shallice, T., and Saffran, E. (1986). Lexical processing in the absence of explicit word identification: evidence from a letter-by-letter reader. *Cogn. Neuropsychol. 3:*429–458.

Shelton, P. A., Bowers, D., Duara, R., and Heilman, K. M. (1994). Apperceptive visual agnosia: a case study. *Brain Cogn. 25:*1–23.

Shoumaker, R. D., Ajax, E. T., and Schenkenberg, T. (1977). Pure word deafness (auditory verbal agnosia). *Dis. Nerv. Syst. 38:*293–299.

Shraberg, D., and Weitzel, W.D. (1979). Prosopagnosia and the Capgras syndrome. *J. Clin. Psychiatry 40:*313–316.

Shuren, J., Geldmacher, D., and Heilman, K. M. (1993). Nonoptic aphasia: aphasia with preserved confrontation naming in Alzheimer's disease. *Neurology 43:*1900–1907.

Shuttleworth, E. C., Syring, V., and Allen, N. (1982). Further observations on the nature of prosopagnosia. *Brain Cogn. 1:*307–322.

Small, S. L., Hart, J., Nguyen, T., and Gordon, B. (1995). Distributed representations of semantic knowledge in the brain. *Brain 118:*441–453.

Sparr, S. A., Jay, M., Drislane, F. W., and Venna, N. (1991). A historic case of visual agnosia revisited after 40 years. *Brain 114:*789–800.

Sprague, J. M., Levy, J. D., and Berlucci, C. (1977). Visual cortical areas mediating form discrimination in the rat. *J. Comp. Neurol. 172:*441–488.

Spreen, O., Benton, A.L., and Fincham, R. (1965). Auditory agnosia without aphasia. *Arch. Neurol. 13:*84–92.

Spreen, O., Benton, A. L., and Van Allen, M. W. (1966). Dissociation of visual and tactile naming in amnesic aphasia. *Neurology 16:*807–814.

Stauffenburg, V. (1914). *Uber Seelenblindheit. Arbeiten aus dem Hirnatomischen Institut in Zurich, Heft 8.* Wiesbaden: Bergman.

Stengel, E. (1948). The syndrome of visual alexia with color agnosia. *J. Ment. Sci. 94:*46–58.

Stockard, J. J., and Rossiter, V. S. (1977). Clinical and pathologic correlates of brainstem auditory response abnormalities. *Neurology 27:*316–325.

Suzuki, K., Nomura, H., Yamadori, A., Nakasato, N., and Takase, S. (1997). "Associative" visual agnosia for objects, pictures, faces and letters with altitudinal hemianopia [in Japanese]. *Rinsho Shinkeigaku* 37:31–36.

Synodinou, C., Christodoulou, G. N., and Tzavaras, A. (1978). Capgras syndrome and prosopagnosia [letter]. *Sr I Psychiatry* 132:413–414.

Taylor, A., and Warrington, E. K. (1971). Visual agnosia: a single case report. *Cortex* 7:152–164.

Teuber, H.-L (1965a). Somatosensory disorders due to cortical lesions. *Neuropsychologia* 3:287–294.

Teuber, H.-L. (1965b). Postscript: some needed revisions of the classical views of agnosia. *Neuropsycholgia* 3:371–378.

Teuber, H.-L. (1968). Alteration of perception and memory in man. In *Analysis of Behavioral Change*, L. Weiskrantz (eds.), New York: Harper and Row,

Tohgi, H., Watanabe, K., Takahashi, H., Yonezawa, H., Hatano, K., and Sasaki, T. (1994). Prosopagnosia without topographagnosia and object agnosia associated with a lesion confined to the right occipitotemporal region. *J. Neurol.* 241:470–474.

Tranel, D. (1991). What has been rediscovered in "rediscovering tactile agnosia"? *Mayo Clin. Proc.* 66:210–214.

Tranel, D., and Damasio, A. R. (1985). Knowledge without awareness: an autonomic index of facial recognition by prosopagnosics. *Science* 228:1453–1454.

Tranel, D., Damasio, A. R., and Damasio, H. (1988). Intact recognition of facial expression, gender, and age in patients with impaired recognition of face identity. *Neurology* 38:690–696.

Tusa, R. J., and Ungerleider, L. G. (1985). The inferior longitudinal fasciculus: a reexamination in humans and monkeys. *Ann. Neurol.* 18:583–591.

Tyler, H. R. (1968). Abnormalities of perception with defective eye movements (Balint's syndrome). *Cortex* 4:154–171.

Tzavaras, A., Hécaen, H., and LeBras, H. (1970). Le probleme de la specificite du deficit de la reconnaisance du visage humans Iors des lesions hemispheriques unilaterales. *Neuropsychologia* 8:403–416.

Ulrich, G. (1978). Interhemispheric functional relationships in auditory agnosia: an analysis of the preconditions and a conceptual model. *Brain Lang.* 5:286–300.

Valentine, T. (1988). Upside down faces: a review of the effects of inversion upon face recognition. *Br. J. Psychol.* 79:471–491.

Van Lancker, D. R., Cummings, J. L., Kreiman, L., and Dobkin, B. H. (1988). Phonagnosia: a dissociation between familiar and unfamiliar voices. *Cortex* 24:195–209.

Van Lancker, D. R., and Kreiman, J. (1988). Unfamiliar voice discrimination and familiar voice recognition are independent and unordered abilities. *Neuropsychologia* 25:829–834.

Van Lancker, D. R., Kreiman, J., and Cummings, J. (1989). voice perception deficits: neuroanatomical correlates of phonagnosia. *J. Clin. Exp. Neuropsychol.* 11:665–674.

Vecera, S. P., and Gilds, K. S. (1998). What processing is impaired in apperceptive agnosia? Evidence from normal subjects. *J. Cogn. Neurosci.* 10:568–580.

Verfaellie, M., and Keane, M. M. (1997). The neural basis of aware and unaware forms of memory. *Semin. Neurol.* 17:153–161.

Verfaellie, M., Rapcsak, S. Z., and Heilman, K. M. (1990). Impaired shifting of attention in Balint's syndrome. *Brain Cogn.* 12:195–204.

Vignolo, L. A. (1969). Auditory agnosia: a review and report of recent evidence. In *Contributions to Clinical Neuropsychology*, A. L. Benton (ed.). Chicago: Aldine.

Von Frey, M. (1895). Beitrage zur Sinnes Physiologie der Haut Berichle u.d. Verhandlungen d.k. Sachs. *Gesell. Wiss.* 2 S:166.

Von Hagen, K. O. (1941). Two cases of mind blindness (visual agnosia), one due to carbon monoxide intoxication, one due to a diffuse degenerative process. *Bull. Los Angeles Neurol. Soc.* 6:191–194.

Wapner, W., Judd, T., and Gardner, H. (1978). Visual agnosia in an artist. *Cortex* 14:343–364.

Warrington, E. K. (1985). Agnosia: the impairment of object recognition. In *Handbook of Clinical Neurology*. P. J. Vinken, G. W. Bruyn, and H. L. Klawans (Eds.). Amsterdam: Elsevier.

Warrington, E. K., and James, M. (1967). An experimental investigation of facial recognition in patients with unilateral cerebral lesions. *Cortex* 3:317–326.

Warrington, E. K., and James, M. (1988). Visual apperceptive agnosia: a clinico-anatomical study of three cases. *Cortex* 24:13–32.

Warrington, E. K., and McCarthy, R. (1987). Categories of knowledge: further fractionation and an attempted integration. *Brain* 110:1273–1296.

Warrington, E. K., and Rabin, P. (1971). Visual span of apprehension in patients with unilateral cerebral lesions. *Q. J. Exp. Psychol.* 23:423–431.

Warrington, E. K., and Shallice, T. (1980). Word-form dyslexia. *Brain* 103:391–403.

Warrington, E. K., and Shallice, T. (1984). Category-specific semantic impairments. *Brain* 107:829–854.

Warrington, E. K., and Taylor, A. M. (1973). The

contribution of the right parietal lobe to visual object recognition. *Cortex 9*:152–164.

Watson, R. T., and Heilman, K. M. (1983). Callosal apraxia. *Brain 106*:391–403.

Watson, R. T., and Rapcsak, S. Z. (1987). Loss of spontaneous blinking in a patient with Balint's syndrome. *Arch. Neurol. 46*:567–570.

Weinstein, S. (1968). Intensive and extensive aspects of tactile sensitivity as a function of body part, sex, and laterality. In *The Skin Senses*. D. R. Kenshalo (ed.). Springfield, IL: Charles C. Thomas, pp. 195–222.

Weiskrantz, L. (1986). *Blindsight: A Case Study and Implications*. New York: Oxford University Press.

Weiskrantz, L., Warrington, E. K., Sanders, M. D., and Marshall, J. (1974). Visual capacity in the hemianopic field following a restricted occipital ablation. *Brain 97*:709–728.

Werner, G., and Whitsel, B. (1973) Functional organization of the somatosensory cortex. In *Somatosensory Systems, Handbook of Sensory Physiology, Vol. 2*, A. Iggo (ed.). New York: Springer-Verlag, pp. 621–700.

Wernicke, C. (1895). Zwei Fälle von Rindenläsion. *Arb. Psychiatr. Klin. Breslau 11*:35.

Wertheim, N. (1969). The amusias. In *Handbook of Clinical Neurology, Vol 4*, P. J. Vinken and G. W. Bruyn (eds.). Amsterdam: North-Holland.

Whiteley, A. M., and Warrington, E. K. (1977). Prosopagnosia: a clinical, psychological, and anatomical study of three patients. *J. Neurol. Neurosurg. Psychiatry 40*:395–403.

Wilbrand, H. (1887). *Die Seelenblindheit als Herderscheinung*. Wiesbaden: Bergmann.

Wohlfart, G., Lindgren, A., and Jernelius, B. (1952). Clinical picture and mobid anatomy in a case of "pure word deafness." *J. Nerv. Ment. Dis. 116*: 818–827.

Wolpert, I. (1924). Die Simultanagnosie: Störung der Gesamtauffassung. *Z. Gesamte Neurol. Psychiatrie 93*:397–413.

Woolsey, C. N. (1952). Cortical localization as efined

by evoked potential and electrical stimulation studies. In *Cerebral Localization and Organization*, G. Schaltenbrand and C. N. Woolsey (eds.). Madison, WI: University of Wisconsin Press, pp. 17–26.

Wortis, S. B., and Pfeffer, A. Z. (1948). Unilateral auditory–spatial agnosia. *J. Nerv. Ment. Dis. 108*: 181–186.

Wyke, M., and Holgate, D. (1973). Color naming defects in dysphasic patients—a qualitative analysis. *Neuropsychologia 8*:451–461.

Yin, R. K. (1969). Looking at upside-down faces. *J. Exp. Psychol. 81*:141–145.

Yin, R. K. (1970). Face recognition by brain-injured patients: a dissociable ability? *Neuropsychologia 8*:395–402.

Young, A. W., de Haan, E. H., and Newcombe, F. (1990). Unawareness of impaired face recognition. *Brain Cogn. 14*:1–18.

Young, A. W., Hellawell, D., and DeHaan, E. H. F. (1988). Cross-domain semantic priming in normal subjects and a prosopagnosic patient. *Q. J. Exp. Psychol. 40A*:561–580.

Young, R. S., and Fishman, G. A. (1980). Loss of color vision and Stiles II, mechanism in a patient with cerebral infarction. *J. Opt. Soc. Am. 170*: 1301–1305.

Zangaladze, A., Epstein, C. M., Grafton, S. T., and Sathian, K. (1999). Involvement of visual cortex in tactile discrimination of orientation. *Nature 401(6753)*:587–590.

Zeki, S. M. (1973). Colour coding in rhesus monkey prestriate cortex. *Brain Res. 53*:422–427.

Zeki, S. M. (1977). Colour coding in the superior temporal sulcus of rhesus monkey visual cortex. *Proc. R. Soc. Lond. B Biol Sci. 197*:195–223.

Ziegler, D. K. (1952). Word deafness and Wernicke's aphasia: report of cases and discussion of the syndrome. *Arch. Neurol. Psychiatry 67*:323–331.

Zihl, J., and Von Cramon, D. (1979). The contribution of the 'second' visual system to directed visual attention in man. *Brain 102*:835–856.

13

Neglect and Related Disorders

KENNETH M. HEILMAN, ROBERT T. WATSON,
AND EDWARD VALENSTEIN

Neglect is the failure to report, respond, or orient to novel or meaningful stimuli presented to the side opposite a brain lesion, when this failure cannot be attributed to either sensory or motor defects (Heilman, 1979). Neglect may be spatial or personal. Spatial neglect may occur in three reference frames: body centered, environmentally centered, and object centered. One may be inattentive to stimuli in space or on the person (attentional or sensory neglect) and one may fail to act in a portion of space, in a spatial direction, or to use a portion of one's body (intentional or motor neglect). Many specific disorders have been described, distinguished by their presumed underlying mechanisms, the distribution of the abnormal behavior, and the means of eliciting the behavior. Different behavioral manifestations may occur at different times, and in some patients certain manifestations are never seen.

The major behavioral manifestations that we will discuss in this chapter include *(1)* inattention or sensory neglect, *(2)* extinction to simultaneous stimuli, *(3)* motor neglect, *(4)* spatial neglect, *(5)* personal neglect, *(6)* allesthesia and allokinesia, and *(7)* anosognosia (unawareness of illness). The first section of this chapter will define specific disorders and describe clinical tests that may be used to assess them.

The second section will discuss pathophysiology, and the third, recovery and treatment.

DEFINITIONS AND TESTS

INATTENTION

Sensory Neglect

Definition. Sensory neglect or *inattention* refers to a deficit in awareness of stimuli contralateral to a lesion that does not involve sensory projection systems or the primary cortical sensory areas to which they project. The distribution of attentional deficits varies from patient to patient, and may vary in the same patient depending on the method of testing. Patients may fail to attend to visual, auditory, or tactile stimuli, and their inattention may be to stimuli in space or to stimuli on the body. It is not unusual for patients with neglect to also be inattentive to stimuli that are ipsilateral to their lesion, but ipsilateral inattention is not as severe as contralateral. In addition to being unaware of stimuli, patients with hemispheric lesions may have difficulty disengaging attention, or shifting attention, especially in a contralesional direction.

When the locus of the lesion is not known, it may be difficult to distinguish sensory neglect from sensory loss. Sometimes instructional cues, novel stimuli, or stimuli with strong motivational value may elicit a response, demonstrating that the primary sensory pathways are intact and that the prior failure to detect stimuli was an attentional deficit. The difficulty of distinguishing sensory neglect from an afferent deficit varies with sensory modality. It is easiest with auditory deficits, where, except for stimuli delivered very close to one ear, failure to report unilateral stimuli usually results from unilateral auditory inattention, for two reasons. First, patients with unilateral hearing loss will usually detect such stimuli, because the sound will project to the good ear. Second, unilateral cerebral lesions do not cause unilateral hearing loss, because the auditory pathways carrying information from each ear project to both cerebral hemispheres. Therefore, patients who neglect or are inattentive to unilateral auditory stimuli most often have unilateral inattention rather than a primary afferent defect.

It is also the case that patients with hemianesthesia from unilateral cortical lesions most likely suffer from inattention rather than deafferentation. Elementary somatic sensation can probably be subserved by the thalamus. Lesions of the ventral posterolateral and ventral posteromedial thalamic nuclei result in hemianesthesia, but lesions in somatosensory cortex should not. Some patients with cortical lesions who appear to have tactile anesthesia can detect contralesional stimuli when cold water is injected into the contralesional ear. This procedure increases orientation toward the side where the cold water is injected, suggesting that the hemianesthesia in fact results from sensory neglect (Vallar et al., 1990). One can also use psychophysiological procedures, such as early evoked potentials and skin conductance responses, to discriminate between inattention and deafferentation.

The distinction between unilateral inattention and deafferentation can be most difficult in the visual modality. Hemianopia is commonly caused by lesions affecting the calcarine (primary visual) cortex, or the geniculocal-

carine pathways that carry visual information from the thalamus to the cerebral cortex. Patients with hemisphere lesions that spare these structures, but produce severe neglect, may act as if they are hemianopic. The ability to point to the location of a stimulus in the blind field or to avoid objects in the hemianopic field does not necessarily indicate an attentional deficit, since patients with hemianopia have been reported to have these abilities, presumably on the basis of subcortical (collicular) visual processing. It is sometimes possible to demonstrate that an apparent hemianopia results from neglect by taking advantage of descrepancies between retinotopic and body frames of reference. The distribution of attention in space depends not only on the position of the stimulus in the visual field but also on the relative position of the stimulus to the patient's body. The retinotopic visual field and the spatial fields defined by head or body position are only congruent when the subject is looking straight ahead. Moving the eyes to one side will result in the retinotopic visual field being different from the head or body spatial field, and moving the head and eyes will result in three noncongruent fields. True hemianopia is not influenced by eye movements, but visual inattention can vary with direction of gaze. For example, patients with body-centered visual inattention may fail to detect stimuli when they gaze straight ahead or to contralesional hemispace, but when their gaze is directed to ipsilesional hemispace, placing the contralateral visual field within the ipsilesional head or body hemispace, they may be able to detect stimuli, even though the stimuli remain at the same locations in their retinotopic visual field (Kooistra and Heilman, 1989; Nadeau and Heilman, 1991).

Testing. Inattention is detected by asking patients where they were stimulated. Language-impaired patients may respond nonverbally, but failure to respond nonverbally may reflect akinesia rather than inattention. Stimuli should be given in each of three modalities: *(1)* visual, *(2)* somesthetic, and *(3)* auditory. These visual, somesthetic, and auditory stimuli should be presented to the abnormal (contralesional) side and to the normal side of the body in random order.

Visual stimuli are presented to each half field with the eyes directed straight ahead, away from the lesion, and towards the lesion. Perimetry and tangent screen examination should be used when possible; however, for bedside testing, confrontation techniques are adequate. Either a cotton-tipped applicator or a finger can be used as the stimulus. The patient may be asked to detect finger movements, or to count fingers in one or both visual fields. To test for somesthetic neglect at the bedside, the patient can be touched with a finger, a cotton applicator, or, if better control of stimulus intensity is desired, von Frei hairs. More elaborate equipment can be used for better control of stimulus intensity, if this is needed for research purposes. Other somatosensory modalities (pin, temperature, etc.) can also be tested. Auditory stimuli for bedside testing may consist of rubbing or snapping the fingers. Audiometric techniques are preferable for rigorous testing.

Extinction to Simultaneous Stimulation

Definition. As patients with inattention improve, they become able to correctly detect and lateralize stimuli contralateral to their lesion, but when presented with bilateral simultaneous stimuli they often fail to report contralesional stimuli. This phenomenon was first noted by Loeb (1885) and Oppenheim (1885) in the tactile modality and by Anton (1899) and Poppelreuter (1917) in the visual modality. It has been called "extinction to double simultaneous stimulation" (or just "extinction"). It may also be seen in the auditory modality (Bender, 1952; Heilman et al., 1970). A patient may have extinction in several modalities (multimodal extinction) or in one modality. Extinction is usually mildest in the auditory modality. Although extinction is most severe when a stimulus presented to the side contralateral to the lesion is paired with a stimulus on the other side, extinction may also occur when both stimuli are on the same side, even when they are both ipsilateral to the lesion (Rapscak et al., 1987).

Testing. If the patient responds normally to unilateral stimulation, bilateral simultaneous stimulation should be given, interspersed with unilateral stimuli. Visual, tactile, or auditory stimuli are presented to the right and left visual fields, sides of the body, or sides of the head, respectively. It is sometimes possible to demonstrate visual or tactile extinction when two stimuli are delivered to the same hemifield or on the same side of the body. Under these testing conditions it is usually the stimulus closer to the contralesional side that is not detected (Rapcsak et al., 1987, Feinberg et al., 1990). Bender (1952) noted that normal subjects may show extinction to simultaneous stimulation when stimuli are delivered to two different (asymmetrical) parts of the body (simultaneous bilateral heterologous stimulation). For example, if the right side of the face and the left hand are stimulated simultaneously, normal subjects sometimes report only the stimulus on the face. Normal subjects do not extinguish symmetrical simultaneous stimuli (simultaneous bilateral homologous stimulation). Simultaneous bilateral heterologous stimulation can sometimes be used to test for milder defects in patients with neglect. For example, when the right face and left hand are stimulated, the patient with left-sided neglect does not report the stimulus on the left hand, but when the left face and right hand are stimulated, the patients reports both stimuli.

Defective Vigilance

Definition. When testing for sensory inattention or extinction, some patients will initially be able to detect contralesional stimuli; however, with repeated stimulation they eventually fail to detect these stimuli.

Testing. Testing for defects in vigilance is similar to that performed for extinction, only in this case the testing is prolonged.

Allesthesia

Definition. When patients without right left confusion are touched on the side opposite their lesion, they may report that they were touched on the same side as their lesion (Obersteiner, 1882). This has been called "allesthesia." A similar defect may be seen in other sensory modalities.

Testing. Testing is the same as that described for sensory inattention. However, to make certain that the defect is one of allesthesia rather than allokinesia, the patient should respond verbally rather than by moving the limb.

INTENTIONAL (MOTOR) NEGLECT

Patients may fail to respond to a stimulus even though they are aware of it, and even when they have the strength to respond. We call the failure to respond in the absence of unawareness or weakness an "action-intentional disorder." In the following sections, we will discuss four types or action-intentional disorder: akinesia, motor extinction, hypokinesia, and motor impersistence.

Akinesia

Definitions. Akinesia is a failure of initiation of movement that cannot be attributed to dysfunction in upper or lower motor neuron systems. Akinesia may involve the eyes, the head, a limb, or the whole body. It may vary, depending on where in space the body part is moved or in what direction it is moved. In directional akinesia, there is a reluctance to move in the direction contralateral to the lesion. Certain forms of gaze palsy are directional akinesias, and there are directional akinesias of the head and even of the arms. Directional akinesia may be associated with a directional motor bias: the eyes may deviate toward the side of the lesion, and, when the patient is asked to point to a spot opposite the sternum with the eyes closed, the arm may also deviate to the side of the lesion (Heilman et al., 1983a).

Akinesia may also depend upon the side in which the action is taken. In the patient described by Meador et al. (1986), the arm contralateral to the lesion was less akinetic in ipsilesional than in contralesional hemispace, independent of the direction of movement.

Movements can be produced in response to an external stimulus or they can occur independently of a stimulus. The former we call

"exogenously evoked" (exo-evoked) and the latter, "endogenously evoked" (endo-evoked). Exo-evoked akinesia is also called "motor neglect." A patient may have both exo- and endo-evoked akinesia.

Testing. Because akinesia may affect different body parts, one should assess movement of the eyes, head, trunk, and limbs. To detect endo-evoked akinesia, it is important to observe spontaneous behavior. Patients with endo-evoked akinesia often have symptoms of abulia (decreased drive, with psychomotor retardation). Patients whose akinesia is principally endo-evoked may respond normally to external stimuli. This has been called "kinesia paradoxica," and is frequently associated with Parkinson's disease.

Exo-evoked akinesia (motor neglect) results in failure to move in response to a stimulus, but failure to respond may also result from an elemental sensory defect or to sensory inattention. To distinguish these deficits, Watson et al. (1978) devised the crossed-response task. Although originally used in monkeys, it can also be used with humans. Monkeys were trained to respond with the right arm to a left-sided stimulus and with the left arm to a right-sided stimulus. An animal was considered to have a sensory deficit or sensory neglect if it did not respond to a contralesional stimulus using the "normal" (ipsilesional) arm. It was considered to have exo-evoked akinesia if it failed to move the contralesional extremity in response to stimulation of the "normal" (ipsilesional) side, despite intact spontaneous movements and normal strength of the contralesional arm. One can use the crossed-response task to test for exo-evoked akinesia of the limbs, the eyes, or the head.

To assess whether the spatial coordinates of actions influence akinesia, one needs to observe directional and hemispatial movements that are both endo-evoked (spontaneous) and exo-evoked (in response to stimuli). When attempting to determine if there is an endo-evoked directional akinesia of the eyes, one should observe spontaneous eye movements to detect eye deviation or bias toward the side of the lesion, or a paresis of gaze to the side opposite the lesion (a failure to look spontaneously into contralesional space). An exo-evoked directional akinesia of the eyes can be assessed by a modification of the Watson et al. (1978) paradigm in which the patient must look either toward or away from ipsi- and contralesional stimuli. The examiner stands directly in front of a patient and positions one hand in the patient's right visual field and the other in the left visual field, at eye level. The patient is instructed to fixate on the examiner's nose, and to look away from a finger if it moves downward and toward the finger if it moves upward. A failure to look at the contralesional finger when it moves upward may be related to sensory defect (e.g., hemianopsia), sensory neglect, or directional akinesia. However, failure to look toward the contralesional finger when the ipsilesional finger moves downward suggests an exo-evoked directional akinesia of the eyes (Butter et al., 1988b).

Similar tests can be used to detect directional and hemispatial akinesia of the head or arm. To test for a directional bias of an arm (similar to eye deviation), patients are asked to close their eyes and point to their sternum. If they are able to point to the sternum, they are then asked to point with the index finger to a point in space perpendicular to their sternum (the midsagittal plane). Patients with a motor (intentional) bias will deviate in the direction of their lesioned hemisphere (Heilman et al., 1983a).

To test for exo-evoked hemispatial akinesia of the arm, patients must be tested with arms crossed and uncrossed. In uncrossed conditions, each hand is placed on a table in compatible hemispace. In the crossed condition, each hand is placed in the opposite hemispace. Patients are instructed to lift their hand on the same side as the moving finger if they see the examiner's finger move up, but to move the hand on the opposite side if they see the examiner's finger move down. After patients are trained on this paradigm (up-same, down-opposite), the examiner randomly moves his or her right or left index finger up or down. When patients fail to move the contralesional arm when it is in contralesional hemispace but moves the arm when it crosses into ipsilesional hemispace, they are considered to have hemispatial limb akinesia (Meador et al., 1986).

To distinguish exo-evoked directional akinesia, hemispatial akinesia or directional hypometria from an ipsilesional attentional bias, Na et al. (1998b) used a video apparatus in such a way that the subjects could not directly see their own hand, but instead observed their hand and the stimulus (a line) on a video monitor. In the direct condition, the hand movements and the line are accurately portrayed; however, in the indirect condition, right and left on the monitor are reversed, so that leftward movements in actual work space appear to be rightward on the monitor and vice versa. Using this paradigm, patients with an ipsilesional attentional bias will reverse the spatial error in the indirect condition but patients with primarily directional akinesia (hypometria) will continue to err in the same direction. Using this same paradigm, Adair et al., 1998 demonstrated that many patients have a combination of attentional and intentional neglect.

To dissociate hemispatial akinesia from hemispatial inattention, Coslett et al. (1990) also had patients view the stimulus (a line) and their own responding hand on a TV monitor. The patient was prevented from viewing the line directly. Both the line (where the action takes place) and the TV monitor were independently placed in either hemispace. A greater ipsilesional bias of line bisection with the TV monitor in contralesional than in ipsilesional hemispace, independent of line placement, indicates a contribution of hemispatial inattention. A greater ipsilesional bias of line bisection when the line is placed in contralesional hemispace than when in ipsilesional hemispace, independent of monitor placement, suggests a contribution of a hemispatial akinesia. Other investigators have used other procedures to dissociate hemispatial and directional akinesia or hypometria from hemispatial sensory neglect or an attention bias. For example, Bisiach et al. (1990) used a pulley with a string, and Tegner and Levander (1991) used a mirror apparatus.

De Renzi et al. (1970) developed a task that can be used to test for endo-evoked directional limb akinesia. In our modification, the patient is blindfolded and small objects such as pennies are randomly scattered on a table to the left and right of the midsagittal plane (both hemispatial fields) within arm's reach. The patient is asked to retrieve as many pennies as possible. The task is endo-evoked because the patient cannot see the pennies and must initiate exploratory behavior in the absence of an external stimulus. Patients with an endo-evoked directional akinesia of the arm may fail to move their arm fully into contralateral hemispace to explore for pennies.

Motor Extinction

Definition. Some patients who do not demonstrate akinesia when they move one limb at a time may demonstrate contralesional akinesia when they must simultaneously move both limbs (Valenstein and Heilman, 1981). We call this "motor extinction."

Testing. Motor extinction is tested by using a method similar to that used to test for sensory extinction; however, the examiner not only requests verbal report as to where the patient was stimulated (e.g., right, left, both), but in other trials requests that the subject move the body part (e.g., hand or arm) on the same side that was stimulated (right, left, both). Patients with sensory extinction will fail to report the contralesional stimulus with simultaneous stimulation and will also fail to move the contralesional limb. Patients with motor extinction will report stimulation of both sides but will move only the ipsilateral limb.

Hypokinesia

Definition. Patients with mild defects in action-intentional systems may not fail to initiate responses, but may initiate them after an abnormally long delay. We have called this "hypokinesia." Since the patient must respond to a stimulus in order to judge whether or not the response is slow, hypokinesia is by definition exo-evoked.

Testing. The same paradigms that are used to test for akinesia of the eyes and limbs can be used to test for hypokinesia. While some patients with hypokinesia have such markedly slowed initiation times that hypokinesia can be

detected easily, others have more subtle defects, necessitating reaction-time paradigms to observe their defects. Reaction times can be slowed for a variety of reasons, including impaired attention, bradyphrenia, or hypokinesia. To detect hypokinesia, one should use simple reaction times that do not require cognition and thus cannot be impaired by bradyphrenia. Similarly, to test for hypokinesia, one has to use stimulus parameters that ensure that inattention cannot masquerade as hypokinesia.

Hypokinesia can be seen both in the limbs and eyes and may be either independent of direction or directionally specific such that there is a greater delay initiating movements in a contralesional direction than in an ipsilesional direction (Heilman et al., 1985). Hypokinesia can also be hemispatial: movements with the same limb may be more slowly initiated in contralesional hemispace than in ipsilesional hemispace (Meador et al., 1986).

Bradyinesia

Definition. Bradykinesia refers to slowness of movement, and is independent of the time to initiate movement (hypokinesia). Bradykinesia may be observed with limb, head, eye, or whole body movements, and it may be directional or hemispatial. Thus, movements of the contralesional limb may be slower than movements of the ipsilesional limb, and contralesional limb movements toward or in contralesional hemispace may be slower than movements of the ipsilesional limb toward or in ipsilesional hemispace (Mattingly et al., 1992)

Testing. To test for limb bradykinesia one can use rapid finger tapping. Special equipment to measure movement times is needed to test for directional bradykinesia of the arm, head, or eyes.

Motor Impersistence

Definition. Motor impersistence is the inability to sustain an act. It is the intentional equivalent of the attentional disorder called "distractibility." It can be demonstrated in a variety of body parts, including the limbs, eyes, eyelids, jaw, and tongue. Like akinesia, it may also be directional (Kertesz et al., 1985) or hemispatial (Roeltgen et al., 1989).

Testing. Limb impersistence can be tested by asking a patient to maintain a limb posture such as arm extension for 20 seconds. Since limb impersistence can be hemispatial (Roeltgen et al., 1989), one can test each limb in its own and in opposite hemispace. To test for directional impersistence, one requests the patient to keep the eyes directed, or the head turned, to the left or right for 20 seconds. Directional impersistence may be worse in one hemispace than the other. Directional impersistence of the arm has not been described. Patients with directional impersistence usually have more difficulty in maintaining motor activation in contralesional hemispace or in the contralesional direction. Whereas all persistence tasks are initially exo-evoked, one can use a signal or instructions to initiate the activity, and then either withdraw the stimulus or allow it to persist throughout the trial.

Allokinesia

Definition. Patients with allokinesia move the incorrect (ipsilesional) extremity or move in the incorrect direction (toward ipsilesional rather than contralesional hemispace).

Testing. When testing subjects for allokinesia one should make certain that the patient does not have right–left confusion or allesthesia. Therefore the patient should give verbal (right–left) as well as nonverbal responses.

SPATIAL NEGLECT

Definitions

When patients with spatial neglect are asked to perform a variety of tasks in space, they neglect

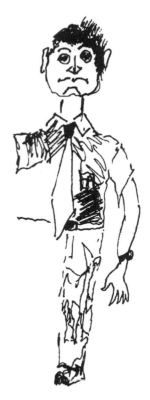

Figure 13–1. Example of left hemispatial neglect (visuospatial agnosia). Patient asked to draw a man. (Provided by Dr. Anna Barrett.)

the hemispace contralateral to their lesion. For example, when asked to draw a picture, they may fail to draw portions of the picture that are in contracesional hemisphere (Fig. 13–1). When asked to bisect a line, they may quarter it instead (Fig. 13–2), or they may fail to cross out lines distributed over a page (Fig. 13–3). The patients appear to be neglecting one-half of visual space. This has been variously termed hemispatial neglect, visuospatial agnosia, hemispatial agnosia, visuospatial neglect, and unilateral spatial neglect.

Although several authors (Battersby et al., 1956; Gainotti et al., 1972) have attributed the original description of hemispatial neglect to

Figure 13–2. Performance of patient with hemisptial neglect on the line bisection task.

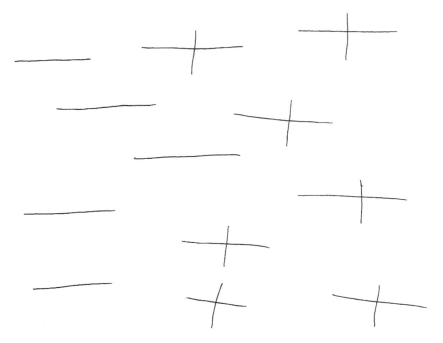

Figure 13–3. Performance by patient with hemispatial neglect on the crossing-out task.

Holmes (1918), Holmes actually reported six patients with disturbed visual orientation from bilateral lesions. It was Riddoch (1935) who reported two patients without any disturbance of central vision who had visual disorientation limited to homonymous half-fields. Brain (1941) also described three patients who had visual disorientation limited to homonymous half-fields not caused by defects in visual acuity. Brain attributed this disorder to inattention of the left half of external space and thought it was similar to the "amnesia" for the left half of the body which may follow a lesion of the right parietal lobe. Paterson and Zangwill (1944), McFie et al. (1950), and Denny-Brown and Banker (1954) demonstrated that patients with unilateral inattention (spatial neglect) not only had visual disorientation limited to a half-field but also omitted material on one side of drawings and failed to eat from one side of their plate.

Patients with hemispatial neglect may fail to read part of a word or a portion of a sentence. For example, they may read the word "cowboy" as "boy." This has been called "neglect paralexia" (Benson and Geschwind, 1969). Pa-

tients may write on only one side of a page, or they may make errors typing letters on the side of a keyboard contralateral to their lesion (Fig. 13–4). This has been termed "neglect paragraphia" (Valenstein and Heilman, 1978).

In addition to horizontal neglect, neglect of lower (Rapcsak et al., 1988) and upper (Shelton et al., 1990) vertical space and neglect of radial space (Shelton et al., 1990) have been reported. Mark and Heilman (1998) demonstrated that many patients with spatial neglect have a combination of horizontal, vertical, and radial neglect. Most commonly this three-dimensional neglect is left-sided, lower vertical, and proximal radial. Halligan and Marshall (1991a) reported a patient who had horizontal neglect when the stimuli were near the body, but did not have neglect when the stimuli were placed far from the body. In contrast, Vuilleumier et al. (1998) reported a patient with a right temporal hematoma who had neglect in far space but no neglect in near space. Neglect may be viewer (body) centered, object centered (allocentric), or environment centered. Viewer-centered neglect may be defined by the trunk, the head, or the eyes.

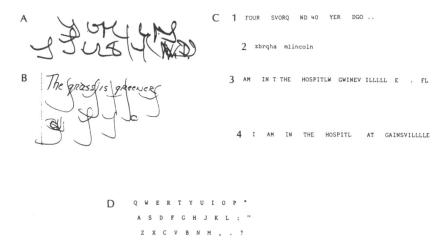

Figure 13–4. *A:* Attempting to write, "You are a doctor." *B:* Copying. *C:* Typing. *1–3:* Typewriter directly in front of patient; *4:* typewriter moved to patient's right. *D:* The typewriter keyboard. Note that the letters missed (A, S, E) are at the left of the keyboard.

Testing

There are many tests for spatial neglect. In the cancellation test described by Albert (1973), lines are drawn in random positions on a sheet of paper. The patient is asked to cancel or cross out all the lines (Fig. 13–3). Patients with spatial neglect may fail to cancel lines on the contralesional side of the page. The cancellation task can be made more difficult and sensitive by asking patients to discriminate between targets and distractors. The more difficult it is to discriminate targets from background distractors, the more sensitive the task (see Rapcsak et al., 1989). Increasing the number of stimuli can also increase the sensitivity of this test (Chatterjee et al., 1999).

The line bisection task is also commonly used to assess patients for spatial neglect. A line 6 to 10 inches long is drawn on a sheet of paper that is placed before the patient. The patient is then asked to bisect this line ("Mark the middle of the line"). Patients with spatial neglect will usually displace their mark to the ipsilesional side (contralateral neglect). Neglect is usually more apparent when longer lines are used (Bisiach et al., 1983; Butter et al., 1988a). Errors in bisection are reduced or even reversed when very short lines are used (Halligan and Marshall, 1991b). Neglect is also usually more apparent when the line is placed in contralesional body or head hemispace (Heilman and Valenstein, 1979). Exceptionally, there are patients who will bisect even very long lines toward contralesional hemispace (Kwon and Heilman, 1991; Na et al., 1998a). This has been called "ipsilateral neglect."

Spatial neglect can also be assessed by asking patients to copy a drawing or to draw spontaneously (Fig. 13–1). If patients fail to draw one side of the object, they may have spatial neglect. Since patients with right hemisphere lesions commonly have visuospatial defects and associated constructional apraxia, they may have difficulty with spontaneous drawing. An alternative test is to have patients place numbers on a clock. Frequently, patients with neglect will write only on one side of the clock. They may write in only the numbers that belong on that side, or they may write all 12 numbers on one side.

Patients with spatial neglect who misbisect lines toward ipsilesional hemispace may be neglecting stimuli on the contralesional side of their body or stimuli on one side of the environment. Thus, experimental paradigms that change the position of the body in relation to gravity may be able to dissociate body- and environment-centered reference systems. If patients who neglect left-sided stimuli in the upright position lie on their right side and continue to neglect stimuli to the left of the body's midsagittal plane, they have body-centered neglect; but if in this recumbent position they are presented with a line oriented parallel to the body's midsagittal plane, and they neglect the side of the line closer to the feet, which is the left side of the line with respect to the environment, they would have environment-centered neglect. Patients might also neglect stimuli both to the left of the body (body- or viewer-centered) and on the left side of the environment (environment-centered) (Ladavas 1987; Farah et al., 1990).

Patients with neglect may also demonstrate a combination of body-centered and object-centered neglect. Rapcsak et al. (1989) asked subjects with left hemispatial neglect to perform a selective cancellation test. On one-half of the trials the subjects were asked to cancel only those stimuli that had a distinctive feature on the left. On the other half of the trials subjects were asked only to cancel those stimuli that had a distinctive feature on the right. As expected, subjects canceled more stimuli on the right side of the page than on the left, but in addition, they canceled more stimuli with distinctive features on the right than on the left, suggesting that in addition to viewer- or environmentally centered neglect, they also had object-centered neglect.

PERSONAL NEGLECT

Definition

Patients with personal neglect (hemi-asomatognosia) may fail to recognize that their contralesional extremities are their own. They may complain that someone else's arm or leg is in bed with them. They may persist in this denial even when confronted with objective evidence. Patients with milder personal neglect may be aware that their extremities belong to them (because they are attached) but still refer to them as though they were objects.

Frequently, patients with this disorder also fail to dress or groom the abnormal side. Although this may be considered a form of dressing apraxia, the pathophysiology may be different from the dressing apraxia seen in patients with visuospatial deficits.

Testing

One of the best means of determining if a patient has personal neglect is to observe their dressing and grooming behavior. However, to more formally test for personal neglect one can ask subjects to point to different parts of their body with their ipsilesional hand (e.g., "Show me your left hand"). One can also blindfold patients and attach small Post-It notes to the left and right side of their trunk and ask them to remove all the pieces of paper. One can also use body bisections (Mark and Heilman, 1990) by putting a large horizontal line in front of patients and asking them to put a mark directly across from their left shoulder, right shoulder, right nipple, left nipple, and sternum.

MEMORY AND REPRESENTATIONAL DEFICITS

Anterograde

Definition. Patients with neglect may be unable to recall stimuli presented in contralesional hemispace even though they can perceive these stimuli. This hemispatial memory deficit has been reported in several modalities.

Testing. We randomly presented consonants through earphones to patients on either the neglected or non-neglected side and asked them to report the stimulus either immediately or after a distraction-filled interval. We found that distraction induced more of a defect in the neglected ear than in the normal ear (Heilman et al., 1974). In the visual modality, Samuels et al. (1971) tested patients with right parietal lesions and found a similar phenomenon, but unfortunately, they did not evaluate their subjects for neglect. We know of no reports of hemispatial memory defects in the somesthetic modality, but this could be tested using a similar paradigm with patients who are able to perceive stimuli in the contralesional hand.

Retrograde-Representational

Definition and Description. Denny-Brown and Banker (1954) described a patient who could not describe from memory the details of the side of a room opposite her cerebral lesion. Bisiach and Luzzatti (1978) also described patients with neglect who were unable to recall left-sided details when imagining themselves facing the cathedral in a square in Milan. However, when asked to imagine that they were facing away from the cathedral, they could now recall details that they were unable to recall when they imagined they were facing in the opposite direction. Whereas most patients with hemispatial representational deficits have hemispatial neglect, there have been reports of patients who have hemispatial neglect but do not appear to have representational neglect. Similarly, there have been reports of patients who have representational neglect who do not appear to have hemispatial neglect.

Testing. Patients can be tested for retrograde hemispatial memory deficits by asking them to recall the buildings they would see if they were driving down a familiar street. The examiner then compares the number of items recalled for each side of the street. To verify that there is a hemispatial defect, one can ask the patient to imagine driving in the opposite direction.

ANOSOGNOSIA AND ANOSODIAPHORIA

Some patients with the neglect syndrome may be unaware or of or deny their hemiparesis. This phenomenon has been called "anosognosia" (Babinski, 1914). Patients may also deny sensory loss or hemianopia. More frequently, patients may admit that they have a neurological impairment but they appear unconcerned about it. This has been termed "anosodiaphoria" (Critchley, 1966). Anosognosia and anosodiaphoria may be associated with conditions other than neglect and hemiparesis (e.g., cortical blindness or Anton's syndrome).

Testing

Because Babinski (1914) defined anosognosia as explicit unawareness of hemiplegia, to assess for anosognosia we ask patients, "Why did you come to the hospital?". This question does not focus patients' attention on their hemiparesis.

If patients are hemiparetic and do not mention their weakness, we then ask, "Do you have any other problems?". If we cannot get patients to tell us about their hemiparesis (grade 1), we then ask, "Are you weak anywhere?" If patients remain unaware of their hemiparesis with this specific question (grade ll), we pick up their arm and move it to the ipsilesional side of their body and ask them if their arm we raised is weak. If they still deny weakness (grade lll), we ask them to attempt to move this arm, and after they attempt to move the arm we again ask if they are weak. Even under these circumstances, some patients fail to recognize that they have a hemiparesis (grade lV).

Anosognosia and its mechanisms are discussed more comprehensively in Chapter 10.

MECHANISMS UNDERLYING NEGLECT AND RELATED DISORDERS

Most of the defects associated with neglect can be attributed to one or more of three basic mechanisms: disorders of attention, disorders of action or intention, and representational or memory disorders. Although the various behavioral manifestations of the neglect syndrome often coexist, patients may not display all of the manifestations, and different manifestations may be present at different times in the same patient. In this section the mechanisms of inattention, extinction, akinesia, representational deficits and hemispatial neglect will be discussed.

MECHANISMS UNDERLYING INATTENTION (SENSORY NEGLECT)

As noted above, patients with neglect may be unaware of novel or meaningful stimuli in one or more modalities. This unawareness of contralesional stimuli has been attributed to disorders of sensation, to complex perceptual deficits including abnormalities of the "body schema," and to disorders of attention.

Sensory Hypotheses

Battersby and associates (1956) thought that neglect in humans resulted from decreased sensory input superimposed on a background of decreased mental function. Sprague et al. (1961) concluded that neglect was caused by loss of patterned sensory input to the forebrain, particularly to the neocortex. Eidelberg and Schwartz (1971) similarly proposed that neglect was a passive phenomenon due to quantitatively asymmetrical sensory input to the two hemispheres. They based this conclusion on the finding that neglect resulted from neospinothalamic lesions but not from medial lemniscal lesions. They claimed that the neospinothalamic tract carries more tactile information to the hemisphere than does the medial lemniscus. However, since lesions in the cerebral cortex may also produce neglect, they postulated that the syndrome could also be caused by a reduced functional mass of one cortical area concerned with somatic sensation relative to another.

Body Schema

Brain (1941) believed that the parietal lobes contain the body schema and mediate spatial perception. Parietal lesions therefore caused patients to fail to recognize not only half of their body but also half of space. Brain thought that allesthesia resulted from severe damage to the schema for one-half of the body, causing events occurring on that half, if perceived at all, to be related in consciousness to the surviving schema representing the normal half.

Amorphosynthesis

Denny-Brown and Banker (1954) proposed that the parietal lobes were important in cortical sensation and that the phenomenon of inattention belonged to the whole class of cortical disorders of sensation: "a loss of fine discrimination . . . an inability to synthesize more than a few properties of a sensory stimulus and a disturbance of synthesis of multiple sensory stimuli." The neglect syndrome was ascribed to a defect in spatial summation that they called "amorphosynthesis."

Attentional Hypotheses

Because patients with neglect and related disorders often appear to be unaware of con-

tralesional stimuli and this unawareness cannot be accounted for by deafferentation, it is thought that many of the symptoms of neglect are related to attentional deficits.

It has often been said that everyone knows what attention is, but no one can fully define it. Perhaps this is so because attention is a mental process rather than a thing. Brains have a limited capacity to process stimuli. Under many circumstances, the brain receives more afferent stimuli than it can possibly process. In addition to external stimuli, humans can activate internal representations. The processing of these internal representations may further tax a limited capacity system and reduce a person's ability to process afferent stimuli. Since organisms, including humans, have a limited processing capacity, they need a means to triage incoming information. Attention is the mental process that permits humans to triage afferent input.

Normally triage depends on the potential importance of the incoming information to the organism. Significance is determined by two major factors: goals or sets and biological drives or needs. Because one cannot know the potential importance of novel stimuli, one must, at least temporarily, attend to novel stimuli until their significance is determined. Therefore, stimuli that are novel or important for a person's goals, sets, needs, or drives will be triaged at a higher level than irrelevant stimuli.

To triage stimuli, organisms must direct their attention to significant stimuli and away from irrelevant stimuli. There are at least two means to direct attention: by sensory modality and by spatial location. One sensory modality may be attended over others. For example, visual information can be attended rather than information carried by touch or audition. Spatial location can be used to direct attention either between sensory modalities or within a sensory modality.

Some of the first references in the neglect syndrome literature referred to defects of attention. Poppelreuter (1917) introduced the word *inattention*. Brain (1941) and Critchley (1966) were also strong proponents of this view. However, Bender and Furlow (1944, 1945) challenged the attentional theory; they felt that inattention could not be important in the pathophysiology of the syndrome because neglect could not be overcome by having the patient "concentrate" on the neglected side.

Heilman and Valenstein (1972) and Watson and associates (1973, 1974) again postulated an attention-arousal hypothesis. These authors argued that the sensory and perceptual hypotheses could not explain all cases of neglect, since neglect was often produced by lesions outside the traditional sensory pathways. Evoked potential studies in animals with unilateral neglect have demonstrated a change in late waves (that are known to be influenced by changes in attention and stimulus significance) but no change in the early (sensory) waves (Watson et al., 1977b). Furthermore, neglect is often multimodal and therefore cannot be explained by a defect in any one sensory modality.

Anatomical Basis of Attention. Unilateral neglect in humans and monkeys can be induced by lesions in many different brain regions. These include cortical areas such as the temporoparietal–occipital junction (Critchley, 1966; Heilman et al., 1970, 1983a) (Fig. 13–5), limbic areas such as the cingulate gyrus (Heilman and Valenstein, 1972; Watson et al., 1973), and subcortical areas such as the thalamus (Fig.

13–6) and mesencephalic reticular formation (Figs. 13–6 and 13–7) (Watson et al., 1974). As we will discuss below, these subcortical areas have been shown to be important in mediating arousal and attention, and the cortical areas are regions that are probably specifically involved in the analysis of the behavioral significance of stimuli and their spatial location. We have proposed that inattention or sensory neglect is an attentional–arousal disorder induced by dysfunction in a corticolimbic reticular formation network (Heilman and Valenstein, 1972; Watson et al., 1973, 1981; Heilman, 1979). Mesulam (1981) has put forth a similar proposal. We will review the evidence for our view, and propose a model or schema to explain sensory neglect (Fig. 13–8).

In monkeys and cats, profound sensory neglect results from discrete lesions of the mesencephalic reticular formation (MRF) (Reeves and Hagaman, 1971; Watson et al., 1974). Stimulation of the MRF is associated with behavioral arousal and also with desynchronization of the electroencephalogram (EEG), a physiological measure of arousal (Moruzzi and Magoun, 1949). In humans the performance of attention-demanding tasks increases the activation of the MRF and the thalamic intralam-

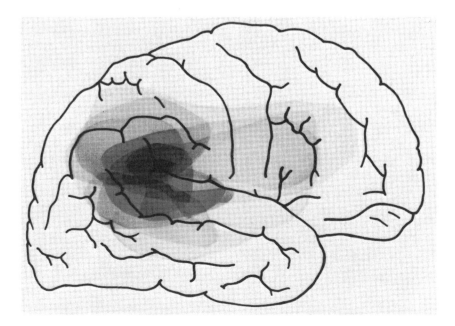

Figure 13–5. Lateral view of the right hemisphere. Lesions (as determined by CT scan) of 10 patients with the neglect syndrome are superimposed.

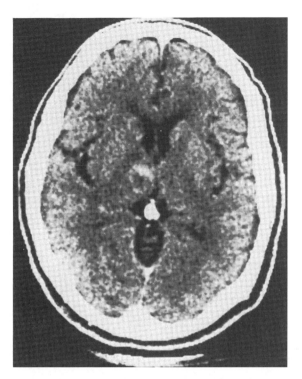

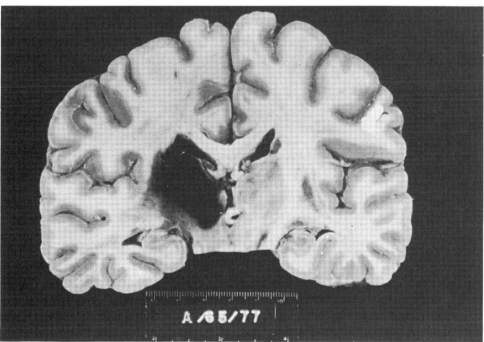

Figure 13–6. *Top:* CT scan demonstrating a contrast-enhancing right thalamic infarction in a patient with the neglect syndrome. *Bottom:* Right thalamic hemorrhage at postmortem examination of a patient who had the neglect syndrome.

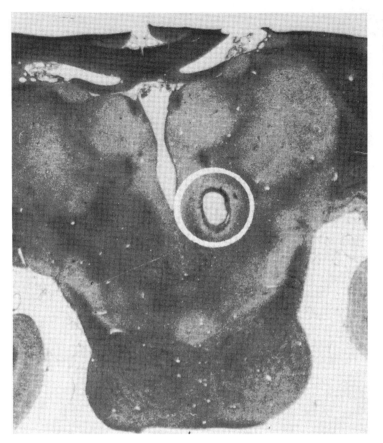

Figure 13–7. Electrolytic lesion in the mesencephalic reticular formation of a monkey who had developed unilateral neglect after the lesion was made.

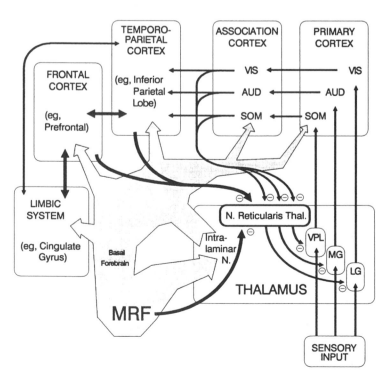

Figure 13–8. Schematic representation of pathways important in sensory attention and tonic arousal. See text for details. AUD, auditory; MRF, mesencephalic reticular formation; SOM, somasthetic; VIS, visual. Within the thalamus, sensory relay nuclei are indicated: LG, lateral geniculate; MG, medial geniculate; VPL, ventralis posterolateralis.

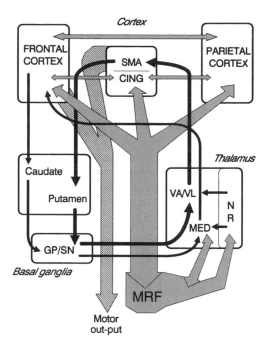

Figure 13–9. Schematic representation of pathways important for motor activation and preparation to respond. See text for details. Two basal ganglia "loops" are indicated: one (thick black arrows) from the supplementary motor area (SMA) to putamen to globus pallidus (GP)/substantia nigra (SN) to ventralis anterior and ventralis lateralis (VA/VL) of thalamus back to the SMA; the other (thin black arrows) from prefrontal cortex to caudate to GP/SN to the medial thalamic nuclei (MED) back to prefrontal cortex. CING, cingulate gyrus; NR, nucleus reticularis thalami.

inar nuclei as determined by positron emission tomography (PET) (Kinomura et al., 1996). Unilateral stimulation of the reticular activating system induces greater EEG desynchronization in the ipsilateral than in the contralateral hemisphere (Moruzzi and Magoun, 1949). Arousal is a physiological state that prepares the organism for sensory and motor processing. Whereas bilateral MRF lesions result in coma, unilateral lesions result in contralateral neglect, which is probably due to unilateral hemispheric hypoarousal (Watson et al., 1974).

Mesencephalic reticular formation influence on the cortex. Many neurons that ascend from the mesencephalic reticular activating system and its environs are monoaminergic. The area of the mesencephalon stimulated by Moruzzi and Magoun (1949) contains ascending catecholamine systems, including the noradrenergic system that projects diffusely from the locus ceruleus to the cortex. Although this norepinephrine system would appear to be ideal for mediating cortical arousal (Jouvet, 1977), destruction or stimulation of the locus coeruleus does not profoundly affect behavioral arousal (Robinson et al., 1977). As mentioned above, Moruzzi and Magoun (1949) demonstrated that unilateral stimulation of the mesencephalic reticular activating system induced greater desynchronization ipsilaterally than contralaterally. We have shown that unilateral lesions in the region of the MRF induce EEG and behavioral changes suggestive of unilateral coma (Watson et al., 1974). Unilateral locus coeruleus lesions do not induce similar behavioral or EEG changes (Deuel, personal communication).

Although unilateral injury to the dopaminergic system may induce neglect because dopamine is critical for mediating intention (see section below on intention), dopamine does not appear to be important in arousal because blockade of dopamine synthesis or of dopamine receptors does not appear to affect desynchronization (Whishaw et al., 1978).

Acetylcholine appears to have a more promising role in the mediation of arousal. Shute and Lewis (1967) described an ascending cholinergic reticular formation. Stimulation of the midbrain mesencephalic reticular activating system not only induces the arousal response but also increases the rate of acetylcholine release from the neocortex (Kanai and Szerb, 1965). Acetylcholine makes some neurons more responsive to sensory input (McCormick, 1989). Cholinergic agonists induce neocortical desynchronization, while antagonists abolish desynchronization (Bradley, 1968). Unfortunately, however, while cholinergic blockers such as atropine interfere with EEG desynchronization, they do not dramatically affect behavioral arousal. Vanderwolf and Robinson (1981) suggested that there may be two types of cholinergic input to the neocortex from the reticular formation, only one of which is atropine sensitive. Therefore, the non–atropine-sensitive cholinergic input may be responsible for behavioral arousal. It is believed that cholinergic projections from the nucleus basalis are responsible for increasing neuronal responsivity (Sato et al., 1987). The nucleus basalis receives a projection from the peripeduncular area of the mesencephalon, which, in turn, receives a projection from the cuneiform area of the mesencephalon (Arnault and Roger, 1987). Mesencephalic stimulation may thus influence cortical cholinergic activity via the nucleus basalis.

The mesencephalic reticular activating system may project to the cortex in a diffuse polysynaptic fashion (Scheibel and Scheibel, 1967) (see Fig. 13–8) and thereby influences cortical processing of sensory stimuli. Steriade and Glenn (1982) found that the centralis lateralis and paracentralis thalamic nuclei also project to widespread cortical regions. Other neurons from these thalamic areas project to the caudate. Thirteen percent of neurons with cortical or caudate projections could be activated by mesencephalic reticular activating system stimulation.

Nucleus reticularis of the thalamus. There is an alternative means through which the mesencephalic reticular activating system may affect cortical processing of sensory stimuli. Sensory information that reaches the cortex is relayed through specific thalamic nuclei. Somatosensory information is transmitted from the ventralis posterolateralis (VPL) to the postcentral gyrus; auditory information is transmitted through the medial geniculate nucleus (MGN) to the supratemporal plane (Heschl's gyrus); and visual information is transmitted through the lateral geniculate nucleus (LGN) to the occipital lobe (area 17) (Fig. 13–8). The nucleus reticularis (NR) thalami, a thin, reticular nucleus enveloping the thalamus, projects to the thalamic relay nuclei and appears to inhibit thalamic relay to the cortex (Scheibel and Scheibel, 1966) (Fig. 13–8). The mesencephalic reticular activating system also projects to the NR. Rapid mesencephalic reticular activating system stimulation or behavioral arousal inhibits the NR and is thereby associated with enhanced thalamic transmission to the cerebral cortex (Singer, 1977). Therefore, unilateral lesions of the MRF may induce neglect not only because the cortex is unprepared

for processing sensory stimuli in the absence of MRF-mediated arousal but also because the thalamic sensory relay nuclei are being inhibited by the NR.

Unimodal sensory association cortex. Lesions of thalamic relay nuclei or of primary sensory cortex induce a sensory defect rather than neglect. Primary cortical sensory areas project to unimodal association cortex (see Fig. 13–8). Association cortex synthesizes multiple features of a complex stimulus within a single sensory modality. Lesions of unimodal association cortex may induce perceptual deficits in a single modality (for example, apperceptive agnosia). Modality-specific association areas may also detect stimulus novelty (modeling) (Sokolov, 1963). When a stimulus is neither novel nor significant, corticifugal projections to the NR may allow habituation to occur by selectively influencing thalamic relay. When a stimulus is novel or significant, corticofugal projections might inhibit the NR and thereby allow the thalamus to relay additional sensory input. This capacity for selective control of sensory input is supported by a study revealing that stimulation of specific areas within NR related to specific thalamic nuclei (e.g., NR lateral geniculate, NR medial geniculate, or NR ventrobasal complex) results in abolition of corresponding (visual, auditory, or tactile) cortical evoked responses (Yingling and Skinner, 1977). Physiologic imaging studies reveal that selectively attending to tactile stimuli may activate primary (somesthetic) cortex (Meyer et al., 1991). This activation may be mediated by corticofugal projections that inhibit the inhibition the NR exerts on thalamic relay nuclei such as VPL.

Polymodal and supramodal association areas. Primary sensory areas project to unimodal sensory association cortex. In the visual system there are many different unimodal association areas, but in general, areas located in ventral occipitotemporal regions are important in processing the visual properties of objects (the "what" system), whereas visual association areas in dorsal (superior) occipitoparietal regions are important in processing the spatial position of stimuli (the "where" system) (Haxby et al., 1991). Patients with ventral ("what" system) lesions may be impaired at recognizing objects (visual object agnosia) and faces (prosopagnosia). In contrast, patients with dorsal ("where" system) lesions may have problems locating objects in space (for example, optic ataxia). Unimodal association areas converge upon polymodal association areas (Fig. 13–8). In the monkey, these are the prefrontal cortex (periarcuate, prearcuate, and orbitofrontal) and both banks of the superior temporal sulcus (STS) (Pandya and Kuypers, 1969). Unimodal association areas may also project directly to the caudal inferior parietal lobule (IPL) or, alternatively, may reach the IPL after a synapse in polymodal convergence areas (e.g., prefrontal cortex and both banks of the STS) (Mesulam et al., 1977). Polymodal convergence areas may subserve cross-modal associations and polymodal sensory synthesis. Polymodal sensory synthesis may also be important in "modeling" (detecting stimulus novelty) and detecting significance. In contrast to the unimodal association cortex that projects to specific parts of the NR and thereby gates sensory input in one modality, these multimodal convergence areas may have a more general inhibitory action on NR and provide further arousal after cortical analysis. These convergence areas also may project directly to the MRF, which either may induce a general state of arousal because of diffuse multisynaptic connections to the cortex or may increase thalamic transmission via connections with the NR, as discussed above, or both.

Evidence that polymodal parietal cortex may be important in enhancing thalamic transmission, by inhibiting the inhibitory thalamic reticular nucleus, comes from the observation that patients with Balint's syndrome from biparietal lesions note that after a few seconds visual stimuli, unless moving, disappear. Mennemeier et al. (1994) suggested and provided support for the hypothesis that visual stimuli disappear because the parietal lobes can no longer inhibit this inhibitory nucleus and visual gaiting occurs. Mennemeier et al. also suggested that whereas the parietal lobes inhibit the inhibitory thalamic reticular nucleus and thereby enhance stimulus transmission, the frontal lobes excite the inhibitory NR, diminish transmission, and promote habituation. To test this hypothesis, Mennemeier et al. studied visual habituation using the Troxlar paradigm. In this paradigm the subject looks at a central fixation point and notes when a dot on the right or left of this fixation point fades from vision. Mennemeier et al. (1994) found that contralateral to parietal lesions there was enhanced habituation (rapid fading) and contralateral to frontal lesions there was delayed habituation.

Evidence that polymodal areas of cortex modulate arousal comes from neurophysiological studies showing that stimulation of select cortical sites induces a generalized arousal response. These sites in monkeys include the frontal prearcuate region and both banks of the STS, which is the precursor of humans' IPL (Segundo et al., 1955). When similar sites are ablated, there is EEG evidence of ipsilateral hypoarousal (Watson et al., 1977a).

Limbic and frontal cortex. Although determination of stimulus novelty may be mediated by sensory association cortex, stimulus significance is determined in part by the needs by the organism (motivational state). Limbic system input into brain regions important for determining stimulus significance might provide information about biological needs. The frontal lobes might provide input about needs related to goals that are neither directly stimulus-dependent nor motivated by an immediate biological need, since the frontal lobes do play a critical role in goal-mediated behavior and in developing sets (see Chapter 15).

Polymodal (e.g., STS) and supramodal (IPL) areas have prominent limbic and frontal connections. Polymodal cortices project to the cingulate gyrus (a portion of the limbic system), and the cingulate gyrus projects to the IPL (Fig. 13–8). The prefrontal cortex, STS, and IPL have strong reciprocal connections. The posterior cingulate cortex (Brodmann's area 23) has more extensive connections with polymodal association areas (prefrontal cortex and STS) and the IPL than does the anterior cingulate cortex (Brodmann's area 24) (Vogt et al., 1979; Baleydier and Maugierre, 1980). These connections provide an anatomic substrate by which motivational states (e.g., biological needs, sets, and long-term goals) may influence stimulus processing.

Physiological Properties of Neurons in the Inferior Parietal Lobe. Investigators have been able to study the physiological function of specific areas of the nervous system by recording from single neurons in awake animals. In this experimental situation, the firing characteristics of individual neurons can be measured in relation to specific sensory stimulation or motor behavior. For example, a single neuron in the visual cortex may respond maximally to a contrast border in a specific region of the visual field, sometimes in a specific orientation. By varying the nature of the stimulus and by training the animal to respond in specific ways, the characteristic patterns of firing of individual neurons can be defined in terms of the optimal stimulus and/or response parameters that cause a maximal change in firing rate. In this fashion, investigators have defined the properties of neurons in the parietal lobe (areas 5 and 7) of the monkey (Mountcastle et al., 1975, 1981; Goldberg and Robinson, 1977; Robinson et al., 1978; Lynch, 1980; Bushnell et al., 1981; Motter and Mountcastle, 1981). Unlike single cells in primary sensory cortex, the activity of many parietal neurons correlates best with stimuli or responses of importance to the animal, while similar stimuli or responses that are unimportant are associated with either no change or a lesser change in neuronal activity (Colby and Goldberg, 1999).

Early investigations identified parietal neurons that responded to visual stimuli of biologic significance, aversive as well as rewarding, suggesting activity that might mediate selective attention (Goldberg and Robinson, 1977; Robinson et al., 1978). Some neurons were active with fixation of non-moving stimuli, some only when the animal was tracking a moving stimulus, and some responded only when stimuli were moving in a specific direction. Most had receptive fields in the contralateral visual field (that is, they responded only to stimuli in a portion of the contralateral visual field), but other neurons had large receptive fields, sometimes spanning both visual fields (Mountcastle et al., 1981).

Subsequent work has revealed a striking specialization of subregions of areas 5 and 7 related to spatial organization (Colby and Goldberg, 1999). Within the intraparietal (IP)

sulcus of the monkey, a lateral region (LIP) contains exclusively visually responsive neurons that are specialized to respond to objects that are beyond the animal's reach and which can only be explored by eye movements. Many neurons in the LIP fire in relation to eye movements, either in anticipation of them, during a delay in a task that entails an eye movement, or after an eye movement has been made. On the opposite bank of the IP sulcus, in the medial intraparietal area (MIP), neurons are found that respond principally to visual or tactile stimuli from objects that are within reach of the animal (Colby and Duhamel, 1991). Ventral to this, in ventral IP (VIP), neurons respond to stimuli in near personal space, which the animal can reach with the mouth. Some bimodal neurons in this region fire in response to tactile stimuli in a region on the face and to moving visual stimuli only when the trajectory of the stimuli would bring them in contact with that region of the face (Colby et al., 1993). Still more anteriorly, in anterior IP (AIP), neurons respond to the shape and orientation of visual or tactile stimuli. These neurons also fire in conjunction with hand movements that grasp the object (Colby and Goldberg, 1999). Thus, within the parietal lobe, there are multiple representations of space that differ with regard to the activity that will target stimuli: eye movements (LIP), touching with the hand (MIP) or face (VIP), or grasping (AIP). Although these spatial representations are doubtless used in the planning of movements, in most instances studied they appear not to program movements directly. Enhancement of response is often independent of the kind of response. Thus, neurons in the LIP will respond equally to a stimulus if the response is an eye movement toward the stimulus, or a bar press without visual fixation (Colby et al., 1996). Because many of the neurons in these regions respond differentially to objects that are of significance to the organism, lesions in these areas can reduce awareness of objects in far or near space, suggesting an anatomic and physiologic basis for the spatial direction of attention. Damage to these areas may therefore result in various distributions of hemispatial neglect. This may be relevant to the production of restricted forms of the neglect syndrome in humans, such as, for example, Vuilleumier et al.'s (1998) report of neglect for far but not near space.

Summary of the Attentional Model. The human brain has a limited capacity to process information, therefore the brain must triage or select information on the basis of its biological significance. To process information, the cortex has to be in a physiological state of readiness, called "arousal." The mesencephalic–diencephalic reticular system mediates arousal. Unilateral inattention will follow unilateral mesencephalic reticular activating system lesions because the MRF does not prepare the cortex for sensory processing, and/or because it no longer inhibits the ipsilateral NR, which then inhibits thalamic transmission of sensory input to the cortex. Corticothalamic collaterals from association cortex to the NR may serve unimodal orienting or habituation. Unilateral lesions of multimodal sensory convergence areas that project to the mesencephalic reticular activating system and the NR, such as the IPL, induce contralateral inattention because the subject cannot be aroused by or process contralateral stimuli. To selectively attend to a biologically significant stimulus one must recognize the stimulus and know its spatial location. The sensory association systems that mediate "what" and "where" sensory analysis converge in the inferior parietal cortex, a process that is critical in spatially directed attention (Watson et al., 1994). Biological significance is determined by immediate needs or drives, mediated by portions of the limbic system such as the cingulate gyrus, or by long-term goals and sets, mediated by dorsolateral frontal lobes. The IPL, cingulate gyrus, and dorsolateral frontal lobe are all highly interconnected, and, with the reticular (arousal) systems, form an attentional network, illustrated in Figure 13–8. A lesion affecting any one of these modules (Watson et al., 1994) or the white matter connections between them (Burcham et al., 1997) can result in unilateral sensory neglect.

MECHANISMS UNDERLYING EXTINCTION

The patient with extinction reports a stimulus presented in isolation, but does not report the same stimulus when another stimulus is presented simultaneously. Most often, the two stimuli are presented on opposite sides of the body, and it is the stimulus contralateral to the lesion that is extinguished. Extinction may be induced by stimuli in the same or different modalities. The nature and complexity of a stimulus may also affect extinction.

Extinction can be seen in normal subjects as well as in patients with central nervous system lesions (Kimura, 1967; Benton and Levin, 1972). The lesions causing extinction are usually in the same areas as lesions that cause inattention. Also, extinction, like inattention, is more commonly associated with right than with left hemisphere dysfunction (Meador et al., 1988). However, certain forms of extinction may also occur after lesions of the corpus callosum (Milner et al., 1968; Sparks and Geschwind, 1968), and left-sided extinction has even been reported to follow left hemisphere lesions (Schwartz et al., 1979). Extinction in normal subjects, extinction in patients with callosal lesions, and extinction in patients with hemisphere lesions may all have different mechanisms. In this section we will primarily discuss the extinction seen with hemisphere lesions.

Extinction in humans is most often reported with parietotemporal lesions (Heilman et al., 1983b). Multimodal extinction may also occur in monkeys with parietotemporal lesions (Heilman et al., 1970). Whereas the ipsilateral extinction reported by Schwartz et al. (1979) required complex stimuli, extinction after parietotemporal lesions can be demonstrated using simple stimuli.

In general, despite many published reports, especially about dichotic listening in normal subjects, the mechanisms underlying extinction are poorly understood. We will discuss several hypotheses that have been advanced to explain extinction.

Sensory Hypothesis

Extinction has been reported to be induced by lesions that affect purely sensory systems. Because patients with partial deafferentation may exhibit extinction, several authors have postulated a sensory mechanism to explain inattention and extinction. Psychophysical methods have been used to demonstrate that in normal subjects the sensory threshold increases on one side when the opposite side is stimulated. This has been called "obscuration," and has been attributed to reciprocal inhibition. If obscuration occurs in patients with an elevated threshold from an afferent lesion, it would appear similar to extinction in patients without deafferentation.

Suppression and Reciprocal Inhibition

Nathan (1946) and Reider (1946) suggested that extinction results from suppression, mediated by transcallosal inhibition. A similar mechanism was proposed by Kinsbourne (1970). Normally, each hemisphere inhibits the other, but the inhibition becomes unbalanced when one hemisphere is damaged. The damaged hemisphere is inhibited more than the undamaged hemisphere. Consequently, stimuli delivered to the side of the body opposite the damaged hemisphere are not perceived when the normal side is stimulated. The notion of transcallosal inhibition thus has bearing on theories of inattention. This is discussed further below (Mechanisms of Hemispatial Neglect).

One can also explain extinction and obscuration on the basis of asymmetric inhibition of thalamic relay. As discussed above, NR thalami normally inhibit thalamic relay nuclei, decreasing sensory transmission to the ipsilateral cortex. The NR is inhibited by ipsilateral sensory association cortex and multimodal cortex (inferior parietal lobe), facilitating sensory transmission to ipsilateral cortex. We postulate that there may be reciprocal facilitation of contralateral NR, resulting in decreased sensory transmission to the contralateral cortex. Therefore, even under normal conditions, a stimulus on one side would increase the threshold for stimuli on the other side. Lesions of association cortex would decrease inhibition of the NR, which in turn would inhibit the thalamic sensory nuclei, thus making the thalamus less sensitive to contralateral stimuli. With bilateral simultaneous stimuli, activated attentional cells in the intact hemisphere would increase contralateral NR activity even more, further inhibiting thalamic sensory nuclei and thereby inducing extinction.

Interference Theory

Birch et al. (1967) proposed that the damaged hemisphere processes information more slowly than the intact hemisphere. Because of this inertia, the damaged side is more subject to interference from the normal side. To support their hypothesis, the authors demonstrated that stimulating the abnormal side (contralesional side) before stimulating the normal side (ipsilateral side) reduced extinction; however, stimulating the normal side before the abnormal side had no effect on extinction.

Limited Attention or Capacity Theory

According to the limited attention or capacity theory, bilateral simultaneous stimuli are normally processed simultaneously, each hemisphere processing the contralateral stimulus and having an attentional bias toward contralateral space or body. However, a damaged hemisphere (usually the right) may be unable to attend to contralateral stimuli. Recovery from unilateral inattention may be mediated by the normal (left) hemisphere. This hemisphere, however, may have not only an attentional bias toward contralateral space and body but also a limited attentional capacity. Therefore, with bilateral simultaneous stimulation, the normal hemisphere's attentional mechanism, biased toward the contralateral stimulus, may be unable to attend to an ipsilateral stimulus (Heilman, 1979).

Evidence for the Different Theories of Extinction

We will briefly review studies that have some bearing on the various theories of extinction. We should note that these theories may not be mutually exclusive: because extinction can be caused by lesions in a variety of anatomically and functionally different areas, the reciprocal inhibition, limited attention, and interference theories could each be correct, but for different lesions.

Benton and Levin (1972) reported that in normal subjects, threshold is raised by presenting a simultaneous stimulus. Because normal persons do not have lesions, Benton and

Levin's findings cannot be explained readily by the limited attention or interference models. Their findings appear to support the reciprocal inhibition model. The findings of Birch et al. (1967) that extinction is reduced when a contralateral stimulus precedes an ipsilateral stimulus, but not when an ipsilateral stimulus precedes a contralateral stimulus, are compatible with both the reciprocal inhibition and limited attention theories. Support for the reciprocal NR gaiting model comes from the work of Staines et al. (2000), who used functional magnetic resonance imaging (fMRI) to study patients with tactile extinction and found there was a reduction of activation in the primary somatosensory cortex. However, Volpe et al. (1979) asked patients with visual extinction to tell whether objects projected into the contralesional field were the same as those presented to the ipsilateral field. Although subjects were unaware of the contralesional stimulus, when presented simultaneously with the ipsilesional stimulus, they could determine if the objects were the same or different. In addition, Beversdorf et al. (personal communication) performed fMRI on a patient with tactile extinction and matched controls. Although the patient was unaware of the contralesional tactile stimulus, when presented with an ipsilesional tactile stimulus, the somatosensory cortex demonstrated activation, suggesting that extinction cannot be entirely explained by thalamic sensory gaiting in all patients. Sevush and Heilman (1981) and Kaplan et al. (1990) showed that a unilateral stimulus preceding a trial with simultaneous stimuli may alter the pattern of extinction in patients with unilateral hemisphere lesions. The subject is more likely to show extinction when a bilateral trial is preceded by a contralateral (e.g., left) stimulus than when a bilateral trial is preceded by an ipsilateral (e.g., right) stimulus. In addition, Rapscak et al. (1987) observed that extinction can occur even within a visual field. These findings cannot be explained by the interference model.

Heilman et al. (1984b) provided additional support for the model of limited attention or capacity. Patients who exhibited extinction were asked to report where they were given a tactile stimulus: on the right, the left, both, or neither. In the "neither" situation, the subject was not stimulated, but was still asked to give a response. Subjects erred by reporting "both" when the arm ipsilateral to the damaged hemisphere was stimulated more than they reported "both" when the contralateral arm was stimulated. Using a similar paradigm, Schwartz et al. (personal communication) found that a patient with left-sided extinction would often report being touched on the left when they were not. One interpretation of these findings is that patients were not sufficiently attentive to their contralesional extremities to realize when they had not been touched. Since the errors consisted of reporting a stimulation that did not occur rather than failing to report a stimulus, these results cannot be explained by the suppression, reciprocal inhibition, or interference theories and are most compatible with the limited attention or capacity theory. Rapscak et al. (1987) demonstrated that capacity is most limited in the contralesional field and becomes progressively reduced as one moves laterally in that field. However, with right hemisphere lesions, capacity may be so reduced that, even when two stimuli are given ipsilaterally either visually (Rapscak et al., 1987) or via the tactile modality (Feinberg, 1990), one is extinguished.

MECHANISMS UNDERLYING ACTION-INTENTIONAL DISORDERS

Unilateral neglect has been described following unilateral dorsolateral frontal lesions in monkeys (Bianchi, 1895; Kennard and Ectors, 1938; Welch and Stuteville, 1958) and humans (Heilman and Valenstein, 1972). Watson et al. (1978) recognized that in most testing paradigms, the animal is required to respond to a stimulus contralateral to the lesion either by orienting to the stimulus or by moving the limbs on the side of the stimulus. Since the animals with frontal lobe lesions were not weak, it was assumed that their failure to make the appropriate response resulted from sensory neglect. Watson et al. (1978) suggested that it could be explained equally well by unilateral akinesia. They therefore trained monkeys to use the left hand to respond to a tactile stimulus on the right leg, and the right hand to respond to a left-sided tactile stimulus. After a unilateral frontal arcuate lesion (Brodmann's

area 8), the monkeys showed contralateral neglect, but when stimulated on their neglected
side, they responded normally with the limb on
the side of the lesion. When stimulated on the
side ipsilateral to the lesion, however, they often failed to respond, or responded by moving
the limb ipsilateral to the lesion. These results
cannot be explained by sensory or perceptual
hypotheses, and are thought to reflect a defect
in intention: an inability to initiate a response
by the contralateral limb in contralesional
hemispace.

Anatomic and Physiological Mechanisms

The region of the arcuate gyrus (periarcuate
region) in monkeys contains the frontal eye
field. Stimulation of the frontal eye field elicits contralateral eye movement, head rotation,
and pupillary dilation resembling attentive orienting (Wagman and Mehler, 1972). The connections of the periarcuate region are important in understanding its possible role in motor
activation or intention. The periarcuate region
has reciprocal connections with auditory,
visual, and somesthetic association cortex
(Chavis and Pandya, 1976). Evoked potential
studies have confirmed this as an area of sensory convergence (Bignell and Imbert, 1969).
The periarcuate region is also reciprocally connected with the cortex on the banks of the STS,
another site of multimodal sensory convergence, and with the cortex on the banks of the
IP sulcus, an area of somatosensory and visual
convergence. There are also connections with
prearcuate cortex. The periarcuate cortex has
reciprocal connections with the following subcortical areas: the paralamellar portion of dorsomedial (DM) nucleus and the adjacent cen-
tromedian-parafascicularis (CM-Pf) complex
(Kievet and Kuypers, 1977; Akert and Von
Monakow, 1980). Just as the periarcuate region
is transitional in architecture between agranular motor cortex and granular prefrontal cortex, the paralamellar-CM-Pf complex is situated between medial thalamus, which projects
to granular cortex, and lateral thalamus, which
projects to agranular cortex. Projections to
MRF (Kuypers and Lawrence, 1967) as well as
nonreciprocal projections to caudate also exist.
Lastly, the periarcuate region also receives in-

put from the limbic system, mainly from the
anterior cingulate gyrus (Baleydier and Mauguiere, 1980).

The neocortical sensory association and sensory convergence area connections provide the
frontal lobes with information about external
stimuli that may call the individual to action.
Limbic connections (from the anterior cingulate gyrus) may provide the frontal lobe with
motivational information. Connections with
the MRF may be important in arousal.

Because the dorsolateral frontal lobe has
sensory association cortex, limbic, and reticular formation connections, it would appear to
be an ideal candidate for mediating a response
to a stimulus to which the subject is attending
(Fig. 13–9). While this area may not be critical for mediating how to respond (e.g., providing instruction for the spatial trajectory and
temporal patterns), it may control when one responds. There is evidence from physiological
studies to support this hypothesis. Recordings
from single cells in the posterior frontal arcuate gyrus reveal responses similar to those of
the superior colliculus, a structure also important in oculomotor control (Goldberg and
Bushnell, 1981). These visually responsive neurons show enhanced activity time-locked to the
onset of stimulus and preceding eye movement. This differs from IPL neurons that respond to visual input independent of behavior:
an IPL neuron whose activity enhances during
a task that requires a saccade also enhances
with tasks that do not require a saccade. Therefore, the IPL neurons seem to be responsible
for selective spatial attention, which is independent of behavior, and any neuron that is enhanced to one type of behavior will also be enhanced to others (Bushnell et al., 1981). The
frontal eye field neurons, however, are linked
to behavior, but only to movements that have
motivational significance. Responses to other
stimulus modalities (e.g., audition) may be controlled by an adjacent group of neurons in the
arcuate gyrus (Whittington and Hepp-
Reymond, 1977).

The dorsolateral frontal lobe has extensive
connections with CM-Pf, one of the "nonspecific" intralaminar thalamic nuclei. Nonsensory
or motor-intentional neglect has also been reported in monkeys after CM-Pf lesions (Wat-

son et al., 1978) and in a patient with an intralaminar lesion (Bogousslavsky et al., 1986). An akinetic state (akinetic mutism) is seen with bilateral CM-Pf lesions in humans (Mills and Swanson, 1978). We have postulated a possible role for CM-Pf in behavior (Watson et al., 1981). This role is based on behavioral, anatomic, and physiological evidence that CM-Pf and periarcuate cortex are involved in mediating responses to meaningful stimuli.

Low-frequency stimulation of CM-Pf induces cortical recruiting responses (Jasper, 1949) and activates the inhibitory NR through a CM-Pf–frontocortical–NR system (Yingling and Skinner, 1975). This NR activation elicits inhibitory postsynaptic potentials in the ventrolateral thalamic nucleus (VL), and thus blocks VL transmission to motor cortex (Purpura, 1970). Transmission in the VL has been shown to be inversely proportional to NR activity (Filion et al., 1971). The VL projects to motor cortex, and may be important in the control of movement initiation. High-frequency stimulation of the CM-Pf or MRF induces inhibition of NR, EEG desynchronization, and behavioral arousal (Moruzzi and Magoun, 1949; Yingling and Skinner, 1975). These manifestations elicited by high-frequency CM-Pf stimulation are predominantly mediated via the MRF-NR system, since they are blocked by a lesion between the CM-Pf and MRF (Weinberger et al., 1965). A lesion of the CM-Pf–frontocortical–NR system also prevents inhibition of the NR response to rapid CM-Pf stimulation, whereas rapid MRF stimulation during this blockade will continue to inhibit the NR (Yingling and Skinner, 1977). This indicates that the NR can be inhibited by either an MRF-NR system or a CM-Pf–frontocortical–NR system and suggests that different types of behavior may be mediated independently by these systems.

Novel or noxious stimuli, or anticipation of a response to a meaningful stimulus, produce inhibition of the NR and a negative surface potential over the frontal cortex (Yingling and Skinner, 1977). This surface-negative potential occurs if a stimulus has acquired behavioral significance (Walter, 1973). Specifically, when a warning stimulus precedes a second stimulus that requires a motor response, a negative

waveform, called the "contingent negative variation" (CNV), appears between stimuli and is thought to reflect motivation, attention, or expectancy.

Skinner and Yingling (1976) demonstrated that in a conditional tone/shock expectancy paradigm, both the frontal negative wave and inhibition of NR elicited by the tone were abolished by blockade of the CM-Pf–frontocortical–NR system, although primitive orienting persisted. Novel or noxious stimuli or rapid MRF stimulation continued to inhibit the NR. In an operant task involving alternate bar press for reward, cooling of the CM-Pf–frontocortical–NR loop sufficient to block cortical recruitment induced incorrect responses to the previously reinforced bar press (i.e., perseveration) (Skinner and Yingling, 1977). Further cooling caused the subject to cease responding altogether. These behavioral observations demonstrated that an appropriate response to a meaningful stimulus in an aroused subject requires an intact CM-Pf–frontocortical–NR system, whereas primitive behavioral orienting elicited by novel or noxious stimuli depends on an intact MRF-NR system. Responding to basic survival stimuli (e.g., food when hungry) may also depend on an MRF-NR system.

Skinner and Yingling (1977) interpreted their data as supporting a role for the MRF-NR system in tonic arousal and the CM-Pf–frontocortical–NR system in "selective" attention. We agree with the hypothesized role of the MRF-NR system in tonic arousal but suggest that the role of the CM-Pf–frontocortical–NR system is preparing the aroused organism to respond to a meaningful stimulus. The demonstration that intralaminar neurons have activity time-locked to either sensory or motor events, depending on the experimental condition, supports the pivotal role of this structure in sensory–motor integration (Schlag-Rey and Schlag, 1980). The periarcuate region and thalamic zone around the lateral aspect of the dorsomedial nucleus and intralaminar nucleus share common anatomic features. In addition to reciprocal connections, there is a complex arc from periarcuate cortex, motor cortex, and CM-Pf to the neostriatum (caudate and putamen), from the neostriatum to globus pallidus to CM-Pf and VL, and from CM-Pf and

VL back to premotor and motor cortex. Not surprisingly, lesions of structures within this loop, including arcuate gyrus (Watson et al., 1978), basal ganglia (Valenstein and Heilman, 1981), VL (Velasco and Velasco, 1979), and CM-Pf (Watson et al., 1978), have induced a deficit in responding to multimodal sensory stimuli (Fig. 13–9). The inferior parietal cortex also has strong projects to the periarcuate region and thus while lesions of parietal cortex are often associated with attentional neglect, lesion in this region can have an intentional component (Valenstein et al., 1982).

Neuropharmocology of Intentional Disorders

Much evidence suggests dopaminergic neurons mediate aspects of intention. Intentional deficits are prominent in patients with Parkinson's disease, which is characterized pathologically by degeneration of ascending dopaminergic neurons. In animals, unilateral lesions in these pathways (Marshall et al., 1971) and unilateral destruction of the dopaminergic system by a toxin (Schneider et al., 1992) cause unilateral neglect. In contrast, stimulation of dopamine (DA) pathways reinforces ongoing behavior (Olds and Milner, 1954; Corbett and Wise, 1980).

Three related dopaminergic pathways have been defined. The nigrostriatal pathway originates in the pars compacta of the substantia nigra (SN), and projects to the neostriatum (caudate and putamen). The mesolimbic pathway originates principally in the ventral tegmental area (VTA) of the midbrain (area A10), just medial to the SN, and terminates in the limbic areas of the basal forebrain (nucleus accumbens septi and olfactory tubercle). The mesocortical pathway originates principally in dopaminergic neurons located more laterally in the midbrain (areas A8 and A9) and project to the frontal and cingulate cortex (Ungerstedt, 1971a; Lindvall et al., 1974; Williams and Goldman-Rakic, 1998).

Ascending dopaminergic (DA) fibers course through the lateral hypothalamus (LH) in the median forebrain bundle. Bilateral lesions in the lateral hypothalamus of rats induce an akinetic state (Teitelbaum and Epstein, 1962). Unilateral LH lesions cause unilateral neglect:

these rats transiently circle toward the side of their lesion; after they recover to the point where spontaneous activity appears symmetrical, they still tend to turn toward their lesioned side when stimulated (e.g., by pinching their tails), and they fail to respond to sensory stimuli delivered to the contralateral side (Marshall et al., 1971). There is considerable evidence that the LH lesions cause neglect by damaging dopaminergic fibers passing through the hypothalamus. Neglect occurs with 6-hydroxydopamine (6-OHDA) lesions of LH that damage dopaminergic fibers relatively selectively (Marshall et al., 1974), but not with kainic acid lesions that damage cell bodies but not fibers of passage (Grossman et al., 1978). Unilateral damage to the same dopaminergic fibers closer to their site of origin in the midbrain also causes unilateral neglect (Ljungberg and Ungerstedt, 1976; Marshall, 1979; Feeney and Wier, 1979). Conversely, unilateral stimulation in the area of ascending dopaminergic fibers (Arbuthnott and Ungerstedt, 1975) or of the striatum (Pycock, 1980) causes animals to turn away from the side of stimulation, as if they are orienting to the opposite side. Normal (nonlesioned) rats spontaneously turn more in one direction. They also have an asymmetry in striatal DA concentration and their direction of turning is generally away from the side of the brain with more DA (Glick et al., 1975).

Lesions of the ascending dopaminergic pathways affect the areas of termination of these pathways in at least two ways. First, degeneration of DA-containing axons depletes these areas of DA. Marshall (1979) has shown that the neglect induced in rats by ventral tegmental 6-OHDA lesions is proportional to the depletion of DA in the neostriatum and, to a lesser extent, in the olfactory tubercle and nucleus accumbens. Second, the target areas attempt to compensate for the depletion of dopaminergic afferents by increasing their responsiveness to DA. This is mediated, at least in part, by an increase in the number of DA receptors (Heikkila et al., 1981), which correlates with behavioral recovery from neglect (Neve et al., 1982).

Changes in DA innervation and in DA receptor sensitivity and number can explain many effects of pharmacological manipulation in animals with unilateral lesions of the ascending dopaminergic pathways. Such lesions result in degeneration of dopaminergic axon terminals on the side of the lesion. Drugs such as L-dopa or amphetamines that increase the release of DA from normal dopaminergic terminals will therefore cause more DA to be released on the unlesioned side than on the lesioned side, resulting in orientation or turning toward the lesioned side (Ungerstedt, 1971b, 1974). Several days after the lesion, when DA receptor concentration on the side of the lesion begins to increase, drugs that directly stimulate DA receptors, such as apomorphine, cause the animal to turn away from the side of the lesion (Ungerstedt; 1971b, 1974).

Although rats have been used in most studies, lesions that probably involve the ascending DA systems have also induced unilateral neglect in cats (Hagamen et al., 1977) and monkeys (Deuel, 1980; Apicella et al., 1991). As mentioned above, bilateral degeneration of the nigrostriatal fibers in humans is associated with Parkinsonism, in which akinesia and hypokinesia are prominent symptoms. Ross and Stewart (1981) described a patient with akinetic mutism secondary to bilateral damage to the anterior hypothalamus. This patient responded to treatment with bromocriptine, a direct DA-receptor agonist. Since the lesion was probably anterior to the site at which nigrostriatal fibers diverge from the median forebrain bundle, the authors suggested that damage to the mesolimbic and mesocortical pathways was critical in causing their patient's hypokinesia.

The evidence summarized above indicates the importance of dopaminergic pathways in mediating intention. Although the neglect induced by LH or VTA lesions has been called "sensory" neglect or inattention, rats trained to respond to unilateral stimulation by turning to the side opposite the side of stimulation respond well to stimulation of their "neglected" side (the side opposite the lesion) but fail to turn when stimulated on their "normal" side (Hoyman et al., 1979). This paradigm is similar to that used by Watson et al. (1978), and demonstrates that lesions in ascending dopaminergic pathways cause a defect of intention.

The striatum, which receives dopaminergic innervation from the substantia nigra, projects to globus pallidus, which in turn has output to three major regions (Fonnum and Walaas, 1979; Grofova, 1979). It projects to subthalamic nucleus, which projects back to the internal segment of the globus pallidus. It projects to the thalamus, as part of the striato-pallidal-thalamo-cortical-striatal loop described above. It also projects to the intralaminar nuclei of the thalamus (Mehler, 1966). In addition, the striatum also projects back to the SN, in part providing feedback to DA neurons, but also connecting the striatum with the targets of SN projections: the intralaminar nuclei of the thalamus, the superior colliculus, and portions of the reticular formation (Anderson and Yoshida, 1977; Herkenham, 1979; Dalsass and Krauthamer, 1981). The intralaminar thalamus, the superior colliculus, and the MRF are all areas that have been implicated in the mediation of attention, and in which lesions can induce unilateral neglect. It appears likely that striatal input into these areas, regulated in part by activity in the ascending dopaminergic pathways, provides information about the intentional state of the organism.

The frontal neocortex and cingulate cortex receive DA input from the ventral tegmental area of the midbrain and adjacent areas (Brown et al., 1979; Williams and Goldman-Rakic, 1998), and the entire neocortex projects strongly to the striatum. This corticostriatal projection is largely glutaminergic (Divac et al., 1977). Stimulation in the motor or visual areas of the cat's cortex causes a release of DA in the striatum (Nieoullon et al., 1978). But in rats, examined 30 days after 6-OHDA lesions of the mesial prefrontal cortex there was an increase of both striatal DA content and striatal DA receptor concentration (Pycock, 1980). Rats with unilateral frontal cortical ablations may turn toward the side of their lesion, and amphetamines initially increase this turning (Avemo et al., 1973). After 1 week, amphetamines induce contralateral turning, while apomorphine causes turning toward the side of the lesion (that is, the opposite of the pharmacological effects seen after unilateral lesions of the ascending dopaminergic pathways). Rats subjected to a previous unilateral 6-OHDA lesion of the ascending dopaminergic pathways and then a unilateral frontal lesion initially reverse their direction of spontaneous turning, but do not change their turning response to amphetamine or apomorphine (Crossman et al., 1977). Monkeys that have recovered from neglect induced by unilateral frontal arcuate lesions do not show asymmetrical behavior when given L-dopa, amphetamine, haloperidol, scopolamine, physostigmine, or bromocriptine, but do show dramatic turning toward the side of their lesion when given apomorphine (Valenstein et al., 1980). This turning is blocked by prior administration of haloperidol. Following unilateral frontal lesions, rats demonstrated contralateral neglect that was reversed by the DA agonist apomorphine (Corwin et al., 1986). This apomorphine-induced reduction of neglect was blocked by the prior administration of the DA blocker spiropiridol. Rats who had neglect induced by ablation of the frontal cortex recover; however, a selective D1 blocker administered to these animals can again induce neglect (Vargo et al., 1989). Humans with neglect have also been treated with DA agonists. This will be discussed in the Treatment section.

Physiological studies of striatal dopaminergic neurons reveal short-latency phasic responses to stimuli that are novel or signal a reward (Shultz, 1998; Redgrave et al., 1999). These neurons may also fire in relation to the preparation, initiation, or execution of movements related to significant stimuli (Shultz et al., 2000). These physiologic studies provide evidence that the activity of dopaminergic neurons is related to the regulation of actions that are triggered by significant environmental stimuli.

MECHANISMS UNDERLYING MEMORY AND REPRESENTATIONAL DEFECTS

William James (1890) noted that "an object once attended will remain in the memory whilst one inattentively allowed to pass will leave no trace behind." The concept of arousal and its relation to learning and retention has received considerable attention (for a review see Eysenck, 1976). For example, direct relationships have been found between phasic skin conductance response amplitude during learning and accuracy of immediate and delayed recall (Stelmack et al., 1983). As discussed in an earlier section (Attentional Hypotheses) neglect may be associated with an attention-arousal deficit. Stimuli presented in the hemispace contralateral to a hemispheric lesion may receive less attention and be associated with less arousal than stimuli presented in ipsilateral hemispace. Because these stimuli are poorly attended and do not induce arousal, they may be poorly encoded and thereby induce a hemispatial antegrade memory deficit.

As discussed earlier in the testing section, Bisiach and Luzzatti (1978) asked two patients with right hemisphere damage to describe from memory a familiar scene (the main square in Milan) from two different spatial perspectives, one facing the cathedral and the other facing away from the cathedral. Regardless of the patients' orientation, more left- than right-sided details were omitted. On the basis of these findings and those of a second study (Bisiach et al., 1979), these investigators postulated that the mental representation of the environment is structured topographically and is mapped across the brain. That is, the mental picture of the environment may be split between the two hemispheres (like the projection of a real scene). Therefore, with right hemisphere damage there is a representational disorder for the left half of this image. The representational map postulated by Bisiach may be hemispatially organized so that left hemispace is represented in the right hemisphere and right hemispace is represented in the left hemisphere.

There are at least three reasons why one side of a mental image could not be envisioned. The first is that the representation may have been destroyed. A failure to represent stimuli may cause both antegrade and retrograde amnesia. The second is that the representation may have been intact but could not be activated so that an image was formed. Finally, the image was formed, but it was not attended to and therefore not correctly inspected. If the representation is destroyed, attentional manipulation should not affect retrieval, but if patients with neglect have an activational or attentional deficit, attentional manipulation may affect retrieval. Meador et al. (1987) replicated Bisiach and Luzzatti's observations and also provided evidence that behavioral manipulations could affect performance. It has been shown that when normal subjects are asked to recall objects in space, they move their eyes to the position the object occupied in space (Kahneman, 1973). Although it is unclear why normal subjects move their eyes during this type of recall task, having patients move their eyes toward neglected hemispace may aid recall because the eye movement induces hemispheric activation or helps direct attention or both. Meador et al. (1987) asked a patient with left hemispatial neglect and defective left hemispatial recall to move his eyes to either the right or left hemispace during recall. The patient's recall of left-sided detail was better when he was looking toward the left than when he looked toward the right. Although this finding provides evidence that hemispatial retrograde amnesia may be induced by an exploratory–attentional deficit or an activation deficit, it does not differentiate between these possibilities. It also does not exclude the possibility that in other cases the representation had been destroyed.

MECHANISMS UNDERLYING HEMISPATIAL NEGLECT

Patients with hemispatial neglect fail to perform on the side of space opposite their lesion, even when using their "normal" ipsilesional hand. For example, they may draw only half a picture, or bisect lines to one side (see Figs. 13–1, 13–2). Although hemianopia may enhance the symptoms of hemispatial neglect, hemianopia by itself cannot entirely account for this deficit, because some patients with hemispatial neglect are not hemianopic (McFie et al., 1950), and some hemianopic patients do not demonstrate hemispatial neglect. Although neglect can be allocentric (the left half of stimuli can be neglected even in ipsilateral hemispace), it is also environmental or viewer or body centered (Heilman and Valenstein, 1979). The abnormal performance of patients in viewer-centered contralateral space suggests that each hemisphere is responsible not only for receiving stimuli from contralateral space and for controlling the contralateral limbs, but also for attending and intending in contralateral hemispace, independent of which hand is used (Heilman, 1979; Bowers and Heilman, 1980).

Hemispace is a complex concept, since it can be defined according to several frames of reference, including the visual half-field (retinotopic), eye position, head position, or trunk position in respect to the environment. With the eyes and head facing directly ahead, the hemispaces defined by these three reference points are congruent. But if the eyes are directed to the far right, for example, the left visual field falls in large part in the right hemispace, as defined by the head and body midline. Similarly, if the head and eyes are turned far to the right, left head and eye hemispace can both be in body right hemispace. There is evidence to suggest that head and body hemispace are important in determining the symptoms of hemispatial neglect (Heilman and Valenstein, 1979; Bowers and Heilman, 1980).

Experimental evidence in normal subjects supports the hypothesis that each hemisphere is organized, at least in part, to interact with stimuli in contralateral hemispace. If a subject fixes his gaze at a midline object, keeps his right arm in right hemispace and his left arm in left hemispace, and receives a stimulus delivered in his right visual half-field, he will respond more rapidly with his right hand than with his left hand. Similarly, if a stimulus is delivered in his left visual half-field, he will respond more rapidly with his left hand than with his right (Anzola et al., 1977). These results were traditionally explained by an anatomic pathway transmission model: the reaction time is longer when the hand opposite the stimulated field responds because in this situation information must be transmitted between hemispheres, and this takes more time than when information can remain in the same hemisphere. But if a choice reaction time paradigm is used, and the hands are crossed so that the left hand is in right hemispace and the right hand is in left hemispace, then the faster reaction times are made by the hand positioned in the same side of space as the stimulus (Anzola et al., 1977), even though in this situation the information must cross the corpus callosum. Clearly, these results cannot be explained by a pathway transmission model.

Cognitive theorists have attributed the stimulus–response compatibility in these crossed-hand studies to a "natural" tendency to respond to a lateralized stimulus with the hand that is in a corresponding spatial position (Craft and Simon, 1970). Alternatively, each hemisphere may be important for intending in the contralateral hemispatial field, independent of which hand is used to respond (Heilman, 1979; Heilman and Valenstein, 1979). According to this hemispatial hypothesis, when each hand works in its own hemispace, the same hemisphere mediates both the sensorimotor system and the intentional system; however, when a hand works in the opposite hemispace, different hemispheres mediate the sensorimotor and intentional systems.

If the cerebral hemispheres are organized hemispatially, a similar compatibility may exist between the visual half-field in which a stimulus is presented and the side of hemispace in which the visual half-field is aligned. Our group (Bowers et al., 1981) has found a hemispace-visual half-field compatibility, which suggests that each hemisphere may be important not only for intending to the contralateral hemispatial field, independent of hand, but also in attending or perceiving stimuli in contralateral hemispace, independent of the visual field to which these stimuli are presented.

According to this hypothesis, when each hand works in its own spatial field, the same hemisphere mediates both the sensorimotor systems and the attentional–intentional systems. However, when a hand (e.g., right) operates in the opposite spatial field (e.g., left), the hemisphere that is contralateral to this hand (e.g., left) controls the sensorimotor apparatus, but the hemisphere ipsilateral to the hand (e.g., right) mediates attention and intention because the hand is crossed and is in left hemispace. Under these conditions, the sensorimotor and attention–intentional system must communicate through the corpus callosum. When patients with callosal disconnection bisect lines in opposite hemispace, each hand errs by gravitating toward its "own" (compatible) hemispace (Heilman et al., 1984a).

Microelectrode studies in alert monkeys support the hypothesis that the brain may be hemispatially organized. Researchers have identified cells with high-frequency activity while the monkey is looking at an interesting target (fixation cells). The activity of these cells depends not only on an appropriate motiva-tional state but also on an appropriate oculomotor state; that is, certain cells become active only when the animals are looking into contralateral hemispace (Lynch, 1980).

These studies support the hypothesis that each hemisphere mediates attention and intention in contralateral viewer-centered hemispace independent of the sensory hemifield or the extremity used. The neural substrate underlying this viewer-centered hemispatial organization of the hemispheres remains unknown. One would expect, for example, that on right lateral gaze there should be a corollary discharge to alert left hemisphere attentional cells to process stimuli that enter the left visual field.

To determine whether patients with neglect have a body-centered hemispatial deficit, we required patients with left-sided neglect to identify a letter at either the right or left end of a line before bisecting the line. The task was given with the lines placed in either right, center, or left hemispace. Even when subjects were required to look to the left before bisecting a line, ensuring that they saw the entire line, performance was significantly better when the line was placed in the right hemispace than in the left hemispace (Heilman and Valenstein, 1979). These observations indicate that patients with hemispatial neglect have a hemispatial defect rather than a hemifield defect.

Several neuropsychological mechanisms have been hypothesized to account for hemispatial neglect: attentional, intentional, exploratory gaze, and representational map.

Attentional Hypothesis

There are at least four attentional hypotheses that have been proposed to explain spatial neglect: *(1)* inattention or unawareness; *(2)* ipsilesional attention bias; *(3)* inability to disengage from right-sided stimuli; and *(4)* reduced sequential attentional capacity or premature habituation. These four hypotheses are not necessarily mutually contradictory.

The inattention hypothesis states that patients with left hemispatial neglect fail to act in left hemispace because they are unaware of stimuli in left hemispace, or because they are inattentive, stimuli in left hemispace appear to have a reduced magnitude. In the cancellation task, for example, patients with neglect fail to cancel targets in left hemispace because they are unaware of them. In the line bisection task, they are unaware of a portion of the left side of the line and only bisect the portion of line of which they are aware, or because they are inattentive, the neglected side of the line appears to be smaller that it actually is. The brain mechanisms that mediate attention have already been discussed. There are several observations that support the attentional hypothesis. The severity of left-sided neglect may be decreased by instructions to attend to a contralesional stimulus, and increased by instructions to attend to an ipsilesional stimulus (Riddoch and Humphreys, 1983). These instructions may modify attention in a "top-down" manner. The severity of neglect may also be modified by novelty, which may influence attention in a "bottom-up" manner. Butter et al. (1990) showed that novel stimuli presented on the contralesional side also reduced spatial neglect. Cues may also be intrinsic to the stimulus. Kartsounis and Warrington (1989) have shown that neglect is less severe when one is drawing meaningful pictures than when drawing meaningless pictures.

On the cancellation task, patients with left-sided neglect often begin to search for targets on the right side of the page (normal people who read European languages usually begin on the left). Ladavas et al. (1990) demonstrated that patients with right parietal lesions have shorter reaction times to right-sided stimuli than to left-sided stimuli, providing evidence of an attentional bias. Kinsbourne (1970) posited that each hemisphere inhibits the opposite hemisphere. When one hemisphere is injured, the other becomes hyperactive, and attention is biased contralaterally. Heilman and Watson (1977) agree that there is an ipsilesional bias, but believe that the bias is not being induced by a hyperactive hemisphere. If normally each hemisphere orients attention in a contralateral direction and one hemisphere is hypoactive, there will also be an attentional bias. A seesaw or teeter-totter may tilt one way because one child is either too heavy (hyperactive hypothesis of Kinsbourne) or because the other child is too light (hypoactive hypothesis of Heilman and Watson).

Support for the hypoactive (vs. Kinsbourne's hyperactive) hemisphere hypothesis comes from both behavioral and physiological studies. Ladavas et al. (1990) found that attentional shifts between vertically aligned stimuli were slower when stimuli were in left (contralesional) hemispace than when they were in right (ipsilesional) hemispace. This slowing cannot be explained by the hyperactive hemisphere hypothesis, which predicts only slowing in the horizontal axis (i.e., left directional shifts of attention should be slower than right shifts) and is therefore supportive of the hypoactive hemisphere theory. Additional support for the hypoactive hypothesis comes from the finding of EEG slowing in the nonlesioned (left) hemisphere (Heilman, 1979) of patients with neglect, and from PET studies that show lower energy metabolism in the uninjured hemisphere (Fiorelli et al., 1991).

Posner et al. (1984) proposed a three-stage model of attention. When one is called upon to shift attention, one must first disengage attention from the stimulus one is currently attending, move attention to the new stimulus, and then engage that stimulus. Posner et al. (1984) studied patients with parietal lesions by providing visual cues as to which side of extrapersonal space the imperative (reaction time) stimulus would appear. The cues could be either valid, indicating the side on which the stimulus would actually appear, or invalid, indicating the opposite side. In normal subjects, valid cues reduce reaction times and invalid cues increase reaction times. Posner et al. found that in patients with parietal lobe lesions, invalid cues indicating that the reaction time stimulus is to appear ipsilesionally resulted in abnormal prolongation of reaction times to contralesional stimuli. These results suggest that one of the functions of the parietal lobe is to disengage attention. Patients may have spatial neglect because they cannot disengage from right-sided (ipsilesional) stimuli.

Mark et al. (1988) tested the disengagement and bias hypothesis of spatial neglect by comparing the performance of patients on a cancellation task in which the subject marked each detected target with their performance on another cancellation task in which the subject erased the targets. If a target is erased, the subject should have no difficulty disengaging from the target. In addition, erasing targets should also systematically reduce bias. They observed that on the standard cancellation task, subjects with neglect would first start canceling targets on the side of the sheet that is ipsilateral to their lesion (right side). Although they could disengage from specific targets, they often returned to these targets and canceled them again. When erasing targets, patients' performance improved (they erased more targets); however, they continued to neglect some targets on the left. These observations suggest a bias rather than a problem with "disengagement." The bias hypothesis accounts for the distribution of neglect: subjects fail to cancel left-sided targets, one could argue, because bias is in part a "top-down" process, and while right-sided stimuli are more likely to "draw" attention than left-sided stimuli, even in the absence of stimuli the subject with left neglect continues to have a right-sided attention bias and is unable to move attention fully leftward.

Chatterjee et al. (1992) requested that a patient who demonstrated left-sided neglect on standard cancellation tasks alternately cancel targets on the right and left side of an array. Using this procedure, the patient was able to overcome her right-sided bias, but she did not cancel more targets. Instead, she now neglected targets in the center of the array. This suggests that, in addition to a spatial attentional bias manifested on the traditional cancellation task, the modified task revealed that there may also be a limited intentional capacity for sequential operations, or inappropriately rapid habituation.

In summary, hemispatial neglect may be induced by an attentional deficit. It appears that patients with neglect have difficulty directing their attention toward contralesional viewer-centered space, and this attentional deficit induces an ipsilesional attention bias.

Motor Intentional Hypothesis

When one is attending to a spatial location, one is also prepared to act in that direction. Therefore, sensory attention and motor intention should be closely linked. However, a patient tested by Heilman and Howell (1980) provides evidence that these processes may be dissocia-

ble. This patient with intermittent right parieto-occipital seizures was monitored by an EEG while he received right, left, and bilateral stimuli. Interictally the patient did not have inattention or extinction; however, while the seizure focus was active, he had left-sided extinction. When asked to bisect lines during two focal seizures, however, rather than neglecting left space, the patient attempted to make a mark to the left of the entire sheet of paper. When asked to bisect lines immediately after a seizure, he bisected the line to the right of midline; this location suggests left hemispatial neglect. However, at this stage no sensory extinction was present. This case illustrates that attention to contralateral stimuli and intention to perform in this contralateral hemispatial field may be dissociable.

The action–intention hypothesis of hemispatial neglect states that while patients may be aware of stimuli in contralateral hemispace, they fail to act on these stimuli because they have either a reduced ability to act (or sustain action) in contralesional hemispace or they have an action–intentional bias to act rightward. There are several observations that support these hypotheses.

Heilman and Valenstein (1979) asked patients to read a letter on the left side of a line prior to bisecting the line. This strategy ensures that the subjects were aware of the entire line. In spite of using this strategy, patients did better when the line was in right (ipsilesional) than in left (contralesional) hemispace, suggesting a reduced ability to act in contralesional hemispace. De Renzi et al. (1970) asked blindfolded patients with hemispatial neglect to search a maze for a target. The subjects failed to explore the left side of the maze. When using the tactile modality to explore, one can only attend to stimuli in a new spatial position after one has moved. Therefore, the failure to explore the left (contralesional) side of the maze cannot be attributed to an attentional deficit and may provide evidence for a hemispatial action–intentional deficit.

The results of a study by Heilman et al. (1983a) suggest that in addition to a hemispatial deficit, patients with unilateral spatial neglect have a rightward motor–intentional bias. Control subjects and patients with left-sided hemispatial neglect were asked to close their eyes, point their right index finger to their sternum, and then point to an imaginary spot in space in the midsagittal plane (perpendicular to their chest). The patients with neglect pointed to the right of midline, whereas the controls pointed slightly to the left of midline. Because this task did not require visual or somesthetic input from left hemispace, the defective performance could not be attributed to hemispatial inattention or attentional bias. Heilman et al. (1983a) also tested the ability of patients with left-sided hemispatial neglect to move a lever toward or away from the side of their lesion. These subjects needed more time to initiate movement toward the neglected left hemispace than to initiate movement toward right hemispace, thus demonstrating a directional hypokinesia. These asymmetries were not found in brain-lesioned controls without neglect. This directional hypokinesia may be related to a motor intentional bias or to an inability for the motor–intentional system to disengage from the right.

To learn if defective attention or defective intention was primarily responsible for the abnormal performance of patients with spatial neglect, Coslett et al. (1990) had patients bisect a line that they only saw displayed on a TV monitor connected to a video camera focused on the patient's hand and line. Using this technique, action and feedback could be dissociated such that the action could take place in left hemispace but the feedback could take place in right hemispace or vice versa. Independent of the position of the line, two of the four subjects improved when the monitor was moved from left (contralesional) to right (ipsilesional) hemispace, which suggests that their primary disturbance was attentional. Performance of the two other subjects was not improved by moving the monitor into right hemispace but was primarily affected by the hemispace in which the action took place. These subjects performed better when the line was in right (ipsilesional) hemispace than when in left (contralesional) hemispace, which suggests that they had primarily a motor–intentional deficit. The two patients who had primarily intentional neglect had frontal lesions and those with attentional neglect had parietal lesions.

That spatial neglect can be associated with a motor–intentional bias is also supported by the work of Bisiach et al. (1990). In their study, they used a loop of string stretched around two pulleys; the string was positioned horizontally, with one pulley on the left and the other on the right, and an arrow was attached to the top segment of string. Subjects with neglect and control subjects were asked to place the arrow midway between the two pulleys. In the congruent condition, the subject held the arrow on the upper string to move it. In the noncongruent condition, the subject moved the arrow by lateral displacement of the lower string, which moved the arrow in the opposite direction. If neglect is caused by a directional hypokinesia, the error in the congruent and noncongruent conditions should be in opposite directions. Six of 13 subjects showed a significant reduction of neglect in the noncongruent condition, which suggests that they had a significant motor–intentional bias.

Na and co-workers (1998b) and Adair et al. (1998) attempted to dissociate attentional and intentional aspects of neglect by having subjects view their performance of a line bisection task on a video monitor on which the task was displayed either normally (direct condition) or right–left reversed (indirect condition). Subjects could not view the workspace directly, but only on the monitor. In the indirect condition, hand movements to the right in the actual work space appeared on the monitor as moving leftward and vice versa. Through this technique, in the indirect condition, the performance of patients with primarily attentional neglect should be influenced by the monitor, so that when they view their performance on the monitor they will bisect lines toward the right, even though in actual work space the line is bisected to the left, a reversal of their usual error. In contrast, the performance of patients with intentional spatial neglect will be influenced primarily by the motor aspects of the task, and they will continue to bisect lines toward the right in the indirect condition, even though this appears on the monitor as a leftward bisection. This technique allows the investigator to determine the relative contribution of attentional and intentional biases in the same subject. For example, if patients reverse their deviation in the indirect condition, but the deviation is less than it was in the direct condition, this suggests an attentional bias, with some lesser contribution of a rightward intentional bias. Using this apparatus, Na et al. (1998b) found that most patients with spatial neglect could be demonstrated to have both intentional and attentional biases, but in patients with frontal lesions the intentional bias dominated, whereas in patients with temporal-parietal lesions the attentional bias predominated. The finding of mixed attentional and intentional bias is consistent with the idea that the networks subserving attention and intention influence one another. Anatomically, the parietal and frontal lobes are involved in both networks. Support of this postulate also comes from Mattingly et al. (1998), who demonstrated that the parietal lobe serves a sensorimotor interface.

Representational Hypothesis

We have already discussed Denny-Brown's and Bisiach's observations that patients can have a deficit in body-centered hemispatial memory or imagery. Bisiach attributed this deficit to destruction of the representation of left space stored in the right hemisphere. Destruction of a representation may account not only for a deficit in imagery and memory but also for hemispatial neglect.

The construct of attention derives from the knowledge that the human brain has a limited capacity to simultaneously process information. The organism, therefore, must select which stimuli to process. Except for stimuli that will be attended to regardless of their significance, such as unexpected moving objects, loud sounds, or bright lights, attention is directed in a "top-down" fashion. Therefore, knowledge or representations must direct the selection process. There are at least two representations that are needed to perform a spatial task such as a cancellation task: a representation of the target and a representation of the environment. Because patients with left-sided spatial neglect are able, in a cancellation task, to detect target stimuli on the right side, their failure to detect stimuli on the left cannot be attributed to a loss of the representation of the target. If the knowledge of left space is stored in the right

hemisphere and these representations are destroyed, attention may not be directed to left space, because the person has no knowledge of this space.

In a similar fashion, mental representations may also direct action. The number of independent actions one can simultaneously perform is also limited. Therefore, just as one selects stimuli to process, one must also select actions to perform. There are at least two pieces of knowledge that guide action: how to move, and where to act. Since patients with spatial neglect know how to act in ipsilesional space, their failure to act in contralesional space cannot be attributed to a loss of the "how" representation. However, if knowledge of contralesional space is lost, one may fail to act in or toward that portion of space.

Therefore, both intentional and attentional defects may be induced by a representational defect. The loss of a representation (knowledge) of one-half of space should be manifested by all the signs we discussed: an attentional deficit, an intentional deficit, a memory deficit, and an imagery deficit. Unless a patient has all these deficits, hemispatial neglect cannot be attributed to a loss of the spatial representation. As we have already discussed, in the clinic we see patients who have primarily a motor–intentional disorder as well as others who have primarily a sensory–attentional disorder. Not all patients with neglect have imagery defects and some patients with imagery defects do not have hemispatial neglect (Guariglia et al., 1993). Therefore, a representational deficit cannot account for all cases of spatial neglect. A representational defect also cannot account for the attentional and intentional biases we have discussed. However, there are patients who are severely inattentive to contralesional stimuli, fail to explore contralesional space, and have a profound contralesional spatial memory defect. Although these patients may have defects in multiple systems, their representation for contralesional space may be destroyed so that they no longer know of its existence.

Exploratory Hypothesis

Chedru et al. (1973) recorded eye movements of patients with left-sided spatial neglect and demonstrated failure to explore the left side of space. This failure to explore could not be accounted for by paralysis, since these patients could voluntarily look leftward. If patients fail to explore the left side of a line, they may never learn the full extent of the line, bisecting only the portion they have explored. Similarly, if they do not fully explore the left side of a sheet, they may fail to cancel targets on the part of the sheet they have failed to explore. However, these defects of visual exploration may all be attributed to the attentional, intentional, or representational defects previously discussed.

MECHANISMS OF IPSILATERAL NEGLECT

The mechanisms of ipsilateral neglect have not been entirely elucidated. Butter and colleagues (1988b) studied the eye movements of a patient with left-sided neglect from a right dorsolateral frontal lesion. In the acute stages of the illness, the patient made rightward but not leftward saccades. To try to determine if this asymmetry in gaze was due to left-sided inattention or to directional ocular akinesia toward the left, Butter et al. modified the crossed-response task of Watson et al. (1978) by asking the patient to move his eyes in the direction opposite a lateralized stimulus. When presented with a left-sided stimulus, he could move his eyes to the right, but when presented with a right-sided stimulus, the patient could not move his eyes to the left, thus suggesting a directional akinesia. As the patient recovered, this directional akinesia abated and the patient was able to look leftward to right-sided stimuli. However, now when presented with a left-sided stimulus, instead of looking to the right the patient first looked to the left. This has been termed a "visual grasp." The patient with ipsilateral neglect reported by Kwon and Heilman (1991) also had a visual grasp from a frontal lesion. Kim et al. (1999) studied a series of patients with ipsilateral neglect and demonstrated that most had frontal lesions. Denny-Brown and Chambers (1958) proposed that the parietal lobes mediate approach behaviors and the frontal lobes mediate avoidance behaviors. Therefore, injury to the frontal lobes disinhibits the parietal lobes and induces aberrant approach. Kwon and Heilman suggested that the left-sided visual grasp and ipsilateral neglect may both be manifestations of inappropriate approach behaviors. Robertson et al. (1994) replicated Kwon and Heilman's observations, but suggested that ipsilateral neglect was related to a learned compensatory strategy. However, some of the patients with ipsilateral neglect reported by Kim et al. (1999) demonstrated this phenomenon almost immediately after their stroke; this suggests that ipsilateral neglect could not be attributed entirely to a compensatory strategy. Na et al. (1998a) also demonstrated that ipsilateral neglect, like contralateral neglect, can be induced by both a contralesional attentional bias and a contralesional intentional bias.

HEMISPHERIC ASYMMETRIES OF NEGLECT

Many early investigators noted that the neglect syndrome was more often associated with right than with left hemisphere lesions (Brain, 1941; McFie et al., 1950; Critchley, 1966). Although Battersby et al. (1956) thought this preponderance of right hemisphere–lesioned patients was the result of a sampling artifact caused by the exclusion of aphasic subjects, more recent studies confirm that lesions in the right hemisphere more often induce elements of the neglect syndrome. Albert (1973), Gainotti et al. (1972), and Costa et al. (1969) demonstrated that hemispatial neglect is more frequent and more severe after right than after left hemisphere lesions. Meador et al. (1988) showed that inattention (extinction) is more common in right than in left hemisphere dysfunction. Studies of limb akinesia (Coslett and Heilman, 1989) and studies of eye movements (De Renzi et al., 1982; Meador et al., 1989) revealed that limb akinesia and directional akinesia are more common after right than after left hemisphere lesions.

Inattention

Most of the attentional cells (or comparator neurons) found in the parietal lobe of monkeys in studies by Lynch (1980) and Robinson et al. (1978) had contralateral receptive fields, but some of these neurons had bilateral receptive fields, and thus responded to stimuli presented in either visual half-field. To account for hemispheric asymmetry of attention in humans, we suggested that the temporoparietal regions of the human brain also have attentional or comparator neurons, but that the cells in the right hemisphere are more likely than cells in the left hemisphere to have bilateral receptive fields (Heilman and Van Den Abell, 1980). Thus, cells in the left hemisphere would be activated predominantly by novel or significant stimuli in right hemispace or the right hemifield, but cells in the right hemisphere would be activated by novel or significant stimuli in either visual field or on either side of hemispace (or both). If this were the case, right hemisphere lesions would cause contralateral inattention more often than left hemisphere lesions. When the left hemisphere is damaged, the right can attend to ipsilateral stimuli, but the left hemisphere cannot attend to ipsilateral stimuli after right-sided damage. If activation of attentional neurons induces local EEG desynchronization (Sokolov, 1963), and if the right hemisphere is dominant for attention, the right hemisphere should desynchronize to stimuli presented in either field, whereas the left hemisphere would desynchronize only to right-sided stimuli. We therefore presented lateralized visual stimuli to normal subjects while recording EEG from the scalp. We found that the right parietal lobe desynchronized equally to right- or left-sided stimuli while the left parietal lobe desynchronized mainly to right-sided stimuli. These observations are compatible with the hypothesis that the right hemisphere (parietal lobe) dominates the attentional processes (Heilman and Van Den Abell, 1980). A similar phenomenon has been demonstrated using PET (Pardo et al. 1991). Using fMRI, Finic and coworkers (2000) had normal subjects perform line bisection judgements and revealed activation of the right inferior parietal lobe. These electrophysiological and imaging studies provide evidence for a special role of the right hemisphere in attention and may also help explain why inattention is more often caused by right hemisphere lesions.

Neglect of environmental stimuli may occur even when these stimuli are presented to the side ipsilateral to right hemisphere lesions (Al-bert, 1973; Heilman and Valenstein, 1979; Weintraub and Mesulam, 1987). Although less severe and less frequent, extinction within ipsilesional visual and tactile fields may be seen with right hemisphere lesions (Rapcsak et al. 1987; Feinberg et al., 1990). These observations suggest that although the left hemisphere can attend rightward, when compared to the right hemisphere, the left hemisphere's attentional capacity is limited even contralaterally.

Arousal

Using the galvanic skin response as a measure of arousal, it has been demonstrated that patients with right temporoparietal lesions have a reduced response when compared to patients with left temporoparietal lesions (Heilman et al., 1978; Schrandt et al., 1989). Yokoyama et al. (1987) obtained similar results using heart rate as a measure of arousal. We also compared the EEG from the nonlesioned hemisphere of awake patients with right or left temporoparietal infarctions. Patients with right-sided lesions showed more theta and delta activity over their nonlesioned hemisphere than patients with left-sided lesions. These studies suggest that the right hemisphere may have a special role in mediating both central and peripheral arousal.

Intention

Patients with right hemisphere lesions more often have contralateral limb akinesia than patients with left hemisphere lesions (Coslett and Heilman, 1989). One can also look at responses of the limb ipsilateral to the lesion, since patients with cerebral lesions confined to a single hemisphere have slower reaction times with the hand ipsilateral to the lesion than do non-lesioned controls using the same hand (Benton and Joynt, 1959). De Renzi and Faglioni (1965) used a simple reaction time task to study patients with unilateral cerebral lesions. Although lesions of either hemisphere slowed the reaction times of the hand ipsilateral to the lesion, right hemisphere lesions caused greater slowing than left hemisphere lesions. De Renzi and Faglioni assumed that this difference in reaction times indicated that patients with right hemisphere injuries had larger lesions that those with left hemisphere injury, but brain imaging was not available at that time to support this claim. Howes and Boller (1975) later confirmed that patients with right hemisphere lesions had slower reaction times, and found that the right hemisphere lesions associated with these deficits were not larger than the left hemisphere lesions. Although Howes and Boller alluded to a loss of topographical sense as perhaps being responsible for these asymmetries, they did not draw any conclusions about the means by which right hemisphere lesions produced slower reaction times. Unfortunately, they did not mention whether the patients with profound ipsilateral slowing had unilateral neglect.

In monkeys, no hemispheric asymmetries in the production of the neglect syndrome have been noted; however, we (Valenstein et al., 1987) found that monkeys with lesions inducing neglect had slower ipsilateral reaction times than monkeys with lesions of equal size that did not induce neglect.

It has been shown that warning stimuli may prepare an individual for action and thereby reduce reaction times (Lansing et al., 1959). Pibram and McGuiness (1975) used the term *activation* to define physiological readiness to respond to environmental stimuli. Because patients with right hemisphere lesions have been shown to have reduced behavioral evidence of activation, we have postulated that, in humans, the right hemisphere may be dominant for mediating the activation process; that is, the left hemisphere prepares the right extremities for action, but the right hemisphere prepares both sides. Therefore, with left-sided lesions, left-side limb akinesia is minimal, but with right-sided lesions there is severe left-limb akinesia. In addition, because the right hemisphere is more involved than the left hemisphere in activating ipsilateral extremities, with right hemisphere lesions there will be more ipsilateral hypokinesia than with left hemisphere lesions.

If the right hemisphere dominates mediation of activation or intention (physiological readiness to respond), normal subjects may show more activation (measured behaviorally by the reaction time) with warning stimuli delivered to the right hemisphere than with warning stimuli delivered to the left hemisphere. We therefore gave normal subjects lateralized warning stimuli followed by central reaction time stimuli. Warning stimuli projected to the right hemisphere reduced reaction times of the right hand more than warning stimuli projected to the left hemisphere reduced left-hand reaction times. Warning stimuli projected to the right hemisphere reduced reaction times of the right hand even more than did warning stimuli projected directly to the left hemisphere. These results support the hypothesis that the right hemisphere dominates activation (Heilman and Van Den Abell, 1979). As we have discussed, motor bias, directional akinesia, and hypokinesia are more common with right than with left hemisphere lesions. This would suggest that the right hemisphere can prepare movement in both directions, but the left hemisphere prepares only for right-sided movements.

Hemispatial Neglect

Gainotti et al. (1972), Albert (1973), and Costa et al. (1969) have shown that hemispatial neglect is both more frequent and more severe with right-sided lesions than with left-sided lesions. In the preceding sections we discussed some of the mechanisms that may underlie hemispatial neglect. The same hypotheses we put forward to explain attentional and intentional asymmetries may also be extended to a representational hypothesis such that the right hemisphere contains representations for both sides of space and the left hemisphere for right space. The right hemisphere has a special role in visuoperceptive, visuospatial, and visuoconstructive processes, and several authors (McFie et al., 1950; Albert, 1973) have proposed that the asymmetries of hemispatial neglect are related to disorders of these processes.

Kinsbourne (1970) proposed that language-induced left hemisphere activation makes neglect more evident with right than with left hemisphere lesions. Behavioral and psychophysiological studies have shown that language may induce left hemisphere activation (Kinsbourne, 1974; Bowers and Heilman, 1976). Patients are usually tested for hemispatial neglect using verbal instructions, and, not being aphasic, they usually think and communicate verbally. To test Kinsbourne's hypothesis, we (Heilman and Watson, 1978) presented patients with left-sided hemispatial neglect a crossing-out task in which the subject was asked either to cross out words or to cross out lines oriented in a specific direction (e.g., horizontal). In the verbal condition, the target words were mixed with two others that were foils, and in the visuospatial condition, the target lines were mixed with other lines (e.g., vertical and diagonal) that acted as foils. All the subjects tested crossed out more lines and went farther to the left on the paper in the nonverbal condition than in the verbal condition. These results give partial support to Kinsbourne's hypothesis. However, Caplan (1985) cold not obtain similar results, suggesting the difference found by Heilman and Watson may be related to differences in attentional demands of the two types of stimuli used in this task (see Rapcsak et al., 1989). However, additional support of Kinsbourne's hypothesis comes from the observation that neglect is less severe when the left hand is used to perform cancellation tasks than when the right hand is used (Halligan and Marshall, 1989).

We have previously discussed the proposal that hemispatial neglect can be induced by hemispatial or directional akinesia, or by hemispatial or directional inattention. In the preceding section, we postulated that the right hemisphere is dominant for intention and attention. That hemispatial neglect occurs more often after right hemisphere lesions may be explained by a similar phenomenon.

NEUROPATHOLOGY OF NEGLECT

Neglect in humans can accompany lesions in the following areas: (1) inferior parietal lobe (Critchley, 1966), (2) dorsolateral frontal lobe (Heilman and Valenstein, 1972), (3) cingulate gyrus (Heilman and Valenstein, 1972), (4) neostriatum (Hier et al., 1977), (5) thalamus and MRF (Watson and Heilman, 1979), and (6) posterior limb of the internal capsule. On the basis of brain imaging, Heilman et al. (1983) and Vallar et al. (1994) concluded that neglect is probably seen most frequently after temporoparietal lesions.

The most common cause of neglect from cortical lesions is cerebral infarction (from either thrombosis or embolus), and the most common cause of subcortical neglect is intracerebral hemorrhage. Neglect can also be seen with tumors. Rapidly growing malignant tumors (e.g., metastatic or glioblastoma) are more likely to produce neglect than are slowly growing tumors. It is unusual to see neglect as the result of a degenerative disease, because the degeneration is most often bilateral and insidious. However, we and others have seen neglect with focal atrophy, and neglect has also been reported with Alzheimer's disease (Ishiai et al., 1996; Mendez et al., 1997; Bartolomeo et al., 1998; Venneri et al., 1998). The akinesia seen with degenerative diseases may be bilateral neglect (Heilman and Valenstein, 1972; Watson et al., 1973), which we believe is the cause of akinetic mutism. We have also seen a transient neglect syndrome as a postictal phenomenon in a patient with idiopathic right temporal lobe seizures, and the transient bilateral akinesia seen with other types of seizures may also be induced by similar mechanisms (Watson et al., 1974). Neglect may also be seen after unilateral (right) electroconvulsive therapy (ECT) (Sackeim, personal communication, 1983).

RECOVERY OF FUNCTION AND TREATMENT

NATURAL HISTORY

After a cerebral infarction, some patients acutely demonstrate a characteristic syndrome that includes neglect of their extremities, limb akinesia, profound sensory inattention or allesthesia, hemispatial neglect, head and eye deviation, and anosognosia for hemiplegia. In a period of weeks to months, profound inattention and allesthesia abate, but extinction can be demonstrated with bilateral simultaneous stimulation. Hemispatial neglect also diminishes, and although anosognosia often disappears, patients continue to be unconcerned about their deficits (anosodiaphoria). Extinction and anosodiaphoria may persist for years. In our experience, it is the motor intentional deficits that are the most persistent disabling aspect of neglect.

Unlike humans, who recover from the neglect syndrome slowly and often incompletely, monkeys rarely show evidence of neglect after 1 month. The neural mechanisms underlying this recovery are poorly understood. One hypothesis is that the undamaged hemisphere plays a role in recovery. It may receive sensory information from the side of the body opposite the lesion, either via ipsilateral sensory pathways or from the damaged hemisphere via the corpus callosum. The uninjured hemisphere might also enhance the injured hemisphere's ability to attend to contralateral sensory information and to initiate contralateral limb movements. In either case, a corpus callosum transection should worsen symptoms of neglect. Crowne et al. (1981) showed that neglect from frontal ablations was worse if the corpus callosum was simultaneously sectioned than if the callosum was intact. Watson et al. (1984) showed that monkeys receiving a frontal arcuate gyrus ablation several months after a corpus callosum transection also had worse neglect than did animals with an intact callosum. These results suggest that the hemispheres are mutually excitatory or compensatory through the corpus callosum.

Although callosal section worsened the severity of neglect, both groups of investigators found that it did not influence the rate of recovery. Subjects with callosal transections recovered completely. This suggests that recovery is an intrahemispheric rather than an interhemispheric process. If the intact hemisphere is responsible for recovery, then a callosal transection, after recovery, should not reinstate neglect. Crowne et al. (1981) did reinstate neglect in three animals undergoing corpus callosum transections. It is possible, however, that extracallosal damage during surgery might be responsible for reinstating neglect. We performed a similar callosal section after a monkey recovered from neglect and did not reinstate neglect. Furthermore, if the intact hemisphere is responsible for recovery in an animal with divided hemispheres, the recovery would have to be mediated through ipsilateral pathways. We have made a unilateral spinal cord lesion to interrupt ipsilateral sensory pathways in one of our recovered subjects without reinstating neglect. Our observations suggest that recovery is occurring within the injured hemisphere. Recent PET studies have supported the postulate that recovery from neglect is primarily intrahemispheric (Pizzamiglio et al., 1998).

Hughlings Jackson (1932) postulated that functions could be mediated at several levels of the nervous system (hierarchical representation). Lesions of higher areas (such as the cortex) would release phylogenetically more primitive areas, which may assume some of the function of the lesioned cortical areas. After cortical lesions disrupt the corticolimbic–reticular network, it is possible that subcortical areas become responsible for mediating responses. Ideally, the area that substitutes for the lesioned area must have similar characteristics. It must have multimodal afferent input, reticular connections, and be capable of inducing activation with stimulation. Lastly, ablation of this area should induce the neglect syndrome, even if transiently. The superior colliculus not only receives optic fibers but also receives somesthetic projections from the spinotectal tract (Sprague and Meikle, 1965) as well as fibers from the medial and lateral lemnisci and the inferior colliculus (Truex and Carpenter, 1964). Sprague and Meikle believe that the superior colliculus is a sensory integrative center, not just a reflex center controlling eye movements. Tectoreticular fibers project to the mesencephalic reticular formation and ipsilateral fibers are more abundant than contralateral fibers (Truex and Carpenter, 1964). Stimulation of the colliculus, like stimulation of the arcuate gyrus or the IPL, produces an arousal response (Jefferson, 1958). Unilateral lesions of the superior colliculus produce a multimodal unilateral neglect syndrome, and combined cortical-collicular lesions produce a more profound disturbance regardless of the order of removal (Sprague and Meikle, 1965). Therefore, it is possible that with injury to the cortico-limbic-reticular system, a collicular-reticular system functionly compensates.

Unlike the neglect induced by cortical lesions in monkeys, the neglect associated with lesions of ascending DA projections in rats can be permanent (Marshall, 1982). The severity and persistence of neglect induced by 6-OHDA injections into the VTA of rats is correlated with the amount of striatal DA depletion: those with more than 95% loss of striatal DA have a permanent deficit. The extent of recovery of these animals is also directly related to the quantity of neostriatal DA present at sacrifice. Unrecovered rats show pronounced contralateral turning after injections of apomorphine, a DA receptor stimulant. Recovered rats given methyl-p-tyrosine, a catecholamine synthesis inhibitor, or spiroperidol, a DA receptor blocking agent, had their deficits reappear. These results suggest that restoration of dopaminergic activity in DA-depleted rats is sufficient to reinstate orientation (Marshall, 1979). Further investigation of these findings indicates that a proliferation of DA receptors may contribute to pharmacological supersensitivity and recovery of function (Neve et al., 1982). Finally, implanting dopaminergic neurons from the ventral tegmental area of fetal rats adjacent to the ipsilesional striatum will induce recovery in rats having unilateral neglect from a 6-OHDA lesion in the ascending DA tracts (Dunnett et al., 1981). This recovery is related to growth of DA-containing neurons into the partially denervated striatum. Corwin et al. (1986) induced neglect in rats by ablating frontal cortex unilaterally. After the rats had recovered from neglect, spiroperidol reinstituted their neglect.

C-14,2-deoxyglucose (2-DG) incorporation permits one to measure metabolic activity. In rats with 6-OHDA lesions of the VTA that had shown no recovery from neglect, the uptake of 2-DG into the neostriatum, nucleus accumbens septi, olfactory tubercle, and central amygdaloid nucleus was significantly less on the denervated side than on the normal side. Rats recovering by 6 weeks showed equivalent 2-DG uptake in the neostriatum and central amygdaloid nucleus on the two sides. Recovery is therefore associated with normalization of neostriatal metabolic activity (Kozlowski and Marshall, 1981).

Similar results have been found in monkeys recovering from frontal arcuate gyrus–induced neglect (Deuel et al., 1979). Animals with neglect showed depression of deoxyglucose in ipsilateral subcortical structures, including the thalamus and basal ganglia. Recovery from neglect occurred concomitantly with a reappearance of symmetrical metabolic activity.

It is possible that cortical lesions in animals induce only transient neglect because these lesions affect only a small portion of a critical neurotransmitter system. Critically placed small subcortical lesions, by contrast, can virtually destroy all of a transmitter system, and can cause a permanent syndrome.

Recovery from cortically induced neglect might also depend on the influence of cortical lesions on subcortical structures. It is likely that just as certain homologous cortical structures are thought to be mutually inhibitory via the corpus callosum, certain pairs of subcortical structures may also be mutually inhibitory. For example, in the study of Watson et al. (1984), a prior corpus callosal lesion worsened neglect from a frontal arcuate lesion. Although this could be explained by loss of an excitatory or compensatory influence from the normal frontal arcuate region on the lesioned hemisphere, it could also be interpreted as a loss of excitation from cortex on a subcortical structure such as the basal ganglia that in turn inhibits the contralateral basal ganglia. The latter is supported by a study showing that anterior callosal section in rats enhances the normal striatal DA asymmetry and increases amphetamine-induced turning (Glick et al., 1975). In addition, Sprague (1966) showed that the loss of visually guided behavior in the visual field contralateral to occipitotemporal lesions in cats could be restored by a contralateral superior colliculus removal or by transection of the collicular commissure. The only way to explain this observation is to assume that the superior colliculi are mutually inhibitory.

The two hemispheres are clearly cooperating in our daily activities. However, it appears that recovery from a central nervous system insult can occur within the injured hemisphere. For the neglect syndrome, this may be secondary to alteration in DA systems. An understanding of interhemispheric cortical and subcortical interactions, and intrahemispheric cortical and subcortical interactions in the normal state and during recovery of function, is one of the most intriguing aspects of the neglect syndrome and holds great promise for pharmacological and possibly even surgical intervention in this syndrome.

TREATMENT

The neglect syndrome is a behavioral manifestation of underlying cerebral disease. The evaluation and treatment of the underlying disease are of primary importance.

There are several things that can be done to manage the symptoms of the neglect syndrome. In the previous edition of this book we wrote, "The patient with neglect should have his bed placed so that his 'good' side faces the area where interpersonal actions are most likely to take place. When he must interact with people or things, these interactions should take place on his good side. When discharged home, his environment should be adjusted in a similar manner." However, Kunkle et al. (1999) treated patients who had a hemiparesis by binding their nonparetic arm and forcing them to use this hemiparetic arm. They found that this procedure induced recovery. It is possible that some of their patients' motor deficit was related to limb akinesia associated with motor neglect, rather than to weakness associated with corticospinal damage. In the last decade, studies, primarily in animals, have demonstrated that experience can change neuronal networks. Therefore, it is possible that stimulation of the contralesional side may induce functional reorganization and thereby reduce the severity of neglect. In contrast, studies of rats suggest that acute sensory depravation, such as being kept in absolute darkness, may induce recovery from neglect (Burcham et al., 1998; Corwin and Vargo, 1993). However, rats are nocturnal, and studies in humans have to be performed to learn if stimulation is beneficial or harmful in the recovery from neglect.

Although we do not know if patients with neglect should be stimulated or sensory deprived, we should not allow them to perform activities that may cause injuries to themselves or others. So long as patients have the neglect syndrome, they should not be allowed to drive or to work with anything that, if neglected, could cause injury to themselves or others. During the acute stages when patients have anosog-

nosia, rehabilitation is difficult; however, in most patients, anosognosia is transient. In addition, because patients with neglect remain inattentive to their left side and in general are poorly motivated, training is laborious and in many cases unrewarding. Diller and Weinberg (1977) were able to train patients with neglect to look to their neglected side; however, it was not clear that these top-down attentional–exploratory treatments generalized to other situations.

In contrast to this top-down treatment, Butter et al. (1990) used a bottom-up treatment. Brainstem structures such as the superior colliculus may play an important role in recovery from neglect. Butter et al. (1990) recognized that since dynamic stimuli readily summon attention in normal subjects and are potent activators of brain structures such as the colliculi, perhaps they could be used to reduce neglect. They tested patients with neglect on a line bisection task and demonstrated that dynamic stimuli presented on the contralesional (left) side reduced neglect. Neglect patients with hemianopia also improved, which suggests that these stimuli affect subcortical structures. Robertson and North (1994) demonstrated that having patients move their contralesional hand in contralesional hemispace can reduce the severity of hemispatial neglect, and these investigators have therefore used a hand movement strategy to manage neglect.

Asymmetrically activating the vestibular system in normal subjects may induce a spatial bias similar to that observed in neglect (Shuren et al., 1998). Rubens (1985) induced asymmetrical vestibular activation in patients with left-sided neglect by injecting cold water into the left ear and noting that unilateral spatial neglect abated. Vallar et al. (1995) reported that vestibular stimulation could help sensory inattention, and Rode et al. (1992) found that vestibular stimulation even helped motor neglect. Inducing optokinetic nystagmus, by having patients look at a series of stimuli moving in a contralesional direction (Pizzamigialo et al., 1990), and using vibration to stimulate muscle afferents from the neck (Karnath, 1995) are also means of reducing neglect. Unfortunately, all these procedures produce only temporary relief.

As we discussed, Coslett et al. (1990) demonstrated that patients with spatial neglect induced by attentional disorders improved when feedback was presented to the ipsilesional side. Rossi et al. (1990) used 15-diopter Fresnel prisms to shift images from the neglected side toward the normal side. After using the prisms for 4 weeks, the treated group performed better than the control group on tasks such as line bisection or cancellation. However, activities of daily living did not improve. Rossetti et al. (1998) had subjects with neglect adapt to prisms by having them repeatedly point straight ahead while wearing the prisms. After this treatment, patients showed a reduction of ipsilesional bias on tests of neglect. The effects of this treatment lasted for 2 hours after the prisms were removed; but it is uncertain how much longer the effects might last, or if this treatment generalizes to other instrumental activities and to activities of daily living.

Neglect associated with cortical lesions may be reduced by destroying the contralesional colliculus or the intercollicular commissure (Sprague, 1966). These findings suggest that the colliculus contralateral to the cortical lesion may be inhibiting the ipsilesional colliculus. Each colliculus gets greater input from the retina of the contralateral eye than it does from the ipsilateral eye. Posner and Rafal (1987) have suggested that patching the ipsilesional eye may reduce neglect because it would deprive the superior colliculus contralateral to the lesioned hemisphere of input and this reduced input may reduce collicular activation. Although some have found this ipsilesional patching procedure useful in reducing the signs of neglect (Butter and Kirsh, 1992), others have found that ipsilateral patching can make neglect more severe (Barrett et al., 2001). Therefore, each eye should be tested before deciding which eye should be patched. The mechanisms underlying reduction in neglect from collicular lesions remain uncertain. Recent studies suggest that interruption of fibers from the substantia nigra pars reticulata to the opposite superior colliculus may account for the reduction in neglect seen with intercollicular commissure section, rather than transection of intercollicular (tecto-tectal) fibers (Wallace et al., 1989, 1990). Reduction in neglect

from lesions in the contralesional superior colliculus may therefore not result from tectotectal inhibition. The underlying mechanisms remain to be elucidated.

Lastly, we discussed the role of DA in neglect and recovery. Neglect in rats with unilateral frontal (Corwin et al., 1986) and parietal lesions (Corwin et al., 1996) were treated with apomorphine, a DA agonist. Dopamine agonist therapy significantly reduced neglect in these animals. Spiroperidol, a DA receptor blocking agent, blocked the therapeutic effect of apomorphine. Fleet et al. (1987) treated two neglect patients with bromocriptine, a DA agonist. Both showed dramatic improvements. Subsequently, other investigators have also shown that DA agonist therapy may be helpful in the treatment of neglect (Geminiani et al., 1998, 1999; Hurford et al., 1998). In addition, Geminiani et al. found that dopaminergic agonist treatment helped both the sensory attentional and motor intentional forms of spatial neglect. Barrett et al. (1999) and Grujic et al. (1998) found, however, that in some patients DA agonist therapy increased rather than decreased the severity of neglect. Barrett et al.'s patient had striatal injury and they suggested that the paradoxical effect seen in their patient may be related to involvement of the basal ganglia. In patients with striatal injury, DA agonists may be unable to activate the striatum on the injured side but instead activate the striatum on the uninjured side and thereby increase the ipsilesional orientation bias.

REFERENCES

Adair, J. C., Na, D. L., Schwartz, R. L., and Heilman, K. M. (1998). Analysis of primary and secondary influences on spatial neglect. *Brain Cogn.* 37:351–367.

Akert, K., and Von Monakow, K. H. (1980). Relationship of precentral, premotor, and prefrontal cortex to the mediodorsal and intralaminar nuclei of the monkey thalamus. *Acta Neurobiol. Exp. (Warsz.) 40:7–25.*

Albert, M. D. (1973). A simple test of visual neglect. *Neurology* 23:658–664.

Anderson, M., and Yoshida, M. (1977). Electrophysiological evidence for branching nigral projections to the thalamus and superior colliculus. *Brain Res.* 137:361–364.

Anton, G. (1899). Uber die Selbstwahrnehmung der Herderkrankungen des Gehirns durch den Kranken der Rindenblindheit und Rindentaubheit. *Arch. Psychiatrie 32*:86–127.

Anzola, G. P., Bertoloni, A., Buchtel, H. A., and Rizzolatti, G. (1977). Spatial compatibility and anatomical factors in simple and choice reaction time. *Neuropsychologia 15*:295–302.

Apicella, P., Legallet, E., Nieoullon, A., and Trouche, E. (1991). Neglect of contralateral visual stimuli in monkeys with unilateral dopamine depletion. *Behav. Brain Res. 46*:187–195.

Arbuthnott, G. W., and Ungerstedt, U. (1975). Turning behavior induced by electrical stimulation of the nigro-striatal system of the rat. *Exp. Neurol. 27*:162–172.

Arnault, P., and Roger, M (1987). The connections of the peripeduncular area studied by retrograde and anterograde transport in the rat. *J. Comp. Neurol. 258*:463–478.

Avemo, A., Antelman, S., and Ungerstedt, U. (1973). Rotational behavior after unilateral frontal cortex lesions in the rat. *Acta Physiol. Scand. Suppl. 396*:77.

Babinski, J. (1914). Contribution a l'etude des troubles mentaux dans l'hemiplegie organique cerebrale (agnosognosie). *Rev. Neurol. (Paris) 27*: 845–847.

Baleydier, C., and Mauguiere, F. (1980). The duality of the cingulate gyrus in monkey—neuroanatomical study and functional hypothesis. *Brain 103*:525–554.

Barrett, A. M., Crucian, G. P., Beversdorf, D. Q., Heilman, K. M. (2001). Monocular patching may worsen sensory-attentional neglect: a case report. *Arch Phys Med Rehab. 84*:516–518.

Barrett, A. M., Crucian, G. P., Schwartz, and R. L., Heilman, K. M. (1999). Adverse effect of dopamine agonist therapy in a patient with motor-intentional neglect. *Arch. Phys. Med. Rehabil. 80*:600–603.

Bartolomeo, P., Dalla Barba, G., Boisse, M. F., Bachout-Levi, A. C., Degos, J. D., and Boller, F. (1998). Right-side neglect in Alzheimer's disease. *Neurology 51*:1207–1209.

Battersby, W. S., Bender, M. B., and Pollack, M. (1956). Unilateral spatial agnosia (inattention) in patients with cerebral lesions. *Brain 79*:68–93.

Bender, M. B. (1952). *Disorders of Perception*. Springfield, IL: C. C. Thomas.

Bender, M. B., and Furlow, C. T. (1944). Phenomenon of visual extinction and binocular rivalry mechanism. *Trans. Am. Neurol. Assoc. 70*:87–93.

Bender, M. B., and Furlow, C. T. (1945). Phenomenon of visual extinction and homonymous fields and psychological principals involved. *Arch. Neurol. Psychiatry 53*:29–33.

Benson, F., and Geschwind, N. (1969). The alexias. In *Handbook of Neurology, Vol. 4*, P. J. Vinken and G. W. Bruyn (eds.). Amsterdam: North-Holland.

Benton, A. L., and Joynt, R. J. (1959). Reaction times in unilateral cerebral disease. *Confin. Neurol. 19*: 147–256.

Benton, A. L., and Levin, H. S. (1972). An experimental study of obscuration. *Neurology 22*:1176 1181.

Bianchi, L. (1895). The functions of the frontal lobes. *Brain 18*:497–522.

Bignall, K. E., and Imbert, M. (1969). Polysensory and cortico-cortical projections to frontal lobe of squirrel and rhesus monkey. *Electroencephalogr. Clin. Neurophysiol. 26*:206–215.

Birch, H. G., Belmont, I., and Karp, E. (1967). Delayed information processing and extinction following cerebral damage. *Brain 90*:113–130.

Bisiach, E., Bulgarelli, C., Sterzi, R., and Vallar, G. (1983). Line bisection and cognitive plasticity of unilateral neglect of space. *Brain Cogn. 2*:32–38.

Bisiach, E., Geminiani, G., Berti, A., and Rusconi, M. L. (1990). Perceptual and premotor factors of unilateral neglect. *Neurology 40*:1278–1281.

Bisiach, E., and Luzzatti, C. (1978). Unilateral neglect of representational space. *Cortex 14*:29–133.

Bisiach, E., Luzzatti, C., and Perani, D. (1979). Unilateral neglect, representational schema and consciousness. *Brain 102*:609–618.

Bogosslavsky, J., Miklossy, J., Deruaz, J. P., Regli, F., and Assai, G. (1986). Unilateral left paramedian infarction of thalamus and midbrain: a clinico-pathological study. *J. Neurol. Neurosurg. Psychiatry 49*:686–694.

Bowers, D., and Heilman, K. M. (1976). Material specific hemispheric arousal. *Neuropsychologia 14*:123–127.

Bowers, D., and Heilman, K. M. (1980). Effects of hemispace on tactile line bisection task. *Neuropsychologia 18*:491–498.

Bowers, D., Heilman, K. M., and Van Den Abell, T. (1981). Hemispace-visual half field compatibility. *Neuropsychologia 19*:757–765.

Bradley, P. B. (1968). The effect of atropine and related drugs on the EEG and behavior. *Prog. Brain Res. 28*:3–13.

Brain, W. R. (1941). Visual disorientation with special reference to lesions of the right cerebral hemisphere. *Brain 64*:224–272.

Brown, R. M., Crane, A. M., and Goldman, P. S. (1979). Regional distribution of monamines in the cerebral cortex and subcortical structures of the rhesus monkey: concentrations and in vivo synthesis rates. *Brain Res. 168:*133–150.

Burcham, K. J., Corwin, J. V., Stoll, M. L., and Reep, R. L. (1997). Disconnection of medial agranular and posterior parietal cortex produces multimodal neglect in rats. *Behav. Brain Res. 86:*41–47.

Burcham, K. J., Corwin, J. V., and Van-Vleet, T. M. (1998). Light deprivation produces a therapeutic effect on neglect induced by unilateral destruction of the posterior parietal cortex in rats. *Behav. Brain Res. 90:*187–197.

Bushnell, M. C., Goldberg, M. E., and Robinson, D. L. (1981). Behavioral enhancement of visual responses in monkey cerebral cortex: I. Modulation if posterior parietal cortex related to selected visual attention. *J. Neurophysiol 46:*755–772.

Butter, C.M., and Kirsch, N. (1992). Combined and separate effects of eye patching and visual stimulation on unilateral neglect following stroke. *Arch. Phys. Med. Rehabil. 73:*1133–1139.

Butter, C. M., Kirsch, N. L., and Reeves, G. (1990). The effect of lateralized dynamic stimuli on unilateral spatial neglect following right hemisphere lesions. *Restorative Neurol. Neurosci. 2:*39–46.

Butter, C. M., Mark, V. W., and Heilman, K. M. (1988a). An experimental analysis of factors underlying neglect in line bisection. *J. Neurol. Neurosurg. Psychiatry 51:*1581–1583.

Butter, C. M., Rapcsak, S. Z., Watson, R. T., and Heilman, K. M. (1988b). Changes in sensory inattention, direction hypokinesia, and release of the fixation reflex following a unilateral frontal lesion: a case report. *Neuropsychologia 26:*533–545.

Caplan, B. (1985). Stimulus effects in unilateral neglect. *Cortex 21:*69–80.

Chatterjee, A., Mennemeier, M., and Heilman, K. M. (1992). Search patterns in neglect. *Neuropsychogia 30:*657–672.

Chatterjee, A., Thompson, K. A., and Ricci, R. (1999). Quantitative analysis of cancellation tasks in neglect. *Cortex 35:*253–262.

Chavis, D. A., and Pandya, D. N. (1976). Further observations on corticofrontal connections in the rhesus monkey. *Brain Res. 117:*369–386.

Chedru, F., Leblanc, M., and Lhermitte, F. (1973). Visual searching in normal and brain-damaged subjects. *Cortex 9:*94–111.

Colby, C. L., and Duhamel, J.-R. (1991). Heterogeneity of extrastriate visual areas and multiple parietal areas in the macaque monkey. *Neuropsychologia 29:*517–537.

Colby, C. L., Duhamel, J.-R., and Goldberg, M. E. (1993). Ventral intraparietal area of the macaque: anatomic location and visual response properties. *J. Neurophysiol. 69:*902–914.

Colby, C. L., Duhamel, J.-R., and Goldberg, M. E. (1996). Visual, presaccadic and cognitive activation of single neurons in monkey lateral intraparietal area. *J. Neurophysiol. 76:*2841–2852.

Colby, C. L., and Goldberg, M. E. (1999). Space and attention in parietal cortex. *Annu. Rev. Neurosci. 22:*319–349.

Corbett, D., and Wise, R. A. (1980). Intracranial self-stimulation in relation to the ascending dopaminergic systems of the midbrain: moveable electrode mapping study. *Brain Res. 185:*1–15.

Corwin, J. V., Burcham, K. J., and Hix, G. I. (1996). Apomorphine produces an acute dose-dependent therapeutic effect on neglect produced by unilateral destruction of the posterior parietal cortex in rats. *Behav. Brain Res. 79:*41–49.

Corwin, J. V., Kanter, S., Watson, R. T., Heilman, K. M., Valenstein, E., and Hashimoto, A. (1986). Apomorphine has a therapeutic effect on neglect produced by unilateral dorsomedial prefrontal cortex lesions in rats. *Exp. Neurol. 36:*683–698.

Corwin, J. V., and Vargo, J. M. (1993). Light deprivation produces accelerated behavioral recovery of function from neglect produced by unilateral medial agranular prefrontal cortex lesions in rats. *Behav. Brain Res. 56:*187–196.

Coslett, H. B., Bowers, D., Fitzpatrick, E., Haws, B., and Heilman, K. M. (1990) Directional hypokinesia and hemispatial inattention in neglect. *Brain 113:*475–486.

Coslett, H. B., and Heilman, K. M. (1989). Hemihypokinesia after right hemisphere strokes. *Brain Cogn. 9:*267–278.

Costa, L. D., Vaughan, H. G., Horowitz, M., and Ritter, W. (1969). Patterns of behavior deficit associated with visual spatial neglect. *Cortex 5:*242–263.

Craft, J., and Simon, J. (1970). Processing symbolic information from a visual display: interference from an irrelevant directional clue. *J. Exp. Psychol. 83:*415–420.

Critchley, M. (1966). *The Parietal Lobes.* New York: Hafner.

Crossman, A. R., Sambrook, M. A., Horwitz, M., and Ritter, W. (1977). The neurological basis of motor asymmetry following unilateral 6-hydroxydopamine lesions in the rat: the effect of motor decortication. *J. Neurol. Sci. 34:*407–414.

Crowne, D. P., Yeo, C. H., and Russell, I. S. (1981). The effects of unilateral frontal eye field lesions in the monkey: visual-motor guidance and avoidance behavior. *Behav. Brain Res.* 2:165–185.

Dalsass, M., and Karuthamer, G. M. (1981). Behavioral alterations and loss of caudate modulation in the CM-PF complex of the cat after electrolytic lesions of the substantia nigra. *Brain Res.* 208:67–79.

Denny-Brown, D., and Banker, B. Q. (1954). Amophosynthesis from left parietal lesions. *Arch. Neurol. Psychiatry* 71:302–313.

Denny-Brown D., and Chambers, R. A. (1958). The parietal lobes and behavior. *Res. Publ. Assoc. Res. Nerv. Ment. Dis.* 36:35–117.

De Renzi, E., Colombo, A., Faglioni, P., and Gilbertoni, M. (1982). Conjugate gaze paralysis in stroke patients with unilateral damage. *Arch. Neurol* 39:482–486.

De Renzi, E., Faglioni, P., and Scotti, G. (1970). Hemispheric contribution to the exploration of space through the visual and tactile modality. *Cortex* 2:191–203.

De Renzi, E., and Faglioni, P. (1965). The comparative efficiency of intelligence and vigilance test detecting hemispheric change. *Cortex* 1:410–433.

Deuel, R. K. (1980). Sensorimotor dysfunction after unilateral hypothalamic lesions in rhesus monkeys. *Neurology* 30:358.

Deuel, R. K., Collins, R. C., Dunlop N., and Caston, T. V. (1979). Recovery from unilateral neglect: behavioral and functional anatomic correlations in monkeys. *Soc. Neurosci. Abstr.* 5:624.

Diller, L., and Weinberg, J. (1977). Hemi-inattention in rehabilitation: The evolution of a rational remediation. *Advances Neurol.* 18:63–82.

Divac, I., Fonnum, F., and Storm-Mathison, J. (1977). High affinity uptake of glutamate in terminals of corticostriatal axons. *Nature* 266:377–378.

Dunnet, S. B., Bjorklund, A. Stenevi, U., and Iverson, S. D. (1981). Behavioral recovery following transplantation of substantia nigra in rats subjected to 6-OHDA lesions of the nigrostriatal pathway. I. Unilateral lesions. *Brain Res.* 215:147–161.

Eidelberg, E., and Schwartz, A. J. (1971). Experimental analysis of the extinction phenomenon in monkeys. *Brain* 94:91–108.

Eysenck, M. W. (1976). Arousal, learning and memory. *Psychol. Bull.* 83:389–404.

Farah, M. J., Brunn, J. L., Wong, A. B., Wallace, M. A., and Carpenter, P. A. (1990). Frames of reference for locating attention to space: evidence from neglect syndrome. *Neuropsychologia* 28:335–347.

Feeney, D. M., and Wier, C. S. (1979). Sensory neglect after lesions of substania nigra on lateral hypothalamus: differential severity and recovery of function. *Brain Res.* 178:329–346.

Feinberg, T. E., Habor, L. D., and Stacy, C. B. (1990). Ipsilateral extinction in the hemineglect syndrome. *Arch. Neurol.* 47:803–804.

Filion, M., Lamarre, Y., and Cordeau, J. P. (1971). Neuronal discharges of the ventrolateral nucleus of the thalamus during sleep and wakefulness in the cat. Evoked activity. *Exp. Brain Res.* 12:499–508.

Finic, G. R., Marshall, J. C., Shah, N. J., Weiss, P. H., Halligan, P. W., Grosse-Ruyken, M., Ziemons, K., Zilles, K., Freund, H. J. (2000). Line bisection judgements implicate right parietal cortex and cerebellum as assessed by fMRI. *Neurology* 54:1324–1331.

Fiorelli, M., Blin, J., Bakchine, S., LaPlane, D., and Baron, J. C. (1991). PET studies of cortical diaschisic in patients with motor hemi-neglect. *J. Neurol. Sci.* 104:135–142.

Fleet, W. S., Valenstein, E., Watson, R. T., and Heilman, K. M. (1987). Dopamine agonist therapy for neglect in humans. *Neurology* 37:1765–1771.

Fonnum, F., and Walaas, I. (1979). Localization of neurotransmitter candidates in neostriatum. In *The Neostriatum*, I. Divac and R. G. E. Oberg (eds.). Oxford: Pergamon Press, pp. 53–69.

Gainotti, G., Messerli, P., and Tissot, R. (1972). Qualitative analysis of unilateral and spatial neglect in relation to laterality of cerebral lesions. *J. Neurol. Neurosurg. Psychiatry* 35:545–550.

Geminiani, G., Bottini, G., and Sterzi, R. (1998). Dopaminergic stimulation in unilateral neglect. *J. Neurol. Neurosurg. Psychiatry* 65:344–347.

Glick, S. D., Cran, A. M., Jerussi, T. P., Fleisher, L. N., and Green, J. P. (1975). Functional and neurochemical correlates to potentiation of striatal asymmetry by callosal section. *Nature* 254:616–617.

Goldberg, M. E., and Bushnell, M. C. (1981). Behavioral enhancement of visual responses in monkey cerebral cortex: II. Modulation in frontal eye fields specifically related saccades. *J. Neurophysiol.* 46:773–787.

Goldberg, M. E., and Robinson, D. C. (1977). Visual responses of neurons in monkey inferior parietal lobule. The physiological substrate of attention and neglect. *Neurology* 27:350.

Grofova, I. (1979). Extrinsic connections of neostriatum. In *The Neostriatum*, I. Divak and R. G. E. Oberg (eds.). Oxford: Pergamon Press, pp. 37–51.

Grossman, S. P., Dacey, D., Halaris, A. E., Collier,

T., and Routtenberg, A. (1978). Aphagia and adipsia after preferential destruction of nerve cell bodies in the hypothalamus. *Science 202:* 537–539.

Grujic, Z., Mapstone, M., Gitelman, D. R., Johnson, N., Weintraub, S., Hays, A., Kwasnica, C., Harvey, R., and Mesulam, M. M. (1998). Dopamine agonists reorient visual exploration away from the neglected hemispace. *Neurology 51:*1395–1398.

Guariglia, C., Padovani, A., Pantano, P., and Pizzamiglio, L. (1993). Unilateral neglect restricted to visual imagery. *Nature 364(6434):*237–237.

Hagamen, T. C., Greeley, H. P., Hagamen, W. D., and Reeves, A. G. (1977). Behavioral asymmetries following olfactory tubercle lesions in cats. *Brain Behav. Evol. 14:*241–250.

Halligan, P. W., and Marshall, J. C. (1989). Laterality of motor response in visuo-spatial neglect: a case study. *Neuropsychologia 27:*1301–1307.

Halligan, P. W., and Marshall, J. C. (1991a). Left neglect for near but not far space in man. *Nature 350(6318):*498–500.

Halligan, P. W., and Marshall, J. C. (1991b). Recovery and regression in visuo-spatial neglect: a case study of learning in line bisection. *Brain Inj. 5:*23–31.

Haxby, J. V., Grady, C. L., Horwitz, B., Ungerleider, L. G., Mishkin, M., Carson, R. E., Herscovitch, P., Schapiro, M. B., and Rapoport, S. I. (1991). Dissociation of object and spatial visual processing pathways in human extrastriate cortex. *Proc. Natl. Acad. Sci. U.S.A. 88:*1621–1625.

Heikkila, R. E., Shapiro, B. S., and Duvoisin, R. C. (1981). The relationship between loss of dopamine nerve terminals, striatal ^{3}H spiroperidol binding and rotational behavior in unilaterally 6-hydroxdopamine-lesioned rats. *Brain Res. 211:* 285–307.

Heilman, K. M. (1979). Neglect and related disorders. In *Clinical Neuropsycology*, K. M. Heilman and E. Valenstein (eds.). New York: Oxford University Press, pp. 268–307.

Heilman, K. M. (1991). Anosognosia: possible neuropsychological mechanisms. In *Awareness of Defect After Brain Injury*, G. Prigatano and D. Schacter (eds.). New York: Oxford University Press.

Heilman, K. M., Bowers, D., and Watson, R. T. (1983a). Performance on hemispatial pointing task by patients with neglect syndrome. *Neurology 33:*661–664.

Heilman, K. M., Bowers, D., and Watson, R. T. (1984a). Pseudoneglect in patients with partial callosal disconnection. *Brain 107:*519–532.

Heilman, K. M., Bowers, D., Coslett, H. B., Whelan, H., and Watson, R. T. (1985). Directional hypokinesia: prolonged reaction times for leftward movements in patients with right hemisphere lesions and neglect. *Neurology 35:*855–860.

Heilman, K. M., and Howell, F. (1980). Seizure-induced neglect. *J. Neurol. Neurosurg. Psychiatry 43:*1035–1040.

Heilman, K. M., Odenheimer, G. L., Watson, R. T., and Valenstein, E. (1984b). Extinction of nontouch. *Neurology 34(Suppl. 1):*188.

Heilman, K. M., Pandya, D. N., and Geschwind, N. (1970). Trimodal inattention following parietal lobe ablations. *Trans. Am. Neurol. Assoc. 95:*259–261.

Heilman, K. M., Schwartz, H. D., and Watson, R. T. (1978). Hypoarousal in patients with neglect syndrome and emotional indifference. *Neurology 28:*229–232.

Heilman, K. M., and Valenstein, E. (1972). Frontal lobe neglect in man. *Neurology 22:*660–664.

Heilman, K. M., and Valenstein, E. (1979). Mechanisms underlying hemispatial neglect. *Ann. Neurol. 5:*166–170.

Heilman, K. M., Valenstein, E., and Watson, R. T. (1983b). Localization of neglect. In *Localization in Neurology*, A. Kertesz (ed.). New York: Academic Press, pp. 471–492.

Heilman, K. M., and Van Den Abell, T. (1979). Right hemispheric dominance for mediating cerebral activation. *Neuropsychologia 17:*315–321.

Heilman, K. M., and Van Den Abell, T. (1980). Right hemisphere dominance for attention: the mechanisms underlying hemispheric asymmetries of inattention (neglect). *Neurology 30:*327–330.

Heilman, K. M., and Watson, R. T. (1977). The neglect syndrome—a unilateral defect of the orienting response. In *Lateralization in the Nervous System*, S. Hardned, R. W. Doty, L. Goldstein, J. Jaynes, and G. Kean Thamer (eds.). New York: Academic Press.

Heilman, K. M., and Watson, R. T. (1978). Changes in the symptoms of neglect induced by changes in task strategy. *Arch. Neurol. 35:*47–49.

Heilman, K. M., Watson, R. T., and Schulman, H. (1974). A unilateral memory deficit. *J. Neurol. Neurosurg. Psychiatry 37:*790–793.

Hier, D. B., Davis, K. R., Richardson, E. T., et al. (1977). Hypertensive putaminal hemorrhage. *Ann. Neurol. 1:*152–159.

Herkenham, M. (1979). The afferent and efferent connections of the ventromedial thalamic nucleus in the rat. *J. Comp. Neurol. 183:*487—518.

Holmes, G. (1918). Disturbances of vision from cerebrel lesions. *Br. J. Opthalmol.* 2:253–384.

Howes, D., and Boller, F. (1975). Evidence for focal impairment from lesions of the right hemisphere. *Brain* 98:317–332.

Hoyman, L., Weese, G. D., and Frommer, G. P. (1979). Tactile discrimination performance deficits following neglect-producing unilateral lateral hypothalamic lesions in the rat. *Physiol. Behav.* 22:139–147.

Hurford, P., Stringer, A. Y., Jann, B. (1998). Neuropharmacologic treatment of hemineglect: a case report comparing bromocriptine and methylphenidate. *Arch Phys Med Rehabil* 79:346–349.

Ishiai, S., Okiyama, R., Koyama, Y., and Seki, K. (1996). Unilateral spatial negelct in Alzheimer's disease. A line bisection study. *Acta Neurol. Scand.* 93:219–224.

Jackson, J. Hughlings (1932). *Selected Writings of John Hughlings Jackson*, J. Taylor (ed.). London: Hodder and Stoughton.

James, W. (1890). *The Principles of Psychology, Vol. 2.* New York: Holt.

Jasper, H. H. (1949). Diffuse projection systems: the intergrative action of the thalamic reticular system. *Electroencephalogr. Clin. Neurophysiol.* 1:405–419.

Jefferson, G. (1958). Substrates for intergrative patterns in the reticular core. In *Reticular Formation*, M. N. E. Scheibel and A. B. Scheibel (eds.). Boston: Little, Brown.

Jouvet, M. (1977). Neuropharmacology of the sleep waking cycle. In *Handbook of Psychopharmacology*, L. L. Iverson, S. D. Iverson, and S. H. Snyder (eds.). New York: Plenum Press, pp. 233–293.

Kahneman, D. (1973). *Eye Movement Attention and Effort.* Englewood Cliffs, NJ: Prentice-Hall.

Kaplan, R. F., Verfaellie, M., DeWitt, D., and Caplan, L. R. (1990). Effects of changes in stimulus contingency on visual extinction. *Neurology* 40:1299–1301.

Kanai, T., and Szerb, J. C. (1965). Mesencephalic reticular activating system and cortical acetylcholine output. *Nature* 205:80–82.

Karnath, H. O. (1995). Transcutaneous electrical stimulation and vibration of neck muscles in neglect. *Exp. Brain. Res.* 105:321–324.

Kartsounis, L. D., and Warrington, E. K. (1989). Unilateral visual neglect overcome by ones implicit in stimulus arrays. *J. Neurol. Neurosurg. Psychiatry* 52:1253–1259.

Kennard, M. A., and Ectors, L. (1938). Forced circling movements in monkeys following lesions of the frontal lobes. *J. Neurophysiol.* 1:45–54.

Kertesz, A., Nicholson, I., Cancelliere, A., Kassa, K., and Black, S. E. (1985). Motor impersistance: a right-hemisphere syndrome. *Neurology* 35:662–666.

Kievet, J., and Kuypers, H. G. J. M. (1977). Organization of the thalamo-cortical connections to the frontal lobe in the rhesus monkey. *Exp. Brain Res.* 29:299–322.

Kim, M., Na, D. L., Kim, G. M., Adair, J. C., Lee, K. H., and Heilman K. M. (1999). Ipsilesional neglect: behavioural and anatomical features. *J. Neurol. Neurosurg. Psychiatry* 67:35–38.

Kimura, D. (1967). Function asymmetry of the brain in dichotic listening. *Cortex* 3:163–178.

Kinomura, S., Larsson, J., Gulyas, B., and Roland, P. E. (1996). Activation by attention of the human reticular formation and thalamic intralaminar nuclei. *Science* 271(5248):512–515.

Kinsbourne, M. (1970). A model for the mechanism of unilateral neglect of space. *Trans. Am. Neurol. Assoc.* 95:143.

Kinsbourne, M. (1974). Direction of gaze and distribution of cerebral thought processes. *Neuropsychologia* 12:270–281.

Kooistra, C. A., and Heilman, K. M. (1989). Hemispatial visual inattention masquerading as hemianopsia. *Neurology* 39:1125–1127.

Kozlowski, M. R., and Marshall, J. F. (1981). Plasticity of neostriatal metabolic activity and behavioral recovery from nigrostriatal injury. *Exp. Neurol.* 74:313–323.

Kunkel, A., Kopp, B., Muller, G., Villringer, K., Villringer, A., Taub, E., and Flor, H. (1999). Constraint-induced movement therapy for motor recovery in chronic stroke patients. *Arch. Phys. Med. Rehabil.* 80:624–628.

Kuypers, H. G. J. M., and Lawrence, D. G. (1967). Cortical projections to the red nucleus and the brain stem in the rhesus monkey. *Brain Res.* 4:151–188.

Kwon, S. E., and Heilman, K. M. (1991). Ipsilateral neglect in patient following a unilateral frontal lesion. *Neurology* 41:2001–2004.

Ladavas, E. (1987). Is the hemispatial deficit produced by right parietal damage associated with retinal or gravitational coordinates. *Brain* 110:167–180.

Ladavas, E., Petronio, A., and Umicta, C. (1990). The deployment of visual attention in the intact field of hemineglect patients. *Cortex* 26:307–312.

Lansing, R. W., Schwartz, E., and Lindsley, D. B. (1959). Reaction time and EEG activation under alerted and nonalerted conditions. *J. Exp. Psychol.* 58:1–7.

Lindvall, O., Bjorklund, A., Morre, R. Y., and

Stenevi, U. (1974). Mesencephalic dopamine-neurons projecting to the neocortex. *Brain Res.* 81:325–331.

Ljungberg, T., and Ungerstedt, U. (1976). Sensory inattention produced by 6-hydroxydopamine-induced degeneration of ascending dopamine neurons in the brain. *Exp. Neurol.* 53:585–600.

Loeb, J. (1885). Die elementaren Störungen einfacher Functionen nach oberflächlicher umschriebener Verletzung des Grosshirns. *Pfluger's Arch. Physiol.* 37:51–56.

Lynch, J. C. (1980). The functional organization of posterior parietal association cortex. *Behav. Brain Sci.* 3:485–534.

Mark V. W., and Heilman, K. M. (1990). Bodily neglect and orientational biases in unilateral neglect syndrome and normal subjects. *Neurology* 40:640–643.

Mark, V. W., and Heilman, K. M. (1998). Diagonal spatial neglect. *J. Neurol. Neurosurg. Psychiatry* 65:348–352.

Mark, V. W., Kooistra, C. A., and Heilman, K. M. (1988). Hemispatial neglect affected by non-neglected stimuli. *Neurology* 38:1207–1211.

Marshall, J. F. (1979). Somatosensory inattention after dopamine-depleting intracerebral 6-OHDA injections: spontaneous recovery and pharmacological control. *Brain Res.* 177:311–324.

Marshall, J. F. (1982). Neurochemistry of attention and attentional disorders. Annual course 214, Behavioral Neurology. Presented at the American Academy of Neurology, April 27, 1982.

Marshall, J. F., Richardson, J. S., and Teitelbaum, P. (1974). Nigrostriatal bundle damage and the lateral hypothalamic damage. *J. Comp. Physiol Psychol.* 87:808–830.

Marshall, J. F., Turner, B. H., and Teitelbaum, P. (1971). Sensory neglect produced by lateral hypothalamic damage. *Science* 174:523–525.

Mattingley, J. B., Bradshaw, J. L., and Phillips, J. G. (1992). Impairments of movement initiation and execution in unilateral neglect. Directional hypokinesia and bradykinesia. *Brain* 115(Pt 6): 1849–1874.

Mattingley, J. B., Husain, M., Rorden, C., Kennard, C., Driver, J. (1998). Motor role of human inferior parietal lobe revealed in unilateral neglect patients. *Nature* 392(6672):179–182.

McCormick, D. A. (1989). Cholinergic and noradrenergic modulation of thalamocortical processing. *Trends Neurol.* 12:215–221.

McFie, J., Piercy, M. F., and Zangwell, O. L. (1950). Visual spatial agnosia associated with lesions of the right hemisphere. *Brain* 73:167–190.

Meador, K., Hammond, E. J., Loring, D. W., Allen,

M., Bowers, D., and Heilman, K. M. (1987). Cognitive evoked potentials and disorders of recent memory. *Neurology* 37:526–529.

Meador, K., Loring, D. W., Lee, G. P., Brooks, B. S., Thompson, W. O., and Heilman, K. M. (1988). Right cerebral specialization for tactile attention as evidenced by intracarotid sodium amytal. *Neurology* 38:1763–1766.

Meador, K., Loring, D. W., Lee, G. P., Brooks, B. S., Nichols, T. T., Thompson, E. E., Thompson, W. O., and Heilman, K. M. (1989). Hemisphere asymmetry for eye gaze mechanism. *Brain* 112:103–111.

Meador, K., Watson, R. T., Bowers, D., and Heilman, K. M., (1986). Hypometria with hemispatial and limb motor neglect. *Brain* 109:293–305.

Mehler, W. R. (1966). Further notes of the center median nucleus of Luys. In *The Thalamus*, D. P. Purpura, and M. D. Yahr (eds.). New York: Columbia University Press, pp. 109–122.

Mendez, M. F., Cherrier, M. M., and Cymerman, J. S. (1997). Hemispatial neglect on visual search tasks in Alzheimer's disease. *Neuropsychiatry Nueropsychol. Behav. Neurol.* 10:203–208.

Mennemeier, M. S., Chatterjee, A., Watson, R. T., Wertman, E., Carter, L. P., and Heilman, K. M. (1994). Contributions of the parietal frontal lobes to sustained attention and habituation. *Neuropsychologia* 32:703–716.

Mesulam, M. M. (1981). A cortical network for directed attention and unilateral neglect. *Ann. Neurol.* 10:309–325.

Mesulam, M., Van Hesen, G. W., Pandya, D. N., and Geschwind, N. (1977). Limbic and sensory connections of the inferior parietal lobule (area PG) in the rhesus monkey: a study with a new method for horseradish perosidase histochemistry. *Brain Res.* 136:393–414.

Meyer, E., Ferguson, S. S. G., Zarorre, R. J., Alivisatos, B., Marrett, S., Evans, A. C., and Hakim, A. M. (1991). Attention modulates somatosensory cerebral blood flow response to vibrotactile stimulation as measured by positron emission tomography. *Ann. Neurol.* 29:440–443.

Mills, R. P., and Swanson, P. D. (1978). Vertical oculomotor apraxia and memory loss. *Ann. Neurol.* 4:149–153.

Milner, B., Taylor, L., and Sperry, R. W. (1968). Lateralized suppression of dichotically presented digits after commissural section in man. *Science* 161:184–186.

Moruzzi, G., and Magoun, H. W. (1949). Brainstem reticular formation and activation of the EEG. *Electroencephalogr. Clin. Neurophysiol.* 1:455–473.

Motter, B. C., and Mountcastle, V. B. (1981). The functional properties of the light sensitive neurons of the posterior parietal cortex studied in waking monkeys: foveal sparing and opponent vector organization. *J. Neurosci.* 1:3–26.

Mountcastle, V. B., Anderson, R. A., and Motter, B. C. (1981). The influence of attentive fixation upon the excitability of the light sensitive neurons of the posterior parietal cortex. *J. Neurosci.* 1:1218–1245.

Mountcastle, V. B., Lynch, J. C., Georgopoulos, A., Sakata, H., and Acuna, C. (1975). Posterior parietal association cortex of the monkey: command function from operations within extrapersonal space. *J. Neurophysiol.* 38:871–908.

Na, D. L., Adair, J. C., Kim, G. M., Seo, D. W., Hong, S. B., and Heilman, K. M. (1998a). Ipsilateral neglect during intracarotid amobarbital test. *Neurology* 51:276–279.

Na, D. L., Adair, J. C., Williamson, D. J., Schwartz, R. L., Haws, B., and Heilman, K. M. (1998b). Dissociation of sensory–attentional from motor–intentional neglect. *J. Neurol. Neurosurg. Psychiatry* 64:331–338.

Nadeau, S. E., and Heilman, K. M. (1991). Gaze-dependent hemianopia without hemispatial neglect. *Neurology* 41:1244–1250.

Nathan, P. W. (1946). On simultaneous bilateral stimulation of the body in a lesion of the parietal lobe. *Brain* 69:325–334.

Neve, K. A., Kozlowski, M. R., and Marshall, J. F. (1982). Plasticity of neostriatal dopamine receptors after nigrostriatal injury: relationship to recovery of sensorimotor functions and behavioral supersensitivity. *Brain Res.* 244:33–44.

Nieoullon, A., Cheramy, A., and Glowinski, J. (1978). Release of dopamine evoked by electrical stimulation of the motor and visual areas of the cerebral cortex in both caudate nuclei and in the substantia nigra in the cat. *Brain Res.* 15:69–83.

Obersteiner, H. (1882). On allochiria—a peculiar sensory disorder. *Brain* 4:153–163.

Olds, J., and Milner, P. (1954). Positive reinforcement produced by electrical stimulation of septal area and other regions of the rat brain. *J. Comp. Physiol. Psychol.* 47:419–427.

Oppenheim, H. (1885). Ueber eine durch eine klinisch bisher nicht verwertete Untersuchungsmethode ermittelte Form der Sensibitatsstorung bei einseitigen Erkrankunger des Grosshirns. *Neurol. Zentrabl.* 4:529–533. Cited by A. L. Benton (1956). Jacques Loeb and the method of double stimulation. *J. Hist. Med. Allied Sci.* 11:47–53.

Pandya, D. M., and Kuypers, H. G. J. M. (1969). Cortico-cortical connections in the rhesus monkey. *Brain Res.* 13:13–36.

Pardo, J. V., Fox, P. T., and Raichle, M. E. (1991). Localization of a human system for sustained attention by positron emission tomography. *Nature* 349:61–64.

Paterson, A., and Zangwill, O. L. (1944). Disorders of visual space perception associated with lesions of the right cerebral hemisphere. *Brain* 67:331–358.

Pibram, K. H., and McGuiness, D. (1975). Arousal, activation and effort in the control of attention. *Psychol. Rev.* 182:116–149.

Pizzamiglio, L., Frasca, R., Guariglia, C., Incoccia, C., and Antonucci, G. (1990). Effect of optokinetic stimulation in patients with visual neglect. *Cortex* 26:535–540.

Posner, M. I., and Rafal, R. D. (1987). Cognitive theories of attention and rehabilitation of attentional deficits. In *Neuropsychological Rehabilitation*, M. J. Mier, A. L. Benton, and L. Diller (eds.). Guilford, New York

Posner, M. I., Walker, J., Friedrich, F. J., and Rafal, R. D. (1984). Effects of parietal lobe injury on covert orienting of visual attention. *J. Neurosci.* 4:163–187.

Poppelreuter, W. L. (1917). *Die psychischen Schadigungen durch Kopfschuss im Krieg 1914–1916: Die Storungen der niederen und hoheren Leistungen durch Verletzungen des Oksipitalhirns.* Vol. 1. Leipzig: Leopold Voss. Referred to by M. Critchley (1949). *Brain* 72:540.

Purpura, D. P. (1970). Operations and processes in thalamic and synaptically related neural subsystemes. In *The Neurosciences, Second Study Program.* F. O. Schmidt (ed.). New York: Rockefeller University Press, pp. 458–470.

Pycock, C. J. (1980). Turning behavior in animals. *Neuroscience* 5:461–514.

Rapcsak, S. Z., Cimino, C. R., and Heilman, K. M. (1988). Altitudinal neglect. *Neurology* 38:277–281.

Rapcsak, S. Z., Fleet, W. S., Verfaellie, M., and Heilman, K. M. (1989). Selective attention in hemispatial neglect. *Arch. Neurol.* 46:178–182.

Rapcsak, S. Z., Watson, R. T., and Heilman, K. M. (1987). Hemispace-visual field interactions in visual extinction. *J. Neurol. Neurosurg. Psychiatry* 50:1117–1124.

Redgrave, P., Prescott, T. J., and Gurney, K. (1999). Is the short-latency dopamine response too short to signal reward error? *Trends Neurosci.* 22:146–151.

Reeves, A. G., and Hagamen, W. D. (1971). Behavioral and EEG asymmetry following unilateral lesions of the forebrain and midbrain of cats. *Electroencephalogr. Clin. Neurophysiol.* 39:83–86.

Reider, N. (1946). Phenomena of sensory suppression. *Arch. Neurol. Psychiatry* 55:583–590.

Riddoch, G. (1935). Visual disorientation in homonymous half-fields. *Brain* 58:376–382.

Riddoch, M. J., and Humphreys, G. (1983). The effect of cuing on unilateral neglect. *Neuropsychologia* 21:589–599.

Robertson, I. H., Halligan, P. W., Bergego, C., Homberg, V., Pizzamiglio, L. Weber, E., and Wilson, B.A. (1994). Right neglect following right hemisphere damage? *Cortex* 30:199–213.

Robertson, I. H., and North, N. T. (1994). One hand is better than two: motor extinction of left hand advantage in unilateral neglect. *Neuropsychologia* 32:1–11.

Robinson, D. L., Goldberg, M. E., and Stanton, G. B. (1978). Parietal association cortex in the primate sensory mechanisms and behavioral modulations. *J. Neurophysiol* 41:910–932.

Robinson, T. E., Vanderwolf, C. H., Pappas, B. A. (1977). Are dorsal noradrenergic bundle projections from locus coerulus important for neocortical or hippocampal activation? *Brain Res.* 138:75–98.

Rode, G., Charles, N., Perenin, M. T., Vighetto, A., Trillet, M., and Aimard, G. (1992). Partial remission of hemiplegia and somatoparaphrenia through vestibular stimulation in a case of unilateral neglect. *Cortex* 28:203–208.

Roeltgen, M. G., Roeltgen, D. P., and Heilman, K. M. (1989). Unilateral motor impersistence and hemispatial neglect from a striatal lesion. *Neuropsychiatry Neuropsychol. Behav. Neurol.* 2:125–135.

Ross, E. D., and Stewart, R. M. (1981). Akinetic mutism from hypothalamic damage: successful treatment with dopamine agonists. *Neurology* 31:1435–1439.

Rossetti, Y., Rode, G., Pisella, L., Farne, A., Ling, L., Boisson, D., and Perenin, M. (1998) Prism adaptation to a rightward optical deviation rehabilitates left hemispatial neglect. *Nature* 395:166–169.

Rossi, P. W., Kheyfets, S., and Reding, M. J. (1990). Fresnel prisms improve visual perception in stroke patients with homonymous hemianopia unilateral visual neglect. *Neurology* 40:1597–1599.

Rubens, A. B. (1985). Caloric stimulation and unilateral visual neglect. *Neurology* 35:1019–1024.

Samuels, I., Butters, N., and Goodglass, H. (1971).

Visual memory defects following cortical limbic lesions: effect of field of presentation. *Physiol. Behav.* 6:447–452.

Sato, H., Hata, Y., Hagihara, K., and Tsumoto, T. (1987). Effects of cholinergic depletion on neuron activities in the cat visual cortex. *J. Neurophysiol.* 58:781–794.

Scheibel, M. E., and Scheibel, A. B. (1966). The organization of the nucleus reticularis thalami: a Golgi study. *Brain Res.* 1:43–62.

Scheibel, M. E., and Scheibel, A. B. (1967). Structural organization of nonspecific thalamic nuclei and their projection toward cortex. *Brain* 6:60–94.

Schlag-Rey, M., and Schlag, J. (1980). Eye movement neurons in the thalamus of monkey. *Invest. Ophthalmol. Vis. Sci.* ARVO supplement, 176.

Schneider, J. S., McLaughlin, W. W., and Roeltgen, D. P. (1992). Motor and nonmotor behavioral deficits in monkeys made hemiparkinsonian by intracarotid MPTP infusion. *Neurology* 42:1565–1572.

Schrandt, N. J., Tranel, D., and Domasio, H. (1989). The effects of total cerebral lesions on skin conductance response to signal stimuli. *Neurology* 39 (Suppl. 1):223.

Schultz, W. (1998). Predictive reward signal of dopamine neurons. *J. Neurophysiology* 80:1–27.

Schultz, W., Tremblay, L., and Hollerman, J. R. (2000). Reward processing in primate orbitofrontal cortex and basal ganglia. *Cereb. Cortex* 10:272–284.

Schwartz, A. S., Marchok, P. L., Kreinick, C. J., and Flynn, R. E. (1979). The asymmetric lateralization of tactile extinction in patients with unilateral cerebral dysfunction. *Brain* 102:669–684.

Segundo, J. P., Naguet, R., and Buser, P. (1955). Effects of cortical stimulation on electrocortial activity in monkeys. *Neurophysiology* 1B:236–245.

Sevush, S., and Heilman, K. M. (1981). Attentional factors in tactile extinction. Presented at a meeting of the International Neuropsychological Society, Atlanta, Georgia.

Shelton, P. A., Bowers, D., and Heilman, K. M. (1990). Peripersonal and vertical neglect. *Brain* 113:191–205.

Shuren, J., Hartley, T., and Heilman, K. M. (1998). The effects of rotation on spatial attention. *Neuropsychiatry Neuropsychol. Behav. Neurol.* 11:72–75.

Shute, C. C. D., and Lewis, P. R. (1967). The ascending cholinergic reticular system, neocortical olfactory and subcortical projections. *Brain* 90:497–520.

Singer, W. (1977). Control of thalamic transmission

by corticofugal and ascending reticular pathways in the visual system. *Physiol. Rev.* 57:386–420.

Skinner, J. E., and Yingling, C. D. (1976). Regulation of slow potential shifts in nucleus reticularis thalami by the mesencephalic reticular formation and the frontal granular cortex. *Electroencephalogr. Clin. Neurophysiol.* 40:288–296.

Skinner, J. E., and Yingling, C. D. (1977). Central gating mechanisms that regulate event-related potentials and behavior—a neural model for attention. In *Progress in Clinical Neurophysiology, Vol. 1,* J. E. Desmedt (ed.). New York: S. Karger, pp. 30–69.

Sokolov, Y. N. (1963). *Perception and the Conditioned Reflex.* Oxford: Pergmon Press.

Sparks, R., and Geschwind N. (1968). Dichotic listening in man after section of the neocortical commissures. *Cortex* 4:3–16.

Sprague, J. M. (1966). Interaction of cortex and superior colliculus in mediation of visually guided behavior in the cat. *Science* 153:1544–1547.

Sprague, J. M., Chambers, W. W., and Stellar, E. (1961). Attentive, affective and adaptive behavior in the cat. *Science* 133:165–173.

Sprague, J. M., and Meikle, T. H. (1965). The role of the superior colliculus in visually guided behavior. *Exp. Neurol.* 11:115–146.

Staines R. T., McIlroy W. E., Graham S. J., Gladstone D. J. and Black S. E. (2000) Somatosensory extinction of simultaneous stimuli is associated with decreased activation of somatosensory cortices. *Neurology* 54(Suppl. 3):A104.

Stelmack, R. M., Plouffe, L. M., and Winogron, H. W. (1983). Recognition memory and the orienting response. An analysis of the encoding of pictures and words. *Biol. Psychol.* 16:49–63.

Steriade, M., and Glenn, L. (1982). Neocortical and caudate projections of intralaminar thalamic neurons and their synaptic excitation from the midbrain reticular core. *J. Neurophysiol.* 48:352–370.

Tegner, R., and Levander, M. (1991). Through a looking glass. A new technique to demonstrate direction hypokinesia in unilateral neglect. *Brain* 114(Pt 4):1943–1951.

Teitelbaum, P., and Epstein, A. N. (1962). The lateral hypothalamic syndrome: recovery of feeding and drinking after lateral hypothalamic lesions. *Psychol. Rev.* 69:74–90.

Truex, R. C., and Carpenter, M. B. (1964). *Human Neuroanatomy.* Baltimore: Williams and Wilkins.

Ungerstedt, U. (1971a). Striatal dopamine release after amphetamine or nerve degeneration revealed by rotational behavior. *Acta Physiol. Scand. Suppl.* 82:49–68.

Ungerstedt, U. (1971b). Post-synaptic supersensitivity of 6-hydroxydopamine induced degeneration of the nigro-striatal dopamine system in the rat brain. *Acta. Physiol. Scand. Suppl.* 82:69–93.

Ungerstedt. U. (1974). Brain dopamine neurons and behavior. In *Neurosciences, Vol. 3,* F. O. Schmidt and F. G. Woren (eds.). Cambridge, MA: MIT Press, pp. 695–703.

Valenstein, E., and Heilman, K. M. (1978). Apraxic agraphia with neglect induced paragraphia. *Arch. Neurol.* 38:506–508.

Valenstein, E., and Heilman, K. M. (1981). Unilateral hypokinesia and motor extinction. *Neurology* 31:445–448.

Valenstein, E., Van den Abell, T., Tankle, R., and Heilman, K. M. (1980). Apomorphine-induced turning after recovery from neglect induced by cortical lesions. *Neurology* 30:358.

Valenstein, E., Van den Abell, T., Watson, R. T., and Heilman, K. M. (1982). Nonsensory neglect from parietotemporal lesions in monkeys. *Neurology* 32:1198–1201.

Valenstein, E., Watson, R. T., Van den Abell, T., Carter, R., and Heilman, K. M. (1987). Response time in monkeys with unilateral neglect. *Arch. Neurol.* 44:517–520.

Vallar, G., Papagno, C., Rusconi, M. L., and Bisiach, E. (1995). Vestibular stimulation, spatial hemineglect and dysphasia, selective effects. *Cortex* 31:589–593.

Vallar, G., Rusconi, M. L., Bignamini, L., Geminiani, G., and Perani, D. (1994). Anatomical correlates of visual and tactile extinction in humans: a clinical CT scan study. *J. Neurol. Neurosurg. Psychiatry* 57:464–470.

Vallar, G., Sterzi, R., Bottini, G., Cappa, S., and Rusconi, L. (1990). Temporary remission of left hemianesthesia after vestibular stimulation: a sensory neglect phenomenon. *Cortex* 26:123–131.

Vanderwolf, C. H., and Robinson, T. E. (1981). Reticulo-cortical activity and behavior: a critique of arousal theory and new synthesis. *Behav. Brain Sci.* 4:459–514.

Vargo, J. M., Lai, H. V., and Marshall, J. F. (1998). Light deprivation accelerates recovery from frontal cortical neglect: relation to locomotion and striatal Fos expression. *Behav. Neurosci.* 112:387–398.

Vargo, J. M., Richard-Smith, M., and Corwin, J. V. (1989). Spiroperidol reinstates asymmetries in neglect in rats recovered from left or right dorsomedial prefrontal cortex lesions. *Behav. Neurosci.* 103:1017–1027.

Velasco, F., and Velasco, M. (1979). A reticulothalamic system mediating proprioceptive attention and tremor in man. *Neurosurgery* 4:30–36.

Venneri, A., Pentore, R., Cotticelli, B., and Della Sala, S. (1998). Unilateral spatial neglect in the late stages of Alzheimer's disease. *Cortex* 34:743–752.

Vogt, B. A., Rosene, D. L., and Pandya, D. N. (1979). Thalamic and cortical afferents differentiate anterior from posterior cingulate cortex in the monkey. *Science* 204:205–207.

Volpe, B. T., Ledoux, J. E., Gazzaniga, M. S. (1979). Information processing of visual stimuli in an "extinguished" field. *Nature* 282:722–724.

Vuilleumier, P., Valenza, N., Mayer, E., Reverdin, A., and Landis, T. (1998). Near and far visual space in unilateral neglect. *Ann. Neurol.* 43: 406–410.

Wagman, I. H., and Mehler, W. R. (1972). Physiology and anatomy of the cortico-oculomotor mechanism. *Prog. Brain Res.* 37:619–635.

Wallace, S. F., Rosenquist, A. C., and Sprague, J. M. (1989). Recovery from cortical blindness mediated by destruction of nontectotectal fibers in the commissure of the superior colliculus in the cat. *J. Comp. Neurol.* 284:429–450.

Wallace, S. F., Rosenquist, A. C., and Sprague, J. M. (1990) Ibotenic acid lesions of the lateral substantia nigra restore visual orientation behavior in the hemianopic cat. *J. Comp. Neurol.* 296:222–252.

Walter, W. G., (1973). Human frontal lobe function in sensory-motor association. In *Psychophysiology of the Frontal Lobes*, K. H. Pribram and A. R. Luria (eds.). New York: Academic Press, pp. 109–122.

Watson, R. T., Andriola, M., and Heilman, K. M. (1977a). The EEG in neglect. *J. Neurol. Sci. 34:* 343–348.

Watson, R. T., and Heilman, K. M. (1979). Thalamic neglect. *Neurology* 29:690–694.

Watson, R. T., Heilman, K. M., Cauthen, J. C., and King, F. A. (1973). Neglect after cingulectomy. *Neurology* 23:1003–1007.

Watson, R. T., Heilman, K. M., Miller, B. D., and King, F. A. (1974). Neglect after mesencephalic reticular formation lesions. *Neurology* 24:294–298.

Watson, R. T., Miller, B. D., and Heilman, K. M. (1977b). Evoked potential in neglect. *Arch. Neurol.* 34:224–227.

Watson, R. T., Miller, B. D., and Heilman, K. M. (1978). Nonsensory neglect. *Ann. Neurol.* 3:505–508.

Watson, R. T., Valenstein, E., and Heilman, K. M. (1981). Thalamic neglect: the possible role of the medial thalamus and nucleus reticularis thalami in behavior. *Arch. Neurol.* 38:501–507.

Watson, R. T., Valenstein, E., Day, A. L., and Heilman, K. M. (1984). The effects of corpus callosum section on unilateral neglect in monkeys. *Neurology 34:*812–815.

Watson, R. T., Valenstein, E., Day, A., and Heilman, K. M. (1994). Posterior neocortical systems subserving awareness and neglect: neglect after superior temporal sucus but not area 7 lesions. *Arch Neurol 51:*1014–1021.

Weinberger, N. M., Velasco, M., and Lindsley, D. B. (1965). Effects of lesions upon thalamically induced electrocortical desynchronization and recruiting. *Electroencephalogr. Clin. Neurophysiol. 18:*369–377.

Weinstein, E. A., and Kahn, R. L. (1955). *Denial of Illness. Symbolic and Physiological Aspects.* Springfield, IL: C. C. Thomas.

Weintraub, S., and Mesulam, M. M. (1987). Right cerebral dominance in spatial attention: further evidence based on ipsilateral neglect. *Arch. Neurol. 44:*621–625.

Welch, K., and Stuteville, P. (1958). Experimental production of neglect in monkeys. *Brain 81:*341–347.

Whittington, D. A., and Hepp-Reymond, M. C. (1977). Eye and head movements to auditory targets. *Neurosci. Abstr. 3:*158

Whishaw, I. Q., Robinson, T. E., Schallert, T., De Ryck, M., Ramirez, U. D. (1978). Electrical activity of the hippocampus and neocortex in rats depleted of brain dopamine and norepinephrine: relations to behavior and effects of atropine. *Exp. Neurol. 62:*748–767.

Williams, S. M., and Goldman-Rakic, P. S. (1998) Widespread origin of the primate mesofrontal dopamine system. *Cereb. Cortex 8:*321–245.

Yingling, C. D., and Skinner, J. E. (1975). Regulation of unit activity in nucleus reticularis thalami by the mesencephalic reticular formation and the frontal granular cortex. *Electroencephalogr. Clin. Neurophysiol. 39:*635–642.

Yingling, C. D., and Skinner, J. E. (1977). Gating of thalamic input to cerebral cortex by nucleus reticularis thalami. In *Progress in Clinical Neurophysiology, Vol. 1*, J. E. Desmedt (ed.). New York: S. Karger, pp. 70–96.

Yokoyama, K. Jennings, R., Ackles, P., Hood, P., and Boller, F. (1987). Lack of heart rate changes during an attention demanding task after right hemisphere lesions. *Neurology 37:*624–630.

14

The Callosal Syndromes

ERAN ZAIDEL, MARCO IACOBONI, DAHLIA W. ZAIDEL,
AND JOSEPH E. BOGEN

The collections of nerve fibers that directly connect one cerebral hemisphere with the other, called the "cerebral commissures," include the corpus callosum, the anterior commissure, and the hippocampal commissures. Of these, the corpus callosum (CC) is by far the largest, with at least 200 million fibers. The 2×10^8 estimate of Tomasch (1954) was based on light microscopy of a few cases. According to Innocenti (personal communication, 1991) measurement by electron microscopy will at least triple the previous estimate (see also Clarke et al., 1989). Aboitiz et al. (1992) conducted a comprehensive analysis of the human CC with light microscopy and a limited analysis with electron microscopy and estimated the total number of fibers in the human CC to be over 200 million.

The posterior and the habenular commissures as well as other commissures of the spinal cord and brainstem are not included among the cerebral commissures.

TERMINOLOGY

Surgical section of all of the cerebral commissures is called "commissurotomy," whereas that of the corpus callosum alone is called "callosotomy." It is now common to use the term "split brain" to refer to cases of callosotomy as well as complete commissurotomy, since both groups of patients manifest most of the same signs and symptoms. The Los Angeles split-brain patients (Bogen and Vogel, 1962, 1975; Bogen et al., 1965, 1988) had complete cerebral commissurotomy (including the anterior commissure, dorsal and ventral hippocampal commissures and, in some cases, the massa intermedia). In the experimental animal, split-brain preparations often include section of all of the cerebral commissures plus the optic chiasm; this makes it possible to restrict visual information to one hemisphere merely by covering one eye. In the human with an intact chiasm, restriction of visual input to one hemisphere requires restriction of the visual stimuli to one or the other visual hemifield.

ETIOLOGY

Surgical section of all or part of the corpus callosum, with or without section of the other cerebral commissures, has been used for treatment of medically intractable, multifocal epilepsy (Reeves, 1984; Spencer et al., 1987). Some seizure disorders respond well to section of only the anterior half or anterior two-thirds of the callosum (the "partial split-brain"). Surgeons may also gain access to deep hemisphere lesions by sectioning a portion of the corpus callosum. Examples are genu section for anterior communicating aneurysm clipping, trunk sections for access to the third ventricle and environs, and splenial section for approaching the pineal region.

Lesions of the corpus callosum also occur naturally. Ischemic strokes affecting the territory of the anterior cerebral artery can destroy the anterior 4/5 of the CC (Foix and Hillemand, 1925; Critchley, 1930; Ethelberg, 1951), and posterior cerebral artery strokes can affect the posterior 1/5 (splenium). Tumors (usually gliomas) can occur anywhere in the callosum, the best studied being tumors of the genu or of the splenium. Multiple sclerosis can cause disconnection signs. Head trauma has also been associated with callosal injury. Toxic and/or infectious lesions of the callosum occasionally occur. From time to time an anterior cerebral artery aneurysm rupture results in hemorrhagic dissection of the CC or spasm with infarction of the CC. These naturally occurring lesions usually result in fractions of the complete callosotomy syndrome that improve over time. Familiarity with the complete syndrome makes identification of the partial varieties easier. Congenital absence of the CC (callosal agenesis) has been intensively studied; it is for the most part not accompanied by disconnection signs, a perplexity that remains elusive to date.

Callosal lesions are often accompanied by damage to neighboring structures. As a result, neighborhood signs may overshadow signs of callosal disconnection. Although any sign after cortical damage (in a region giving rise to callosal fibers) could be suspected of being partially callosal in origin, small lesions of the callosum rarely can be reliably correlated with any behavioral deficit.

HISTORICAL BACKGROUND

THE HUMORAL ANATOMISTS

By "humoral anatomists" we mean those writers of antiquity whose concepts of brain function emphasized the contents of the brain cavities and the flow of various fluids such as air, phlegm, cerebrospinal fluid (CSF), blood, etc. For them, the CC seemed largely a supporting structure. Even that original Renaissance genius, Vesalius, believed that the CC served mainly as a mechanical support, maintaining the integrity of the various cavities.

THE TRAFFIC ANATOMISTS

The "traffic anatomists" took a major step forward toward our understanding of brain function. As indicated by Joynt (1974), it was at about the time of Willis (1664) that anatomists began thinking more in terms of a traffic or communication between the more solid parts of the brain. This view became quite explicit in the statement of Viq d'Azyr, who wrote in 1784: "It seems to me that the commissures are intended to establish sympathetic communications between different parts of the brain, just as the nerves do between different organs and the brain itself" (Clarke and O'Malley, 1968, p. 592).

THE CLASSICAL NEUROLOGISTS

In the closing decades of the nineteenth century (or more broadly construed, in the period between the American Civil War and the First World War), there emerged a group of neurologists whose discoveries and formulations are still the core of current clinical knowledge; many issues debated among themselves remain live issues today. Among these investigators were several, including Wernicke, Liepmann, Dejerine, and Goldstein, who interpreted various neurological symptoms as resulting from disconnection, including interruption of information flow through the CC.

The concept of callosal apraxia was developed by Liepmann and Maas (1907), who described a right-hander whose callosal lesion caused a left limb apraxia as well as a left-hand agraphia in the absence of aphasia. These disabilities have subsequently been observed many times. Unilateral apraxia and unilateral agraphia are not always present, and they may subside as a stroke victim progressively recovers, but they remain prominent signs of hemisphere disconnection. Liepmann's callosal concept is now hardly doubted. But this was not always the case.

THE CRITICS

Even during the time of Liepmann, there were critics and doubters of his theories who became progressively more influential in the ensuing decades. In an extensive review, Ironside and Guttmacher (1929) concluded: "Taking into account the completeness of the case records, our series of tumor cases would lead us to believe that apraxia is not a common symptom of tumors of the CC. . . . The symptoms in CC tumors are largely of the 'neighborhood' type and arise from involvement of, or pressure on, adjacent structures by the growth" (p. 454).

In addition to the criticism of hemisphere disconnection as a cause of symptoms, the situation was clouded by certain distractions that we shall consider briefly before returning to the central theme of disconnection.

Mental Symptoms

These distractions arose as the result of attempts to correlate lesions, especially tumors of the CC, with mental symptoms. Most of the symptoms attributed to the corpus callosum were neighborhood signs, relating principally to deficits that we now recognize as resulting from frontal lobe damage (Botez, 1974; Barbizet et al., 1977; Damasio, 1985; Stuss and Benson, 1986; Fuster, 1989; Levin et al., 1991). For example, a mental callosal syndrome was formulated by Raymond et al. (1906) and their views were widely accepted for many years. They observed a certain loss of connectedness of ideas but no delirium, a difficulty with recent memory, a "bizarreness" of manner, and a lability of mood.

Alpers (1936) redescribed the callosal syndrome, emphasizing "imperviousness," or a certain indifference to stimuli as if the threshold were elevated; difficulties in concentration; and a lack of elaboration of thought. After reviewing the relevant literature, and on the basis of personal cases, Brihaye (in Bremer et al., 1956) agreed with the observation of Le Beau (1943) that "[t]here is a certain apathy, that is

to say, a clouding without somnolence which is possibly very specific."[1] We are now inclined to attribute this symptom not to involvement of the genu of the CC (which, to be sure, is involved) but rather to involvement of the medial aspects of the frontal lobes including the anterior cingulate gyri. It is frequently seen in glioblastomas of the anterior corpus callosum, called "butterfly gliomas" because they spread their wings into both frontal lobes. This apathy or imperviousness may be a milder form of akinesia, often approaching a mute immobility, seen in patients with "the subfrontal syndrome" consequent to bleeding from an anterior cerebral artery aneurysm, or with a third ventricle tumor (also see Chapters 13 and 15).

Neighborhood signs have also been noted with posterior callosal lesions, with involvement of the hippocampi. Escourolle et al. (1975) reported that "[a] certain number of our tumors of the splenium [twice as common as genu gliomas] were accompanied by memory dysfunction, whereas the anterior tumors were more often manifested by akinetic states with mutism, probably because of bilateral anterior cingulate involvement" (p. 48; translation ours).

Disconnection Signs Were Not Often Seen with Naturally Occurring Lesions

The eclipse of Liepmann's understanding of the CC was only partly attributable to a clouding of the issue with neighborhood signs: mainly it was from an unwillingness to accept as meaningful such disconnection signs as unilateral apraxia, unilateral agraphia, and hemialexia. The objections raised included the following three points:

1. Callosal lesions are rarely, if ever, isolated, so deficits attributed to such lesions may well result, at least in part, from associated damage. This problem is real enough; the only solution is to obtain a sufficient variety of cases so that one can reasonably attribute to their common anatomic aspects those clinical features that they also have in common.
2. Signs attributable to callosal lesions often subside or disappear altogether. This crit-

icism is correct, especially for younger patients with unimanual dyspraxia and unimanual dysgraphia. But it does not apply to all callosal signs, notably the unilateral anomia and the hemialexia following callosotomy. Even if it did, subsidence does not mean that a sign was without significance, any more than the frequent subsidence of aphasia means that it is not a reliable sign (in right-handers) of a left hemisphere (LH) lesion. Progressive compensation following focal damage is a characteristic feature of the brain.

3. In numerous cases of callosal disease, including toxic degeneration of the CC (Marchiafava-Bignami disease) as well as the far more common cases of callosal tumor or callosal infarction, the expected disconnection signs are not elicited. In the massive revised edition of his neurology text, Gowers (1903) reasonably concluded: "we do not yet know of any symptoms that are the result of the damage to the callosal fibers" (p. 314). However, the definitive (in English) neurology text of S. A. K. Wilson (Wilson and Bruce, 1940) not so reasonably reaffirmed, on the basis of tumor cases, much the same conclusion. Wilson mentioned apraxia as an inconstant symptom, emphasized certain mental symptoms such as lack of spontaneity, and concluded: "In fact, the claim might be advanced that all 'callosal' symptoms are of a neighboring or distant kind" (p. 1235). Wilson's discussion refers to studies by Bristowe, Ransom, Tooth, Guillain, Alpers and Grant, Voriz and Adson, Dyke and Davidoff, and the book by Mingazzini (1922), as well as the article by Ironside and Guttmacher (1929) quoted above in The Critics. He does not refer to Liepmann.

Some of these negative findings can be attributed to inadequate testing. One must perform specific tests to detect signs of callosal disconnection, and, in particular, one must prevent cross-cueing. When patients with malfunction of the CC are appropriately tested, such signs as unilateral anomia and dyspraxia have been found (Geschwind and Kaplan,

1962; Lhermitte et al., 1977; Barbizet et al., 1978).

Callosal Section in Animal Experiments Does Not Produce Significant Deficits

The negative experiments of Zinn (in 1748), Magendie, Muratow, Roussy, Franck, and Pitres; Koranyi, Dotto, and Pusateri; Lo Monaco; and Baldi were all reviewed by Lévy-Valensi (1910), whose own monkey experiments were (to his dismay) also negative, as were the experiments of Lafora and Prados (1923), Hartmann and Trendelenberg (1927), Seletzky and Gilula (1928), and Kennard and Watts (1934) (all cited by Bremer et al., 1956). In retrospect, these negative results can be attributed to a lack of relevant testing. Besides, the more striking signs and symptoms seen in human patients are attributable to hemispheric specialization which is less evident in rats, cats, dogs, or even monkeys (Warren and Nonneman, 1976; Dewson, 1977; Doty and Overman, 1977; Hamilton, 1977, Harnad et al., 1977; Stamm et al., 1977; Denenberg, 1981; Hamilton and Vermeire, 1982, 1988; Overmann and Doty, 1982).

Surgical Section of the Corpus Callosum in Humans Is Often Asymptomatic

Walter Dandy went so far as to say the following in 1936: "The corpus callosum is split longitudinally . . . [and] no symptoms follow its division. This simple experiment at once disposes of the extravagant claims to the functions of the corpus callosum." (p. 40). Even more persuasive was the negative testing by Akelaitis (1944–45) of patients who had had callosal section. These results were acknowledged by Tomasch (1954, 1957), whose interest in the CC and anterior commissure led him to make his widely known estimates of their fiber content. Of the Akelaitis results he wrote: "They showed very clearly and in accordance with some earlier authors like Dandy, Foerster, Meagher and Barre, whose material however was not so extensive, that the corpus callosum is hardly connected with any psychological functions at all." Finally, after an extensive review of the literature, Ethelberg (1951), concluded: "It may be premature to consider the recent clinical, surgical, and experimental observations an obituary of Liepmann's concepts as to the role played by the corpus callosum in the development of 'true' apraxia. But they certainly suggest the need of some hesitance in accepting them" (p. 117).

About the same time, Fessard (1954) summarized the view that was then generally accepted:

[T]here is a great deal of data showing [that] section of important associative white tracts such as the corpus callosum does not seem to affect mental performances. Other similar observations in man or animals are now accumulated in great number and variety. These results are so disturbing that one may be tempted to admit the irrational statement that a heterogeneous system of activities in the nervous system could form a whole in the absence of any identified liaison (pp. 207–208).

Meanwhile, we now realize that most of the negative findings after surgical section of the CC resulted from two sources. As already mentioned, when surgical section of the commissures is incomplete, a remarkable capacity for maintaining cross-communication between the hemispheres may be retained with commissural remnants, particularly when the part remaining is the splenium. Second, negative findings often result from the use of inappropriate or insensitive testing techniques. What one finds depends on what one looks for; whereas Dandy (1936) said that callosal section produces no observable deficits, among his own patients was the one reported by Trescher and Ford to have hemialexia.

THE TWO-BRAIN THEORISTS

In the nineteenth century, the consideration that the cerebrum was a "double brain" was espoused by Wigan (1844), Jackson (1874), and a multitude of others, as described in detail by Harrington (1987). But such ideas, along with Liepmann's callosal concept, fell far out of favor by the end of World War I and remained so for many decades. A distinct reversal of opinion occurred during the 1960s, following publication of the split-brain experiments, and the concept of a "double brain" again became popular (Dimond, 1972).

Current views on callosal function are attributable in large part to studies, under the aegis of R. W. Sperry, of our patients with surgical section of the cerebral commissures. These patients are indeed without, in Dandy's words, "any deficits" in the ordinary social situation, or even as determined by most of a routine neurological examination (Bogen and Vogel, 1975; Botez and Bogen, 1976). In specially devised testing situations, however, they can be shown to have a wide variety of deficits in interhemispheric communication (Gazzaniga, et al., 1962, 1963, 1965, 1967; Sperry and Gazzaniga 1967; Sperry, 1968, 1970, 1974, 1982; Sperry et al., 1969; Gazzaniga, 1970; Zaidel, 1973, 1983; Zaidel et al., 1990; Bogen, 1998).

Animal Experiments

The split-brain humans confirmed in a particularly striking way the importance of commissural fibers for interhemispheric communication. But the essential fact had already been described in animal experiments during the 1950s, initiated by Ronald Myers and Sperry (1953, 1958; Myers, 1956). It was found that each hemisphere of a cat or monkey could learn solutions to a problem different from (even conflicting with) the solutions learned by the other hemisphere. This made it clear that effective functioning could occur independently in the two hemispheres. As Sperry (1961) put it:

Callosum-sectioned cats and monkeys are virtually indistinguishable from their normal cagemates under most tests and training conditions. [But] if one studies such a split-brain monkey more carefully, under special training and testing conditions where the inflow of sensory information to the divided hemispheres can be separately restricted and controlled, one finds that each of the divided hemispheres now has its own independent mental sphere or cognitive system—that is, its own independent perceptual, learning, memory and other mental processes . . . [I]t is as if the animals had two separate brains (p. 1749).

It is important to understand that the duality of minds seen after hemisphere disconnection is not an inference solely from certain striking clinical cases and a handful of surgical patients, as sometimes said. Split-brain experiments have been carried out with many different species by hundreds of investigators around the world. They are virtually unanimous in concluding that each of the disconnected hemispheres can act independently of the other (Bogen, 1977).

The split-brain experiments started with the problem of interocular transfer (Sperry and Clark, 1949). That is, if one learns with one eye how to solve a problem, then with that eye covered and using the other eye, one readily solves the problem without further learning. This is called "interocular transfer of learning." Of course, the learning is not *in* the eye and then transferred to the other eye, but that is the way it is usually described. In this case the question is: how can the learning with one eye appear with use of the other? Experiments showed that the transfer required the CC. Sperry's scheme was to split the optic chiasm so that the right eye goes to the right cerebral hemisphere and the left eye to the LH and also to cut the CC between the two hemispheres. This is a "split-brain cat." The cat can be trained with the right eye to choose a cross rather than a square, while the left eye is covered. The cat chooses one of two doors at the end of a runway, the cross and square being attached to the doors randomly, only the door with cross leading to a food reward. After the cat has learned the problem (regularly picks whichever door has the cross), one can test the left eye with the right eye covered; the split-brain cat has to learn all over again, that is, it starts at 50% (chance). For each cat the learning curve for the left eye (and LH) is very similar to the learning curve for the right eye. Since a split-brain cat has to learn all over from the beginning with the second eye, the cat can be trained to pick the square instead of the cross when using the second eye. The choice the cat makes then depends on which eye is open. Thus, each hemisphere has developed a different memory about what is correct; that is to say, each hemisphere has its own semantic system (i.e., a system that gives meaning to symbols). That the two hemispheres could be so disparate, giving different, even opposite meanings to symbols (cross and square) may be surprising since the two thalami in a cat are quite tightly coupled

anatomically. The anatomical coupling of thalami in a monkey is a bit less, hence one might expect a similar duality of mentation in split-brain monkeys, whose visual system is more similar to that of humans than to that of cats, who learn much faster, and who have a considerable capacity for fine finger manipulation. Indeed, monkeys show even more than cats a duality of mentation (Sperry, 1964). Two monkey experiments exemplify the large literature on this subject.

One of the most reliable signs of a bilateral prefrontal lobectomy in monkeys is their inability to do delayed-alternation tasks (Jacobsen and Nissen, 1937; Sawaguchi and Goldman-Rakic, 1991; Fuster, 1997). It was long supposed that this inability might be explained as the result of the hyperactivity and/or distractibility that is also characteristic of such monkeys. This supposition can be tested in a split-brain monkey, where each hemisphere can function separately. If one hemisphere has a prefrontal lobectomy, it performs poorly on the delayed-alternation task. This poor performance by the lobectomized hemisphere is not accompanied by hyperactivity or distractibility. Apparently, the remaining frontal lobe keeps the monkey quiet and attentive, even though the intact hemisphere is not participating in the recognition of various stimuli or the evaluation of their significance (Glickstein et al., 1963).

A truly dramatic example occurs when only one hemisphere of a split-brain monkey has had a temporal lobectomy. A bitemporal monkey manifests the Klüver-Bucy syndrome, which includes difficulties in the visual identification of objects, orality (often mouthing inappropriate objects), hypersexuality, hypomotility, and tameness in the presence of humans. When the intact hemisphere can see, the split-brain rhesus monkey behaves in the usual rhesus manner, manifesting a fierce fear of humans. But if only the temporal lobectomized hemisphere receives the visual information, the split-brain animal acts like a Klüver-Bucy monkey, particularly as regards its relative tameness. When this was reported (Downer, 1961, 1962) it was so amazing that many of us doubted the results, although we were already convinced of the duality of mind in the split-brain monkey. Little room for doubt remains because this finding has, in its essentials, been reported by a number of other investigators (Bossom et al., 1961; Barrett, 1969; Doty et al., 1971, 1973; Horel and Keating, 1972; Doty and Overman, 1977).

It was knowledge of the split-brain experiments in laboratory animals that alerted Geschwind and Kaplan (1962) to the possibility of a hemisphere-disconnection syndrome in the human. When a suitable patient appeared, they searched for the disconnection effects. From a complex, evolving clinical picture, they teased out the relevant phenomena.

One of the first things Geschwind and Kaplan found was that although the patient wrote clearly with his right hand, he wrote "aphasically" with his left (and was astonished by what he had written). Among other things, they found that an object placed in his left hand was handled correctly and was correctly retrieved by feel, but it could not be named; nor could it be retrieved by feel with his right hand. Geschwind and Kaplan reported that "he behaved as if his two cerebral hemispheres were functioning nearly autonomously. Thus, we found that so long as we confined stimulation and response within the same hemisphere, the patient showed correct performance." In contrast, the patient performed incorrectly when the stimulus was provided to one hemisphere and the response required from the other. They concluded that the best explanation was to suppose that his hemispheres were disconnected by a lesion of the CC. Their anatomic prediction was eventually confirmed by autopsy. And their conclusions were soon amply confirmed by surgical cases, discussed later in the chapter.

Liepmann's callosal concept has been resurrected. There is now widespread acceptance of an idea long ignored, an interesting example of what Kuhn (1962) has called a paradigm shift. Geschwind (1974) wrote: "What was astonishing was the fact that this work had been so grossly neglected, . . . that important confirmed scientific observations could almost be expunged from the knowledge of contemporary scientists" (p. 19). As Harrington (1987) put it, ways of thinking about the brain (i.e., laterality and duality) which seem natural enough now had "vanished from the working world

view" for nearly 50 years. Chapter 9 of her book is devoted to the causes of this half-century eclipse, which include "neurology's rediscovery of the 'whole' " led by Marie (1906), Head (1926), Goldstein (1939), and, in the laboratory, Lashley (1929, 1951). She is particularly critical of Henry Head, whose highly selective reference to Jackson "borders on intellectual dishonesty." Concurrent was a "trend toward psychologism in psychiatry," including the work of Bleuler and, especially, Freud.

Geschwind (1964) has suggested in correspondence that, with the rise of psychoanalysis, there was a widespread revulsion against attempts to link brain to behavior. He also had a sociological explanation:

Henry Head had been shrewd enough to point out that much of the great German growth of neurology had been related to their victory in the Franco-Prussian war. He was not shrewd enough to apply this valuable historical lesson to his own time and to realize that perhaps the decline of the vigor and influence of German neurology was strongly related to the defeat of Germany in World War I and the shift of the center of gravity of intellectual life to the English-speaking world, rather than necessarily to any defects in the ideas of German scholars (p. 63).

But there were other factors. One thing missing was a widespread conviction that the essential facts could be observed repeatedly in humans under controlled, prospective circumstances. Such observations (described below) are possible with persons who have had a complete cerebral commissurotomy or, short of that, a complete callosotomy.

Meanwhile, it is useful to mention briefly some objections to the two-brain view that have been resurrected in the past few years.

THE REVISIONISTS

The two-brain view, recognizing a significant degree of cerebral hemisphere independence (including in cats and monkeys) and conspicuous hemispheric specialization (in most humans) caught the public eye in the 1970s. The media pushed the popularity of the "right brain/left brain" story to fad proportions reaching an almost frenzied peak by 1980. This led not only to simplistic degradation, probably inevitable with popularization, but also to exploitation. Commercially motivated entrepreneurs promised to educate people's right hemispheres (RHs) in short order, sometimes even overnight, ignoring the lengthy, arduous training necessary for any mature competence. This was followed by a reaction or backlash, which itself served to confuse nonspecialists hoping to distinguish replicable fact from speculation. Much of the reaction involved the debunking of extravagant claims. Some of it, however, was more revisionist. By this we mean work by writers who challenged the basic observations by emphasizing limitations on hemispheric independence and by pointing out the relative nature of hemispheric specialization, as well as emphasizing the obvious point that for intact individuals, most activities involve hemispheric interaction. A notable example is the extreme denigration of hemispheric specialization by Efron (1990).

THE DISCONNECTION SYNDROME FOLLOWING COMPLETE CEREBRAL COMMISSUROTOMY

SYNOPSIS OF THE HUMAN SPLIT-BRAIN SYNDROME

When patients who have had a complete callosotomy have recovered from the acute operative effects and reach a fairly stable state, they manifest a variety of phenomena that can be grouped under four headings:

1. *Social ordinariness*. One of the most remarkable results is that in ordinary social situations the patients are indistinguishable from normal individuals. Special testing methods, usually involving the lateralization of input, are needed to expose their deficits.
2. *Lack of interhemispheric transfer*. A wide variety of situations (described below) have been contrived to show that the human subjects are in this respect the same as split-brain cats and monkeys. A typical example is the inability to identify with

one hand an object palpated with the other.
3. *Hemispheric specialization effects*. The hemispheric specialization typical of human subjects results in phenomena not seen in split-brain animals. A typical example is the inability of right-handers to name or describe an object in the left hand, even when it is being appropriately manipulated.
4. *Compensatory phenomena*. Split-brain subjects progressively acquire a variety of strategies for circumventing their interhemispheric transfer deficits. A common example is for the patient to speak out loud the name of an object palpated in the right hand; because the RH can recognize many individual words, the object can then be identified with the left hand.

In this section, after discussing the acute effects of commissurotomy, the human split-brain syndrome will be analyzed in its various domains. Within each domain, the patient's behavior can reflect lack of interhemispheric transfer, hemisphere specialization, or compensatory phenomena, as discussed above. In this and subsequent sections frequent reference is made to specific split-brain patients. The case histories of the most commonly studied patients are summarized in Table 14–1.

ACUTE EFFECTS OF COMMISSUROTOMY

In the immediate postoperative period and diminishing for weeks after, behavioral deficits may be related to injury to the RH from retraction during surgery, such as left-sided weakness and focal clonic seizures; to *diaschisis*, the dysfunction of undamaged brain regions related to the loss of contact with other regions resulting from the sudden destruction of millions of commissural fibers; and to disconnection effects that will eventually be compensated. It may be difficult to know which factor or factors account for any specific deficit.

During the first few days after complete cerebral commissurotomy in right-handers operated on from the right side, patients commonly respond reasonably well with their right limbs to simple commands. But they are eas-

Table 14–1. Summary of Case Histories

Patient	Gender	Handedness	Surgery	Age at Surgery (years)	Age at Onset of Symptoms (years)	IQ HISTORY Preoperative	IQ HISTORY Postoperative	Lesion Localization	Predominant Extracallosal Damage
N.G.	F	R	Complete cerebral commissurotomy: single-stage midline section of anterior commissure, corpus callosum, massa intermedia, and right fornix. Surgical approach by retraction of RH	30	18	Weschler-Bellvue 76 (79, 74) at age 30	WAIS, 77 (83, 71) at age 35	L posterior temporal R central	RH (BI)
L.B.	M	R	As above, but massa intermedia was not visualized	13	3:6	WISC 113 (119,108) at age 13	WAIS 106 (110, 100) at age 16	R central	RH (BI)
R.Y.	M	R	As above (normal cerebral development until age 13)	43	17	—	WAIS 90 (99, 79) at age 45	R posterior?	RH
N.W.	F	R	As above. Massa intermedia divided. Partial damage to left fornix	36	8	WAIS 93 (97, 89) at age 36	WAIS 93 (97, 89) at age 36	R temporal, parietal	RH (BI)
C.C.	M	R	As above. Surgical approach by LH retraction. Very difficult operation and slow recovery	13	10	WISC 76 (73, 83) at age 13	WAIS 72 (72, 75) at age 16:8	L temporal, parietal	LH
A.A.	M	R	As above. Difficult operation	14	5:6	WAIS 74 (80, 72) at age 14	WAIS 78 (77, 82) at age 17:8	L frontoparietal; birth injury to R arm area R frontal	LH (BI)
P.S.	M	R	Callosotomy, two-stage, anterior first	15	2	WAIS 89 (83, 99)	WAIS 89	L temporal	LH
V.P.	F	R	Callosotomy, two-stage, anterior first	27	6		WAIS-R 91	Bilateral L temporal	LH (BI)
D.R.	F	R	Callosotomy, single-stage	38	17	WAIS 117 (114, 100) at age 52	WAIS-R 89 (105, 72)	R temporal	RH
J.W.	M	R	Callosotomy, two-stage, posterior first	25	19	WAIS-R 95 (97, 95) at age 34	WAIS-R 95 (97, 95) at age 34	R anterior L frontoparietal	BI
V.J.	F	L	Callosotomy, two-stage, anterior first	42	16	WAIS-R 80 (88, 75)	WAIS-R 88 (96, 73)		

BI, bilateral; L, left; LH, left hemisphere; R, right; RH, right hemisphere; WAIS, Wechsler Adult Intelligence Scale; WISC, Wechsler Intelligence Scale for Children. WAIS-R, Wechsler Intelligence Scale Revised ily confused by three- or even two-part commands, each part of which is obviously understood. These patients often lie quietly and may seem mildly "akinetic," although they cooperate when stimulated. There is sometimes an imperviousness resembling that often seen with naturally occurring genu lesions. The patients are often mute, even when willing to write short (usually one-word) answers (Bogen, 1976). Failure of left-side responses to verbal command is usually severe and can be mistaken for hemiplegia. With improvement, well-coordinated but repetitive reaching, groping, and grasping with the left hand sometimes resembles a grasp reflex; grasp reflexes may actually be present bilaterally for a day or two after surgery. When forced grasping cannot be elicited (by inserting two fingers into the patient's palm and drawing them out across the web between the thumb and index finger), it is nevertheless possible in most cases to demonstrate a proximal traction response; that is, the patient is unable to relax the hand grip when the examiner pulls so as to exert traction on the elbow and shoulder flexors (Twitchell, 1951). As the patient improves, there may be competitive movements between the left and right hands. These patients commonly have bilateral Babinski signs as well as bilaterally absent superficial abdominal reflexes.

Left arm hypotonia, left arm positive traction response, bilateral Babinski responses, and mutism were regularly observed in our cases; but there was considerable variation from one patient to another, both in our series and in others' (Wilson et al., 1975, 1977; Holtzman et al., 1981; McKeever et al., 1981; Ferguson et al., 1985; Reeves, 1991; Sass et al., 1991). At one extreme, our first patient, W.J., had preoperative right-frontal atrophy, was oldest at the time of brain injury (age 30) and at the time of operation (45), and subsequently showed the most severe apraxic and related symptoms. At the other end of the spectrum, L.B., a 13-year-old boy (see Bogen et al., 1988, for MRI status), had relatively little brain damage before surgery, had brain injury at birth, was youngest at the time of operation, and subsequently had the smoothest postoperative course and minimal left-hand apraxia.

Within a few months after operation, the symptoms of hemisphere disconnection tend to be compensated to a remarkable degree. In personality, in social situations, and in most of a routine neurologic exam the patient appears much as before. However, with appropriate tests using lateralized input the disconnected hemispheres can be shown to operate independently to a large extent. Each of the hemispheres appears to have its own learning processes and its own separate memories, many of which are largely inaccessible to the other hemisphere.

THE CHRONIC, STABILIZED SYNDROME OF HEMISPHERE DISCONNECTION: DISSOCIATIVE PHENOMENA

Phenomena that suggest volitional ambivalence may be elicited by history or, less commonly, observed in the clinic. There may be a disparity between facial expression and verbalization, or between what the left hand is doing and what the patient is saying. Or there may be a dissociation between general bodily actions (rising, walking, etc.) and what is being done by either hand or what is being said. Such dissociations have occurred sufficiently often following callosal section in animals (Trevarthen, 1965) and in humans that they should arouse suspicion of hemisphere disconnection. Indeed, there may be some substance to the notion that such conative or volitional ambivalence, when it occurs in normal subjects, might be attributable, at least on some occasions, to altered information transfer by anatomically intact commissures (Galin, 1974; Hoppe, 1977).

In contrast with volitional ambivalence, emotional ambivalence (such as the report by the patient of possessing two conflicting internal feelings simultaneously) has not been a symptom of commissurotomy nor of most reported natural cases. Indeed, individuals with cerebral commissurotomy are less apt than normal individuals to discuss their feelings, conflicting or otherwise (Hoppe and Bogen, 1977). This condition, *callosal alexithymia* (TenHouten et al., 1986), may be explained by a defect in right-to-left callosal conduction (Speedie et al., 1984; Klouda et al., 1988), or in RH function. (We may generalize callosal alexithymia to the normal brain and predict that individuals with higher scores on an alexithymia scale will show a greater RH deficit and weaker callosal transfer in an emotionality judgment task. However, Tabibnia et al. [2001] found that this was not the case.)

Intermanual Conflict

The dissociative phenomenon most clearly identifiable with hemisphere disconnection is intermanual conflict, in which the hands act at cross purposes. Almost all of the complete commissurotomy patients in the Los Angeles series, manifested some degree of intermanual conflict in the early postoperative period. For example, a few weeks after one patient (R.Y.) underwent surgery, his physiotherapist said, "You should have seen R.Y. yesterday—one hand was buttoning up his shirt and the other hand was coming along right behind it undoing the buttons!" (Bogen, 1979). Another patient (A.M.) exhibited similar conflicts during Bogen's follow-up examination in February 1973: "when attempting a Jendrassik reinforcement, the patient reached with his right hand to hold his left but the left hand actually pushed his right hand away. While testing finger-to-nose test (with the patient sitting), his left hand suddenly started slapping his chest like Tarzan."

Similar phenomena after callosotomy have been observed by others (Wilson et al., 1977; Ferguson et al., 1985; Reeves, 1991; Sass et al., 1991) as well as by Akelaitis (1944–45), who called it "diagonistic dyspraxia." Intermanual conflict has been described in many individual case reports of callosal infarcts or tumors (Fisher, 1963; Schaltenbrand, 1964; Joynt, 1977; Barbizet et al., 1978; Beukelman et al., 1980: Watson and Heilman, 1983; Sine at al., 1984; Degos et al., 1987; Levin et al., 1987; Tanaka et al., 1990; Della Sala et al., 1991, 1994; Schwartz et al., 1991; Baynes et al., 1997).

Intermanual conflict usually subsides soon after callosotomy, probably because other integrative mechanisms supplement or replace commissural function. In rare cases it may persist for years, for reasons still poorly understood (Ferguson et al., 1985; Reeves, 1991).

The Anarchic (Alien) Hand

Related to intermanual conflict is a circumstance in which one of the patient's hands, usually the left hand in the right-handed patient, behaves in a way that the patient finds "foreign," "alien," or at least uncooperative. Della Sala et al. (1991) point out that such patients rarely deny that the troublesome hand belongs to them; hence, they prefer the term "anarchic" to "alien." The anarchic hand (AH) often leads to intermanual conflict, and has been seen consequent to callosal lesions at least since the report of Goldstein (1908). Even our youngest patient (L.B.), who had no long-term appreciable apraxia to verbal command, manifested this phenomenon 3 weeks after surgery: while doing the block design test unimanually with his right hand, his left hand came up from beneath the table and was reaching for the blocks when he slapped it with his right hand and said, "That will keep it quiet for a while." Among our patients it has been most persistent in a subject (N.W.) with a rather flamboyant personality which we believe contributed to her frequent complaints about "my little sister" in referring to whomever or whatever it was that made her left hand behave peculiarly. Evidence has been steadily accumulating that the AH, to be persistent, depends upon mesial frontal cortical dysfunction (Goldberg et al., 1981; McNabb et al., 1988; Banks et al., 1989; Leiguarda et al., 1989; Starkstein et al., 1990; and Tanaka et al., 1990). Della Sala et al. (1991) suggest that, in its persistent form, AH results from a loss of inhibition originating in mesial frontal cortex (presumably of actions organized or "programmed" elsewhere). This can help us understand anarchic behavior of either hand, or even both hands (Mark et al., 1991).

Autocriticism

In a related phenomenon, described by Brion and Jedynak (1975), and which they called "l'autocritique interhémisphérique," the patient expresses fairly frequent astonishment at the capacity of the left hand to behave independently. When the left hand makes some choice among objects, the patient may say that "my hand did that," rather than taking the responsibility. A patient was described by Sweet (1945) as saying, "Now you want me to put my left index finger on my nose." She then put that finger into her mouth and said, "That's funny; why won't it go up to my nose?" (p. 88).

Split-brain patients soon accept the idea that they have capacities of which they are not aware, such as left hand retrieval of objects not nameable. They may quickly rationalize such acts, sometimes in a transparently erroneous way (Gazzaniga and LeDoux, 1978). But even many years after surgery, these patients will occasionally be surprised or even irritated when some well-coordinated or obviously well-informed act has just been carried out by the left hand. This is particularly common under conditions of continuously lateralized input (Zaidel, 1977, 1978a; Zaidel and Peters, 1981). Praised by the examiner following successful performance by L.B.'s disconnected right hemisphere (DRH) on difficult language tasks, he would sometimes exclaim: "How can I be correct when I don't know what I just did." But it occurs even in social situations. In the summer of 1989, L.B. (then 24 years postoperative) was having lunch between testing sessions with two investigators. One of them asked about his attitude toward his left hand. He replied, "I hardly ever use it." The other examiner (Bogen) then pointed out that he was, at that moment, holding up a cup of juice in his left hand and had just taken a drink from the cup. "Sure enough," he said, looking at it, "I guess it is good for something."

Signs of Release from Frontal Control

We can distinguish between behaviors of increasing complexity and/or appropriateness in the affected (but nonparetic, nonataxic) upper limb. Relatively simple is forced grasping. However, there may also be groping movements, called "impulsive grasping" if they are followed by grasping upon contact. Visual guidance may give an appearance of purposefulness, as in "magnetic apraxia" (Denny-Brown, 1958) or, when more complex, "utilization behavior" (Lhermitte, 1983; Lhermitte et al., 1986; LaPlane et al., 1989; Shallice et al., 1989). Frontal infarction (or transient dys-

function), even if insufficient to cause forced grasping, may release synergic effects. A related but less severe deficit is an inability to keep the thumb extended while exerting a forceful grip (Wartenberg, 1953). Automatic (i.e., reliably elicited by the examiner) actions should be distinguished from well-coordinated behavior that is autonomous, that is, behavior that occurs without obvious external stimulus (i.e., is spontaneous). The distinctions "exogenous vs. endogenous" and "induced vs. incidental" have also been offered. Behavior that is stereotyped and repetitive can be distinguished from well-directed movement sequences adapted to the surroundings of a particular moment. Any of these behaviors may be accompanied (or not) by verbal denial, simple recognition, elaborate rationalization, or even appreciation.

The Alien Hand: Terminology and Pathogenesis

The term "alien hand" was erroneously introduced (Bogen, 1979) as the result of Bogen's misreading of Brion and Jedynak (1975). We disapprove of the use of this term. A recent rereading makes clear that Brion and Jedynak used the term "la main étrangère" to describe a misidentification resulting from failure of interhemispheric *sensory* transfer, whereas they used the term "l'autocritique interhémisphérique" to describe seemingly purposeful *actions* disavowed by the patients.

The emphasis by Brion and Jedynak (1975) and by Bogen (1979) on callosal disconnection as the cause of AH was challenged by Goldberg et al. (1981), who reported two right-handed patients with a right AH subsequent to left mesial frontal infarction. The role of mesial frontal damage is difficult to evaluate since such lesions typically also involve the CC. The necessity for callosal disconnection (particularly for persisting cases) thus resulting in hemispheric independence would be disproved if AH emerged in hemispherectomized individuals suffering subsequent frontal damage. This debate is unresolved. It has been suggested (Feinberg et al., 1992) that there are two forms of AH, one callosal and the other mesiofrontal. To the extent that a callosal lesion is essential (Geschwind et al., 1995) the AH supports the idea of an "other mind" (Bogen, 2000). Alternatively, it may be that the behavioral dissociation (between hand action and verbalization) is the result of interhemispheric disconnection of visually guided motor planning from verbal awareness (Milner and Goodale, 1995; Bogen, 1997).

Marchetti and Della Sala (in press) argue that the "anarchic hand" is not associated with an (anterior) callosal lesion but is attributable to damage to the contralateral Supplementary Motor Area in the mesial frontal lobe. In this view, the SMA converts intentions to self-initiated actions, and damage to it leads to failure to modulate and inhibit externally-triggered action generated by the Premotor Area on the same side.

The literature refers to a variety of phenomena with the term "alien hand." All share the occurrence of involuntary movements, but the types of movement differ. In the callosal form, there are purposeful complex movements of the nondominant hand. In the frontal form, there is grasping and utilization behavior of the dominant hand. Forced grasping occurs about equally often with either the right or the left hand; it is usually a stereotyped response following stimulation; and it is typically a sign of contralateral frontal lobe dysfunction, requiring no direct callosal involvement in the lesion. The alien hand associated with cortical–basal degeneration is characterized by what appears to be spontaneous elevations of an arm, and a better term for this phenomenon might be "wayward" or "wandering" hand. It is misleading to describe any form of AH as alien because (as pointed out by Della Sala et al., 1994) the patients do not ascribe the hand to someone else but recognize it as their own, although out of control. While all three forms (callosal, frontal, basal-ganglionic) involve loss of motor control, only the callosal form involves denial of purposeful movement and the occurrence of intermanual conflict which can be termed "alien." We therefore propose that the different forms represent distinct syndromes and should be so named. For the type of movement that is well-coordinated, seemingly purposeful, and commonly effective, we prefer to use "autonomous hand."

THE CHRONIC, STABILIZED SYNDROME OF HEMISPHERE DISCONNECTION: SYMPTOMS, SIGNS, AND METHODS OF TESTING IN SPECIFIC DOMAINS

The testing of split-brain patients in the psychology laboratory has become progressively more sophisticated, and is often unfamiliar even to otherwise experienced neuropsychologists (Zaidel, et al., 1990). Thus, we will first emphasize simple maneuvers that can be used in the clinic when hemisphere disconnection is suspected. The general logic for studying hemispheric specialization in split-brain patients is to restrict sensory input and motor response to one hemisphere at a time, and compare latency or accuracy in the two conditions. In the case of visual and somesthetic input, predominantly contralateral innervation guarantees that left visual field (LVF) and left-hand information, respectively, will reach the RH, whereas right visual field (RVF) and right-hand input will reach the LH. In the case of auditory stimuli, contralateral input can be assumed only when two acoustically similar, but not identical, stimuli reach both ears simultaneously (dichotic listening). For motor responses, it is assumed that each hemisphere has better control of the contralateral hand, especially at distal movements, but in the chronic disconnection syndrome, both hemispheres develop ipsilateral motor control sufficient for simple actions, such as binary choices. Consequently, experiments should rely on complete or partial lateralization at the input side. Given the emergence of speech in some disconnected right hemispheres, it should not be assumed without further testing that verbal output reflects responses by the disconnected left hemisphere (DLH).

The descriptions provided here apply to right-handers. In left-handers the situation is rarely a simple reversal. Usually it is quite complex, as can be seen in the case histories described in the literature (Liepmann, 1900; Hécaen and Ajuriaguerra, 1964; Botez and Crighel, 1971; Tzavaras et al., 1971; Heilman et al., 1973; Schott et al., 1974; Aptman et al.,

1977; Hirose et al., 1977; Poncet et al., 1978; Herron, 1980; Hécaen et al., 1981; Gur et al., 1984; Joseph, 1986; Baynes et al., 1998; Spencer et al., 1988).

Olfaction: Unilateral Verbal Anosmia

Unlike most other sensory pathways, the olfactory pathways are almost exclusively uncrossed. Berlucchi and Aglioti (1999) describe the pathways as follows: "Information from primary sensory neurons in the olfactory epithelium of each nostril is transmitted to the olfactory bulb of the same side. The axons of the projection neurons of the olfactory bulb form the lateral olfactory tract that reaches the ipsilateral olfactory cortex consisting of paleocortical (prepiriform and periamigdaloid areas) and mesocortical components (entorhinal area)" (p. 656). The anterior olfactory nucleus, which receives input from the second-order bulbar neurons, may then send information across the anterior commissure, and cortical olfactory areas, such as the piriform cortex, may also project across the splenium of the corpus callosum. Berlucchi and Aglioti (1999) believe that "the interhemispheric transmission of olfactory information does not involve the CC and relies upon the anterior and hippocampal commissures" (p. 656).

Following complete cerebral commissurotomy, the patient is unable to name odors presented to the right nostril, even when they can be named quite readily when presented to the left nostril. This is not a unilateral defect of smell, since the patient can select, by feeling with the left hand, an object that corresponds to the odor presented to the right nostril, such as selecting a plastic banana or a plastic fish after having smelled the related odor (Gordon and Sperry, 1969).

The original study of commissurotomy subjects found that odor identification (using a nonlinguistic task and response mode) was superior using the left nostril as compared to using the right (Gordon and Sperry, 1969). A subsequent study of callosotomy patients found left hemispheric specialization for odor memory, although not for odor identification (Eskenazi et al., 1988). Other populations suggest the opposite pattern of laterality. Some studies show more impairment in olfactory ability among patients with right- rather than left-sided brain damage or temporal lobectomy (e.g., West and Doty, 1995), although others have found no differences (Zatorre and Jones-Gotman, 1991). Tasks designed to measure the olfactory ability of each hemisphere in normal subjects have also suggested RH specialization (e.g., Hummel et al., 1998), but brain activation studies are conflicting (Zald and Pardo, 1997; Dade et al., 1998; Sobel et al., 1999).

Regardless of the relative abilities of the hemispheres, there are two lines of evidence which suggest that the hemispheres normally work together in olfaction. The first is that, among normal individuals, using both nostrils (birhinal presentation) increases the perceived intensity of odors relative to using only one nostril (unirhinal presentation) (Cain, 1977; Garcia Medina and Cain, 1982) and facilitates odor memory (Bromley and Doty, 1995), but it does not affect detection threshold (Doty et al., 1992). Second, patients who lack interhemispheric fibers suffer olfactory deficits. In a study by Eskenazi et al. (1988), two callosotomy patients had severe impairments in odor discrimination and identification. These patients were also epileptic, which appears to cause a generalized decrease in olfactory function (West and Doty, 1995), but although performance was indeed subnormal in the one patient tested presurgically, it was further reduced following callosotomy.

Is it possible for olfactory information to transfer between the hemispheres at all in the absence of the CC and anterior commissure? Previous experiments have addressed this question by testing the ability of split-brain patients to verbally name unirhinally presented odors. Gordon and Sperry (1969) found that four of five complete commissurotomy patients could name odors presented to the left nostril, but not those presented to the right. This suggests that information was generally unable to cross from the right olfactory cortex to exclusively left-sided speech centers. However, the fifth subject in this study (patient N.G.) was able to name right nostril items above chance in one of four well-controlled blocks, which suggests that some transfer may still occur. Of the two interhemispheric connections in the olfactory system, the anterior commissure appears to be more important. The three callosotomy patients studied by Risse et al. (1978) and the two patients of Eskenazi et al. (1988) were all able to name odors presented to the right nostril. In sharp contrast to the commissurotomy patients studied by Gordon and Sperry (1969), some of these patients with intact anterior commissures showed no difference between nostrils or even better naming of stimuli presented to the right nostril than the left.

In a recent study, Allison and Zaidel (2000) examined three commissurotomy patients from the Los Angeles series (L.B., N.G., and A.A.), one agenesis patient with an intact anterior commissure, and an epileptic control. They used a standardized set of olfactory stimuli ("scratch and sniff" strips) from the University of Pennsylvania Smell Identification Test (UPSIT; Doty et al., 1984). The first finding of this study was that there is a consistent impairment of odor identification among individuals lacking the CC, as in previous studies of patients with callosotomy (Eskenazi et al., 1988) and callosal agenesis (Kessler et al., 1991). Second, the results do not provide support for the hypothesis that there is hemispheric specialization for olfaction. Third, patients in whom the CC failed to form during development showed no disadvantage when the odors to be discriminated were presented to separate hemispheres. In contrast, both of the commissurotomy patients who could do the task at all were significantly worse during this between-hemisphere condition than when the odors were presented to the same hemisphere. Patient A.A., however, was still able to compare odors between hemispheres above chance. When tested by Gordon and Sperry (1969), patient N.G. was also sometimes able to name odors presented to the RH. This suggests that some subcallosal routes may be able to convey information about odors. Subcallosal routes may exist for other sensory modalities as well, and these routes appear to vary across individual patients (Clarke and Zaidel, 1989).

Taste

The lateral organization of the gustatory pathway in humans is incompletely understood.

Most studies support an uncrossed projection from each side of the tongue to the cortex, but reports of a crossed organization continue to appear. The afferent gustatory fibers from each half of the tongue are known to travel via the VIIth and IXth cranial nerves to the ipsilateral nucleus of the solitary tract (NST). This projects to the parvocellular part of the ventroposteromedial nucleus of the thalamus (VPMpc), which in turn projects ipsilaterally to the primary gustatory cortex in the frontal operculum and anterior insula (Kobayakawa et al., 1996). The unsolved question is whether the projection from NST to VPMpc is crossed or uncrossed. Following unilateral brain lesions, gustatory impairments such as ageusias, hypogeusias, or dysgeusias can be localized to one side of the tongue. But both subcortical and cortical lesions give conflicting results (reviewed in Aglioti et al., 2001).

Aglioti et al. (2000) studied the lateral organization of the gustatory pathway in normal controls, a man with a complete callosal agenesis, and a man with a complete section of the CC, a right anterior frontal lesion, and language in the LH. Sapid solutions were applied to one or the other side of the tongue and subjects reported the taste of the stimulus either verbally or by manually pointing to the name of the taste. There were no differences in accuracy and reaction time (RT) between the right and left hemitongues of the controls and the acallosal subject. By contrast, the callosotomy subject showed a constant marked advantage of the left hemitongue over the right for both accuracy and speed of response, though performance with right stimuli was clearly above chance. Assuming LH control of speech in the callosotomy patient, the results reject an exclusively crossed organization of the gustatory pathway from tongue to cortex, and favor a bilaterally distributed organization of this pathway, with a marked predominance of the uncrossed over the crossed component. These results, however, cannot rule out an exclusively uncrossed organization.

Berlucchi (personal communication, 2000) has since confirmed these results in two more callosotomy patients without cortical lesions. Still needed is a demonstration that the uncrossed gustatory component is stronger than the crossed one in the disconnected right hemisphere as well. There may also be individual differences in the relative magnitude of the uncrossed and crossed gustatory components, and these differences might explain the conflicts in the neurological literature.

Vision

Methods. To restrict sensory visual information to one hemisphere, lateralized visual stimuli are presented for <150 msec. This prevents the confounding effects of involuntary saccadic eye movements, which have a latency of about 180 msec. To avoid possible confounds due to predominance of crossed over uncrossed fibers at the chiasm, binocular vision is used. Although humans are believed to show negligible bihemispheric anatomic overlap around the vertical meridian (on the order of minutes of arc), it is prudent to present stimuli with their outermost edge at least 1°–2° away from fixation. Although electroencephalographic (EEG) recording is often used to monitor eye movements (Jordan et al., 1998), adequate fixation can usually be ascertained by videotaping or direct inspection. Currently, hemifield tachistoscopy is usually implemented on personal computers.

To study processing of continuous visual stimuli restricted to one hemisphere, E. Zaidel (1973) developed a contact lens system that is effective but requires individual fitting. Other investigators used part-opaque contact lenses (Dimond et al., 1975) or goggles (Francks et al., 1985), which are imprecise. Instead of yoking the hemifield occluder directly to the eye via a contact lens, it is possible to track eye movements noninvasively and use the horizontal component of the eye movements to control hemifield occlusion, either optically–mechanically (Zaidel and Frazier, 1977) or on a video monitor (Wittling, 1990). The critical needs are to separate eye movements from head movements, obtain an accurate measure of eye movements (with an error of <30 minutes of arc) within a relatively wide visual scanning area (about 10° of arc), and ensure occlusion in real time. No fully operational eye tracker–based system for simulating hemianopsia currently exists.

Failure of Interhemispheric Transfer: Double Hemianopia. Stimuli confined to one visual half-field will reach only the contralateral hemisphere. Callosal section will prevent the hemisphere ipsilateral to the stimulus from having access to this stimulus. Therefore, only one hemisphere can reliably report the presence of the stimulus. Although tachistoscopic presentation is ideal for confining the stimulus to one hemisphere, the disconnection can sometimes be demonstrated with simple confrontation testing of the visual fields. The patient is allowed to have both eyes open but does not speak, and is allowed to use only one hand to respond (sitting on the other hand, for example). Using the free hand, the subject indicates the onset of a stimulus, such as the wiggling of the examiner's fingers. With such testing there may appear to be an homonymous hemianopia contralateral to the indicating hand (the patient reliably points to the right half-field stimulus with the right hand but not to a left half-field stimulus). When the patient is tested with the other hand there seems to be an homonymous hemianopia in the other half-field. One can also test for this deficit by holding up one or more fingers in one half-field, and asking the patient to show the same number of fingers using the hand ipsilateral or contralateral to the stimulus, or by asking the patient to demonstrate a hand posture shown to only one hemisphere.

Compensatory Strategies. Most patients eventually achieve a condition in which no field defect can be demonstrated by the confrontation technique. This depends mainly upon the ability of each hemisphere to direct the head and eyes toward the visual target; this can signal the hemisphere ipsilateral to the stimulus to respond. If turning of the head is prevented, a lateral glance will suffice to cue the patient. Some patients learn to "cheat:" for example, as soon as it is apparent that there is no suitable stimulus in the right visual half-field, the right hand may point to the left visual half-field. This cheating can sometimes be detected by providing no stimulus at all on some trials.

Each hemisphere, especially the left, can exert a modicum of ipsilateral control, especially for gross arm movements. As a result, stimuli in the right half-field (seen only by the LH) may be pointed to when the patient is using only the left hand, and similarly for the left half-field stimuli when only the right hand is available. But such pointing is less reliable and accurate, as compared with the dependable response and precise localization possible when the patient is using the hand contralateral to the stimulated hemisphere.

Visual Deficits Related to Hemisphere Specialization

Verbal report of left visual field stimuli: left hemi-anomia. Since verbal output is controlled almost exclusively by the LH, there may be no verbal report to stimuli confined to the left half-field, which access only the RH. If stimuli are presented simultaneously in both visual half-fields, only the stimulus in the right half-field is described by the patient, that is, by the LH. There is usually no verbal response to the stimulus in the left visual half-field until the LH realizes that the patient's left hand is also in action, pointing to the left half-field stimulus.

Split-brain patients may be unable to name aloud objects presented in the left half-field. This problem is usually not evident in patients with left hemi-alexia from acquired splenial lesions (usually with right hemianopia from a left posterior cerebral artery territory infarction), but see Poeck (1984), whose patient with alexia was also unable to name objects, i.e., had optic anomia as well as hemialexia.

Left hemi-alexia. In the absence of hemianopia, subjects with left hemialexia cannot read individual words flashed to the left half-field. This is true not only for complete callosotomy but also for patients with section of only the splenium (Trescher and Ford, 1937; Maspes, 1948; Gazzaniga and Freedman, 1973; Damasio et al., 1980; Sugishita et al., 1986; Sugishita and Yoshioka, 1987). It is sometimes possible to demonstrate left hemialexia by the brief presentations of cards, showing printed letters or short words, in the left half-field. Patients are often unable to read a card presented this way, although they can readily read it when it is presented in the right half-field. Although eye movements are

usually too active for such simple testing methods, hemialexia was, in fact, observed using such methods, long before its demonstration by tachistoscopic presentation (Trescher and Ford, 1937). Hemialexia has been intensively studied with both tachistoscopic and computerized techniques by Sugishita et al. (1986, 1987; see also Grüsser and Landis, 1991).

Compensation. There is some apparent recovery over the years, part of which is attributable to semantic transfer; that is, the word in the LVF is recognized by the RH and this semantic information somehow transfers to the speaking LH, which can then approximate the stimulus word. Indeed, if the stimuli are known and not too numerous, the diffuse semantic information may be used to identify the word (Myers and Sperry, 1985; Sidtis et al., 1981a; Cronin-Golomb, 1986b; Sugishita et al., 1986; Zaidel et al., 1990).

Audition

Left Hemisphere Suppression of Ipsilateral Verbal Input. Auditory information to each ear crosses at the level of the superior olive and the midbrain (inferior colliculus); however, there are also ipsilateral projections, so that even in the split-brain patient, each hemisphere receives input from both ears. Monaural stimulation therefore projects to both hemispheres. Dichotic stimulation, in which distinct but acoustically similar stimuli are presented simultaneously to each ear, suppresses the ipsilateral projections and reveals an advantage for the contralateral ear–hemisphere projections in normal subjects. Which of the competing two stimuli is identified depends upon the degree to which the ipsilateral stimulus is suppressed by the stronger contralateral auditory projections, and also upon hemisphere specialization for processing the specific type of auditory input. Thus when verbal stimuli are used, there is a right ear advantage in normal subjects, because the LH preferentially analyzes the verbal stimuli, and contralateral (right ear) projections to the LH dominate weaker ipsilateral (left ear) and cross-callosal projections. In split-brain subjects, this right ear advantage becomes much more pronounced (Milner et al., 1968; Sparks and Geschwind, 1968; Gordon, 1975; Springer and Gazzaniga, 1975; Zaidel, 1976, 1983; Zaidel et al., 1990), suggesting that interruption of callosal transfer prevents the LH from accessing auditory information from the left ear via the RH. Both ipsilateral suppression and hemispheric competence can be assessed in the split-brain patient by using lateralized visual probes to be matched with the sound in either ear (Zaidel, 1983). Although left ear words are poorly reported verbally, their perception by the RH is occasionally evidenced by appropriate actions of the left hand (Gordon, 1973).

Left ear extinction has also been found in patients with lesions of the LH, if the lesions are fairly deep, where they are apt to interrupt commissural fibers. Since LH lesions are usually associated with suppression of the right ear, the suppression of the left ear by a LH lesion has been called "paradoxical ipsilateral extinction" (Sparks et al., 1970). Further observations support the conclusion that lesions close to the midline in either hemisphere cause suppression of left ear stimuli by interrupting interhemispheric pathways (Michel and Péronnet, 1975; Damasio and Damasio, 1979; Cambier et al., 1984; Rubens et al., 1985; Rao et al., 1989; Pujol et al., 1991). Because paracallosal lesions can also result in right ear extinction for nonverbal material such as complex pitch discrimination, it has been suggested that the so-called paradoxical loss would better be termed "callosal extinction" (Sidtis et al., 1989).

Right Hemisphere Suppression of Nonverbal Ipsilateral Auditory Input. We have tested patient L.B. on a verbal identification version of Ley and Bryden's dichotic words/emotions test (1982). This test consists of four rhyming consonant-vowel-consonant (CVC) words spoken in four different emotional prosodies. The word identification task yielded a massive right ear advantage whereas the emotional identification test yielded a massive left ear advantage, consistent with complementary hemispheric specialization for words and emotions observed in normal subjects. The simplest account of this pattern of results is that (*1*) there is good ipsilateral suppression for both tasks in both hemispheres; (*2*) the LH specializes for and domi-

nates the identification of the words, exhibiting an expected massive right ear advantage; (*3*) the RH specializes for and dominates the identification of emotional prosody, yielding a massive left ear advantage; and (*4*) verbal identification of the emotions reflects either RH speech or else LH verbalization of the emotion or a code identifying it which is transferred subcallosally from the RH to the LH.

Sidtis (1988) demonstrated an apparent advantage in the DRH for complex pitch discrimination. Tramo and Barucha (1991) found an advantage for the DRH for harmonic progression and associative auditory function.

Somesthesis

Somatosensory projections to the hemispheres are more lateralized than auditory projections, but not as completely contralateral as visual projections. The medial lemniscus system, which is mainly involved in the transmission of tactile and proprioceptive input, and even more the spinothalamic system, which mainly transmits thermal and pain sensations, project not only contralaterally but also ipsilaterally. While the ipsilateral connections from distal body parts are almost absent, those from axial and proximal body parts are dense. Moreover, somesthetic afferents from the face go to both ipsi- and contralateral cortical areas (Berlucchi and Aglioti, 1999).

Failure of Interhemispheric Transfer. The lack of interhemispheric transfer following brain bisection can be demonstrated with respect to somesthesis (including touch, pressure, and proprioception) in a variety of ways.

Cross-retrieval of small test objects. The patient is given an object to feel with one hand, and then asked to retrieve the same object from among a number of objects. Such a collection is most conveniently placed in a paper plate about 15 cm in diameter, around which the subject can shuffle the objects with one hand while exploring for the test object. What distinguishes the split-brain patients from normals is that their excellent same-hand retrieval (with either hand) is not accompanied by ability to retrieve with one hand objects felt with the other.

Cross-replication of hand postures. Specific postures impressed on one (unseen) hand by the examiners cannot be mimicked by the patient's opposite hand. But if more proximal stimuli are used, it may be difficult to demonstrate any failure of interhemispheric communication, probably because of ipsilateral hemispheric projections of sensory stimuli.

Intermanual point localization. After complete cerebral commissurotomy there is a partial loss of the ability to name exact points stimulated on the left side of the body. This defect is least apparent, if at all, on the face and it is most apparent on the distal extremities, especially the fingertips. This deficit is not dependent on language as it can be done in a nonverbal fashion and in both directions (right to left and vice versa).

Young children also have difficulty in cross-localizing or cross-matching (Galin et al., 1977, 1979; but cf. Pipe, 1991), possibly because their commissures are not yet fully functioning (Yakovlev and Lecours, 1967; but cf. Brody et al., 1987; Baierl et al., 1988). Immaturity of transcallosal inhibition has been suggested as the source of unnecessary duplication during simple reaching (Lehman, 1978).

Hemispheric Specialization: Left Tactile Anomia. One of the most convincing ways to demonstrate hemisphere disconnection is to ask the patient to feel with one hand and then to name various small, common objects, in the absence of vision. Unilateral anomia is a reliable and persistent sign following callosotomy. Of the many maneuvers developed in the laboratory to test split-brain patients, this is the principal one to be adopted as part of a routine neurological examination.

Patients with extensive callosal lesions are commonly unable to name or describe an object held in the left hand, although they readily name objects held in the right hand. Sometimes a recovering patient can give a vague description of the object but still be unable to name it. After a patient with a callosal lesion (e.g., a callosally dissecting hemorrhage) has regained the ability to name objects in the left hand, this ability may extinguish (Mayer et al., 1988) with dichaptic stimulation, i.e., by placing an object in each hand simultaneously (Witelson, 1974).

To establish hemisphere disconnection, it is necessary to exclude other causes of unilateral anomia, particularly astereognosis (or even a gross sensory deficit), as may occur with a right parietal lesion. The best way to exclude astereognosis or tactile agnosia (Caselli, 1991) is to show that the object has in fact been recognized even though it cannot be verbally identified or described, by retrieving it correctly from a collection of similar objects, as described above.

Compensatory Mechanisms. In testing for anomia, one must be aware, in certain clever patients, of strategies for circumventing the defect. For example, the patient may drop an object or may manipulate it in some other way (such as running a fingernail down the teeth of a comb) to produce a characteristic noise by which the object can be identified. In the same vein, a subject may identify a pipe or some other object by a characteristic smell and thus circumvent the inability of the LH to identify, by palpation alone, an object in the left hand.

With time, it may be increasingly difficult to demonstrate any hemispheric disconnection, even using distal stimuli. E. Zaidel (1998b) found that persisting deficits in tests of stereognosis reflected extracallosal damage more than failure of interhemispheric transfer.

Neuroimaging. Fabri et al. (1999) imaged normal controls and callosotomy patients from the Ancona series with functional magnetic resonance imaging (fMRI) during unilateral somatosensory stimulation. Normal subjects showed contralateral activation in S1, posterior parietal cortex, and parietal opercular cortex, as well as ipsilateral activation in homologous posterior parietal and parietal opercular cortex. In patients with anterior callosal section up to and including the posterior body, ipsilateral activation was missing, implicating the posterior third of the body of the CC in the transfer.

Motor Functions

Information Transfer. We have performed several studies on how motor information is transferred through the CC in visuomotor integration tasks. The task is a simple reaction time

(SRT) to lateralized flashes (Poffenberger, 1912). When subjects respond with the hand ipsilateral to the visual stimulus, the same hemisphere processes the visual stimulus and initiates the motor response, and therefore there is no need for transferring information through the CC. In contrast, when the stimulus is contralteral to the responding hand, the visual stimulus is received by the hemisphere opposite to the one controlling the responding hand, and thus a transfer of information through callosal fibers is needed. The difference in reaction times between crossed responses and uncrossed responses is an estimate of the conduction time through callosal fibers. Typically, in normal subjects this difference, called the "crossed–uncrossed difference" (CUD), is 3–4 msec, whereas in split brain patients it is 30–60 msec and in callosal agenesis patients it is 15–20 msec (Clarke and Zaidel, 1989; Marzi et al., 1991).

What kind of information is transferred through callosal fibers—motor, visual, or cognitive? Our series of studies support the conclusion that it is motor. Only visual areas representing the vertical meridian have direct callosal connections, so that eccentric stimuli that require additional synaptic connections should produce a longer CUD. Thus visual transfer should be sensitive to stimulus eccentricity. More generally, only visual transfer should be sensitive to visual parameters, such as brightness. By the same token, motor transfer should be sensitive to motor parameters of the SRT paradigm, such as changing response finger or alternating finger responses. We studied a patient before and after partial callosotomy sparing the splenium of the CC. The splenium should support visual and not motor transfer. Changing visual parameters of the stimulus produced no change in the CUD before partial callosotomy, which suggests that, normally in this task callosal transfer is not visual but motor. After surgery, when the transfer of information was likely only visual, there was a change in the CUD with changing visual parameters (Iacoboni et al., 1994).

In a later study we manipulated motor and visual parameters in both normal subjects and split-brain patients. If the transfer that determines the behavioral CUD occurs at motor level, the motor manipulation should affect the

CUD in normal subjects, whereas the visual manipulation should not. Furthermore, if the effect of the motor manipulation is truly mediated by interhemispheric corticocortical connections, this effect should not be visible in split-brain patients. Again, the empirical results supported both predictions (Iacoboni and Zaidel, 1995).

As mentioned above, auditory pathways from the brainstem access both hemispheres, whereas visual projections are almost exclusively to the hemisphere opposite the visual half-field stimulated. If auditory stimuli are used instead of visual stimuli in the SRT task, one would predict no effect of crossed stimulation/response because both hemispheres receive the sensory information simultaneously, so that all conditions are actually "uncrossed." To test this hypothesis, we performed a study on a split-brain patient in which we compared the CUD obtained with SRTs to lateralized flashes and the CUD obtained with SRTs to lateralized auditory stimuli. As predicted, a very long CUD was obtained when the subject responded to visual stimuli, but almost no difference at all was observed when comparing crossed and uncrossed responses to auditory stimuli (Iacoboni and Zaidel, 1999).

Bimanual Motor Control. If the LH controls the right hand and the RH controls the left hand, how then does bimanual motor control happen and what is the role of the CC in organizing it? Classic and recent studies on callosal involvement in bimanual motor control both suggest that overlearned bimanual motor sequences, including either parallel or alternating sequences, do not require intact callosal fibers, whereas novel bimanual motor sequences, such as those requiring interdependent bimanual control, cannot be learned if callosal fibers are transected, whether in the presence of vision or in the absence of visual guidance (Zaidel and Sperry, 1977; Franz et al., 2000).

With regard to temporal and spatial characteristics of bimanual movements, it seems that the CC is important in coordinating the spatial aspects of bimanual movements and in desynchronizing bimanual movements requiring a complex temporal pattern. Franz et al. (1996) have shown that normal subjects produce trajectory errors when the spatial demands of the task differ between the two hands. Remarkably, callosal patients were not impaired in this task. Temporal synchrony, however, was similar in normal subjects and in split-brain patients, which suggests that spatial control and temporal synchronization are dissociable. In an earlier study, Tuller and Kelso (1989) demonstrated that phase-locked bimanual movements are very stable in split-brain patients, whereas intermediate states between in-phase and antiphase coordinated patterns are severely affected. This suggests that complex temporal patterns between the two hands require the desynchronizing function of callosal fibers.

More recently, Ivry and Hazeltine (1999) looked at the synchronization of manual responses to acoustic timing signals in a callosotomy patient. The task required the patient to synchronize bimanual or unimanual responses to auditory tones. Both normal subjects and the patient tested demonstrated less temporal variability in the bimanual condition, suggesting that motor commands are not integrated by callosal fibers in this task.

Deficits Due to Hemispheric Specialization. Following callosal section, right-handed patients are often unable to correctly execute those movements on verbal command with the left hand that they can readily and accurately execute with the right hand. Historically, this was the first callosal symptom described. In the absence of an elemental motor deficit, a pronounced inability to perform certain movements in the left hand to verbal command is strong evidence for a callosal lesion. There are two other explanations for this deficit, not mutually exclusive. First, it can reflect RH disconnection from LH language comprehension: the RH (left hand) cannot perform the commanded movement because it has not comprehended the command. Second, it may reflect LH dominance for motor control: the disconnected RH may understand the command, but may not have the ability to execute the command correctly. Nonverbal tasks such as imitation or the use of three-dimensional objects may help separate verbal comprehension from motor programming deficits.

The study of motor control in absence of the CC is important to better understand theoretical aspects of motor behavior and to design better interventions in clinical populations. The first systematic study of motor control in the split brain was reported by D. Zaidel and Sperry (1977) for patients in the Los Angeles series. The insight obtained from studying split-brain patients or patients born without the CC is often surprisingly different from that obtained from studying patients with unilateral brain damage. For instance, behavioral neurology studies suggest that the LH is dominant for praxis (see, for instance Chapter 11). This belief has been challenged by observations in split-brain patients. Tachistoscopic presentations of drawings of hand postures to the two visual hemifields of split-brain patients have shown that they can actually imitate hand postures with both hands, as long as the hand used for imitation is ipsilateral to the visual hemifield of presentation (Sperry, 1974). Earlier studies found no substantial difference in imitative performance between the right and the left hand (Sperry, 1974; Volpe, 1982). However, more recently, Lausberg et al. (in press) found selective left hand apraxia in pantomime to visually presented objects in split brain patients.

Compensatory Mechanisms. Immediately after surgery all of our patients were unable to perform actions to verbal commands such as "Wiggle your left toes," or "Make a fist with your left hand." The degree of left hand (and left foot) deficit is subject to individual differences. The left limb dyspraxia is attributable to the simultaneous presence of two deficits: poor comprehension by the RH (which has good control of the left hand), and poor ipsilateral control by the LH (which understands very well). Subsidence of the dyspraxia can therefore result from two compensatory mechanisms: increased RH comprehension of words, and increased LH control of the left hand. The capacity of either hemisphere, and particularly the LH, to control the ipsilateral hand varies from one patient to another both in the immediate postoperative period and many years later. The extent of ipsilateral motor control can be tested by flashing to the right or left visual half-field sketches of thumb and fingers in different postures, for the subject to mimic with one or the other hand. Responses are poor with the hand on the side opposite the visual input, with simple postures such as a closed fist or an open hand being attainable after further recovery. As recovery proceeds, good ipsilateral control is first attained for responses carried out by the more proximal musculature. After several months, most of these patients can form a variety of hand and finger postures with either hand to verbal instructions such as "Make a circle with your thumb and little finger," and the like.

Subsidence of the apraxia continues but even many years later, left-sided apraxia to verbal command can still be demonstrated (Zaidel and Sperry, 1977; Trope et al., 1987), sometimes under paradoxical circumstances. Thus, split-brain patients are sometimes unable to follow verbal commands with the left hand even though they can demonstrate separately, recognition of the printed verb and of the pictured action (cf., Zaidel, 2001).

Language

The split-brain person provides a unique perspective on the independent contribution of each cerebral hemisphere to language processing and on the role of interhemispheric interaction in normal language function. However, although the absence of the CC reduces interhemispheric facilitation, inhibition, and cooperation, it does not eliminate them completely. We will consider descriptive clinical observations of language in the acute and chronically split-brain patient, followed by an analysis of RH capacities in language comprehension and production.

Clinical Impression

Postcallosotomy mutism. It was first thought that mutism following callosotomy was simply a neighborhood sign, a partial form of akinetic mutism (without the akinesia) that resulted from retraction around the anterior end of the third ventricle during section of the anterior commissure (Cairns, 1952; Ross and Stewart, 1981; Lebrun, 1990), or retraction of medial frontal lobe (Fuiks et al., 1991; Reeves, 1991).

But there is evidence to suggest that more persistent mutism may in fact result from hemispheric disconnection rather than from medial frontal extracallosal damage. Bogen

(1998) has had a number of patients who did not have mutism, despite extensive retraction of either anterior third ventricle or mesial right frontal cortex or both. In these patients commissural section spared the splenium. Rayport et al. (1983; personal communication to J. E. Bogen from S. Ferguson in 1991) observed in three of eight cases with staged callosotomy a marked decrease in spontaneous speech without paraphasia or comprehension deficit or inability to sing. This deficit occurred only after the second stage of surgery. Notable was the absence of any mutism after the first stage (rostrum, genu, and most of the trunk); the mutism appeared only after the second stage (splenium and remainder of the trunk). It had been proposed that hemispheric disconnection may lead to mutism because of an unusual interdependence of the hemispheres in language function secondary to early brain injury. This may lead to anomalous (including bilateral) speech representation (Bogen and Vogel, 1975; Bogen, 1976; Sussman et al., 1983; Sass et al., 1990), and particularly to discordant manual and speech dominance (Ferguson et al., 1985; Spencer et al., 1988), which creates unusual dependence on interhemispheric interaction for speech programming. Mutism may thus result from interhemispheric conflict (possibly at a brainstem level) or from a bilateral diaschisis that affects speech much more than writing (Bogen, 1976; Ferguson et al., 1985).

Quattrini et al. (1997) reviewed post-callosotomy mutism in 36 patients of the Ancona series. Two out of 8 patients with complete two-stage sections and 8 out of 27 with anterior callosotomies had transient mutism lasting from 4 to 25 days. One patient with a splenial section had no mutism. The two patients with complete callosotomy had mutism after both the initial anterior and the subsequent posterior callosal sections. Mutism was accompanied by good comprehension, following of verbal commands, and writing. Recovery from mutism was always complete. Mutism was not associated with left-handedness, but it was associated with more complex surgical manipulation.

Mild pragmatic deficit. Though seemingly normal on clinical aphasiological tests, more subtle observation reveals persistent lacunae in the language repertoires of patients with cerebral commissurotomy. These lacunae include chronic impoverishment of verbal description of personal emotional experience (alexithymia, cf. TenHouten et al., 1986), failure to sustain adequate comprehension when reading paragraphs or extended text (Zaidel, 1982), and deficits in conversational interaction. The lacunae involve pragmatics, rather than phonology and syntax, and are highly variable across patients. They include social inappropriateness by failing to follow leads, using inappropriate rules of politeness, and a tendency to rationalize mistakes and confabulate reasons for strange behavior.

Formal testing of the pragmatic ability of (the LH of) commissurotomy patients L.B., N.G., A.A., and R.Y. with the RH Communication Battery (Gardner and Brownell, 1986) showed consistently severe deficits across all patients in three tests: appreciation of prosody, the understanding of pictorial metaphors, and the retelling of stories, reflecting impaired recognition of emotion, nonliteral language, and integrative processes (discourse), respectively. This suggests selective normal RH contribution to those subtests (Spence et al., 1990). To varying degrees, however, all four patients showed a consistent and frequent use of humor in conversation. They also used common idioms and proverbs appropriately and frequently, and their gestures and intonation seemed normal.

Clinical and Experimental Assessment of Language in the Disconnected Right Hemisphere. Auditory comprehension of nouns by the DRH is suggested by the subject's ability to retrieve with the left hand various objects named aloud by the examiner. Visual comprehension of printed words by the DRH is often present, especially short, concrete, high-frequency words. For example, after a printed noun is flashed to the left visual half-field, the subjects are typically able to retrieve with the left hand the designated item from among an array of objects hidden from view. Ipsilateral control by the DLH in these tests is excluded because incorrect verbal descriptions given by the subject immediately after a correct response by the left hand show that only the DRH knew the answer.

There follows a more detailed consideration of observations in two series of callosotomy patients: the Los Angeles series (Zaidel's lab) and the Dartmouth-Toledo series (Gazzaniga's lab). The two laboratories use somewhat different methodologies and one should exercise caution in making comparisons between them.

The Los Angeles Series. Experimental studies of RH language in patients with complete commissurotomy have focused on detailed case studies of L.B. and N.G. using a contact lens system for presenting extended displays and permitting free ocular scanning by one hemisphere at a time (Zaidel, 1975). But occasional studies reported some language competence in the DRHs of other patients as well. Those reports include auditory comprehension by A.A. (Nebes, 1971; Nebes and Sperry, 1971), RH execution of verbal commands by R.Y. (Gordon, 1980), phonological encoding in the RH of CC (Levy and Trevarthen, 1977), and auditory comprehension by the RH in N.W. and R.M. (Bogen, 1979).

Phonetics/phonology, syntax, lexical semantics, and pragmatics. The DRHs have poor auditory discrimination (Zaidel, 1978b) and poor phonetic identification (Zaidel, 1983) (e.g., dichotic listening to nonsense stop consonant-vowel [CV] syllables). They also have a poor short-term verbal memory (Token Test; Zaidel, 1977) with a capacity of 3 ± 1 items, similar to anterior aphasics. The DRH cannot match words for rhyming, i.e., it has no grapheme–phoneme conversion rules (Zaidel and Peters, 1981), and must read words through a lexical route (Zaidel, 1998a).

The DRH has access to some rudimentary syntactic structures, such as passives or negatives, it finds grammatical categories easier than syntactic structures, and it finds lexicalized morphological constructions easier than inflected ones. When processing syntax, it seems particularly constrained by memory load (Zaidel, 2001).

The DRH has a rich and diverse auditory lexicon and it recognizes a variety of semantic relations. It has linguistic access to both episodic and semantic information, and its semantic network is organized connotatively. The visual lexicon is smaller and organized differently. The DRH has abstract letter identities (Eviatar and Zaidel, 1994). It can perform lexical decision, and it exhibits sensitivity to word frequency (Zaidel, 2001) and concreteness (Eviatar et al., 1990) but not to grapheme–phoneme regularity (Zaidel and Peters, 1981; Zaidel, 2001). It is sensitive to format distortion (zigzag, vertical), especially for words (Zaidel, 2001).

Developmental profile. The DRH does not exhibit a uniform mental age profile in a sample of auditory language functions (Zaidel, 1978b). Its competence tends to be in the range of normal 3- to 6-year-olds, but it has little or no speech, and its auditory vocabulary can reach an adult level (Zaidel, 1976).

The Dartmouth-Toledo Series

Phonetics/phonology, syntax, and lexical semantics. Patient V.P. showed RH ability to discriminate CV syllables (Sidtis et al., 1981b), and patient J.W. showed phonetic competence in the DRH by being able to combine visual and auditory cues to produce the McGurk Illusion (Baynes et al., 1994). All five patients (P.S., V.P., J.W., D.R. and V.J.) showed good comprehension of single spoken words in the DRH. Those tested (P.S., V.P., J.W.) showed some grammatical competence. V.P. and J.W. could perform grammaticality judgments and disambiguate syntactically ambiguous sentences but not identify passive sentences. Thus, their DRHs have some grammatical competence but poor grammatical performance, similar to the California patients.

All five patients could read single words, some (J.W., D.R.) as many as they could comprehend aurally. P.S. and V.P. but not J.W. had grapheme–phoneme conversion in the DRH. All five patients displayed considerable lexical semantic flexibility in the DRH.

Writing. The acute disconnection syndrome usually includes left hand agraphia. Only P.S. and V.P. could write with the left hand. V.J.'s most severe postoperative language deficit was bilateral agraphia (Baynes et al., 1998). V.J. was left-handed and LH dominant for speech. She had two-stage callosotomy at age 41 with loss

of writing in either hand (Baynes et al., 1998). Although V.J. was LH dominant for speech, she had reduced speech output after callosotomy. Agraphia has been reported as a consequence of callosotomy in other patients discordant for speech and manual dominance (Spencer et al., 1988), but not universally (Gur et al., 1984). V.J.'s LH could speak and understand, read and spell aloud. Thus it could control both spoken and written language. V.J.'s RH could not speak but it could understand spoken and written language and make lexical decision, i.e., it is similar to the DRH of L.B. It could copy but not write spontaneously to dictation or the name of a picture in the LVF. Thus, the writing deficit of the LH appears peripheral, at the level of "allographs." V.J.'s RH, in turn, had no "output graphemic buffer" (Margolin, 1984).

Right Hemisphere Speech. One of the most important recent developments in the study of language in the DRH is arguably the emergence of RH speech. The data on RH speech from the California and Dartmouth-Toledo series can be summarized as follows (Table 14–2):

1. RH speech is most likely to occur soon after surgery and to show the greatest range in patients with early damage to language cortex in the LH.
2. Evidence for apparent RH speech is more likely to occur in patients who show evidence for linguistic transfer between the hemispheres.
3. Right hemisphere speech may develop or emerge gradually over the long term and then it may assume or lose control periodically.
4. In most patients RH speech never emerges or develops at all.

Left Agraphia. Right-handers can write legibly, if not fluently, with the left hand. This ability is commonly lost with callosal lesions, especially (but not always) those that cause unilateral apraxia (Gersh and Damasio, 1981). Inability to write to dictation is common with LH lesions (also see Chapter 7), but the deficit is almost always present in both hands. In con-

Table 14–2. Summary of Language Abilities of Right Hemispheres of Split-brain Patients from the California and Dartmouth-Toledo Series

Patient	AUDITORY LANGUAGE COMPREHENSION			READING						ACTIONS WITH LEFT HAND				
	Phonetics	Words	Sentences	Words	Sentences	GPC	Lex. Dec.	Lexical Semantics	Grammar	Pictures	Auditory	Written	Writing	Speech
L.B.	+[a]	+	–	+	–	–	+	+	+[d]	+	+[d]	+[d]	–	+[f]
N.G.	+[a]	+	–	+	–	–	+[d]	+	+[d]	+	+[d]	+[d]	–	–
R.Y.	–	+	0	+	–	–	+[d]	0	0	0	+[d]	0	–	–
A.A.	–	+	0	+	–	–	+[d]	0	0	0	+[d]	0	–	–
N.W.	0	+	0	0	0	0	0	0	0	0	+[d]	0	–	–
C.C.	0	0	0	0	0	0	0	0	0	0	+[d]	0	–	–
P.S.	0	+	+	+	0	+	0	+	+	+[c]	+[c]	+	+	+
V.P.	+[a]	+	0	+	0	+	+[d]	+	+[e]	0	+[c]	+[d]	+	+[f]
J.W.	+	+	0	+[b]	0	–	+[d]	+	+[d,e]	+	+[c]	+[d]	–	–
D.R.	0	+	0	+	–[c]	0	+[d]	+	0	0	–[f]	–[c]	–	–
V.J.	0	+	0	+	0	0	+	0	0	0	0	0	–	–

GPC, grapheme–phoneme correspondance rules; +, present; –, absent; 0, not tested.

[a]Phoneme discrimination, not identification. [b]Slow. [c]Assumed. [d]Limited. [e]Grammatically judgment but not grammatical comprehension. [f]Occasionally.

trast, patients with callosal disconnection are able to copy simple or even complex geometric figures with their left hand despite being unable to write with the left hand or even copy writing previously made with their own right hand (Bogen and Gazzaniga, 1965; Bogen, 1969a; Kumar, 1977; Zaidel and Sperry, 1977; Della Sala et al., 1991). Copying of block letters may be present when the copying of cursive writing is not; this may not represent printing with the left hand but rather only copying of geometric figures that happen also to have linguistic content.

Summary. Whereas more behavioral data are needed to characterize RH speech and more physiological data are needed to delineate the conditions under which it is expressed, the overwhelming neuropsychological evidence suggests that the DRH has a unique linguistic profile, although different experimental populations yield somewhat different profiles, and there are considerable individual differences. When the RH is disconnected from the LH, the emerging RH language profile is characterized by the following: *(1)* much better language comprehension than speech; *(2)* better auditory comprehension than reading; *(3)* visual word recognition which proceeds via (abstract) ideography or through orthographic rules, but without grapheme–phoneme translation, so that lexical representations are "addressed" rather than "assembled"; *(4)* a rich lexical semantic system but poor phonology and an impoverished syntax; and *(5)* paralinguistic competence in appreciating the communicative significance of prosody and facial expressions.

Table 14–3 shows four patterns of lexical language in the DRH. All patients have a sub-stantial auditory lexicon and at least a moderate reading vocabulary. The difference in patterns across individual patients is in terms of speech and writing. First, some patients, such as P.S. and V.P., have early evidence for rich RH speech and writing. Second, some patients, such as L.B. and J.W., develop some intermittent RH control of speech. Third, most patients, such as N.G., R.Y., A.A., and D.R., never develop RH speech. Finally, left-handed patients with LH language dominance, such as V.J., may suffer some loss of fluency and may be agraphic in both hands. The fact that all DRHs understand at least some spoken language is important to the clinician: testing of the DRH can be facilitated with verbal instructions. However, every effort should be made to illustrate the task nonverbally so as not to bias the results in favor of the DLH.

Visospatial, Visuoperceptual, and Visuoconstructive Functions

Stereopsis. Only midline stereopsis requires interhemispheric integration. Thus, off the midsagittal plane in front of or behind the fixation point, callosal section does not affect stereopsis (Gazzaniga et al., 1965). Split-brain patients show significant midline deficits with random dot stereograms with disparities ranging from 15 to 180 minute arc within 1° to 3° off the vertical meridian (Hamilton and Vermeire, 1986). In contrast, Lassonde (1986) described a deficit in tachistoscopic depth perception in commissurotomy patients over the entire field, attributable to loss of nonspecific diffuse callosal contributions (but see Rivest et al., 1994).

Table 14–3. Lexical Language in the Disconnected Right Hemisphere

Patients	Auditory Comprehension	Reading	Speech	Writing
Early RH speech: P.S., V.P.	+	+	+	+
Late, occasional RH speech: L.B., J.W.	+	+	~+	−
No RH speech: N.G., R.Y., A.A., D.R.	+	+	−	−
Left-handed, LH dominant for speech: V.J.	+	+	−	−

RH, right hemisphere; +, present; −, absent.

Space. The DRH was found to be superior to the DLH in part/whole and gestalt completion tasks (Nebes, 1974), on modified forms of standardized spatial relations tests, such as the Differential Aptitude Test (Levy, 1974; Kumar, 1977), on the use of perspective cues to assist in accurate perception (Cronin-Golomb, 1986a), and on tests of geometric invariance (Euclidean, Affine, projective, and topological) (Franco and Sperry, 1977). The DLH was found to be superior in figure–ground disembedding (Zaidel, 1978a).

More recently, Funnell et al. (1999) found that the DRH of callosotomy patient J.W. from the Dartmouth-Toledo series was superior to the DLH in matching of mirror-reversed stimuli. From their findings they concluded that both disconnected hemispheres (DHs) can perform pattern recognition, but that the DRH is specialized for processing spatial information. Corballis et al. (1999) studied illusory contours and amodal completion in two callosotomy patients from the Dartmouth-Toledo series (J.W. and V.P.) and found equal bilateral perception of illusory contours in the DHs but better amodal completion in the DRH. They concluded that illusory contours might be attributed to low-level visual processes common to both hemispheres, whereas amodal completion reflects a higher-level, lateralized process.

Because of large individual differences, results obtained from a few patients should be interpreted with caution until they are confirmed in larger samples of callosum-sectioned patients, or better, in lateralized paradigms with normal subjects.

Visual Imagery. Different components of visual imagery are differentially lateralized. Mental rotation shows superiority in the DRH (Farah et al., 1985; Corballis and Sergent, 1988). Image generation shows superiority in the DLH (Farah et al., 1985; Corballis and Sergent, 1988).

Hierarchic Perception. It has been suggested that the LH is specialized for local processing (details) or the analysis of patterns with relatively high spatial frequency, whereas the RH is specialized for global processing (wholes) or the analysis of patterns with relatively low spa-

tial frequency (Hellige, 1993). Left hemisphere perception then proceeds bottom-up, RH perception proceeds top-down, and the two streams are integrated via the CC. This conceptualization is often operationalized in the Navon paradigm (Navon, 1977). When large *H*'s or *S*'s made up of little *H*'s or *S*'s are presented peripherally to normal subjects who are required to identify the large (global) or small (local) letter (*H* or *S*). Subjects exhibit three effects: *(1)* it is easier to identify the large letters than the small letters ("global precedence" or "the level effect"); *(2)* consistent stimuli in which the large and small elements are the same (e.g., a large *H* made up of small *H*'s) are easier to identify than inconsistent stimuli in which the large and small elements are different (e.g., a large *S* made up of small *H*'s) ("the consistency effect"); and *(3)* the consistency effect is stronger for local identification ("global interference") than for global identification ("local interference"). We refer to the latter as the "asymmetric consistency effect," and it is reflected in a significant Level × Consistency interaction. In normal subjects, some find RVF specialization for identifying local targets and, less frequently LVF specialization for global targets (van Kleek, 1989). On the basis of findings in patients with unilateral temporoparietal lesions, Robertson and colleagues (1988) speculated that the consistency effect, and particularly the asymmetric consistency effect, is mediated by the CC. This predicts that the effect should be absent in patients with complete cerebral commissurotomy (Robertson and Lamb, 1991).

Robertson et al. (1993) presented hierarchic patterns in the LVF or RVF, or the same pattern simultaneously in both VFs (BVF) of commissurotomy patients L.B., N.G., and A.A., and Weekes et al. (1997) conducted a follow-up study with two of the same commissurotomy patients, using very similar stimuli and conditions. Together, the two studies observed instances of unilateral consistency effects and asymmetric effects. Three conclusions can be drawn from these results. First, the absence a Level × VF interaction is not a necessary consequence of disconnection. Second, consistency effects can occur in the absence of the CC. Third, the asymmetric consistency effect can occur in the split brain. Both disconnected hemispheres could process both local and global stimuli and each could therefore exhibit consistency effects.

Right Constructional Apraxia. By "constructional praxis" we mean the ability to put together a meaningful configuration, such as an object (three dimensions) or a complex drawing (two dimensions). *Constructional dyspraxia* is the inability to organize several parts into a configuration despite a normal ability to handle or draw the individual parts (Benton, 1962; Benton and Fogel, 1962; Warrington, 1969; De Renzi, 1982). Constructional dyspraxia can occur from lesions in either hemisphere. Left lesions may result in an absence of some of the parts and in simplified versions of a model, and RH lesions tend to result in inappropriate relationships among the parts, including a loss of perspective in drawings intended to represent three dimensions (Paterson and Zangwill, 1944; Warrington et al., 1966; Benton, 1967; Hécaen and Assal, 1970; Gainotti et al., 1977).

Constructional apraxia can be quite prominent in the right hand of right-handers with callosal lesions. Hemisphere disconnection (in a right-hander) is strongly suggested if the patient can copy designs better with the left hand than with the right (Bogen, 1969b; Yamadori et al., 1983). Of course, if a callosal lesion is accompanied by RH involvement, the left hand may be paretic or ataxic so that the patient does no better with the left hand than with the right.

Spatial Acalculia. Because of spatial disability when using the right hand, the patient with hemisphere disconnection may have difficulties using pencil and paper to solve arithmetic problems (Dahmen et al., 1982). Our patients with complete cerebral commissurotomy had some difficulty with written arithmetic, a deficit that progressively receded (Bogen, 1969a, p. 92). We were surprised to note that sometimes a patient following complete commisurotomy would have difficulty in doing arithmetic on paper whereas comparable problems could be done by mental calculation.

Attention

Attention in the split brain can be viewed more generally as a model system for the problem of intermodular communication. How can anatomically and functionally separate "modules" maintain their independence to permit parallel processing at one time, but communicate at other times?

Sleep. Sleep is controlled by the diencephalon and brainstem with ascending brainstem systems that project diffusely to both hemispheres, and it is therefore not surprising that split-brain patients are said to have normal sleep–wake cycles and synchronous EEG indices of sleep onset and arousal in the two hemispheres (Sperry, 1974).

Vigilance. There is some controversy about whether the split-brain syndrome includes abnormal gaps in vigilance and about whether the DRH is more vigilant than the DLH (Dimond, 1979) or not (Ellenberg and Sperry, 1979).

Focused Attention in Dichotic Listening. We have administered to commissurotomy patients a dichotic listening test with CV syllables (*bee, dee, gee, pee, tee, kee*) using lateralized visual probes and attention instructions (left ear, right ear, divided) (Zaidel, 1983). We found (1) exclusive LH specialization for the task and (2) ipsilateral suppression of the left ear signal in the LH. We thus inferred (3) that in the normal brain, the left ear signal is relayed from the RH to the LH vial the CC prior to processing. We found no effect of focussed attention to either ear on the right ear advantage in normal subjects but a substantial effect in a split-brain patient (L.B.). In the DLH, attention to the right ear had no effect but attention to the left ear increased the left ear score and decreased the right ear score. Similarly, in the DRH, attention to the left ear had no effect but attention to the right ear reduced the left ear score and increased the right ear score. Taken together, the data suggest that focussed attention in the split brain activates attention-specific subcallosal interhemispheric auditory channels. In the normal brain, these subcallosal channels are presumably superceded by callosal channels that are less sensitive to spatial attention.

Dichotic listening tests vary widely in the degree of temporal and acoustic overlap between left and right ear signals. The greater the overlap, the greater the ipsilateral suppression and the less susceptible is the ear advantage to modulation by focussed attention.

Covert Orienting of Spatial Attention. If each cerebral hemisphere is an independent cognitive system, then each has an independent control system, i.e., an independent attentional mechanism that regulates the resources and operations of the hemisphere. But split-brain patients largely behave as well-integrated and coordinated organisms, and this suggests that there is an overall, shared attentional system that coordinates the interaction of the two disconnected hemispheres. This creates a puzzle: is attention in the split brain divided or shared? Four interrelated solutions have been proposed.

1. Stage of processing. The two disconnected hemispheres can select stimuli, encode them, decode and select responses independently, but they share response execution mechanisms to avoid behavioral conflict. Thus, early stages of processing show attentional disconnection, whereas late stages of processing are attentionally unified (Reuter-Lorenz, in press).

2. Automatic vs. controlled attention. One distinguishes fast automatic orienting due to peripheral cues that are not informative from slow strategic orienting due to central cues when valid cues predominate (cf. Briand and Klein, 1987). Automatic orienting of spatial attention is believed to be controlled by the parietal–putamen–superior colliculus complex (Posner and Dehaene, 1994). By contrast, controlled orienting of spatial attention may also engage the frontal lobe in an executive role (Mesulam, 1990). Reuter-Lorenz (in press) argues that when spatial attention is oriented automatically via a peripheral cue, there is evidence for independent and parallel attentional systems in the two disconnected hemispheres,

whereas when attention is oriented strategically via a central cue, there is evidence for a shared attentional system.

3. Location- vs. object-based attention. Corballis (1995) argues that location-based attention, as in covert orienting in space, is unified, whereas object-based attention is divided. He argues that location-based attention is mediated subcortically by the superior colliculus and the second visual system just mentioned, also believed to mediate unconscious "blind sight" and projecting via the pulvinar to extra striate cortex. In the split brain, this system applies to spatial information in the periphery as well as close to fixation, and it does not require sustained input. Object-based attention, by contrast, is cortically mediated via the geniculostriate system and is necessary for conscious identification of form information.

Cortically vs. subcortically mediated attention. The subcortical system is unified via the intercollicular commissure or perhaps via the diencephalon, midbrain, or cerebellum (Trevarthen, 1991), whereas the cortical system is divided. The cortical–subcortical distinction applies both to attention and to perception (Corballis, 1995). Thus, it is not the case simply that attention is integrated in the split brain while perception is divided, as originally claimed by Gazzaniga (1987). None of the four views completely accounts for all available data. Some key experiments are reviewed below.

Spatial Cueing

Simple reaction time (SRT). In Posner's cue paradigm (1980), two or more positions across the vertical meridian are predesignated as potential target locations. One of these locations is cued centrally (symbolically, e.g., a letter *L* or *R*) or peripherally (at the location of the target, e.g., a box around the stimulus location) before the onset of the target. The task is an SRT with unimanual button presses. Responses to cued targets are usually faster than responses to uncued targets. Cued targets usually yield a small facilitation (benefit) relative to a neutral cue (e.g., cueing all the targets).

Uncued targets usually exhibit a (larger) inhibition (cost) relative to the neutral cue. The cost and benefit are often conceptualized as being due to shifts of attention in space. Recall that one distinguishes fast (<350 msec between cue and target) automatic priming due to uninformative (mostly invalid) peripheral cues from controlled slow priming (>350 msec) due to central informative (mostly valid) cues. What would we predict about valid vs. invalid cueing across the vertical meridian in the split brain? If the two hemispheres have independent attentional systems, then the most straightforward prediction is that there should be no benefit or cost to such cues. Any validity–invalidity effect across the vertical meridian in the split brain is presumably mediated by a unified attentional system that represents both VFs, a system that has access to ipsilateral visual cue information or to other subcallosal interhemispheric cue information. But would such validity/invalidity, benefits/costs be greater or smaller in the split brain than in the normal brain? The simplest prediction is that they should be smaller. Otherwise, subcallosal channels must have spatial orienting functions that are normally suppressed by the CC but released following callosal section.

Reuter-Lorenz and Fendrich (1990) used a Posner paradigm with informative peripheral cues with long stimulus onset asynchrony (SOAs) and observed unified attention in patients with complete callosotomies. By contrast, Arguin et al. (2000) used informative central cues and intermediate SOAs and found that some but not all callosotomy patients showed attentional disconnection and some anterior callosotomy patients also showed attentional disconnection. Thus, conflict in the literature exists and there is a need for a common methodology. Nonetheless, two conclusions emerge. First, attention can be split in the disconnection syndrome Second, some subcallosal channels can mediate attentional interactions in the split brain.

Passarotti et al. (unpublished data; Zaidel, 1994) administered to commissurotomy patients L.B. and N.G. different versions of the Posner experiment with both peripheral and semi-central informative cues and SOAs ranging from 150 to 250 msec. Targets appeared in one of four boxes in the corners of a square centered at fixation. In this way we could compare neutral and valid trials to invalid trials crossing the horizontal meridian, invalid trials crossing the vertical meridian, and invalid trials crossing both. The results with both paradigms showed complex attentional interactions between the two VFs, both facilitatory and inhibitory, consistent with unified attention. These data are consistent with a model which assumes that (1) the RH has as attentional map that includes both VFs, whereas the LH has an attentional map that includes only the RVF; (2) the LH controls attention to RVF targets and the RH controls attention to LVF targets; (3) the two hemispheres show different patterns of costs and benefits, with the RH more likely than the LH to show costs due to invalid cues; (4) the two attentional systems can maintain independence in the normal brain; (5) the attentional system in the RH has both callosal and subcallosal access to RVF information; (6) both the callosal and subcallosal interhemispheric attentional effects include facilitatory as well as inhibitory components; and (7) there are large individual differences across split-brain patients in the nature of subcallosal attention effects present. In particular, the data from L.B. together with the data from normal subjects suggest that there is an asymmetric, callosally mediated mirror image facilitation from the RVF to the LVF, as well as a subcallosally mediated mirror image inhibition in the same direction. In the normal brain, callosal facilitation dominates, whereas the split brain unmasks subcallosal inhibition. Our data suggest that, contrary to Reuter-Lorenz's hypothesis, automatic attention can be unified between the two disconnected hemispheres.

Spatial cueing in choice reaction time. Similar discrepancies are reported for spatial cueing in choice RT tasks. Thus, Holtzman (1984) found evidence for shared attention, whereas Mangun et al. (1994) found evidence for independent attentional systems in the disconnected hemispheres. In both experiments, subjects made binary choices of cued lateralized targets. Holtzman used central cues and large (1500 msec) SOAs, whereas Mangun et al. used peripheral cues and shorter SOAs (150–600 msec). Thus, different attentional systems may have been engaged in the two tasks. It is important to note that even though invalid cues crossing the vertical meridian had an effect, demonstrating some unification of attention between the two disconnected hemispheres, it is nonetheless the case that invalid cues crossing the midline affected target detection in the other hemisphere rather differently (more extremely) than invalid cues within the same hemisphere as the target. Thus, unification is far from normal. The CC appears to be necessary for modulating some of the extreme effects of orienting to peripheral stimuli in the split brain.

Visual Search. Search of visual targets among distractors engages controlled attention and its speed is negatively correlated with the number of distractors when it requires feature conjunction, i.e., when the target is composed of a conjunction of features that are also present in the distractors (Treisman and Gelade, 1980). Is visual search in one visual hemifield sensitive to distractors in the other visual hemifield? Luck et al. (1989) showed that, unlike normal subjects, one callosotomy patient (J.W.) and one commissurotomy patient (L.B.) exhibited search times for targets in one VF which were independent of the number of distractors in the other. This then is an example of divided, controlled attentional systems, arguing against the automatic–controlled, divided–unified hypothesis of Reuter-Lorenz. The results are consistent with the location- vs. object-based and subcortical–cortical hypotheses of Corballis (1995), since the visual search task of Luck et al. is most likely object based and cortically mediated.

An opposite result was obtained by Pollmann and Zaidel (1998), who studied the effects of ipsilateral and contralateral distractors on lateralized visual search in two commissurotomy patients N.G. and L.B. Targets and distractors varied in relative salience. In general, distractors slowed down the search for contralateral targets, showing that, contrary to Luck et al., the search was not independent in the two hemispheres. This effect was equally true for low-salience targets with high-salience distractors and for high-salience targets with low-salience distractors, arguing against the automaticity hypothesis of Reuter-Lorenz. However, the response arrangement was unique: patients were asked to press a button with their left finger if a target was present in the LVF and to press another button with the right hand if a target was present in the RVF. Thus, both hemispheric response systems were poised to respond, and this may have activated interhemispheric interaction to prevent conflict. By contrast, Luck et al. used bimanual responses, which may not invoke a strategic response competition (Reuter-Lorenz, in press).

Pollmann (1996) had demonstrated earlier an extinction-like asymmetry in the search task using low-salience targets and high-salience distractors in the normal brain: RVF distractors interfered with LVF targets but not vice versa. This effect was reversed in commissurotomy patient L.B., who is not able to transfer visual form information between the hemispheres, but not in N.G., who is able to transfer such information. This is another example of attentional interdependence, albeit abnormal, between the disconnected hemispheres. Pollman and E. Zaidel, moreover, proposed a model for the interdependence. They considered two competing models for the contralateral distractor asymmetry in normal subjects: (1) Kinsbourne and Bruce's (1987) proposal that the LH orienting system is dominant, and (2) Heilman et al.'s (1987) and Mesulam's (1981) proposal that the RH has a more bilateral coverage in space, together with (3) the proposal that the RH is dominant for spatial orienting (Heilman and Van Den Abell, 1980). The search data in splits support elements from both of the earlier proposals. They are consistent with a model of an attentional gradient for the whole field in each hemisphere, but one that is steeper in the LH. This explains the reversed contralateral distractor asymmetry in L.B. by absence of ipsilateral visual information rather than by subcallosal inhibition. The model assumes that there are independent attentional systems in the two disconnected hemispheres, but it does not assume that they interact directly. The model suggests that the CC has a limited role in spatial orienting during search, and this may help explain the absence of neglect phenomenon in the disconnected hemispheres (Plourde and Sperry, 1984). (Several split-brain studies have even reported rightward attentional biases in visual tasks; see Proverbio et al., 1994; Reuter-Lorenz et al., 1995; Berlucchi et al., 1997).

Hemispheric specialization. Pollmann and E. Zaidel's (1998) controlled visual search experiments (with targets, nontargets, and distractors) revealed a LH advantage in L.B. for both low- and high-effort searching, with and without ipsilateral distractors. N.G. showed no hemispheric difference. By contrast, Pollmann and E. Zaidel's (1999) controlled visual search experiments (with targets and nontargets only) suggested an RH advantage in L.B. and an LH advantage for N.G. for both low- and high-effort searching. Kingstone et al. (1995) asked whether there is a consistent hemispheric specialization for *guided* visual search, where (effortful, controlled) conjunction search is constrained to a subset of items that share a target feature, thus rendering the search more efficient. They used "congruent responding" (press a right-hand key when a target is present in the RVF, etc.) and long presentations while monitoring eye fixation. The task was administered to callosotomy patients J.W., V.P., and D.R. All patients scanned bilateral arrays twice as fast as unilateral arrays with the same number of stimuli, thus confirming Luck et al.'s evidence of divided attention. J.W. and D.R. exhibited a RVF advantage for the standard conjunction search and a selective RVF benefit from guided search. VP exhibited a LVF advantage for standard search and no advantage from the guided search. Kingstone et al. concluded that guided search is specialized in the LH and attribute VP's discrepancy to individual differences. Taken together, the data from both series of patients suggest dramatic individual differences in hemispheric specialization for attentional tasks and individual shifts across tasks. Generalization from a limited group of patients and tasks is therefore unwise.

In sum, there is abundant evidence for interhemispheric attentional effects in the split brain. It appears that some levels of processing automatically engage interhemispheric integration by interactions between the two attentional systems, even in the split brain. Other levels of processing permit hemispheric independence in cognition by also segregating the attentional systems of the two disconnected (and normal) hemispheres.

Dual Tasks. Two early experiments showed that hemispheric disconnection can produce superior performance of two concurrent tasks. Gazzaniga and Sperry (1966) required subjects to perform two different visual discriminations simultaneously in the two VFs. Unlike normal subjects, commissurotomy patients performed the tasks equally well concurrently and alone. Ellenberg and Sperry (1979) reported similar results from a tactile sorting task performed either unimanually or bimanually without visual guidance, even when opposite sorting rules applied for the two VF-response hand combinations. Franz et al. (1996) showed an analogous effect in a drawing task.

Other studies of dual tasks show dominance by the hemisphere that is specialized for processing the stimuli or by the hemisphere that controls the response mode (Levy et al., 1972). This is consistent with the stage-of-processing hypothesis of Reuter-Lorenz.

Experiments on the psychological refractory period (PRP) suggest that the attentional systems of the two disconnected hemispheres are unified. In the typical PRP paradigm, subjects are required to perform two different tasks in a fixed order. Typically, the RT for task 2 increases as the SOA between stimuli in the two tasks decreases. It is believed that the PRP effect reflects a bottleneck in response selection or movement production for task 2 (Reuter-Lorenz, in press). Contrary to expectation, the PRP in callosotomy patient J.W. was robust and similar to that in normal subjects (Pashler et al., 1995), even when the tasks were felicitous for each hemisphere (Ivry et al., 1998). Unlike normal subjects, however, the PRP in J.W. was not affected by the consistency of stimulus–response (S-R) mapping in the two VFs (Ivry et al., 1998). Taken together, this implies that each disconnected hemisphere can maintain distinct rules for S-R mapping and can select the appropriate response without interference from the other hemisphere, but the two hemispheres cannot initiate independent responses (Reuter-Lorenz, in press). This pattern would be consistent with the stage-of-processing hypothesis of Reuter-Lorenz.

Redundant Target Effects. Detection or identification of targets is facilitated when redundant copies of the target appear. This phenomenon is called the "redundant target effect" (RTE) and it reflects parallel processing with unlimited resources. There are at least two possible mechanisms for the RTE: *(1)* a horse race between two independent equal processes that operate at the stage of response generation (probability summation); and *(2)* neural interaction/co-activation between the stimulus copies, leading to hyper-priming that surpasses a horse race and operates at an early processing stage, presumably at a secondary sensory area (neural summation) (Miller, 1982). One may expect a similar RTE within a VF in a normal and a split brain, but a reduced RTE between the two VFs in split-brain patients compared to normal subjects. Instead, when the redundant targets occur in both VFs, there is a standard RTE (which does not exceed a horse race) in the normal brain but there may be a paradoxically large hyper-RTE (which shows neural summation) in the split brain. This was shown both for SRT (Reuter-Lorenz et al., 1995) and for controlled visual search (Pollmann and E. Zaidel, 1999). Iacoboni and E. Zaidel (in press) found that the hyper-RTE in the split brain was greater when bilateral targets were blocked than when they alternated randomly with unilateral targets or with redundant targets in the same VF. This means that the neural summation can emerge in a single trial but that it can be enhanced by repetition in time.

The hyper-redundant target effect. Iacoboni et al. (2000) examined the RTE in SRT in two patients with complete commissurotomy (L.B. and N.G.), two patients with complete callosotomy (D.T. and G.C.), three patients with anterior callosal section (B.M., J.P., and D.W.), and two patients with agenesis of the CC (M.M. and J.L.). The occurrence of a hyper-RTE (violation of the horse race inequality), signaling neural summation, was not associated with a specific callosal pathology: two patients with complete commissurotomy, one patient with complete callosotomy, and one patient with agenesis of the CC exhibited a hyper-RTE. Instead, the hyper-RTE was associated with long CUDs, exceeding 15 msec (Fig. 14–1). This must be the time window that permits neural co-activation.

The selective susceptibility of the split brain to redundant targets appears to be a useful clinical tool for establishing structural disconnection because it is unconscious. Unfortunately, it provides a sufficient but not a necessary sign. The RTE is certainly a useful test for implicit perception and has been used in blindsight, in hemianopsia due to hemispherectomy (Tomaiuolo et al., 1997), in neglect (Marzi et al., 1996), and in cortical blindness (Iacoboni et al., 1996b). The hyper-RTE appears to include an attentional release phenomenon due to removal of callosal function and it may lead to special skills in target detection but also increased distractibility in such cognitive activities as reading.

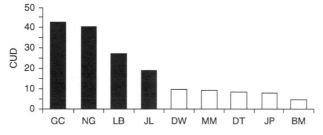

Figure 14–1. The crossed–uncrossed difference in simple reaction time (SRT) to lateralized flashes as a measure of interhemispheric transfer time in patients with callosal involvement. Black bars, patients who show a hyper-redundant target effect in SRT; white bars, patients who do not show a hyper-redundant RTE. G.C. and D.T. had complete callosotomy. N.G. and L.B. had complete commissurotomy. D.W., B.M., and J.P. had an anterior callosal section. J.L. and M.M. had agenesis of the corpus callosum. Iacoboni et al. (2000). Reprinted with permission from Oxford University Press.

An fMRI experiment with an agenesis patient (J.L.) showed that neural summation was associated with activation in medial and lateral right extrastriate regions (Iacoboni et al., 2000). We interpreted this as sensory cortical modulation of collicular activity. It is consistent with the view that neural summation occurs at a sensory level. Indeed, Corballis (1998) observed a hyper-RTE in split-brain patients when the targets and background were different in luminance, but this reduced to a "standard" RTE with equiluminant targets and background. This implicates the superior colliculus in the hyper-RTE because that structure is believed to modulate luminance but not color information. By contrast, fMRI of the standard RTE in the normal brain was associated with bilateral premotor activation (Iacoboni and E. Zaidel, unpublished data), consistent with the view that probability summation occurs at a late stage of response programming.

Pollmann and E. Zaidel (1999) observed a hyper-RTE during a controlled visual search in patient L.B. and in N.G. The hyper-RTE occurred in a more effortful search with high-salience distractors and low-salience targets but not in a less effortful search with high-salience targets and low-salience distractors. Patients responded unimanually with response hand fixed within trial blocks. The hyper-RTE occurred for the slower hemisphere (hand-visual hemifield) of both patients. This argues against the tonic-inhibition-of-response model of the RTE proposed by Reuter-Lorenz et al. (1995), which is indifferent to response hand.

Corballis (1998) noted that even while equiluminance reduced the RTE, it did not universally affect the CUD, arguing for an independence of the CUD and RTE, allegedly counter to Iacoboni et al. (2000). However, Iacoboni and E. Zaidel's argument that the hyper-RTE occurs for "callosally challenged" patients with CUDs larger than ~15 msec applies to midbrain-mediated neural summation, which is precluded in Corballis's second experiment.

The Effect of Response Mode. Lateralized hemifield testing of split brain patients in simple or choice RT tasks usually takes one of three forms: *(1)* blocked unimanual responses;

(2) congruent field–hand responses, where subjects respond to LVF targets with the left hand and to RVF targets with the right hand; and *(3)* simultaneous bimanual responses. These different modes can be expected to engage different degrees of attentional interhemispheric interaction and the experimenter should choose among them carefully. One may expect congruent responding to increase hemispheric independence and bimanual responding to increase interhemispheric interaction. Instead, Luck et al. (1989) found evidence for divided attention during visual search using bimanual responses, whereas Pollmann and E. Zaidel (1998) found evidence for unified attention during visual search using congruent responses. Thus, task demands can override response mode in engaging independent attentional systems in the two disconnected hemispheres. However, one may expect blocked unimanual responses to increase interhemispheric interaction, and that is what we found. Pollmann and E. Zaidel (1999) found an interhemispheric hyper-RTE in L.B. using visual search with high attentional demands when employing unimanual responses but not when employing congruent responses (Pollmann and E. Zaidel, unpublished data). Taking the interhemispheric hyper-RTE as an index of unified attention, this means that unimanual responses increase interhemispheric interaction relative to congruent responses. We conclude that the three response modes engage unified attention decreasingly in the following order: unimanual > congruent > bimanual.

Brain Imaging of Response Selection. A different perspective on motor control issues in the split brain is derived from neuroimaging studies. For example, deoxyglucose mapping of the macaque brain has shown that reaches toward visual targets in split-brain monkeys are largely controlled by the contralateral hemisphere and involve a large network of visual, motor, and integrative areas (see review in Savaki and Dalezios, 1999). With regard to the role played by callosal fibers in transhemispheric motor inhibition, a series of studies had previously shown that the primary motor activation in one hemisphere is associated with primary motor inhibition in the opposite hemisphere (Meyer et al., 1998; Allison et al., 2000, and references therein). However, transhemispheric motor inhibition may be in principle mediated by cortico-subcortico-cortical pathways rather than by callosal pathways. To test this hypothesis, we recently performed an fMRI study on a chronic commissurotomy patient and on normal controls. Subjects were required to perform unimanual movements with the right hand in response to visual stimuli. Normal subjects demonstrated the expected pattern of activation of the contralateral motor cortex and inhibition of the ipsilateral motor cortex. In the split-brain patients, however, we observed only a contralateral primary motor activation during unimanual right-hand movements (Iacoboni et al., unpublished observation). This suggests that the transhemispheric motor inhibition observed during unimanual movements in normal subjects is callosally mediated.

Memory

Short- and Long-term Memory in Complete and Partial Commissurotomy Patients. Sectioning the CC alone or in conjunction with other neocortical commissures leads to impairments in recent memory (reviewed in (D. Zaidel, 1990b), but in the absence of extensive extracallosal damage, no amnesia-like symptoms are observed. The forebrain commissures are most likely important in the encoding rather than in the retrieval stages. Semantic knowledge (D. Zaidel, 1994; Cronin-Golomb, 1995) or episodic events occurring before surgery are remembered (Sperry et al., 1979; D. Zaidel, 1994). Explicit and implicit memory, verbal or visual processes are functional after surgery (Huppert, 1981; Cronin-Golomb et al., 1996), as is procedural memory for motor skills (D. Zaidel and Sperry, 1977), albeit all at a level lower than normal. Unilateral memory, even when hemispheric specialization for the material is dominant, is impaired (Milner and Taylor, 1972; Milner et al., 1990). The first systematic memory study following surgical section of the CC, and to date still with the greatest number of cases ($N = 10$), was of eight patients with single-stage, complete commissurotomy (CC, anterior, and hippocampal com-

missures) and two with partial commissurotomy of the CC (splenium left intact and anterior commissure sectioned) in the Bogen-Vogel (Caltech) series (D. Zaidel and Sperry, 1974; D. Zaidel, 1990b). Previously, a mild though persistent recent memory impairment following the surgery had been noted by family members. Severe amnesia has never been observed. Memory for personal or historical events occurring prior to surgery continued to be intact after surgery (Sperry et al., 1979; D. Zaidel, 1993). Memory deficit on a specific test in the same patients was also confirmed by Milner and Taylor (1972). These patients were given six standardized tests of recent memory postoperatively, including the Wechsler Memory Scale (WMS). This battery tested memory for pictured objects, nonverbal visual designs, sequential and temporal–spatial order, verbal paired-associates, digit span, and other related measures (for a detailed review, see D. Zaidel, 1990b). The findings revealed that the most substantial decrement in recent memory was seen in patients with complete commissurotomy, but even when the disconnection syndrome is absent, as was the case with the two partial commissurotomy patients, memory scores were below normal. There were no systematic tests of memory preoperatively in this group. But because patients suffer from a high rate of epileptic seizures and receive high doses of anticonvulsant medication preoperatively, and surgery often reduces both the need for anticonvulsant medication and the frequency of seizures, it is unlikely that comparison of pre- vs. postoperative testing can validly assess the contribution of comissurotomy to memory loss.

Mild to moderate memory impairments have also been documented in patients who have undergone callosotomy (CC section alone) to control intractable epilepsy (LeDoux et al., 1977; Ferguson et al., 1985; Phelps et al., 1991). In the Wilson-Dartmouth series, a case report was published of a 15-year-old boy with RH atrophy and substantial right temporal lobe damage incurred at age 10 with reportedly no memory impairment (LeDoux et al., 1977). Close scrutiny of this report, however, reveals below-normal performance on the story passages of the WMS, the scores being closely similar to those obtained by the two partial commissurotomy patients in the Bogen-Vogel series described above.

Subsequently, standardized memory tests were administered to a few additional patients in the Wilson-Dartmouth series, some with partial and some with complete callosotomy (Phelps et al., 1991). The patients with complete collosotomy and those with posterior callosal sections were found to have consistent memory deficits, but not those with anterior callosotomy. In contrast to these findings, a published report described seven patients with anterior callosotomy due to aneurysms of the conjuctival and pericallosal arteries who developed memory disturbances following surgery (Simernitskaia and Rurua, 1989).

Role of the Fornix in Memory. In none of the 10 cases of the Bogen-Vogel series is there bilateral fornix damage, as judged by surgical estimates; in several cases there is no damage at all, and in some there is only partial unilateral interruption. It is hardly plausible to attribute the results of the memory tests administered to these patients to the status of the fornix, as others have erroneousely suggested (LeDoux et al., 1977; Clark and Geffen, 1989; Berlucchi and Aglioti, 1999).

Role of the Hippocampal Commissure in Memory. The hippocampal commissure connects the left and right hippocampi. It is just beneath the posterior portion of the CC. In humans it is relatively much smaller than in monkeys, cats, or rats (Amaral et al., 1984) and its functionality in humans has been questioned (Wilson et al., 1987). It was sectioned in the eight complete commissurotomy patients but not in partial commissurotomy cases or in partial callosotomy patients in whom the splenium was left intact. And yet memory deficits were found in two patients with partial commissurotomy. Thus, attributing anterograde memory problems in callosum-sectioned patients to the status of the hippocampal commissure (Clarke et al., 1989; Phelps et al., 1991; Berlucchi et al., 1995;Baynes and Gazzaniga, 2000) may not be justified.

Role of the Anterior Commissure in Memory. The role of the anterior commissure alone in the memory scores is difficult to assess in the

Bogen-Vogel cases since it was sectioned in all cases, and there are few reports of sections restricted to this commissure. However, judging from the split-brain work with monkeys by Doty and colleagues (1994), this commissure alone does not seem to play a critical role in human memory.

Conclusions about the Role of Corpus Callosum in Memory. When posterior regions of the callosum are damaged, memory for visual material suffers, regardless of whether the patients have had complete callosal section (D. Zaidel and Sperry, 1974; D. Zaidel, 1990a) or only section of the posterior callosal regions (Phelps et al., 1991; Rudge and Warrington, 1991). Multiple variables may affect scores on memory tests. Even so, three observations are worth pointing out:

1. Some memory decrement, varying from mild to substantial in severity, is often present following section of the CC alone, or following only a small lesion in the CC.
2. Single, as opposed to serial, section does not appear to affect occurrence of memory impairment.
3. The word association and story passages subtests of the WMS appear to be sensitive to partial or complete forebrain commissurotomy. These tasks most likely depend on intact interhemispheric integration. The mechanism for the integration is a matter for speculation at this point.

In humans, unilateral hemisphere lesions may be associated with memory loss, whereas in animals bilateral lesions are required. We may speculate that in humans, asymmetry in the memory functions of the two hemispheres (see D. Zaidel, 1990a, 1994; Beardsworth and D. Zaidel, 1994), increases the need for mechanisms of integration between the hemispheres. Whereas evidence suggests a progressive phylogenetic reduction in hippocampal commissural connections from rats to cats to monkeys and to humans (Amaral et al., 1984; Pandya and Rosene, 1985; Rosene and Van Hoesen, 1987; Wilson et al., 1990), we suggest that the CC may function to integrate the specialized memory functions of the two hemispheres.

INTERHEMISPHERIC TRANSFER

In spite of complete disconnection, residual transfer of information, ranging from sensory to abstract, has been repeatedly reported. The classic test of transfer is verbalization of stimuli presented to the nonverbal (right) hemisphere. There are many possible explanations for this, including *(1)* ipsilateral projection of sensory information from the LVF to the LH where verbalization occurs; *(2)* improper lateralization of stimuli; *(3)* transfer of cognitive information sufficient to identify the stimulus to the LH following recognition by the RH; *(4)* cross-cueing from the RH to the LH, using shared perceptual space (e.g., the RH may fixate on a related item in the room, thus identifying it to the LH, or it may trace the shape of the object in question with the head so the movement can be "read off" by the LH) (Bogen, 1998); or *(5)* if all other alternatives are ruled out, RH speech (see above).

SENSORY INFORMATION

Ambient (Peripheral) Vision

Trevarthen and Sperry (1973) described residual transfer following complete cerebral commissurotomy of gross peripheral changes in *(1)* movement, *(2)* orientation, *(3)* position, *(4)* size, and *(5)* brightness. They attributed it to a subcortically mediated, "second," extrageniculostriate and primitive ambient visual system. This system, which is dedicated to space around the body, involves projections from the superior colliculus to the pulvinar and visual association areas of the cortex, and allows for transfer between sides via brainstem commissures following cerebral commissurotomy. Trevarthen contrasted the subcortical, peripheral, space-based ambient system with the cortical, foveal, object-based focal geniculostriate system which mediates shape perception and is disconnected by the surgery. Use of the contact lens for hemispheric scanning (Zaidel, 1975) provides optimal conditions to test for interhemispheric transfer and did disclose shape transfer (verbalization of LVF stimuli) of simple binary sensory features, such as curved vs. straight, long or short, single or two parts.

Focal (Parafoveal) Vision

More recent experiments suggest that foveal visuospatial information can also transfer in the split brain. Holtzman (1984) showed that callosotomized patients could direct their eyes to a *location* in one VF on the basis of a location cue in the other VF. However, they could not direct their eyes to a *shape* in one VF on the basis of a shape cue in the other VF. Sergent (1987) showed transfer of orientation, alignment (location + orientation), and angle, and Corballis (1984) refined these findings. Ramachandran et al. (1986) found that commissurotomized subjects experienced apparent motion when two stimuli in different locations were presented in rapid succession, even when the stimuli were distributed across the midline. This finding was disputed by Gazzaniga (1987) but confirmed by Naikar and Corballis (1996). Naikar (1999) showed that the direction but not the color of bilateral apparent motion stimuli can be perceived in the split brain, arguing for a superior–collicular mediation of apparent motion across the vertical meridian. Apparent motion is presumably inferred from subcortically based shifts of attention (Naikar and Corballis, 1996).

Sergent (1991) also showed transfer of area size (large/small), and spatial direction (left/right, above/below), but the task included only three levels in each stimulus dimension and the results can be explained by subcortical transfer or cross-cueing of one bit of information. For example, the cue may be a subtle raising or lowering of the tongue inside the mouth (Corballis, 1995).

TRANSFER OF ABSTRACT CONCEPTS

There are many examples of subcortical transfer of abstract semantic features of the stimulus, generally without making complete identification possible. Those features include affective and connotative information (e.g., happy, sad) (E. Zaidel, 1976; Sperry et al., 1979), associative features, both perceptual and semantic (Myers and Sperry, 1985), categorical information (e.g., "animals that go in the water," where one picture is shown to each VF simultaneously), functional features (e.g., "shoe-sock") and abstract semantic relations (e.g., communication: envelope-telephone) (Cronin-Golomb, 1986b).

Sergent argued that some commissurotomy patients could transfer the concept of a "vowel" (Sergent, 1983), of "green" (Sergent, 1986), "odd or even" (Sergent, 1987), or "add up to less than 10" (Sergent, 1987). But these can all be explained by a simple guessing strategy based on the information in one VF, or by the transfer of binary information (Corballis, 1995). Sergent (1987) also found that split-brain patients could determine whether four-letter strings straddling the midline were words or not, although they could not identify them. However, Corballis and Trudel (1993) could not replicate this with a larger set of stimuli that precluded cross-cueing. Sergent (1990) further reported that commissurotomy patients could compare digits across the vertical meridian under certain instructions (press one key if either digit is higher than the other, and press another key if they are equal) but not with other instructions (same–different judgment). Again, appropriate strategies and binary transfer can explain some success, but Corballis (1995) failed to replicate the findings with the same patients and Seymour et al. (1994) failed to replicate them with others. Overall, then, Sergent's data provide little support for the transfer of high-level information about shape or quantity, or for sophisticated transfer at an implicit rather than an explicit level.

For one of the patients tested by Sergent, N.G., we now have evidence that, although she cannot name LVF stimuli, N.G. can integrate surprisingly complex form information across the midline. She was able to compare meaningless Vanderplas shapes just as well between as within the hemispheres (Zaidel, 1994), independent of the visual complexity of the stimuli (Clarke, 1990). She could compare letters across the midline by shape (A-A or a-a) but not by name (A-a) (Eviatar and Zaidel, 1994). She could compare primary colors or shades of colors between the two hemifields but only when luminance was not equal (Weems and Zaidel, unpublished data). Finally, she could match across the two VFs two faces with identical views but not with rotated views (Weems and Zaidel, unpublished data). Thus, she seemed unable to transfer person identity nodes. We can take N.G.'s transfer to be automatic and unconscious (correct same–different judgment but no identification) and thus identify the information-processing locus of attention/consciousness. In N.G. that locus is quite late or deep.

DOUBLE DISSOCIATION BETWEEN LEFT HEMI-ANOMIA AND CROSS-HEMISPHERE COMPARISONS

The two classical symptoms of the disconnection syndrome, namely, LVF anomia and failure of cross-integration across the midline, can show double dissociation in the chronic condition. On the one hand, L.B. can name some LVF pictures, letters, or words without being able to make same–different judgments about the same stimuli across the vertical meridian (see RH speech). On the other hand, N.G. can make accurate same–different judgments about visual stimuli in the two visual hemifields, without being able to name the same stimuli in the LVF.

It is important to notice that neither misnaming of LVF stimuli alone nor failure at cross-matching alone is sufficient to establish complete disconnection. For example, cross-matching may fail in the absence of disconnection because of a tendency to neglect one hemifield with bilateral presentation even while accurate verbalizing of LVF stimuli is preserved. Conversely, verbalizing of LVF stimuli may fail in the absence of disconnection, where cross-matching is present, because the transferred code may be so degraded as to be sufficient only for visual pattern matching but not for stimulus identification.

Intriligator et al. (1995) reported a pattern similar to L.B.'s in A.C., a patient who had a lesion of the posterior third of his CC. He could name unilateral or bilateral stimuli in both VFs, ranging in complexity from sine wave gratings to faces and objects. He could not, however, compare (same–different) the same stimuli across the vertical meridian, although he could compare them within either VF. This implies that interhemispheric transfer for visual comparisons and for naming is carried out by different callosal channels, the former more posterior than the latter.

IMPLICIT TRANSFER

We define interhemispheric transfer in the split brain as being implicit if both verbalization of LVF stimuli and cross-matching on demand fail (i.e., disconnection is present), but there is nonetheless some automatic influence of the unattended stimulus in one VF (the distractor) on a conscious decision of an attended stimulus in the other (the target). Given L.B.'s and J.W.'s ability to name some LVF pictures or words (see RH speech) and N.G.'s ability to compare shapes across the vertical meridian, the preconditions for implicit transfer may not be satisfied and may need to be assessed for each task and patient on a case-by-case basis. The canonical case for implicit priming in the split brain would require *(1)* evidence for failure of explicit transfer, *(2)* information about priming within each disconnected hemisphere, and *(3)* evidence for significant priming between the disconnected hemispheres. We may even require converging evidence from the normal brain. Several examples of alleged implicit priming follow.

Lambert (1993) showed presumed *negative priming* of a RVF target by a LVF prime in a lexical categorization task in both normal subjects and L.B. However, this result awaits confirmation because the targets that showed inhibition were different from those that did not, and various control conditions were not reported.

Iacoboni and E. Zaidel (1996) used a lateralized lexical decision task with simultaneous bilateral stimulus strings and with unilateral targets cued peripherally. Normal subjects exhibit three distinct distractor effects of a letter string in the unattended field on the decision of the target in the attended field. First, there is a *lexicality priming effect*, such that unattended word distractors enhance decision of word targets relative to unattended nonword distractors, especially in the LVF (Iacoboni and Zaidel, 1996). This effect persists in the split brain (L.B.) although it is mediated by different, subcallosal channels (Zaidel, 1994). Sec-

ond, there is a bilateral loss that is selective for words, i.e., lexical decision of unilateral word targets is more accurate than of word targets accompanied by *different* word or nonword distractors (Iacoboni and Zaidel, 1996). This effect is absent or dramatically reduced in the split brain (L.B.). Third, bilateral presentation of the *same* target speeds up RVF decisions of word targets in normal subjects (Mohr et al., 1994) but not in L.B. (Mohr et al., 1994a). Taken together, the results suggest that the split brain prevents the normal implicit sharing of lexical resources between the two hemispheres, but nonetheless permits implicit transfer of postlexical decision codes.

Weekes and E. Zaidel (1996) used a version of the Stroop task with spatially separate color patches and color words and with unimanual rather than verbal responses. The spatial separation permits a comparison of the Stroop effects within and between the hemispheres; and unimanual responses (pressing one of three keys) permit probing of either hemisphere. Both the spatial separation and the unimanual responses dilute the Stroop effect but do not eliminate it (Weekes and Zaidel, 1996). Both N.G. and L.B. showed significant Stroop effects within and between the hemispheres (Zaidel, 1994; Weekes and Zaidel, unpublished data).

Complex implicit facilitatory and inhibitory subcallosal effects occur in covert orienting of spatial attention using the Posner paradigm of cueing in SRT (see Attention, above).

Finally, perhaps the most dramatic example of implicit transfer in the split brains is the enhanced redundant target effects (hyper-RTE) in SRT and choice RT (see Attention, above). Some callosal patients show co-activation of detection or identification of unilateral targets by bilateral copies in the other VF, and this fails to occur in the normal brain. It appears that the CC normally serves to modulate or inhibit some of these automatic interactions.

In sum, complete cerebral commissurotomy allows explicit and implicit transfer of information about location, orientation, size, and movement through the collicular visual system. There are large individual differences, however, in the transfer of object (shape) information. Color information is least likely to transfer. Response codes in choice tasks can also transfer, even for abstract decisions. Some semantic, especially affective, information can transfer. Thus, it is critical for the investigator to assess transfer before measuring hemispheric competence along some experimental variable in the disconnected hemispheres on a case-by-case basis.

PARTIAL DISCONNECTION

The effects of partial disconnection are not yet completely understood. Some conflict exists between the symptoms following surgical disconnection and those following disconnection due to traumatic or cerebrovascular accidents. Symptoms tend to be more dramatic with natural lesions, perhaps because of associated extracallosal damage.

Anatomical (Aboitiz et al., 1992), physiological (Chen, 1986), and behavioral/clinical data (see below) support the view that the CC contains modality-, material-, and function-specific channels for communication and control that interconnect homotopic regions in the two cerebral hemispheres (Zaidel et al., 1990; Zaidel and Iacoboni, in press) (Fig. 14–2). The anteroposterior arrangement of those channels respects the anteroposterior arrangement of the corresponding cortical regions: going in a caudal–rostral direction the splenium interconnects visual cortices, the isthmus probably interconnects auditory cortices and superior temporal lobes, the posterior midbody interconnects somatosensory cortices, the anterior midbody interconnects motor cortices, and the genu interconnects frontal cortices. Aboitiz et al. (1992) compared the number of small unmyelinated fibers that predominantly interconnect association cortex with the number of myelinated fibers that predominantly interconnect sensory motor cortex. They found complementary distributions for the two types of fibers: small fibers predominated in anterior and posterior callosal regions, whereas large fibers predominated in the posterior midbody and locally in the posterior splenium. Assignment of callosal channels to specific tasks has barely been attempted. Clarke and E. Zaidel

(1994) explored the conjecture (Galaburda et al., 1990) that the connectivity of callosal channels is inversely proportional to the asymmetry of the module that they interconnect. Using both anatomical morphometric callosal measures and lateralized behavioral data in normal subjects, they concluded that lexical access is processed in superior–posterior temporal regions that interconnect through the isthmus, whereas phonetic perception is processed in frontal regions that interconnect through the anterior callosum.

THE ANTERIOR COMMISSURE

Patients with complete callosotomy sparing the anterior commissure are said to exhibit a generalized but not the complete disconnection syndrome (Sidtis et al., 1981b). They exhibit somatosensory auditory, and, usually but not always, visual disconnection. Left hemialexia/hemianomia may (Risse et al., 1978) or may not (McKeever et al., 1981) be present. They do not exhibit olfactory disconnection (Risse et al., 1989).

DiVirglio et al. (1999) found interhemispheric inferotemporal and occipital projections through the anterior commissure in humans and suggested that they may mediate visuosemantic information. Indeed, Laura-Grotto et al. (submitted) describe a callosotomy patient, M.E., with a right prefrontal lesion who was unable to read LVF words but could name some LVF pictures and make semantic decisions about LVF pictures. The authors attributed these symptoms to visuosemantic transfer via the anterior commissure in a patient with LH speech.

THE SPLENIUM

Complete section of the splenium is necessary and sufficient for visual disconnection (Maspes, 1948), but hemianomia or hemialexia are not invariably present. The splenium appears to contain several different channels. The posterior splenium may transfer nonverbal visual information, whereas the anterior splenium may transfer verbal visual information (Damasio and Damasio, 1983). The posterior splenium (and genu) was severed in a Japanese pa-

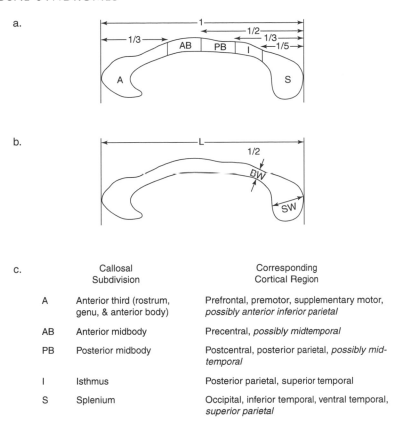

Figure 14–2. *a,b:* Scheme for partitioning the midsagittal cross-sectional area of the human corpus callosum (Witelson, 1989). BW, minimum body width; L, total anterior–posterior callosum length; SW, maximum splenial width. *c:* Putative topographic relationships between five callosum subdivisions and corresponding cortical regions are based on findings from the rhesus monkey (Pandya and Seltzer, 1986) and human (de Lacoste et al., 1985). *c:* Italicized cortical regions represent potentially positive findings in the human that were not found in the rhesus monkey. Positive findings in the rhesus monkey were not found in the human case studied by Degos et al. (1987). (Adapted from Clarke, 1990.)

tient who attempted suicide with an ice pick (Abe et al., 1986). This resulted in a more severe left hemialexia for Kana (phonological script) than for Kanji (logographical script). Cohen and Dehaene (1996) described a patient with an infarct in the posterior half of the CC. There was a disconnection for Arabic digits and for numerosity but transfer for approximate magnitude of the digits.

THE ISTHMUS

Section of the isthmus of the CC usually (Alexander and Warren, 1988) but not always (Sugishita et al., 1995) results in auditory disconnection. This is best demonstrated by a massive right ear advantage (left ear suppression) in dichotic listening to stop consonant-vowel syllables (see Audition). The anterior splenium may subserve auditory interhemispheric transfer in some subjects (Sugishita et al., 1995).

THE BODY

Lesions in the body of the CC often result in more or less severe tactile or motor disconnection (Jeeves, 1979; Bentin et al., 1984; Mayer et al., 1988). Tactile disconnection consists of failure of interhemispheric tactile transfer and results in left hand tactile anomia. Section of the anterior body may result in left hand apraxia to verbal command (see above). Section of the posterior body may result in left hand agraphia.

ANTERIOR CALLOSOTOMY SPARING THE SPLENIUM

Surgical section of the anterior two-thirds of the CC may paradoxically result in few or no disconnection symptoms. Auditory disconnection may be present depending on the posterior extent of the lesion. There may be mild deficit in bimanual coordination and in tactile or motor transfer. Memory for new events may also be impaired (Gordon, 1990). This contrasts with natural lesions to those parts, which may prevent cross-modal associations and may result in left unilateral agraphia and apraxia.

CONSCIOUSNESS

Descartes (1649) believed that the special structure for consciousness should be "in the middle," "n'est nullement le coeur, ni aussi tout le cerveau, mais seulement la plus intérieure de ses parties, qui est une certaine glande fort petite, située *dans le milieu* de sa substance." [emphasis added]. ["it is neither the heart nor the entire cerebrum, but the most interior of its parts, which is a certain very small gland situated in the middle of its substance."] No such midline structure, however, exists (the pituitary and pineal no longer being credible candidates).

Each disconnected hemisphere possesses not only a separate sensory-motor interface with the environment, its own perceptual, mnestic, cognitive, and linguistic repertoires, but also a distinct personality and distinct feelings, as well as characteristic preferences and dislikes (Zaidel, 1994). Thus, the two hemispheres have similar, but not identical, concepts of self, past and future, family, social culture, and history. Sperry et al. (1979) studied the reactions of the two disconnected hemispheres of L.B. and N.G. to pictures of self, relatives, pets, and belongings, and of public, historical, and religious figures and personalities from the entertainment world. They found

a characteristic social, political, personal, and self-awareness roughly comparable in the two sides of the same subject. However, Schiffer et al. (1998) probed more deeply into the psychological status of the two hemispheres of L.B. and A.A. and found that they have different perspectives on the world, especially with regard to self-image and childhood memories. Informal testing (E. Zaidel, unpublished data) suggests that the DRH has a rather conventional self-image ("super ego"), akin to RH affinity for conventional scenes and stereotypical concepts (D.W. Zaidel, 1990a; see Memory, above).

The experience of dreams may be affected by commissurotomy. E. Zaidel found that N.G. and L.B. from the Los Angeles series do not report dreams (unpublished data), but Greenwood et al. (1977) found normal dream report in some callosotomy patients from the Dartmouth series. Hoppe (1977) interviewed 12 commissurotomy patients and found that their dreams lacked condensation, displacement, and symbolization, and that their fantasies were unimaginative, utilitarian, and tied to reality. Their symbolizations were concrete, discursive, and rigid.

Each hemisphere can adapt to new situations and solve complex reasoning problems (Zaidel, 1981; Zaidel et al., 1981). After some testing experience with patients, examiners spontaneously refer to the two hemispheres as if they were distinct people, e.g., "the LH was upset at the RH responses today." While such references may be regarded as shorthand for patterns of behavior with specific lateralized stimuli and responses, they nonetheless express a strong phenomenological sense of two coexisting streams of consciousness. Both hemispheres can probably be simultaneously and independently conscious; both can simultaneously possess conflicting wills so that the split brain can exhibit two distinct, and possibly incompatible, loci of moral responsibility (Iacoboni et al., 1996a; but see MacKay and MacKay, 1982).

Recognizing that the DRH is conscious provides additional evidence that language is not necessary for human consciousness. More important, using the split brain as a model for the normal mind, a normal individual's consciousness can then be viewed as the net result of an interaction among at least two distinct states of consciousness. The question then arises why the normal person with an intact brain experiences consciousness as unified rather than dual. Sperry reasoned that normal consciousness is a higher emergent entity that transcends the separate awareness in the connected LH and RH, supersedes them in controlling thought and action, and integrates their activity. Instead, we argue that normal consciousness is also dual, with partially separate parallel processing in the two hemispheres that sometimes results in subjective feelings of conflict. This implies a duality of the mechanisms for consciousness (Bogen, 1995a, 1995b, 1997, 2000). Moreover, some normal subjects behave like split-brain patients during lateralized tests, thus demonstrating spontaneous or dynamic functional disconnection (Iacoboni et al., 1996a).

It can be argued that consciousness presupposes adaptive problem solving and complex cognition, and that, other things being equal, more complex cognition entails greater consciousness. Since the CC is important for modulating cognition (e.g., Weekes and E. Zaidel, 1995a,b, 1997), it follows that consciousness in the unified brain is different from the sum of each consciousness of the two disconnected hemispheres together. The normal CC permits hemispheric dominance by callosal inhibition as well as interhemispheric interaction by callosal facilitation. Thus, the cognitive repertoire of the unified brain is richer than the sum of the cognitive repertoires of the two disconnected hemispheres.

It is noteworthy that the two chronically disconnected hemispheres generally do not engage in overt conflict. This is partly explained by characteristic RH passivity, LH dominance, and a unified system of motor control, as well as shared subcortical structures. Intermanual conflict has usually been observed in the acute stage following surgical disconnection and in partial disconnection due to natural lesions, as in cases of the alien (anarchic) hand syndrome. However, even in the chronic stage we often encounter LH disbelief of intentional RH output.

In sum, each disconnected hemisphere is a model of a whole brain, complete with representations of the self and of the environment and the perceptual–cognitive repertoire to manipulate them. Each disconnected hemisphere is also separately conscious. How and where their separate sets of consciousness are integrated remains a major challenge for cognitive neuroscience. Especially promising is a research program aimed at characterizing the self-concept in each disconnected (and normal) hemisphere and discovering how the interaction of the two gives rise to a unified individual self-concept.

NOTES

1. When we actually read Le Beau, we find that the rest of his sentence is "but this, in any case, is insufficient to permit more than a clinical suspicion of localization in the CC. Most of the time, there is nothing of the sort" (p. 1370). And on the very first page of his extensive article, Le Beau says, "The clinical diagnosis of these tumors is hardly possible, because there is no callosal syndrome" (p. 1365). Finally, in his summary he states, "in particular there is no characteristic mental deficit and no apraxia" (p. 1381).

REFERENCES

Abe, T., Nakamura, N., Sugishita, M., Kato, Y., and Iwata, M. (1986). Partial disconnection syndrome following penetrating stab wound of the brain. *Eur. Neur.* 25:233–239.

Aboitiz, F., Scheibel, A. B., Fisher, R. S., and Zaidel, E. (1992). Fiber composition of the human corpus callosum. *Brain Res.* 598:143–153.

Aglioti, S., Tassinari, G., Corballis, M. C., and Berlucchi, G. (2000). Incomplete gustatory lateralization as shown by analysis of taste discrimination after callosotomy. *J. Cogn. Neurosci..* 12:238–245.

Aglioti, S., Tassinari, G., Fabri, M., Del Pesce, M., Quattrini, A., Manzoni, T., and Berlucchi, G. (2001). Taste laterality in the split brain. *Eur. J. Neurosci.,* 13:1–8.

Akelaitis, A. J. (1944–45). Studies on the corpus callosum, IV: Diagnostic dyspraxia in epileptics following partial and complete section of the corpus callosum. *Am. J. Psychiatry 101*:594–599.

Alexander, M. P. and Warren, R. L. (1988). Localization of callosal auditory pathways: a CT case study. *Neurology 38*:802–804.

Allison, J. D., Meador, K. J., Loring, D. W., Figueroa, R. E., and Wright, J. C. (2000). Functional MRI cerebral activation and deactivation during finger movement. *Neurology* 54:135–142.

Allison, T., and Zaidel, E. (2000). Complete commissurotomy abolishes interhemispheric olfactory transfer. *J. Int. Neuropsychol. Soc.* 6:179.

Alpers, B. J. (1936). The mental syndrome of tumors of the corpus callosum. *Arch. Neurol. Psychiatry* 35:911–912.

Amaral, D. G., Insausti, R., and Cowan, W. M. (1984). The commissural connections of the monkey hippocampal formation. *J. Comp. Neurol.* 224:307–336.

Aptman, M., Levin, H., and Senelick, R. C. (1977). Alexia without agraphia in a left-handed patient with prosopagnosia. *Neurology* 27:533–536.

Arguin, M., Lassonde, M., Quattrini, A., Del Pesce, M., Foschi, N., and Papo, I. (2000). Divided visuospatial attention systems with total and anterior callosotomy. *Neuropsychologia* 38:283–291.

Baierl, P., Förster, C., Fendel, H., Naegele, M., Fink, U., and Kenn, W. (1988). Magnetic resonance imaging of normal and pathological white matter maturation. *Pediatr. Radiol.* 18:183–189.

Banks, G., Short, P., Martinez, A. J., Latchaw, R., Ratcliff, G., and Boller, F. (1989). The Alien hand syndrome: clinical and postmortem findings. *Arch. Neurol.* 46:456–459.

Barbizet, J., Degos, J. D., Leeune, A., and Leroy, A. (1978). Syndrome de dysconnection interhémisphérique avec dyspraxie diagonistique aucours d'une maladie de Marchafava-Bignami. *Rev. Neurol. (Paris)* 134:781–789.

Barbizet, J., Duizabo, P., Bouchareine, A., Degos, J. D., and Poirier, J. (1977). *Abrégé de Neuropsychologie*. Paris: Masson.

Barrett, T. W. (1969). Studies of the function of the amygdaloid complex in *Macaca mulatta*. *Neuropsychologia* 7:1–12.

Baynes, K., Eliassen, J. C., Lutsep, H. L., and Gazzaniga, M. S. (1998). Modular organization of cognitive systems masked by interhemispheric integration. *Science* 280:902–905.

Baynes, K., Funnell, M. G., and Fowler, C. A. (1994). Hemispheric contributions to the integration of visual and auditory information in speech perception. *Percept. Psychophys.* 55:633–641.

Baynes, K., and Gazzaniga, M. S. (2000). Callosal disconnection. In *Patient-Based Approaches to Cognitive Neuroscience*, M. J. Farah and T. E. Feinberg (eds.). Cambridge, MA: MIT Press, pp. 327–333.

Baynes, K., Tramo, M. J., Reeves, A. G., and Gazzaniga, M. S. (1997). Isolation of a right hemisphere cognitive system in a patient with anar-

chi (alien) hand sign. *Neuropsychologia* 8:1159–1173.

Beardsworth, E., and Zaidel, D. W. (1994). Memory for faces in epileptic children before and after unilateral temporal lobectomy. *J. Clin. Exp. Neuropsychol.* 16:738–748.

Bentin, S., Sahar, A., and Moscovitch, M. (1984). Interhemispheric information transfer in patients with lesions in the trunk of the corpus callosum. *Neuropsychologia* 22:601–611.

Benton, A. L. (1962). The visual retention test as a constructional praxis task. *Confin. Neurol.* 22:141–155.

Benton, A. L. (1967). Constructional apraxia and the minor hemisphere. *Confin. Neurol.* 29:1–16.

Benton, A. L., and Fogel, M. L. (1962). Three-dimensional constructional praxis. *Arch. Neurol.* 7:347–354.

Berlucchi, G., and Aglioti, S. (1999). Interhemispheric disconnecton syndrome. In *Handbook of Clinical and Experimental Neuropsychology*, G. Denes and L. Pizzamiglio (eds.). Psychology Press, East Sussex, pp. 635–670.

Berlucchi, G., Aglioti, S., Marzi, C. A., and Tassinari, G. (1995). Corpus callosum and simple visuomotor integration. *Neuropsychologia* 33:923–936.

Beukelman, D. R., Flowers, C. R., and Swanson, P. D. (1980). Cerebral disconnection associated with anterior communicating artery aneurysm: implications for evaluation of symptoms. *Arch. Phys. Med. Rehabil.* 61:18–23.

Bogen, J. E. (1969a). The other side of the brain. I: Dysgraphia and dyscopia following cerebral commissurotomy. *Bull. Los Angeles Neurol. Soc.* 34:73–105.

Bogen, J. E. (1969b). The other side of the brain. II: An appositional mind. *Bull. Los Angeles Neurol. Soc.* 34:135–162.

Bogen, J. E. (1976). Language function in the short term following cerebral commissurotomy. In *Current Trends in Neurolinguistics*, H. Avakian-Whitaker and N. A. Whitaker (eds.). New York: Academic Press, pp. 193–224.

Bogen, J. E. (1977). Further discussion on split-brains and hemispheric capabilities. *Br. J. Phil. Sci.* 28:281–286.

Bogen, J. E. (1979). A systematic quantitative study of anomia, tactile cross-retrieval and verbal cross-cueing in the long term following complete cerebral commissurotomy. Invited address, Academy of Aphasia, San Diego.

Bogen, J. E. (1995a). On the neurophysiology of consciousness. Part 1: Overview. *Conscious. Cogn.* 4:52–62.

Bogen, J. E. (1995b). On the neurophysiology of consciousness. Part 2: Constraining the semantic problem. *Conscious. Cogn.* 4:137–158.

Bogen, J. E. (1997). Some neurophysiologic aspects of consciousness. *Semin. Neurol.* 17:95–103.

Bogen, J. E. (1998). Physiological consequences of complete or partial commissural section. In *Surgery of the Third Ventricle, 2nd ed.*, M. L. J. Apuzzo (ed.). Baltimore: Williams and Wilkins, pp. 167–186.

Bogen, J. E. (2000). Split-brain basics: relevance for the concept of one's other mind. *J. Am. Acad. Psychoanal.* 28(2):341–369.

Bogen, J. E., Fisher, E. D., and Vogel, P. J. (1965). Cerebral commissurotomy: a second case report. *JAMA* 194:1328–1329.

Bogen, J. E. and Gazzaniga, M. S. (1965). Cerebral commissurotomy in man: minor hemisphere dominance for certain visuospatial functions. *J. Neurosurg.* 23:394–399.

Bogen, J. E., Schultz, D. H., and Vogel, P. J. (1988). Completeness of callosotomy shown by magnetic resonance imaging in the long term. *Arch. Neurol.* 45:1203–1205.

Bogen, J. E., and Vogel, P. J. (1962). Cerebral commissurotomy in man. *Bull. Los Angeles Neurol. Soc.* 27:169–172.

Bogen, J. E., and Vogel, P. J. (1975). Neurologic status in the long term following cerebral commissurotomy. In *Les Syndromes de Disconnexion Calleuse Chez L'Homme*, F. Michel and B. Schott (eds.). Lyon: Hopital Neurologique, pp. 227–251.

Bossom, J., Sperry, R. W., and Arora, H. (1961). Division of emotional behavior patterns in split-brain monkeys. *Caltech. Biol. Ann. Rep.* p. 127.

Botez, M. (1974). Frontal lobe tumours. In *Handbook of Clinical Neurology, Vol. 17*. In P. J. Vinken and G. U. Bruyn, (eds.) North Holland, pp. 234–280.

Botez, M. I., and Bogen, J. E. (1976). The grasp reflex of the foot and related phenomena in the absence of other reflex abnormalities following cerebral commissurotomy. *Acta Neurol. Scand.* 54:453–463.

Botez, M. I., and Crighel, E. (1971). Partial disconnexion syndrome in an ambidextrous patient. *Brain* 94:487–494.

Bremer, F., Brihaye, J., and André-Balisaux, G. (1956). Physiologie et pathologie du corps calleux. *Arch. Suisses Neurol. Psychiatrie* 78:31–87.

Briand, K. A., and Klein, R. M. (1987). Is Posner's "beam" the same as Treisman's "glue?" On the relation between visual orienting and feature integration theory. *J. Exp. Psychol. Hum. Percept. Perform.* 13:228–241.

Brion, S., and Jedynak, C. P. (1975). *Les Troubles du Transfert Interhémisphérique*. Paris: Masson.

Brody, B. A., Kinney, H. C., Kloman, A. S., and Gilles, F. H. (1987). Sequence of central nervous system myelination in human infancy. I. An autopsy study of myelination. *J. Neuropathol. Exp. Neurol.* 46:283–301.

Bromley, S. M., and Doty, R. L. (1995). Odor recognition memory is better under bilateral than unilateral test conditions. *Cortex* 31:25–40.

Cain, W. S. (1977). Bilateral interaction in olfaction. *Nature* 268:50–52.

Cairns, H. R. (1952). Disturbances of consciousness with lesions of the brainstem and diencephalon. *Brain* 75:109–146.

Cambier, J., Elghozi, D., Graveleau, P., and Lubetzki, C. (1984). Hemisomatagnosie droite et sentiment d'amputation par lésion gauche sous-corticale. Rôle de la disconnexion calleuse. *Rev. Neurol. (Paris)* 140:256–262.

Caselli, R. J. (1991). Rediscovering tactile agnosia. *Mayo Clin. Proc.* 66:129–142.

Chen, B. H. (1986). Selective corpus callosotomy for the treatment of intractable generalized epilepsy. *Chin. J. Neurosurg.* 1:197.

Clark, C. R., and Geffen, G. M. (1989). Corpus callosum surgery and recent memory. *Brain* 112:165–175.

Clarke, E., and O'Malley, C. D. (1968). *The Human Brain and Spinal Cord*. Berkeley: University of California Press.

Clarke, J. M. (1990). Interhemispheric functions in humans: relationships between anatomical measures of the corpus callosum, behavioral laterality effects and cognitive profiles. Unpublished doctoral dissertation, University of California, Los Angeles.

Clarke, J. M., and Zaidel, E. (1989). Simple reaction times to lateralized flashes: varieties of interhemispheric communication routes. *Brain* 112:849–870.

Clarke, J. M., and Zaidel, E. (1994). Anatomical-behavioral relationships: corpus callosum morphometry and hemispheric specialization. *Behav. Brain Res.* 64:185–202.

Clarke, S., Kraftsik, R., Van Der Loos, H., and Innocenti, G. M. (1989). Forms and measures of adult and developing human corpus callosum: is there sexual dimorpism? *J. Comp. Neurol.* 280:213–230.

Cohen, L., and Dehaene, S. (1996). Cerebral networks for number processing: evidence from a case of posterior callosal lesion. *Neurocase* 2:155–174.

Corballis, M. C. (1984). Human laterality: matters of pedigree. *Behav. Brain Sci.* 7:734–735.

Corballis, M. C. (1995). Visual integration in the split brain. *Neuropsychologia* 33:937–959.

Corballis, M. C. (1998). Interhemispheric neural summation in the absence of the corpus callosum. *Brain* 121:1795–1807.

Corballis, M. C., and Sergent, J. (1988). Imagery in a commissurotomized patient. *Neuropsychologia* 26:13–26.

Corballis, M. C., and Trudel, C. I. (1993). The role of the forebrain commissures in interhemispheric integration. *Neuropsychology* 7:306–324.

Corballis, P. M., Fendrich, R., Shapley, R. M., and Gazzaniga, M. S. (1999). Illusory contour perception and amodal boundary completion: evidence of a dissociation following callosotomy. *Journal of Cognitive Neuroscience* 11:459–466.

Critchley, M. (1930). The anterior cerebral artery and its syndromes. *Brain* 53:120–165.

Cronin-Golomb, A. (1986b). Subcortical transfer of cognitive information in subjects with complete forebrain commissurotomy. *Cortex* 22:499–519.

Cronin-Golomb, A. (1986a). Figure–background perception in right and left hemispheres of human commissurotomy subjects. *Perception* 15:95–109.

Cronin-Golomb, A. (1995). Semantic networks in the divided cerebral hemispheres. *Psychol. Sci.* 6:212–218.

Cronin-Golomb, A., Gabrieli, J. D. E., and Keane, M. M. (1996). Implicit and explicit memory retrieval within and across the disconnected cerebral hemispheres. *Neuropsychology* 10:254–262.

Dade, L. A., Jones-Gotman, M., Zatorre, R. J., and Evans, A. C. (1998). Human brain function during odor encoding and recognition. A PET activation study. *Ann. N.Y. Acad. Sci.* 855:572–574.

Dahmen, W., Hartje, W., Bussing, A., and Sturm, W. (1982). Disorders of calculation in aphasic patients: spatial and verbal components. *Neuropsychologia* 20:145–153.

Dandy, W. E. (1936). Operative experience in cases of pineal tumor. *Arch. Surg.* 33:19–46.

Damasio, A. R. (1985). The frontal lobes. In *Clinical Neuropsychology, 2nd ed.*, K. M. Heilman and E. Valenstein, (eds.). New York: Oxford University Press, pp. 339–375.

Damasio, A. R., Chui, H. C., Corbett, J., and Kassel, N. (1980). Posterior callosal section in a nonepileptic patient. *J. Neurol. Neurosurg. Psychiatry* 43:351–356.

Damasio, A. R., and Damasio, H. (1983). The anatomic basis of pure alexia. *Neurology (Cleveland)* 33:1573–1583.

Damasio, H., and Damasio, A. (1979). "Paradoxic" ear extinction in dichotic listening: possible anatomic significance. *Neurology* 29:644–653.

Degos, J. D., Gray, F., Louarn, F., Ansquer, J. C.,

Poirier, J., and Barbizet, J. (1987). Posterior callosal infarction. *Brain* 110:1155–1171.

Della Sala, S., Marchetti, C., and Spinnler, H. (1991). Right-sided anarchic (alien) hand: a longitudinal study. *Neuropsychologia* 29:1113–1127.

Della Sala, S., Marchetti, C., and Spinnler, H. (1994). The anarchic hand: a fronto-mesial sign. In *Handbook of Neuropsychology, Vol. 9*, F. Boller, and J. Grafman (eds.). Amsterdam Elsevier Science, pp. 233–255.

Denenberg, V. H. (1981). Hemispheric laterality in animals and the effects of early experience. *Behav. Brain Sci.* 4:1–49.

Denny-Brown, D. (1958). The nature of apraxia. *J. Nerv. Ment. Dis.* 126:9–32.

De Renzi, E. (1982). *Disorders of Space Exploration and Cognition*. New York: John Wiley and Sons.

Descartes, R. (1649). Les passions de l'ame. In *Descartes: Oeuvres et Lettres* (Bibliothèque de la Pléiade), A. Bridoux, (ed.). Gallimard. 1969, p. 710.

Dewson, J. H., III. (1977). Preliminary evidence of hemispheric asymmetry of auditory function in monkeys. In *Lateralization in the Nervous System*, S. Harnad et al. (eds.). New York: Academic Press, pp. 63–71.

Dimond, S. J. (1972). *The Double Brain*. London: Churchill Livingstone.

Dimond, S. J. (1979). Performance by split-brain humans on lateralized vigilance tasks. *Cortex* 15: 43–50.

Dimond, S. J., Bures, J., Farrington, L.J., and Brouwers, E. Y. M. (1975). The use of contact lenses for the lateralization of visual input in man. *Acta Psychol.* 39:341–349.

DiVirgilio, G., Clarke, S., Pizzolato, G., and Schaffner, T. (1999). Cortical regions contributing to the anterior commissure in man. *Exp. Brain Res.* 124:1–7.

Doty, R. L., Stern, M. B., Pfeiffer, C., Gollomp, S. M., and Hurtig, H. I. (1992). Bilateral olfactory dysfunction in early stage treated and untreated idiopathic Parkinson's disease. *J. Neurol. Neurosurg. Psychiatry* 55:138–142.

Doty, R. W., Negrào, N., and Yamaga, K. (1973). The unilateral engram. *Acta Neurobiol. Exp.* 33:711–728.

Doty, R. W., and Overman, W. H. (1977). Mnemonic role of forebrain commissures in macaques. In *Lateralization in the Nervous System*, S. Harnad et al. (eds.). New York: Academic Press, pp. 75–88.

Doty, R. W., Ringo, J. L., and Lewine, J. D. (1994). Interhemispheric sharing of visual memory in macaques. *Behav. Brain Res.* 20:79–84.

Doty, R. L., Shaman, P., and Dann, M. (1984). Development of the University of Pennsylvania

Smell Identification Test: a standardized microencapsulated test of olfactory function. *Physiol Behav.* 32:489–502.

Doty, R. W., Yamaga, K., and Negrào, N. (1971). Mediation of visual fear via the corpus callosum. *Proc. Soc. Neurosci.* 1:104.

Downer, J. L. de C. (1961). Changes in visual gnostic functions and emotional behavior following unilateral temporal pole damage in the split-brain monkey. *Nature 191:*50–51.

Downer, J. L. de C. (1962). Interhemispheric integration in the visual system. In *Interhemispheric Relations and Cerebral Dominance*, V. B. Mountcastle, (ed.). Baltimore: Johns Hopkins University Press, pp. 87–129.

Efron, R. (1990). *The Decline and Fall of Hemispheric Specialization.* Hillsdale, NJ: Lawrence Erlbaum Associates.

Ellenberg, L., and Sperry, R. W. (1979). Capacity for holding sustained attention following commissurotomy. *Cortex* 15:421–438.

Ellenberg L., and Sperry, R. W. (1980). Lateralized division of attention in the commissurotomized and intact brain. *Neuropsychologia* 18:411–418.

Escourolle, R., Hauw, J. J., Gray, F., and Henin, D. (1975). Aspects neuropathologiques des lésions du corps calleux. In *Les Syndromes de Disconnexion Calleuse Chez L'Homme*, F. Michel and B. Schott (eds.). Lyon: Hôpital Neurologique, pp. 41–51.

Eskenazi, B., Cain, W. S., Lipsitt, E. D., and Novelly, R. A. (1988). Olfactory functioning and callosotomy: a report of two cases. *Yale J. Biol. Med.* 61:447–456.

Ethelberg, S. (1951). Changes in circulation through the anterior cerebral artery. *Acta Psychiatr. Neurol. Suppl.* 75:3–211.

Eviatar, Z., Menn, L., and Zaidel, E. (1990). Concreteness: nouns, verbs and hemispheres. *Cortex 26:*611–624.

Eviatar, Z., and Zaidel, E. (1994). Letter matching within and between the disconnected hemispheres. *Brain Cogn.* 25:128–137.

Fabri, M., Polonara, G., Quattrini, A., Salvolini, U., Del Pesce, M., and Manzoni, T. (1999). Role of the corpus callosus in the somatosensory activation of the ipsilateral cerebral cortex: an fMRI study of callosotomized patients. *Eur. J. Neurosci.* 11:3983–3994.

Farah, M. J., Gazzaniga, M. S., Holtzman, J. D., and Kosslyn, S. M. (1985). A left hemisphere basis for visual mental imagery? *Neuropsychologia* 23:115–118.

Feinberg, T. E., Schindler, R. J., Glanagan, N. G., and Haber, L. D. (1992). Two alien hand syndromes. *Neurology* 42:19–24.

Ferguson, S. M., Rayport, M., and Corrie, W. S. (1985). Neuropsychiatric observations on behavioral consequences of corpus callosum section for seizure control. In *Epilepsy and the Corpus Callosum*, M. A. Reeves (ed.). New York: Plenum Press, pp. 501–514.

Fessard, A. E. (1954). Mechanisms of nervous integration and conscious experience. In *Brain Mechanisms and Consciousness*, J. F. Delafresnaye (ed.). Springfield, IL: C. C. Thomas, pp. 200–236.

Fisher, C. M. (1963). Symmetrical mirror movements and left ideomotor apraxia. *Trans. Am. Neurol. Assoc.* 88:214–216.

Foix, C., and Hillemand, P. (1925). Les syndromes de l'artère cérèbrale antérieure. *Encéphale* 20:209–232.

Francks, J. B., Smith, S. M., and Ward, T. M. (1985). The use of goggles for testing hemispheric asymmetry. *Bull. Psychon. Soc.* 23:487–488.

Franco, L., and Sperry, R. W. (1977). Hemisphere lateralization for cognitive processing of geometry. *Neuropsychologia* 15:107–114.

Franz, E. A., Eliassen, J. C., Ivry, R. B., and Gazzaniga, M. S. (1996). Dissociation of spatial and temporal coupling in the bimanual movements of callosotomy patients. *Psychol. Sci.* 7:306–310.

Franz, E. A., Waldie, K. E., and Smith, M. J. (2000). The effect of callosotomy on novel versus familiar bimanual actions: a neural dissociation between controlled and automatic processes? *Psychol. Sci.* 11:82–85.

Fuiks, K. S., Wyler, A. R., Hermann, B. P., and Somes, G. (1991). Seizure outcome from anterior and complete corpus callosotomy [see comments]. *J. Neurosurg.* 74:573–578.

Funnell, M. G., Corballis P. M., and Gazzaniga, M. S. (1999). A deficit in perceptual matching in the left hemisphere of a callosotomy patient. *Neuropsychologia* 37:1163–1154.

Fuster, J. M. (1989). *The Prefrontal Cortex: Anatomy, Physiology and Neuropsychology of the Frontal Lobe.* New York: Raven Press.

Fuster, J. M. (1997). Network memory. *Trends Neurosci.* 20:451–459.

Gainotti, G., Miceli, G., and Caltagirone, C. (1977). Constructional apraxia in left brain-damaged patients: a planning disorder? *Cortex 13:*109–118.

Galaburda, A. M., Rosen, G. D., and Sherman, G. F. (1990). Individual variability in cortical organization: its relationship to brain laterality and implications to function. *Neuropsychologia 28:* 529–546.

Galin, D. (1974). Implications for psychiatry of left and right cerebral specialization. *Arch. Gen. Psychiatry* 31:572–583.

Galin, D., Diamond, R., and Herron, J. (1977). Development of crossed and uncrossed tactile localization on the fingers. *Brain Lang. 4*:588–590.

Galin, D., Johnstone, J., Nakell, L., and Herron, J. (1979). Development of the capacity for tactile information transfer between hemispheres in normal children. *Science 204*:1330–1332.

Garcia Medina, M. R., and Cain, W. S. (1982). Bilateral integration in the common chemical sense. *Physiol. Behav. 29*:349–353.

Gardner, H., and Brownell, H. H. (1986). Hemispheric Communication Battery. VAMC, Boston Psychology Service.

Gazzaniga, M. S. (1970). *The Bisected Brain*. New York: Appleton.

Gazzaniga, M. S. (1987). Perceptual and attentional processes following callosal section in humans. *Neuropsychologia 25*:119–133.

Gazzaniga, M. S., Bogen, J. E., and Sperry, R. W. (1962). Some functional effects of sectioning the cerebral commissures in man. *Proc. Natl. Acad. Sci. U.S.A. 48*:1765–1769.

Gazzaniga, M. S., Bogen, J. E., and Sperry, R. W. (1963). Laterality effects in somesthesis following cerebral commissurotomy in man. *Neuropsychologia 1*:209–215.

Gazzaniga, M. S., Bogen, J. E., and Sperry, R. W. (1965). Observations on visual perception after disconnexion of the cerebral hemispheres in man. *Brain 88*:221–236.

Gazzaniga, M. S., Bogen, J. E., and Sperry, R. W. (1967). Dyspraxia following division of the cerebral commissures. *Arch. Neurol. 16*:606–612.

Gazzaniga, M. S., and Freedman, H. (1973). Observations on visual processes after posterior callosal section. *Neurology 23*:1126–1130.

Gazzaniga, M. S., and LeDoux, J. E. (1978). *The Integrated Mind*. New York: Plenum Press.

Gazzaniga, M. S., and Sperry, R. W. (1966). Simultaneous double discrimination response following brain bisection. *Psychon. Sci. 4*:261–262.

Gersh, F., and Damasio, A. R. (1981). Praxis and writing of the left hand may be served by different callosal pathways. *Arch. Neurol. 38*:634–636.

Geschwind, D. H., Iacoboni, M., Mega, M. S., Zaidel, D. W., Cloughesy, T., and Zaidel, E. (1995). The alien hand syndrome: interhemispheric motor disconnection due to a lesion in the midbody of the corpus callosum. *Neurology 45*:802–808.

Geschwind, N. (1964). The development of the brain and the evolution of language. In *Monograph Series on Language and Linguistics, Vol. 17*, C. I. J. M. Stuart (ed.). Washington, DC: Georgetown University Press, pp. 155–169.

Geschwind, N. (1974). *Selected Papers on Language and the Brain*. Boston: Reidel.

Geschwind, N., and Kaplan, E. (1962). A human cerebral deconnection syndrome: a preliminary report. *Neurology 12*:675–685.

Glickstein, M., Arora, H. A., and Sperry, R. W. (1963). Delayed/response performance following optic tract section, unilateral frontal lesion, and commissurotomy. *J. Comp. Physiol. Psychol. 56*:11–18.

Goldberg, G., Mayer, N. H., and Toglia, J. U. (1981). Medial frontal cortex infarction and the alien hand sign. *Arch. Neurol. 38*:683–686.

Goldstein, K. (1908). Zur Lehre von der motorischen Apraxie. *J. Physiol. Neurol. XI(4/5)*: 169–187 (cited by Brion and Jedynak [1975]).

Goldstein, K. (1939). *The Organism*. New York: American Book Co.

Gordon, H. W. (1973). Verbal and non-verbal cerebral processing in man for audition. Thesis, California Institute of Technology.

Gordon, H. W. (1975). Comparison of ipsilateral and contralateral auditory pathways in callosum-sectioned patients by use of a response-time technique. *Neuropsychologia 13*:9–18.

Gordon, H. W. (1980). Right hemisphere comprehension of verbs in patients with complete forebrain commissurotomy: use of the dichotic method and manual performance. *Brain Lang. 11*:76–86.

Gordon, H. W. (1990). Neuropsychological sequelae of partial of partial commissurotomy. In *Handbook of Neuropsychology, Vol. 4*, F. Boller and J. Grafman (eds.). Amsterdam: Elsevier, pp. 85–97.

Gordon, H. W., and Sperry, R. W. (1969). Lateralization of olfactory perception in the surgically separated hemispheres of man. *Neuropsychologia 7*:111–120.

Gowers, W. R. (1903). *A Manual of Diseases of the Nervous System, Vol. II (2nd ed.)*. Philadelphia: P. Blakiston's Son and Co.

Greenwood, P., Wilson, D. H., and Gazzaniga, M. S. (1977). Dream report following commissurotomy. *Cortex 13*:311–316.

Grüsser, O. J., and Landis, T. (1991). *Visual Agnosias and Other Disturbances of Visual Perception and Cognition*. London: Macmillan Press.

Gur, R. E., Gur, R. C., Sussman, N. M., O'Connor, M. J., and Vey, M. M. (1984). Hemispheric control of the writing hand: the effect of calosotomy in a left-hander. *Neurology 34*:904–908.

Hamilton, C. R. (1977). Investigations of perceptual and mnemonic lateralization in monkeys. In *Lateralization in the Nervous System*, S. Harnad et al. (eds.). New York: Academic Press, pp. 45–62.

Hamilton, C. R., and Vermeire, B. A. (1982). Hemispheric differences in split-brain monkeys learning sequential comparisons. *Neuropsychologia* 20:691–698.

Hamilton, C. R., and Vermeire, B. A. (1986). Localization of visual functions with partially split-brain monkeys. In *Two Hemispheres—One Brain: Functions of the Corpus Callosum*, F. Lepore, and M. Ptito, and H. H. Jasper (eds.). New York: Alan R. Liss, pp. 315–333.

Hamilton, C. R., and Vermeire, B. A. (1988). Complementary hemispheric specialization in monkeys. *Science* 242:1691–1694.

Harnad, S., Doty, R. W., Goldstein, L., Jaynes, J., and Krauthamer, G. (1977). *Lateralization in the Nervous System*. New York: Academic Press.

Harrington, A. (1987). *Medicine, Mind, and the Double Brain*. Princeton, NJ: Princeton University Press.

Hécaen, H., and Ajuriaguerra, J. (1964). *Left Handedness*. New York: Grune and Stratton.

Hécaen, H., and Assal, G. (1970). A comparison of constructive deficits following right and left hemispheric lesions. *Neuropsychologia* 8:289–303.

Hécaen, H., De Agostini, M., and Monzon-Montes, A. (1981). Cerebral organization in left-handers. *Brain Lang.* 12:261–284.

Head, H. (1926, reprinted in 1963). *Aphasia and Kindred Disorders of Speech, Vol. I*. New York: Hafner.

Heilman, K. M., Bowers, D., Valenstein, E., and Watson, R. T. (1987). Hemispace and hemispatial neglect. In *Neurophysiological and Neuropsychological Aspects of Spatial Neglect*, E. Marc Jeannerod and (eds.). Amsterdam: pp. 115–150.

Heilman, K. M., Coyle, J. M., Gonyea, E. F., and Geschwind, N. (1973). Apraxia and agraphia in a left-hander. *Brain* 96:21–28.

Heilman, K. M., and Van Den Abell, T. (1980). Right hemisphere dominance for attention: the mechanisms underlying hemispheric asymmetries of inattention (neglect). *Neurology* 30:327–330.

Hellige, J. B. (1993). Hemispheric asymmetry: what's right and what's left. Cambridge, MA: Harvard University Press.

Herron, J. (ed.(, (1980). *Neuropsychology of Left-Handedness*. Academic Press: New York.

Hirose, G., Kin, T., and Murakami, E. (1977). Alexia without agraphia associated with right occipital lesion. *J. Neurol. Neurosurg. Psychiatry* 40:225–227.

Holtzman, J. D. (1984). Interactions between cortical and subcortical visual areas: evidence from human commissurotomy patients. *Vision Res.* 24:801–813.

Holtzman, J. D., Sidtis, J. J., Volpe, B. T., Wilson, D. H., and Gazzaniga, M. S. (1981). Dissociation of spatial information for stimulus localization and the control of attention. *Brain* 104:861–872.

Hoppe, K. D. (1977). Split brains and psychoanalysis. *Psychoanal. Q.* 46:220–244.

Hoppe, K., and Bogen, J. E. (1977). Alexithymia in 12 commissurotomized patients. *Psychother. Psychosom.* 28:148–155.

Horel, J. A, and Keating, E. G. (1972). Recovery from a partial Klüver-Bucy syndrome in the monkey produced by disconnection. *J. Comp. Physiol. Psychol.* 79:105–114.

Hummel, T., Mohammadian, P., and Kobal, G. (1998). Handedness is a determining factor in lateralized olfactory discrimination. *Chem. Senses* 23:541–544.

Huppert, F. A. (1981). Memory in split-brain patients: a comparison with organic amnesic syndromes. *Cortex* 17:303–311.

Iacoboni, M., Fried, I., and Zaidel, E. (1994). Callosal transmision time before and after partial commissurotomy. *Neuroreport* 5:2521–2524.

Iacoboni, M., Ptito, A., Weekes, N. Y., and Zaidel, E. (2000). Parallel visuomotor processing in the split brain: cortico-subcortical interactions. *Brain* 123:759–769.

Iacoboni, M., Rayman, J., and Zaidel, E. (1996a). Left brain says yes, right brain says no: normative duality in the split brain. In *Toward a Scientific Basis of Consciousness*, S. R. Hameroff, A. W. Kasniak, and A. C. Scott (eds.). Cambridge, MA: MIT Press, pp. 197–202.

Iacoboni M., Saver J. L., and Zaidel, E. (1996b). Second visual system and blindsight: evidence from simple reaction times to bimodal (auditory and visual) stimuli. *Eur. J. Neurol. 3 (Suppl. 5)*:167–168.

Iacoboni, M., and Zaidel, E. (1995). Channels of the corpus callosum: evidence from simple reaction times to lateralized flashes in the normal and the split brain. *Brain* 118:779–788.

Iacoboni, M., and Zaidel, E. (1996). Hemispheric independence in word recognition: evidence from unilateral and bilateral presentations. *Brain Lang.* 53:121–140.

Iacoboni, M., and Zaidel, E. (1999). The crossed-uncrossed difference in simple reaction times to lateralized auditory stimuli is not a measure of interhemispheric transmission time: evidence from the split brain. *Exp. Brain Res.* 128:421–424.

Iacoboni, M., and Zaidel, E. (in press). Stable and variable aspects of callosal channels: lessons from partial disconnection. In *The Parallel Brain: The Cognitive Neuroscience of the Cor-*

pus Callosum, E. Zaidel and M. Iacoboni (eds.). Cambridge, MA: MIT Press, pp. 301–306.

Intriligator, J., Hanaff, M. A., and Michel, F. (1995). A patient suffering from damage to the posterior portion of the corpus callosum can name items in both visual fields but cannot report whether they are the same or different. *Soc. Neurosci. Abstr.* 36:5470.

Ironside, R., and Guttmacher, M. (1929). The corpus callosum and its tumours. *Brain* 52:442–483.

Ivry, R. B., Franz, E. A., Kingstone, A., Johnston, J. C. (1998). The PRP effect following callosotomy: uncoupling of lateralized response codes. *J. Exp. Psychol. Hum. Percept. Perform.* 24:463–480.

Ivry, R. B., and Hazeltine, E. (1999). Subcortical locus of temporal coupling in the bimanual movements of a callosotomy patient. *Hum. Move. Sci.* 18:345–375.

Jackson, J. H. (1874). On the nature of the duality of the brain. *Med. Press Circular.* 1:19, 41, 63. Reprinted in *Brain* 1915, and in *Selected Writings of John Hughlings Jackson, Vol. 2*, J. Taylor (ed.). London: Hodder and Stoughton, 1932, pp. 129–145.

Jacobsen, C. F., and Nissen, H. W. (1937). Studies of cerebral function in primates. IV: The effects of frontal lobe lesions on the delayed alternation habit in monkeys. *J. Comp. Physiol. Psychol.* 23: 101–112.

Jeeves, M. A. (1979). Some limits to interhemispheric integration in cases of callosal agenesis and partial commissurotomy. In *Structure and Function of Cerebral Commissures*, I. S. Russell, M. W. van Hof, and G. Berlucchi (eds.). Baltimore: University Park Press, pp. 449–474.

Jordan, T. R., Patching, G. R., and Milner, A. D. (1998). Central fixations are inadequately controlled by instructions alone: implications for studying cerebral asymmetry. *Q. J. Exp. Psychol.* 51A:371–391.

Joseph, R. (1986). Reversal of cerebral dominance for language and emotion in a corpus callosotomy patient. *J. Neurol. Neurosurg. Psychiatry* 49:628–634.

Joynt, R. J. (1974). The corpus callosum: history of thought regarding its function. In *Hemispheric Disconnection and Cerebral Function*, M. Kinsbourne and W. L. Smith (eds.). Springfield, IL: C. C. Thomas, pp. 117–125.

Joynt, R. J. (1977). Inattention syndromes in split-brain man. In *Hemi-Inattention and Hemisphere Specialization*, E. A. Weinstein and R. P. Friedland (eds.). New York: Raven Press, pp. 33–39.

Kessler, J., Huber, M., Pawlik, G., Heiss, W. D., and Markowitsch, H. J. (1991). Complex sensory cross-integration deficits in a case of corpus callosum agenesis with bilateral language representation: positron-emission-tomography and neuropsychological findings. *Int. J. Neurosci.* 58: 275–282.

Kingstone, A., Enns, J. T., Mangun, G. R., and Gazzaniga, M. S. (1995). Guided visual search is a left-hemisphere process in split-brain patients. *Psychol. Sci.* 6:11–121.

Kinsbourne, M., and Bruce, R. (1987). Shift in visual laterality within blocks of trials. *Acta Psychol.* 66:159–166.

Klouda, R. V., Robin, D. A., Graff-Radford, N. R., and Cooper, W. E. (1988). The role of callosal connections in speech prosody. *Brain Lang.* 35:154–171.

Kobayakawa T., Endo, H., Ayabe-Kanamura, S., Kumagai, T., Yamaguchi, Y., Kikuchi, Y., Takeda T., Saito, S., and Ogawa H. (1996). The primary gustatory area in human cerebral cortex studied by magnetoencephalography. *Neurosci. Lett.* 212: 155–158.

Kuhn, T. S. (1962). *The Structure of Scientific Revolutions*. Chicago: University of Chicago Press.

Kumar, S. (1977). Short-term memory for a non-verbal tactual task after cerebral commissurotomy. *Cortex* 13:55–61.

Lambert, A. J. (1993). Attentional interaction in the split-brain: evidence from negative priming. *Neuropsychologia* 31:313–324.

LaPlane, D., Levasseur, M., Pillon, B., Dubois, B., Baulac, M., Mazoyer, B., Tran Dinh, S., Sette, G., Danze, F., and Baron, J. C. (1989). Obsessive-compulsive and other behavioural changes with bilateral basal ganglia lesions. *Brain 112:* 699–725.

Lashley, K. (1929). *Brain Mechanisms and Intelligence*. Chicago: University of Chicago Press.

Lashley, K. (1951, reprinted in 1967). The problem of serial order in behavior. In *Cerebral Mechanisms in Behavior*, L. A. Jeffress (ed.). New York: Hafner, pp. 112.

Lassonde, M. (1986). The facilitatory influence of the corpus callosum on intrahemispheric processing. In *Two Hemispheres—One Brain: Functions of the Corpus Callosum*, F. Lepore, M. Ptito, and H. H. Jasper (eds.). New York: Alan R. Liss, pp. 385–401.

Lauro-Grotto, R., Tassinari, G., and Shallice, T. (submitted). Interhemispheric transfer of visual-semantic information in the callostomized brain.

Lausberg, H., Cruz, R. F., Kita, S., Zaidel, E., and Ptito, A. (in press). Pantomime to visual presentation of objects: left hand dyspraxia with complete callostomy. *Brain*.

Le Beau, J. (1943). Sur la chirurgie des tumeurs du corps calleux. *Union Med. Can.* 72:1365–1381.

Lebrun, Y. (1990). *Mutism*. London: Whurr.

LeDoux, J. E., Risse, G. L., Springer, S. P., Wilson, D. H., and Gazzaniga, M. S. (1977). Cognition and commissurotomy. *Brain 100:*87–104.

Lehman, R. A. W. (1978). The handedness of rhesus monkeys. II: Concurrent reaching. *Cortex 14:*190–196.

Leiguarda, R., Starkstein, S., and Berthier, M. (1989). Anterior callosal haemorrhage: a partial interhemispheric disconnection syndrome. *Brain 112:*1019–1037.

Levin, H. S., Eisenberg, H. M., and Benton, A. L. (eds.). (1991). *Frontal Lobe Function and Dysfunction*. New York: Oxford University Press.

Levin, H. S., Goldstein, F. C., Ghostine, S. Y., Weiner, R. L., Crofford, M. J., and Eisenberg, H. M. (1987). Hemispheric disconnection syndrome persisting after anterior cerebral artery aneurysm rupture. *Neurosurgery 21:*831–838.

Levy, J. (1974). Cerebral asymmetries as manifested in split-brain man. In *Hemispheric Disconnection and Cerebral Function,* M. Kinsbourne and W. L. Smith (eds.). Springfield, IL: C. C. Thomas, pp. 165–183.

Levy, J., and Trevarthen, C. (1977). Perceptual, semantic and phonetic aspects of elementary language processes in split-brain patients. *Brain 100:*105–118.

Levy, J., Trevarthen, C. and Sperry, R. W. (1972). Perception of bilateral chimeric figures following hemispheric deconnection. *Brain 95:*61–78.

Lévy-Valensi, J. (1910). *Le Corps Calleux* (Paris theses 448). Paris: G. Steinheil.

Ley, R. G., and Bryden, M. P. (1982). A dissociation of right and left hemispheric effects for recognizing emotional tone and verbal content. *Brain Cogn. 1:*3–9.

Lhermitte, F. (1983). "Utilization behaviour" and its relation to lesions of the frontal lobes. *Brain 106:*237–255.

Lhermitte, F., Marteau, R., Serdaru, M., and Chedru, F. (1977). Signs of interhemispheric disconnection in Marchiafava-Bignami disease. *Arch. Neurol. 34:*254.

Lhermitte, F., Pillon, B., Serdaru, M. (1986). Human autonomy and the frontal lobes. Part I: Imitation and utilization behavior: a neuropsychological study of 75 patients. *Ann. Neurol. 19:*326–334.

Liepmann, H. (1900). Das Krankheitsbild der Apraxie (motorische Asymbolie) auf Grund eines Falles von einseitiger Apraxie. *Monatsschr. Psychiatr. Neurol. 8:*182–197.

Liepmann, H., and Maas, O. (1907). Fall von linksseitiger Agraphie und Apraxie bei rechtsseitiger Lahmung. *J. Psychol. Neurol. 10:*214–227.

Luck, S. J., Hillyard, S. A., Mangun, G. R., and Gazzaniga, M. S. (1989). Independent hemispheric attentional systems mediate visual search in split-brain patients. *Nature 342:*543–545.

MacKay, D. M., and MacKay, V. (1982). Explicit dialogue between left and right half-systems of split brains. *Nature 295:*690–691.

Mangun, G. R., Luck, S. J., Plager, R., and Loftus, W. (1994). Monitoring the visual world: hemispheric asymmetries and subcortical processes in attention. *J. Cogn. Neurosci. 6:*267–275.

Marchetti, C. and Della Sala (1998). Disentangling alien hand and anarchic hand. *Cog. Neuropsychiatry 3(3):*191–207.

Margolin, D. I. (1984). The neuropsychology of writing and spelling: semantic, phonological, motor, and perceptual processes. *Q. J. Exp. Psychol. 36:*459–489.

Marie, P. (1906, reprinted in 1971). The third left frontal convolution plays no special role in the function of language. *Semaine Méd 26:*241–247. Reprinted in *Pierre Marie's Papers on Speech Disorders*, M. F. Cole and M. Cole (eds.). New York: Hafner, pp. 51–71.

Mark, V. W., McAlaster, R., and Laser, K. L. (1991). Bilateral alien hand. *Neurology 41(Supp. 1):*302.

Marzi, C. A., Bisiacchi, P., and Nicoletti, R. (1991). Is interhemispheric transfer of visuomotor information asymmetric? Evidence from a meta-analysis. *Neuropsychologia 29:*1163–1177.

Marzi, C. A., Smania, N., Martini, C., Gambina, G., Tomelleri, G., Palamara, A., Alessandrini, F., and Prior, M. (1996). Implicit redundant-targets effect in visual extinction. *Neuropsychologia 34:*9–22.

Maspes, P. E. (1948). Le syndrome expérimental chez l'homme de la section du splénium du corps calleux: alexie visuelle pure heminnopisque. Rev Neurol. (Paris). *80:*100–113.

Mayer, E., Koenig, O., Panchaud, A. (1988). Tactual extinction without anomia: evidence of attentional factors in a patient with a partial callosal disconnection. *Neuropsychologia 26:*851–868.

McKeever, W. F., Sullivan, K. F., Ferguson, S. M., and Rayport, M. (1981). Typical cerebral hemisphere disconnection deficits following corpus callosum section despite sparing of the anterior commissure. *Neuropsychologia 19:*745–755.

McNabb, A. W., Carroll, W. M., and Mastaglia, F. L. (1988). "Alien hand" and loss of bimanual coordination after dominant anterior cerebral artery territory infarction. *J. Neurol. Neurosurg. Psychiatry 51:*218–222.

Mesulam, M. M. (1981). A cortical network for directed attention and unilateral neglect. *Ann. Neurol. 10:*309–325.

Mesulam, M. M. (1990). Large-scale neurocognitive networks and distributed processing for attention, language, and memory. *Ann. Neurol. 28:* 597–613.

Meyer B.-U., Roricht S., and Woiciechowsky, C. (1998). Topography of fibers in the human corpus callosum mediating interhemispheric inhibition between the motor cortices. *Ann. Neurol. 43:*360–369.

Michel, F., and Peronnet, F. (1975). Extinction gauche au test dichotique: lésion hémisphérique ou lésion commissurale? In *Les Syndromes de Disconnexion Calleuse Chez L'Homme*, F. Michel and B. Schott (eds.). Lyon: Hôpital Neurologique, pp. 85–117.

Miller, J. (1982). Divided attention: evidence for coactivation with redundant signals. *Cogn. Psychol. 14:*247–279.

Milner, A. D., and Goodale, M. A. (1995). *The Visual Brain in Action*. Oxford, UK: Oxford University Press.

Milner, B., and Taylor, L. (1972). Right-hemisphere superiority in tactile pattern-recognition after cerebral commissurotomy: evidence for nonverbal memory. *Neuropsychologia 10:*1–15.

Milner, B., Taylor, L., and Jones-Gorman, M. (1990). Lessons from cerebral commissurotomy: auditory attention, haptic memory, and visual images in verbal associative learning. In *Brain Functions and Circuits of the Mind*, C. B. Trevarthen (ed.). Cambridge, UK: Cambridge University Press, pp. 293–303.

Milner, B., Taylor, L., and Sperry, R. W. (1968). Lateralized suppression of dichotically presented digits after commissural section in man. *Science 161:*184–186.

Mingazzini, G. (1922). *Der Balken*. Berlin: Springer-Verlag.

Mohr, B., Pulvermuller, F., Rayman, J., and Zaidel, E. (1994a). Interhemispheric cooperation during lexical processing is mediated by the corpus callosum: evidence from a split-brain patient. *Neuroreport 181:*17–21.

Mohr, B., Pulvermuller, F., and Zaidel, E. (1994b). Lexical decision after left, right and bilateral presentation of function words, content words and non-words: evidence for interhemispheric interaction. *Neuropsychologia 32:*105–124.

Myers, R. E. (1956). Function of the corpus callosum in interocular transfer. *Brain 79:*358–363.

Myers, R. E., and Sperry, R. W. (1953). Interocular transfer of visual form discrimination habit in cats after section of the optic chiasma and corpus callosum. *Anat. Rec. 115:*351–352.

Myers, R. E., and Sperry, R. W. (1958). Interhemispheric communication through the corpus callosum: mnemonic carry-over between the hemispheres. *Arch. Neurol. Psychiatry 80:*298–303.

Myers, J. J., and Sperry, R. W. (1985). Interhemispheric communication after section of the forebrain commissures. *Cortex 21:*249–260.

Naikar, N. (1999). Same/different judgements about the direction and colour of apparent-motion stimuli after commissurotomy. *Neuropsychologia 37:*485–493.

Naikar, N., and Corballis, M. C. (1996). Perception of apparent motion across the retinal midline following commissurotomy. *Neuropsychologia 34:* 297–309.

Navon, D. (1977). Forest before trees: the precedence of global features in visual perception. *Cogn. Psychol. 9:*353–383.

Nebes, R. D. (1971). Priority of the minor hemisphere in commissurotomized man for the perception of part–whole relations. *Cortex 11:* 333–349.

Nebes, R. D. (1974). Hemispheric specialization in commissurotomized man. *Psychol. Bull. 81:*1–14.

Nebes, R. D., and Sperry, R. W. (1971). Hemispheric deconnection syndrome with cerebral birth injury in the dominant arm area. *Neuropsychologia 9:*247–259.

Overman, W. H., and Doty, R. W. (1982). Hemispheric specialization displayed by man but not by macaques for analysis of faces. *Neuropsychologia 20:*113–128.

Pandya, D. N., and Rosene, D. F. (1985). Some observations on trajectories and topography of commissural fibers. In *Epilepsy and the Corpus Callosum*, A. G. Reeves (ed.). New York: Plenum Press, pp. 21–39.

Pashler, H., Luck, S. L., Hillyard, S. A., Mangun, G. R., O'Brien, S., and Gazzaniga, M. S. (1995). Sequential operation of disconnected cerebral hemispheres in split-brain patients. *Neuroreport 5:*2381–2384.

Paterson, A., and Zangwill, O. L. (1944). Disorders of visual space perception associated with lesions of the right cerebral hemisphere. *Brain 67:* 331–358.

Phelps, E. A., Hirst, W., and Gazzaniga, M. S. (1991). Deficits in recall following partial and complete commissurotomy. *Cereb. Cortex* 492–498.

Pipe, M. (1991). Developmental changes in finger localization. *Neuropsychologia 29:*339–342.

Plourde, G., and Sperry, R. W. (1984). Left hemisphere involvement in left spatial neglect from right-sided lesions: a commissurotomy study. *Brain 107:*95–106.

Poeck, K. (1984). Neuropsychological demonstration of splenial interhemispheric disconnection in a case of "optic anomia." *Neuropsychologia* 22:707–713.

Poffenberger, A. (1912). Reaction time to retinal stimulation with special reference to the time lost in conduction through nervous centers. *Arch. Psychol.* 23:1–73.

Pollmann, S. (1996). A pop-out induced extinction-like phenomenon in neurologically intact subjects. *Neuropsychologia* 34:413–425.

Pollmann, S., and Zaidel, E. (1998). The role of the corpus callosum in visual orienting: importance of interhemispheric visual transfer. *Neuropsychologia* 36:763–774.

Pollmann, S., and Zaidel, E. (1999). Redundancy gains for visual search after complete commissurotomy. *Neuropsychology* 13:246–258.

Poncet, M., Ali Chérif, A., Choux, M., Boudo-uresques, J., and Lhermitte, F. (1978). Étude neuropsychologique d'un syndrome de déconnexion calleuse totale avec hémianopsie latérale homonyme droite. *Rev. Neurol. (Paris)* 11:633–653.

Posner, M. I. (1980). Orienting of attention. *Q. J. Exp. Psychol.* 32:3–25.

Posner, M. I., and Dehaene, S. (1994). Attentional networks. *Trends Neurosci.* 17:75–79.

Proverbio, A. M., Zani, A., Gazzaniga, M. S., and Mangun, G. R. (1994). ERP and RT signs of a rightward bias for spatial orienting in a split-brain patient. *Neuroreport* 5:2457–2461.

Pujol, J., Junqué, C., Vendrell, P., Garcia, P., Capdevila, A., and Martí-Vilalta, J. L., (1991). Left-ear extinction in patients with MRI periventricular lesions. *Neuropsychologia* 29:177–184.

Quattrini, A., Del Pesce, M., Provinciali, L., Cesarano, R., Ortenzi, A., Paggi, A., Rychlicki, F., Fioravanti, P., and Papo, I. (1997). Mutism in 36 patients who underwent callosotomy for drug-resistant epilepsy. *J. Neurosurg. Sci.* 41:93–96.

Ramachandran, V. S., Cronin-Golomb, A., and Myers, J. J. (1986). Perception of apparent motion by commissurotomy patients. *Nature* 320:358–359.

Rao, S. M., Bernardin, L., Leo, G. J., Ellington, L., Ryan, S. B., and Burg, L. S. (1989). Cerebral disconnection in multiple sclerosis: relationship to atrophy of the corpus callosum. *Arch. Neurol.* 46:918–920.

Raymond, F., Lejonne, P., and Lhermitte, J. (1906). Tumeurs du corps calleux. *Encéphale* 1:533–565.

Rayport, M., Ferguson, S. M., and Corrie, W. S. (1983). Outcomes and indications of corpus callosum section for intractable seizure control. *Appl. Neurophysiol.* 46:47–51.

Reeves, A. G. (ed.) (1984). *Epilepsy and the Corpus Callosum*. New York: Plenum Press.

Reeves, A. G. (1991). Behavioral changes following corpus callosotomy. In *Advances in Neurology, Vol. 55*, D. Smith, D. Treiman, and M. Trimble (eds.). New York: Raven Press, pp. 293–300.

Reuter-Lorenz, P. A. (in press). Parallel processing in the bisected brain: implications for callosal functions. In E. Zaidel and M. Iacoboni (eds.). *The Parallel Brain: The Cognitive Neuroscience of the Corpus Callosum*. Cambridge, MA: MIT Press, pp. 341–354.

Reuter-Lorenz, P. A., and Fendrich, R. (1990). Orienting attention across the vertical meridian: evidence from callosotomy patients. *J. Cogn. Neurosci.* 2:232–238.

Reuter-Lorenz, P. A., Nozawa, G., Gazzaniga, M. S., and Hughes, H. C. (1995). Fate of neglected targets: a chronometric analysis of redundant target effects in the bisected brain. *J. Exp. Psychol. Hum. Percept. Perform.* 21:211–230.

Risse, G., Gates, J., Lund, G., Maxwell, R., and Rubens, A. (1989). Interhemispheric transfer in patients with incomplete section of the corpus callosum. *Arch. Neurol.* 46:437–443.

Risse, G. L., LeDoux, J., Springer, S. P., Wilson, D. H., and Gazzaniga, M. S. (1978). The anterior commissure in man: functional variation in a multisensory system. *Neuropsychologia* 16:23–31.

Rivest, J., Cavanagh, P., and Lassonde, M. (1994). Interhemispheric depth judgment. *Neuropsychologia* 32:69–76.

Robertson, L. C., and Lamb, M. R. (1991). Neuropsychological contributions to theories of part/whole organization. *Cogn. Psychol.* 23:299–330.

Robertson, L. C., Lamb, M. R., and Knight, R. T. (1988). Effects of lesions of temporal-parietal junction on perceptual and attentional processing in humans. *J. Neurosci.* 8:3757–3769.

Robertson, L. C., Lamb, M. R., and Zaidel, E. (1993). Interhemispheric relations in processing hierarchical patterns: evidence from normal and commissurotomized subjects. *Neuropsychology* 7:325–342.

Rosene, D. L., and Van Hoesen, G. W. (1987). The hippocampal formation of the primate brain. In *Cerebral Cortex*. E. G. Jones and A. Peters (eds.). New York: Plenum Press, pp. 345–456.

Ross, E. D., and Rush, A. J. (1981). Diagnosis and neuroanatomical correlates of depression in brain-damaged patients. *Arch. Gen. Psychiatry* 38:1344–1354.

Ross, E. D., and Stewart, R. M. (1981). Akinetic mutism from hypothalamic damage: successful treatment with dopamine agonists. *Neurology* 31:1435–1439.

Rubens, A. B., Froehling, B., Slater, G., and Anderson, D. (1985). Left ear suppression on verbal dichotic tests in patients with multiple sclerosis. *Ann. Neurol.* 18:459–463.

Rudge, P., and Warrington, E. K. (1991). Selective impairment of memory and visual perception in splenial tumours. *Brain* 114:349–360.

Sass, K. J., Lencz, T., Westerveld, M., Novelly, R. A., Spencer, D. D., and Kim, J. H. (1991). The neural substrate of memory impairment demonstrated by the intracarotid amobarbital procedure. *Arch. Neuol.* 48:48–52.

Sass, K. J., Novelly, R. A., Spencer, D. D., and Spencer, S. S. (1990). Postcallosotomy language impairments in patients with crossed cerebral dominance. *J. Neurosurg.* 72:85–90.

Savaki, H., and Dalezios, Y. (1999). 14C-deoxyglucose mapping of the monkey brain during reaching to visual targets. *Prog. Neurobiol.* 58:473–540.

Sawaguchi, T., and Goldman-Rakic, P. S. (1991). D1 dopamine receptors in prefrontal cortex: involvement in working memory. *Science* 251:947–950.

Schaltenbrand, G. (1964). Discussion. In *Cerebral Localization and Organization*, G. Schaltenbrand and C. N. Woolsey (eds.). Madison: University of Wisconsin Press, p. 41.

Schiffer, F., Zaidel, E., Bogen, J., and Chasan-Taber, S. (1998). Different psychological status in the two hemispheres of two split-brain patients. *Neuropsychiatry Neuropsychol. Behav. Neurol.* 11:151–156.

Schott, B.,Trillet, M., Michel, F., and Tommasi, M. (1974). Le Syndrome de disconnexion calleuse chez l'ambidextre et le gaucher. In *Les Syndromes de Disconnexion Calleuse Chez L'Homme*, F. Michel and B. Schott (eds.). Lyon: Hôpital Neurologique, pp. 343–346.

Schwartz, M. F., Reed, E. S., Montgomery, M., Palmer, C., and Mayer, N. H. (1991). The quantitative description of action disorganisation after brain damage: a case study. *Cogn. Neuropsychol.* 8:381–414.

Sergent, J. (1983). Unified response to bilateral hemispheric stimulation by a split-brain patient. *Nature* 305:800–802.

Sergent, J. (1986). Subcortical coordination of hemisphere activity in commissurotomized patients. *Brain* 109:357–369.

Sergent, J. (1987). A new look at the human split brain. *Brain* 110:1375–1392.

Sergent, J. (1990). Furtive incursions into bicameral minds: integrative and coordinating role of subcortical structures. *Brain* 113:537–568.

Sergent, J. (1991). Processing of spatial relations within and between the disconnected cerebral hemispheres. *Brain* 114:1025–1043.

Seymour, S. E., Reuter-Lorenz, P. A., and Gazzaniga, M. S. (1994). The disconnection syndrome: basic findings reaffirmed. *Brain* 117:105–115.

Shallice, T., Burgess, P. W., Schon, F., and Baxter, D. M. (1989). The origins of utilization behaviour. *Brain* 112:1587–1598.

Sidtis, J. J. (1988). Dichotic listening after commissurotomy. In *Handbook of Dichotic Listening: Theory, Methods and Research*, K. Hugdahl (ed.). New York: John Wiley and Sons, pp. 161–184.

Sidtis, J. J., Sadler, A. E., and Nass, R. D. (1989). Double disconnection effects resulting from infiltrating tumors. *Neuropsychologia* 27:1415–1420.

Sidtis, J. J., Volpe, B. T., Holtzman, J. D., Wilson, D. H., and Gazzaniga, M. S. (1981a). Cognitive interaction after staged callosal section: Evidence for transfer of semantic activation. *Science* 212:344–346.

Sidtis, J. J., Volpe, B. T., Wilson, D. H., Rayport, M., Gazzaniga, M. S. (1981b). Variability in right hemisphere language function after callosal section: evidence for a continuum of generative capacity. *J. Neurosci.* 1:323–331.

Simernitskaia, E. G., and Rurua, V. G. (1989). Memory disorders in lesions of the corpus callosum in man [in Russian]. *Zh. Vyssh. Nerv. Delat. Im. I P Pavlova* 39:995–1002.

Sine, R. D., Soufi, A., and Shah, M. (1984). The callosal syndrome: implications for stroke. *Arch. Phys. Med.* 65:606–610.

Sobel, N., Prabhakaran, V., Hartley, C. A., Desmond, J. E., Glover, G. H., Sullivan, E. V., and Gabrieli, J. D. (1999). Blind smell: brain activation induced by an undetected air-borne chemical. *Brain* 122(Pt 2):209–217.

Sparks, R., and Geschwind, N. (1968). Dichotic listening in man after section of neocortical commissures. *Cortex* 4:3–16.

Sparks, R., Goodglass, H., and Nickel, B. (1970). Ipsilateral versus contralateral extinction in dichotic listening from hemispheric lesions. *Cortex* 6:249–260.

Speedie, L. J., Coslett, H. B., and Heilman, K. M. (1984). Repetition of affective prosody in mixed transcortical aphasia. *Arch. Neurol.* 41:268–270.

Spence, S. J., Zaidel, E., and Kasher, A. (1990). The right hemisphere communication battery: results from commissurotomy patients and normal subjects reveal only partial right hemisphere contribution. *J. Clin. Exp. Neuropsychol.* 12:42–43.

Spencer, S. S., Gates, J. R., Reeves, A. R., Spencer, D. D., Maxwell, R. E., and Roberts D. (1987). Corpus callosum section. In *Surgical Treatment of the Epilepsies*, J. Engel, Jr. (ed.). New York, Raven Press, pp. 425–444.

Spencer, S. S., Spencer, D. D., Williamson, P. D.,

Sass, K. J., Novelly, R. A., and Mattson, R. H. (1988). Corpus callosotomy for epilepsy. II. Neuropsychological outcome. *Neurology* 38:24–28.

Sperry, R. W. (1961). Cerebral organization and behavior. *Science 133*:1749–1757.

Sperry, R. W. (1964). The great cerebral commissure. *Sci. Am. 210*:42–52.

Sperry, R. W. (1968). Mental unity following surgical disconnection of the cerebral hemispheres. *Harv. Lect. 62*:293–323.

Sperry, R. W. (1970). Perception in the absence of the neocortical commissures. *Assoc. Res. Nerv. Ment. Dis. 48*:123–138.

Sperry, R. W. (1974). Lateral specialization in the surgically separated hemispheres. In *Neuroscience 3rd Study Prog.*, F. O. Schmitt and F. G. Worden (eds.). Cambridge, MA: MIT Press, pp. 5–19.

Sperry, R. W. (1982). Some effects of disconnecting the cerebral hemispheres. *Science 217*:1223–1226.

Sperry, R. W., and Clark, E. (1949). Interocular transfer of visual discrimination habits in teleost fish. *Physiol. Zool. 22*:372–378.

Sperry, R. W., and Gazzaniga, M. S. (1967). Language following surgical disconnection of the hemispheres. In *Brain Mechanisms Underlying Speech and Language*. C. H. Millikan and F. L. Darley eds. New York: Grune and Stratton, pp. 177–184.

Sperry, R. W., Gazzaniga, M. S., and Bogen, J. E. (1969). Interhemispheric relationships: the neocortical commissures; syndromes of hemisphere disconnection. *In* Handbook of Clinical Neurology, Vol. 4. P. J. Vinken and G. W. Bruyn eds. North Holland: pp. 273–290.

Sperry, R. W., Zaidel, E., and Zaidel, D. (1979). Self recognition and social awareness in the deconnected minor hemisphere. *Neuropsychologia 17*:153–166.

Springer, S. P., and Gazzaniga, M. S. (1975). Dichotic testing of partial and complete split-brain subjects. *Neuropsychologia 13*:341–346.

Stamm, J. S., Rosen, S. C., and Godotti, A. (1977). Lateralization of functions in the monkey's frontal cortex. In *Lateralization in the Nervous System*, S. Harnad, R. W. Doty, L. Goldstein, J. Jaynes, and G. Krauthamer (eds.). New York: Academic Press, pp. 385–402.

Starkstein, S. F., Berthier, M. L., Fedoroff, P., Price, T. R., and Robinson, R. G. (1990). Anosognosia and major depression in 2 patients with cerebrovascular lesions. *Neurology 40*:1380–1382.

Stuss, D. T., and Benson, D. F. (1986). *The Frontal Lobes.* New York: Raven Press.

Sugishita, M., Otomo, K., Yamazaki, K., Shimizu, H. Yoshioka, M., and Shinohara, A. (1995). Dichotic listening in patients with partial section of the corpus callosum. *Brain 118*:417–427.

Sugishita, M., and Yoshioka, M. (1987). Visual processes in a hemialexic patient with posterior callosal section. *Neuropsychologia 25*:329–339.

Sugishita, M., Yoshioka, M., and Kawamura, M. (1986). Recovery from hemialexia. *Brain Lang. 29*:106–118.

Sussman, N. M., Gur, R. C., Gur, R. E., and O'Connor, M. J. (1983). Mutism as a consequence of callosotomy. *J. Neurosurg. 59*:514–519.

Sweet, W. H. (1945). Seeping intracranial aneurysm simulating neoplasm: syndrome of the corpus callosum. *Arch. Neurol. Psychiatry 45*:86–104.

Tabibnia, A., Kee-Rose, K., Rickels, W., and Zaidel, E. (2001). Hemispheric specialization, emotion, and alexithymia. *Cogn. Neurosci. Soc. Abstr.* 8:30.

Tanaka, Y., Iwasa, H., and Yoshida, M. (1990). Diagonistic dyspraxia: case report and movement-related potentials. *Neurology 40*:657–661.

TenHouten, W. D., Hoppe, K. D., Bogen, J. E., and Walter, D. O. (1986). Alexithymia: an experimental study of cerebral commissurotomy patients and normal control subjects. *Am. J. Psychiatry 143*:312–316.

Tomaiuolo, F., Ptito, M., Marzi, C. A., Paus, T., and Ptito, A. (1997). Blindsight in hemispherectomized patients as revealed by spatial summation across the vertical meridian. *Brain 120*: 795–803.

Tomasch, J. (1954). Size, distribution, and number of fibres in the human corpus callosum. *Anat. Rec. 119*:7–19.

Tomasch, J. (1957). A quantitative analysis of the human anterior commissure. *Acta Anat. 30*:902–906

Tramo, M. J., and Bharucha, J. J. (1991). Musical priming by the right hemisphere post-callosotomy. *Neuropsychologia 29*:313–325.

Treisman, A. M., and Gelade, G. (1980). A feature-integration theory of attention. *Cogn. Psychol. 12*:97–136.

Trescher, H. H., and Ford, F. R. (1937). Colloid cyst of the third ventricle; report of a case: operative removal with section of posterior half of corpus callosum. *Arch. Neurol. Psychiatry 37*:959–973.

Trevarthen, C. (1965). Functional interactions between the cerebral hemispheres of the split-brain monkey. In *Functions of the Corpus Callosum*, E. G. Ettlinger (ed.). London: Churchill, pp. 24–40.

Trevarthen, C. (1991). Integrative functions of the cerebral commissures. In *Handbook of Neuropsychology, Vol. 4: The Commissurotomized Brain*, R. D. Nebes (ed.). Oxford: Elsevier, pp. 49–83.

Trevarthen, C., and Sperry, R. W. (1973). Perceptual unity of the ambient visual field in human commissurotomy patients. *Brain* 96:547–570.

Trope, I., Fishman, B., Gur, R. C., Sussman, N. M., and Gur, R. E. (1987). Contralateral and ipsilateral control of fingers following callosotomy. *Neuropsychologia* 25:287–291.

Tuller, B., and Kelso, J. A. (1989). Environmentally specified patterns of movement coordination in normal and split-brain subjects. *Exp. Brain Res.* 75:306–316.

Twitchell, T. E. (1951). The restoration of motor function following hemiplegia in man. *Brain* 74:443–480.

Tzavaras, A., Hécaen, H., and Le Bras, H. (1971). Troubles de la reconnaissance du visage humain et latéralisation hémisphérique lésionnelle chez les sujets gauchers. *Neuropsychologia* 9:475–477.

Van Kleek, M. (1989). Hemisphere differences in global versus local processing of hierarchical visual stimuli by normal subjects: new data and a meta-analysis of previous studies. *Neuropsychologia* 27:1165–1178.

Volpe, B. T. (1982). Cortical mechanisms involved in praxis: observations following partial and complete section of the corpus callosum in man. *Neurology* 32:645–650.

Warren, J. M., and Nonneman, A. J. (1976). The search for cerebral dominance in monkeys. *Ann. N.Y. Acad. Sci.* 280:732–744.

Warrington, E. K. (1969). Constructional apraxia. *Handbook of Clinical Neurolology, Vol. 4.* P. J. Vinken and G. W. Bruyn eds. North Holland: pp. 67–83.

Warrington, E. K., James, M., and Kinsbourne, M. (1966). Drawing disability in relation to laterality of cerebral lesion. *Brain* 89:53–82.

Wartenberg, R. (1953). *Diagnostic Tests in Neurology.* Chicago: Yearbook Publishers.

Watson, R. T., and Heilman, K. M. (1983). Callosal apraxia. *Brain* 106:391–403.

Weekes, N., Ptito, A., and Zaidel, E. (submitted). Perceptual and hemispheric relationships in a hierarchical perception task.

Weekes, N. Y., and Zaidel, E. (1995). The effects of hormonal and psychological levels of masculinity in females on neuropsychological functioning. *JINS* 1:175.

Weekes, N. Y., and Zaidel, E. (1995). The effects of steroid hormones on interhemispheric interactions: Between- and within-subjects analyses. *JINS* 1:187.

Weekes, N. Y., Carusi, D., and Zaidel, E. (1997). Interhemispheric relations in hierarchical perception: A second look. *Neuropsychologia* 35:37–44.

Weekes, N. Y., and Zaidel, E. (1997). The effects of masculinity and menstrual stage on cognition. *JINS* 3:35.

Weekes, N. Y., and Zaidel, E. (1996). The effects of procedural variations on lateralized Stroop effects. *Brain Cogn.* 31:308–330.

West, S. E., and Doty, R. L. (1995). Influence of epilepsy and temporal lobe resection on olfactory function. *Epilepsia* 36:531–542.

Wigan, A. L. (1844). The Duality of the Mind. London: Longman, Brown, Green and Longmans. Republished in 1985 by Joseph Simon, Malibu, CA.

Wilson, C. L., Isokawa-Akesson, M., Babb, T. L., and Crandall, P. H. (1990). Functional connections in the human temporal lobe: I. Analysis of limbic system pathways using neuronal activity evoked by electrical stimulation. *Exp. Brain Res.* 82:279–292.

Wilson, C. L., Isokawa-Akesson, M., Babb, T. L., Engle, J. J., Cahan, L. D., and Crandall, and P. H. (1987). A comparative view of local and interhemispheric limbic pathways in humans: an evoked potential analysis. In *Fundamental Mechanisms of Human Brain Function* J. Engle Jr. (ed.), New York: Raven Press, pp. 27–38.

Wilson, D. H., Culver, C., Waddington, M., and Gazzaniga, M. (1975). Disconnection of the cerebral hemispheres. *Neurology* 25:1149–1153.

Wilson, D. H., Reeves, A., Gazzaniga, M., and Culver, C. (1977). Cerebral commissurotomy for control of intractable seizures. *Neurology* 7:708–715.

Wilson, S. A. K., and Bruce, A. N. (1940). *Neurology, Vol. I.* Baltimore: Williams and Wilkins.

Witelson, S. F. (1974). Hemispheric specialization for linguistic and nonlinguistic tactual perception using a dichotomous stimulation technique. *Cortex* 10:3–17.

Witelson, S. F. (1989). Hand and sex differences in the isthmus and genu of the human corpus callosum. *Brain* 112:799–835.

Wittling, W. (1990). Psychophysiological correlates of human brain asymmetry: blood pressure changes during lateralized presentation of an emotionally laden film. *Neuropsychologia* 28:457–470.

Yakovlev, P. I., and Lecours, A. R. (1967). The myelogenetic cycles of regional maturation of the brain. In *Regional Development of the Brain in Early Life*, A. Minkowski, (ed.). Edinburgh: Blackwell, pp. 3–70.

Yamadori, A., Nagashima, T., and Tamaki, N. (1983). Ideogram writing in a disconnection syndrome. *Brain Lang.* 19:346–356.

Zaidel, D., and Sperry, R. W. (1974). Memory impairment after commissurotomy in man. *Brain* 97:263–272.

Zaidel, D., and Sperry, R. W. (1977). Some long-term motor effects of cerebral commissurotomy in man. *Neuropsychologia* 15:193–204.

Zaidel, D. W. (1990a). Long-term semantic memory in the two cerebral hemispheres. In *Brain*

Circuits and Functions of the Mind, C. Trevarthen (ed.). New York: Cambridge University Press, pp. 266–280.

Zaidel, D. W. (1990b). Memory and spatial cognition following commissurotomy. In *Handbook of Neuropsychology, Vol. 4*. F. Boller and J. Grafman (eds.). Amsterdam: Elsevier, pp. 151–166.

Zaidel, D. W. (1993). View of the world from a split-brain perspective. In *Neurological Boundaries of Reality*, E. M. R. Critchley (eds.). London: Farrand Press, pp. 161–174.

Zaidel, D. W. (1994). Worlds apart: pictorial semantics in the left and right cerebral hemispheres. *Curr. Direct. Psychol. Sci.* 3:5–8.

Zaidel, E. (1973). Linguistic competence and related functions in the right hemisphere of man following commissurotomy and hemispherectomy. Ph.D. thesis, California Institute of Technology. Dissertation Abstracts International. 34:2350B (University Microfilms 73–26, 481).

Zaidel, E. (1975). A technique for presenting lateralized visual input with prolonged exposure. *Vision Res.* 15:283–289.

Zaidel, E. (1976). Auditory vocabulary of the right hemisphere following brain bisection or hemidecortication. *Cortex* 12:191–211.

Zaidel, E. (1977). Unilateral auditory language comprehension on the token test following cerebral commissurotomy and hemispherectomy. *Neuropsychologia* 15:1–17.

Zaidel, E. (1978a). Concepts of cerebral dominance in the split-brain. In *Cerebral Correlates of Conscious Experience*, P. Buser and A. Rougeul-Buser (eds.). Amsterdam: Elsevier, pp. 263–284.

Zaidel, E. (1978b). Lexical organization in the right hemisphere. In *Cerebral Correlates of Conscious Experience*, P. Buser and A. Rougeul-Buser (eds.). Amsterdam: Elsevier, pp. 263–284.

Zaidel, E. (1981). Hemispheric intelligence: the case of the Raven Progressive Matrices. In *Intelligence and Learning*, M. P. Friedman, J. P. Das, and N. O'Connor (eds.). New York: Plenum Press, pp. 531–552.

Zaidel, E. (1982). Reading in the disconnected right hemisphere: an aphasiological perspective. In *Dyslexia: Neuronal, Cognitive and Linguistic Aspects*, Y. Zotterman (ed.). Oxford: Pergamon Press, pp. 67–91.

Zaidel, E. (1983). Disconnection syndrome as a model for laterality effects in the normal brain. In *Cerebral Hemisphere Asymmetry: Method, Theory and Application*, J. Hellige (ed.). New York: Praeger, pp. 95–151.

Zaidel, E. (1994). Interhemisppheric transfer in the split brain: long-term status following complete cerebral commissurotomy. In *Brain Asymmetry*, R. J. Davidson and K. Hughdal (eds.). Cambridge, MA: MIT Press, pp. 491–532.

Zaidel, E. (1998a). Language in the right hemisphere following callosal disconnection. In *Handbook of Neurolinguistics*, B. Stemmer and H. Whitaker (eds.). San Diego: Academic Press, pp. 369–383.

Zaidel, E. (1998b). Stereognosis in the chronic split brain: hemispheric differences, ipsilateral control and sensory integration across the midline. *Neuropsychologia* 36:1033–1047.

Zaidel, E. (2001). Hemispheric specialization for language in the split brain. In *Handbook of Neuropsychology, 2nd ed., Vol. 2, Language and Aphasia*, R. Berndt (vol. eds.), F. Boller and J. Grafman (series eds.). Elsevier: Amsterdam, pp. 393–418.

Zaidel, E., Clarke, J. M. and Suyenobu, B. (1990). Hemispheric independence: a paradigm case for cognitive neuroscience. In *Neurobiology of Higher Cognitive Functions*, A. B. Scheibel and A. F. Wechsler (eds.). New York: Guilford Press, pp. 297–355.

Zaidel, E., and Frazer, R. E. (1977). A universal half-field occluder for laterality research. *Caltech Biol. Ann. Rep.* 137–138.

Zaidel, E., and Iacoboni, M. (in press.). Sensory-motor integration in the split brain. In *The Parallel Brain: The Cognitive Neuroscience of the Corpus Callosum*, E. Zaidel and M. Iacoboni (eds.). Massachusetts: MIT Press, pp. 319–336.

Zaidel, E., and Peters, A. M. (1981). Phonological encoding and ideographic reading by the disconnected right hemisphere: two case studies. *Brain Lang.* 14:205–234.

Zaidel, E., Zaidel, D. W., and Bogen, J. E. (1990). Testing the commissurotomy patient. In *Neuromethods, Vol. 15: Neuropsychology*. A. A. Boulton, G. B. Baker and M. Hiscock (eds.). Clifton, NJ: Humana Press, pp. 147–201.

Zaidel, E., Zaidel, D. W., and Sperry, R. W. (1981). Left and right intelligence: case studies of Raven's Progressive Matrices following brain bisection and hemidecortication. *Cortex* 17:167–186.

Zald, D. H., and Pardo, J. V. (1997). Emotion, olfaction, and the human amygdala: amygdala activation during aversive olfactory stimulation. *Proc. Natl. Acad. Sci. U.S.A.* 94:4119–4124.

Zatorre, R. J., and Jones-Gotman, M. (1991). Human olfactory discrimination after unilateral frontal or temporal lobectomy. *Brain* 114(Pt 1A):71–84.

15

The Frontal Lobes

ANTONIO R. DAMASIO AND STEVEN W. ANDERSON

Although this is a time of unprecedented progress in cognitive neuroscience, clinicians who evaluate and treat frontal lobe dysfunction still face many of the frustrations encountered by prior generations. Damage to the frontal lobes can disrupt in various ways a set of very complex neuroanatomical and functional systems, which for the most part remain incompletely understood. The frontal lobes make up over one-third of the human cerebral cortex and have diverse anatomical units, each with distinct connections to other cortical and subcortical regions and to each other. Although we have made progress in elucidating the connectional pattern and physiology of some of its subregions in nonhuman primates (see below), we have not had a means to map the equivalent complexity in the human brain. Paralleling the challenges presented by the anatomical complexity of the frontal lobes are those which stem from the nature of the signs and symptoms of frontal damage, since they do not lend themselves easily to quantitative analysis in a laboratory setting. Nonetheless, new findings on frontal lobe dysfunction are appearing regularly, and have provided support for some long-held suppositions as well as new ideas regarding the operations of the frontal lobes. The central role of the frontal lobes in higher cognitive activities is not in question, and there is

growing evidence that frontal dysfunction may contribute to certain psychiatric disorders.

The purpose of this chapter is to review important cognitive and behavioral changes which result from damage to the human frontal lobes. Selected findings from research with nonhuman primates and functional imaging studies of normal persons are also included. In light of the limited sensitivity and specificity of established clinical neuropsychological probes to the cognitive and behavioral defects which result from frontal lobe damage, it is particularly important for clinicians to be aware of experimental findings regarding frontal lobe dysfunction. Attention to such research will not only allow for more sophisticated conceptualizations of the behavioral problems seen in patients with frontal lobe damage, but may also provide clues to help guide development of the next generation of clinical measures.

NEUROANATOMICAL OVERVIEW

Knowledge of neuroanatomy is necessary to the understanding of frontal lobe functions and a prerequisite for the interpretation of the investigations discussed later in this chapter. For that reason, a brief review of frontal lobe morphology is presented at this point.

FRONTAL CORTEX

Inspection of the external surface of the lobe reveals three important natural borders—the Rolandic sulcus, the Sylvian fissure, and the corpus callosum—and three large expansions of cortex—in the lateral convexity, in the mesial flat aspect that faces the opposite lobe, and in the inferior concave aspect that covers the roof of the orbit. Traditional anatomy has divided this cortex into the following principal regions: the precentral cortex, the prefrontal cortex, and the limbic cortex (Fig. 15–1).

The *precentral cortex* corresponds to the long gyrus immediately anterior to the rolandic fissure, forming its anterior bank and depth. This area continues over the mesial lip of the lobe, forming the anterior part of the paracentral lobule. Histologically it is a region of agranular cortex and its function as the primary motor area is well known. The presence of Betz cells is a distinguishing feature. In Brodmann's map (Fig. 15–1), it corresponds to field 4. Anterior and parallel to this region lies the *premotor cortex*, which in humans corresponds to the posterior portion of the three horizontally placed frontal gyri. Histologically, this is a transitional cortex, the function of which is closely related to motor activity. For the most part, this is field 6 in Brodmann's map, but the lower region, which comprises a portion of the third (inferior) frontal gyrus, is referenced as field 44 and presumably corresponds to Broca's area. Field 45 is closely connected to 44, both anatomically and, in all probability, functionally. In the mesial prolongation of the premotor zone, which also approximates the cingulate sulcus, lies the supplementary motor area. A cingulate motor area with a topographically organized body map lies in the depths and lower bank of the cingulate sulcus. Like the primary and supplementary motor cortices, it gives rise to corticospinal axons.

Anterior to both the precentral and premotor regions lies the *prefrontal cortex*, which makes up most of the frontal cortex and encompasses the pole of the lobe. Macroscopically, three major aspects may be distinguished: mesial, dorsolateral, and orbital. Histologically much of this is granular cortex that corresponds in Brodmann's map to fields

8, 9, 10, 11, 12, 46, and 47. This is the enigmatic area that most authors have in mind when they speak of the frontal lobe in relation to behavior. Little is known about the contribution of each of these separate areas, with the exception of area 8, the so-called eye field, which presumably serves a central role in relation to eye and head movements. Limbic system parts of the frontal lobe correspond to areas 24, 25, and 32 (the anterior and subgenual portions of the cingulate gyrus) and to areas 13 and 14 (the posterior parts of the orbitofrontal area and the gyrus rectus). Technically, these are agranular cortices; however, they are probably related in essential ways to both the granular and agranular cortices.

FRONTAL LOBE CONNECTIONS

Understanding the prefrontal lobe depends upon knowledge of the company it keeps, that is, its afferent and efferent connections. Some of these connections are with other neocortical structures, mainly from and to association areas in the temporal, parietal, and occipital lobes, including special areas of multimodal convergence. The prefrontal cortex is also connected to the premotor region and thus indirectly to motor cortex. There are significant connections with limbic and motor subcortical structures, as well as with the cingulate motor area, giving prefrontal cortex direct access to neurons that give rise to corticobulbar and corticospinal axons. Some projections are unidirectional, such as those to the caudate and putamen. Some seem to be bidirectional, such as those with the nucleus medialis dorsalis of the thalamus. The latter is a particularly important connection, so much so that some authors have defined the prefrontal cortex as that region which is coextensive with projections from the nucleus medialis dorsalis. The arrangement of projections is quite specific: the orbital aspect is linked with the pars magnocellularis, the dorsolateral cortex with the pars parvocellularis. Other major subcortical connections are with the hippocampus by way of the cingulate and parahippocampal gyri, with the amygdala by way of the uncinate fasciculus, and with the hypothalamus, the

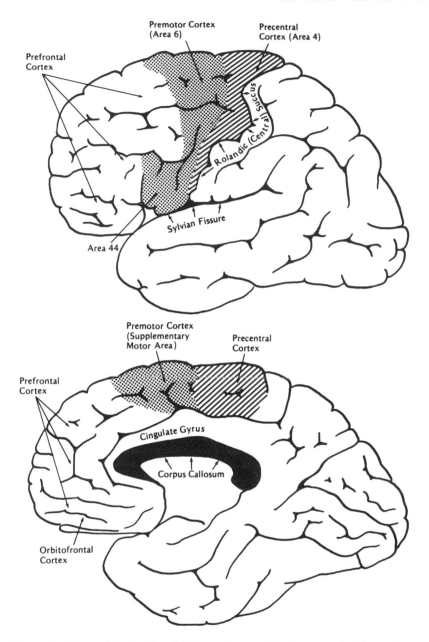

Figure 15–1. Lateral (*top*) and medial (*bottom*) views of the human cerebral hemisphere.

septum, and the mesencephalon by direct pathways.

The prefrontal cortex thus receives input, by more than one channel, from the sensory association regions of the cortex, it is closely woven with the limbic system, and it can affect the motor system in multiple ways. The functionally central position of the frontal lobe can be made more clear by a brief review of its ef-

ferent and afferent connections in nonhuman primates. The frontal lobe of the monkey is roughly comparable to that of humans in shape, limits, connections, and cytoarchitecture. Important differences, other than size, are apparent in the dorsolateral aspect, where instead of the three horizontally oriented gyri of the human frontal lobe, there are two fields placed in a dorsal and ventral position in relation to a single sulcus, the principalis (Fig. 15–1). One other major sulcus, the arcuate, arch-shaped and more or less vertically oriented, represents the seam between the monkey's prefrontal and premotor cortex. It is in this transition zone, particularly in the rostral bank of the sulcus, that Brodmann's field 8 is located. Sources used in the following description of subcortical and cortical projections are Ward and McCulloch (1947); Bailey and Von Bonin (1951); Pribram and MacLean (1953); Pribram et al. (1953); Whitlock and Nauta (1956); Crosby et al. (1962); Nauta (1962, 1964); Akert (1964); De Vito and Smith (1964); Kuypers et al. (1965); Powell et al. (1965); Valverde (1965); Johnson et al. (1968); Nauta and Haymaker (1969); Pandya et al. (1969, 1971); Pandya and Kuypers (1969); Pandya and Vignolo, 1971; Kievit and Kuypers (1974); Chavis and Pandya (1976); Rosene et al. (1976); Goldman and Nauta (1977); Yeterian and Van Hoesen (1977); Goldman (1978); Potter and Nauta (1979); Damasio and Van Hoesen (1980); Barbas and Mesulam (1981, 1985); Porrino et al. (1981); Goldman-Rakic and Schwartz (1982); Porrino and Goldman-Rakic (1982); Petrides and Pandya (1984, 1988); Barbas and Pandya (1987, 1989); Goldman-Rakic (1987); Moran et al. (1987); Pandya and Barnes (1987); Cavada and Goldman-Rakic (1989); Seltzer and Pandya (1989); Di Pellegrino and Wise (1991); Goldman-Rakic and Friedman (1991); Preuss and Goldman-Rakic (1991); Morecraft and Van Hoesen (1993); Barbas (1995); Fuster (1997); and Price (1999a, 1999b).

SUBCORTICAL CONNECTIONS

Projections from the Hypothalamus

Direct projections from the hypothalamus have not been as easy to identify as the ones in the opposite direction, which may possibly reflect a different functional significance. At any rate, there is some evidence that there are such projections to several regions above and below the arcuate sulcus and to the rostral part of the principal sulcus. These projections may be parallel to the monoaminergic projections arising in the mesencephalic tegmentum and may in-

deed be interwoven with them, since the latter are known to travel in the lateral hypothalamic region.

Projections from the Amygdala and Hippocampus

There are strong projections from the amygdala and hippocampus to the orbital cortex, particularly in its most posterior and medial region, but the amygdala also projects to the mesial aspect of the frontal lobe, particularly into areas such as the gyrus rectus and the subcallosal portion of the cingulate gyrus and the anterior parts of the cingulate gyrus (Brodmann's areas 25 and 24, respectively). The amygdala, as does the hippocampus, projects to areas of the diencephalon and mesencephalon to which the prefrontal lobe itself strongly projects.

Projections from the Thalamus

The afferent projections from the thalamus originate mostly in the regions where the efferent projections from the prefrontal cortex terminate, that is, in both the medial and lateral aspects of the dorsomedial nucleus. The medial thalamus thus appears as a transforming station for inputs from the prefrontal regions. Projections of the medial pulvinar to area 8 have also been described, and it is now known that other projections from the thalamic association nuclei, midline nuclei, and intralaminar nuclei exist. These link the prefrontal cortex to ascending reticular, visceral, and autonomic systems.

Projections to the Amygdala and Hippocampus

These arise mostly from the mesial and orbital aspects and partly from the inferior ventral dorsolateral aspect and travel in the cingulum and uncinate fasciculus. Many go directly to the amygdala, although others go to rostral temporal cortex, which in turn projects to the amygdala. Projection to the hippocampus is indirect via the limbic cortex of the cingulate and hippocampal gyri (retrosplenial and perirhinal cortices, respectively).

Projections to the Hypothalamus

Direct connections to various hypothalamic nuclei have been mentioned for a long time, and only recently have been described with certainty in monkeys. Almost in continuum with the latter, there are projections to the mesencephalic tegmentum, namely, to the anterior half of the periaqueductal gray matter. These are areas to which both the hippocampus and the anygdala send strong projections.

Projections to the Septum

In the monkey, these probably arise from the upper bank of the sulcus principalis. A reciprocal connection is probably involved. As with hypothalamic projections, further investigations of these potentially important prefrontal efferents are needed.

Projections to the Thalamus

Other than the well-known projections to the nucleus dorsalis medialis, fibers also terminate in the intraluminar thalamic complex and pulvinar.

Projections to the Striatum

Projections to the caudate and the putamen but not the pallidum have been identified. The projections from the cingulate gyrus and supplementary motor area are especially strong. It was once thought that the frontocaudate projection was limited to the head of the caudate, but it has recently been shown that the prefrontal cortex projects to the whole caudate. Of particular interest is the fact that regions of the cortex with which the frontal lobe is reciprocally innervated, e.g., the parietal lobe, seem to project to the caudate in approximately the same area. This integrates corticostriate neural systems with corticocortical neural systems.

Projections to the Claustrum, Subthalamic Regions, and Mesencephalon

Projections to the claustrum travel in the uncinate fasciculus and external capsule and originate in the orbital and inferior dorsolateral aspects. Projections to the regions of the subthalamic nucleus and the red nucleus also seem to come primarily from the orbital aspects. Some projections to the central gray seem to come from the convexity, but a strong contingent arises from orbitofrontal and medial frontal cortices.

CORTICAL CONNECTIONS

Projections from Visual, Auditory, and Somatosencory Cortex

Practically all areas of the association cortex project to the frontal lobe. In the rhesus monkey these projections have been studied in relation to two distinct regions: the periarcuate cortex, which surrounds the arcuate sulcus, and the prearcuate cortex, which includes all of the frontal pole lying anterior to the former region and which encompasses the region of the sulcus principalis.

Projections terminating in the periarcuate cortex arise from the caudal portion of the superior temporal gyrus, the lateral peristriate belt, the superior parietal lobule, and the anterior portion of the inferior parietal lobule. Projections terminating in the prearcuate cortex arise from the middle region of the superior temporal gyrus, the caudal and inferior temporal cortex, and the middle portion of the inferior bank of the intraparietal sulcus.

Direct projections to the orbital cortex come mainly from the anterior region of the superior temporal gyrus, but there are also indirect projections that reach this area by way of the mediodorsal thalamus: they originate in the middle and inferior temporal gyri and share the same route of projections from the olfactory cortex.

Considerable overlap takes place in relation to these connections, for instance, between the first-order visual and auditory projections in the periarcuate region and between second-order visual, auditory, and somatosensory projections in prearcuate cortex.

Projections from Olfactory Cortex and Olfactory Bulb

The piriform cortex projects to the frontal lobe indirectly by way of the mediodorsal nucleus of the thalamus. In this way, olfactory information joins that of the other senses to create a convergence absent in the posterior sensory cortex. There are direct connections from the olfactory bulb to the posterior orbitofrontal cortex.

Projections to Temporal Cortex

The temporal cortex receives projections from regions of the sulcus principalis in a well-organized fashion. The anterior third projects mainly to the anterior third of the superior temporal sulcus and the superior temporal gyrus. The middle third connects with both the anterior and the middle portions of the superior temporal sulcus. The posterior third projects mainly to the more caudal region of the superior temporal sulcus. The orbital aspect of the frontal lobe also projects to the rostral area of the temporal lobe and especially the temporal polar cortex.

Projections to Posterior Sensory Cortex

These are mainly directed to the inferior parietal lobule and originate in the posterior third of the sulcus principalis and in the arcuate sulcus.

Projections to Nonmotor Limbic Cortex

Both the anterior and middle thirds of the sulcus principalis project to the lower part of the cingulate gyrus, the latter in a more intense fashion, as do areas in the concavity of the arcuate sulcus. This is an interesting projection that courses all along the cingulate, distributing fibers to the overlying cortex but then continuing as a bundle to reach the parahippocampal gyrus.

PATHOPHYSIOLOGY

Two problems frequently complicate the evaluation of frontal lobe damage: (1) the concept of a single "frontal lobe syndrome," and (2) the failure to consider the multitude of pathophysiological, individual, and environmental variables that can influence the expression of frontal lobe dysfunction. The notion that there

is a unitary frontal lobe syndrome is not supported by anatomical or neuropsychological evidence. The locus of a lesion within the frontal lobe is a crucial factor in the profile of frontal lobe signs. Side of lesion, for instance, is important, as there is evidence that some lesions of the dominant frontal lobe interfere with verbal behavior more so than corresponding nondominant lesions, and certain emotional changes are related to the left–right dichotomy. Bilateral lesions may produce yet a different clinical picture, both quantitatively and qualitatively. Regional effects within a lobe may determine distinctive clinical configurations and allow the prediction of whether the involvement is predominantly mesial or dorsolateral or inferior orbital. Depth of lesion is also an important variable, probably as much so as surface extent of damage. Many signs of frontal lobe dysfunction result from severed subcortical connections, which a deep lesion has a better chance of destroying.

Analysis of the behavioral effects of different loci of damage must also take account of the nature of the lesion. The clinical presentation of the various pathophysiological processes that can cause damage to the frontal lobes can be quite different from one another. Vascular disorders, tumors, and traumatic injury are among the most common causes of structural damage in the frontal lobes.

The vascular syndromes are the most distinctive, particularly those related to the anterior cerebral artery. Bilateral as well as unilateral involvement is a common cause of mutism with or without akinesia. Personality changes are also frequently found, and a characteristic amnesic syndrome has been identified with lesions in this vascular distribution (Damasio et al., 1985). Damage is predominantly to the ventromedial and mesial aspects of the frontal lobe. The most common cause of these abnormalities is rupture of an aneurysm of the anterior communicating artery or of the anterior cerebral artery itself. In other cases, the frontal branches of the middle cerebral artery may be involved, the more frequent causes being embolism and thrombosis. Damage is almost always unilateral and predominantly affects the dorsolateral aspect of the lobe, giving rise to various speech and language impairments when the dominant hemisphere is involved and to affective and spatial alterations when the nondominant hemisphere is injured.

The syndromes caused by tumors naturally vary with location and histological nature. Extrinsic tumors, such as meningiomas, are frequently located subfrontally or at the cerebral falx, where they involve the mesial aspect of the frontal lobes and often cause bilateral changes. They may also have a more lateral origin and compress the dorsolateral aspect of one frontal lobe only. Intrinsic tumors may show up unilaterally or bilaterally. The distinction often depends on time, as an originally unilateral glioma may invade the corpus callosum and cross to the opposite side.

Not uncommonly, frontal lobe tumors present with major intellectual and affective impairment that justifies the use of the term "dementia," so pervasive is the disorganization of normal behavior (e.g., Strauss and Keschner, 1935). For this reason, the diagnosis of frontal lobe tumor should always be considered in the study of a dementia syndrome. Confusional states are also frequently associated with tumors of the frontal lobe, perhaps more so than with tumors anywhere else in the central nervous system (Hécaen, 1964). Disturbances of mood and character, although less frequent than confusion or dementia, were noted almost as frequently in Hécaen's study.

Wounds caused by head injury—whose clinical pictures were vividly described by Kleist (1936) and Goldstein (1948)—may have a preponderant frontal involvement and present with a combination of frontal lobe signs. The orbital surface of the frontal lobes and the frontal poles are particularly susceptible to damage from traumatic head injury, because of contact of these structures with the skull. Although the consequences of head injury typically reflect the combined effects of damage to multiple brain areas, many of the sequelae that prove to be most disruptive are similar to those seen following focal damage in frontal cortex.

The rate of development of a lesion and the time elapsed since peak development are additional factors that interact with lesion type to influence the clinical picture. Worsening, stabilization, or recovery depend on the nature of the underlying pathological process. Most patients with cerebrovascular lesions tend to stabilize and then improve gradually, whereas the course of patients with tumors is a function of the degree of cytological and mechanical malignancy of the tumor and of the type of surgical or medical management adopted. Patients with severe symptomatology from a vascular event or traumatic injury will often have a remarkable remission within a period of weeks. Patients with slowly growing tumors that infiltrate neural tissue without grossly disrupting its function, by contrast, may fail to show measurable behavioral defects, in spite of the considerable size of their malignancies (Anderson et al., 1989).

Another important factor is the age at which the dysfunction begins. There is evidence that the effects of lesions starting in childhood or adolescence are different from those caused by lesions starting in adulthood (Grattan and Eslinger, 1991; Anderson et al., 1999). If these factors are not taken into account, it will not be possible to make an adequate clinical evaluation of patients and clinical research may produce paradoxical results.

The results of prefrontal leucotomy and prefrontal lobotomy, which were a source of early information on frontal lobe physiology, have also been a consistent source of controversy. Although Moniz (1936, 1949) was impressed by the lack of pronounced defects of motor, sensory, and language function in cases of frontal lobe lesion, it is clear that he attributed several important functions to the frontal lobe. He reasoned that in cases of schizophrenic thought disorder or of obsessive-compulsive disease, the wrongly learned and abnormally repetitive thinking processes were dependent on frontal lobe function and based on reverberating circuitry connecting the frontal lobe to midline subcortical structures and to the posterior cortical areas. Such "repetitive linkages" called for surgical interruption. He also hypothesized a relation between the aberrant thought process and the accompanying emotional status of the patient and assumed that a lesion that altered one would also alter the other. He recalled the frequent observation of affective indifference in frontal lobe patients, as well as the remarkable affective changes shown in Jacobsen's chimpanzees (Fulton and Jacobsen, 1935) after frontal lobe surgery. It seems that Moniz conceived of the frontal lobes as important for higher cognition and for the regulation of emotion (Fulton, 1951). Far from designing an innocuous intervention, he planned the creation of particular defects which might benefit patients whose previous abnormality was thoroughly incapacitating.

Objective assessment of the results of prefrontal surgery is hard to come by. The original Moniz method, apparently one of the most effective and least damaging, was not used in this country. Several other surgical methods have been devised involving various amounts of damage to different structures. All cases suffered from preexisting psychiatric disease or intractable pain, generally of considerable severity and duration. Finally, the methods of behavioral assessment have been varied in scope and quality. It is evident, however, that bilateral, surgically controlled frontal lobe damage, particularly when it involves the mesial and inferior orbital cortices or their connections, causes modifications in the affective and emotional sphere. Leaving aside any discussion of the value of this approach in psychiatry, it is important for neuropsychologists to know that even minor psychosurgery may be a factor in their patients' behavior. For a modern appraisal of the measurable neuropsychologic disturbances associated with leucotomy see Stuss et al. (1981).

Frontal lobe damage may also play a prominent role in many progressive demential syndromes. For example, Van Hoesen et al. (2000) found extensive distribution of neurofibrillary tangles throughout the orbitofrontal cortex of patients with Alzheimer's disease. It is likely that this damage contributes to some of the non-memory behavioral disorders which are common in Alzheimer's disease. In light of recent findings of orbitofrontal activation in normal adults during memory tasks (Frey and Petrides, 2000), it also is possible that neurofibrillary tangles in this region contribute to the memory defects in Alzheimer's disease. In other demential syndromes, frontal lobe dysfunction is the most important feature. Progressive impairments of behavioral regulation, attention, and emotion, in the context of relatively preserved memory, characterize the frontal variant of frontotemporal dementia

(e.g., Neary et al., 1988; Rahman et al., 1999; Perry and Hodges, 2000). The behavior of these patients gradually deteriorates to resemble that of persons with macroscopic lesions in the frontal lobes. The insidious onset of the behavioral abnormalities in the absence of an identifiable neurological event presents particular challenges for diagnosis and management.

NEUROLOGICAL FINDINGS

CHANGES IN AROUSAL AND ORIENTING RESPONSE

Patients who move little or not at all often pay limited attention to new stimuli. The possibility that akinesia associated with frontal lobe lesions goes pari passu with severe bilateral neglect is an interesting one. Thus, changes in motor and affective processing may be associated with changes in the mechanisms of arousal. The type of abnormality described by Fisher (1968) as "intermittent interruption of behavior" in cases of anterior cerebral artery infarction is another good example of the coexistence of such changes.

There is little doubt that orienting responses are impaired after dorsolateral and cingulate gyrus damage. The changes frequently appear in the setting of neglect to stimuli arriving in the space contralateral to the lesion, with associated hypomobility of the neglected side (Heilman and Valenstein, 1972; Damasio et al., 1980). Lesions in the arcuate region in primates cause unilateral neglect (Kennard and Ectors, 1938; Welch and Stuteville, 1958), not unlike that determined by lesions of multimodal parietal association areas (Heilman et al., 1971), and the same applies to the cingulate gyrus (Watson et al., 1973). Lesions in non–frontal lobe structures—including the thalamus, hypothalamus, and midbrain—can also cause neglect in both humans and animals (Segarra and Angelo, 1970; Marshall et al., 1971; Marshall and Teitelbaum, 1974; Watson et al., 1974).

ABNORMAL REFLEXES

The more significant abnormal reflexes are the grasp reflex, the groping reflex, and the snout and sucking reflexes. Traditionally these abnormal responses have been termed "psychomotor signs," calling attention to the fact that they almost invariably appear in the setting of an abnormal mental status.

The most useful of the group is the *grasp reflex* (the prehension reflex of Kleist, the forced grasping of Adie and Critchley), which may appear unilaterally or bilaterally, in the hands or in the feet. It consists of a more or less forceful prehension of an object that has come into contact with the palm or the sole. It can be elicited by touching or by stroking the skin, particularly in the region between the thumb and index finger. Most maneuvers used to elicit the plantar reflex may produce a grasp reaction of the foot and may even mask an abnormal extensor response, which, in that case, may be obtained from stimulation of the lateral side of the foot. The degree of the grasp reflex varies from patient to patient and is generally more intense in cases with impaired mentation. In more alert states, it is characteristic that the patient cannot release the prehension even if told to do so and even if she or he wishes to do so. The reflex may extinguish after repeated stimulation and reappear after a period of rest. Classic descriptions used to refer to changes in lateralization induced by positioning of the head and body, but such changes are not reliable and should not be used for clinical localization.

The *groping reflex* is less frequent than the grasp reflex and generally appears in conjunction with the latter. The hand of the patient, as well as the eyes, tend to follow an object or the fingers of the examiner. For a brief period, the patient behaves as if stimulus bound.

The *sucking reflex* is elicited by touching the lips of the patient with a cotton swab, and the *snout reflex* is obtained by tapping the skin of the upper perioral region with a finger or hammer. These responses are often present in patients with disease confined to the frontal lobe, but, more so than the grasp reflex, they appear in a wide variety of demential syndromes associated with more wide-ranging damage. Furthermore, the snout reflex, just like the palmomental reflex, may appear in patients with basal ganglia disorders and even in normal older individuals.

Traditionally, these signs have been interpreted as an indication of release of primitive forms of reflex response, kept in abeyance by normal inhibitory function of frontal lobe structures. This view seems entirely valid.

ABNORMAL TONE

Patients with lesions in the prefrontal areas often show changes in muscle tone. These may be more closely associated with lesions in the dorsolateral aspect of the frontal lobes, particularly near the premotor regions. The most characteristic sign is Kleist's *Gegenhalten*, also referred to as counterpull, paratonia, opposition, or the Mayer-Reisch phenomenon. This is another of the so-called psychomotor signs and may be wrongly interpreted as a deliberate negative attitude on the part of the patient. When the examiner tries to assess tone by passively moving the arm, he or she may find a sudden resistance to the extension maneuver and note that the counteracting flexion movement actually increases in intensity in an attempt to neutralize the action. The patient may or may not be aware of this development and, as with the grasp reflex, will be unable to suppress the reflex even if desiring to do so. Rigidity may also be present, but since it is not associated with tremor, it will not have "cogwheel" characteristics. The degree of rigidity may show little consistency and may vary between observations. It is best described as plastic. Periodic hypotonia resembling cataplexy is quite rare (Ethelberg, 1949).

ABNORMAL GAIT AND POSTURE

Patients with severe frontal lobe damage often show abnormalities of gait. A wide range of characteristic changes may be present, including walking with short steps but without festination, loss of balance with retropulsion, or inability to walk (as in cases of gait apraxia). The latter may be seen in a variety of conditions, most frequently in the syndrome of normal-pressure hydrocephalus, which is, in effect, a frontal lobe syndrome consequent to periodically raised intraventricular pressure. In diagnosing gait apraxia, an effort should be made to demonstrate that the patient can execute while recumbent all the movements he or she is unable to perform while standing.

The designation "frontal ataxia" probably does not cover a manifestation typical of frontal lobe lesions, as even Bruns admitted when he coined the term. A tendency to fall backward rather than to the side and a predominance of deficits in the trunk rather than in the extremities are evident in some cases.

Abnormalities of posture are possible, though not pathognomic or frequent. In some cases, the examiner is able to place the arms of the patient in various bizarre positions and note the waxy flexibility with which the patient will remain in those unlikely positions. True catalepsy and sudden freezing of posture have also been described but seem rare.

CHANGES IN CONTROL OF EYE MOVEMENT

The control of eye and head movements is part of a highly developed system tuned to orient the organism toward possibly important stimuli and therefore aid perception of the environment. The role of the frontal eye fields, located bilaterally in area 8 of Brodmann, in the control of these movements is still a matter of controversy. The paucity of spontaneous head and eye movement toward new stimuli, which is commonly described in connection with the impairment of orienting responses of frontal lobe patients, is possibly related to eye field function. On the whole, however, the value of eye movement defects in the assessment of higher levels of behavior disturbance is limited.

Frontal seizures, originating in lesions in or near one eye field, may be characterized by a turning of the eye and head away from the side of the lesion. Structural damage of one eye field, however, particularly if acute, produces a turning of eyes and head toward the side of the lesion.

Clear anomalies of conjugate gaze mechanism have their greatest value in the assessment of the comatose patient, where their relation to a concomitant paresis may decide whether the damage is in the frontal lobe or in the brainstem.

OLFACTORY DISTURBANCES

Anatomical and electrophysiological studies in the monkey have suggested that the prefrontal cortex may be involved in qualitative olfactory discrimination (Tanabe et al., 1975a, 1975b; Potter and Nauta, 1979). Potter and Butters (1980) have reported that damage to the orbital region of the frontal lobe can lead to impaired odor-quality discrimination without a significant decrease in odor detection. Projections from the temporal lobe directly to orbitofrontal cortex as well as by way of the thalamus were hypothesized to carry olfactory information in a hierarchical system of "odor-quality analyzers." Damage to thalamic and prefrontal lobe structures has also been found to impair odor-quality discrimination in non-primates without influencing odor detection (Eichenbaum et al., 1980; Sapolsky and Eichenbaum, 1980). The findings suggest that selective frontal lobe damage can be associated with deficits in a cognitive task of odor-quality discrimination without decreasing odor-detection ability. Although olfactory identification impairments can arise from damage to right or left orbitofrontal cortex, lesions of the right orbitofrontal cortex may produce greater deficits in olfactory processing than comparable damage on the left (e.g., Zatorre and Jones-Gotman, 1991; Jones-Gotman and Zatorre, 1993). Recent functional imaging studies have also provided support for the notion that human frontal cortex, particularly pyriform and orbital regions, plays an integral role in olfaction (Kobal and Kettenmann, 2000; Zald and Pardo, 2000). The orbitofrontal cortex also may be important for taste, and representation of the reward value of taste and odors may be linked to more general representation of punishment and reward (Rolls, 2000).

CHANGES IN SPHINCTER CONTROL

It is often noted that patients with frontal lobe damage have disturbances of sphincter control. The patient shows little concern about urinating or even defecating in socially unacceptable situations. Bilateral involvement of the mesial aspect of the frontal lobe is the rule in these cases. Resection of an underlying tumor often improves sphincter disturbances, which tend to recover spontaneously in cases of stroke. Extensive lesions of the white matter may also produce incontinence, as the early techniques of frontal lobotomy demonstrated. This defect is probably the result of loss of the inhibitory action that the frontal lobe presumably exerts over the spinal detrusor reflex.

COGNITION AND BEHAVIOR

Although patients with frontal lobe damage may exhibit any of the neurologic signs noted above, it is not uncommon for the neurological examination to be entirely normal except for a history of behavioral disturbance. Evaluation of the consequences of frontal lobe damage is arguably the most challenging task faced by clinical neuropsychologists, because the laboratory manifestations of frontal lobe damage are often subtle. Standard psychological or neuropsychological evaluations may reveal few unequivocal defects, even in patients who are no longer able to behave normally in real life. Nevertheless, comprehensive evaluations can disclose a variety of signs suggestive of dysfunction in frontal cortices.

INTELLIGENCE

When we consider the role of the frontal lobes in human intellect, it is necessary to distinguish between intelligence as a global capacity to engage in adaptive, goal-directed behavior, and intelligence as defined by performance on standard psychometric instruments. There is little controversy regarding the idea that the frontal cortices constitute a necessary anatomical substrate for human intelligence as a global adaptive capacity. By contrast, extensive frontal lobe damage may have little or no impact on the abilities measured by intelligence tests.

Although not originally designed as neuropsychological instruments, standardized intelligence tests, and the Wechsler Scales in particular, are among the most frequently administered measures of cognitive function (Benton, 1991b; Tranel, 1992). There is general agreement that summary IQ scores provide limited information for the purposes of most neuropsychological evaluations (Lezak,

1988), but the analysis of performances on selected subtests remains a cornerstone of clinical evaluation for neuropsychologists. Early indications that standardized intelligence tests do not address the type of cognitive ability lost by frontal lobe patients were provided by Hebb's patient, who obtained an IQ of 98, and by Brickner's patient A., who obtained an IQ of 80 on Terman's revision of the Binet-Simon 1 year after operation and an IQ of 99 when he was retested 12 months later.

The preservation of psychometric intelligence in patients with frontal lobe damage appears to be a consistent finding. For example, Milner (1963) reported a mean loss of 7.2 IQ points following dorsolateral frontal lobectomies, with mean postoperative IQ scores remaining in the average range, and Black (1976) found a mean Wechsler Adult Intelligence Scale (WAIS) Verbal IQ of 99.1 and a mean Performance IQ of 99.5 in a group of 44 Vietnam veterans who had sustained unilateral frontal lobe shrapnel injuries. Likewise, Janowsky et al. (1989) described seven subjects with various focal frontal lobe lesions who obtained a mean WAIS-R Full Scale IQ of 101.

We presented WAIS-R data from patients with focal frontal lobe lesions in the prior edition of this volume which made the same point. Shown in Table 15–1 are the WAIS-III performances of seven patients with focal lesions in the frontal lobes caused by stroke (Fig. 15–2). All subjects were studied at least 3 months after the event. As with our findings on the prior version of these scales, the most notable feature of the scores is the consistent preservation of the cognitive abilities required to perform the various intellectual tasks.

We have examined the possibility that the new Matrix Reasoning subtest of the WAIS-III, as a measure of "fluid intelligence" (i.e., the ability to solve novel abstract problems), would provide a more sensitive index of frontal lobe dysfunction, but again found no impairment in patients with frontal lobe lesions and no difference in performance between patients with prefrontal and those with nonfrontal lesions (Anderson and Manzel, 2001). In sum, with the exception of patients who present with confusion or dementia, impairments of cognitive ability measured by standard intelligence tests are not striking in patients with frontal lobe lesions,

Table 15–1. WAIS-III Subtest Performances of Patients with Frontal Lobe Damage

Subject	1	2	3	4	5	6	7
Age (years)	58	88	55	62	26	51	51
Education	16	16	8	12	16	14	16
Vocabulary	14	—	9	8	12	11	—
Similarities	12	—	8	9	9	11	—
Arithmetic	12	—	8	10	12	10	—
Digit Span	13	—	9	11	13	13	—
Information	16	—	7	10	15	10	—
Comprehension	12	—	8	8	12	14	—
Letter–Number	12	—	6	10	15	13	—
Picture Completion	6	9	12	11	11	9	11
Digit Symbol	5	7	8	5	7	14	6
Matrix Reasoning	13	11	8	10	11	10	15
Block Design	12	12	11	11	7	11	14
Picture Arranging	10	12	9	8	7	8	10
Symbol Search	6	—	10	8	15	14	9

Note: WAIS-III scores are age-corrected scaled scores. Subjects 2 and 7 were too aphasic to complete the verbal subtests.

even when bilateral. And yet, frontal lobe patients often behave in a most unintelligent way.

Many of the real-life problems encountered by patients with frontal lobe lesions are in social situations, raising the possibility of a selective defect in some aspect of "social intelligence." One possible mechanism for the impairment of social behavior is that frontal lobe damage alters the ability to generate an appropriate array of response options and an adequate representation of the future consequences. Another possible mechanism is that these patients are able to conjure up adequate response options and consequences, yet fail to select the most advantageous choice. Saver and Damasio (1991) administered to subject E.V.R.

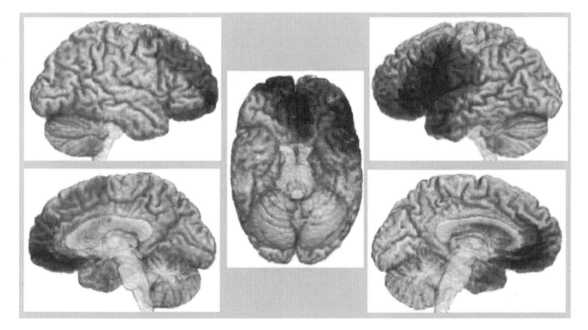

Figure 15–2. Subjects with prefrontal damage and Wechsler Adult Intelligence Scale–III (WAIS-III) evaluation shown in Table 15–1. The location and overlap of lesions in the seven subjects is depicted on a normal reference brain. Lesions of individual subjects were transferred onto the reference brain using MAP-3 (Frank et al., 1997).

a series of standardized measures designed to examine the manipulation of response options and projected outcomes to social stimuli. E.V.R. demonstrated normal or superior performances on tasks that required the generation of response options to social situations, consideration of the future consequences of pursuing particular responses, and moral reasoning, and this was replicated in additional subjects with adult-onset damage to the frontal lobes (Anderson et al., 1999). These findings suggest that the defect in these patients does not result from deficient social knowledge or an inability to reason regarding social situations, although some patients with frontal lobe lesions have been found to be impaired in rating the effectiveness of solutions to social problems (Dimitrov et al., 1996).

This mismatch between intelligence measured in a laboratory and intelligence applied to real-life behaviors remains one of the most compelling challenges in frontal lobe research. It is evident that real-life intelligent behavior requires more than basic problem-solving rules. In real-life problems, unlike most artificial problems posed by neuropsychological tasks, the relevant issues, rules of engagement, and end points are not always clearly identified. Real-life behaviors often introduce heavy time processing and working memory demands, and there is a requirement for the prioritization and weighing of multiple options and possible outcomes.

ATTENTION AND MEMORY

Although frontal lobe damage usually does not cause amnesia in the conventional sense, it can disrupt mnemonic processes at several stages. Ever since Jacobsen's (1935) demonstration of impairments on a delayed-response task by monkeys with frontal lobe ablations, investigators have been attempting to explicate the memory defects that follow damage to the frontal lobes. As reviewed earlier, the anatomical connections of the frontal lobes are certainly consistent with the notion that the frontal cortices are involved in memory. Bidirectional connections with sensory association cortices, thalamic nuclei, and the amygdalohippocampal region provide a framework by which the frontal cortices could play a role in the formation and activation of stored representations.

Many of the reasoning abilities considered uniquely characteristic of humans, such as long-term planning, hypothetical reasoning, and reorganization of complex concepts, require *working memory*, or the transient maintenance of representations in an activated or accessible state while the reasoning is taking place. Working memory is not a unitary process and likely is an essential function of many nonfrontal brain regions. However, the frontal cortex appears to be important for working memory tasks that involve bridging of temporally separate elements and the comparison or manipulation of several pieces of information (e.g., Goldman-Rakic, 1984; Petrides, 1995; Fuster, 1997; Kim and Shadlen, 1999). Functional imaging studies have linked different subregions of the dorsolateral cortex to working memory for different types of stimulus material, such as stimulus identity, spatial location, and aspects of verbal processing (e.g., Cohen et al., 1994; Smith et al., 1996; Crossen et al., 1999). Despite evidence of prefrontal involvement in working memory, patients with damage in this area generally do not have impairments on standard measures of working memory, such as verbal or spatial span, although delayed response performance can be impaired under certain conditions (e.g., Ghent et al., 1962; Chorover and Cole, 1966; D'Esposito and Postle, 1999). Milner et al. (1985) noted that the ability to solve such problems through verbal mediation so alters the task requirements that they may not be appropriate paradigms for human subjects. Also, there is growing reason to think that much of the contribution of the frontal lobes to working memory task performance may be in executive control over mnemonic processing, rather than working memory per se (Robbins, 1996; Postle et al., 1999). Consistent with this idea, activation of anterior dorsolateral frontal regions, on the left and right, has been found in normal persons when the task requires both keeping in mind a main goal (working memory) and allocating attention during dual task performance (Koechlin et al., 1999).

We examined performance on delayed-response and delayed-non–matching-to-sample tasks in patients with lesions in ventromedial (VM) or dorsolateral/high mesial (DL/M) prefrontal areas (Bechara et al., 1998). Only patients with right DL/M or posterior VM lesions (with likely involvement of the basal forebrain) were impaired on these spatial working memory tasks. The posterior VM patients, but not the DL/M patients, were impaired on an experimental decision-making task, and patients with VM lesions were able to perform normally on the working memory tasks despite impairments of decision making. These findings suggest a dissociation of working memory and decision making in the human prefrontal cortex. Within the prefrontal region, damage to dorsolateral cortex appears to have the greatest impact on working memory, possibly through disrupted regulation of posterior regions more directly involved in memory encoding and storage. It has also been found that frontal lobe patients with impaired working memory may show impairments of procedural learning (Beldarrain et al., 1999).

While aspects of working memory may be disturbed, anterograde memory tends to be less affected. When damage is limited to the frontal lobes, there typically appears to be little or no impairment on most standardized neuropsychological memory tests (e.g., Black, 1976; Stuss et al., 1982; Janowsky et al., 1989; Damasio and Anderson, 1993; Swick and Knight, 1996). However, in some instances free recall of recently presented or remote information may be defective (e.g., Dimitrov et al., 1999). At least in part, this appears to be due to reduced executive control of active learning and recall strategies (Eslinger and Grattan, 1994; Gershberg and Shimamura, 1995; Mangels et al., 1996; Fletcher et al., 1998). Damage to the frontal lobes has also been linked to high rates of false recognition and confabulation (e.g., Stuss et al., 1978; Parkin et al., 1996; Schacter et al., 1996; Rapcsak et al., 1998), suggestive of a defect in monitoring or evaluating mnemonic operations. Recent positron emission tomographic (PET) evidence from normal subjects has supported the notion that the posterior orbitomesial frontal region is involved in distinguishing between memories that are or are not relevant to ongoing reality (Schnider et al., 2000). Neural pathways exist that could pro-

vide a substrate for prefrontal influence on memory. Neurons in prefrontal cortex project to the hippocampal region via at least two distinct routes (Goldman-Rakic, 1984), and recent neurophysiological studies in monkeys have supported the concept of prefrontal "top-down" control of mesial temporal lobe memory functions (Tomita et al., 1999).

The relatives and caretakers of patients with frontal lobe damage often describe them as forgetful in the execution of daily activities, despite relatively normal scores on standard tests of anterograde memory. One factor contributing to this discrepancy is impairment in various aspects of attention (e.g., Stuss et al., 1999; Metzler and Parkin, 2000). Norman and Shallice (1986) provided a detailed model of a supervisory attentional system based in the frontal lobes, which is involved primarily in allocating attention in non-routine situations. There is evidence that frontal lobe damage results in diminished attention to novel events and increased susceptibility to distraction (Malmo, 1942; Milner, 1964; Stuss et al., 1982; Knight, 1984; Daffner et al., 2000). The acquisition of new, functionally relevant information requires the filtering or gating of irrelevant stimuli, and prefrontal cortex appears to contribute to this process by exerting inhibitory effects on posterior brain regions involved in perception. Holmes (1938) argued that an important role of the frontal lobes was suppression of reflexive ocular behavior, and damage to inferior dorsolateral prefrontal cortex has been associated with impairments on the "antisaccade" paradigm, which requires inhibition of reflexive glances to peripheral stimuli (Guitton et al., 1985; Walker et al., 1998).

Patients with frontal lesions show heightened vulnerability to distracting stimuli in other modalities, as well as electrophysiological evidence of disinhibition in sensory regions. For example, Chao and Knight (1998) found that patients with frontal lesions generated enhanced event-related potentials in primary auditory cortex in response to distracting noises. It has been proposed that the dependency on immediately present environmental cues shown by some patients with frontal lobe damage may be due to release of parietal lobe activity resulting from loss of frontal lobe inhibition (Lhermitte et al., 1986). Dias et al. (1997) have provided evidence suggesting that dorsolateral prefrontal damage in primates may have a greater impact on inhibitory control of attention selection, while orbitofrontal damage may have a greater effect on affectively related inhibition. Impairment of inhibitory control following frontal lobe damage appears to be a common mechanism affecting not just allocation of attention but also several aspects of cognition and behavior.

Defects in working memory, attention, or executive control may result in major dissociations between well-preserved memory capacity (as demonstrated by normal performances on standardized memory tests) and severely impaired utilization of those abilities in real-life situations. A telling example of this dissociation was provided by a patient studied in our laboratory following a large right dorsolateral frontal lobe lesion caused by stroke (#1331) (Fig. 15–3). Six months after the event, this 56-year-old former industrial engineer obtained a Wechsler Memory Scale MQ of 132 and correctly identified 29 of 30 words (15 targets and 15 foils) on a 30-minute delayed-recognition version of the Auditory–Verbal Learning Test. However, the patient's wife described him as extremely forgetful in his normal daily activities. In contrast to his formerly conscientious behavior, the patient would now repeatedly misplace his keys and other personal effects, and would regularly leave the television and lights on when he would leave a room. He was known to forget to turn off his car engine after parking and occasionally leave it running for hours. This "failure to remember" remained a constant feature of his behavior.

The distinction of which memory defects are or are not attributable to frontal damage is an important one. For instance, the proximity of the basal forebrain region to the ventromedial frontal lobe makes it likely that both frontal and basal forebrain areas are damaged by the same lesion. The problem is made more difficult by the fact that the basal forebrain region, due to its location and size, is often difficult to visualize. This region contains the largest concentration of cholinergic neurons (including those in the nucleus basalis of Meynert), along with major neurotransmitter projections en route from brainstem to cerebral cortex. Lesions here result in an amnesic syndrome (Damasio et al., 1985). Such lesions are commonly caused by infarcts secondary to rupture of aneurysms on the anterior communicating or anterior cerebral arteries.

Temporal Organization of Memory

It was noted earlier that part of the reason for failure on the delayed-response and delayed-alternation tasks by monkeys with dorsolateral frontal lobe lesions may be related to temporal aspects of the task requirements (see Fuster, 1997, for discussion). Also pointing to a specific role of the frontal lobes in aspects of temporal contextual memory are studies that

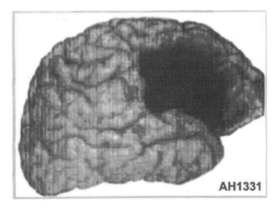

Figure 15–3. Three-dimensional reconstruction of the brain of subject 1331, obtained from thin-cut MRI slices using Brainvox (Frank et al., 1997).

have documented impairments of the ability to make judgments of relative recency or frequency (e.g., Milner, 1971; Smith and Milner, 1988; Milner et al., 1991; Butters et al., 1994). In the recency task, the subject is presented with a series of stimuli (e.g., words or abstract designs). Mixed in with the stimulus items are test items where two stimuli are presented; these are either two stimuli that have been presented previously or one previous item paired with a novel item. The subject is required to judge which of the two items was seen most recently. In the original studies, subjects with frontal cortical excisions for treatment of epilepsy were able to discriminate between novel and familiar items, but were impaired in the ability to judge the relative recency of two familiar items (Corsi and Milner, reported in Milner, 1971; Milner et al., 1991). In contrast, subjects with unilateral temporal lobectomies showed material-specific recognition problems, but normal recency judgements. The defect may be primarily due to defects in strategic, rather than automatic, processing of temporal information (Mangels, 1997). Impairment of the ability to judge the relative frequency of occurrence of nonverbal items has also been demonstrated in subjects with right frontal lobe damage (Smith and Milner, 1988). Impairments of memory for recency and frequency also can occur in the context of pathology outside of the frontal lobes (e.g., Parkin and Hunkin, 1993; Stanhope et al., 1998); although the defects do dissociate from standard anterograde memory impairments. For example, it has been shown that patient H.M. has relatively preserved recency and frequency judgments despite severely impaired item recognition (Sagar et al., 1990).

Kinesthetic Memory

Teuber's (1964, 1966) contribution to the problem of frontal lobe function is of special interest. At a time when researchers were primarily looking at the sensory aspect of the problem, he emphasized the motor end of the process and introduced the concept of *corollary discharge*. In brief, this is defined as the preparatory action that the motor system exerts on the sensory system to announce the in-

tention of incoming movement, correct for displacement of perception, and assure smooth perceptual continuity once movement is carried out. Teuber viewed this mechanism as being dependent on frontal lobe structures and considered it to be a basic physiological function of the frontal lobe. In keeping with this idea, he hypothesized that most signs of frontal lobe dysfunction in animals and humans were derived from impairment of the corollary discharge mechanism. Indications of dysfunction as disparate as delayed-response deficits in monkeys, perseveration, and the inability to handle sorting tasks were seen as resulting from the absence of a motor sensory alerting signal.

There is no doubt that some mechanism of corollary discharge exists and is essential for the continuity of perception, but it is not clear that frontal lobe structures are indispensable to corollary information processes. Nor does it seem probable that a single impaired mechanism can explain the variety of clinical and experimental signs of frontal lobe damage.

The observations that led Teuber to his concept of corollary discharge were made in patients with penetrating gunshot wounds involving the frontal lobes. Objective evidence of dysfunction in Teuber's patients was reflected in impairment on a series of perceptuomotor tasks that included tests of visuopostural orientation, visual-search, body orientation, and reversal-of-perspective ability. The visuopostural task (Teuber and Mishkin, 1954) called for the mechanical setting of a brightly luminous rod in the vertical position. The test was conducted in a dark room with the patient under different conditions of body tilt. Frontal lobe subjects did poorly on this task, displacing the rod to the right when tilted left, and displacing it to the left when tilted right. However, if the task was strictly visual and no visuoproprioceptive conflict was established, the subjects performed normally. Teuber interpreted displacement of the line in the direction opposite the side of the tilt as compensation for the tilt of the body. Exaggeration of this normal compensatory effect by patients with frontal damage only under conditions of altered proprioception was seen as a consequence of dysfunction in the corollary discharge mechanism. The visual-search task involved active head and eye movement in the search for certain patterns, and the body orientation task involved rapidly shifting left-to-right pointing responses on the patient's body. The reversal-of-perspective task was performed with two Necker cubes. The patient was requested to signify perception of left or right perspective reversal by pressing levers placed to the left and to the right. Impairment on these tasks was also interpreted as a failure in the integration of motor with perceptual activity due to dysfunctional corollary discharge. According to this view, disruption of feedback from anterior motor systems to posterior sensory cortices during the movements required to perform each task resulted in impairment on subsequent responses. Since all of these tasks are difficult for a normal person and probably more so for a brain-damaged individual, the strength of the results lies in the verification that patients with nonfrontal brain damage perform consistently better than those with frontal disease. The preliminary results of Teuber and co-workers suggested that this was so.

SPEECH AND LANGUAGE

Aphasia

One of the most influential discoveries in the early history of brain–behavior relationships was Paul Broca's (1861) description of an infarction in left posterior inferior frontal cortex in a patient whose speech was limited to repetitive production of a single syllable. It is now known that various sectors of left dorsolateral frontal lobe interface with posterior cortices and subcortical structures to provide the substrate for linguistic formulation and comprehension. The left frontal lobe appears to play an important role in aspects of language processing that involve combinatorial assembly, e.g., the combination of phonemes into morphemes, and of morphemes into sentences (Damasio, 1992). Other frontal regions, namely the cingulate gyrus and supplementary motor area, are involved in the affective and motor control of speech production. Although Broca's aphasia remains the best known language defect associated with frontal lobe damage, it is

becoming increasingly evident that this clinical diagnostic category encompasses various interactions of several dissociable impairments, including defects of linguistic formulation, motor programming, and the initiation and maintenance of output (Alexander et al., 1989). Correspondingly, damage to posterior inferior frontal cortex alone does not produce the full syndrome, but rather Broca's aphasia is caused by extensive and varied damage to several neighboring brain areas (e.g., Mohr, 1976). Because discussion of Broca's aphasia, transcortical motor aphasia, and speech apraxia are provided elsewhere in this volume, we will not go into further detail here. There are, however, several other aspects of frontal lobe involvement in speech and language which warrant comment.

Mutism

Mutism, generally associated with some degree of both akinesia and bradykinesia, is a frequent sign of frontal lobe dysfunction. It denotes involvement of the mesial cortex of the frontal lobe or of its connections, unilaterally or bilaterally. Current evidence indicates that lesions in the cingulate gyrus or the supplementary motor area (often in both) are crucial for the appearance of mutism and akinesia. Bilateral damage tends to cause longer-lasting changes. Unilateral damage, in vascular cases or in ablations, permits recovery in a matter of weeks. There is no evidence that side of lesion plays a major role here, and dominant as well as nondominant lesions cause much the same results, providing further evidence that the areas in question are related to affective and motor control but not to linguistic processing, thus being capable of interfering with speech (and all other movement, purposeful or automatic) but not language. The most frequent cause for the lesions that cause mutism is impairment in the blood supply of the anterior cerebral artery territories. Rupture of aneurysms of the anterior communicating or anterior cerebral artery is the usual antecedent event. The patient is mostly silent and motionless or nearly so, but tracking movements of the eyes and blinking are almost always preserved. The ability to walk is maintained in patients who do not have concomitant paraparesis from involvement of the mesial aspect of the motor areas. Often patients make many purposeful movements, such as those needed to adjust clothes or eat. The facial expression is empty, and the patient makes no effort to communicate verbally or by gesture. Rare isolated utterances may be produced, and repetition of single words and short sentences can occasionally be performed under coaxing. Whatever the amount of verbal output, patients do not produce paraphasias and have well-articulated though often hypophonic speech (Damasio and Van Hoesen, 1980, 1983).

The diagnosis of mutism should be made only after careful judgment of accompanying signs and of the whole context of the clinical presentation. Patients with mutism often evoke psychiatric disease, and if it were not for a clarifying previous history, a primarily neurological nature could go unnoticed. Mutism must be distinguished from anarthria and aphemia, conditions in which the inability to speak (or to speak without phonetic errors) is accompanied by a frustrated intent to communicate verbally and in which attempts to communicate by gesture or facial expression are often successful. These features also help distinguish mutism from the transcortical motor aphasias, in which speech is sparse and nonfluent, and in which word and sentence repetition are preserved.

Verbal Fluency

Verbal fluency, as measured by verbal association tests, often is impaired by frontal lobe damage. This may be noted in the absence of any detectable change in speech output. A curious instance is Brickner's patient A. He spoke fluent and well-articulated speech, often at a high rate, manifesting a free flow of verbal association of almost manic nature. However, when given a certain word, his ability to produce morphologically similar words by changing a letter or letter positions was impaired.

Using Thurstone's Word Fluency Test, Milner (1964) showed that patients with left frontal lobectomies that spared Broca's area scored very poorly on this test, despite there being no evidence of aphasia. Controls with

temporal lobectomies performed as well as patients with right frontal lobectomies. Interestingly, both left frontal– and right frontal–damaged patients performed at the same level in a task of verbal memory, suggesting the relative independence of the mechanism underlying fluency. The temporal lobe controls did poorly on the verbal memory task.

Benton (1968) arrived at the same conclusions studying a group of patients with left, right, and bilateral frontal damage. The task used to test fluency was an oral version of the Thurstone test, in which the patient is requested to say as many words beginning with a given letter of the alphabet as come to mind. Not only did the left hemisphere patients do remarkably worse than the right hemisphere ones, but bilaterally damaged patients also performed more poorly than those with right hemisphere damage only. A number of subsequent studies have replicated this basic pattern, although fluency may also be affected by nonfrontal lesions in the left hemisphere or by diffuse damage. Recently, Baldo and Shimamura (1998) found that frontal lobe damage affected both letter and category fluency. Stuss et al. (1998) examined the effects on verbal fluency of damage to various subregions of the frontal lobes, and found that left dorsolateral and superior mesial lesions on the left or right affected letter fluency. Category fluency was impaired by damage to these same regions, as well as by damage to right dorsolateral and inferior medial regions.

These findings generally support the classic views of Feuchtwanger (1923) and Kleist (1936), according to which "dominant" frontal lesions, but not "minor" frontal ones, interfere with verbal processes, particularly with respect to spontaneity and the ability to maintain a flow of verbal evocation without actually producing one of the typical aphasias. These views are in opposition to the views of Jefferson (1937) and Rylander (1940), who denied any lateralization of defect after frontal lobectomies.

Several functional imaging studies have reported left inferior frontal gyrus activation when normal subjects are shown concrete nouns and required to generate semantically appropriate verbs (the so-called verb generate task), but the exact role of this brain region in the task has not been clear (e.g., Petersen et al., 1989; Raichle et al., 1994). Thompson-Schill et al. (1998) found that patients with lesions in the left inferior frontal gyrus were impaired on the verb generation task when there were high demands for selection among competing responses, but not when there were low selection demands (i.e., in response to nouns with only one commonly associated verb, such as "scissors"). This suggests that the role of the inferior frontal gyrus in verb generation tasks may not be in semantic retrieval per se, but rather in the process of selection among multiple competing sources of information, a function that may apply across a wider range of tasks.

Nonvocal Language

The role of the frontal lobes in language is not limited to the auditory–vocal channel. Impairments of visuogestural language, reading comprehension, and writing have been documented in patients with focal damage in left premotor and prefrontal cortex. Damage to the left frontal lobe has been shown to result in breakdowns of signed language that have similarities to the patterns of aphasia in spoken language following damage to this area, with agrammatism and halting, effortful signing (Bellugi et al., 1989).

Damage to the left frontal lobe has long been associated with alexia in the setting of Broca's aphasia (Lichtheim, 1885; Dejerine and Mirallie, 1895; Nielsen, 1938, 1946). Benson (1977) reported that 51 of 61 patients (84%) with Broca's aphasia and no evidence of posterior lesions had at least mild alexia, and that these patients had particular difficulty in decoding words by grapheme-to-phoneme conversion. It has also been noted that oral reading and reading comprehension of Broca's aphasia may mirror the typical patterns of language breakdown in these patients, in that concrete nouns may be more likely to be read correctly than function words such as conjunctions, prepositions, pronouns, and articles (Gardner and Zurif, 1975; Kaplan and Goodglass, 1981).

Exner (1881) is usually credited with first describing agraphia following lesions in the superior aspect of the left premotor cortex ("Exner's area" in area 6, above areas 44 and 45). Other cases of agraphia associated with left dorsolateral frontal lesions have been described by Gordinier (1899), Penfield and Roberts (1959), and Rapscak et al. (1988). We have studied a case with isolated alexia and agraphia associated with a circumscribed surgical lesion in Exner's area (Anderson et al., 1990). This patient was not aphasic or hemiparetic, but was virtually unable to write any words or letters, with her writing attempts showing severe spatial distortion. Reading of single letters, words, and sentences was also severely impaired, but she could occasionally recognize single words in a gestalt fashion. The impairments of reading and writing were limited to the domain of letters; she could read and write numbers and perform written calculations without difficulty.

Further evidence that Exner's area may be involved in reading is provided by a case of reading epilepsy associated with a focal lesion in this region (Rittacio et al., 1992). The patient was a 24-year-old college student who underwent removal of a left frontal arteriovenous malformation. He was left without neurologic or cognitive defects except for seizures that occurred only when reading. In a series of controlled laboratory experiments, silent reading while subvocalizing was the most reliable means of eliciting seizure activity. Electrophysiological studies suggested that the epileptogenic zone was just anterior to the postsurgical lesion in Exner's area.

MOTOR FUNCTION AND VISUAL PERCEPTION

Axons from neurons in primary motor cortex and premotor cortex run through the corticospinal tract, providing the major substrate for cortical control of movement. In addition to motor dysfunction due to primary motor cortex damage, lesion studies in humans and monkeys have documented a variety of motor impairments associated with frontal lobe damage, including motor neglect, hypokinesia, motor impersistence, and perseveration (for a review, see Heilman and Watson, 1991). Elementary defects in reflexes, muscle tone, and eye movements resulting from frontal lobe damage were briefly reviewed earlier in this chapter.

Frontal lobe damage, especially that involving the left hemisphere, has long been associated with ideomotor apraxia (Liepmann, 1908), although this apraxia is generally of less severity and occurs less frequently than that with parietal lobe damage (e.g., Kolb and Milner, 1981; De Renzi et al., 1983). Defects also can be found on other visuomotor tasks with significant demands for generation or organization of motor behavior. For example, Benton (1968) demonstrated that performance of patients with right frontal or bilateral frontal lobe lesions was inferior to that of patients with left frontal lobe lesions on tests of three-dimensional block construction and copying designs, and Jones-Gotman and Milner (1977) found that subjects with right frontal lobe damage were impaired relative to subjects with temporal lobe or left frontal lobe damage on a task requiring the rapid generation of original abstract drawings.

Although visuoperceptual defects are more commonly associated with dysfunction in posterior cortical regions, visuoperception may also be affected by frontal lesions. Infarction of the middle cerebral artery often results in combined damage to the dorsolateral frontal lobe and the anterior parietal lobe, with a high probability of contralateral neglect if the damage is on the right. Damage limited to the frontal lobes has been shown to cause both contralateral and ipsilateral neglect (Heilman and Valenstein, 1972; Kwon and Heilman, 1991).

In cases of frontal lobe stroke or traumatic injury, considerable recovery of voluntary movement and perception usually occurs in the weeks or months following onset, particularly when the damage is unilateral. Focal frontal lobe damage usually results in little or no long-term impairment on most standardized tests of visual perception or construction. This is illustrated in Table 15–2, which provides the scores of eight subjects with focal damage to various frontal regions, including left and right dorsolateral frontal cortex and bilateral ventromedial areas. The tests include (1) The Facial Recognition Test (Benton et al., 1983), which requires discrimination between black and white photographs of faces which are similar in gender and age, (2) Judgment of Line Orientation (Benton et al., 1983), which requires the

Table 15–2. Visual Perception and Constructional Function

ID No.	Facial Recognition	Line Orientation	Complex Figure
318	43	30	36
414	50	22	30
468	44	30	34
534	46	21	31
1065	43	25	33
1173	47	20	32
1198	47	22	31
1331	50	23	33

Note: Data for Facial Recognition and Line Orientation are presented as corrected scores, and data for the Complex Figure are presented as raw scores.

matching of lines positioned at the same angle, and (3) the Rey-Osterrieth Complex Figure Test (Spreen and Strauss, 1991; Lezak, 1993), which requires the drawing of an abstract geometric figure from a model. All performances were within normal limits. When the area of dysfunction is limited to the prefrontal cortex, performances on perceptual and motor tasks with limited higher-order demands tend not to be significantly affected.

EMOTION AND PERSONALITY

Alterations of emotion and personality, including changes in characteristic behavioral response patterns, mood, and attitudes, are frequent consequences of frontal lobe damage and among the most difficult to evaluate. The assessment of changes at this level of behavior implies a notion of the limits or normal variation of several aspects of human personality. Naturally, only an approximation is possible, taking into account the patient's age, educational level, social and cultural group, and previous achievements. Alterations of personality and emotion following prefrontal damage are not independent of cognitive impairments. It is possible for elementary cognitive defects resulting from frontal lobe damage to have an impact on behaviors considered to be aspects of personality. For example, Deutsch et al. (1979) found that patients with frontal lobe damage who were rated as having a tendency toward social isolation showed defective orientation to other people who entered a room, and Daffner et al. (2000) found strong correlations between measures of visual attention to novel stimuli by a group of patients with frontal lobe damage and rating of apathy in their daily activities. Also, as described later, disruption of emotion is likely to play a key role in impairments of judgement and decision making following prefrontal damage (Damasio, 1994).

Affect

Butter et al. (1963, 1968) observed that monkeys with orbital ablations showed marked and long-lasting changes in emotional behavior that seemed to be related to an increase in aversive reactions and a concomitant decrease in aggressive reactions. They followed these observations with a careful study of aversive and aggressive behaviors in two groups of monkeys, one with orbital lesions, the other with temporal lesions (Butter et al., 1970). The orbital lesions produced a clear reduction in aggressive behaviors, a change that could still be seen after 10 months. This reduction seemed to be situational, as there were noticeable differences in the way the animals reacted to different potentially threatening stimuli, and the animals could still demonstrate aggression when brought back to the colony where they had been dominant figures. This suggests that a regulatory mechanism of aggression had been impaired and that the capacity to display aggression had not been eliminated. The authors point out that the dependence on environmental configuration and the variety of possible emotional responses are not consistent with a permanent state of "bluntness of affect" used to describe similar changes in animals or in patients, even if the animals do appear tame in many situations.

Anatomical study of the experimental lesions indicated that damage to the posteromedial sector of the orbital frontal lobe was closely correlated with the reported changes. This area of the cortex is intimately connected to the amygdala, and along with the dorsomedial nucleus of the thalamus, the amygdala and posteromedial orbital cortex project to roughly the same regions of the hypothalamus. The combination of behavioral and anatomical data sup-

ports the conjecture that these structures are part of a system involved in certain types of emotional reaction.

The standard descriptions of affective and emotional changes in frontal lobe patients include *witzelsucht*, a term coined by Oppenheim (1889) to describe the facetiousness of these patients, and *moria*, a term coined by Jastrowitz (1888) to denote a sort of caustic euphoric state that is almost inseparable from witzelsucht. Phenomena resembling such descriptions are occasionally found, especially in the acute presentation of cases, but it should be understood that in no patient are such changes permanent. Indeed, a patient who appears facetious and boastful will look apathetic and indifferent at some later time or else may show a sudden burst of short-lived anger. The instability of humor also applies to the traditional and somewhat misleading descriptions of "tameness" and "bluntness" of emotion, which may be quite changeable and actually give way to unbridled aggressive behavior against a background of flat affect. External circumstances, particularly if they are stressful, as during an examining session, may "set" the patient's emotional tone. Frequently, the reaction will be found inappropriate to the circumstances but not necessarily in a consistent or predictable manner.

When facetiousness is present, it often has a sexual content, but the inappropriate acts usually are verbal, and rarely do patients attempt to behave according to the wishes or judgments expressed in their profane remarks. The lack of appreciation of social rules is usually evident, but even so there tends to be little or no intentional viciousness. Nor is there any indication that facetiousness produces pleasure: indeed, affect tends to be shallow. Limited ability to enjoy pleasurable stimulation, particularly if it involves social, intellectual, and aesthetic situations, is probably characteristic of such patients and accompanies a restricted response to punishment. Both of these underscore the elementary disorder of emotion.

The association of changes in affect and in emotional control with predominant involvement of a specific region of the frontal lobe is still unsettled. Nonetheless, there is little doubt that the ventral and medial aspects of the frontal lobe are especially involved in many patients presenting with emotional changes. Also, patients with mesial frontal lobe lesions often appear to have blunted emotional responses, as if their affect had been neutralized (Damasio and Van Hoesen, 1983). Damasio et al. (1990) found that subjects with bilateral ventromedial frontal lobe lesions had abnormal autonomic responses to socially meaningful stimuli, despite normal autonomic responses to elementary and unconditioned stimuli. These findings suggest that such stimuli failed to activate somatic states previously associated with specific social situations, and which marked the anticipated outcomes of response options as advantageous or not.

Although patients with ventral and medial frontal lobe damage rarely show the concern and preoccupation that depressed patients do, damage to the dorsolateral prefrontal region, particularly on the left, has been associated with depression. Blumer and Benson (1975) referred to a pseudodepressed syndrome with decreased self-initiation following dorsolateral frontal lobe damage, and Cummings (1985) described apathy, indifference, and psychomotor retardation as frequent features. Depressive symptomatology and social unease were found to be common in patients 3 months after dorsolateral prefrontal damage from stroke or trauma (Paradiso et al., 1999). Patients with lesions on the left appear to have the greatest chance of developing depression (Robinson et al., 1984, 1985). Damage to the left dorsolateral frontal region, for example, resulting from stroke in the anterior distribution of the middle cerebral artery, often has devastating consequences (paresis of the dominant side, aphasia), and unlike comparable lesions on the right, generally does not impair awareness for the acquired impairments. However, during the acute phase following a stroke, depression cannot be fully explained by these factors, suggesting a neurophysiological basis for the relationship between left dorsolateral prefrontal damage and depression. Reaction to functional impairments is likely to play a more important role in depression that begins 6 months or more after a stroke (Robinson et al., 1987).

The emotional consequences of focal damage to the right dorsolateral frontal cortex have not been well characterized, but may include both restriction of affect and emotional dyscontrol. Damage to the right frontal lobe may also contribute to anosognosia for hemiparesis and unawareness of acquired cognitive impairments. Self-awareness has been described as the highest cognitive attribute of the frontal lobes (Stuss and Benson, 1987). A lack of awareness regarding alterations in behavior, emotions, and thought processes is a common consequence of frontal lobe dysfunction, and one which has major implications for assessment and rehabilitation. Interviews with patients may suggest that all is normal, in contrast to descriptions of marked behavioral dysfunction provided by relatives and caretakers. In addition to the lack of appreciation of changes from the premorbid state, frontal lobe damage may impair the ability to gain insight on specific cognitive abilities. For example, Janowsky et al. (1989) found that subjects with frontal lobe lesions were impaired on a task in which they had to judge the probability that they would recognize the correct answer to a multiple-choice question.

Patients with limited awareness of acquired impairments tend not to be motivated to improve their behavior in rehabilitation settings. A major component of interventions directed at impairments of social behavior, impulse control, and decision making involves training patients to become increasingly aware of their dysfunctional behaviors. These patients often have a more general problem with evaluating the consequences and implications of their own behavior. Patients with frontal lobe damage may fail to see the significance of their decisions for themselves and for those around them. Their behavior suggests difficulty assessing the value of each new action, or lack of action, in terms of goals that are not overtly specified in the immediate environment.

The perception or comprehension of emotional information also appears to be altered in some patients with frontal lobe damage (e.g., Grattan et al., 1994). The families of patients with frontal lobe injuries often complain that the patient has impaired empathy, but little is known regarding anatomical–functional correlations for this deficit. Damage to right somatosensory cortex appears to be the most important factor contributing to impairments in the recognition of emotional facial expressions (Adolphs et al., 2000), but damage to various sectors of prefrontal cortex also may disrupt empathic processing. Eslinger (1998) has raised the possibility that damage to dorsolateral frontal areas may impair certain cognitive aspects of empathy (e.g., perspective taking), while orbital damage may have more of an impact on emotional aspects of empathy. In another example of disrupted processing of social–emotional information, damage to the right frontal lobe has been associated with impaired appreciation of humor, possibly through disruption of component processes such as emotional reactivity and abstract thought (Shammi and Stuss, 1999). Finally, we should note that patients with some right prefrontal lesions, especially if these lesions are located in the white matter and disrupt the cross-talk between ventromedial and dorsolateral regions, develop changes in emotion and decision making similar to those we have reported in patients with bilateral ventromedial damage.

Hallmark Case Studies

A number of detailed case studies have helped to characterize the personality changes that can result from frontal lobe damage. The famous patient Gage, described by Harlow (1848, 1868), provides the first solid reference to specific injury of the frontal lobes and its relation to disturbances of complex behavior. The other important observations were added in this century. They include the case studies of Brickner (1934; 1936), Hebb (Hebb and Penfield, 1940), Benton (Ackerly and Benton, 1948), and Damasio (Eslinger and Damasio, 1985; Damasio et al., 1991; Saver and Damasio, 1991). For a review of the early history of clinical investigations into frontal lobe damage, see Benton (1991a).

Brickner's patient, known as A., was a 39-year-old New York stockbroker who, until 1 year before surgery, led a normal life. Slowly progressive headaches, which became more and more severe, and finally the sudden onset of mental obtundation brought him to medical attention. A diagnosis of frontal tumor was made, which, at surgery, proved to be a volu-minous meningioma of the falx compressing both frontal lobes. The neurosurgeon, Walter Dandy, had to perform an extensive bilateral resection of frontal tissue in two stages. On the left side all the frontal tissue rostral to Broca's area was removed. On the right, the excision was even larger and included all the brain anterior to the motor area. The patient's condition gradually stabilized and no motor or sensory defect could be detected. For months there were frequent periods of restlessness, but akinesia or changes in tone were never noted, nor were there any signs of motor perseveration. Orientation to person, place, and time seemed intact as well as remote and recent memory. A. was able to understand the circumstances of his illness and the surgical intervention to which he had been subject, and he was aware of the efforts of his family and physician to have him recover as much as possible. The range of his intellectual ability could be inferred from his capacity to play checkers, sometimes at a quick and expert pace; to explain the meaning of proverbs; and, occasionally, to discuss with lucidity the meaning of his predicament for himself, his relatives, and his friends. On the negative side, his behavior had undergone a marked deterioration. He was unable to adjust his emotional reactions appropriately. Furthermore, his affect was shallow. He became boastful, constantly insisting on his professional, physical, and sexual prowess, and showed little restraint, not only in describing his mythical adventures but in verbalizing judgments about people and circumstances surrounding him. His train of thought was hypomanic, with facetious remarks to match, but he could suddenly become aggressive if frustrated. Frequently he tried to be witty, generally at the expense of others. He was particularly nasty toward his wife. Prior to surgery he had always been kind to her, although not unusually considerate. His sex life, which his wife described as normal before the operation, changed radically. He became impotent and after a few frustrated attempts at intercourse, never again sought her or indeed any other partner, although much of his conversation would revolve around his sexual exploits. Ability to plan daily activity meaningfully had been lost and so had his initiative and creativity. Although he constantly spoke of returning to work, he never made any effort to do so and continued living in close dependence on his relatives. Certain levels of learning ability, however, both verbal and nonverbal, seemed intact. For example, in the face of his constant distractibility and lack of interest, he was taught how to operate proficiently a complex printing machine, on which he produced visiting cards. Moreover, when faced with strangers in a reasonably nondemanding situation, he would be charming, display impeccable manners, and be considerably restrained. Independent examiners, including neurologists, would then be unable to detect any abnormality even after fairly long conversations.

Brickner's painstaking description produced different impressions on the readers of the time. The overall view was that the intervention had a crippling effect on A.'s mental ability, but for Egas Moniz, the enterprising pioneer of frontal leucotomy (1936), A.'s case was remarkable in that it proved bilateral frontal damage to be compatible with maintenance of major operational abilities and especially because it demonstrated a change in affect and emotional response with pronounced reduction of anxiety. This view is likely to have played a role in the theorization behind the leucotomy project.

In view of the location and size of the tumor, damage to the septal and hypothalamic regions was a possibility, and, although the autopsy report on this case (Brickner, 1952) mentioned no such evidence, there may have been microscopic basal forebrain changes. The report is clear in noting that the cortical territory of the anterior cerebral arteries was intact (which might have been predicted from the patient's lack of crural paresis). Nevertheless, the autopsy did becloud the issue by revealing several meningiomas, one of which was of significant size and located in the right occipital area. In retrospect, it seems clear that the latter tumor had not grown yet at the time of operation because the patient developed a new set of symptoms 6 to 7 years after surgery. Such findings should not be used to minimize the significance of this case, as it is unlikely that they played any role in the patient's behavior.

Hebb and Penfield (1940) described an example of relatively successful bilateral removal of frontal tissue with a more straightforward possibility of a clinicoanatomical correlation. This patient had been normal until age 16, when he sustained a compounded frontal fracture that damaged both frontal lobes, produced the formation of scar tissue, and resulted in a severe convulsive disorder. At age 28, the patient was operated on and the frontal lobes were extensively resected bilaterally, exposing both orbital plates back to the lesser wing of the sphenoid and transecting the frontal horns of the lateral ventricles. The anterior cerebral arteries were spared. At least a third of the frontal lobes was removed. In terms of the anatomical result the intervention was not very different from that of Brickner's patient, but, unlike A., this patient's brain had not been distorted and edematous prior to resection and the ablation took place under optimal surgical circumstances. In the postoperative period, seizures practically stopped and the behavioral disturbances associated with interictal periods disappeared. The authors suggest that the patient's personality actually improved (from the time he had sustained the fracture) and that his intellectual ability was probably better than before the surgical intervention. We take this to mean that comparison with the period of convulsive disorder was favorable. Comparison with the period prior to the initial damage would certainly not be as favorable, as we believe this patient's intellectual and emotional maturation had been considerably affected by his frontal lobe lesion. Even if he is described as relatively independent, socially adequate, and intellectually intact, some observers have felt that his personality development seemed arrested at the age of the accident, and a certain resemblance with the patient of Ackerly and Benton has been indicated. In a later study, Hebb (1945) conceded that, in spite of the patient's apparently good adjustment, his long-term planning and initiative were impaired.

The patient of Ackerly and Benton (1948), by contrast, sustained bilateral frontal lobe damage either at birth or during the perinatal period. A neurosurgical exploration was performed at age 20 years and revealed cystic degeneration of the left frontal lobe and absence of the right one, probably as a result of atrophy. This patient's history was marked throughout childhood and adolescence by severe be-havioral problems, in school and at home. He could not hold a job, generally because after some days of being an obedient and even charming employee, he would suddenly show bursts of bad temper, lose interest in his activ-ity, and often end up stealing or being disor-derly. He reacted badly to frustration, and de-parture from routine would easily frustrate him. Except for periods of frustration and cat-astrophic reaction, his docility, quietness, and polite manners were quite impressive. His gen-eral health seems to have been good. His sex-ual interests were dim, and he never had an emotional involvement with any partner al-though, for a time, he did have occasional sex with prostitutes. As a whole, his behavior was described as stereotyped, unimaginative, and lacking in initiative. He never developed any particular professional skill or hobby. He also failed to plan for the future, either immediate or long range, and reward and punishment did not seem to influence the course of his behav-ior. His memory was described as capricious, showing at times a remarkable capacity (such as his ability to remember the makes of auto-mobiles) and at other times an inaccurate rep-resentation of events. There was no evidence of the common varieties of neurotic disorder, of somatization or deliberate antisocial behav-ior, or of addictive behaviors. Apparently, he could not be described as being joyful or happy, and it looked like both pleasure and pain were short-lived and directly related to the presence or absence of frustration.

When he was reevaluated 15 years later, there had been no remarkable personality changes except for a higher frustration thresh-old. Intellectually, however, recent memory deficits were now noticeable and an inability to perform the Wisconsin Card Sorting Test was recorded.

For the past 20 years we have had the op-portunity to study in detail patient E.V.R. (Es-linger and Damasio, 1985). The patient grew up as the oldest of five children, an excellent student and a role model for many friends and siblings. After high school he married and com-pleted a business college degree in accounting. By age 30, he was the father of two children and a church elder and had come through the ranks of his company to a supervisory post. In 1973 his family and employers began to notice a variety of personality changes. He became unreliable, could not seem to complete his usual work, and experienced marital difficul-ties. He was suspended from his job. In 1975 a large orbitofrontal meningioma compressing both frontal lobes was removed. After his post-operative recovery, E.V.R. returned to ac-counting with a small home construction busi-ness. He soon established a partnership with a man of questionable reputation and went into business, against sound advice. The venture proved catastrophic. E.V.R. had to declare bankruptcy and lost his entire personal invest-ment. Next, he tried several different jobs (warehouse laborer, apartment complex man-ager, accountant) but was consistently fired from all of them when it became clear that he could not keep reliable standards. His wife left home with the children and filed for a divorce. When he was reevaluated 2 years later, a CT excluded a recurrence of tumor and the neu-rological examination was normal except for slight incoordination in the left upper extrem-ity and bilateral anosmia. Psychometric evalu-ation at that time revealed a verbal IQ of 120 (91st percentile), a performance IQ of 108 (70th percentile), and a Wechsler memory quotient of 140. A Minnesota Multiphasic Per-sonality Inventory (MMPI) was valid and en-tirely within the normal range.

E.V.R.'s problems persisted. He was fired from two additional jobs. The reasons given in-cluded tardiness and lack of productivity. He remarried within a month after his first divorce, against the advice of his relatives. The second marriage ended in divorce 2 years later. Fur-ther neurological and psychological evaluation of E.V.R. at a private psychiatric institution in September 1981 revealed "no evidence of or-ganic brain syndrome or frontal dysfunction." Assessment with the WAIS disclosed a Verbal IQ of 125 (95th percentile) and a Performance IQ of 124 (94th percentile). His Wechsler Memory Quotient was 148, and the Halstead-Reitan Battery revealed average to superior ability on every subtest. An MMPI was once again valid with no evidence of psychopathol-ogy on the clinical scales. Psychiatric evaluation suggested only psychological adjustment problems which should be amenable to psychotherapy. To this day, E.V.R.'s basic neuropsychological test performances remain normal.

Neuroanatomical analysis of E.V.R.'s neuroimaging studies reveals the structural correlate of his behavioral defect. Computed tomography shows clear evidence of bilateral damage to frontal cortices, especially marked in the ventromedial area, and more so on the right than on the left. The dorsolateral sectors, the cingulate gyri, and the motor and supplementary motor regions are intact.

Reflection on these cases is most rewarding. The patients of Hebb and Benton shared a rigid, perseverative attitude in their approach to life, and both had the courteous manner described as "English valet politeness," though in the judgment of several examiners, Hebb's patient led a clearly more productive but not fully independent existence. The evolution of the personality in Hebb's patient seems to have been arrested at the time of his accident, when he was 16, while in Ackerly's patient the defect came early in development. The patients of Brickner and of Damasio, on the other hand, had normal development and sustained frontal lobe damage in adult life. The fact that their lesions came at an age when plasticity of the nervous system was more limited may account for some differences of outcome. Nonetheless, the patients share a number of features: inability to organize future activity and hold gainful employment; tendency to present a favorable view of themselves; stereotyped but correct manners; diminished ability to respond to punishment and experience pleasure; diminished sexual and exploratory drives; lack of motor, sensory, or communication defects; and overall intelligence within expectations based on educational and occupational background. With the exception of Damasio's patient, all patients showed lack of originality and creativity, inability to focus attention, recent memory vulnerable to interference, and a tendency to display inappropriate emotional reactions. The cluster of these features constitutes one of the more typical frontal lobe syndromes, and perhaps the one that easily comes to mind when there is a reference to "frontal lobe syndrome." Let us point out again that many patients with frontal lobe damage have no such defects.

The generalizability of the conclusions regarding personality changes and frontal lobe damage drawn from the individual case studies and clinical lore is supported by findings from a recent group study. For a large sample of subjects with chronic focal adult-onset lesions, Barrash et al. (2000) obtained standardized ratings of a wide range of personality characteristics from informants who knew the patients well both before and after lesion onset. It was found that bilateral lesions in the orbital and mesial frontal cortex were reliably associated with a number of specific, highly disruptive, and persistent emotional and personality alterations, including blunted emotional experience, low emotional expressivity, apathy, indecisiveness, poor judgement, lack of planning, lack of initiative, social inappropriateness, and lack of insight.

BEHAVIORAL GUIDANCE

Regulation of Arousal and Behavior

Luria's contribution to the study of frontal lobe function encompasses many years of extensive investigation of patients and normal subjects (Luria, 1966, 1969; Luria and Homskaya, 1964). As in so many other studies on the frontal lobe, the importance of the results is somewhat limited by the choice of the subjects for experimentation. Most of the patients studied by Luria and co-workers had large frontal tumors, some intrinsic and some extrinsic. Some involved subcortical limbic-system structures, such as the septum. Some had associated hydrocephalus and some did not. Most patients had associated nonfrontal dysfunction, due to mass effect or compromise of vascular supply elsewhere in the brain. The location within the frontal lobe was also varied. Nevertheless, Luria's concept of frontal lobe function and dysfunction is quite stimulating.

His interpretation emphasizes the verbally mediated activating and regulatory role of the frontal lobes and their role in problem solving. He suggests that the orienting reaction, as measured by galvanic skin response or suppression of the alpha rhythm in the EEG, cannot be stabilized by verbal stimuli in patients with frontal lobe lesions. In normal subjects, the presentation of verbally meaningful instructions is expected to prevent habituation to stimuli and therefore prevent the orienting response from disappearing (Homskaya, 1966). Apparently nonaphasic patients with tumors, gunshot wounds, or stroke involving the posterior sensory cortex behave as normals in terms of verbal stabilization of the orienting responses even in the presence of praxic and gnosic defects. In patients with frontal lobe lesions, however, the verbal signal does not prevent habituation. Moreover, subjects with damage to the frontal poles and to the mesial and basal aspects of the frontal structures tend to be more affected than those with dorsolateral involvement.

Additional evidence for altered orienting responses in frontal lobe patients comes from studies of visual potentials evoked by verbally tagged stimuli. Stimuli that would have increased the amplitude of visual evoked potentials in normals failed to do so in patients with frontal lobe damage (Simernitskaya and Homskaya, 1966; Simernitskaya, 1970). Animal studies have also supported the idea that frontal lobe damage produces changes in the processing of information by altering the orienting response (e.g., Grueninger et al., 1965; Kimble et al., 1965), but as noted earlier, the impact of frontal lobe damage on attention is not limited to immediate orienting responses.

Another aspect of frontal lobe dysfunction concerns the possibility of directing the execution of complex actions by verbal mediation. Kaczmarek (1987) documented impairments in several aspects of the linguistic formulations of patients with frontal lobe damage, particularly in the production of propositional statements and descriptions of relationships among objects, and suggested that these impairments may contribute to a defect of regulatory behavior. Several authors have pointed out that frontal lobe patients may be able to repeat correctly the instructions for a given task while making no use whatever of the information in performing a task. Thus, while performing a sorting task, subjects may make perseverative sorting errors even while verbalizing the correct strategy. The same has been said regarding the utilization of perceived error: patients will verbally admit the mistake but fail to correct it. Luria has repeatedly called attention to

this type of defect and considers it one of the hallmarks of frontal lobe dysfunction. He attempted to objectify the defect in a series of experiments in which patients were requested to follow progressively more complex verbal instructions. He noted that patients were able to perform only the more direct and simple commands and would fail to carry out more complex instructions, particularly if they involved some change in principle or some conflict with additional cues provided by the examiner. Since the patient would still be able to repeat the initial verbal instruction, Luria concluded that the primary difficulty was one of verbal guidance of actions (Luria and Homskaya, 1964). Again, the weakness of these studies resides in the subjects used for the observations, i.e., patients with massive bilateral tumors of the frontal lobes. Attempts at replication have met with difficulties (Drewe, 1975). Some defects of the kind reported by Luria were found, but the dissociation between verbal and motor ability was not verified and the author considered it unlikely that a loss of verbal regulatory action was the mechanism underlying impaired performance.

A similar objection may be raised about Luria's description of the changes in problem-solving behavior that attend massive lesions of the frontal lobes. A state of confusion seems to underlie many of the disturbances of planning and calculation exhibited by his patients. Naturally, one can respond to this argument by stating that an element of confusion is part of some frontal lobe syndromes to begin with, but confusion can be caused by central nervous system changes that have little to do with frontal lobe dysfunction, although they may coincide with it and derive from a common cause. Also, confusion is not a necessary accompaniment of frontal lobe damage; it is associated with acute and massive damage of frontal tissue and clearly improves with time as adaptation to the pathological process occurs.

Nonetheless, Luria's observations are very suggestive and his proposals have heuristic value. The ideas that patients have trouble in the choice of programs of action, that their strategy for gathering information necessary for the solution of the problem is impoverished, and that they seldom verify whether their actions meet the original intent, are interesting interpretations of defects that can often be found in frontal lobe damage. In addition, it is our impression that even when these defects cannot be demonstrated by an experimental task in the immediate and consistent manner claimed by Luria, one can still encounter them at more complex levels of behavior, for instance, in goal-oriented decision making during long-term planning operations.

Response to Changing Contingencies

Failure to adjust behavior adequately in response to environmental conditions may play an important role in the cognitive/behavioral defects seen after frontal lobe damage. Socially inappropriate behavior and nonadaptive decision making by patients with frontal lobe damage may reflect dysfunction of the neural system by which the consequences of past actions affect the on-line guidance of behavior. It has long been known that monkeys with frontal lobe ablations are unable to make normal adjustments of behavior in response to changing contingencies (Settlage et al., 1948).

Testing for the ability to initiate, stop, and modify behavior in response to changing stimuli has traditionally been part of the evaluation for frontal lobe dysfunction. Depending on the circumstances, the evaluation may involve observation of performances on bedside "go–no go" tasks or more sophisticated psychometric assessment. The Wisconsin Card Sorting Test (WCST) was developed by Berg (1948) and Grant and Berg (1948) to provide a measure of the ability to identify abstract categories and shift cognitive set, and has been widely applied in the assessment of frontal lobe damage. The test requires patients to sort a deck of response cards according to various stimulus dimensions. The patient is not informed of the sorting principles, but rather must infer these from information given by the examiner after each response. Further complicating the patient's task is the fact that the sorting principles change throughout the test without any clue other than the changing pattern of feedback. Although there have been several variations on the original methodology, certain features have remained generally constant (see Heaton, 1981,

for a complete description of the test). Each response card contains from one to four identical figures (stars, crosses, triangles, or circles), in one of four colors. These figures provide the basis for the three sorting principles: color, form, and number. At the beginning of the test, four stimulus cards are placed before the patient (one red triangle, two green stars, three yellow crosses, and four blue circles). The patient is instructed to place each consecutive response card in front of one of the stimulus cards, wherever it appears to match best. The patient is not informed of the correct sorting principle, but is told only if each response is right or wrong. After the patient has made 10 consecutive correct sorts, the initial sorting principle (color) is changed (to form) without warning. Again, after 10 correct sorts, the sorting principle is changed without warning from form to number. This procedure continues until either five shifts of sorting category have been completed, or the two decks of 64 cards have been sorted.

The requirements of the WCST for cognitive abstraction and flexibility in response to changing contingencies make it an attractive instrument for investigating the consequences of frontal lobe damage. In a pioneering study, Milner (1963) documented a consistent and severe impairment on the WCST in patients who had undergone prefrontal lobectomies for treatment of epilepsy. None of her subjects were able to complete more than two shifts of set (three categories). The findings were interpreted as suggesting that the ability to shift from one strategy to another in a sorting task is more compromised by frontal lobe damage than by rolandic or posterior sensory cortex damage. The manifest perseveration that made patients rigidly adhere to one criterion and ignore the examiner's guiding information was interpreted as an inability to overcome an established response set.

Although some subsequent studies also found that, as a group, frontal lobe–damaged subjects tended to perform worse than subjects with focal nonfrontal damage, these investigations showed substantial variability in WCST performance across subjects with frontal lobe damage (Drewe, 1974; Heaton, 1981), and one study using a slightly modified procedure found that patients with posterior lesions performed worse than patients with anterior lesions (Teuber et al., 1951). We examined the WCST performances of 91 subjects with focal brain lesions caused by stroke or tumor resection, and found no differences between those subjects with frontal and those with nonfrontal lesions (Anderson et al., 1991). Consistent with most prior studies, there was considerable variability in WCST performances across subjects with frontal damage. Some subjects with extensive frontal lobe damage performed the task with ease and made virtually no errors, while others with comparable lesions were severely defective. Likewise, many subjects with nonfrontal lesions had defective performances. Within the frontal lobe group, performances on the WCST did not appear to be related to the specific area of damage (e.g., dorsolateral vs. ventromedial). Along similar lines, a large-scale study of Vietnam war veterans found no difference in WCST performances between subjects with frontal lobe damage and those with posterior damage (Grafman et al., 1990). Regional cerebral blood flow studies have indicated that performance on the WCST is associated with relative increase in physiological activity in the prefrontal area, but that several other areas also show increased activity relative to a resting state (Weinberger et al., 1986). Clearly, scores on the WCST must be interpreted in a broad neuropsychological context. Performances are correlated with age, education, and IQ, and the combined findings of several studies suggest that time since onset is a critical factor, with considerable improvement occurring over time (see Stuss et al., 2000).

The performance measure from the WCST that has proven most sensitive to prefrontal damage has been the number of perseverative errors committed. Perseveration at multiple levels of behavioral organization may be observed in some patients with frontal lobe damage, but the localizing value of perseveration is limited (e.g., Goldberg, 1986). Decreased ability to inhibit repetition of ineffective responses appears to be one of the basic defects arising from frontal lobe damage, affecting performance on a variety of tasks. It is possible that variations in inhibitory control may underlie important cognitive differences between humans and other species, as well as differences

that arise during the course of human development (Hauser, 1999).

Frontal lobe damage may cause impairments on conditional learning tasks other than those on the WCST. For example, patients with frontal lobe tumors were found to be impaired relative to those with posterior tumors on a task in which they were required to generate hypotheses regarding the relevance of certain stimulus dimensions, and then modify the hypotheses on the basis of repeated feedback (Cicerone et al., 1983). The subjects with frontal lobe tumors showed a tendency to repeat responses despite negative feedback. In a series of studies with nonhuman primates and human subjects with frontal lobe ablations, Petrides has investigated the ability to select, from a number of possible alternative responses, the correct response given the current stimulus. Each of the alternative responses is correct only in the presence of one particular stimulus, and the subject must discover on the basis of information given by the examiner after each response which is the appropriate response for each one of the set of stimuli. Petrides (1985) found that patients with unilateral frontal lobe excisions were impaired, relative to patients with temporal lobe excisions, on tasks that required the subject to point to different locations or display various hand shapes in response to specific stimuli. This basic finding was replicated with a task in which the subjects learned to associate various abstract designs with various colored lights (Petrides, 1990), suggesting that the defect in conditional learning following frontal damage is a general one not limited to situations requiring selection between distinct movements or spatial locations. The subjects involved in these studies had undergone extensive prefrontal lobectomies, with lesions generally involving dorsolateral as well as ventral or medial cortices. However, parallel research with nonhuman primates has suggested that the posterior dorsolateral frontal cortex may be the critical region for performance on the conditional association tasks (Petrides, 1987).

Planning and Sequencing

The ability to plan short- and long-term future behaviors often seems to be devastated in patients with frontal lobe damage. In our experience, the modal response of these patients to questions regarding plans for the upcoming days or months is a recitation of the activities of the past several days. Consistent with this, their daily behavior often becomes a highly repetitious routine if left to their own devices. Other patients may describe, generally in vague terms, long-term goals that are typically fanciful, unrealistic, or illogical. These verbalizations provide scant evidence of planning, and seem to have little or no impact on the guidance of behavior.

The relationship of planning defects to frontal lobe damage is due in part to the major working memory and temporal sequencing demands of planning (Sirigu et al., 1995; Owen, 1997). Recent neurophysiological evidence from monkeys also indicates that neurons in prefrontal cortex are involved in prospective coding of anticipated reward and expected objects (Watanabe, 1996; Rainer et al., 1999), and functional imaging in normal humans has suggested that anterior dorsolateral prefrontal cortex may have a unique role in maintaining goals in working memory while proceeding with subgoals (Koechlin et al., 1999).

Much of the evidence for an impairment of planning following prefrontal damage has been based on the "Tower" tasks (e.g., Tower of Hanoi, Tower of London), which require movement of a set of disks to a goal position, following certain rules that require planning of a series of steps (Shallice, 1982; Owen et al., 1990; Carlin et al., 2000). The linkage between performance on such tasks and frontal activity has been supported by functional imaging studies (e.g., Dagher et al., 1999). Goel and Grafman (1995) have pointed out that the Tower of Hanoi (TOH) task may have different cognitive demands than the Tower of London, with the critical step in TOH being the ability to see and resolve a goal–subgoal conflict (i.e., to perform a counterintuitive backward move), rather than planning.

Although there appears to be an association between dorsolateral frontal damage and impairments on laboratory tests involving planning, Sarazin et al. (1998) have provided evidence that orbital prefrontal dysfunction is most highly correlated with planning defects in real-world activities. Planning clearly is not a single cognitive operation. Rather, planning involves conflation of multiple component processes and occurs over a broad range of circumstances involving widely divergent time frames, levels of complexity and intentionality, and methods of execution. It appears that broad sectors of the frontal lobes, including dorsolateral and orbital prefrontal regions, in addition to premotor cortex, are involved in aspects of planning. An important research challenge at this point is delineation of component cognitive processes and their linkage to specific regions of the prefrontal cortex (Goel et al., 1997).

Petrides and Milner (1982) contrasted the effect of lesions in the frontal lobe with the effect of lesions in the temporal lobe on four self-ordered tasks that required the organization of the sequence of pointing responses. In these sequential tasks, subjects are free to choose their own order of response but are prevented from giving the same response twice. Patients with frontal lobe excisions had significant impairments in all four tasks, whereas the patients with temporal excisions either had no impairment or, when their lesions encompassed the hippocampus, exhibited material-specific deficits. It is of interest that the patients with left frontal lobe excisions were impaired in performing both verbal and nonverbal tasks, whereas the patients with right frontal lobe excisions were impaired only in nonverbal ones. Petrides and Milner (1982) pointed out how this disparity is compatible with the notion of left hemisphere dominance for the programming of voluntary actions.

Learning to maneuver through a spatial maze requires that a sequence of behaviors be performed in a particular order, and subjects with frontal lobe lesions have been found to be defective in various maze-learning tasks (e.g., Porteus et al., 1944; Milner, 1965; Canavan, 1983). Milner (1965) noted that the frontal lobe subjects repeatedly failed to return to the correct path despite feedback regarding their error. Consistent with this, Karnath et al. (1991) used a computerized maze task to demonstrate that, relative to normal control subjects, subjects with medial frontal lobe lesions showed greater rule-breaking behavior on the second trial through the mazes. The finding that subjects with frontal lobe damage are slower to benefit from experience for the guidance of maze learning is reminiscent of Petrides' findings on learning conditional associations. Additional information regarding the effects of frontal lesions on maze learning comes from a recent study by Winocur and Moscovitch (1990). Rats with bilateral prefrontal lesions were impaired in learning the general skill of maze learning, despite good memory for information regarding the specific maze they had experience with. The opposite pattern was found in rats with bilateral hippocampal lesions.

Strategy Application

The complexity of real-world problem solving and decision making is not approximated by standard clinical or laboratory tasks, which typically are characterized by having a single explicit problem, brief trials, and clear cues for task initiation and completion. Problem solving and decision making in the real world involve integration of information from diverse sources over extended time frames, a seemingly unlimited choice of response options, and often an absence of specific criteria for adequate task performance. It appears likely that much of the dissociation between standardized test performance and real-world dysfunction may arise because prefrontal cortex damage leaves relatively preserved an ability to respond appropriately when sufficient constraints and structure are provided by immediately present environmental stimuli. Cummings (1995) has emphasized the role of increased environmental dependency as a key organizing theme for understanding frontal lobe dysfunction. In its most extreme form, environmental dependency can be expressed as a near compulsion to grasp and use immediately present items, the so-called utilization behavior (Lhermitte et al., 1986; Shallice et al., 1989; Brazzelli and Spinnier, 1998). In milder forms, environmental dependency may set the stage for deceptively good problem solving, provided the necessary components for the task are placed on the table in front of the patient. This factor introduces a fundamental conflict between the format of most standardized testing and the nature of the impairments that arise from prefrontal damage.

Goldberg and Podell (2000) have emphasized the additional distinction between veridical problem solving (tapped by most neuropsychological tests) and adaptive problem solving, which incorporates the organism's priorities and more closely resembles real-world activity. The have developed the Cognitive Bias Test, which requires response selection based on the subject's preferences rather than external criteria. Measures reflecting the extent to which responses in an ambiguous situation were guided by context appeared to be sensitive to hemispheric and gender differences.

Shallice and Burgess (1991) developed a quantifiable analog of the type of relatively unstructured, open-ended, multiple subgoal tasks which seem to cause so much difficulty in the daily life of patients with frontal lobe damage. Subjects were required to complete a set of everyday tasks (e.g., buy a certain item, meet someone at a given time, obtain basic meteorological and consumer information), which were designed to place limited demands on non-executive cognitive functions. They found that three patients with traumatic head injuries involving prefrontal damage approached the tasks inefficiently and tended to violate rules (task imposed and societal norms). We have replicated this experiment in a group of 34 patients with focal brain lesions caused by stroke or surgery (17 prefrontal, 17 nonfrontal). The tasks are performed in a complex real-world environment presenting myriad options (i.e., a shopping mall). We found that the behavior of patients with prefrontal lesions was marked by inefficiencies, failure to complete tasks, and rule infractions (Anderson et al., 2000). The impairments tended to be most severe in patients with damage to orbital prefrontal regions, although dorsolateral lesions also resulted in impairments of lesser severity. These findings help substantiate the linkage between frontal lobe dysfunction and impairment in meeting the exigencies of normal daily life, and highlight some of the behavioral and environmental factors that may contribute to the defect.

Decision Making

A hallmark of frontal lobe dysfunction is difficulty making decisions that are in the long-term best interests of the patient. Clearly there are many cognitive factors that contribute to adaptive decision making. For instance, to make a selection among multiple options with several possible outcomes, both immediate and future, it is necessary to operate on many premises, some just perceived, some recalled from previous experiences, and some recalled from imagined future scenarios. The process of analysis requires the relatively simultaneous holding of numerous sites of neural activity, in widespread regions of the cerebral cortex across long delays of many thousands of milliseconds, i.e., working memory. However, significant decision-making defects occur in patients with no apparent defect in other cognitive abilities, including working memory (e.g., Bechara et al., 1998).

In an effort to detect and measure this impairment, Bechara et al. (1994) developed a card task that mimics real-life decision making in the way it factors uncertainty, reward, and punishment. Subjects are given a loan of play money, shown four decks of cards (face down), and asked to draw cards in a manner to lose the least amount of money and win the most. Turning each card results in an immediate reward ($100 for decks A and B, and $50 for decks C and D). At unpredictable points, the turning of some cards results in a financial penalty (larger for decks A and B, and smaller in decks C and D). Playing mostly from the decks with the larger initial payoff (A and B) is disadvantageous over the long run because of the larger penalties. Playing mostly from decks C and D, with the smaller initial reward, turns out to be advantageous, i.e., leading to financial gain. There is no way for a subject to predict when a penalty will arise or to calculate with precision the net gain or loss from each deck. Normal subjects and subjects with damage to nonfrontal brain areas tend to initially sample from all decks, but choose significantly more from decks C and D while avoiding A and B over the course of 100 card selections. In contrast, subjects with frontal lobe damage select more from the disadvantageous decks (A and B) than from the advantageous decks (C and D). These findings suggest that performance on this task by patients with ventromedial frontal lobe damage is comparable to their real-life inability to guide behavior on the basis of previous mistakes, despite normal intelligence and memory. Functional imaging studies in persons without brain damage have supported the notion that this brain region is involved in decision making, particularly if uncertainty and reward are involved (Rogers et al., 1999; Elliot et al., 2000).

An important part of the mechanism underlying the impairment of decision making in patients with frontal lobe damage is tied to the disruption of emotion noted earlier. Damasio (1994; Damasio et al., 1991) has proposed that a major factor (albeit not the only one) in the appearance of the abnormal social conduct which repeatedly leads to punishing consequences is the defective activation of somatic states linked to punishment. The primary signal used to guide response selection is a somatic marker, i.e., a somatic state consisting of a combination of the state of viscera, internal milieu, and skeletal musculature, that is temporally correlated with a particular representation that is "marked" by it. Those states ought to have been reenacted in connection with the representation of negative future outcomes related to a given response option. The failure of their reactivation deprives patients of an alarm signal marking the representation of negative consequences for options that might, nonetheless, produce an immediate reward. (Note that positive somatic states may also mark future advantageous outcomes relative to responses that might bring immediate pain). The activation of somatic markers works at both conscious and nonconscious levels. At a conscious level it draws attention to future negative consequences and promotes the deliberate suppression of the options leading to a negative outcome. At a nonconscious level, somatic markers or signals related to them would trigger inhibition of response states. Subcortical neurotransmitter systems linked to appetitive or aversive behaviors would be involved in this covert level processing. The neural systems necessary for somatic state activation include the cortices in the ventromedial frontal region, whose damage is the main correlate of these behavioral changes.

In support of this model, it was found that patients with frontal lobe damage did not generate the anticipatory skin conductance responses (SCRs) that normal subjects produced prior to making risky decisions in the Gambling

Task (Bechara et al., 1997). When normal subjects performed the task, they developed anticipatory SCRs prior to choosing from the disadvantageous decks even before they could explicitly identify these choices as risky. These covert biases appear to be important in avoiding disadvantageous behavior.

There are many reasons, discussed elsewhere, why we place such an emphasis on somatic states. First, and most obvious, is that the human acquisition of appropriate behavioral guidance, especially in the social setting, occurs during the process of education and acculturation, under the control of punishment and reward. There are repeated interactions that occur during childhood and adolescence during which social events are paired with somatic states, at both the time of the event, and at the time at which future consequences take place. Second, it is apparent that event/somatic state conjunctions have been important for the behavior of nonhuman species, and that those species seem to have an automatic signaling system alerting individuals for immediate potential danger, and immediate opportunities for food, sex, and shelter. Such a system has been especially important in those species in which representational capacity and intelligence are limited. We believe there is an equivalent automated device in humans but that it is tuned to future outcomes. The human somatic markers would thus mark future outcome rather than immediate outcome. In subhuman species, the critical conjunction is between response option and immediate outcome and the somatic marker thus tags immediate outcome. We also believe that in humans such an automated decision-making system is then overlaid by cognitive strategy systems that perform cost/benefit analyses but remain connected, neurophysiologically, to the primitive systems. In other words, the systems that humans use for deliberate decision making and planning of future are rooted in the primitive automated systems that other species have long used for their immediate decision making. The neural architecture of the former is connected to the neural architecture of the latter. When the primitive part of the system fails, superimposed levels cannot operate efficiently.

CONCLUDING REMARKS

In conclusion, the manifestations of frontal lobe dysfunction are varied, ranging from akinesia and mutism to major changes in personality. Often there are no apparent defects of movement, perception, or intelligence. Depending on the cause and location of the lesion, a variety of frontal lobe symptom clusters can thus appear. There is no single frontal lobe syndrome.

In general, the vast set of cerebral cortices collectively known as the frontal lobes appear to have evolved to guide response selection in order to offer the organism its best chance of long-term survival. It is probable that this overall goal was implemented first in simple social environments, dominated by the needs for food, sex, and the avoidance of predators. Other contingencies, in ever more complex environments, were later connected with those original contingencies so that the basic neural mechanism for response selection was incorporated in the decision-making mechanisms developed for newer and more challenging environments. Damage to this system disrupts many of the cognitive and behavioral abilities that have come to define humanity.

ACKNOWLEDGMENTS

We thank Hanna Damasio for providing the illustrations and Gary W. Van Hoesen for review of the manuscript and editorial suggestions. This work was supported by NINDS Program Project Grant NS 19632.

REFERENCES

Ackerly, S. S., and Benton, A. L. (1948). Report of a case of bilateral frontal lobe defect. *Res. Publ. Assoc. Res. Nerv. Ment. Dis.* 27:479–504.

Adolphs, R., Damasio, H., Tranel, D., Cooper, G., and Damasio, A. R. (2000). A role for somatosensory cortices in the visual recognition of emotion as revealed by three-dimensional lesion mapping. *J. Neurosci.* 20:2683–2690.

Akert, K. (1964). Comparative anatomy of frontal cortex and thalamofrontal connections. In *The Frontal Granular Cortex and Behavior*, J. M. Warren and K. Akert (eds.). New York: McGraw-Hill, pp. 372–396.

Alexander, M. P., Benson, D. F., and Stuss, D. T.

(1989). Frontal lobes and language. *Brain Lang.* 37:656–691.

Anderson, S. W., Bechara, A., Damasio, H., Tranel, D., and Damasio, A. R. (1999). Impairment of social and moral behavior related to early damage in the human prefrontal cortex. *Nat. Neurosci.* 2:1032–1037.

Anderson, S. W., Damasio, A. R., and Damasio, H. (1990). Troubled letters but not numbers: domain specific cognitive impairments following focal damage in frontal cortex. *Brain* 113:749–766.

Anderson, S. W., Damasio, H., Jones, R. D., and Tranel, D. (1991). Wisconsin Card Sorting Test performance as a measure of frontal lobe damage. *J. Clin. Exp. Neuropsychol.* 13:909–922.

Anderson, S. W., Damasio, H., and Tranel, D. (1989). Neuropsychological profiles associated with lesions caused by tumor or stroke. *Arch. Neurol.* 47:397–405.

Anderson, S. W., Hathaway-Nepple, J., Tranel, D., and Damasio, H. (2000). Impairments of strategy application following focal prefrontal lesions. *J. Int. Neuropsychol. Soc.* 6:205.

Anderson, S. W., and Manzel, K. (2001). Matrix reasoning as an index of fluid intelligence following frontal lobe damage. *J. Int. Neuropsychol. Soc.* 7:234–235.

Bailey, P., and Von Bonin, G. (1951). *The Isocortex of Man.* Urbana, IL: University of Illinois Press.

Barbas, H. (1995). Anatomic basis of cognitive–emotional interactions in the primate prefrontal cortex. *Neurosci. Biobehav. Rev.* 19:499–510.

Barbas, H., and Mesulam, M. M. (1981). Organization of afferent input of subdivisions of area 8 in the rhesus monkey. *J. Comp. Neurol.* 200:407–431.

Barbas, H., and Mesulam, M. M. (1985). Cortical afferent input to the principalis region of the rhesus monkey. *Neuroscience* 15:619–637.

Barbas, H., and Pandya, D. N. (1987). Architecture and frontal cortical connections of the premotor cortex (area 6) in the rhesus monkey. *J. Comp. Neurol.* 256:211–228.

Barbas, H., and Pandya, D. N. (1989). Architecture and intrinsic connections of the prefrontal cortex in the rhesus monkey. *J. Comp. Neurol.* 286:353–375.

Barrash, J., Tranel, D., and Anderson, S. W. (2000). Acquired sociopathy: characteristic personality changes following ventromedial frontal lobe damage. *Dev. Neuropsychol.* 18:355–381.

Bechara, A., Damasio, A. R., Damasio, H., and Anderson, S. W. (1994). Insensitivity to future consequences following damage to prefrontal cortex. *Cognition* 50:7–15.

Bechara, A., Damasio, H., Tranel, D., and Anderson, S. W. (1998). Dissociation of working memory from decision-making within the human prefrontal cortex. *J. Neurosci.* 18:428–437.

Bechara, A., Damasio, H., Tranel, D., and Damasio, A. R. (1997). Deciding advantageously before knowing the advantageous strategy. *Science* 275:1293–1295.

Beldarrain, G., Grafman, J., Pascual-Leone, A., and Garcia-Monco, J. C. (1999). Procedural learning is impaired in patients with prefrontal lesions. *Neurology* 52:1853–1860.

Bellugi, U., Poizner, H., and Klima, E. S. (1989). Language, modality and the brain. *Trends Neurosci.* 12:380–388.

Benson, D. F. (1977). The third alexia. *Arch. Neurol. (Chicago)* 34:327–331.

Benton, A. L. (1968). Differential behavioral effects in frontal lobe disease. *Neuropsychologia* 6:53–60.

Benton, A. L. (1991a). The prefrontal region: its early history. In *Frontal Lobe Function and Dysfunction*, H. S. Levin, H. M Eisenberg, and A. L. Benton (eds.). New York: Oxford University Press, pp. 3–34.

Benton, A. L. (1991b). Basic approaches to neuropsychological assessment. In *Handbook of Schizophrenia, Vol. 5: Neuropsychology, Psychophysiology, and Information Processing,* S. R. Steinhauer, J. J. Gruzelier, and J. Zubin (eds.). Amsterdam: Elsevier, pp. 505–523.

Benton A. L., Hamsher, K., Varney, N. R., and Spreen, O. (1983). *Contributions to Neuropsychological Assessment: A Clinical Manual.* New York: Oxford University Press.

Berg, E. A. (1948). A simple objective technique for measuring flexibility in thinking. *J. Genet. Psychol.* 39:15–22.

Black, F. W. (1976). Cognitive deficits in patients with unilateral war-related frontal lobe lesions. *J. Clin. Psychol.* 32:366–372.

Blumer, D., and Benson, D. F. (1975). Personality changes with frontal and temporal lobe lesions. In *Psychiatric Aspects of Neurologic Disease,* D. F. Benson and D. Blumer (eds.). New York: Grune and Stratton, pp. 151–169.

Brazelli, M., and Spinnler, H. (1998). An example of lack of frontal inhibition: the 'utilization behavior'. *Eur. J. Neurol.* 5:347–353.

Brickner, R. M. (1934). An interpretation of frontal lobe function based upon the study of a case of partial bilateral frontal lobectomy. *Res. Publ. Assoc. Res. Nerv. Ment. Dis.* 13:259–351.

Brickner, R. M. (1936). *The Intellectual Functions of the Frontal Lobes: Study Based upon Obser-*

vation of a Man After Partial Bilateral Frontal Lobectomy. New York: Macmillan.

Brickner, R. M. (1952). Brain of patient "A" after bilateral frontal lobectomy: status of frontal lobe problem. *Arch. Neurol. Psychiatry* 68:293–313.

Broca, P. (1861). Remarques sur le siege de la faculte du langage articule, suivies d'une observation d'aphemie (perte de la parole). *Bull. Soc. Anat. (Paris)* 36:330–357.

Butter, C. M., Mishkin, M., and Mirsky, A. F. (1968). Emotional responses toward humans in monkeys with selective frontal lesions. *Physiol. Behav.* 3:213–215.

Butter, C. M., Mishkin, M., and Rosvold, H. E. (1963). Conditioning and extinction of a food-rewarded response after selective ablations of frontal cortex in rhesus monkeys. *Exp. Neurol.* 7:65–75.

Butter, C. M., Snyder, D. R., and McDonald, J. A. (1970). Effects of orbital frontal lesions on aversive and aggressive behaviors in rhesus monkeys. *J. Comp. Physiol. Psychol.* 72:132–144.

Butters, M. A., Kaszniak, A. W., Glisky, E. L., Eslinger, P. J., and Schacter, D. L. (1994). Recency discrimination deficits in frontal lobe patients. *Neuropsychology* 8:343–353.

Canavan, A. G. M. (1983). Stylus-maze performance in patients with frontal-lobe lesions: effects of signal valency and relationship to verbal and spatial abilities. *Neuropsychologia* 21:375–382.

Carlin, D., Bonerba, J., Phipps, M., Alexander, G., Shapiro, M., and Grafman, J. (2000). Planning impairments in frontal lobe dementia and frontal lobe lesion patients. *Neuropsychologia* 38:655–665.

Cavada, C., and Goldman-Rakic, P. S. (1989). Posterior parietal cortex in rhesus monkey: II. Evidence for segregated corticocortical networks linking sensory and limbic areas with the frontal lobe. *J. Comp. Neurol.* 287:422–445.

Chao, L. L., and Knight, R. T. (1998). Contribution of human prefrontal cortex to delay performance. *J. Cogn. Neurosci.* 10:167–177.

Chavis, D. A., and Pandya, D. N. (1976). Further observations on corticofrontal connections in the rhesus monkey. *Brain Res.* 117:369–386.

Chorover, S. L., and Cole, M. (1966). Delayed alternation performance in patients with cerebral lesions. *Neuropsychologia* 4:1–7.

Cicerone, K. D., Lazar, R. M., and Shapiro, W. R. (1983). Effects of frontal lobe lesions on hypothesis sampling during concept formation. *Neuropsychologia* 21:513–524.

Cohen, J. D., Forman, S. D., Braver, T. S., Casey, B. J., Servan-Schreiber, D., and Noll, D. C. (1994). Activation of the prefrontal cortex in a nonspatial working memory task with functional MRI. *Hum. Brain Mapping* 1:293–304.

Crosby, E. C., Humphrey, T., and Lauer, E. W. (1962). *Correlative Anatomy of the Nervous System.* New York: Macmillan.

Crosson, B., Rao, S. M., Woodley, S. J., Rosen, A. C., Bobholz, J. A., Mayer, A., Cunningham, J. M., Hammeke, T. A., Fuller, S. A., Binder, J. R., Cox, R. W., and Stein, E. A. (1999). Mapping of semantic phonological and orthographic verbal working memory in normal adults with functional magnetic resonance imaging. *Neuropsychology* 13:171–187.

Cummings, J. L. (1985). *Clinical Neuropsychiatry.* New York: Grune and Stratton.

Cummings, J. L. (1995). Anatomic and behavioral aspects of frontal-subcortical circuits. *Ann. N. Y. Acad. Sci.* 769:1–14.

Daffner, K. R., Mesulan, M. M., Scinto, L. F. M., Acar, D., Calvo, V., Faust, R. Chabrerie, A., Kennedy, B., and Holcomb, P. (2000). The central role of the prefrontal cortex in directing attention to novel events. *Brain* 123:927–939.

Dagher, A., Owen, A. M., Boecker, H., and Brooks, D. J. (1999). Mapping the network for planning: a correlational PET activation study with the Tower of London task. *Brain* 122:1973–1987.

Damasio, A. R. (1992). Aphasia. *N. Engl. J. Med.* 326:531–539.

Damasio, A.R. (1994). *Descartes' Error: Emotion, Reason, and the Human Brain.* New York: Grosset/Putnam.

Damasio, A. R., and Anderson, S. W. (1993). The frontal lobes. In *Clinical Neuropsychology, Third Edition,* K. M. Heilman and E. Valenstein (eds.). New York: Oxford, pp. 409–460.

Damasio, A. R., Damasio, H., and Chui, H. C. (1980). Neglect following damage to frontal lobe or basal ganglia. *Neuropsychologia* 18:123–132.

Damasio, A. R., Eslinger, P., Damasio, H., Van Hoesen, G. W., and Cornell, S. (1985). Multimodal amnesic syndrome following bilateral temporal and basal forebrain damage. *Arch. Neurol.* 42:252–259.

Damasio, A. R., Tranel, D., and Damasio, H. (1990). Individuals with sociopathic behavior caused by frontal damage fail to respond autonomically to social stimuli. *Behav. Brain Res.* 41:81–94.

Damasio, A. R., Tranel, D., and Damasio, H. (1991). Somatic markers and the guidance of behavior: theory and preliminary testing. In *Frontal Lobe Function and Dysfunction,* H. S. Levin, H. M. Eisenberg, and A. L. Benton (eds.). New York: Oxford University Press, pp. 217–229.

Damasio, A. R., and Van Hoesen, G. W. (1980). Structure and function of the supplementary motor area. *Neurology* 30:359.

Damasio, A. R., and Van Hoesen, G. W. (1983). Emotional disturbances associated with focal lesions of the frontal lobe. In *The Neurophysiology of Human Emotion: Recent Advances*, K. Heilman and P. Satz (eds.). New York: Guilford Press, pp. 85–108.

Dejerine, J., and Mirallie, C. (1895). Sur les alterations de la lecture mentale chez les aphasiques moteurs corticaux. *C R Seances Memoires Soc. Biol., Paris 10th ser.(ii)*:523–527.

De Renzi, E., Faglioni, P., Lodesani, M., and Vecchi, A. (1983). Impairment of left brain–damaged patients on imitation of single movements and motor sequences: frontal and parietal injured patients compared. *Cortex* 19:333–343.

D'Esposito, M., and Postle, B. R. (1999). The dependence of span and delayed-response performance on prefrontal cortex. *Neuropsychologia* 37:1303–1315.

Deutsch, R. D., Kling, A., and Steklis, H. D. (1979). Influence of frontal lobe lesions on behavioral interactions in man. *Res. Commun. Psychol. Psychiatry Behav.* 4:415–431.

De Vito, J. L., and Smith, O. E. (1964). Subcortical projections of the prefrontal lobe of the monkey. *J. Comp. Neurol.* 123:413.

Dias, R., Robbins, T. W., and Roberts, A. C. (1997). Dissociable forms of inhibitory control within prefrontal cortex with an analog of the Wisconsin card sort test: restriction to novel situations and independence from "on-line" processing. *J. Neurosci.* 17:9285–9297.

Dimitrov, M., Grafman, J., and Hollnagel, C. (1996). The effects of frontal lobe damage on everyday problem solving. *Cortex* 32:357–366.

Dimitrov, M., Granetz, J., Peterson, M., Hollnagel, C., Alexander, G., and Grafman, J. (1999). Associative learning impairments in patients with frontal lobe damage. *Brain Cogn.* 41:213–230.

Di Pellegrino, G., and Wise, S. P. (1991). A neurophysiological comparison of three distinct regions of the primate frontal lobe. *Brain* 114:951–978.

Drewe, E. A. (1974). The effect of type and area of brain lesion on Wisconsin Card Sorting Test performance. *Cortex* 10:159–170.

Drewe, E. A. (1975). An experimental investigation of Luria's theory on the effects of frontal lobe lesions in man. *Neuropsychologia* 13:421–429.

Eichenbaum, H., Shedlack, K. J., and Eckmann, K. W. (1980). Thalamocortical mechanisms in odor-guided behavior. I: Effects of lesions of the mediodorsal thalamic nucleus and frontal cortex on olfactory discrimination in the rat. *Brain Behav. Evol.* 17:225–275.

Elliot, R., Dolan, R. J., and Frith, C. D. (2000). Dissociable functions in the medial and lateral orbitofrontal cortex: evidence from human neuroimaging studies. *Cereb. Cortex* 10:308–317.

Eslinger, P. J. (1998). Neurological and neuropsychological bases of empathy. *Eur. Neurol.* 39:193–199.

Eslinger, P. J., and Damasio, A. R. (1985). Severe disturbance of higher cognition after bilateral frontal lobe ablation: patient EVR. *Neurology* 35:1731–1741.

Eslinger, P. J., and Grattan, L. M. (1994). Altered serial position learning after frontal lobe lesion. *Neuropsychologia* 32:729–739.

Ethelberg, S. (1949). On "cataplexy" in a case of frontal lobe tumor. *Acta Psychiatr. Neurol.* 24:421–427.

Exner, S. (1881). *Untersuchungen uber die Localisation der Functionen in der Grosshirnrinde des Menschen*. Vienna: W. Braumuller.

Feuchtwanger, E. (1923). Die Funktionen des Stirnhirns. In *Monographien aus dem Gesamtgebiete der Neurologie und Psychiatrie*, O. Forster and K. Willmanns (eds.). Berlin: Springer-Verlag.

Fisher, C. M. (1968). Intermittent interruption of behavior. *Trans. Am. Neurol. Assoc.* 93:209–210.

Fletcher, P. C., Shallice, T., and Dolan, R. J. (1998). The functional roles of prefrontal cortex in episodic memory. *Brain* 121:1239–1248.

Frank, R. J., Damasio, H., and Grabowski, T. J. (1997). Brainvox: an interactive multimodal visualization and analysis system for neuroanatomical imaging. *Neuroimage* 5:13–30.

Frey, S., and Petrides, M. (2000). Orbitofrontal cortex: a key prefrontal region for encoding information. *Proc. Natl. Acad. Sci. U.S.A.* 97:8723–8727.

Fulton, J. F. (1951). *Frontal Lobotomy and Affective Behavior*. New York: Norton.

Fulton, J. F., and Jacobsen, C. F. (1935). The functions of the frontal lobes: a comparative study in monkeys, chimpanzees and man. *Adv. Mod. Biol. (Moscow)* 4:113–123.

Fuster, J. M. (1997). *The Prefrontal Cortex: Anatomy, Physiology, and Neuropsychology of the Frontal Lobe*. New York: Lippincott-Raven.

Gardner, H., and Zurif, E. (1975). Bee but not be: oral reading of single words in aphasia and alexia. *Neuropsychologia* 13:181–190.

Gershberg, F. B., and Shimamura, A. P. (1995). Impaired use of organizational strategies in free recall following frontal lobe damage. *Neuropsychologia* 13:1305–1333.

Ghent, L., Mishkin, M., and Teuber, H. L. (1962). Short-term memory after frontal-lobe injury in man. *J. Comp. Physiol. Psychol.* 55:705–709.

Goel, V., and Grafman, J. (1995). Are the frontal lobes implicated in "planning" functions? Interpreting data from the Tower of Hanoi. *Neuropsychologia* 33:623–642.

Goel, V., Grafman, J., Tajik, J., Gana, S., and Danto, D. (1997). A study of the performance of patients with frontal lobe lesions in a financial planning task. *Brain 120:*1805–1822.

Goldberg, E. (1986). Varieties of perseveration: a comparison of two taxonomies. *J. Clin. Exp. Neuropsychol.* 8:710–726.

Goldberg, E., and Podell, K. (2000). Adaptive decision making, ecological validity, and the frontal lobes. *J. Clin. Exp. Neuropsychol.* 22:56–68.

Goldman, P. S. (1978). Neuronal plasticity in primate telencephalon: anomalous projections induced by prenatal removal of frontal cortex. *Science* 202:768–770.

Goldman, P. S., and Nauta, W. J. H. (1977). An intricately patterned prefrontocaudate projection in the rhesus monkey. *J. Comp. Neurol. 171:*369–386.

Goldman-Rakic, P. S. (1984). Modular organization of the prefrontal cortex. *Trends Neurosci. 7:*419–424.

Goldman-Rakic, P. S. (1987). Circuitry of primate prefrontal cortex and regulation of behavior by representational memory. In *Handbook of Physiology: The Nervous System, Vol. 5,* F. Plum (ed.). Bethesda: American Physiological Society, pp. 373–401.

Goldman-Rakic, P. S., and Friedman, H. R. (1991). The circuitry of working memory revealed by anatomy and metabolic imaging. In *Frontal Lobe Function and Dysfunction,* H. S. Levin, H. M. Eisenberg, and A. L. Benton (eds.). New York: Oxford University Press, pp. 72–91.

Goldman-Rakic, P. S., and Schwartz, M. L. (1982). Interdigitation of contralateral and ipsilateral columnar projections to frontal association cortex in primates. *Science 216:*755–757.

Goldstein, K. (1948). *Aftereffects of Brain Injuries in War.* New York: Grune and Stratton.

Gordinier, H. C. (1899). A case of brain tumor at the base of the second left frontal convolution. *Am. J. Med. Sci. 117:*526–535.

Grafman, J., Jonas, B., and Salazar, A. (1990). Wisconsin Card Sorting Test performance based on location and size of neuroanatomical lesion in Vietnam veterans with penetrating head injury. *Percept. Mot. Skills 71:*1120–1122.

Grant, D. A., and Berg, E. A. (1948). A behavioral analysis of degree of reinforcement and ease of shifting to new responses in a Weigl-type card-sorting problem. *J. Exp. Psychol.* 38:404–411.

Grattan, L. M., Bloomer, R. H., Archambault, F. X., and Eslinger, P. J. (1994). Cognitive flexibility and empathy after frontal lobe lesion. *Neuropsychiatry Neuropsychol. Behav. Neurol.* 7:251–259.

Grattan, L. M., and Eslinger, P. J. (1991). Frontal lobe damage in children and adults: a comparative review. *Dev. Neuropsychol.* 7:283–326.

Grueninger, W. E., Kimble, D. P., Grueninger, J., and Levine, S. E. (1965). GSR and corticosteroid response in monkeys with frontal ablations. *Neuropsychologia* 3:205–216.

Guitton, D., Buchtel, H. A., and Douglas, R. M. (1985). Frontal lobe lesions in man cause difficulties in suppressing reflexive glances and in generation of goal directed saccades. *Exp. Brain Res. 58:*455–472.

Harlow, J. M. (1848). Passage of an iron rod through the head. *Boston Med. Surg. J. 39:*389–393.

Harlow, J. M. (1868). Recovery from the passage of an iron bar through the head. *Publ. Mass. Med. Soc. 2:*327–347.

Hauser, M. D. (1999). Perseveration, inhibition and the prefrontal cortex: a new look. *Curr. Opin. Neurobiol. 9:*214–222.

Heaton, R.K. (1981). *Wisconsin Card Sorting Test Manual.* Odessa, FL: Psychological Assessment Resources, Inc.

Hebb, D. O. (1945). Man's frontal lobes: a critical review. *Arch. Neurol. Psychiatry* 54:421–438.

Hebb, D. O., and Penfield, W. (1940). Human behavior after extensive bilateral removals from the frontal lobes. *Arch. Neurol. Psychiatry 44:*421–438.

Hécaen, H. (1964). Mental symptoms associated with tumors of the frontal lobe. In *The Frontal Granular Cortex and Behavior,* J. M. Warren and K. Akert (eds.). New York: McGraw-Hill, pp. 335–352.

Heilman, K. M., Pandya, D. N., Karol, E. A., and Geschwind, N. (1971). Auditory inattention. *Arch. Neurol. 24:*323–325.

Heilman, K. M., and Valenstein, E. (1972). Frontal lobe neglect in man. *Neurology 22:*660–664.

Heilman, K. M., and Watson, R. T. (1991). Intentional motor disorders. In *Frontal Lobe Function and Dysfunction,* H. S. Levin, H. L. Eisenburg, and A. L. Benton (eds.). New York: Oxford University Press, pp. 199–216.

Holmes, G. (1938). The cerebral integration of ocular movements. *BMJ 2:*107–112.

Homskaya, E. D. (1966). Vegetative components of the orienting reflex to indifferent and significant stimuli in patients with lesions of the frontal lobes. In *Frontal Lobes and Regulation of Psychological Processes*, A. R. Luria and E. D. Homskaya (eds.). Moscow: Moscow University Press.

Jacobsen, C. F. (1935). Functions of the frontal association area in primates. *Arch. Neurol. Psychiatry* 33:558–569.

Janowsky, J. S., Shimamura, A. P., Kritchevsky, M., and Squire, L. R. (1989). Cognitive impairments following frontal lobe damage and its relevance to human amnesia. *Behav. Neurosci. 103*:548–560.

Janowsky, J. S., Shimamura, A. P., and Squire, L. R. (1989). Memory and metamemory: comparisons between patients with frontal lobe lesions and amnesic patients. *Psychobiology 17*:3–11.

Jastrowitz, M. (1888). Beitrage zur Localisation im Grosshirn and uber deren praktische Verwerthung. *Dtsch. Med. Wochenschr. 14*:81.

Jefferson, G. (1937). Removal of right or left frontal lobes in man. *BMJ* 2:199.

Johnson, T. N., Rosvold, H. E., and Mishkin, M. (1968). Projections from behaviorally defined sectors of the prefrontal cortex to the basal ganglia, septum, and diencephalon of the monkey. *Esp. Neurol. 21*:20.

Jones-Gotman, M., and Milner, B. (1977). Design fluency: the invention of nonsense drawings after focal cortical lesions. *Neuropsychologia 15*:653–674.

Jones-Gotman, M., and Zatorre, R. J. (1993). Odor recognition memory in humans: role of right temporal and orbitofrontal regions. *Brain Cogn. 22*:182–198.

Kaplan, E., and Goodglass, H. (1981). Aphasia related disorders. In *Acquired Aphasia*, M. T. Sarno (ed.). New York: Academic Press, pp. 303–326.

Kaczmarek, B. L. J. (1987). Regulatory function of the frontal lobes: a neurolinguistic perspective. In *The Frontal Lobes Revisited*, E. Perecman (ed.). Hillsdale, NJ: Lawrence Erlbaum Associates, pp. 225–240.

Karnath, H. O., Wallesch, C. W., and Zimmerman, P. (1991). Mental planning and anticipatory processes with acute and chronic frontal lobe lesions: a comparison of maze performance in routine and non-routine situations. *Neuropsychologia 29*:271–290.

Kennard, M. A., and Ectors, L. (1938). Forced circling movements in monkeys following lesions of the frontal lobes. *J. Neurophysiol. 1*:45–54.

Kievit, J., and Kuypers, H. G. J. M. (1974). Basal forebrain and hypothalamic connections to frontal and parietal cortex in the rhesus monkey. *Science 187*:660–662.

Kim, J.-N. and Shadlen, M. N. (1999). Neural correlates of a decision in the dorsolateral prefrontal cortex of the macaque. *Nat. Neurosci.* 2:176–185.

Kimble, D. P., Bagshaw, M. H., and Pribram, K. H. (1965). The GSR of monkeys during orienting and habituation after selective partial ablations of the cingulate and frontal cortex. *Neuropsychologia 3*:121–128.

Kleist, K. (1936). *Gehirnpatholgie*. Leipzig: Barth.

Knight, R. T. (1984). Decreased response to novel stimuli after prefrontal lesions in man. *Electroencephalogr. Clin. Neurophysiol. 59*:9–20.

Kobal, G., and Kettenmann, B. (2000). Olfactory functional imaging and physiology. *Int. J. Psychophysiol. 36*:157–163.

Koechlin, E., Basso, G., Peitrini, P., Panzer, S., and Grafman, J. (1999). The role of the anterior prefrontal cortex in human cognition. *Nature 399*: 148–151.

Kolb, B., and Milner, B. (1981). Performance of complex arm and facial movements after focal brain lesions. *Neuropsychologia 19*:491–503.

Kuypers, H. G. J. M., Szwarobart, M. K., and Mishkin, M. (1965). Occipitotemporal corticocortical connections in the rhesus monkey. *Exp. Neurol. 11*:245.

Kwon, S. E., and Heilman, K. M. (1991). Ipsilateral neglect in a patient following a unilateral frontal lesion. *Neurology 41*:2001–2004.

Lezak, M .D. (1988). IQ: RIP. *J. Clin. Exp. Neuropsychol. 10*:351–361.

Lezak, M. D. (1993). *Neuropsychological Assessment, 3rd ed*. New York: Oxford University Press.

Lhermitte, F., Pillon, B., and Serdaru, M. (1986). Human autonomy and the frontal lobes. Part 1: Imitation and utilization behavior. *Ann. Neurol. 19*:326–334.

Lichtheim, L. (1885). On aphasia. *Brain 7*:433–484.

Liepmann, H. (1908). *Drei Aufsatze aus dem Apraxiegebiet*. Berlin: Karger.

Luria, A. R. (1966). *Human Brain and Psychological Processes*. New York: Harper and Row.

Luria, A. R. (1969). Frontal lobe syndrome. In *Handbook of Clinical Neurology, Vol. 2*, P. J. Vinkin and G. W. Bruyn (eds.). Amsterdam: North-Holland.

Luria, A. R., and Homskaya, E. D. (1964). Disturbances in the regulative role of speech with frontal lobe lesions. In *The Frontal Granular Cortex and Behavior*, J. M. Warren and K. Akert (eds.). New York: McGraw-Hill, pp. 353–371.

Malmo, R. B. (1942). Interference factors in delayed response in monkeys after removal of frontal lobes. *J. Neurophysiol. 5*:295–308.

Mangels, J. A. (1997). Strategic processing and memory for temporal order in patients with frontal lobe lesions. *Neuropsychology* 11:207–221.

Mangels, J. A., Gershberg, F. B., Shimamura, A. P., and Knight, R. T. (1996). Impaired retrieval from remote memory in patients with frontal lobe damage. *Neuropsychology* 10:32–41.

Marshall, J. F., and Teitelbaum, P. (1974). Further analysis of sensory inattention allowing lateral hypothalamic damage in rats. *J. Comp. Physiol. Psychol.* 86:375–395.

Marshall, J. F., Turner, B. H., and Teitelbaum, P. (1971). Sensory neglect produced by lateral hypothalamic damage. *Science* 174:523–525.

Metzler, C., and Parkin, A. J. (2000). Reversed negative priming following frontal lobe lesions. *Neuropsychologia* 38:363–379.

Milner, B. (1963). Effects of different brain lesions on card sorting. *Arch. Neurol.* 9:90–100.

Milner, B. (1964). Some effects of frontal lobectomy in man. In *The Frontal Granular Cortex and Behavior*, J. M. Warren and K. Akert (eds.). New York: McGraw-Hill, pp. 313–334.

Milner, B. (1965). Visually guided maze learning in man: effects of bilateral hippocampal, bilateral frontal, and unilateral cerebral lesions. *Neuropsychologia* 3:317–338.

Milner, B. (1971). Interhemispheric differences in the localisation of psychological processes in man. *Br. Med. Bull.* 27:272–277.

Milner, B., Corsi, P., and Leonard, G. (1991). Frontal-lobe contribution to recency judgements. *Neuropsychologia* 29:601–618.

Milner, B., Petrides, M., and Smith, M. L. (1985). Frontal lobes and the temporal organization of memory. *Hum. Neurobiol.* 4:137–142.

Mohr, J. P. (1976). Broca's area and Broca's aphasia. In *Studies in Neurolinguistics, Vol. 1*, H. Whitaker and H. A. Whitaker (eds.). New York: Academic Press.

Moniz, E. (1936). *Tentatives Operatoires dans le Traitement de Certaines Psychoses*. Paris: Masson et Cie.

Moniz, E. (1949). *Confidencias de um Investigador Cientifico*. Lisbon: Livraria Atica.

Moran, M. A., Mufson, E. J., and Mesulam, M. M. (1987). Neural inputs into the temporopolar cortex of the rhesus monkey. *J. Comp. Neurol.* 256: 88–103.

Morecraft, R. J., and Van Hoesen, G. W. (1993). Frontal granular cortex input to the cingulate (M3), supplementary (M2) and primary (M1) motor cortices in the rhesus monkey. *J. Comp. Neurol.* 337:669–689.

Nauta, W. J. H. (1962). Neural associations of the

amygdaloid complex in the monkey. *Brain* 85:505–520.

Nauta, W. J. H. (1964). Some efferent connections of the prefrontal cortex in the monkey. In *The Frontal Granular Cortex and Behavior*, J. M. Warren and K. Akert (ed.). New York: McGraw-Hill, pp. 397–409.

Nauta, W. J. H., and Haymaker, W. (1969). *The Hypothalamus*. Springfield, IL: C.C. Thomas.

Neary, D., Snowden, J. S., Northen, B., and Goulding, P. (1988). Dementia of frontal lobe type. *J. Neurol. Neurosurg. Psychiatry* 51:353–361.

Nielsen, J. M. (1938). The unsolved problems in aphasia. I. Alexia in motor aphasia. *Bull. Los Angeles Neurol. Soc.* 4:114–122.

Nielsen, J. M. (1946). *Agnosia, Apraxia, Aphasia. Their Value in Cerebral Localization*. New York: P.B. Hoeber.

Norman, D. A., and Shallice, T. (1986). Attention to action: willed and automatic control of behaviour. In *Consciousness and Self-regulation: Advances in Research and Theory, Vol. 4*, R. J. Davidson, G. E. Schwartz, and D. Shapiro (eds.). New York: Plenum Press, pp. 1–18.

Oppenheim, H. (1889). Zur Pathologie der Grosshirngeschwulste. *Arch. Psychiatrie* 21.560.

Owen, A. M. (1997). Cognitive planning in humans: neuropsychological, neuroanatomical and neuropharmacological perspectives. *Prog. Neurobiol.* 53:431–450.

Owen, A. M., Downes, J. D., Sahakian, B. J., Polkey, C. E. and Robbins, T. W. (1990). Planning and spatial working memory following frontal lobe lesions in man. *Neuropsychologia* 28:1021–1034.

Pandya, D. N. and Barnes, C. L. (1987). Architecture and connections of the frontal lobe. In *The Frontal Lobes Revisited*, E. Perecman (ed.). Hillsdale, NJ: Lawrence Erlbaum Associates, pp. 41–72.

Pandya, D. N., Dye, P., and Butters, N. (1971). Efferent cortico-cortical projections of the prefrontal cortex in the rhesus monkey. *Brain Res.* 31:35–46.

Pandya, D. N., Hallett, M., and Mukherjee, S. K. (1969). Intra- and interhemispheric connections of the neocortical auditory system in the rhesus monkey. *Brain Res.* 13:49.

Pandya, D. N., and Kuypers, H. G. J. M. (1969). Cortico-cortical connections in the rhesus monkey. *Brain Res.* 13:13.

Pandya, D. N., and Vignolo, L. A. (1971). Intra- and interhemispheric projections of the precentral, premotor and arcuate areas in the rhesus monkey. *Brain Res.* 26:217–233.

Paradiso, S., Chemerinski, E., Yazici, K. M., Tartaro,

A., and Robinson, R. G. (1999). Frontal lobe syndrome reassessed: comparison of patients with lateral or medial frontal brain damage. *J. Neurol. Neurosurg. Psychiatry* 67:664–667.

Parkin, A. J., Bindschaedler, C., Harsent, L., and Metzler, C. (1996). Pathological false alarm rates following damage to the left frontal cortex. *Brain Cogn.* 32:14–27.

Parkin, A. J., and Hunkin, N. M. (1993). Impaired temporal context memory on anterograde but not retrograde tests in the absence of frontal pathology. *Cortex* 29:267–280.

Penfield, W., and Roberts, L. (1959). *Speech and Brain Mechanisms*. Princeton, NJ: Princeton University Press.

Perry, R. J., and Hodges, J. R. (2000). Differentiating frontal and temporal variant frontotemporal dementia from AD. *Neurology* 54:2277–2284.

Petersen, S. E., Fox, P. T., Posner, M. I., Mintun, M. A., and Raichle, M. A. (1989). *J. Cogn. Neurosci.* 1:153–170.

Petrides, M. (1985). Deficits on conditional associative-learning tasks after frontal- and temporal-lobe lesions in man. *Neuropsychologia* 23:601–614.

Petrides, M. (1987). Conditional learning and the primate frontal cortex. In The *Frontal Lobes Revisited*, E. Perecman (ed.). Hillsdale, NJ: Lawrence Erlbaum Associates, pp. 91–108.

Petrides, M. (1990). Nonspatial conditional learning impaired in patients with unilateral frontal but not unilateral temporal lobe excisions. *Neuropsychologia* 28:137–149.

Petrides, M. (1995). Functional organization of the human frontal cortex for mnemonic processing. *Ann. N. Y. Acad. Sci.* 769:85–96.

Petrides, M., and Milner, B. (1982). Deficits on subject-ordered tasks after frontal- and temporal-lobe lesions in man. *Neuropsychologia* 20:259–262.

Petrides, M., and Pandya, D. N. (1984). Projections to the frontal cortex from the posterior parietal region in the rhesus monkey. *J. Comp. Neurol.* 228:105–116.

Petrides, M., and Pandya, D.N. (1988). Association fiber pathways to the frontal cortex from the superior temporal region in the rhesus monkey. *J. Comp. Neurol.* 310:507–549.

Porrino, J. J., and Goldman-Rakic, P. S. (1982). Brainstem innervation of prefrontal and anterior cingulate cortex in the rhesus monkey revealed by retrograde transport of HRP. *J. Comp. Neurol.* 205:63–76.

Porrino, L. J., Craine, A. M., and Goldman-Rakic, P. S. (1981). Direct and indirect pathways from the amygdala to the frontal lobe in rhesus monkeys. *J. Comp. Neurol.* 198:121–136.

Porteus, S. D., De Monbrun, R., and Kepner, M. D. (1944). Mental changes after bilateral prefrontal leucotomy. *Genet. Psychol. Monogr.* 29:3–115.

Postle, B. R., Berger, J. S., and D'Esposito, M. (1999). Functional neuroanatomical double dissociation of mnemonic and executive control processes contributing to working memory performance. *Proc. Natl. Acad. Sci. U.S.A.* 96:12959–12964.

Potter, H., and Butters, N. (1980). An assessment of olfactory deficits in patients with damage to prefrontal cortex. *Neuropsychologia* 18:621–628.

Potter, H., and Nauta, W. J. H. (1979). A note on the problem of olfactory associations of the orbitofrontal cortex in the monkey. *Neuroscience* 4:316–367.

Powell, T. P. S., Cowan, W. M., and Raisman, G. (1965). The central olfactory connexions. *J. Anat. (London)* 99:791.

Preuss, T. M., and Goldman-Rakic, P. S. (1991). Ipsilateral cortical connections of the granular frontal cortex in the Strepsirhine primate Galago, with comparative comments on anthropoid primates. *J. Comp. Neurol.* 310:507–549.

Pribram, K. H., Chow, K. L., and Semmes, J. (1953). Limit and organization of the cortical projection from the medial thalamic nucleus in monkey. *J. Comp. Neurol.* 98:433–448.

Pribram, K. H., and MacLean, P. D. (1953). Neuronographic analysis of medial and basal cerebral cortex. II: Monkey. *J. Neurophysiol.* 16:324–340.

Price, J. L. (1999a). Networks within the orbital and medial prefrontal cortex. *Neurocase* 5:231–241.

Price, J. L. (1999b). Prefrontal cortical networks related to visceral function and mood. *Ann. N. Y. Acad. Sci.* 877:383–396.

Rahman, S., Sahakian, B. J., Hodges, J. R., Rogers, R. D., and Robbins, T. W. (1999). Specific cognitive deficits in mild frontal variant frontotemporal dementia. *Brain* 122:1469–1493.

Raichle, M. E., Fiez, J. A., Videen, T. O., MacLeod, A. M., Pardo, J. V., Fox, P. T., and Petersen, S. E. (1994). Practice-related changes in human brain functional anatomy during nonmotor learning. *Cereb. Cortex* 4:8–26.

Rainer, G., Rao, S. C., and Miller, E. K. (1999). Prospective coding for object in primate prefrontal cortex. *J. Neurosci.* 19:5493–5505.

Rapcsak, S. Z., Arthur, S. A., and Rubens, A. B. (1988). Lexical agraphia from focal lesion of the left precentral gyrus. *Neurology* 38:1119–1123.

Rapcsak, S. Z., Kaszniak, A. W., Reminger, S. L., Glisky, M. L., Glisky, E. L., and Comer, J. F. (1998). Dissociation between verbal and autonomic measures of memory following frontal lobe damage. *Neurology 50*:1259–1265.

Ritacciao, A. L., Hickling, E. J., and Ramani, V. (1992). The role of dominant premotor cortex and grapheme to phoneme transformation in reading epilepsy. *Arch. Neurol. 49*:933–939.

Robbins, T. W. (1996). Dissociating executive functions of the prefrontal cortex. *Phil. Trans. R. Soc. Lond. Biol. Sci. 351*:1463–1470.

Robinson, R. G., Bolduc, P. L., and Price, T. R. (1987). Two-year longitudinal study of poststroke mood disorders: diagnosis and outcome at one and two years. *Stroke 18*:837–843.

Robinson, R. G., Kubos, K. L., Starr, L. B., Rao, K., and Price, T. R. (1984). Mood disorders in stroke patients. Importance of location of lesion. *Brain 107*:81–93.

Robinson, R. G., Starr, L. B., Lipsey, J. R., Rao, K., and Price, T. R. (1985). A 2-year longitudinal study of poststroke mood disorders: in-hospital prognostic factors associated with 6-month outcome. *J. Nerv. Ment. Dis. 173*:221–226.

Rogers, R. D., Owen, A. M., Middleton, H. C., Williams, E. J., Pickard, J. D., Sahakian, B. J., and Robbins, T. W. (1999). Choosing between small, likely rewards and large, unlikely rewards activates inferior and orbital prefrontal cortex. *J. Neurosci. 20*:9029–9038.

Rolls, E. T. (2000). The orbitofrontal cortex and reward. *Cereb. Cortex 10*:284–294.

Rosene, D. L., Mesulam, M. M., and Van Hoesen, G. W. (1976). Afferents to area FL of the medial frontal cortex from the amygdala and hippocampus of the rhesus monkey. In *Neuroscience Abstracts*, *Vol. 2, Part 1*. Bethesda: Society for Neuroscience.

Rylander, G. (1940). *Personality Changes After Operations on the Frontal Lobes*. Copenhagen: Munksgaard.

Sagar, H. J., Gabrieli, J. D. E., Sullivan, E. V., and Corkin, S. (1990). Recency and frequency discrimination in the amnesic patient H.M. *Brain 113*:581–602.

Sapolsky, R. M., and Eichenbaum, H. (1980). Thalamocortical mechanisms in odor guided behavior. II: Effects of lesions of the mediodorsal thalamic nucleus and frontal cortex on odor preferences and sexual behavior in the hamster. *Brain Behav. Evol. 17*:276–290.

Sarazin, M., Pillon, B., Giannakopoulos, P., Rancurel, G., Samson, Y., and Dubois, B. (1998). Clinicometabolic dissociation of cognitive functions and social behavior in frontal lobe lesions. *Neurology 51*:142–148.

Saver, J. L., and Damasio, A. R. (1991). Preserved access and precessing of social knowledge in a patient with acquired sociopathy due to ventromedial frontal damage. *Neuropsychologia 29*:1241–1249.

Schacter, D. L., Curran, T., Gallucio, L., Millberg, W. P., and Bates, J. F. (1996). False recognition and the right frontal lobe: a case study. *Neuropsychologia 34*:793–808.

Schnider, A., Treyer, V., and Buck, A. (2000). Selection of currently relevant memories by the human posterior medial orbitofrontal cortex. *J. Neurosci. 20*:5880–5884.

Segarra, J., and Angelo, J. (1970). Anatomical determinants of behavioral change. In *Behavioral Change in Cerebrovascular Disease*, A. L. Benton (ed.). New York: Harper and Row.

Seltzer, B., and Pandya, D. N. (1989). Frontal lobe connections of the superior temporal sulcus in the rhesus monkey. *J. Comp. Neurol. 281*:97–113.

Settlage, P., Zable, M., and Harlow, H. F. (1948). Problem solving by monkeys following bilateral removal of the prefrontal areas: VI. Performance on tests requiring contradictory reactions to similar and identical stimuli. *J. Exp. Psychol. 38*:50–65.

Shallice, T. (1982). Specific impairments of planning. *Phil. Trans. R. Soc. Lond. 298*:199–209.

Shallice, T., and Burgess, W. P. (1991). Deficits in strategy application following frontal lobe damage in man. *Brain 114*:727–741.

Shallice, T., Burgess, W. P., Schon, F., and Baxter, M. D. (1989). The origin of utilization behaviour. *Brain 112*:1587–1598.

Shammi, P., and Stuss, D. T. (1999). Humour appreciation: a role of the right frontal lobe. *Brain 122*:657–666.

Simernitskaya, E. G. (1970). *Evoked Potentials as an Indicator of the Active Process*. Moscow: Moscow University Press.

Simernitskaya, E. G., and Homskaya, E. D. (1966). Changes in evoked potentials to significant stimuli in normal subjects and in lesions of the frontal lobes. In *Frontal Lobes and Regulation of Psychological Processes*, A. R. Luria and E. D. Homskaya (eds.). Moscow: Moscow University Press.

Sirigu, A., Zalla, T., Pillon, B., Grafman, J., Dubois, B., and Agid, Y. (1995). Planning and script analysis following prefrontal lobe lesions. *Ann. N. Y. Acad. Sci. 769*:277–288.

Smith, E. E., Jonides, J., and Koeppe, J. R. A. (1996). Dissociating verbal and spatial working memory using PET. *Cereb. Cortex 6*:11–20.

Smith, M. L., and Milner, B. (1988). Estimation of frequency of occurrence of abstract designs after frontal or temporal lobectomy. *Neuropsychologia* 26:297–306.

Spreen, O., and Strauss, E. (1991). *A Compendium of Neuropsychological Tests*. New York: Oxford University Press.

Stanhope, N., Guinan, E., and Kopelman, M. D. (1998). Frequency judgements of abstract designs by patients with diencephalic, temporal lobe or frontal lobe lesions. *Neuropsychologia* 26:1387–1396.

Strauss, I., and Keschner, M. (1935). Mental symptoms in cases of tumor of the frontal lobe. *Arch. Neurol. Psychiatry* 33:986–1007.

Stuss, D. T., Alexander, M. P., Hamer, L., Palumbo, C., Dempster, R., Binns, M., Levine, B., and Izukawa, D. (1998). The effects of focal anterior and posterior brain lesions on verbal fluency. *J. Int. Neuropsychol. Soc.* 4:265–278.

Stuss, D. T., Alexander, M. P., Lieberman, A., and Levine H. (1978). An extraordinary form of confabulation. *Neurology* 28:1166–1172.

Stuss, D. T. and Benson, D. F. (1987). The frontal lobes and control of cognition and memory. In *The Frontal Lobes Revisited*, E. Perecman (ed.). Hillsdale, NJ: Lawrence Erlbaum Associates, pp. 141–158.

Stuss, D. T., Kaplan, E. F., Benson, D. F., Weir, W. S., Chiulli, S., and Sarazin, F. F. (1982). Evidence for the involvement of orbitofrontal cortex in memory functions: an interference effect. *J. Comp. Physiol. Psychol.* 96:913–925.

Stuss, D. T., Kaplan, E. F., Benson, D. F., Weir, W. S., Naeser, M. A., and Levine, H. L. (1981). Long term effects of prefrontal leucotomy: An overview of neuropsychologic residuals. *J. Clin. Neuropsychol.* 3:13–32.

Stuss, D. T., Levine, B., Alexander, M. P., Hong, J., Palumbo, C., Hamer, L., Murphy, K. J., and Izukawa, D. (2000). Wisconsin Card Sorting Test performance in patients with focal frontal and posterior brain damage: effects of lesion location and test structure on separable cognitive process. *Neuropsychologia* 38:388–402.

Stuss, D. T., Toth, J. P., Franchi, D., Alexander, M. P., Tipper, S., and Craik, F. (1999). Dissociation of attentional processes in patients with focal frontal and posterior lesions. *Neuropsychologia* 37:1005–1027.

Swick, D., and Knight, R. T. (1996). Is prefrontal cortex involved in cued recall? A neuropsychological test of PET findings. *Neuropsychologia* 34:1019–1028.

Tanabe, T., Iino, M., and Takogi, S. F. (1975a). Discrimination of odors in olfactory bulb, pyriform-amygdaloid areas, and orbitofrontal cortex of the monkey. *J. Neurophysiol.* 38:1284–1296.

Tanabe, T., Yarita, H., Iino, M., Ooshima, Y., and Takagi, S. F. (1975b). An olfactory projection area in orbitofrontal cortex of the monkey. *J. Neurophysiol.* 38:1269–1283.

Teuber, H. L. (1964). The riddle of frontal lobe function in man. In *The Frontal Granular Cortex and Behavior*, J. M. Warren and K. Akert (eds.). New York: McGraw-Hill, pp. 410–444.

Teuber, H. L. (1966). The frontal lobes and their function. Further observations on rodents, carnivores, subhuman primates, and man. *Int. J. Neurol.* 6:282–300.

Teuber, H. L., Battersby, W. S., and Bender, M. B. (1951). Performance of complex visual tasks after cerebral lesions. *J. Nerv. Ment. Dis.* 114:413–429.

Teuber, H. L., and Mishkin, M. (1954). Judgment of visual and postural vertical after brain injury. *J. Psychol.* 38:161–175.

Thompson-Schill, S. L., Swick, D., Farah, M., D'Esposito, M., Kan, I. P., and Knight, R. T. (1998). Verb generation in patients with focal frontal lesions: a neuropsychological test of neuroimaging findings. *Proc. Natl. Acad. Sci. U.S.A.* 95:15855–15860.

Tomita, H., Ohbayashi, M., Nakahara, K., Hasegawa, I., and Miyashita, Y. (1999). Top-down signal from prefrontal cortex in executive control of memory retrieval. *Nature* 401:699–703.

Tranel, D. (1992). Neuropsychological assessment. In *Psychiatric Clinics of North America: The Interface of Psychiatry and Neurology*, J. Biller and R. Kathol (eds.). Philadelphia: W. B. Saunders, pp. 283–299.

Valverde, F. (1965). *Studies on the Piriform Lobe*. Cambridge, MA: Harvard University Press.

Van Hoesen, G. W., Parvizi, J., and Chu, C.-C. (2000). Orbitofrontal cortex pathology in Alzheimer's disease. *Cereb. Cortex* 10:243–251.

Walker, R., Husain, M., Hodgson, T. L., Harrison, J., and Kennard, C. (1998). Saccadic eye movement and working memory deficits following damage to human prefrontal cortex. *Neuropsychologia* 26:1141–1159.

Ward, A. A., and McCulloch, W. S. (1947). The projection of the frontal lobe on the hypothalamus. *J. Neurophysiol.* 10:309–314.

Watanabe, M. (1996). Reward expectancy in primate prefrontal neurons. *Nature* 382:629–632.

Watson, R. T., Heilman, K. M., Cauthen, J. C., and King, F. A. (1973). Neglect after cingulectomy. *Neurology* 23:1003–1007.

Watson, R. T., Heilman, K. M., Miller, B. D., and

King, F. A. (1974). Neglect after mesencephalic reticular formation lesions. *Neurology 24*:294–298.

Weinberger, D. R., Berman, K. F., and Zec, R. F. (1986). Physiologic dysfunction of dorsolateral prefrontal cortex in schizophrenia. *Arch. Gen. Psychiatry 43*:114–124.

Welch, K., and Stuteville, P. (1958). Experimental production of neglect in monkeys. *Brain 81*:341–347.

Whitlock, D. C., and Nauta, W. J. H. (1956). Subcortical projections from the temporal neocortex in *Macaca mulatta. J. Comp. Neurol. 106*:183–212.

Winocur, G., and Moscovitch, M. (1990). Hippocampal and prefrontal cortex contribution to learning and memory: analysis of lesion and aging effects on maze learning in rats. *Behav. Neurosci. 104*:544–551.

Yeterian, E. H., and Van Hoesen, G. W. (1977). Cortico-striate projections in the rhesus monkey. The organization of certain cortico-caudate connections. *Brain Res. 139*:43–63.

Zald, D. H., and Pardo, J. V. (2000). Functional neuroimaging of the olfactory system in humans. *Int. J. Psychophysiol. 36*:165–181.

Zatorre, R. J., and Jones-Gotman, M. (1991). Human olfactory discrimination after unilateral frontal or temporal lobectomy. *Brain 114*:71–84.

16

Emotional Disorders Associated with Neurological Diseases

KENNETH M. HEILMAN, LEE X. BLONDER, DAWN BOWERS, AND EDWARD VALENSTEIN

In this chapter we will discuss changes in emotional experience and behavior that are caused directly by diseases of the central nervous system. These disorders interfere with brain mechanisms that underlie emotion. There are other ways in which neurological disorders and emotions may interact: patients with neurological diseases may have an emotional response to their illness (e.g., they may get depressed because they are disabled); emotional states may enhance neurological symptoms (e.g., anxiety may aggravate tremor); and emotional states may induce neurological symptoms (e.g., stress may cause headaches). Emotional response to disease, emotional enhancement of symptoms, and emotion-induced disorders are not unique to neurology, and are not discussed in this chapter. It has long been recognized that several disorders traditionally in the realm of psychiatry, such schizophrenia, are probably caused by abnormalities in the brain. However, this chapter is limited to traditional neurological illnesses.

Our approach in this chapter is primarily anatomic. We first consider emotional changes that result from lesions in the cerebral hemispheres. These may result from interference with specific neocortically mediated cognitive processes, such as stimulus appraisal, or from disruption of cortical modulation of limbic or other subcortical regions. The frontal lobes have particularly strong limbic connections, and frontal lobe lesions can cause prominent emotional changes. These are treated primarily in Chapter 15. After discussing emotional changes resulting from dysfunction of either cerebral hemisphere, we consider changes associated with limbic and basal ganglia disorders. Finally, we discuss the pseudobulbar state, in which inappropriate emotional expression occurs despite appropriate emotional experience.

Emotions can be divided into three major domains: emotional experiences, emotional memories, and emotional behaviors. Emotions may be transient or prolonged. Prolonged emotional experiences are called "moods." Ross (1994) also divides emotions into primary (e.g., happy, sad, angry, fearful) and social (e.g., embarrassed) emotions. Our discussion will mainly address the primary emotions. Throughout this chapter, we emphasize information gained from studies of humans with brain dysfunction, because most of our knowledge comes from the investigation of pathological states in humans. We also consider animal studies when they pertain to observations in humans, but we do not attempt to summarize the extensive literature on animals.

HEMISPHERIC DYSFUNCTION

Hemispheric dysfunction may affect emotion in several ways. There may be behavioral changes, including receptive and expressive communicative disorders, changes in the viscera, and changes in the autonomic nervous system. Hemisphere dysfunction may cause changes in emotional experience and mood as well as changes in emotional memory. Each of these will be discussed separately.

COMMUNICATIVE DEFECTS

Receptive

Visual Nonverbal Processes. The development of an appropriate emotional state may depend on perceiving and comprehending visual stimuli such as facial expressions, gestures, and scenes. DeKosky et al. (1980) gave facial affective recognition tasks to patients with left or right hemisphere lesions as well as to control subjects without hemispheric disease. There were several subtests in this study. Patients were asked to determine if a pair of neutral faces was from the same person or from two different people, to name the emotion expressed by a face (happy, sad, angry, indifferent), to select from a multiple-choice array of faces a "target" emotion ("Point to the happy face"), and to determine whether two pictures of the same person's face expressed the same or a different emotion. When compared to control subjects, patients with right hemisphere disease were markedly impaired in their ability to discriminate between pairs of neutral faces, as previously reported by Benton and Van Allen (1968). Although both the right and left hemisphere–damaged patients had difficulty naming and selecting emotional faces, patients with right hemisphere disease performed more poorly on these two tasks than patients with left hemisphere disease. In addition, patients with right hemisphere disease were more impaired in making same–different discriminations between emotional faces. When performance across these various emotional facial recognition tasks was covaried for neutral facial discrimination (a visuoperceptual nonemotional task), differences between the two

groups disappeared. This finding suggests that a visuoperceptual disturbance may underlie the poor performance of right hemisphere–damaged patients on facial affect tasks. However, the poor facial discrimination by the right hemisphere group did not entirely correlate with their ability to recognize and discriminate between emotional faces. Retrospective review of the individual cases revealed that about one-third of the patients with right hemisphere disease performed poorly on both the neutral facial task and the emotional faces tasks, whereas about one-third performed well on both. The remaining patients with right hemisphere disease, however, performed relatively well on neutral facial discrimination but poorly on the emotional faces tasks. This observation suggests that visuoperceptual deficits do not account for impaired affective processing in all right hemisphere–damaged patients and that some of these patients do have an impairment of processing emotional facial expressions.

Some of the facial emotion tasks used by the DeKosky group could be performed by using strategies that involved no knowledge of the emotion expressed on faces. One such task required subjects to judge whether two faces depicted the same or different emotions. Because the same actor was used for both pictures, subjects could have accurately made this determination merely by deciding whether the two faces had identical physiognomic/structural configurations, without any regard to emotionality on the face. This is what might be referred to as a "perceptual" rather than an "associative" emotion judgment. To circumvent the use of pure perceptual "template matching" in making judgments about the similarity of two facial expressions, two different actors would have to be used, sometimes displaying the same emotion and sometimes displaying different emotions. The faces of two actors have inherently unique physiognomic properties (i.e., faceprints) and therefore must be matched by comparing the similarity of their emotional expressions.

Taking these considerations in mind, Bowers and co-workers (1985) assessed stroke patients with hemispheric lesions and control subjects across a series of seven perceptual and associative facial affect tasks. When the patient groups were statistically equated for visuoperceptual ability, the right hemisphere–damaged group was impaired on three of the facial affect tasks, including naming, selecting, and discriminating facial emotions across two different actors. The critical factor distinguishing these three tasks from those that did not give rise to hemispheric asymmetries was related to the underlying task demand of "categorizing" facial emotions. These findings suggest that the disorders of facial affect recognition among right hemisphere–damaged patients cannot be solely attributed to defects in visuoperceptual processing, and that a right hemisphere superiority for processing facial affect exists above and beyond its superiority for processing faces in general. Investigators from other laboratories have also reported that right hemisphere–damaged stroke patients are more impaired than their left hemisphere counterparts in recognizing or categorizing facial emotions (Cicone et al., 1980; Etcoff, 1984; Borod et al., 1986). In general, these defects in identifying facial affect by right hemisphere–damaged patients are not valence-dependent and extend to all categories of emotion (but see Mandel et al., 1991).

In addition to stroke patients, hemispheric asymmetries in the evaluation of facial emotional expressions have also been described in split-brain patients and in individuals undergoing Wada testing. Benowitz and colleagues (1983) presented filmed facial expressions from the Profile of Nonverbal Sensitivity Test (PONS) to each hemisphere of a split-brain patient. This patient was fitted with a special contact lens that restricted visual input to one hemisphere. The patient had no difficulty identifying facial expressions when they were directed to the isolated right hemisphere, but was impaired when the facial expressions were directed to the isolated left hemisphere. Comparable findings have also been reported in patients undergoing intracarotid sodium amytal procedures (Ahern et al., 1991). Ahern and colleagues found that affective faces were rated as less emotionally intense (as compared to baseline ratings) when they were shown to patients whose nondominant language hemisphere (usually right) was anesthestized. Such an effect was not observed with anesthetization of the language-dominant hemisphere. Studies of normals have also implicated the right hemisphere in processing affective faces. Tachistoscopic studies have generally found that affective faces are responded to more accurately and/or more quickly when presented to the left visual field (right hemisphere) than to the right visual field (Suberi and McKeever, 1977; Ley and Bryden, 1979; Strauss and Moscovitch, 1981). Reuter-Lorenz and Davidson (1981) reported hemispheric-specific valence effects, in that happy faces were responded to more quickly in the right visual field and sad faces were responded to more quickly in the left visual field. Subsequent investigators have failed to replicate this finding (Duda and Brown, 1984; McLaren and Bryson, 1987; Bryson et al., 1991).

Other studies using chimeric and/or composite face stimuli with normal subjects have found that the side of the face on the viewer's left influences judgments of emotionality more than the side of the face on the viewer's right (Campbell, 1978; Heller and Levy, 1981). On the basis of these studies with both normal and neurologically impaired subjects, we believe that the right hemisphere is important for perceiving both faces and facial expressions. In particular, we have argued that the right hemisphere may contain a "store of facial emotion icons" or representations (Bowers and Heilman, 1984). Support for this representational hypothesis comes from the research of Blonder and colleagues (1991a), who found that right hemisphere–damaged patients were impaired relative to left hemisphere–damaged patients and normal controls in identifying the emotion associated with a verbal description of a nonverbal signal. The subjects were read brief sentences describing facial ("His face whitened"), vocal ("She raised her voice"), and gestural signals ("He shook his fist"). Because these signals were described verbally, the poor performance of the right hemisphere–damaged group could not be attributed to a perceptual disturbance. Furthermore, their poor performance was not due to a general derangement in emotional knowledge in that these patients performed normally on another task in which they had to make inferences about emotions that are linked to various situational contexts (i.e., "The children track dirt over your white carpet"). Rather, the poor performance of the right hemisphere–damaged patients in assigning an emotion to a verbally described nonverbal signal is consistent with the view that the right hemisphere normally contains representations of species-typical facial expressions. Further evidence that the right hemisphere contains representations of species-typical facial expressions comes from a study in which right and left hemisphere–damaged patients were evaluated on two imaging tasks (Bowers et al., 1991). One involved imagery for facial emotional expressions and the other involved imagery for common objects. On both tasks, the subjects were asked to image a target (i.e., frowning face) and were then asked a series of yes–no questions regarding the structural characteristics of the face (i.e., "Are the outer lips pulled down?"). The right hemisphere–damaged group was more impaired on the facial emotion imagery task than on the object imagery task, whereas the left hemisphere group showed the opposite pattern. That some of these right hemisphere–damaged patients were also more impaired at recognizing visible facial emotions (i.e., a recognition task, rather than an imagery task) than the left hemisphere–damaged group suggests that the right hemisphere contains a hypothetical "store of facial emotional representations" that had been destroyed in these individuals. Bowers et al. (1991) also described a patient with a ventral temporal-occipital lesion of the right hemisphere who could recognize emotional faces but could not image them. This case suggests that the mechanism underlying emotion imagery generation is at least in part mediated by the posterior ventral area, and that the facial emotional representations are anatomically distinct from the areas that either generate, display, or immediately inspect the image.

Work from Roll's laboratory, in which single-cell recordings were used, has identified visual neurons in the temporal cortex and amygdala of monkeys that respond selectively to faces and facial expressions (Baylis et al., 1985; Leonard et al., 1985). Similar findings have been reported during intraoperative recordings of awake humans while undergoing epilepsy surgery (Fried et al., 1982). Bowers and Heilman (1984) described a patient with a category-specific visual verbal discrimination deficit that was confined to facial emotion. The patient had a tumor in the region of the forceps major (the white matter tract leading into the corpus callosum). This patient was unable to both name emotional facial displays and point to the emotional faces named by the examiner. In contrast, the patient could determine if two faces displayed the same or different emotions, and performed normally across an array of other affect tasks, including prosody, gesture, and narration. It was posited that the tumor induced a callosal disconnection such that the speech and language areas of the left hemisphere were unable to access the emotional facial icons (and vice versa), thus causing a verbal–emotional face disconnection. A similar case has been described by Rapscak et al. (1989).

Auditory Nonverbal Processes. "It was not what you said, but how you said it." This sentence conveys that speech may simultaneously communicate propositional and emotional messages. The propositional message is conveyed by a complex code requiring semantic, lexical, syntactic, and phonemic decoding. Although prosody, which includes pitch, tempo, and rhythm, may also convey linguistic content (e.g., declarative vs. interrogative sentences), prosody is more important in conveying emotional content (Paul, 1909; Monrad-Krohn, 1947). In more than 90% of people the left hemisphere is superior to the right when decoding the propositional message. To learn if the right hemisphere was superior to the left in decoding the emotional prosody of speech, Heilman et al. (1975) and Tucker et al. (1977) presented sentences with propositionally neutral content, using four different emotional prosodies (happy, sad, angry, and indifferent), to patients with right hemisphere infarctions and to aphasic patients with left hemisphere infarctions. The patients were asked to identify the emotional tone of the speaker, not on the basis of what was said, but rather according to how it was said. Patients with right hemisphere lesions performed worse on this task than those with left hemisphere lesions, a finding suggesting that the right hemisphere is more involved in processing the emotional intonations of speech than the left hemisphere. Similar findings were reported by Ross (1981). Schlanger and colleagues (1976) failed to find any differences between right and left hemisphere–damaged patients in the comprehension of emotional prosody, but only 3 of the 20 right hemisphere patients in the Schlanger et al. study had lesions involving temporoparietal areas. Further evidence for the dominant role of the right hemisphere in comprehending affective intonation comes from studies that demonstrate preserved abilities in patients with left hemisphere lesions. We examined a patient with pure word deafness (normal speech output and reading but impaired speech comprehension) from a left hemisphere lesion. In patients with pure word deafness, the left auditory cortex is thought to be destroyed and the right auditory cortex is disconnected from Wernicke's area in the left hemisphere; however, the right auditory area and its connections to the right hemisphere are intact. Although this patient comprehended speech very poorly, he had no difficulty recognizing either environmental sounds or emotional intonations of speech.

Weintraub et al. (1981) reported that, relative to normal controls, right hemisphere–damaged patients have difficulty determining whether prosodically intoned sentences were statements, commands, or questions. On the basis of these findings, they suggested that a generalized prosodic disturbance might be associated with right hemisphere damage. However, a left hemisphere–damaged group was not tested in this study. Heilman and colleagues (1984) compared right and left hemisphere–damaged patients for comprehension of emotional (happy, sad, angry) or non-emotional prosody (questions, commands, statements). Compared to normal controls, both the right hemisphere–damaged and the left hemisphere–damaged groups were equally impaired on the non-emotional (syntactic-propositional) prosody task. However, on the emotional prosody task, the right hemisphere–damaged patients performed significantly worse than the left hemisphere–damaged patients. This finding suggests that, whereas both hemispheres may be important in comprehending syntactic-propositional prosody, the right hemisphere plays a dominant role in comprehending emotional prosody. Us-

ing dichotic listening tasks in which two different auditory messages were simultaneously presented to the right and left ears of normal subjects who were asked to recall what they heard, Kimura (1967) found that words were recalled best from the right ear (left hemisphere). However, the moods of the speaker, as determined by affective intonation, were better recalled from the left ear (right hemisphere) (Haggard and Parkinson, 1971).

The defect underlying the impaired ability of patients with right hemisphere disease to identify affective intonations in speech is not entirely clear. It may be related to a cognitive disability whereby these patients fail to verbally denote or name prosodic stimuli. It could also be related to an inability to discriminate between different affective intonations in speech. Tucker et al. (1977) attempted to determine whether patients with right hemisphere disease could in fact discriminate between affective intonations of speech without having to verbally classify or denote these intonations. Patients were required to listen to identical pairs of sentences spoken with either the same or different emotional prosody. The patients did not have to verbally denote or name the emotional prosody, but had to indicate whether the prosody associated with the sentences sounded the same or different. Patients with right hemisphere disease performed more poorly on this task than patients with left hemisphere disease. We suspect that the right hemisphere contains not only representations of species-typical facial expressions but also representations of species-typical affective prosodic expressions. Destruction of these representations or an inability to access them could impair both comprehension and discrimination of emotional prosody.

In normal conversation and in experimental tasks, emotional prosody is often superimposed on propositional speech. Another possible explanation for the poor performance of right hemisphere–damaged patients on emotional prosody tasks is that these patients are "distracted" by the propositional-semantic message of affectively intoned sentences. Findings from studies of hemispheric asymmetries of attention in normal adults demonstrate that each hemisphere is more disrupted by stimuli it normally processes (Heilman et al., 1977), the left hemisphere being more disrupted by speech distractors (i.e., running conversation), and the right hemisphere being more disrupted by music distractors. After right hemisphere damage, perhaps the "intact" left hemisphere can comprehend emotional prosody, but in our tasks, it is distracted by the propositional-semantic message. To test this hypothesis, we presented right and left hemisphere–damaged subjects with an emotional prosody task that varied in the degree of conflict between the emotional message conveyed by the prosody and that conveyed by the propositional content (Bowers et al., 1987). If right hemisphere–damaged patients were distracted by the propositional content, then their comprehension of emotional prosody should be worse when the propositional content and prosody messages are strongly conflicting (i.e., "all the puppies are dead" said in a happy tone of voice). We found that the right hemisphere–damaged group was more disrupted when the propositional and prosodic emotional messages were highly conflicting than when they were less conflicting. The left hemisphere–damaged group was unaffected by increasing the discrepancy between the two messages. These results suggest that, at least in part, the defect in comprehending emotional prosody by right hemisphere–damaged patients is related to distraction, by which they are pulled to the propositional-semantic content of emotionally intoned sentences. However, this distraction defect cannot entirely account for their poor performance, in that right hemisphere–damaged patients remained impaired in identifying emotional prosody even when the semantic content was rendered completely unintelligible by speech filtering (Bowers et al., 1987). In summary, these studies suggest that right hemisphere–damaged patients have both processing and distraction defects that contribute to their poor performance on emotional prosody tasks. The coexistence of these defects might emerge when a right hemisphere lesion induces defective processing or miscategorization of emotional prosody due to disruption of right hemisphere prosodic processors. Defective processing of emotional prosody may render the right hemisphere–damaged patients

more susceptible to the distracting effects of propositional semantic stimuli. They may not hear how it was said, but only what was said.

Visual and Auditory Verbal Processes. While the preceding sections dealt with the evaluation of nonverbal communicative signals of emotion, the focus here is on emotional meaning that is derived from verbal-propositional language. Emotional messages can be conveyed at the single word level (i.e., fear, joy), or by sentences or lengthier narratives that describe contextual situations that are associated with specific emotional states. One obvious question concerns whether the right hemisphere plays a critical role in deriving emotional meaning from propositional language, as it appears to do for nonverbal affective signals. Historically, this question has been addressed from several perspectives.

Reading and auditory comprehension by aphasic left hemisphere–damaged patients is improved when emotional words or phrases are used (Boller et al., 1979; Landis et al., 1982; Reuterskiold, 1991). Landis and colleagues (1982) reported that emotional words were read and written more accurately than nonemotional words by left hemisphere–damaged aphasics. Improvements in auditory comprehension have been reported for aphasics with severe comprehension defects when emotional vs. nonemotional words (object names, actions) are presented (Reuterskiold, 1991). Such improvements may suggest that the right hemisphere has a lexical semantic system that can process emotional words.

Alternatively, the increased arousal that typically accompanies emotional stimuli may be the critical factor. Several studies have directly assessed the comprehension of emotional words, sentences, and narratives by patients with right hemisphere lesions. Borod and co-workers (1992) tested right and left hemisphere–injured patients with emotional and non-emotional sentence and word discrimination tests. In the emotional condition the right hemisphere–damaged subjects were more impaired that those subjects with left hemisphere damage. However, others could not find these asymmetries. For example, Morris and colleagues (1992) found no differences between right hemisphere–damaged and left hemisphere–damaged patients in their ability to comprehend the denotative or connotative meaning of emotional vs. non-emotional words. Etcoff (1984) presented pairs of emotional words to right and left hemisphere–damaged subjects who were required to judge the similarity of the emotional states conveyed by these words. Using multidimensional scaling techniques, she found that right hemisphere–damaged patients did not differ from controls in their scaling solutions for emotion words, nor in the strategies they described for judging the similarity of the emotions conveyed in words. Other studies have indicated that right hemisphere–damaged patients are not impaired in their understanding of the emotionality of short propositional sentences (Cicone et al., 1980; Heilman et al., 1984). This is true even when the sentences contain no specific emotion words and the emotional meaning must be derived from the situational context (e.g., "the children tracked over your white carpet") (Blonder et al., 1991a). A different pattern of findings emerges when right hemisphere–damaged patients are presented with lengthier and more complex narratives. Several investigators have found that these patients are impaired in understanding the affective-emotional content of stories and in appreciating humor (Gardner et al., 1975; Brownell et al., 1983). Such problems, however, do not appear to be specific to emotion per se, but are related to more general difficulties that right hemisphere–damaged patients have in drawing inferences and logical reasoning (Brownell et al., 1986; McDonald and Wales, 1986; Blonder et al., 1991b) and in interpreting figures of speech. Taken together, these studies suggest that lesions of the right hemisphere do not specifically disrupt lexical semantic knowledge about emotions or emotional situations, at least when conveyed by short verbal descriptions. Patients with right hemisphere lesions appear to have intact conceptual knowledge about emotions that are communicated verbally, as long as this communication does not involve verbal descriptions of nonverbal affect signals (Blonder et al., 1991a) or does not entail higher-level inferential processes (Brownell et al., 1986). Left

hemisphere–damaged patients, especially those with word deafness or Wernicke's, global, transcortical sensory, or mixed transcortical aphasia, may have defects in comprehending propositional speech. If the development of an appropriate cognitive state were dependent on propositional language, patients with these aphasias would not be able to do so. Patients with Broca's and conduction aphasia may have difficulty comprehending emotional messages conveyed by propositional speech if these messages contain complex syntax or require a large memory store (see Chapter 2).

Although left hemisphere–damaged aphasic and word-deaf patients may have difficulty comprehending propositional speech, some of these patients can comprehend emotional intonations, and their comprehension of propositional speech may be aided by these intonations (Heilman et al., 1975; Coslett et al., 1984). Finally, some support for the role of the right hemisphere in comprehending emotional verbal language comes from studies of normal subjects. Graves et al. (1981) found a relative superiority in the left visual field for the recognition of emotional words over non-emotional words. However, Strauss (1983) was unable to replicate these findings.

Expressive Defects

Speech and Writing. We attempted to determine whether patients with right hemisphere disease could express emotionally intoned speech (Tucker et al., 1977). The patients were asked to say semantically neutral sentences (e.g., "The boy went to the store") using a happy, sad, angry, or indifferent prosody. These patients were severely impaired. Typically, they spoke the sentences in a flat monotone and often denoted the target affect (e.g., "The boy went to the store and he was sad"). Similar findings have been reported by Borod et al. (1985). Ross and Mesulam (1979) described two patients who could not express affectively intoned speech but could comprehend affective speech. Ross (1981) also described patients who could not comprehend affective intonation but could repeat affectively intoned speech. He postulated that right hemisphere lesions might disrupt the comprehension, repetition, or production of affective speech in the same manner that left hemisphere lesions disrupt propositional speech.

Although there is no evidence to suggest that patients with right hemisphere dysfunction are impaired at expressing emotions when they use propositional speech or writing, Bloom et al. (1992) reported that right hemisphere–damaged patients used fewer words when denoting emotions in their spontaneous speech. However, depending on the type of aphasia, patients with left hemisphere disease may have difficulty expressing emotions when these emotions are expressed as a spoken or written propositional message. Hughlings Jackson (1932) observed that even nonfluent aphasic patients could imbue their simple utterances with emotional content by using affective intonation. In addition, some nonfluent aphasics may be very fluent when using expletives. Jackson postulated that the right hemisphere might be mediating these activities. Roeltgen et al. (1983) demonstrated that aphasic patients with agraphia were able to write emotional words better than non-emotional words. Similar findings were reported by Landis et al. (1982). However, the role of the right hemisphere in these cases remains uncertain.

Normally, propositional speech is colored by affective intonation that is governed by mood. Whereas the left hemisphere is responsible for mediating the propositional aspect of speech, there is parallel processing in the right hemisphere that is responsible for the emotional prosodic element of speech. Speedie et al. (1984) provided evidence that this propositional and affective prosodic mixing occurs interhemispherically.

Facial Expressions. Although it is well established that lesions of the right hemisphere disrupt the perception and evaluation of nonverbal affective signals, controversy exists regarding the role right hemisphere plays in expressing facial emotions. Some investigators have found that right hemisphere–damaged patients are more impaired than left hemisphere–damaged patients in expressing facial emotions. In an initial study, Buck and Duffy (1980) reported that right hemisphere–

damaged patients were less facially expressive than left hemisphere–damaged patients when viewing slides of familiar people, unpleasant scenes, and unusual pictures. Subsequent research, much of it from Borod's laboratory, has replicated these right–left differences in facial expressiveness across a series of studies on stroke patients with focal lesions involving both spontaneous and voluntarily expressed emotions (Borod et al., 1985, 1986, 1988; Kent et al., 1988; Richardson et al., 1992). Similar deficits have also been observed in more naturalistic settings outside the laboratory. Blonder and colleagues (1993) videotaped interviews with patients and their spouses in their homes and found that patients with right hemisphere damage were rated less facially expressive than left hemisphere–damaged patients and normal controls. They also smiled and laughed less. A study of deaf signers (Bellugi et al., 1988) found that right hemisphere lesions are associated with dramatic impairments in the spontaneous use of affective facial expressions in the context of preserved use of linguistic facial expressions. The opposite pattern is observed in deaf signers with left hemisphere lesions.

In contrast, other investigators have reported no differences in facial emotion expressiveness between right and left hemisphere–damaged patients, using the facial action scoring system (FACS) (Mammucari et al., 1988; Caltagirone et al., 1989). Still others have found that lesions that extend into the frontal lobes, regardless of whether the right or left hemispheres are involved, are critical for a reduction of facial expression (Kolb and Milner, 1981; Weddell et al., 1990). The basis for these discrepant findings is unclear (see Buck, 1990). In part, they may relate to subject factors, intrahemispheric lesion location, and the different methods used across laboratories for quantifying facial expressions. Some systems involve scoring the movements of various muscle groups that appear pathognomic of certain emotional facial expressions (i.e., FACS of Ekman and Friesen, 1978), whereas others involve subjective judgments by raters about intended facial expressions, including their intensity and frequency. Another factor may relate to the manner through which facial expressions are elicited. Richardson and colleagues (1992) found that while right hemisphere–damaged patients were overall less accurate than left hemisphere–damaged patients and normal control subjects in communicating target facial emotions, their expressive deficits were most salient in response to affective pictures, affective prosody, and other affective faces. There were no differences among the groups in producing facial expressions on verbal command or in response to the emotional meaning of sentences. These findings have direct implications for studies that use emotional scenes or films for eliciting spontaneous facial expressions, in that defects in fully evaluating the affective meaning of such stimuli could directly reduce one's responsivity to them. This observation, however, cannot readily account for the diminished facial expressiveness of right hemisphere–damaged patients in more naturalistic settings (Blonder et al., 1993) or the asymmetries seen in normal subjects. In general, normal subjects express emotions more intensely on the left side of the face (Campbell, 1978; Sackheim et al., 1978; Heller and Levy, 1981; Moreno et al., 1990).

EMOTIONAL EXPERIENCES AND MOOD

Clinical Descriptions

Babinski (1914) noted that patients with right hemisphere disease often appeared indifferent or euphoric. Hécaen et al. (1951) and Denny-Brown et al. (1952) also noted that patients with right hemisphere lesions were often inappropriately indifferent. Gainotti's (1972) study of 160 patients with lateralized brain damage supported these earlier clinical observations: right hemisphere lesions were often associated with indifference. Terzian (1964) and Rossi and Rosadini (1967) studied the emotional reactions of patients recovering from barbiturate-induced hemispheric anesthesia produced by left or right carotid artery injections (Wada test). They observed that right carotid injections were associated with a euphoric-manic response. Milner (1974), however, was unable to replicate these findings. In contrast to the flattened emotional response or inappropriate euphoric mood associated with right hemisphere damage, Goldstein (1948) noted that many patients with left hemisphere lesions and aphasia appeared anxious, agitated, and sad, which Goldstein called the "catastrophic reaction." Gainotti (1972) confirmed Goldstein's (1948) observations. Terzian (1964) and Rossi and Rosadini (1967) observed that barbiturate injections into the left carotid artery could induce a catastrophic reaction. Gainotti (1972) thought that the indifference reaction was an abnormal mood associated with denial of illness (anosognosia) but that the catastrophic reaction was a normal response to a serious physical or cognitive deficit. However, there are several studies and observations that are incompatible with Gainotti's hypothesis. The Wada test causes only a transient aphasia with hemiparesis and would therefore be unlikely to cause a reactive depression in patients who are undergoing a diagnostic test. Anosognosia is the verbal explicit denial of a hemiplegia (see Chapter 10). We see right hemisphere–damaged patients in the clinic who also appear to be indifferent but do not demonstrate anosognosia. Critchley (1953) has termed this "anosodiaphoria." It is not clear if these patients' propensity to be unconcerned about their own illness is related to a general emotional flattening or if anosodiaphoria is a mild form of anosognosia and their indifference is related to defective evaluation of their own illness. The depressive reaction associated with left hemisphere disease is usually seen in nonfluent aphasic patients with anterior perisylvian lesions (Benson, 1979; Robinson and Sztela, 1981; Starkstein and Robinson, 1990). As discussed earlier, Hughlings Jackson (1932) noted that left hemisphere lesions induced deficits in propositional language, and the nonfluent aphasics who could not express themselves with propositional speech could express feelings by using expletives and by intoning simple verbal utterances. Hughlings Jackson postulated that the right hemisphere might be mediating this activity. His postulate was supported by the observations of Tucker et al. (1977) and Ross and Mesulam (1979). Because left hemisphere–damaged patients are unable to use propositional speech, they may rely more on right hemisphere nonpropositional-affective systems by more heavily intoning their speech and by using more facial expression. As we discussed, patients with right hemisphere disease have more difficulty than patients with left-hemisphere disease in comprehending and expressing affectively intoned speech as well as comprehending and expressing emotional facial expressions. Patients with right-hemisphere disease may also have more difficulty comprehending or remembering emotionally charged speech. These perceptual, cognitive, and expressive deficits might underlie and account for the flattened emotional reaction of patients with right-hemisphere lesions (i.e., indifference reactions), as previously described by clinical investigators. Alternatively, these perceptual, cognitive, and expressive deficits may not reflect the patients' underlying mood.

Although defects of affective communication may account for some of the behavioral symptoms discussed by Goldstein (1948), Babinski (1914), and Gainotti (1972), they cannot explain the results of Gasparrini et al. (1978), who administered the Minnesota Multiphasic Inventory (MMPI) to patients with unilateral hemisphere lesions. The MMPI has been widely used as an index of underlying affective experience, and the completion of this inventory does not require the perception of affectively intoned speech or the perception of emotional facial expressions. Patients with left hemisphere disease showed a marked elevation on the depression scale of this inventory, whereas patients with right hemisphere disease did not. This finding suggests that the differences in emotional reactions of patients after right vs. left hemisphere disease cannot be attributed entirely to difficulties in perceiving or expressing affective stimuli. In Starkstein et al.'s (1987) study of stroke and depression, they found that about one-third of stroke patients had a major depression and long-lasting depressions were associated with both cortical lesions and subcortical lesions. They also found that the left frontal and left caudate lesions were most frequently associated with severe depression: the closer to the frontal pole, the more severe the depression. Many of the patients with depression, and especially those with cortical lesions, were anxious. In contrast, in the acute post-stroke period, right frontal le-

sions were associated with indifference and even euphoria. When patients with right hemisphere damage had depression, they were more likely to have parietal lesions.

Not all investigators agree that there are hemispheric asymmetries in depression. House and colleagues (1990) believe that depression associated with right hemisphere disease may be underdiagnosed because right hemisphere–damaged patients may have an emotional communicative disorder.

Possible Mechanisms of Changes in Mood and Emotional Experience Associated with Hemispheric Dysfunction

If the observation that left hemisphere–damaged patients are depressed (or anxious) and right hemisphere–damaged patients are indifferent (or euphoric) is correct, how can these asymmetries be explained? Unfortunately, the brain mechanisms underlying mood have not been entirely elucidated. However, we will briefly review some of the major theories. We will also discuss their relative merits and how well they explain clinical observations. Theories of emotional experience can be divided into two major types: feedback theories and central theories. Because feedback and central theories both have explanatory value, we will discuss both.

Feedback Theories

Facial. Emotional experiences are also called emotional "feelings." In general, in order to feel something, one must have sensory or afferent input into the brain. Because emotional experience is associated with feelings, emotional experience may also require afferent input. However, emotional feelings are unlike traditional sensory experiences (e.g., visual, tactile, auditory) in that they do not rely directly on the physical characteristics of the external stimulus. Rather, they may rely on the pattern of neural activity that the stimulus is eliciting. Emotional feelings may even occur in the absence of an external stimulus, which suggests that afferent activity must have been induced by efferent activity. This efferent activity may not only be important for emotional expression, but feedback of this expression to the brain may be responsible for emotional feelings.

There are two major feedback hypotheses: the facial theory of Charles Darwin and the visceral theory of William James. Darwin (1872) noted that the free expression by outward signs of an emotion intensifies it. The repression, as far as possible, of all outward signs, however, softens our emotions. "He who gives violent gesture increases his rage." Darwin also thought that emotional expression is innate. Izard (1977) and Ekman et al. (1969), using cross-cultural studies, provided support for Darwin's hypothesis that emotional expression is innate. Tomkins (1962, 1963) thought that sensory receptors in the face provide afferent activity to the brain and that it was self-perception of the facial expression that induced emotion. Laird (1974) experimentally manipulated facial expression, and these manipulations induced emotional experience. Because patients with right hemisphere lesions may be impaired in expressing emotions, including facial expression, they may have reduced facial feedback and therefore appear indifferent. However, the facial feedback theory cannot explain why patients with left hemisphere disease are anxious and depressed. There are many other unresolved problems with the facial feedback theory. If one is feeling a strong emotion (e.g., sadness), one cannot entirely change this emotion to happiness by voluntarily smiling. Therefore, one can express one emotion while feeling another. Patients with pseudobulbar affect (see the final section in this chapter) may express strong facial emotions that they are not feeling. Although it is possible that feedback is interrupted in these patients, we reported a patient with no facial mobility from a polyneuritis (Guillain-Barre syndrome) who reported feeling emotions (Keillor et al., 2002). Therefore, while facial expressions may influence emotions as Darwin suggested, the facial feedback theory cannot alone account for emotional experience.

Visceral-Autonomic Feedback. William James (1890) proposed that emotion-provoking stimuli induced bodily changes and that the self-perception of these changes as they occur produced the emotional feeling or experience. James, however, noted that there were also "cerebral" forms of pleasure and displeasure that did not require bodily changes or perception of these changes. James's model was challenged by Cannon (1927), who argued that the separation of the viscera from the brain does not eliminate emotional feelings. This argument was supported by observations that patients with cervical spinal cord transections continued to experience emotions. For example, Hohmann (1966) found that patients with either high or low spinal cord transections experienced emotions, but patients with lower lesions reported stronger emotions than those with higher lesions. In addition, because the vagus nerve contains visceral afferents, cord transection at any level may not fully interfere with feedback. Cannon also noted that pharmacologically induced visceral activation does not produce emotion. Maránon (1924) injected epinephrine into subjects and then inquired whether or not these injections induced an emotion. He found that these injections produced only "as if" feelings. Schachter and Singer (1962) also found that pharmacologically induced visceral activation did not produce an emotion, unless this arousal was accompanied by a cognitive set. Schachter thus modified William James's postulate and proposed the cognitive-arousal or attribution theory of emotions. According to this theory, the experience of emotion involves specific cognitive attributions superimposed on a state of diffuse physiologic arousal; that is, a primary determinant of felt emotion is the environmental context within which arousal occurs. Cannon thought that the visceral feedback theory could not account for a variety of emotions because the same visceral responses occur with different emotions. While Schachter's modification of James's theory could also deal with this critique, Ax (1953) and Ekman et al. (1969) have demonstrated that different bodily reactions can be associated with different emotions. It has not been shown, however, that feedback of these different bodily reactions can induce different emotional experiences. Regarding Cannon's critique that the viscera have insufficient afferent input to the brain, contemporary researchers have examined the role of autonomic feedback in emotional experience using the heartbeat detection paradigm. Katkin et al. (1982) found that some normal subjects can accurately detect their heartbeats, and it was those individuals who had a stronger emotional response to negative slides as determined by self-report (Hantas et al., 1982). Further support for the importance of autonomic feedback comes from other observations. Experiments in animals demonstrate that sympathectomy may retard aversive conditioning (DiGiusto and King, 1972), most likely because sympathectomy reduces fear. Taken together, not only do Cannon's critiques fail to refute the feedback theory, but there is also evidence that would support a role of visceral feedback in emotional experience. In order for feedback to occur, there must be a means for the viscera and autonomic nervous system to become activated. We will use the term *feedforward* to refer to the brain's ability to activate the autonomic nervous system and viscera. In humans, the cortex plays a critical role in the analysis and interpretation of various stimuli, including those that induce emotional feeling and autonomic-visceral responses. Consequently, feedforward systems must exist to enable the cortex to control the autonomic nervous system and the viscera, such as the heart (visceral *efferents*). Similarly, if visceral activity can be detected by subjects, there must be neuronal pathways that support the feedback system and bring this information back to the brain (visceral *afferents*). As we briefly mentioned, the major nerve that carries visceral afferent information is the vagus. The vagus nerve(s) afferents terminate in the medulla, primarily in the nucleus of the solitary tract. The nucleus of the solitary tract projects to the central nucleus of the amygdala (as well as to several hypothalamic nuclei), which in turn projects to other amygdala nuclei and to the insula. Electrical stimulation of the vagus nerve also produces excitation of the insula and amygdala. The amygdala and insula project to several cortical areas, including temporal, parietal, and frontal regions. It is possible that the vagal–solitary tract nucleus–amygdala–insula–cortical pathway may be responsible for visceral feedback.

Emotions can be expressed by both the striated muscles and the autonomic nervous system–controlled viscera. We have already discussed the facial feedback theory. James did not believe that muscle and facial feedback was critical for emotional experience. Viscera, such as the heart, are controlled by the autonomic nervous system. The autonomic nervous system has two major components, the sympathetic and parasympathetic. The *sympathetic* nerves originate in the spinal cord (intermediolateral). The major *parasympathetic* nerves that innervate the viscera are the vagus nerves that originate in the brainstem (dorsal motor nucleus). Sympathetic neurons in the spinal cord receive projections from the hypothalamus as well as from cells in the ventrolateral pons and medulla. However, the ventrolateral medulla also receives projections from the hypothalamus (e.g., paraventricular and lateral nuclei). While the hypothalamus receives projections from many "limbic" areas, one of the strongest projections comes from the amygdala. The amygdala not only appears to influence the sympathetic nervous system via the hypothalamus, but also sends direct projections to the nucleus of the solitary tract and the dorsal motor nucleus and, therefore, may also directly influence the parasympathetic system. While there are more widespread projections from the amygdala to the cortex than vice versa, the amygdala does receive cortical input. The insula also receives projections from the neocortex, and stimulation of the insula induces autonomic and visceral changes. In humans, stimuli that induce emotional behavior must be analyzed and interpreted by the cortex, including such areas as the temporoparietal association cortex. Stimuli that induce emotion do cause changes in the autonomic nervous system and the viscera. Although it is not clear which limbic area or areas are critical for transcoding the knowledge gained from the emotional stimuli into changes of the autonomic nervous system and viscera, the amygdala and insula would appear to be ideal candidates. The visceral afferent and efferent pathways discussed above are bilateral. However, several studies suggest that there may be asymmetries both in the control of the autonomic nervous system and viscera as well as in the monitoring of the autonomic nervous system.

To investigate the efferent control of the autonomic nervous system (i.e., feedforward system), Heilman et al. (1978) studied skin conductance responses (SCR) to mildly noxious stimuli in patients with right or left hemisphere lesions. The SCR, which results from phasic changes in eccrine sweat gland activity, is almost entirely mediated by the sympathetic branch of the autonomic nervous system. When compared to both normal controls and subjects with left hemisphere lesions, those with right hemisphere damage had decreased SCRs. In contrast, when compared to controls, the left hemisphere–damaged patients had increased responsivity. While Morrow et al. (1981) also found decreased SCR to emotional stimuli in patients with right hemisphere damage, they did not find an increased SCR in patients with left hemisphere damage. Yokoyama et al. (1987) measured heart rate changes in response to an attention-demanding task. These authors found that right hemisphere–damaged patients had reduced heart rate responses, whereas left hemisphere–damaged patients had increased responsivity. The exact parts of the brain that induced these autonomic changes are not known. Although Heilman et al. (1978) suspected the parietal and temporal regions, high-quality neuroimaging was not available when they did this study. In Yokoyama's study, the lesion loci were noted in the Methods section, but no mention is made of the relationship between lesion locus and changes in heart rate. However, Schrandt et al. (1989) reported a study in which they measured SCR to emotional slides. Within the right hemisphere–damaged group, only those patients whose lesions involved the right parietal lobe showed reduced SCR. Luria and Simernitskaya (1977) proposed that the right hemisphere might be more important than the left in perceiving visceral changes (i.e., feedback system). To our knowledge, however, visceral perception (e.g., heart rate detection) has not been systematically studied in brain-impaired subjects.

There have been several studies in normal subjects that suggest that the right hemisphere may play a special role in visceral perception.

For example, Davidson and co-workers (1981) gave a variety of tapping tests to normal individuals to assess whether the left or right hand was more influenced by heartbeat. They found that the left hand was more influenced by heart rate than was the right hand, suggesting that the right hemisphere might be superior at detecting heartbeat. However, other investigators could not replicate this left-hand superiority in the detection of heartbeat. Hantas et al. (1984) used a signal detection technique to learn if normal subjects could detect their own heartbeat. They also assessed cerebral lateral preference by judging conjugate lateral eye movements and found that left movers (who were "right hemisphere preferent") were better at detecting their own heartbeat than were those who were right movers. If the right hemisphere plays a dominant role in visceral autonomic activation and a dominant role in perceiving visceral changes, and if this feedback is critical to emotional experience, it would follow that right hemisphere lesions that damage critical cortical and limbic areas should be associated with reduced emotional feeling or indifference even in those patients who are aware of their deficits. Left hemisphere lesions may not only spare the right hemisphere feedforward and feedback systems, but the left hemisphere may help regulate or control the feedforward systems such that, with left hemisphere lesions, there is increased visceral-autonomic activation (Heilman et al., 1978; Yokoyama et al., 1987). Therefore, the heightened autonomic-visceral activity found in patients with left hemisphere injuries, together with their knowledge that they are impaired (e.g., aphasic and hemiparetic), may lead to the anxiety associated with left hemisphere lesions.

Central Theories

Diencephalic. One of the first central theories was that of Walter Cannon (1927), who proposed that stimuli that enter the brain by way of the thalamus activate the hypothalamus. The hypothalamus controls the endocrine systems and also controls the autonomic nervous system. The endocrine and autonomic nervous systems can induce physiological changes in almost all organ systems. Cannon posited that hypothalamic-induced changes in organ systems are adaptive in that they aid survival. Cannon also thought that the hypothalamus activated the cerebral cortex, and it was this cerebral activation that was responsible for the conscious experience of emotion. Although Cannon believed that the cortex normally inhibits the hypothalamus and a loss of this inhibition was responsible for a loss of appropriate emotional control, such as seen in sham rage, he did not suggest a critical role for the cortex in the interpretation of stimuli.

Limbic System. In 1878, Broca designated a group of anatomically related structures on the medial wall of the cerebral hemisphere "le grand lobe limbique." Because these structures are in proximity to structures of the olfactory system, it was assumed that they all have olfactory or related functions. In 1901, Ramon y Cajal (1965) concluded, on the basis of histological studies, that portions of the limbic lobe (the hippocampal–fornix system) had no more than a neighborly relationship with the olfactory apparatus. Papez (1937) postulated that a "circuit" in the limbic lobe (cingulate–hippocampus–fornix–mammillary bodies–anterior thalamus–cingulate) was an important component of the central mechanism subserving emotional feeling and expression. After Bard (1934) demonstrated that the hypothalamus was important in mediating the rage response, Papez (1937) postulated that the hypothalamus was the effector of emotion. In 1948, Yakovlev added the basolateral components (orbitofrontal, insular, and anterior temporal lobe cortex, the amygdala, and the dorsomedial nucleus of the thalamus) to the medial system, and together these were designated as the "limbic system" (MacLean, 1952). Although the cortex influences the hypothalamus, both inhibiting and activating it, the cortex does not have strong, direct projections to the hypothalamus. Most of the cortical projections that influence the hypothalamus are mediated by the limbic system. In addition, as we will discuss in a later section, patients who are stimulated in limbic areas or have seizures that emanate from limbic areas may experience an emotion. As demonstrated by Kluver and Bucy

(1937), monkeys with a portion of their limbic system ablated (e.g., amygdala) have decreased emotions. On the basis of these seminal observations, it would appear that Cannon's hypothalamic cortical model is insufficient. However, LeDoux and co-workers (1990) have modified Cannon's diencephalic circuit to include the amygdala in fear conditioning. In their study, animals were conditioned by associating a nociceptive stimulus with an auditory stimulus. Whereas ablation of the auditory thalamus and amygdala interrupted the behavioral response to the conditioned stimulus, ablation of auditory cortex did not change the animal's response.

We agree with Cannon that emotions are adaptive and many of the physiologic changes associated with adaptation are mediated by the hypothalamus. We also agree with LeDoux that conditioned fear may not require cortical mediation. However, as we pointed out earlier in this chapter, it is the cortex, rather than the thalamus or hypothalamus, that appears to be critical in the interpretation of the complex stimuli, and it is complex stimuli that most commonly induce emotions in humans. The diencephalic theories of Cannon and the limbic–diencephalic theory of LeDoux also fail to explain how humans can experience a variety of emotions.

Modular Theory of Emotion. In 1903 Wundt proposed that emotional experiences vary in three dimensions: quality (good or bad), excitement (arousal), and activity. Osgood et al. (1957) had normal subjects verbally assess emotions and then performed a factor analysis on these judgments. These investigators found three major factors that were similar to those of Wundt, but instead of activity, these investigators found that the third factor was control (in control/out of control). However, Frijda (1987), who also explored the cognitive structure of emotion, found, as Wundt (1903) posited, that action readiness, instead of control, was the third factor. This dimensional view of emotional experience was supported by psychophysiological studies (Greenwald et al., 1989). On the basis of this dimensional view of emotions, Heilman (1994) suggested that the conscious experience of emotion may be mediated by three anatomically distributed modular networks: one that determines quality or valence (positive or negative), a second that mediates arousal (high or low), and a third that mediates motor activation (approach or avoid).

Valence. In regard to valence or quality, we have previously discussed the observations that after left hemisphere injury, patients appear to be more depressed than after right hemisphere injury. In addition to these clinical data, several functional imaging studies performed on patients with depression suggested that the left hemisphere appeared hypoactive (Phelps et al., 1984; Bench et al. 1992). Lastly, using electrophysiological techniques, Davidson et al. (1979) and Tucker (1981) demonstrated in normal subjects that, whereas the left hemisphere mediates emotions with positive valence, the right hemisphere mediates emotions with negative valence. The mechanism by which each hemisphere mediates valence is unknown. Since the time of Hippocrates, it has been postulated that body humors can influence mood. Tucker and Williamson (1984) suggested that hemispheric valence asymmetries might be related to asymmetrical control of neuropharmocologic systems. This hypothesis was supported by a study using positron emission tomographic (PET) imaging. Robinson and Starkstein (1989) reported that after left hemisphere stroke there was reduced serotonergic receptor binding and that after a right hemisphere stroke there was increased serotonergic binding. The also found that the lower the serotonergic binding, the worse the depression. Although clinical psychiatry has provided strong evidence that depression is associated with a reduction of serotonin, it remains unclear how these neuropharmacological changes induce the emotional experiences associated with a depressed or happy mood.

Arousal. The term *arousal*, like the terms *attention* and *emotion*, is difficult to define. Behaviorally, an aroused organism is awake, alert, and prepared to process stimuli, whereas an unaroused organism is lethargic or comatose and not prepared to process stimuli. Physiologically arousal has several definitions. In the central nervous system arousal usually refers to

the excitatory state of neurons or the propensity of neurons to discharge when appropriately activated. In functional imaging arousal is usually measured by increases of blood flow and electrophysiologically it is measured by desynchronization of the electroencephalogram (EEG) or by the amplitude and latency of evoked potentials. Outside the central nervous system arousal usually refers to activation of the sympathetic nervous system and to increased visceral activity, such as heart rate.

The neural substrate of arousal and attention is discussed in detail in Chapter 13. Briefly, arousal and attention are intimately linked and appear to be mediated by a cortical limbic reticular modular network (Heilman, 1979; Watson, 1981). Sensory information relayed through the thalamus is processed in primary sensory cortices, and then in unimodal sensory association cortices, which in turn converge upon polymodal sensory cortex in frontal cortex and on both banks of the superior temporal sulcus (Pandya and Kuypers, 1969). Both of these sensory polymodal convergence areas project to the supramodal inferior parietal lobe (Mesulam et al., 1977). Whereas the determination of stimulus novelty may be mediated by modality-specific sensory association cortex, stimulus significance requires knowledge as to both the meaning of the stimulus and the motivational state of the organism. The motivational state is dependent on at least two factors: immediate biological needs and long-term goals. It has been demonstrated that portions of the limbic system, together with the hypothalamus, monitor the internal milieu and develop drive states. Therefore, limbic input into regions important in determining stimulus significance may provide information about immediate biological needs. Information about long-term goals that are not motivated by immediate biological needs is provided by the frontal lobes, which have been demonstrated to play a major role in goal-oriented behavior and set development (Stuss and Benson, 1986; Damasio and Anderson, 1993). Studies of cortical connectivity in monkeys have demonstrated that the temporoparietal region has strong connections with not only portions of the limbic system (i.e., cingulate gyrus) but also the frontal cortex.

Polymodal and supramodal cortex not only determine stimulus significance but also modulate arousal by influencing the mesencephalic reticular formation (MRF) (Segundo et al., 1955). Stimulation of the MRF in animals induces behavioral and physiological arousal (Moruzzi and Magoun, 1949). In contrast, bilateral lesions of the MRF induce coma, and unilateral lesions cause ipsilateral hemispheric hypoarousal (Watson et al., 1974). The exact means by which these cortical areas influence the MRF and the MRF influences the cortex remain unknown. There are at least three mechanisms by which the MRF may influence cortical processing. The first is by projections to the nucleus basalis of the basal forebrain, which has cholinergic projections to the entire cortex. These cholinergic projections appear to be important for increasing neuronal responsivity (Sato et al., 1987). Second, MRF stimulation activates specific thalamic nuclei such as centralis lateralis and paracentralis that project to widespread cortical regions (Steriade and Glenn, 1982). Third, gating of sensory input through thalamic relay nuclei is accomplished via the thalamic nucleus reticularis (NR). This thin nucleus envelops the thalamus and projects to all the sensory thalamic relay nuclei. Physiologically, the NR inhibits the thalamic relay of sensory information (Scheibel and Scheibel, 1966). However, when cortical limbic networks determine that a stimulus is significant or novel, corticofugal projections may inhibit the inhibitory NR, thereby allowing the thalamic sensory nuclei to relay sensory information to the cortex.

The level of arousal in the central nervous system is usually mirrored by activity of the peripheral autonomic nervous system. Hand sweating, as measured by the galvanic skin response (GSR), is one means of measuring peripheral autonomic arousal. Heilman et al. (1978) measured GSR in patients with right and left hemisphere damage as well as normal controls. Patients with right hemisphere lesions had a reduced GSR response to a nonpainful electric shock when compared to normals and left hemisphere–damaged controls. Subsequently, other investigators reported similar findings (Morrow et al., 1981; Schrandt et al.,

1989). However, Heilman and co-workers reported another interesting finding: when compared to normal subjects, patients with left hemisphere lesions appeared to have a greater autonomic response (Heilman et al., 1978). Using changes in heart rate as a peripheral measure of arousal, Yokoyama et al. (1987) obtained similar results. Using physiological imaging, Perani et al. (1993) found metabolic depression of the left hemisphere in cases of right hemisphere stroke. Unfortunately, left hemisphere–damaged control patients were not reported.

The mechanisms underlying the asymmetrical hemispheric control of arousal remains unknown. Because lesions restricted to the right hemisphere could not directly interfere with the left hemisphere's corticofugal projections to the reticular systems or the reticular system's corticipetal influence of the left hemisphere, one would have to propose that the right hemisphere's control of arousal may be related to privileged communication that the right hemisphere has with the reticular activating system. Alternatively, portions of the right hemisphere may play a dominant role in computing stimulus significance. The increased arousal associated with left hemisphere lesions also remains unexplained. Perhaps the left hemisphere maintains inhibitory control over the right hemisphere or the reticular activating system.

Motor activation. Some emotions do not call for action (e.g. sadness, satisfaction), but others do (e.g. anger, fear, joy, surprise). The stimulus that induces the emotion may be approached or avoided. In general, one would like to avoid situations that induce unpleasant emotions and approach situations that induce pleasant emotions. Thus, as a rule, we avoid stimuli that induce fear and approach stimuli that induce joy; however, sometimes we approach stimuli that induce negative emotions, as when we approach a stimulus that has made us angry. In the following discussion of approach and avoidance, we refer to the behavior associated with the emotion, rather than one's ideal plans for structuring behavior (which, for example, would be to avoid stimuli that induce anger).

We have posited that motor activation or intention is mediated by a modular network that includes portions of the cerebral cortex, basal ganglia and limbic system (see Chapter 13 for a detailed review). The dorsolateral frontal lobe appears to be the fulcrum of this motor preparatory network (Watson et al., 1978, 1981). Physiological recording from cells in the dorsolateral frontal lobe reveals neurons that have enhanced activity when the animal is presented with a stimulus that is meaningful and predicts movement (Goldberg and Bushnell, 1981). The dorsolateral frontal lobes receive input from the cingulate gyrus and from unimodal, polymodal, and supramodal posterior cortical association areas. Input from these posterior neocortical areas may provide the frontal lobes with information about the stimulus, including its meaning and spatial location. The cingulate gyrus, which is not only part of Papez' circuit but also receives input from Yakolov's basolateral circuit, may provide information as to the organism's motivational state. The dorsolateral frontal lobes participate in a cortical–basal ganglia–thalamo–cortical loop (dorsolateral frontal cortex → neostriatum (caudate and putamen) → globus pallidus → thalamus → frontal cortex) (Alexander et al., 1986), and also have extensive connections with the nonspecific intralaminar nuclei of the thalamus (centromedian and parafasicularis). The intralaminar nuclei may gait motor activation by their influence on the basal ganglia, especially the putamen, or by influencing the thalamic portion of motor circuits (ventralis lateralis pars oralis). Lastly, the dorsolateral frontal lobes have strong input into premotor areas. The observation that lesions of the dorsolateral frontal lobe, the cingulate gyrus, the basal ganglia, the intralaminar nuclei, and the ventrolateral thalamus may all cause akinesia supports the postulate that this system mediates motor activation.

The right hemisphere appears to play a special role in motor activation or intention. Coslett and Heilman (1984) demonstrated that right hemisphere lesions are more likely to be associated with contralateral akinesia than lesions of the left hemisphere. Howes and Boller (1975) measured reaction times (a measure of the time taken to initiate a response) of the hand ipsilateral to a hemispheric lesion and demonstrated that right hemisphere lesions were associated with slower reaction times than left hemisphere lesions. However, as previously discussed, this finding may be related to the important role of the right hemisphere in mediating attention-arousal. Heilman and Van Den Abell (1979) measured the reduction of reaction times of normal subjects who received warning stimuli directed to either their right or left hemisphere. They found that independent of the hand used, warning stimuli delivered to the right hemisphere reduced reaction times to midline imperative stimuli more than warning stimuli delivered to the left hemisphere.

Summary. In summary we propose, as did Wundt, that there are three major components of emotional experience: *(1)* emotional cognition, *(2)* arousal, and *(3)* motor intention-activation. Emotional experience is a "top-down" process. Except in conditioned responses where direct thalamic–amygdala connections appear important (Iwata et al., 1986), cognitive interpretation of stimuli helps determine the type of emotion, including its valence (positive–negative). The valence decision is based on whether the stimulus is beneficial (positive) or detrimental (negative) to the well-being of the organism, its family, or species. Positive or negative emotions can be associated with high (joy, fear) or low (satisfaction, sadness) arousal. Certain negative emotions are associated with preparation for action (e.g., fear and anger) and others are associated with reduced intention–activation (e.g., sadness, satisfaction). Certain positive emotions may also be associated with preparations for action (joy and surprise) and others may not (satisfaction). The negative emotions associated with high arousal are usually associated with action: anger is associated with approach behaviors and fear with avoidance. As we have discussed, depending on the nature of the stimulus (e.g., verbal or nonverbal), the left or right hemisphere determines the type of emotion. The frontal lobes play a critical role in mediating valence—the left mediating positive valence, and the right negative. The right hemisphere, and especially the parietal lobe, appears to have a strong excitatory role on arousal, and the left hemisphere, an inhibitory role. Arousal is mediated by the mesencephalic and diencephalic portions of the reticular activating system. However, the cortex, and especially the right inferior parietal cortex, appears to modulate these arousal systems. The dorsolateral and medial frontal lobes form a recurrent circuit with the basal ganglia and thalamus. This system appears to be important in motor activation, with the right frontal lobe playing a dominant role in motor activation.

The cortical areas discussed above are extensively interconnected. In addition, they are strongly connected with the limbic system (e.g. amygdala), basal ganglia, thalamus, and reticular system. Therefore, the anatomic modules that mediate valence, arousal, and activation systems are richly interconnected and form a modular network. Emotional experience depends on the patterns of neural activation of this modular network.

EMOTIONAL MEMORY

There are only a limited number of studies that have examined the ability of right and left hemisphere–damaged patients to recall emotional memories. Wechsler (1973) studied right and left hemisphere–damaged patients' ability to recall neutral and emotionally charged stories. The left hemisphere–damaged patients recalled more portions of the emotional story than those of the neutral story. The right hemisphere–damaged patients did not show this enhanced recall. Since the story was sad, this finding was compatible with both a valence–mood congruence and right hemisphere–dominance hypotheses. Cimino and co-workers (1991) examined the ability of right hemisphere–damaged patients and normal controls to recall personal episodic memories. The autobiographical memories of the right hemisphere–damaged patients were less emotional and less detailed than those of the controls. There were no valence effects. Borod et al. (1996) also studied right and left hemisphere–damaged subjects' recall of emotional experiences and found that the recall of right hemisphere–damaged patients was less intense than that of those with left hemisphere damage.

LIMBIC SYSTEM DYSFUNCTION

COMMUNICATIVE DEFICITS

It is unusual to observe communicative deficits in patients with limbic system dysfunction. However, bilateral injury to the amygdala is associated with impairment in processing emotional faces (Adolphs and Tranel, 1999). Functional imaging studies also support a role of the amygdala in the processing of emotional faces (Breiter et al., 1996). When compared with cortically medicated perception, the amygdala may play a more direct role in preparing the autonomic nervous and endocrine systems via the hypothalamus for fight or flight. It also might play a role in adverse conditioning to faces (Le Doux et al., 1990).

EMOTIONAL EXPERIENCE

Animal Studies

Myriad stimulation and ablation experiments in animals have attempted to define the role of the limbic system in regulating emotion (Valenstein, 1973). Many of these studies have provided confusing and contradictory results. Some of the difficulty in interpreting these studies results from the complex functional differentiation within each component of the limbic system (Isaacson, 1982). Adding to this is the difficulty of measuring emotional experience in animals; most experiments use techniques such as active or passive avoidance and infer the emotional state from the animal's behavior. Finally, species differences may be significant, even in phylogenetically older portions of the cerebral hemispheres. Therefore, we will provide only a brief review of these studies.

One of the earliest and most important animal observations was that bilateral ablation of the anterior temporal lobe changes the aggressive rhesus monkey into a tame animal (Kluver and Bucy, 1937). Such animals also demonstrated hypersexuality and visual agnosia. Akert et al. (1961) demonstrated that the removal of the temporal lobe neocortex did not produce this tameness. Ursin (1960) stimulated the amygdaloid nucleus and produced a ragelike response and an increase in emotional behavior. Amygdala ablation (Woods, 1956) produced placid animals. Septal lesions in animals produced a ragelike state (Brady and Nauta, 1955), and septal stimulation produced what appeared to be a pleasant state, in which animals stimulated themselves without additional reward (Olds, 1958). Decortication in animals produced a state of pathological rage ("sham rage"). In a series of experiments, Bard (1934) demonstrated that the caudal hypothalamus was mediating this response. Both the amygdala (a component of the basolateral circuit) and the septal region (a portion of both limbic circuits) have strong input into the hypothalamus (Yakovlev, 1948). MacLean (1952) proposed that the septal pathway is important for species preservation (that is, social–sexual behavior) and that the amygdala circuit is more important for self-preservation (fight and flight).

Human Studies

Lesions. Some of the findings in humans have been analogous to the results reported in animals. In humans, for example, tumors in the septal region have been reported to produce ragelike attacks and increased irritability (Zeman and King, 1958; Poeck and Pilleri, 1961). Bilateral temporal lobe lesions in humans entailing the destruction of the amygdala, uncus, and hippocampal gyrus have been reported to produce placidity (Poeck, 1969). In aggressive patients, stereotactic amygdaloidectomy has been reported to reduce rage (Mark, 1973). Anterior temporal lobectomy for seizure disorders has been reported to increase sexuality (Blumer and Walker, 1975).

Inflammation. Several inflammatory and viral diseases can affect the limbic system. Herpes simplex encephalitis has a predilection for the orbitofrontal and anterior temporal regions and thus selectively destroys much of the limbic system. Impulsivity, memory loss, and abnormalities of emotional behavior are frequently early manifestations of this infection. Limbic encephalitis may be a remote effect of cancer. In this condition there is inflammation and in-

jury to the amygdaloid nuclei, hippocampi, and cingulate gyri, as well as to other structures. Clinically, the picture is similar to that of herpes infection, with memory loss and abnormalities of emotional behavior occurring, including depression, agitation, and anxiety (Corsellis et al., 1968). Rabies also has a predilection for limbic structures and may be associated with prominent emotional symptoms, including profound anxiety and agitation.

Seizures. Partial (focal) seizures with complex symptomatology (temporal lobe epilepsy, psychomotor epilepsy) are known to produce emotional symptoms. These symptoms may be seen with a seizure (ictal phenomena), immediately after a seizure (postictal phenomena), or between seizures (interictal behavior). We will discuss each of these separately.

Ictal phenomena. One of the strongest arguments supporting the notion that the limbic system is important in mediating emotional behavior is the observation that emotional change as a manifestation of a seizure discharge is highly correlated with foci in or near the limbic system, particularly with foci in the anteromedial temporal lobes.

- *Sexuality.* Currier et al. (1971) described patients who had ictal behavior that resembled sexual intercourse. Undressing and exhibitionism have been described with temporal lobe seizures (Hooshmand and Brawley, 1969; Rodin, 1973). In general, however, ictal sexual behavior is not purposeful. Remillard et al. (1983) reported 12 women with temporal lobe epilepsy who had sexual arousal or orgasm as part of their seizures. In their review of 14 other cases, they found that most cases had right-sided foci, and most were women. Spencer et al. (1983) reported sexual automatisms in four patients with seizure foci in the orbitofrontal cortex. They proposed that sexual experiences were more likely to occur with temporal lobe foci, whereas sexual automatisms occurred with frontal foci.
- *Gelastic and dacrystic seizures. Gelastic epilepsy* refers to seizures in which laugh-

ter is a prominent ictal event (Daly and Mulder, 1957). Sackeim et al. (1982) reviewed 91 reported cases of gelastic epilepsy and found that of 59 cases with lateralized foci, 40 were left-sided. Gascon and Lombroso (1971) described 10 patients with gelastic epilepsy; 5 had bilateral synchronous spike-and-wave abnormalities, and 2 of these had diencephalic pathology; the other 5 had right temporal lobe foci. Gascon and Lombroso thought they could differentiate two types of laughter: the diencephalic group appeared to have automatic laughter without affect and the temporal lobe group had more affective components (including pleasurable auras). The diencephalic lesion most often associated with gelastic epilepsy is a hypothalamic hamartoma.

Crying as an ictal manifestation, termed *dacrystic epilepsy* (Offen et al., 1976), is much less common than laughing. Of the six cases reviewed by Offen et al., four probably had right-sided pathology, one had left-sided pathology, and in one the site of pathology was uncertain.

• *Aggression*. Ictal aggression is rare. Ashford et al. (1980b) documented nonpurposeful violent behavior as an ictal event. The relationship between epileptic seizures and directed, purposeful violence is controversial. Mark and Ervin (1970) are among the strongest proponents of such a relationship, finding a high incidence of epilepsy in a group of violent prisoners. Pincus (1980) reviewed other studies showing a similar relationship; however, Stevens and Hermann (1981) found that controlled studies did not support this view. Many neurologists who have cared for large numbers of temporal lobe epileptics have never seen directed, purposeful violence as an ictal phenomenon. This clinical impression is supported by careful analysis of larger groups of epileptic patients (Delgado-Escueta et al., 1981; Trieman and Delgado-Esqueta, 1983).

• *Fear and anxiety*. Fear is the affect most frequently associated with a temporal lobe seizure (Williams, 1956). Ictal fear may be found equally with right- and left-sided dysfunction (Williams, 1956; Strauss et al., 1982). A prolonged attack of fear has been associated with right-sided temporal lobe status (McLachlan and Blume, 1980). Although fear responses are usually associated with temporal lobe seizures, they may also be associated with seizures emanating from the cingulate gyrus (Daly, 1958). The amygdala appears to be the critical structure in the induction of the fear response (Gloor, 1972), and volumetric MRI studies have associated ictal fear with amygdala atrophy (Cendes et al., 1994).

• *Depression and euphoria*. Williams (1956) described patients who became very sad and others who had extreme feelings of well-being.

Postictal phenomena. Many patients are confused, restless, and combative after a seizure, especially after a temporal lobe seizure. Instances of aggression in this state are common but usually consist only of the patient's struggling with persons who are trying to restrain him or her. Depression may last for several days after a seizure.

Interictal phenomena. The postulate that seizures directly induce interictal behavioral changes has proved to be the most difficult of issues and has yet to be resolved.

• *Anxiety, fear, and depression*. Currier et al. (1971) found that 44% of patients with temporal lobe epilepsy had psychiatric complications. The most common were anxiety and depression. Men with left-sided foci reported more fear than men with right sided foci. Patients with left-sided foci reported more fear of social and sexual situations (Strauss et al., 1982). There is an increased risk of suicide in epileptics (Hawton et al., 1980). Flor-Henry (1969) found a relationship between right temporal lobe seizure foci and affective disorders. McIntyre et al. (1976) and Bear and Fedio (1977) also showed that patients with right-hemisphere foci are more likely to show emotional tendencies. However, according to some studies, patients with left-sided foci score higher on depression scales than do patients with right-sided foci (Robertson et al., 1987). Bear (1979) has suggested that a sensory–limbic hyperconnection may account for interictal behavioral aberrations. Hermann and Chhabria (1980) postulated that classical conditioning might mediate an overinvestment of affective significance. The unconditioned response is the emotion caused by the firing of a limbic focus. Environmental stimuli coincidentally paired with this firing result in the conditioned response of inappropriate emotional significance attributed to environmental stimuli.

- *Sexuality.* Hyposexuality has been associated with temporal lobe epilepsy (Gastaut and Colomb, 1954). Taylor (1969) studied patients with temporal lobe seizures and found that 72% had a decreased sexual drive. Pritchard (1980) was able to confirm that reduced libido and impotence were associated with temporal lobe seizures. The side of the epileptic focus, type of drug therapy, and seizure control did not seem to be related to the hyposexuality. The location of the focus did, however, appear important. A seizure focus in the mesobasal area of the temporal lobe appears to be most often associated with decreased libido. However, increased libido has also been reported to be associated with seizures (Cogen et al., 1979).

The medial temporal lobe structures, including the amygdala, have a close anatomic and physiological relationship with the hypothalamus. Pritchard (1980) found that endocrine changes could be demonstrated in patients with seizures, including eugonadotropic, hypogonadotropic, and hypergonadotropic hypogonadism. Herzog et al. (1982) also demonstrated endocrine changes and suggested that hypothalamic–pituitary control of gonadotropin secretion may be altered in patients with temporal lobe epilepsy. Further studies have suggested a relationship between the laterality of discharge and the type of endocrine pathology (Herzog, 1993). Pritchard et al. (1981) found elevation of prolactin following complex partial seizures. Hyperprolactinemia may be associated with impotence in males. Taylor (1969) and Cogen et al. (1979) noted that temporal lobectomy may restore normal sexual function.

- *Aggressiveness.* Interictal aggressiveness, like ictal aggressiveness, remains controversial and has many medicolegal implications. Taylor (1969) found that about one-third of patients with temporal lobe epilepsy were aggressive interictally. Williams (1969) reviewed the EEGs of aggressive criminals, many of whom had committed acts of violence. Abnormal EEGs were five times more common in this group than in the general population. However, Stevens and Hermann (1981) note that this observation has not been validated by detailed controlled studies. Treiman (1991) reported that interictal violence tends to occur in young men of subnormal intelligence, with character disorders, a history of early and severe seizures, and associated neurological deficits. When patients with psychiatric disorders or subnormal intelligence are removed from a series, there is no increased evidence of violence.

- *Other interictal changes.* Patients with temporal lobe epilepsy are said to have a dramatic, and possibly specific, disorder of personality (Blumer and Benson, 1975). Slater and Beard (1963) described "schizophreniform" psychosis in patients with temporal lobe epilepsy, but they described selected cases and could not comment on the incidence of this disorder in temporal lobe epileptics. Other studies (Currie et al., 1971) have failed to show a higher than expected incidence of psychosis in temporal lobe epileptics, but it can still be maintained that less severe psychiatric abnormalities could have eluded these investigators. Studies that claim to show no difference in emotional makeup between temporal lobe and other epileptics (Guerrant et al., 1962; Stevens, 1966) have been reinterpreted (Blumer,

1975) to indicate that there is, in fact, a difference: temporal lobe epileptics are more likely to have more serious forms of emotional disturbance. The "typical personality" of the temporal lobe epileptic has been described in roughly similar terms over many years (Blumer and Benson, 1975; Geschwind, 1975, 1977; Blumer, 1999). These patients are said to have a deepening of emotions; they ascribe great significance to commonplace events. This can be manifested as a tendency to take a cosmic view; hyperreligiosity (or intensely professed atheism) is said to be common. Concern with minor details results in slowness of thought and circumstantiality, and can also be manifested by hypergraphia, a tendency of such patients to record in writing minute details of their lives (Waxman and Geschwind, 1974). In the extreme, psychosis, often with prominent paranoid qualities, can be seen (the schizophreniform psychosis noted above), but, unlike schizophrenics, these patients do not have a flat affect and tend to maintain interpersonal relationships. McIntyre et al. (1976) demonstrated that, whereas patients with left temporal lobe foci demonstrate a reflective conceptual approach, patients with right temporal lobe foci are more impulsive. Bear and Fedio (1977) designed a questionnaire specifically to detect personality features, and found that these personality changes are significantly more common among temporal lobe epileptics than among normal subjects. Patients with right hemisphere foci are more likely to show emotional tendencies and denial, and patients with left temporal lobe foci show ideational aberrations (paranoia, sense of personal destiny) and dyssocial behavior. Since a control population with seizure foci in other sites was not used, the specificity of these changes to limbic regions can still be questioned. Attempts to replicate Bear and Fedio's findings have failed to define a personality profile specific to temporal lobe epilepsy (Hermann and Riel, 1981; Mungas, 1982; Brandt et al., 1985; Weiser,

1986). Several studies have suggested that patients with limbic temporal lobe foci are more likely to have abnormal personality traits than patients with lateral temporal lobe foci (Nielsen and Kristensen, 1981; Hermann et al., 1982; Weiser, 1986). Much of this literature has been reviewed by Strauss (1989), Blumer (1999), and Devinsky and Najjar (1999).

BASAL GANGLIA DYSFUNCTION

Basal ganglia disorders are commonly thought to be primarily motor disorders; however, patients with basal ganglia disorders frequently have emotional communicative and mood disorders.

PARKINSON'S DISEASE

Communicative Defects

Parkinson's disease is characterized by akinesia, rigidity, and resting tremor. There may be other associated signs and symptoms, including disorders of gait and intellectual deterioration. Patients with Parkinson's disease often demonstrate a decrease of emotional facial expressions. In addition, these patients may have problems with discriminating emotional faces (Jacobs et al., 1995). Patients with Parkinson's disease may also have impaired production and comprehension of emotional prosody (Blonder et al., 1989).

Emotional Experience

Parkinson (1938) noted that his patients were unhappy. Depression has subsequently been found to be a frequent part of the Parkinson's complex. Mayeux et al. (1981), for example, studied well-functioning outpatients, and using the Beck Depression Index, found that 47% of these patients were depressed. Other investigators have also found a high rate of depression among Parkinson's patients (Warburton, 1967; Mindham, 1970; Celesia and Wanamaker, 1972, Cummings 1992). The depression may be reactive or a part of the parkinsonian syndrome or both. Support for the hypothesis that it is not entirely reactive comes from the observation that the motor impairment and the depression correlate poorly. Patients who are more severely disabled are often less depressed (Robins, 1976), and in many patients, depression is noted prior to the onset of motor symptoms (Mindham, 1970; Mayeux et al., 1981). Patients with Parkinson's disease may also have anxiety and panic associated with their depression. As might be expected from the poor correlation between depression and motor impairment, the depression in parkinsonism responds poorly to the drugs that help the motor symptoms.

Many of the motor symptoms are primarily induced by deficits in the nigrostriatal dopaminergic system. Although L-dopa replacement therapy improves the motor symptoms, it may not reduce depression (Marsh and Markham, 1973; Mayeux et al., 1981). Parkinson's disease may be associated with cell loss in both the Raphe nuclei and locus coeruleus, and the depression associated with Parkinson's disease may be related to defects in the serotonergic or noradrenergic systems. However, Maricle et al. (1995) reported patients who had elevation of mood with dopaminergic treatment. Therefore, the mechanisms underlying mood changes associated with Parkinson's disease need to be further elucidated.

HUNTINGTON'S DISEASE

Communicative Deficits

Huntington's disease, or Huntington's chorea, is characterized by involuntary movements and intellectual decline. Patients with Huntington's disease may have impaired comprehension of emotional prosody (Speedie et al., 1990) and of emotional faces (Jacobs et al., 1995; Sprengelmeyer et al., 1996). The brain mechanisms underlying the deficits are not well understood.

Emotional Experience

Huntington (1872) noted that many patients with this disease have severe emotional disorders and that there is a tendency toward suicide. Almost every patient who develops Huntington's disease has emotional or psychiatric

signs and symptoms (Mayeux, 1983). Although it is possible that some of the emotional signs and symptoms are a reaction to the disease, in many cases they precede motor and cognitive dysfunction (Heathfield, 1967). The emotional changes are variable and include mania and depression (Folstein et al., 1979), apathy, aggressiveness, irritability, promiscuity, and irresponsibility. Different emotional symptoms may be manifested at different times during the course of the disease. In general, however, the apathy is usually seen later in the course, when there are signs of intellectual deterioration. The pathophysiology of the emotional disorders associated with Huntington's disease is unclear. In general, patients have cell loss in the neostriatum and especially in the caudate. There is also cortical cell loss. However, other areas of the brain may also show degenerative changes. Many of the signs displayed by patients with Huntington's disease are similar to those seen with frontal lobe dysfunction (e.g., apathy), and frontal lobe atrophy may be responsible for these signs (see Chapter 19). However, there are profound neurochemical changes associated with Huntington's disease. For example, gamma-aminobutyric acid (GABA) and acetylcholine levels are reduced in the basal ganglia. Mayberg et al. (1992) studied patients with Huntington's disease using functional imaging. They found that patients with depression, compared to patients who were not depressed, had reduced activation of the inferior and orbitofrontal portions of the frontal cortex. The frontal cortex modulates the activity of the locus ceruleus, the source of norepinephrine. Studies suggest that reduction of norepinephrine may be important in depression.

PSEUDOBULBAR PALSY

Wilson (1924) postulated a pontobulbar area responsible for emotional facial expressions. Lesions that interrupt the corticobulbar motor pathways bilaterally release reflex mechanisms for facial expression from cortical control. This was called "pseudobulbar palsy," to distinguish it from motor deficits (palsy) resulting from lower motor neuron (bulbar) dysfunction, a common occurrence when polio was prevalent.

The syndrome consists of involuntary laughing or crying (or both). As with many forms of release phenomena, this excess of emotional expression is stereotypic, lacking variation in quality or modulation of intensity of expression. It can be triggered by a wide variety of stimuli but cannot be initiated or stopped voluntarily. Examination usually shows weakness of voluntary facial movements and increase in the facial and jaw stretch reflexes. The location of the centers for the control of facial expression is not known, and although Wilson postulated it to be in the lower brainstem, Poeck (1969) has postulated centers in the thalamus and hypothalamus. Although bilateral lesions are usually responsible, the syndrome has been described with unilateral lesions on either side (Bruyn and Gaithier, 1969).

Patients with pseudobulbar palsy usually consistently either laugh or cry. Sackeim et al. (1982) noted that, although most patients with pseudobulbar crying or laughing have bilateral lesions, the larger lesion is usually in the right hemisphere when there is laughter and in the left when there is crying. Patients with this syndrome report feeling normal emotions, despite the abnormality of expression. Commonly, their family and physicians speak of them as being emotionally labile, implying that they no longer have appropriate internal emotional feeling. It is important to make the distinction between true emotional lability (as may be seen with bilateral frontal lobe disturbance) and pseudobulbar lability of emotional expression (with normal inner emotions).

REFERENCES

Adolphs, R., and Tranel, D. (1999). Preferences for visual stimuli following amygdala damage. *J. Cogn. Neurosci.* 6:610–616.

Ahern, G., Schumer, D., Kleefield, J., Blume, H., Cosgrove, G., Weintraub, S., and Mesalum, M. (1991). Right hemisphere advantage in evaluating emotional facial expressions. *Cortex* 27:193–202.

Akert, K., Greusen, R. A., Woosley, C. N., and Meyer, D. R. (1961). Kluver-Bucy syndrome in monkeys with neocortical ablations of temporal lobe. *Brain* 84:480–498.

Alexander, G. E., DeLong, M. R., and Strick, P. L. (1986). Parallel organization of functionally seg-regated circuits linking basal ganglia and cortex. *Ann. Rev. Neurosci.* 9:357–381.

Ashford, J. W., Aabro, E., Gulmann, N., Hjelmsted, A., and Pedersen, H. E. (1980a). Antidepressive treatment in Parkinson's disease. *Acta Neurol. Scand.* 62:210–219.

Ashford, J. W., Schulz, C., and Walsh, G. O. (1980b). Violent automatism in a partial complex seizure. Report of a case. *Arch. Neurol.* 37:120–122.

Ax, A. F. (1953). The physiological differentiation between fear and anger in humans. *Psychosom. Med.* 15:433–442.

Babinski, J. (1914). Contribution á l'etude des troubles mentaux dans l'hemisplegie organique cerebrale (anosognosie). *Rev. Neurol.* 27:845–848.

Bard, P. (1934). On emotional expression after decortication with some remarks on certain theoretical views. *J. Neurophysiol.* 41:309–329, 424–449.

Baylis, G., Rolls, E., and Leonard, C. (1985). Selectivity between faces in the responses of a population of neurons in the superior temporal sulcus of the monkey. *Brain Res.* 342:91–102.

Bear, D. M. (1979). Temporal lobe, epilepsy: a syndrome of sensory-limbic hyperconnection. *Cortex* 15:357–384.

Bear, D. M., and Fedio, P. (1977). Quantitative analysis of interictal behavior in temporal lobe epilepsy. *Arch. Neurol.* 34:454–467.

Bellugi, U., Corina, D., Normal, F., Klima, E., and Reilly, J. (1988). Differential specialization for linguistic facial expressions in left and right lesioned deaf singers. Presented at the 27th Annual Meeting of the Academy of Aphasia,

Bench, C. J., Friston, K. J., Brown, R. G., Scott, L. C., Frackowiak, R. S., and Dolan, R. J. (1992). The anatomy of melancholia—focal abnormalities of cerebral blood flow in major depression. *Psychol. Med.* 22:607–615.

Benowitz, L., Bear, D., Mesulam, M., Rosenthal, R., Zaidel, E., and Sperry, W. (1983). Nonverbal sensitivity following lateralized cerebral injury. *Cortex* 19:5–12.

Benson, D. F. (1973). Psychiatric aspects of aphasia. *British J. Psychiatry* 123:555–566.

Benton, A. L., and Van Allen, M. W. (1968). Impairment in facial recognition in patients with cerebral disease. *Cortex* 4:344–358.

Blonder, L. X., Bowers, D., and Heilman, K. M. (1991a). The role of the right hemisphere on emotional communication. *Brain* 114:1115–1127.

Blonder, L., Bowers, D., and Heilman, K. (1991b). Logical inferences following right hemisphere damage [abstract]. *J. Clin. Exp. Neuropsychol.* 13:39.

Blonder, L. X., Burns, A., Bowers, D., Moore,

R. W., and Heilman, K. M. (1993). Right hemisphere facial expressivity during natural conversation. *Brain Cogn.* 21:44–56.

Blonder, L. X., Gur, R. E., and Gur, R. C. (1989). The effects of right and left hemiparkinsonism on prosody. *Brain Lang.* 36:193–207.

Bloom, R., Borod, J. C., Obler, L., and Gerstman, L. (1992). Impact of emotional content on discourse production in patients with unilateral brain damage. *Brain Lang.* 42:153–164.

Blumer, D. (1975). Temporal lobe epilepsy and its psychiatric significance. In *Psychiatric Aspects of Neurological Disease*, D. F. Benson and D. Blumer (eds.). New York: Grune and Stratton.

Blumer, D. (1999). Evidence supporting the temporal lobe epilepsy personality syndrome. *Neurology 53(Suppl 2)*:S9–S12.

Blumer, D., and Benson, D. F. (1975). Personality changes with frontal and temporal lobe lesions. In *Psychiatric Aspects of Neurological Disease*, D.F. Benson and D. Blumer (eds.). New York: Grune & Stratton.

Blumer, D., and Walker, A. E. (1975). The neural basis of sexual behavior. In Psychiatric Aspects of Neurological Disease, D. F. Benson and D. Blumer (eds.). New York: Grune and Stratton.

Boller, F., Cole, M., Vtunski, P., Patterson, M., and Kim, Y. (1979). Paralinguistic aspects of auditory comprehension in aphasia. *Brain Lang.* 7:164–174.

Borod, J. C., Andelman, F., Obler, L. K., Tweedy, J. R., and Welkowitz, J. (1992). Right hemisphere specialization for the identification of emotional words and sentences: evidence from stroke patients. *Neuropsychologia 30*:827–844.

Borod, J. C., Koff, E., Lorch, M. P., and Nicholas, M. (1985). Channels of emotional communication in patients with unilateral brain damage. *Arch. Neurol.* 42:345–348.

Borod, J., Koff, E., Perlman-Lorch, J., and Nicholas, M. (1986). The expression and perception of facial emotions in brain-damaged patients. *Neuropsychologia* 24:169–180.

Borod, J., Koff, E., Perlman-Lorch, M., Nicholas, M., and Welkowitz, J. (1988). Emotional and nonemotional facial behavior in patients with unilateral brain damage. *J. Neurol. Neurosurg. Psychiatry* 51:826–832.

Borod, J. C., Rorie, K. D., Haywood, C. S., Andelman, F., Obler, L. K., Welkowitz, J., Bloom, R. L., and Tweedy, J. R. (1996). Hemispheric specialization for discourse reports of emotional experiences: relationships to demographic, neurological, and perceptual variables. *Neuropsychologia 34*:351–359.

Bowers, D., Bauer, R. M., Coslett, H. B., and Heilman, K. M. (1985). Processing of faces by patients with unilateral hemispheric lesions. I. Dissociation between judgments of facial affect and facial identity. *Brain Cogn.* 4:258–272.

Bowers, D., Blonder, L. X., Feinberg, T., and Heilman, K. M. (1991). Differential impact of right and left hemisphere lesions on facial emotion and object imagery. *Brain 114*:2593–2609.

Bowers, D., Coslett, H. B., Bauer, R. M., Speedie, L. J., and Heilman, K. M. (1987). Comprehension of emotional prosody following unilateral hemispheric lesions: processing defect vs. distraction defect. *Neuropsychologia 25*:317–328.

Bowers, D., and Heilman, K. M. (1984). Dissociation of affective and nonaffective faces: a case study. *J. Clin. Neuropsychol.* 6:367–379.

Brady, J. V., and Nauta, W. J. (1955). Subcortical mechanisms in control of behavior. *J. Comp. Physiol. Psychol.* 48:412–420.

Brandt, J., Seidman, L. J., and Kohl, D. (1985). Personality characteristics of epileptic patients: a controlled study of generalized and temporal lobe cases. *J. Clin. Exp. Neuropsychol.* 7:25–38.

Breiter, H. C., Etcoff, N. L., Whalen, P. J., Kennedy, W. A., Rauch, S. L., Buckner, R. L., Strauss, M. M., Hyman, S. E., and Rosen, B. R. (1996): Response and habituation of the human amygdala during visual processing of facial expression. *Neuron 17*:875–887.

Broca, P. (1878). Anatomie comparee des enconvolutions cerebrales: le grand lobe limbique et al scissure limbique dans la seire des mammiferes. *Rev. Antrop.* 1:385–498.

Brownell, H., Michel, D., Powelson, J., and Gardner, H. (1983). Surprise but not coherence: sensitivity to verbal humor in right hemisphere patients. *Brain Lang.* 18:20–27.

Brownell, H., Potter, H., and Birhle, A. (1986). Inferences deficits in right brain–damaged patients. *Brain Lang.* 27:310–321.

Bruyn, G. W., and Gaither, J. C. (1969). The opercular syndrome. In *Handbook of Clinical Neurology, Vol. 1*, P. J. Vincken and G. W. Bruyn (eds.). Amsterdam: North-Holland, pp. 776–783.

Bryson, S., McLaren, J., Wadden, N., and Maclean, M. (1991). Differential asymmetries for positive and negative emotions: hemisphere or stimulus effects. *Cortex 27*:359–365.

Buck, R. (1990). Using FACS versus communication scores to measure spontaneous facial expression of emotion in brain damaged patients. *Cortex 26*:275–280.

Buck, R., and Duffy, R. J. (1980). Nonverbal communication of affect in brain damaged patients. *Cortex* 16:351–362.

Caltagirone, C., Ekman, P., Friesen, W., Gainotti, G., Mammucari, A., Pizzamiglio, L., and Zoccolatti, P. (1989). Posed emotional facial expressions in brain damaged patients. *Cortex* 25:653–663.

Campbell, R. (1978). Asymmetries in interpreting and expressing a posed facial expression. *Cortex* 14:327–342.

Cannon, W. B. (1927). The James-Lange theory of emotion: a critical examination and an alternative theory. *Am. J. Psychol.* 39:106–124.

Celesia, G. G., and Wanamaker, W. M. (1972). Psychiatric disturbances in Parkinson's disease. *Dis. Nerv. System* 33:577–583.

Cendes, F., Andermann, F., Gloor, P., Gambardella, A., Lopes-Cendes, I., Watson, C., Evans, A., Carpenter, S., and Olivier, A. (1994). Relationship between atrophy of the amygdala and ictal fear in temporal lobe epilepsy. *Brain* 117:739–746.

Cicone, M., Waper, W., and Gardner, H. (1980). Sensitivity to emotional expressions and situation in organic patients. *Cortex* 16.145–158.

Cimino, C. R., Verfaellie, M., Bowers, D., and Heilman, K. M. (1991). Autobiographical memory with influence of right hemisphere damage on emotionality and specificity. *Brain Cogn.* 15:106–118.

Cogen, P. H., Antunes, J. L., and Correll, J. W. (1979). Reproductive function in temporal lobe epilepsy: the effect of temporal lobe lobectomy. *Surg. Neurol.* 12:243–246.

Corsellis, J. A. N., Goldberg, G. J., and Norton, A. R. (1968). Limbic encephalitis and its association with carcinoma. *Brain* 91:481–496.

Coslett, H. B., Brasher, H. R., and Heilman, K. M. (1984). Pure word deafness after bilateral primary auditory cortex infarcts. *Neurology* 34:347–352.

Coslett, H. B., and Heilman, K. M. (1987). Hemihypokinesia after right hemisphere strokes. *Brain and Cognition* 9:267–278.

Critchley, M. (1953). *The Parietal Lobes*. London: E. Arnold.

Currie, S., Heathfield, K.W.G., Henson, R. A., and Scott, D. F. (1971). Clinical course and prognosis of temporal lobe epilepsy: a survey of 666 patients. *Brain* 94:173–190.

Cummings, J. L. (1992). Depression and Parkinson's disease: a review. *Am. J. Psychiatry* 149:443–454.

Currier, R. D., Little, S. C., Suess, J. F., and Andy, O. J. (1971). Sexual seizures. *Arch. Neurol.* 25:260–264.

Daly, D. (1958). Ictal affect. *Am. J. Psychiatry* 115:97–108.

Daly, D. D., and Mulder, D. W. (1957). Gelastic epilepsy. *Neurology* 7:189–192.

Damasio, A. R., and Anderson, S. W. (1993). The frontal lobes. In K. M. Heilman and E. Valenstein (Eds), *Clinical Neuropsychology*, 3rd ed. New York: Oxford University Press, pp. 409–460.

Darwin, C. (1872). *The Expression of Emotion in Man and Animals*. London: John Murray.

Davidson, R. J., Horowitz, M. E., Schwartz, G. E., and Goodman, D. M. (1981). Lateral differences in the latency between finger tapping and heart beat. *Psychophysiology* 18:36–41.

Davidson, R. J., Schwartz, G. E., Saron, C., Bennett, J., and Goldman, D. J. (1979). Frontal versus parietal EEG asymmetry during positive and negative affect. *Psychophysiology* 16:202–203.

DeKosky, S., Heilman, K. M., Bowers, D., and Valenstein, E. (1980). Recognition and discrimination of emotional faces and pictures. *Brain Lang.* 9:206–214.

Delgade-Escueta, A. V., Mattson, R. H., King, L., Goldensohn, E. S., Spiegel, H., Madsen, J., Crandall, P., Dreifus, F., and Porter, R. J. (1981). The nature of aggression during epileptic seizures. *N. Engl. J. Med.* 305:711–716.

Denny-Brown, D., Meyer, J. S., and Horenstein, S. (1952). The significance of perceptual rivalry resulting from parietal lesions. *Brain* 75:434–471.

Devinsky, O., and Najjar, S. (1999). Evidence against the existence of a temporal lobe epilepsy personality syndrome. *Neurology* 53(Suppl 2):S13–S25.

DiGuisto, E. L., and King, M. G. (1972). Chemical sympathectomy and avoidance learning. *Natl. J. Comp. Physiol. Psychol.* 81:491–500.

Duda, P., and Brown, J. (1984). Lateral asymmetry of positive and negative emotions. *Cortex* 20:253–261.

Ekman, P., and Friesen, W. V. (1978). *Facial Action Coding System*. Palo Alto, CA: Consulting Psychologists Press.

Ekman, P., Sorenson, E. R., and Friesen, W. V. (1969). Pancultural elements in facial displays of emotions. *Science* 164:86–88.

Etcoff, N. (1984). Perceptual and conceptual organization of facial emotions. *Brain Cogn.* 3:385–412.

Flor-Henry, P. (1969). Psychosis and temporal lobe epilepsy: a controlled investigation. *Epilepsia* 10:363–395.

Folstein, S. E., Folstein, M. F., and McHugh, P. R.

(1979). Psychiatric syndromes in Huntington's disease. *Adv. Neurol.* 23:281–289.

Fried, I., Mateer, C., Ojemann, G., Wohns, R., and Fedio, P. (1982). Organization of visuospatial functions in human cortex. *Brain* 105:349–371.

Frijda, N. H. (1987). Emotion, cognitive structure and action tendency. *Cognition and Emotion* 1:115–143.

Gainotti, G. (1972). Emotional behavior and hemispheric side of lesion. *Cortex* 8:41–55.

Gardner, H., Ling, P. K., Flam, I., and Silverman, J. (1975). Comprehension and appreciation of humorous material following brain damage. *Brain* 98:399–412.

Gascon, G. G., and Lombroso, C. T. (1971). Epileptic (gelastic) laughter. *Epilepsia* 12:63–76.

Gasparrini, W. G., Spatz, P., Heilman, K. M., and Coolidge, F. L. (1978). Hemispheric asymmetries of affective processing as determined by the Minnesota Multiphasic Personality Inventory. *J. Neurol. Neurosurg. Psychiatry* 41:470–473.

Gaustaut, H., and Colomb, H. (1954). Étude du comportement sexuel chez les ipieptiques psychomoteurs. *Ann. Med. Psychol. (Paris) 112*:659–696.

Geschwind, N. (1979). Behavioral changes in temporal lobe epilepsy. *Psychological Medicine* 9:217–219.

Geschwind, N. (1977). Behavioral changes in temporal lobe epilepsy. *Arch. Neurol. 34*:453.

Gloor, P. (1972). Temporal lobe epilepsy. In *Advances in Behavioral Biology, Vol. 2*, B. Eleftheriou (ed.). New York: Plenum Press, pp. 423–427.

Goldberg, M. E., and Bushnell, B. C. (1981). Behavioral enhancement of visual responses in monkey cerebral cortex: II. Modulation in frontal eye fields specifically to related saccades. *J. Neurophysiol.* 46:773–787.

Goldstein, K. (1948). *Language and Language Disturbances*. New York: Grune and Stratton.

Graves, R., Landis, T., and Goodglass, H. (1981). Laterality and sex differences for visual recognition of emotional and nonemotional words. *Neuropsychologia* 19:95–102.

Greenwald, M. K., Cook, E. W., Lang, P. J. (1989). Affective judgement and psychophysiological response: Dimension co-variation in the evaluation of pictorial stimuli. *J. Psychophysiology* 3:51–64.

Guerrant, J., Anderson, W. W., Fischer, A., Weinstein, M. R., Janos, R. M., and Deskins, A. (1962). *Personality in Epilepsy*. Springfield, IL: Charles C. Thomas.

Haggard, M. P., and Parkinson, A. M. (1971). Stimulus and task factors as determinants of ear advantages. *Q. J. Exp. Psychol.* 23:168–177.

Hantas, M., Katkin, E. S., and Blasovich, J. (1982). Relationship between heartbeat discrimination and subjective experience of affective state. *Psychophysiology* 19:563.

Hantas, M., Katkin, E. S., and Reed, S. D. (1984). Heartbeat discrimination training and cerebral lateralization. *Psychophysiology* 21:274–278.

Hawton, K., Fagg, J., and Marsack, P. (1980). Association between epilepsy and attempted suicide. *J. Neurol. Neurosurg. Psychiatry* 43:168–170.

Heathfield, K. W. G. (1967). Huntington's chorea. *Brain* 90:203–232.

Hécaen, H., Ajuriagurra, J., and de Massonet, J. (1951). Les troubles visuoconstuctifs par lesion parieto-occipitale droit. *Encephale 40*:122–179.

Heilman, K. M. (1979). Neglect and related syndromes. In *Clinical Neuropsychology*, K. M. Heilman and E. Valenstein (eds.). New York: Oxford University Press.

Heilman, K. M. (1979). Neglect and related disorders. In K. M. Heilman & E. Valenstein (Eds), *Clinical Neuropsychology*. New York: Oxford University Press, pp. 268–307.

Heilman, K. M. (1994). Emotion and the brain: A distributed modular network mediating emotional experience. In: Zaidel, D. W., ed. *Neuropsychology: Handbook of Perception and Cognition* (2nd ed.). San Diego: Academic Press, pp. 139–158.

Heilman, K. M., Bowers, D., Rasbury, W., and Ray, R. (1977). Ear asymmetries on a selective attention task. *Brain Lang.* 4:390–395.

Heilman, K. M., Bowers, D., Speedie, L., and Coslett, B. (1984). Comprehension of affective and nonaffective speech. *Neurology* 34:917–921.

Heilman, K. M., Scholes, R., and Watson, R. T. (1975). Auditory affective agnosia: disturbed comprehension of affective speech. *J. Neurol. Neurosurg. Psychiatry* 38:69–72.

Heilman, K. M., Schwartz, H., and Watson, R. T. (1978). Hypoarousal in patients with the neglect syndrome and emotional indifference. *Neurology* 28:229–232.

Heilman, K. M., and Van Den Abell, T. (1979). Right hemispheric dominance for mediating cerebral activation. *Neuropsychologia* 17:315–321.

Heller, W., and Levy, J. (1981). Perception and expression of emotion in right handers and left handers. *Neuropsychologia* 19:263–272.

Hermann, B. P., and Chhabria, S. (1980). Interictal psychopathology in patients with ictal fear: examples of sensory-limbic hyperconnection? *Arch. Neurol.* 37:667–668.

Hermann, B. P., Dikmen, S., and Wilensky, A. (1982). Increased psychopathology associated with multiple seizure types: fact or artifact? *Epilepsia* 23:587–596.

Hermann, B. P., and Riel, P. (1981). Interictal personality and behavioral traits in temporal lobe and generalized epilepsy. *Cortex* 17:125–128.

Herzog, A. G. (1993). A relationship between particular reproductive endocrine disorders and the laterality of epileptiform discharges in women with epilepsy. *Neurology* 43:1907–1910.

Herzog, A. G., Russell, V., Vaitukatis, J. L., and Geschwind, N. (1982). Neuroendocrine dysfunction in temporal lobe epilepsy. *Arch. Neurol.* 39:133–135.

Hohmann, G. (1966). Some effects of spinal cord lesions on experimental emotional feelings. *Psychophysiology* 3:143–156.

Hooshmand, H., and Brawley, B. W. (1969). Temporal lobe seizures and exhibitionism. *Neurology* 19:119–124.

House, A., Dennis, M., Warlow, C., Hawton, K., and Molyneux, A. (1990). Mood disorders after stroke and their relation to lesion location. *Brain* 113:1113–1120.

Howes, D. and Boller, F. (1975). Evidence for focal impairment from lesions of the right hemisphere. *Brain* 98:317–332.

Hughlings Jackson, J. (1932) *Selected Writings of John Hughlings Jackson*, J. Taylor (ed.). London: Hodder and Stoughton.

Huntington, G. W. (1872). On chorea. *Med. Surg. Rep.* 26:317–321.

Isaacson, R. L. (1982). *The Limbic System*, 2nd ed. New York: Plenum Press.

Iwata, J., LeDoux, J. E., Meeley, M. P., Arneric, S., and Reis, D. J. (1986). Intrinsic neurons in the amygdaloid field projected to by the medial geniculate body mediate emotional responses conditioned to acoustic stimuli. *Brain Res.* 383:195–214.

Izard, C. E. (1977). *Human Emotions*. New York: Plenum Press.

Jacobs, D. H. (1995). Emotional facial imagery, perception, and expression in Parkinson's disease. *Neurology* 45:1696–1702.

James, W. (1890, reprinted 1950). *The Principles of Psychology, Vol. 2*. New York: Dover Publications.

Katkin, E. S., Morrell, M. A., Goldband, S., Bernstein, G. L., and Wise, J. A. (1982). Individual differences in heartbeat discrimination. *Psychophysiology* 19:160–166.

Keillor, J. M., Barrett, A. M., Crucian, G. P., Kortenkamp, S., and Heilman, K. M. (2002). Emotional experience and perception in the absence of facial feedback. *J. Int. Neuropsychol. Soc.* 8:130–355.

Kent, J., Borod, J. C., Koff, E., Welkowitz, J., and Alpert, M. (1988). Posed facial emotional expression in brain-damaged patients. *Int. J. Neurosci.* 43:81–87.

Kimura, D. (1967). Functional asymmetry of the brain in dichotic listening. *Cortex* 3:163–178.

Kluver, H., and Bucy, P. C. (1937). "Psychic blindness" and other symptoms following bilateral temporal lobe lobectomy in rhesus monkeys. *Am. J. Physiol.* 119:352–353.

Kolb, B., and Milner, B. (1981). Observations on spontaneous facial expression after focal cerebral excisions and after intracarotid injection of sodium amytal. *Neuropsychologia* 19:505–514.

Laird, J. D. (1974). Self-attribution of emotion: the effects of expressive behavior on the quality of emotional experience. *J. Pers. Soc. Psychol.* 29:475–486.

Landis, T., Graves, R., and Goodglass, H. (1982). Aphasic reading and writing: possible evidence for right hemisphere participation. *Cortex* 18:105–122.

LeDoux, J. E., Cicchetti, P., Xagoraris, A., and Romanski, L. M. (1990). The lateral amygdaloid nucleus: sensory interface of the amygdala in fear conditioning. *J. Neurosci.* 10:1062–1069.

Leonard, C., Rolls, E., and Wilson, A. (1985). Neurons in the amygdala of the monkey with responses selective for faces. *Behav. Brain Res.* 15:159–176.

Ley, R., and Bryden, M. (1979). Hemispheric differences in recognizing faces and emotions. *Brain Lang.* 1:127–138.

Luria, A. R., and Simernitskaya, E. G. (1977). Interhemispheric relations and the functions of the minor hemisphere. *Neuropsychologia* 15:175–178.

MacLean, P. D. (1952). Some psychiatric implications of physiological studies of the frontotemporal portion of the limbic system (visceral brain). *Electroencephalogr. Clin. Neurophysiol.* 4:407–418.

Mammucari, A., Caltagirone, C., Ekman, P., Friesen, W., Gainotti, G., Pizzamiglio, L., and Zoccolatti, P. (1988). Spontaneous facial expression of emotions in brain-damaged patients. *Cortex* 24:521–533.

Mandel, M., Tandon, S., and Asthana, H. (1991). Right brain damage impairs recognition of negative emotions. *Cortex* 27:247–253.

Marátnon, G. (1924). Contribution a l'entude de l'action emotive de l'adrenaline. *Rev. Fr. Endocrinol.* 2:301–325.

Maricle, R. A., Nutt, J. G., Valentine, R. J., and Carter, J. H. (1995). Dose–response relationship of levodopa with mood and anxiety in fluctuating Parkinson's disease: a double-blind, placebo-controlled study. *Neurology* 45:1757–1760.

Mark, V. H., and Ervin, F. R. (1970). *Violence and the Brain*. New York: Harper and Row.

Mark, V. H. (1973). Brain surgery in agressive epileptics: Social and ethical implications. *JAMA* 226:765–772.

Marsh, G. G., and Markham, C. H. (1973). Does levodopa alter depression and psychopathology in parkinsonism patients? *J. Neurol. Neurosurg. Psychiatry* 36:935.

Mayberg, H. S., Starkstein, S. E., Peyser, C. E., Brandt, J., Dannals, R. F., and Folstein, S. E. (1992). Paralimbic frontal lobe hypometabolism in depression associated with Huntington's disease. *Neurology* 42:1791–1797.

Mayeux, R. (1983). Emotional changes associated with basal ganglia disorders. In *Neuropsychology of Human Emotion*, K. M. Heilman and P. Satz (eds.). New York: Guilford Press, pp. 141–164.

Mayeux, R., Stern, Y., Rosen, J., and Leventhal, J. (1981). Depression, intellectual impairment, and Parkinson disease. *Neurology* 31:645–650.

McDonald, S., and Wales, R. (1986). An investigation of the ability to process inferences in language following right hemisphere brain damage. *Brain Lang.* 29:68.

McIntyre, M., Pritchard, P. B., and Lombroso, C. T. (1976). Left and right temporal lobe epileptics: a controlled investigation of some psychological differences. *Epilepsia* 17:377–386.

McLachlan, R. S., and Blume, W. T. (1980). Isolated fear in complex partial status epilepticus. *Ann. Neurol.* 8:639–641.

McLaren, J., and Bryson, S. (1987). Hemispheric asymmetry in the perception of emotional and neutral faces. *Cortex* 23:645–654.

Mesulam, M. M., Van Hesen, G. W., Pandya, D. N., et al. (1977). Limbic and sensory connections of the inferior parietal lobule (area PG) in the rhesus monkey: a study with a new method for horseradish peroxidase histochemistry. *Brain Res.* 136:393–414.

Milner, B. (1974). Hemispheric specialization: scope and limits. In *The Neurosciences: Third Study Program*, F. O. Schmitt and F. G. Worden (eds.). Cambridge, MA: MIT Press.

Mindham, H. S. (1970). Psychiatric syndromes in Parkinsonism. *J. Neurol. Neurosurg. Psychiatry* 30:188–191.

Monrad-Krohn, G. (1947). The prosodic quality of speech and its disorders. *Acta Psychol. Scand.* 22:225–265.

Moreno, C. R., Borod, J., Welkowitz, J., and Alpert, M. (1990). Lateralization for the expression and perception of facial emotion as a function of age. *Neuropsychologia* 28:119–209.

Morris, M., Bowers, D., Verfaellie, M., Blonder, L., Cimino, C., Bauer, R., and Heilman, K. (1992). Lexical denotation and connotation in right and left hemisphere damaged patients [Abstract]. *J. Clin. Exp. Neuropsychol.* 14:105.

Morris, M. K., Bradley, M., Bowers, D., Lang, P. J., and Heilman, K. M. (1991). Valence-specific hypoarousal following right temporal lobectomy. Presented at the 19th Annual Meeting of the International Neuropsychology Society, San Antonio, TX.

Morrow, L., Vrtunski, P. B., Kim, Y., and Boller, F. (1981). Arousal responses to emotional stimuli and laterality of lesions. *Neuropsychologia* 19:65–71.

Moruzzi, G. and Magoun, H. W. (1949). Brainstem reticular formation and activation of the EEG. *Electroencephalography Clin. Neurophysiol.* 1:455–473.

Mungas, D. (1982). Interictal behavior abnormality in temporal lobe epilepsy: a specific syndrome or nonspecific psychopathology? *Arch. Gen. Psychiatry* 39:108–111.

Nielsen, H., and Kristensen, O. (1981). Personality correlates of sphenoidal EEG foci in temporal lobe epilepsy. *Acta Neurol. Scand.* 64:289–300.

Offen, M. L., Davidoff, R. A., Troost, B. T., and Richey, E. T. (1976). Dacrystic epilepsy. *J. Neurol. Neurosurg. Psychiatry* 39:829–834.

Olds, J. (1958). Self-stimulation of the brain. *Science* 127:315–324.

Osgood, C., Suci, G., Tannenbaum, P. (1971). The measure of meaning: Urbana University of Illinois Press.

Pandya, D. M. and Kuypers, H. G. (1969). Cortico-cortical connections in the rhesus monkey. *Brain Res.* 13:13–36.

Papez, J. W. (1937). A proposed mechanism of emotion. *Arch. Neurol Psychiatry* 38:725–743.

Parkinson, J. (1938). An essay of the shaking palsy, 1817. *Med. Classics* 2:964–997.

Paul, H. (1909). *Principien der Sprachgeschichte*, 4th ed. Niemeyer.

Perani, D., Vallar, G., Paulesu, E., et al. (1993). Left and right hemisphere contributions to recovery from neglect after right hemisphere damage. *Neuropsychologia* 31:115–125.

Phelps, M. E., Mazziotta, J. C., Baxter, L., and Gerner, R. (1984). Positron emission tomographic study of affective disorders: problems and strategies. *Ann. Neurol. 15(Suppl):*S149–S156.

Pincus, J. H. (1980). Can violence be a manifestation of epilepsy? *Neurology 30:*304–307.

Poeck, K. (1969). Pathophysiology of emotional disorders associated with brain damage. In *Handbook of Neurology, Vol. 3,* P. J. Vinken and G. W. Bruyn (eds.). New York: Elsevier, pp. 343–367.

Poeck, K., and Pilleri, G. (1961). Wutverhalten and pathologischer Schlaf bei Tumor dervorderen Mitellinie. *Arch. Psychiatr. Nervenkr. 201:*593–604.

Pritchard, P. B. (1980). Hyposexuality: a complication of complex partial epilepsy. *Trans. Am. Neurol. Assoc. 105:*193–195.

Pritchard, P. B., Wannamaker, B. B., Sagel, J., and deVillier, C. (1981). Post-ictal hyperprolactinemia in complex partial epilepsy. *Ann. Neurol. 10:*81–82.

Rámon y Cajal, S. (1965). *Studies on the Cerebral Cortex (Limbic Structures),* L. M. Kraft (trans.). London: Lloyd-Luke.

Rapscak, S., Kasniak, A., and Rubins, A. (1989). Anomia for facial expressions: evidence for a category specific visual verbal disconnection. *Neuropsychologia 27:*1031–1041.

Remillard, G. M., Andermann, F., Testa, G. F., Gloor, P., Aube, M., Martin, J. B., Feindel, W., Guberman, A., and Simpson, C. (1983). Sexual manifestations predominate in a woman with temporal lobe epilepsy: a finding suggesting sexual dimorphism in the human brain. *Neurology 33:*3–30.

Reuter-Lorenz, P., and Davidson, R. (1981). Differential contributions of the two cerebral hemispheres for perception of happy and sad faces. *Neuropsychologia 19:*609–614.

Reuterskiold, C. (1991). The effects of emotionality on auditory comprehension in aphasia. *Cortex 27:*595–604.

Richardson, C., Bowers, D., Eyeler, L., and Heilman, K. (1992). Asymmetrical control of facial emotional expression depends on the means of elicitation. Presented at the Meeting of the International Neuropsychology Society, San Diego, CA.

Robertson, M. M., Trimble, M. R., and Townsend, H. R. (1987). Phenomenology of depression in epilepsy. *Epilepsia 28:*364–372.

Robins, A. H. (1976). Depression in patients with Parkinsonism. *Br. J. Psychol. 128:*141–145.

Robinson, R. G., and Starkstein, S. E. (1989).

Robinson, R. G., and Sztela, B. (1981). Mood change

following left hemisphere brain injury. *Ann. Neurol. 9:*447–453.

Rodin, E. A. (1973). Psychomotor epilepsy and aggressive behavior. *Arch. Gen. Psychiatry 28:*210–213.

Roeltgen, D. P., Sevush, S., and Heilman, K. M. (1983). Ponological agraphia: writing by the lexical semantic route. *Neurology 33:*755–765.

Ross, E. D. (1981). The aprosodias: functional–anatomic organization of the affective components of language in the right hemisphere. *Ann. Neurol. 38:*561–589.

Ross, E. D., and Mesulam, M. M. (1979). Dominant language functions of the right hemisphere? Prosody and emotional gesturing. *Arch. Neurol. 36:*144–148.

Ross, E. D., Homan, R. W., Buck, R. (1994). Differential hemispheric lateralization of primary and social emotions. *Neuropsychiatry Neuropsychology and Behavioral Neurology 7:*1–19.

Rossi, G. S., and Rodadini, G. (1967). Experimental analysis of cerebral dominance in man. In *Brain Mechanisms Underlying Speech and Language,* C. Millikan and F. L. Darley (eds.). New York: Grune & Stratton.

Sackeim, H., Gur, R., and Saucy, M. (1978). Emotions are expressed more intensely on the left side of the face. *Science 202:*434–436.

Sackeim, H. A., Greenberg, M. S., Weiman, A. L., Gur, R. C., Hungerbuhler, J. P., and Geschwind, N. (1982). Hemispheric asymmetry in the expression of positive and negative emotion: neurologic evidence. *Arch. Neurol. 39:*210–218.

Sato, H., Hata, Y., Hagihara, K., et al. (1987). Effects of cholinergic depletion on neuron activities in the cat visual cortex. *J. Neurophysiol. 58:*781–794.

Schacter, S., and Singer, J. E. (1962). Cognitive, social, and physiological determinants of emotional state. *Psychol. Rev. 69:*379–399.

Scheibel, M. E. and Scheibel, A. B. (1966). The organization of the nucleus reticularis thal-

Schlanger, B. B., Schlanger, P., and Gerstmann, L. J. (1976). The perception of emotionally toned sentences by right-hemisphere damaged and aphasic subjects. *Brain Lang. 3:*396–403.

Schrandt, N. J., Tranel, D., and Damasio, H. (1989). The effects of total cerebral lesions on skin conductance response to signal stimuli. *Neurology 39 (Suppl.)* 1:223.

Segundo, J. P., Naguet, R., and Buser, P. (1955). Effects of cortical stimulation on electrocortical activity in monkeys. *Neurophysiology, 1B:*236–245.

Slater, E., and Beard, A. W. (1963). The schizophrenia-like psychoses of epilepsy. *Br. J. Psychiatry* 109:95–150.

Speedie, L. J., Broke, N., Folstein, S. E., Bowers, D., and Heilman, K. M. (1990). Comprehension of prosody in Huntington's disease. *J. Neurol. Neurosurg. Psychiatry* 53:607–610.

Speedie, L. J., Coslett, H. B., and Heilman, K. M. (1984). Repetition of affective prosody in mixed transcortical aphasia. *Arch. Neurol.* 41:268–270.

Spencer, S. S., Spencer, D. D., Williamson, P. D., and Mattson, R. H. (1983). Sexual automatisms in complex parital seizures. *Neurology* 33:527–533.

Sprengelmeyer, R., Young, A. W., Calder, A. J., Karnat, A., Lange, H., Homberg, V., Perrett, D. I., and Rowland, D. (1996). Loss of disgust. Perception of faces and emotions in Huntington's disease. *Brain* 118:1647–1665.

Starkstein, S. E., and Robinson, R. G. (1989). Affective disorders and cerebral vascular disease. *Br. J. Psychiatry* 154:170–182.

Starkstein, S., and Robinson, R. (1990). Depression following cerebrovascular lesions. *Semin. Neurol.* 10:247.

Starkstein, S. E., Robinson, R. G., and Price, T. R. (1987). Comparison of cortical and subcortical lesions in the production of poststroke mood disorders. *Brain* 110:1045–1059.

Steriade, M. and Glenn, L. (1982). Neocortical and caudate projections of intralaminar thalamic neurons and their synaptic excitation from the midbrain reticular core. *J. Neurophysiol.* 48:352–370.

Stevens, J. R. (1966). Psychiatric implications of psychomotor epilepsy. *Arch. Gen. Psychiatry* 14:461–471.

Stevens, J. R., and Hermann, B. P. (1981). Temporal lobe epilepsy, psychopathology and violence: the state of evidence. *Neurology* 31:1127–1132.

Strauss, E. (1983). Perception of emotional words. *Neuropsychologia* 21:99–103.

Strauss, E. (1989). Ictal and interictal manifestations of emotions in epilepsy. In *Handbook of Neuropsychology, Vol. 3*, F. Boller and J. Grafman (eds.). Amsterdam: Elsevier, pp. 315–344.

Strauss, E., and Moscovitch, M. (1981). Perception of facial expressions. *Brain & Language* 13:308–332.

Strauss, E., Risser, A., and Jones, M. W. (1982). Fear responses in patients with epilepsy. *Neurology* 39:626–630.

Stuss, D. T. and Benson, D. F. (1986). *The Frontal Lobes*. New York: Raven Press.

Suberi, M., and McKeever, W. (1977). Differential right hemisphere memory storage of emotional and nonemotional faces. *Neuropsychologia* 15:757–768.

Taylor, D. C. (1969). Aggression and epilepsy. *J. Psychiatr. Res.* 13:229–236.

Terzian, H. (1964). Behavioral and EEG effects of intracarotid sodium amytal injections. *Acta Neurochirugica (Vienna)* 12:230–240.

Tomkins, S. S. (1962). *Affect, Imagery, Consciousness, Vol. 1, The Positive Affect*. New York: Springer-Verlag.

Tomkins, S. S. (1963). *Affect, Imagery, Consciousness, Vol. 2, The Negative Affects*. New York: Springer-Verlag.

Treiman, D. M. (1991). Psychobiology of ictal aggression. In *Neurobehavioral Problems in Epilepsy Advances in Neurology* 55:341–356.

Trieman, D. M., and Delgado-Escueta, A. V. (1983). Violence and epilepsy: a critical review. In *Recent Advances in Epilepsy, Vol. 1*, T. A. Pedley and B. S. Meldrum (eds.). London: Churchill Livingstone, pp. 179–209.

Tucker, D. M. (1981). Lateral brain function, emotion and conceptualization. *Psychol. Bull.* 89:19–46.

Tucker, D. M., Watson, R. T., and Heilman, K. M. (1977). Affective discrimination and evocation in patients with right parietal disease. *Neurology* 17:947–950.

Tucker, D. M., and Williamson, P. A. (1984). Asymmetric neural control in human self-regulation. *Psychol. Rev.* 91:185–215.

Ursin, II. (1960). The temporal lobe substrate of fear and anger. *Acta Psychiatr. Scand.* 35:378–396.

Valenstein, E. S. (1973). *Brain Control: A Critical Examination of Brain Stimulation and Psychosurgery*. New York: Wiley-Interscience.

Warburton, J. W. (1967). Depressive symptoms in Parkinson patients referred for thalamotomy. *J. Neurol. Neurosurg. Psychiatry* 30:368–370.

Watson, R. T., Valenstein, E. and Heilman, K. M. (1981). Thalamic neglect: the possible role of the medial thalamus and nucleus reticularis thalami in behavior. *Arch. Neurol.* 38:501–507.

Watson, R. T., Heilman, K. M., Miller, B. D., et al. (1974). Neglect after mesencephalic reticular formation lesions. *Neurology* 24:294–298.

Watson, R. T., Miller, B. D., and Heilman, K. M. (1978). Nonsensory neglect. *Ann Neurol.* 3:505–508.

Waxman, S. G., and Geschwind, N. (1974). Hypergraphia in temporal lobe epilepsy. *Neurology* 24:629–636.

Wechsler, A. F. (1973). The effect of organic brain disease on recall of emotionally charged versus neutral narrative texts. *Neurology* 23:130–135.

Weddell, R., Miller, R., and Trevarthen, C. (1990). Voluntary emotional facial expressions in patients with focal cerebral lesions. *Neuropsychologia* 28:49–60.

Weintraub, S., Mesulam, M. M., and Kramer, L. (1981). Disturbances in prosody. *Arch. Neurol.* 38:742–744.

Wieser, H. G. (1986). Selective amygdalohippocampectomy: indication, investigative technique and results. *Adv. Techn. Stand. Neurosurg.* 13:39–133.

Williams, D. (1956). The structure of emotions reflected in epileptic experiences. *Brain* 79:29–67.

Williams, D. (1969). Neural factors related to habitual aggression. *Brain* 92:503–520.

Woods, J. W. (1956). Taming of the wild in Norway rat by rhinocephalic lesions. *Nature* 170:869.

Wundt, W. (1903). Grundriss der Psychologie. Stuttgart, Engelmann.

Yakovlev, P. I. (1948). Motility, behavior and the brain: stereodynamic organization and neural coordinates in behavior. *J. Nerv. Ment. Dis.* 107:313–335.

Yokoyama, K., Jennings, R., Ackles, P., Hood, P., and Boller, F. (1987). Lack of heart rate changes during an attention-demanding task after right hemisphere lesions. *Neurology* 37:624–630.

17

Hallucinations and Related Conditions

SIBEL TEKIN AND JEFFREY L. CUMMINGS

Hallucinations are common symptoms of a variety of neurologic, psychiatric, or medical conditions. Although hallucinations have traditionally been considered to be manifestations of psychiatric disorders, they are known to occur with space-occupying lesions, strokes, trauma, central nervous system (CNS) infections, seizures, neurodegenerative disorders, deprivation states, sleep disorders, and delirium. It is important to recognize and distinguish the characteristics of hallucinations, since they may be informative for the differential diagnosis of these conditions (Cummings and Miller, 1987).

In this chapter, we shall first define hallucinations and related symptoms. We then systematically discuss the different clinical conditions associated with visual and nonvisual hallucinations, and the related phenomena of illusions and misidentification syndromes. Finally, we review pathogenetic mechanisms and treatment strategies.

DEFINITIONS

Hallucinations are defined as false perceptual experiences in the absence of a sensory stimulus (Benson and Gorman, 1996). Hallucinations may be experienced in different modalities, including visual, auditory, olfactory, gustatory, tactile, and visceral (Carter, 1992).

They may be unformed (simple) or formed (complex). Photopsias, phosphenes, scintillating scotomas, geometric forms, or checkerboard patterns are examples of *unformed* visual hallucinations, whereas images of people, objects, animals, scenes or landscapes are *formed* visual hallucinations. The term *multimodal hallucinations* has been suggested for hallucinations experienced in more than one modality at the same time (Chesterman and Boast, 1994). Hallucinations must be distinguished from illusions which are misinterpretations of an existing stimulus.

Delusions are persistent false beliefs that are held despite contrary evidence. The basic distinction between hallucinations and delusions is the content. Hallucinations are sensory experiences, whereas delusions are abnormal ideas or beliefs (Benson and Gorman, 1996). *Misidentifications* are delusional beliefs of reduplication of objects, people, or places (Ellis et al., 1994; Roane et al., 1998). Hallucinations comprise a hallucinatory–delusional complex if the patient endorses the hallucination content as veridical.

VISUAL HALLUCINATIONS

Visual hallucinations may be associated with ophthalmologic diseases, neurologic disorders, toxic or metabolic disturbances, or psychiatric disor-

Table 17–1. Causes of Visual Hallucinations

Ophthalmologic Diseases

Enucleation
Cataract formation
Retinal disease
Choroidal disorder
Macular abnormalities
Glaucoma

Neurologic Disorders

Optic nerve disorders
Brainstem lesions
Hemispheric lesions
Epilepsy
Migraine
Narcolepsy

Neurodegenerative Disorders

Alzheimer's disease
Dementia with Lewy bodies
Parkinson's disease

Toxic and Metabolic Conditions

Toxic–metabolic encephalopathies
Drug and alcohol withdrawal syndromes
Hallucinogenic agents

Psychiatric Disorders

Schizophrenia
Bipolar disorders
Psychotic depression
Conversion reactions

Hallucinations in Normal Circumstances

Imagery playmates of children
Visual deprivations
Grief reaction
Fatigue
Emotional distress
Hypnagogic hallucinations
Sleep deprivation
Hypnosis
Dreams

ders, but may also occur in normal persons (Brasic, 1998). The common etiologies of visual hallucinations are summarized in Table 17–1.

VISUAL LOSS (BLINDNESS)

Visual hallucinations may accompany visual impairment due to eye trauma, cataracts, macular degeneration, choroidal neovascularization, or retinal diseases, such as retinal detachment, retinal traction, central retinal vein occlusion, or central serous retinopathy (Olbrich et al.,

1987; Brown and Murphy, 1992; Barodawala and Mulley, 1997). Glaucoma can also be a cause of visual hallucinations (White, 1980; Brown and Murphy, 1992).

In cases of vitreous detachment or retinal traction, patients may experience vertical bands of light in the temporal visual fields during eye movement, known as *Moore's lightning streaks*. Saccadic eye movements may cause flick *phosphenes*, which are streaks of light occurring in the central field (Newman, 1992). Visual hallucinations following eye enucleation have been likened to phantom pains experienced after losing a limb and have been called "phantom vision" (Cohn, 1971; Palmowski and Ruprecht, 1994; Gross et al., 1997). Phantom vision was found by Lepore (1990) in 57% of 104 patients with acute visual loss. In the same group of patients, unformed (simple) hallucinations were twice as common as formed (complex) hallucinations. Hallucinations after visual loss are rare in the young (White and Jan, 1992; Lanska and Lanska, 1993).

Visual hallucinations in the elderly unrelated to psychopathology or an altered state of consciousness define the *Charles Bonnet syndrome* (Teunisse et al., 1995; Schultz et al., 1996; Fernandez et al., 1997). Although most cases are associated with visual deprivation, it is controversial whether eye or brain disease should be included in the diagnostic criteria of this syndrome. Patients with the Charles Bonnet syndrome usually have insight to their hallucinations. The hallucinations are commonly pleasant formed images, lasting for a few seconds to a whole day, and may disappear when the patients close their eyes.

Entopic phenomena arise from particles floating in the vitreous, nerve bundles swollen with macular edema or elements of one's own retinal circulation (Scheere's phenomenon). These experiences are not considered hallucinatory experiences since they represent actual visual experiences based on stimulation external to the visual system (Cummings and Miller, 1987; Newman, 1992; Benson and Gorman, 1996).

OPTIC NERVE DISEASES

Primary optic nerve disorders usually cause unformed visual hallucinations. Phosphenes are commonly associated with optic neuritis or compressive and ischemic optic neuropathy. They usually occur during horizontal eye movements, when the eyes are closed or in dim illumination (Newman, 1992). In patients with optic nerve disorders, light flashes can occasionally be evoked by sudden sounds, a phenomenon known as *auditory–visual synesthesia* (Jacobs et al., 1981).

PEDUNCULAR HALLUCINOSIS

Brainstem lesions produce a distinctive type of formed hallucination called "peduncular hallucinosis." Peduncular hallucinosis may occur after vertebral artery angiography, posterior cerebral artery occlusions, hypoxia, cardiac surgery, or pituitary tumors extending posteriorly. The associated lesions are usually located in posterior occipital regions, cerebral peduncles, midbrain, fornices, and medial thalami (Robinson, 1995). Infarction of rostral brainstem and cerebral hemispheric regions supplied by the distal basilar artery causes the clinical syndrome known as "top-of-the-basilar syndrome" (Caplan, 1980). Peduncular hallucinosis is one

of the findings of this syndrome. Peduncular hallucinations are usually vivid and full of motion including small (Lilliputian) people, animals, objects, or kaleidoscopic scenes of landscape (Cummings and Miller, 1987). They commonly occur at twilight or in the evening. Most episodes last for a few seconds or minutes over a period of days to weeks. Visual fields and visual acuity are not affected. The hallucinatory experiences are usually pleasant, but sometimes they may lead to anxiety. Peduncular hallucinations may be associated with impaired ocular movement, disturbed sleep–wake cycle, variation in the level of consciousness, and coordination disorders. Imbalance between serotonergic and dopaminergic activity in the thalami and mesencephalic reticular nuclei have been hypothesized as the cause of these hallucinations (Kölmel, 1991).

RELEASE HALLUCINATIONS WITH HOMONYMOUS HEMIANOPIA

Release hallucinations develop when sensory loss disengages higher neural networks. Visual release hallucinations may be due to pathology

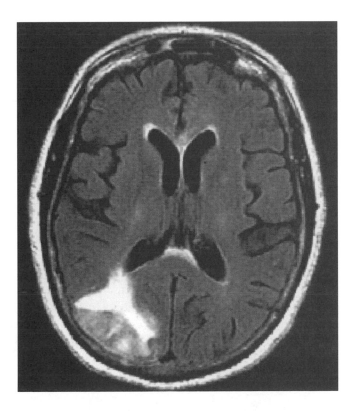

Figure 17–1. Magnetic resonance imaging scan (T2-weighted, TE: 12, TR: 4200) of a patient with release hallucinations due to an infarction in the right temporooccipital area.

involving any portion of visual pathway from retina to occipital cortex and are associated with visual field defects (Vaphiades et al., 1996). The lesion is most commonly an infarct, hemorrhage, or a space-occupying lesion. Visual release hallucinations are reported in 13% of patients with infarction involving the postchiasmal visual pathways (Kölmel, 1985). They usually last minutes to hours and consist of complex visual patterns, colored patterns, or formed images confined to the area of visual field defect (Kölmel, 1984; Anderson and Rizzo, 1994). They may be modified by environmental factors such as opening or closing the eyes. The type of image does not correlate with the anatomic site involved. Although visual release hallucinations have been reported more often with right-sided lesions, they may occur with lesions of either side (Fig. 17–1). A complex form of visual release hallucination has recently been reported in a fully aware patient with right parietoccipital infarction (Benegas et al., 1996). This patient complained of seeing people milling about in the lower left quadrant of her visual field, while vision remained normal in the remainder of the visual field. This was called the "picture-within-a-picture" sign.

EPILEPSY

Nearly 20% of patients with temporal lobe seizures experience visual hallucinations as a part of the ictus (Luciano, 1993). Epileptic visual hallucinations are usually brief and stereotyped, and may be associated with automatisms. Visual hallucinations may also be a part of ictal or postictal psychotic phenomena. They may be either formed or unformed. Formed or complex visual hallucinations, such as remembered scenes, usually arise from seizures that originate in parietal or temporal visual association cortex (VanNess et al., 1998). The initial clinical symptoms in seizures arising in the occipital lobes are usually unformed hallucinations (Aykut-Bingöl et al., 1998). Later they may transform into complex visual hallucinations. Seizures arising in calcarine cortex usually produce simple visual hallucinations such as colored lights, weaving patterns, zig-zag lights, spots, or ictal amaurosis.

MIGRAINE

Migraine is a well-recognized cause of unformed visual hallucinations. Simple flashes of light or color, scintillating scotomas, and zig-zag lines often with a scotoma called "fortification spectra" are among the most common types of hallucinations (Asaad and Shapiro, 1986; Cummings and Miller, 1987). Formed hallucinations may also be experienced. Visual reproductions of the self or parts of the body in external space, called "autoscopic phenomena," may occur in migraine. Hallucinations usually precede the headache. The characteristics of migrainous unformed hallucinations help to distinguish them from hallucinations due to occipital lobe epileptic foci. Visual epileptic seizures are reported predominantly as multicolored circular or spherical patterns differing from the black and white zigzag linear patterns described by patients with migraine (Panayiotopoulos, 1994). Migrainous hallucinations tend to last longer than epileptic hallucinations.

NARCOLEPSY

Visual hallucinations are common and usually transitory manifestations of narcolepsy (Autret et al., 1994). They are observed in 15%–50% of patients with narcolepsy. They are usually experienced either just as one is falling asleep (hypnagogic) or awakening (hypnopompic). They have a dreamlike quality. Visual hallucinations during narcolepsy may be unformed, like colored circles or parts of objects, or formed, such as an image of a person or an animal. Hypnopompic hallucinations are usually accompanied by sleep paralysis, a condition in which patients find themselves unable to move their extremities, speak, open their eyes, or even breath deeply even though they are fully awake (Robinson and Guilleminault, 1999).

DEGENERATIVE DISORDERS

Hallucinations can be observed in a variety of neurodegenerative disorders including Alzheimer's disease (AD), Parkinson's disease (PD), and dementia with Lewy bodies (DLB).

Parkinson's Disease

Hallucinations are commonly present in parkinsonian psychosis (Doraiswamy et al., 1995). About 30% of patients with idiopathic PD develop hallucinations during therapy with levodopa, dopaminergic agonists, and/or anticholinergic agents, typically after about 10 years of treatment (Cummings, 1991, 1992). They may be evident during the treatment with both short-acting and slow-release levodopa/carbidopa preparations. The hallucinations are most commonly visual (63%), followed by auditory (9.7%), tactile (3%), or combined (26%) (Sanchez-Ramos et al., 1996; Klein et al., 1997; Inzelberg et al., 1998). Visual hallucinations are typically realistic images of familiar or strange people or of domestic animals or insects and are nonthreatening. Visual misidentifications such as abnormal perception of distance or inverted visions may occur. The duration of hallucinatory episodes may vary from several minutes to a few hours. They usually occur at the end of the day and insight is usually preserved. They are commonly associated with sleep disturbances and vivid dreams. The associated factors most commonly reported are age and cognitive decline (Cummings, 1991; Sanchez-Ramos et al., 1996). Dementia is present in at least one-third of PD patients who have hallucinations (Miyoshi et al., 1996). Hallucinations in PD are more commonly observed in the seventh and eighth decades of life. Diederich et al. (1998) reported an association with deficient visual discrimination of color and contrast. Miyoshi et al. (1996) classified visual hallucinations in PD into simple and complex types. They concluded that simple hallucinations more frequently occur in advanced stages whereas complex-type hallucinations are more common in early stages of the disease. In a group of 129 PD patients, Graham et al. (1997) identified two groups of patients susceptible to developing hallucinations. The first group included patients with the disease duration of 5 years or less, with early motor complications, and the second group comprised patients with disease duration of more than 5 years. Patients in the first group usually had no cognitive impairment, whereas the second group of patients developed hallucinations with cognitive impairment. The group with early-onset hallucinations commonly progressed to non-PD syndromes such as DLB. Tanner et al. (1983) found that age, multiple-drug therapy, and anticholinergic treatment are risk factors for hallucinosis in PD patients, whereas disease duration, severity of disease, and dyskinetic side effects are not associated. The cholinergic deficit present in most patients with PD and cognitive impairment may render the patient vulnerable to treatment-associated hallucinations.

Alzheimer's Disease

Hallucinations are reported in 15%–20% of patients with AD (Mendez et al., 1990a, 1990b). Among patients in acute-care facilities, the frequency of hallucinations is as high as 67% (Molcan et al., 1995). In 80%–90% of hallucinating patients, the hallucinations are visual. Visual hallucinations are usually in color, lilliputian, animate, and formed. They may be frightening or pleasant. Hallucinations decrease in frequency as the cognitive impairment increases in the course of AD (Gilley et al., 1991; Mega et al., 1996). Hallucinations in AD patients have also been found to be related to aggressive behavior (Aarsland et al., 1996). In a longitudinal study by Drevets and Rubin (1989), it was shown that hallucinating AD patients deteriorated much faster in cognitive and functional ability than nonhallucinating patients. Lerner et al. (1994) found associations between visual hallucinations and deficits in complex visual processing. It has been hypothesized that changes throughout the retinocalcarine pathway and visual association cortex may contribute to visual hallucinations in AD (Cronin-Golomb et al., 1991). In a prospective study, McShane et al. (1995) suggested that in patients with AD, the existence of cortical Lewy bodies was associated with more persistent and severe hallucinations, independent of the severity of cognitive decline. He also claimed that poor eyesight contributed to the severity but not the persistence of hallucinations. Hallucinations in multi-infarct dementia and AD are similar (Cummings et al., 1987).

Dementia with Lewy Bodies

Hallucinations are one of the defining clinical manifestations of DLB. It has been reported that 23%–80% of patients with this type of dementia have hallucinations (Kuzuhara and Yoshimura, 1993; Papka et al., 1998). According to the Consensus Criteria for the diagnosis of DLB, recurrent visual hallucinations are one of the three essential elements, along with parkinsonism and fluctuating consciousness (McKeith et al., 1996). The presence of hallucinations in the early course of a dementing state has significance in differentiating DLB from AD (Ala et al., 1997). Neurochemical alterations have been related to hallucinations in DLB: Perry et al. (1990) found lower levels of choline acetyltransferase activity in patients with DLB than in normal subjects and levels were 50%–55% further reduced in the hallucinating patients. They suggested that cortical interactions between different neurotransmitter systems and the relative hyperserotonergic/hypocholinergic state may distinguish hallucinating cases of DLB (Perry et al., 1990, 1993).

DELIRIUM

Visual hallucinations are one of the most prominent symptoms of delirious states caused by toxic or metabolic disorders such as cardiopulmonary insufficiency, uremia, hepatic disease, endocrine disturbances, vitamin deficiencies, and inflammatory or infectious diseases. Toxic levels of carbon dioxide, mercury, bromide, and many other substances can produce hallucinations. Systemic lupus erythematosis, temporal arteritis, and CNS infections such as meningitis and encephalitis can present with hallucinations (Mize, 1980; Dunn et al., 1983; Cummings and Miller, 1987).

Withdrawal from alcohol can cause visual hallucinations as part of the delirium tremens syndrome. Symptoms usually appear on the second or third day following the cessation of alcohol intake, during the period of declining blood ethanol levels (Barodawala and Mulley, 1997). The hallucinations are typically images of animals, but Lilliputian hallucinations may also occur. Hallucinations in other modalities may accompany the visual experiences. Initially the visual

hallucinations are typically brief without alterations in consciousness, but in later stages continuous hallucinations may appear. They are usually auditory (see below), but they can be visual. When hallucinosis becomes chronic, it may be difficult to differentiate it from schizophrenia with concurrent alcohol abuse.

Barbiturates and benzodiazepines cause a chronic dependence state and sudden cessation may be associated with symptoms similar to alcohol withdrawal. Patients may develop tremor, insomnia, anxiety, visual hallucinations, or seizures.

HALLUCINOGENS

Hallucinogens are substances that produce hallucinations when administered below toxic doses. They may have an effect on mood and thought content, but insight is usually preserved. Hallucinations produced by hallucinogenic substances occur in a state of full wakefulness and alertness, whereas hallucinations occurring with drug intoxication are associated with confusion and disorientation. Drug-induced visual hallucinations tend to be exacerbated by eye closure. Lysergic acid diethylamide (LSD) is the most potent hallucinogen. Visual hallucinations caused by LSD are usually geometric colors or audiovisual synesthesias. Other well-known hallucinogens include mescaline, phencyclidine, cannabis derivatives, cocaine, and amphetamine. The hallucinogenic potential of these drugs has been shown to correlate with their serotonergic activity. Both LSD and mescaline are 5-hydroxytryptamine receptor agonists. Cocaine acts on 5-hydroxytryptamine–type 3 (5-HT$_3$) receptors, which are mainly localized in the limbic system, and also on dopamine receptors (Jacobs and Azmitia, 1992). Specific agents may not always produce the same type of hallucination. Effects vary according to person, dose, mood, social setting, and physical condition. After repeated ingestion of drugs, spontaneous recurrences of illusions and visual hallucinations may appear as "flashback" phenomena, during the drug-free period, even months after the last drug use (Ashaad and Shapiro, 1986).

A list of drugs associated with visual hallucinations is given in Table 17–2.

Table 17–2. Drugs Associated with Visual Hallucinations

Hallucinogens	***Anticonvulsants***
Dimethltryptamine	Ethosuximide
Harmine	Phenobarbital
Ketamine hydrochloride	Phenytoin
LSD	Primidone
Mescaline	
Nitrous oxide	***Cardiovascular Agents***
Phencyclidine (PCP)	Digitalis
Psilocybin	Disopyramide
Tetrahydrocannibinol sodium	Methyldopa
	Propranolol hydrochloride
Stimulants	Quinidine
Amphetamine	Reserpine
Cocaine	Timolol
Methylphenidate	
	Miscellaneous Agents
Antiparkinsonian Agents	Antimalarial agents
Amantadine hydrochloride	Baclofen
Amoxapine	Bromide
	Cimetidine
Antibiotics	Clonazepam
Antimalarial agents	Disulfiram
Cycloserine	Ephedrine
Isoniazid	Heavy metals
Podophyllum resin	Hexamethylamine
Procaine penicillin	Metrizamide
Sulfonamides	Ranitidine
Tetracycline	Solvents
	Vincristine
Hormonal Agents	Volatile hydrocarbons
Levothyroxine	
Steroidal agents	
Analgesics and NSAI Agents	
Salicylates	
Indomethacin	
Nalorphine	
Narcotic agents	
Phenacetin	
Psychotropic Agents	
Amitryptiline hydrochloride	
Amoxapine	
Bupropion hydrochloride	
Doxepin hydrochloride	
Imipramine hydrochloride	
Phenelzine sulfate	

NSAI, nonsteroidal anti-inflammatory.

PSYCHIATRIC DISORDERS

Hallucinations may accompany several idiopathic psychiatric disorders, such as schizophrenia, bipolar disorder, major depression, or dissociative states.

Auditory hallucinations are typical of schizophrenia, but visual hallucinations also are occur. They are usually images of people, animals, or events. Lilliputian hallucinations have been reported (Hendrickson, 1996). Visual hallucinations in schizophrenia appear suddenly, in a psychological setting of intense affect or delusional preoccupation. Unlike visual hallucinations induced by drugs, the hallucinations in schizophrenia do not get worse with eye closure (Weller and Wiedemann, 1989). Hallucinations in affective disorders are mood-congruent, but hallucinations occurring in bipolar disorder (manic states), psychotic depression, or with neurologic disorders do not have other characteristic findings that will help differentiate them from schizophrenia (Lowe, 1973; Asaad and Shapiro, 1986; Manford and Andermann, 1998). Visual hallucinations may also occur as a conversion symptom in patients with conversion reactions. Recently, visual and auditory hallucinations have been reported in patients with borderline personality disorder (Suzuki et al., 1998).

HALLUCINATIONS IN NORMAL INDIVIDUALS

Under certain conditions, hallucinations may occur in normal individuals and do not imply a pathological state. In some cultures, hallucinations may be experienced in the course of religious or ritualistic activities such as trance states or hysterical possessions and are considered within the cultural norms. Some children may have imaginary play objects or companions whom they visualize. Eidetic imagery is described as "projection of a mental image into external perceptual visual space," usually as a memory, and is experienced as a vivid, colorful hallucination. During grief reactions, some people may experience hallucinations of seeing or hearing the deceased. It has been suggested by Hobson (1997) that visual hallucinosis is one of the components of dreaming that occasionally occurs in the waking state. When normal people are subject to prolonged isolation and sensory or sleep deprivation, hallucinations may occur (Babkoff, 1989; Cummings and Miller, 1987). Hallucinations may be experienced during hypnosis. Hypnagogic hallucinations can occur in some healthy people just before falling asleep (Ribstein, 1976).

NONVISUAL HALLUCINATIONS

Various etiologies of nonvisual hallucinations are summarized in Table 17–3.

Table 17–3. Causes of Nonvisual Hallucinations

Auditory Hallucinations

Alcohol withdrawal
Brainstem lesions
Diencephalic lesions
Temporal lobe lesions
Epilepsy
Hearing impairment
Meningitis
Alzheimer's disease
Parkinson's disease
Dementia with Lewy bodies
Schizophrenia
Intoxications
   Amphetamine
   Cannabis
   Cocaine
   Phencyclidine hydrochloride (PCP)
   Amoxycillin
   Cimetidine
   Ciprofloxacin
   Clonidine
   Maprotiline
   Pentoxifiline
   Propranolol
Migraine
Narcolepsy

Olfactory Hallucinations

Migraine
Epilepsy
Temporal lobe lesions
Depression
Schizophrenia
Alzheimer's disease
Parkinson's disease
Intoxication
   Cocaine

Gustatory Hallucinations

Temporal lobe lesions
Epilepsy
Migraine
Schizophrenia
Intoxication
   Cocaine

Tactile Hallucinations

Intoxications
   Amphetamine
   Cannabis
   Cocaine
   Phencyclidine
Alcohol withdrawal
Drugs
   Amoxycillin
   Maprotiline
   Paroxetine
Alzheimer's disease

Visceral Hallucinations

Schizophrenia

AUDITORY HALLUCINATIONS

Although auditory hallucinations typically indicate the presence of a psychiatric disorder, a number of neurologic and systemic disorders or sensory deprivation states may lead to auditory hallucinations. Psychiatric disorders commonly associated with auditory hallucinations are schizophrenia, psychotic depression, and mania. Auditory hallucinations in schizophrenia are usually formed hallucinations including words or sentences. The voices may be heard as coming from inside the head or from outside. The voices may converse or quarrel with the patient. Most of the time they are unpleasant, accusatory, or obscene. Sometimes they may echo the patients' thoughts. Command auditory hallucinations in schizophrenia have been reported to be associated with a high risk of suicide or destructive behavior. Positron emission tomography (PET) studies on schizophrenic patients with auditory hallucinations reveal decreased activity in the left middle temporal gyrus and bilateral rostral supplementary motor area, whereas a single photon emission computerized tomography (SPECT) study showed decreased regional cerebral flow in the left orbitofrontal region and a relative increase in the right lateral temporal region (McGuire et al., 1995; Kawasaki et al., 1996).

Auditory hallucinations have also been reported in personality disorders, as auras of temporal lobe epilepsy, or during alcohol withdrawal. In epileptic patients, ictal auditory hallucinations may be unformed, such as buzzing, clicking, or ringing sounds. They usually arise from foci in the area of Heschl's gyrus. Alcoholic hallucinosis is mainly characterized by auditory hallucinations. The voices are unpleasant and patients may harm themselves or others following auditory commands. Hallucinations in alcoholic hallucinosis usually last a few hours to days, but sometimes may continue for several months (Manford and Anderman, 1998). Auditory hallucinations such as collections of sounds or melodies may also be experienced in narcolepsy. Occasionally, auditory hallucinations may accompany sensory deprivation states. Rubin et al. (1988) reported auditory hallucinations in AD, usually experienced as conversational voices or command

hallucinations. Auditory hallucinations are also reported in PD patients, particularly those who have visual hallucinations and some degree of cognitive impairment (Inzelberg et al., 1998)

Auditory hallucinations may sometimes occur unilaterally, indicating ipsilateral hearing loss or contralateral cerebral lesions (Almeida et al., 1993). Patients with impaired hearing may experience tinnitus as a complex series of sounds which can lead to paranoid states in severe cases.

Musical hallucinations are a variation of release hallucinations. They usually occur in deafness, neurological disorders including encephalitis, epilepsy, and structural lesions involving the brainstem and temporal lobes. Depression or schizophrenia may also produce musical hallucinations.

TACTILE HALLUCINATIONS

Tactile hallucinations occur in most patients who have limb amputations. The feeling that the limb is still present is known as *phantom limb* sensation. Pain in the amputated phantom limb is common. Children born without limbs may also have phantom hallucinations, leading to the hypothesis that the brain contains a genetically inherited template of the body image (Melzac, 1990). Phantom hallucinations generally diminish or disappear over time. Sometimes amputated body parts may be perceived as moving. This phenomenon is known as *kinesthetic hallucination*. Following surgery, cutting or crampy-type pain hallucinations may be experienced.

Tactile hallucinations may also be observed in drug withdrawal delirium, schizophrenia, or complex partial seizures or during the use of hallucinogens, such as cocaine or amphetamine. They may be in the form of formification hallucinations, which is the feeling of bugs crawling over the skin. Unilateral formification hallucinations may be associated with parietal or thalamic lesions. Tactile hallucinations may in some cases be a sign of paraneoplastic syndrome. Tactile hallucinations such as pinching, rubbing, light touching, or some peculiar extracorporial experiences described as "feeling up above bed and seeing own body below" have also been reported in narcolepsy (Robinson and Guilleminault, 1999).

OLFACTORY HALLUCINATIONS

Olfactory hallucinations are usually associated with structural lesions involving olfactory bulb, third ventricle, parietal cortex, or temporal areas. They may be experienced as an aura of migraine or of complex partial seizures originating from basal frontal olfactory cortex, posterior medial orbitofrontal cortex, uncus, or anterior temporal lobe (Luciano, 1993). They may be observed in patients with drug abuse and rarely in AD (Burns et al., 1990; Molcan et al., 1995).

GUSTATORY HALLUCINATIONS

Gustatory hallucinations are most commonly associated with temporal lobe lesions, especially uncinate gyrus seizures. Patients report experiencing bitter, sweet, salty, tobacco-like, metallic, or indescribable strange tastes. They are found in 4% of seizure patients with temporal lobe foci, but may also be a part of seizures originating from the parietal opercular region (Hauser-Hauw and Bancaud, 1987).

VISCERAL HALLUCINATIONS

Visceral hallucinations are common in complex partial seizures. Patients may experience a feeling such as butterflies in the abdomen rising up into the head as an aura. Abnormal sensations sometimes involve the genitalia and have the quality of a sexual experience. Unusual visceral sensations may also be experienced in schizophrenia. These hallucinations may involve feelings of burning in the brain, urine passing through the ureters, or blood coursing through one's own vessels (Carter, 1992).

Nihilistic delusions of bodily death or nonexistence, usually observed in psychotic depression (Cotard's syndrome), may be confused with visceral hallucinations.

ILLUSIONS AND RELATED SYMPTOMS

Illusions are misinterpretations of an actual existing stimulus. The image may be altered in size (micropsia or macropsia), shape (metamorphopsia), position (telopsia), number (polyopia),

color, or movement. Illusions commonly are associated with macular diseases, migraine, or epileptic disorders. Illusions related to seizures are usually experienced in the form of micropsia, macropsia, or distortions in shape, color, motion, or distance. The right hemisphere has been reported to be involved more than the left in illusions with temporal lobe seizures (Palmini and Gloor, 1992). Visual illusions including macropsia and micropsia, as in the Alice in Wonderland syndrome, may also occur during migraine attacks. The Alice in Wonderland syndrome, named for the Alice stories written by Lewis Carroll (Takaoka and Takata, 1999) includes the symptoms of body image disturbances with macropsia, micropsia, illusory feelings of levitation, and depersonalization. Illusions may also occur rarely in patients with neurodegenerative disorders such as AD or as a complication of drug treatment in PD. Metamorphopsia has been reported in bilateral occipital or occipitotemporal lesions as a part of the top of the basilar artery syndrome.

The persistence or recurrence of an image after the cessation of stimulus is termed "palinopsia." In classical palinopsia, the image can appear for up to several hours or days in the same visual field as that wherever the patient directs the gaze. Palinopsia is considered to be a variant of release hallucinations (Cummings et al., 1982). It usually occurs in patients with visual field defects due to occipital or parietal lobe lesions mostly in the right hemisphere, but it may also occur during nonketotic hyperglycemia, cocaine abuse, or occipital lobe seizures. Illusions may be experienced in other sensory modalities such as auditory or tactile illusions. *Palinacusis*, which is the persistence of prior auditory perception, may be related to temporal lobe seizures. In some cases, palinacusis and musical hallucinations may be experienced together (Takeshi and Matsunaga, 1999).

MISIDENTIFICATION SYNDROMES

Misidentification syndromes are defined as delusional conditions in which patients incorrectly identify and reduplicate people, places, objects, or events (Feinberg and Roane, 1997).

The most commonly reported misidentification syndrome is *Capgras syndrome*, which is the delusional belief that a person usually close to the patient has been replaced by a double or imposter. Capgras delusions are usually associated with psychiatric disorders, such as schizophrenia, coupled with depersonalization and derealization phenomena. They may occur in mood disorders and in some neurodegenerative diseases, especially AD, PD, or DLB (Cummings and Victorof, 1990). Misidentification syndromes in PD are thought to be due to a combination of frontal lobe dysfunction and levodopa psychosis, and they correlate with the severity of disease (Roane et al., 1998). Dementia patients with delusional misidentification have more severe impairment of recent memory and receptive language functions (Ballard et al., 1995).

A related type of misidentification is the Fregoli syndrome. In this disorder, patients believe that a person whom they know well is impersonating another, taking on the appearance of a stranger. In the syndrome of intermetamorphosis, people known to the patient are believed to have exchanged identities with each other.

Drug intoxication, withdrawal syndromes, infectious diseases, head trauma, epilepsy, stroke or endocrine abnormalities may be the cause of misidentification syndromes (Förstl et al., 1991). Misidentification syndromes have also been reported after electroconvulsive therapy (Hay, 1986).

Patients with misidentification syndromes have a tendency toward confabulation, and abnormal comprehension of sensory information is an important factor in misidentification syndromes. It has been suggested that misidentification syndromes are the result of disconnection of right temporal and limbic areas from the frontal lobes, which prevents patients from properly utilizing information regarding places, people, or objects (Alexander et al., 1979). Impaired frontal lobe functioning with lack of judgement may be a contributing factor to delusional misidentification.

The phantom boarder sign is the false belief that imaginary guests are living in the patient's house, and the mirror sign is the patient's misidentification of her or his own mirror image as someone else's. The picture sign is the patient's misidentification of television images or photographs as real, present individuals. Some patients may also have a strong belief that their house is not their actual home. In a study by Förstl et al. (1994), 34% of AD patients had delusional misidentification syndromes, Capgras syndrome being the most frequent sign (16%), followed by phantom boarder (12%), mirror sign (4%), and picture sign (4%). These patients showed more severe right frontal lobe atrophy and quantitative electroencephalograms (EEG) showed significantly higher delta power over the right hemisphere (Förstl et al., 1994). The relationship of the misidentification syndromes to visual agnosia, prosopagnosia, and amnesia remains to be determined.

Delusional misidentification syndromes may be related to reduplicative paramnesia, which is usually the result of neurologic disorders involving confusion and memory loss. In contrast to Capgras syndrome, it usually involves misidentification of places rather than people.

PATHOGENIC MECHANISMS OF HALLUCINATIONS

Several basic pathogenic mechanisms are responsible for different types of hallucinations. Hallucination may emerge when there is decreased sensory stimulation, as in the Charles-Bonnet disease, enucleation, amputations (phantom limb), or structural lesions in occipital lobe. In the absence of sensory input, remembered perceptions may enter consciousness and be experienced as hallucinations. The perceptual release theory was proposed by West (1962), who suggested that a sustained level of sensory input was required to inhibit the emergence of previous percepts or memory traces within the brain. When sensory input decreases below a certain threshold, previously recorded sensory perceptions emerge into awareness in the form of hallucinations. This mechanism may also be responsible for hallucinations associated with decreased arousal, as in narcolepsy, confusional states, or hypnosis (Cummings and Miller, 1987).

Other studies suggest that hallucinations may result from hyperexcitement of the CNS. It has been known that electrical stimulation of specific cortical and subcortical structures can cause hallucinations. Ictal hallucinations experienced during complex partial seizures or migraine headaches may be consistent with this mechanism. Release hallucinations are found to be more continuous and nonstereotyped than ictal hallucinations.

Electroencephalographic studies provide some evidence that abnormalities of sleep or dreaming may be associated with hallucinations. Rapid eye movement (REM) sleep abnormalities have been associated with a higher risk of hallucinations in PD patients (Fenelon et al., 2000). The diurnal pattern of peduncular hallucinations also suggests that they may be related to sleep and dream mechanisms. Dream intrusions into wakefulness have been encountered in hypnagogic and hypnopompic hallucinations of narcolepsy and during withdrawal from alcohol.

Biochemical changes have also been related to hallucinatory experiences. There is evidence that dopaminergic transmission is involved in the pathogenesis of hallucinations. Dopamine receptor agonists and L-dopa induce hallucinations during treatment of patients with PD. One of the potent hallucinogenic agents, amphetamine, has indirect dopamine agonistic properties (Weller and Wiedemann, 1989). Antipsychotic medications exert their effects mainly by blocking central dopaminergic activity. Hyperactivity of the mesolimbic dopaminergic system has been suggested to be responsible for visual hallucinations in PD.

It has been shown that patients with DLB have a deficiency of choline acetyltransferase activity and there is some evidence that PD patients with hallucinations also have cholinergic dysfunction. They are more susceptible to cognitive side effects of anticholinergic agents than age-matched subjects and hallucinations are common in PD patients with dementia, many of whom have an associated choline acetyltransferase deficiency (Perry et al., 1991).

Serotonergic systems have also been proposed to be involved in the neurochemistry of hallucinations. Powerful hallucinogens such as LSD and mescaline act mainly on serotonergic receptors in median raphJ nuclei. The interaction between cholinergic and serotonergic systems may have an important role in hallucinogenesis. It has been shown that there are reciprocal connections between serotonergic and cholinergic systems in raphJ nuclei and pedunculopontine tegmental nuclei, which often are affected in peduncular hallucinosis (Jones, 1994). Although the cholinergic system is affected in AD, the cholinergic neurons of pedunculopontine tegmental nucleus are spared, and serotonergic neurons are less affected than in DLB (Manford and Andermann, 1998). Thus hallucinations are relatively less common in AD than in DLB.

Perceptual release, ictal phenomenon, dream intrusions, and neurochemical effects on brainstem and limbic system structures comprise the principal basic mechanisms correlating with hallucinations in a variety of clinical conditions.

TREATMENT OF HALLUCINATIONS

The treatment of hallucinations is based mainly on the resolution of underlying cause.

Monoamine oxidase inhibitors have been reported to relieve hypnagogic hallucinations of narcolepsy by blocking REM sleep. Clomipramine and protryptiline, which influence 5-HT_2 receptors, also delay onset of REM sleep and may be beneficial for narcolepsy-related hallucinations. 5-HT_2 receptor antagonists such as pizotifen and methysergide are known to prevent migraine auras with hallucinations (Manford and Andermann, 1998).

Antipsychotic agents are widely used for symptomatic treatment of hallucinations (Leysen et al., 1998). Hallucinations in schizophrenic patients respond well to antipsychotic medications. Clozapine, which has strong antiserotonergic properties mainly at 5-HT_2 receptor sites as well as dopamine antagonist activity at D_4 receptors, is especially effective against hallucinations in schizophrenia. Lithium and anxiolytics may be used as adjuvant therapies for increasing the potency of neuroleptics in schizophrenic patients. Hallucinations in patients with psychotic depression are treated with combinations of antidepressants and neuroleptics. In refractory cases of schizophrenia or mania, electroconvulsive therapy may be helpful. Alternative approaches to treatment of hallucinations in patients with schizophrenia may include behavioral and conditioning techniques or increasing external sensory stimuli (Carter, 1992).

Antipsychotic agents have seizure threshold–lowering effects, therefore they are not used in treatment of hallucinations related to complex partial seizures. Also, low-potency neuroleptics, with anticholinergic side effects, may cause paradoxical exacerbations when used in patients with delirium, AD, or DLB.

Hallucinations occurring in PD patients as a complication of therapy are best managed by rearranging the drug regimen. Anticholinergics should be eliminated, followed by amantadine, selegiline, dopamine agonists, and carbidopa-levodopa (Lieberman, 1998). Serotonin antagonists have also been reported to be effective for hallucinations in PD. When the symptoms are severe, clozapine, olanzapine, and quetiapine are the drugs of choice among atypical neuroleptics (Graham et al., 1998; Stoppe et al., 1999). Since sleep disturbance is a predisposing factor to hallucinations in PD, benzodiazepines are suggested for REM sleep behavior disorder (Trenkwalder, 1998).

Visual hallucinations are among the behavioral symptoms most responsive to treatment with cholinesterase inhibitors such as rivastiamine in DLB patients (Cummings, 2000; McKeith, 2001). Xanomeline, a selective muscarinic agonist, also has been shown to reduce hallucinations in AD patients (Bodick et al., 1997; Levy et al., 1999).

Hallucinations associated with epilepsy are primarily treated with antiepileptic agents. Valproic acid and carbamazepine have been shown to have beneficial effects on psychotic findings of schizophrenia and neurodegenerative disorders. Kraft et al. (1984) reported carbamazepine-responsive auditory hallucinations in a depressed patient. Antiepileptic agents may also be helpful in management of alcohol withdrawal syndrome.

REFERENCES

Aarsland, D., Cummings, J. L., Yener, G., and Miller, B. (1996). Relationship of aggressive behaviour to other neuropsychiatric symptoms in patients with Alzheimer's disease. *Am. J. Psychiatry* 153:243–247.

Ala, T. A., Yang, K-H., Sung, J. H., and Frey, W. H. (1997). Hallucinations and signs of parkinsonism help distinguish patients with dementia and cortical Lewy bodies from patients with Alzheimer's diseaseat presentation: a clinicopathological study. *J. Neurol. Neurosurg. Psychiatry* 62:16–21.

Alexander, M. P., Stuss, D. T., and Benson, D. F. (1979). Capgras syndrome: a reduplicative phenomenon. *Neurology* 29:334–339.

Almeida, O. P., Förstl, H., Howard, R., and David, A. S. (1993). Unilateral auditory hallucinations. *Br. J. Psychiatry* 162:262–264.

Anderson, S. W., and Rizzo, M. (1994). Hallucinations following occipital lobe damage: the pathological activation of visual representations. *J. Clin. Exp. Neuropschol.* 16:651–663.

Asaad, G., and Shapiro, B. (1986). Hallucinations: theoretical and clinical overview. *Am. J. Psychiatry* 143:1088–1097.

Autret, A., Lucas, B., and Henry-Lebras, F. (1994). Symptomatic narcolepsies. *Sleep* 17:21–24.

Aykut-Bingöl, C., Bronen, A. R., Kim, H. J., Spencer, D. D., and Spencer, S. S. (1998). Surgical outcome in occipital lobe epilepsy: implications for pathophysiology. *Ann. Neurol.* 44:60–69.

Babkoff, H. (1989). Perceptual distortions and hallucinations reported during the course of sleep deprivation. *Percept. Mot. Skills* 68:787–798.

Ballard, C. G., Bannister, C. L., Patel, A., Graham, C., Oyebode, F., Wilcock, G., and Chung, M. C. (1995). Classification of psychotic symptoms in dementia sufferers. Acta Psychiatr. Scand. 92:63–68.

Barodawala, S., and Mulley, G. P. (1997). Visual hallucinations. *J. R. Coll. Phys. Lond.* 31:42–48.

Benegas, M. N., Liu, G. T., Volpe, N. J., and Galetta, S. L. (1996). "Picture within a picture" visual hallucinations. *Neurology* 47:1347–1348.

Benson, D. F., and Gorman, D. G. (1996). Hallucinations and delusional thinking. In *Neuropsyhiatry*, B. S. Fogel, R. B. Schiffer, and S. Rao (eds.). Baltimore: Williams and Wilkins, pp. 309–323.

Bodick, N. C., Offen, W. W., Lewey, A. I., Cutler, N. R., Gauthier, S. G., Satlin, A., Shannon, H. E., Tollefson, G. D., Rasmussen, K., Bymaster, F. P., Hurley, D.J., Potter, W. Z., and Paul, S. M. (1997). Xanomeline, a selective muscarinic receptor agonist on cognitive function and behavioural symptoms in Alzheimer disease. *Arch. Neurol.* 54:465–473.

Brasic, R. B. (1998). Hallucinations. *Percept. Motor Skills* 86:851–877.

Brown, G. C., and Murphy, R. P. (1992). Visual symptoms associated with choroidal neovascularization-photopsias and the Charles Bonnet syndrome. *Arch. Ophthalmol.* 110:1251–1256.

Burns, A., Jacoby, R., and Levy, R. (1990). Psychiatric phenomena in Alzheimer's disease. II: Disorders of perception. *Br. J. Psychiatry* 157: 76–81.

Caplan, L. R. (1980). "Top of the basilar" syndrome. *Neurology* 30:72–79.

Carter, J. L. (1992). Visual, somatosensory, olfacory and gustatory hallucinations. *Psychiatr. Clin. North Am.* 15:347–358.

Chesterman, L. P., and Boast, N. (1994). Multi-modal hallucinations. *Psychopathology* 27:273–280.

Cohn, R. (1971). Phantom vision. *Arch. Neurol.* 25:468–471.

Cronin-Golomb, A., Corkin, S., Rizzo, J. F., Cohen, J., Growdon, J. H., and Banks, K. S. (1991). Visual dysfunction in Alzheimer's disease: relation to normal aging. *Ann. Neurol.* 29:41–52.

Cummings, J. L. (1991). Behavioural complications of drug treatment of Parkinson's disease. *J. Am. Geriatr. Soc.* 39:708–716.

Cummings, J. L. (1992). Neuropsychiatric complications of drug treatment of Parkinson's disease. In *Parkinson's Disease. Neurobehavioural Aspects*, S. J. Huber and J. L. Cummings (eds.). New York: Oxford University Press, pp. 313–327.

Cummings, J. L. (2000). Cholinesterase inhibitors: a new class of psychotropic compounds. *Am. J. Psychiatry* 157:4–15.

Cummings, J. L., and Miller, B. (1987). Visual hallucinations. Clinical occurrence and use in differential diagnosis. *West. J. Med.* 146:46–51.

Cummings, J. L., Miller, B., Hill, M. A., and Neshkes, R. (1987). Neuropsychiatric aspects of multi-infarct dementia and dementia of Alzheimer type. *Arch. Neurol.* 44:389–393.

Cummings, J. L., Syndulko, K., and Goldberg, Z. (1982) Palinopsia reconsidered. *Neurology* 32:444–447.

Cummings, J. L., and Victoroff, J. (1990). Noncognitive neuropsychiatric syndromes in Alzheimer's disease. *J. Neuropsyhiatry Neuropsychol. Behav. Neurol.* 2:140–158.

Diederich, N. J., Goetz, G. C., Raman, R., Pappert, E., Leurgans, S., and Piery, V. (1998). Poor visual discrimination and visual hallucinations in Parkinson's disease. *Clin. Neuropharmacol.* 21:289–295.

Doraiswamy, M., Martin, W., Metz, A., and Deveaugh-Geiss, J. (1995). Psychosis in Parkinson's disease: diagnosis and treatment. *Prog. Neuropsychopharmacol. Biol. Psychiatry* 19:835–846.

Drevets, W. C., and Rubin, E. T. (1989). Psychotic symptoms and the longitudinal course of senile dementia of Alzheimer type. *Biol. Psychiatry* 25:39–48.

Dunn, D. W., Weisberg, L. A., and Nadell, J. (1983). Peduncular hallucinations caused by brainstem compression. *Neurology* 33:1360–1361.

Ellis, H. D., Luaute, J., and Retterstol, N. (1994). Delusional misidentification syndromes. *Psychopathology* 27:117–120.

Feinberg, T. E., and Roane, D. M. (1997). Missidentification syndromes. In *Behavioural Neurology and Neuropsychology*, T. E. Feinberg and M. J. Farah (eds.). New York: McGraw Hill, pp. 391–397.

Fenelon, G., Mahieux, F., Huon, R., and Ziegler, M. (2000). Hallucinations in Parkinson's disease: pathophysiology, phenomenology and risk factors. *Brain* 123:733–745.

Fernandez, A., Lichtshein, G., and Vieweg, V. R. (1997). The Charles Bonnet syndrome: a review. *J. Nerv. Ment. Dis.* 185:195–200.

Förstl, H., Almeida, O. P., Owen, A. M., Burns, A., and Howard, R. (1991). Psychiatric, neurological and medical aspects of misidentification syndromes: a review of 260 cases. *Psychol. Med.* 21:905–910.

Förstl, H., Besthorn, C., Geiger-Kabisch, C., Levy, R., and Sattel, A. (1994). Delusional misidentification in Alzheimer's disease: a summary of clinical and biological aspects. *Psychopathology* 27:194–199.

Gilley, D. W., Whalen, M. E., Wilson, R. S., and Bennet, D. A. (1991). Hallucinations and associated factors in Alzheimer's disease. *J. Neuropsychiatry Clin. Neurosci.* 3:371–376.

Graham, J. M., Grunewald, R. A., and Sagar, H. J. (1997). Hallucinosis in idiopathic Parkinson's disease. *J. Neurol. Neurosurg. Psychiatry* 63: 434–440.

Graham, J. M., Sussman, J. D., Ford, K. S., and Sagar, H. J. (1998). Olanzapine in the treatment of hallucinosis in idiopathic parkinson's disease: a cautionary note. *J. Neurol. Neurosurg. Psychiatry* 65:774–777.

Gross, N. D., Wilson, D. J., and Roger, A. D. (1997). Visual hallucinations after enucleation. *Ophthal. Plast. Reconstr. Surg.* 13:221–225.

Hauser-Hauw, C., and Bancaud, J. (1987). Gustatory hallucinations in epileptic seizures. *Brain* 110:339–359.

Hay, G. G. (1986). Electroconvulsive therapy as a contributor to the production of delusional misidentification. *Br. J. Psychiatry* 148:667–669.

Hendrickson, J. (1996). Lilliputian hallucinations in

schizophrenia: case report and review of literature. *Psychopathology* 29:35–38.

Hobson, J. A. (1997). Dreaming as delirium: a mental status analysis of our nightly madness. *Semin. Neurol.* 17:121–128.

Inzelberg, R., Kipervasser, S., and Korzyn, A. (1998). Auditory hallucinations in Parkinson's disease. *J. Neurol. Neurosurg. Psychiatry* 64: 533–535.

Jacobs, B. L., and Azmitia, E. C. (1992). Structure and function of the brain serotonin system. *Physiol. Rev.* 72:165–229.

Jacobs, L. Karpik, A., Bozian, D., and Gothgen S. (1981). Auditory–visual synesthesia. Sound-induced photisms. *Arch. Neurol.* 38:211–216.

Jones, B. E. (1994). Basic mechanisms of sleep-wake states. In: *Principles and Practice of Sleep Medicine*, M. H. Kryger, T. H. Roth, and W. C. Derevet (eds.). Philadelphia: W. B. Saunders.

Kawasaki, Y., Maeda, Y., Sakai, N., Higashima, M., Yamaguchi, N., Koshino, Y., Hisado, K., Suzuki, M., and Matsuda, H. (1996). Regional cerebral blood flow in patients with schizophrenia: relevance to symptom structures. *Psychiatry Res.* 67:49–58.

Klein, C., Kompf, D, Pulkowski, U., Moser, A., and Vieregge, P. (1997). A study of visual hallucinations in patients with Parkinson's disease. *J. Neurol.* 244:371–377.

Kölmel, H. W. (1984). Colored patterns in hemianopic fields. *Brain* 107:155–167.

Kölmel, H. W. (1985). Complex visual hallucinations in the hemianopic field. *J. Neurol. Neurosurg. Psychiatry* 48:29–38.

Kölmel, H. W. (1991). Peduncular hallucinations. *J. Neurol* 238:457–459.

Kraft, M. A., Hassenfeld, N. I., and Zarr, M. (1984). Response of functional hallucinations to carbamazepine. *Am. J. Psychiatry* 141:1018.

Kuzuhara, S., and Yoshimura, M. (1993). Clinical and neuropathological aspects of diffuse Lewy body disease in the elderly. *Adv. Neurol.* 60:464–469.

Lanska, D. J., and Lanska, M. (1993). Visual release hallucinations in juvenile neuronal ceroid lipofuscinosis. *Pediatr. Neurol.* 9:316–317.

Lepore, F. E. (1990). Spontaneous visual phenomea with visual loss. *Neurology* 40:444–447.

Lerner, A. J., Koss, E., Patterson, M. B., Ownby, R. L., Hedera, P., Friedland, R. P., and Whitehouse, P. J. (1994). Concomitants of visual hallucinations in Alzheimer's disease. *Neurology* 44:523–527.

Levy, M. L., Cummings, J. L., and Kahn-Rose, R. (1999). Neuropsychiatric symptoms and cholinergic therapy for Alzheimer's disease. *Gerontology* 45(Suppl 1):15–22.

Leysen, J. E., Janssen, P. M. F., Heylen, L., Gompel, P. V., Lesage, A. S., Megens, A. A., and Schotte, A. (1998). Receptor interactions of new antipsychotics: relation to pharmacodynamic and clinical effects. *Int. J. Psychiatry Clin. Pract.* 2:3–17.

Lieberman, A. (1998). Managing the neuropsychiatric symptoms of Parkinson's disease. *Neurology* 50(Suppl. 6):33–38.

Lowe, G. R. (1973). The phenomenology of hallucinations as an aid to differential diagnosis. *Br. J. Psychiatry* 123:621–633.

Luciano, D. (1993). Partial seizures of frontal and temporal lobe origin. *Neurol. Clin.* 11:805–822.

Manford, M., and Andermann, F. (1998). Complex visual hallucinations. Clinical and neurobiological insights. *Brain* 121:1819–1840.

McGuire, P. K., Silbersweig, D. A., Wright, I., Murray, R. M., David, A. S., Frackowiak, R. S., and Frith, C. P. (1995). Abnormal monitoring of inner speech: a physiological basis for auditory hallucinations. *Lancet* 346:596–600.

McKeith, I. G., Galasko, D., Kosaka, K., Perry, E. K., Dickson, D.W., et al. (1996). Consensus guidelines for the clinical and pathological diagnosis of dementia with Lewy bodies (DLB): report of the Consortium on DLB International Workshop. *Neurology* 47:1113–1124.

McKeith, I., Delser, T., Spano P., Emre, M., et al. (2000). *Lancet* 356:2031–2036.

McShane, R., Gedling, K., Reading, M., McDonald B., Esiri, M. M., and Hope, T. (1995). Prospective study of relations between cortical Lewy bodies, poor eyesight, and hallucinations in Alzheimer's disease. *J. Neurol. Neurosurg. Psychiatry* 59:185–188.

Mega, M. S., Cummings, J. L., Fiorello, T., and Gorbein, J. (1996). The spectrum of behavioral changes in Alzheimer's disease. *Neurology* 46:130–135.

Melzack, R. (1990). Phantom limbs and the concept of a neuromatrix. *Trends Neurosci.* 13:88–92.

Mendez, M. F., Martin, R. M., Smyth, K. A., and Whitehouse, P. J. (1990a). Psychiatric symptoms associated with Alzheimer's disease. *J. Neuropsychiatry Clin. Neurosci.* 2:28–33.

Mendez, M. F., Tomsak, R. L., and Remler, G. (1990b). Disorders of the visual system in Alzheimer's disease. *J. Clin. Neuroophthalmol.* 10: 62–69.

Miyoshi, K., Ueki, A., and Nagano, O. (1996). Management of psychiatric symptoms of Parkinson's disease. *Eur. Neurol.* 36(Suppl. 1):49–54.

Mize, K. (1980). Visual hallucinations following viral encephalitis: a self-report. *Neuropsychologia* 18:193–202.

Molcan, S. E., Little, J. T., Cantillon, M., and Sunderland, T. (1995). Psyhosis. In *Behavioral Complications in Alzheimer's Disease,* B. Lawlor (ed.). Washington, DC: American Psychiatric Press, pp. 55–73.

Newman, N. M. (1992). Photopsias, entopias, illusions, and hallucinations. In *Neuro-ophthalmology. A Practical Text.* Norwolk: Appleton & Lange, pp. 161–167.

Olbrich, H. M., Engelmeier, M. P., Pauleikhoff, D., and Waubke, T. (1987). Visual hallucinations in ophthalmology. *Graefe's Arch. Clin. Exp. Ophthalmol.* 225:217–220.

Palmini, A., and Gloor, P. (1992). A prospective and retrospective study. *Neurology* 42:801–808.

Palmowski, A., and Ruprecht, K.W. (1994). Paranoid hallucinations following ocular surgery. *Ophthalmologica* 208:44–45.

Panayiotopoulos, C. P. (1994). Elementary visual hallucinations in migraine and epilepsy. *J. Neurol. Neurosurg. Psychiatry* 57:1371–1374.

Papka, M., Rubio, A., and Schiffer, R. B. (1998). A review of Lewy Body disease, an emerging concept of cortical dementia. *J. Neuropsychiatry Clin. Neurosci.* 10:267–279.

Perry, E. K., Marshall, E., Kerwin, J. M., Smith, C. J., Jabeen, S., Cheng, A. V., and Perry, R. H. (1990). Evidence of monoaminergic–cholinergic imbalance related to visual hallucinations in Lewy Body dementia. *J. Neurochem.* 55:1454–1456.

Perry, E. K., Marshall, E., Thompson P., McKeith, I. G., Collerton, D., Fairbairn, A. F., Ferrier, I. N., Irving, D., and Perry, R. H. (1993). Monoaminergic activities in Lewy body dementia: relation to hallucinosis and extrapyramidal features. *J. Neural Transm.* 6:167–177.

Perry, E. K., McKeith, I., Thompson, P., Marshall, E., Kerwin, J., and Jabeen, S. (1991). Topography, extent and clinical relevance of neurochemical defisits in dementia of Lewy body type, Parkinson's disease and Alzheimer's disease. *Ann. N.Y. Acad. Sci.* 640:197–202.

Ribstein, M. (1976). Hypnagogic hallucinations. *Adv. Sleep Res.* 3:145–160.

Roane, D. M., Rogers, J. R., Robinson, J. H., and Feinberg, T. (1998). Delusional misidentifications in association with parkinsonism. *J. Neuropsychiatry Clin. Neurosci.* 10:194–198.

Robinson, A., and Guilleminault, C. (1999). Narcolepsy. In: *Sleep Disorders Medicine,* Chokroverty, S. (ed.). Boston: Butterworth, Heinemann, pp. 427–440.

Robinson, R. G. (1995). Psychiatric syndromes following stroke. In *Stroke Syndromes,* J. Bogousslavski and L. Caplan (eds.). Cambridge, UK: Cambridge University Press, pp. 188–199.

Rubin, E. H., Drevets, W. C., and Burke, W. J. (1988). The nature of psychotic symptoms in senile dementia of Alzheimer type. *Geriatr Psychiatry Neurol* 1:16–20.

Sanchez-Ramos, J. R., Ortoll, R., and Paulson, G. W. (1996). Visual hallucinations associated with Parkinson's disease. *Arch. Neurol* 53:1265–1268.

Schultz, G., Needham, W., Taylor, R., Shindell, S., and Melzack, R. (1996). Properties of complex hallucinations associated with deficits in vision. *Perception* 25:715–726.

Stoppe, G., Brandt, C. A., and Staedt, J. H. (1999). Behavioral problems associated with dementia. *Drugs Aging* 14:41–54.

Suzuki, H., Tsukamoto, C., Nakano, Y., Aoki, S., and Kuroda, S. (1998). Delusions and hallucinations in patients with borderline personality disorder. *Psychiatry Clin. Neurosci.* 52:605–610.

Takaoka, K., and Takata, T. (1999) 'Alice in Wonderland' syndrome and lilliputian hallucinations in a patient with a substance-related disorder. *Psychopathology* 32:47–49.

Takeshi, T., and Matsunaga, K. (1999). Musical hallucinations and palinacousis. *Psychopathology* 32:57–59.

Tanner, C. M., Vogel, C., and Goetz, C. G. (1983). Hallucinations in Parkinson's disease. *Ann. Neurol.* 14:136–138.

Teunisse, R. J., Cruysberg, J. R. M., Verbeek, A., and Zitman, F. G. (1995). The Charles Bonnet syndrome: a large prospective study in The Netherlands. *Br. J. Psychiatry* 166:254–257.

Trenwalder, C. (1998). Sleep dysfunction in Parkinson's disease. *Clin. Neurosci.* 5:107–114.

VanNess, P. C., Lesser, R. P., and Duchowny, S. M. (1998) Sensory seizures. In: *Epilepsy—A Comprehensive Textbook,* J. Engel and T. A. Pedley (eds.). New York: Lippincott-Raven Press, pp. 533–555.

Vaphiades, M. S., Celesia, G. G., and Brigell, M. G. (1996) Positive spontaneous visual phenomena limited to the hemianopic field in lesions of central visual pathways. *Neurology* 47:408–417.

Weller, M., and Wiedemann, P. (1989) Visual hallucinations. An outline of etiological and pathogenetic concepts. *Int. Ophthalmol.* 13:193–199.

West, L. J. (1962). A general theory of hallucinations and dreams. In *Hallucinations,* L. J. West (ed.) New York: Grunn and Stratton, pp. 275–291.

White, C. P., and Jan, J. E. (1992). Visual hallucinations after acute visual loss in a young child. *Dev. Med. Child Neurol.* 34:252–265.

White, N. J. (1980). Complex visual hallucinations in partial blindness due to eye disease. *Br. J. Psychiatry* 136:284–286.

18

Amnesic Disorders

RUSSELL M. BAUER, LAURA GRANDE, AND EDWARD VALENSTEIN

During the past five decades, our understanding of disorders of memory and of normal memory processes has increased dramatically. In 1950, very little was known about the localization of brain lesions causing amnesia. Despite a few clues in earlier literature, it came as a complete surprise in the early 1950s that bilateral medial temporal resection caused amnesia. The importance of the thalamus in memory was hardly suspected until the 1970s and the basal forebrain was an area virtually unknown to clinicians before the 1980s. An animal model of the amnesic syndrome was not developed until the 1970s.

During this same period, neuropsychological characteristics of amnesia were being uncovered through intense research efforts with clinical populations. The amnesic syndrome has been a topic of fundamental interest to neuropsychologists, neuroscientists, and cognitive psychologists (Baddeley, 1982); the resulting literature in many respects reflects a model system for the interdisciplinary activity that some refer to as "cognitive neuropsychology" (Caramazza, 1992; Kosslyn and Intriligator, 1992) or "cognitive neuroscience" (Kosslyn and Koenig, 1992; Schacter et al., 1998). As a result of this explosion of activity, we no longer consider memory to be a unitary phenomenon. The amnesic syndrome does not affect all kinds of memory, and memory-disordered patients without full-blown amnesia (e.g., patients with frontal lesions) may nonetheless have qualitative impairment in cognitive processes that support remembering. The idea that there is a core amnesic syndrome can also be called into question, but we will use this term to describe the behavioral characteristics of memory disorders that follow medial temporal lobe destruction and the substantially similar disorders associated with diencephalic and basal forebrain lesions.

In this chapter we begin by summarizing the most salient features of this syndrome and by briefly describing methods of evaluating amnesia in the clinic. The neuropsychological abilities that are normally impaired, or spared, in amnesia are then given detailed discussion. Lesion data relevant to the anatomic localization of memory functions are then reviewed. The next sections consider the disorders that commonly present with amnesia, and the chapter concludes with brief reviews of key principles in memory rehabilitation and of recent functional imaging studies of memory.

CLINICAL CHARACTERISTICS OF THE AMNESIC SYNDROME

The amnesic disorders caused by different diseases, or by lesions in different parts of the brain have common characteristics considered to comprise the amnesic syndrome. In many cases, it is possible to provide relatively precise estimates of the date of onset of the illness. Loss of memory for events occurring after illness onset is referred to as *anterograde amnesia*. Many amnesics have difficulty recalling some events that occurred prior to the onset of amnesia, a phenomenon known as *retrograde amnesia*. Finally, many amnesic patients show preservation of certain cognitive abilities, and these preserved abilities also help to define the syndrome.

ANTEROGRADE AMNESIA

The hallmark of the amnesic syndrome is a profound defect in new learning. In the literature, the deficit is variously described as involving recent or long-term memory; the essential feature of the deficit is that that patient is impaired in the conscious, deliberate recall of information initially learned after illness onset. The defect is disclosed in practically any situation in which the recall burden exceeds the immediate memory span, or in which a delay with distraction ensues between information exposure and the memory test. Anterograde memory loss prevents the patient from establishing new, permanent memories from the time of illness onset. Amnesic patients are severely impaired in everyday life and their learning deficit is apparent on even casual observation. Such patients may fail to learn the names of hospital staff and will fail to recognize newly encountered persons after brief delays. They may appear disoriented in place or time because they have failed to learn their location or have lost the ability to monitor and keep track of ongoing events. Amnesic patients are frequently capable of maintaining adequate conversation, but their deficit may become obvious when they are asked to recall an event that occurred only hours or minutes before. Instructions to remember such events for later recall rarely result in measurable improvement. Although such deficits are apparent in the patient's everyday behavior, they may be more precisely documented by objective tests of delayed free recall, cued recall, and recognition.

RETROGRADE AMNESIA AND REMOTE MEMORY DISTURBANCE

In addition to defects of new learning, the amnesic patient usually also has difficulty in recalling events that occurred prior to illness onset. In many cases, this impairment is worse for relatively recent events than for events that occurred in the very remote past. The deficit typically involves autobiographical information from the patient's specific past (e.g., the circumstances surrounding an important relative's death), as well as more public information (e.g., which American president was recently impeached). It has been suggested (Kapur, 1999) that autobiographical memory for past personal events is both anatomically and functionally distinct from remote semantic knowledge and fact memory. Autobiographical defects are commonly seen after lesions to the medial temporal and diencephalic structures, while defects in remote semantic memory result more commonly from neocortical damage.

Three patterns of remote memory impairment in amnesic subjects have been described in the literature. The first is an impairment that is temporally limited, involving primarily the few years prior to the onset of amnesia with complete or near-complete sparing of more remote time periods. This has been documented in the amnesic patient H.M. (Milner et al., 1968; Marslen-Wilson and Teuber, 1974; Corkin, 1984), in patients receiving electroconvulsive therapy (ECT) for depression (Squire et al., 1975; Squire and Fox, 1980), and in recent cases of remote memory impairment after language-dominant temporal lobectomy (Barr et al., 1990). The second pattern involves an impairment that is temporally graded, affecting all time periods, with greater impairment of memories derived from recent time periods. This pattern of remote memory disturbance is said to be typical of patients with alcoholic Korsakoff's syndrome (Seltzer and Benson, 1974; Albert et al., 1979; Meudell et al., 1980; Cohen and Squire, 1981; Squire and Cohen, 1984; Squire et al., 1989a), and has been reported in patients with basal forebrain damage (Gade and Mortensen, 1990). The third pattern, a decade-nonspecific impairment, affecting all time periods equally, has been described in patients surviving herpes simplex encephalitis (Cermak and O'Connor, 1983; Butters et al., 1984; Damasio et al., 1985a,b; Kopelman et al., 1999) and in certain other amnesic subjects (Sanders and Warrington, 1971) as well as in patients with Huntington's disease (Albert et al., 1981).

OTHER CHARACTERISTICS OF THE AMNESIC SYNDROME

Amnesic patients, despite significant impairments in new learning and remote memory, often score normally or near normally on psychometric tests of intelligence (e.g., Wechsler Scales) and perform normally on measures of immediate memory, provided that the amount of information they are required to learn is within their attention span (Drachman and Arbit, 1966). Thus, amnesia cannot be explained on the basis of poor attention span or generalized intellectual loss. However, other cognitive deficits can be seen in some amnesic patients and may contribute to their deficits in memory. A good example is the patient with alcoholic Korsakoff's syndrome, in whom visuospatial and visuoperceptual deficits (Kapur and Butters, 1977) and impairment on tests of executive skill and strategy formation (Moscovitch, 1982; Squire, 1982b; Kopelman, 1995) are commonly found.

Classically defined, the anterograde and retrograde deficits that characterize the amnesic syndrome are multimodal. Such a pattern likely results from bilateral or midline involvement of a memory system that is not itself organized in a modality-specific way. However, modality-specific impairments in new learning have been described in patients with circumscribed vascular lesions affecting cortico-cortical pathways linking sensory association cortices with the medial temporal memory system (Ross, 1980, 1982). Also, patients with unilateral lesions may have a modality-independent amnesia that is nevertheless material-specific: patients with language-dominant (usually left hemisphere) lesions usually have more difficulty with verbal than with nonverbal memory,

while the reverse tends to be true (though less strongly) of patients with language-nondominant (usually right hemisphere) lesions.

Finally, even densely amnesic patients show certain spared memory capacities in addition to their spared attentional and intellectual skills. When memory is indexed indirectly by changes in performance rather than by direct, conscious recollection, amnesics often show normal or near-normal new learning capacity. These intact capabilities are reflected in (a) the acquisition of new motor, perceptual, and cognitive skills (Cohen and Squire, 1980; Schmidtke et al., 1996; Cohen et al., 1997; Beaunieux et al., 1998), (b) the intact facilitation ("priming") of performance (as measured by increased accuracy or response speed) when specific stimuli or stimulus contexts are repeated after initial presentation (e.g., Cermak et al., 1985; Hamann and Squire, 1997), and (c) intact "noncognitive" forms of learning such as classical conditioning in some amnesics (Woodruff Pak, 1993; Gabrieli et al., 1995a; Schugens and Daum, 1999).

EVALUATING THE AMNESIC PATIENT

The two main goals of memory assessment of amnesic patients are to (1) establish the severity of the memory defect in the context of other cognitive complaints and (2) characterize the nature of the memory impairment and its basis in encoding, storage, and retrieval operations.

The first goal is best achieved by embedding memory testing in a comprehensive mental status or neuropsychological examination that includes assessment of general intellectual capacity, language functions, visuoperceptual/ visuospatial skill, frontal-executive skills, and motor functions, and an evaluation of psychopathology and emotional dysfunction. While brief screening evaluations are often useful for determining whether a memory disorder is present, detailed prescriptive and rehabilitative recommendations require the kind of data only supplied by comprehensive neuropsychological evaluation.

The second goal is achieved by assessing memory functions relevant to the diagnostic or descriptive task faced by the clinician. Historically, there have been two general approaches to the neuropsychological examination of memory deficits. The first approach, the *global achievement model* (Delis, 1989), is primarily designed to quantify the severity of a memory deficit by subjecting a patient to a variety of tests and by representing the patient's performance in terms of a single overall score. For example, the original Wechsler Memory Scale (WMS; Wechsler, 1945) yielded an overall Memory Quotient (MQ), which was intended as an omnibus index of memory ability that could be compared with the IQ. Subsequent editions of the WMS have tended to de-emphasize this approach because, in representing performance by a single numerical score, it fails to account for qualitative differences among patients who score at about the same level (Kaplan, 1983). In the second approach, the *cognitive science model* by Delis (1989), methods of memory assessment derived from the cognitive information-processing literature are applied to the clinical evaluation of memory-disordered patients. As such, this endeavor represents an intersection between cognitive psychology and psychometrics. Determination of which of the two approaches to use depends to some extent on the goals of memory assessment. In some clinical settings, where the goal is to detect rather than to characterize a memory defect, a global achievement approach with a valid (sensitive and selective) measure may be quite appropriate. However, in other settings, more specific information about the nature of a patient's memory disorder is needed; in this case, an extended assessment with a flexible battery of memory tests may be required.

Such a battery should broadly evaluate immediate, recent, and remote memory; should incorporate different types of material (e.g., verbal and nonverbal); should evaluate the manner in which the patient learns complex material (e.g., short passages, word lists, complex nonverbal designs); and should test for memory using a variety of testing formats (e.g., free recall, cued recall, recognition). A detailed description of the various clinical memory tests available is given by Lezak (1995), and other reviews of the memory assessment enterprise

include those by Delis (1989), Larrabee and Crook, (1995), Loring and Papanicolaou (1987), and Russell (1981).

IMMEDIATE MEMORY SPAN

As indicated above, the classic amnesic patient performs normally on tasks that require the repetition of information immediately after it is presented. Normal performance, however, is not characteristic of patients with impaired attention secondary to psychiatric illness, degenerative dementia, or other forms of brain dysfunction in which there is increased distractibility. Diseases that interfere with rehearsal, such as certain forms of aphasia, can also impair immediate memory. Tests of immediate memory are given to determine whether a patient's memory impairment can be explained by disturbances of attention or rehearsal. The most widely used span tests are the Digit Span subtests of the Wechsler Intelligence Scales and the Wechsler Memory Scale (in its various editions). These tests are actually two tests in one: a digits-forward and a digits-backwards test, the latter of which likely places more demand on effort, vigilance, and mental control, and may also involve a visual scanning component (Weinberg et al., 1972). Separate scores for digits forward and digits backwards are available on the Wechsler Memory Scale II and III (WMS-R; Wechsler, 1987). Nonverbal pointing span can be evaluated with a recent modification of the Corsi Blocks (Kaplan et al., 1991) that has been incorporated into the WMS-III. Tests evaluating memory for increasingly long sequences of words (Miller, 1973) or sentences (Benton and Hamsher, 1976) are also available.

TESTS OF ANTEROGRADE LEARNING

Memory for Word Lists and Stories

By far the most widely used clinical memory tests are those that require the patient to verbally recall or recognize information presented in list or story format. The most useful tests are those which include both immediate- and delayed-recall probes. Prominent examples of list-learning tasks include the Rey Auditory

Verbal Learning Test (RAVLT; Lezak, 1983), the California Verbal Learning Test-II (CVLT-II; Delis et al., 2000), the Selective Reminding Procedure (Bushke and Fuld, 1974), and the Hopkins Verbal Learning Test (Brandt, 1991). Examples of story recall tests include the WMS Logical Memory subtest (Wechsler, 1945, and subsequent revisions), the Babcock-Levy Story (Babcock, 1930), and the Randt Memory Test (Randt and Brown, 1983). The Warrington Recognition Memory Test (RMT; Warrington, 1984) provides a relatively sensitive (but nonspecific) test of verbal (word) and nonverbal (face) recognition using a forced-choice format. This test can be used for documenting material specificity (e.g., verbal vs. nonverbal memory deficits) in memory performance after unilateral brain lesions, although its use in this context should be considered in conjunction with other memory performances.

The CVLT-II is particularly useful in documenting the manner in which the patient goes about learning a supraspan list. It consists of 16 shopping items, arranged into four categories (animals, furniture, ways of traveling, vegetables). The items are randomly presented to the subject, who must recall as many as possible in any order. After five repetitions of the list, a second list is introduced and recall is probed once. Free and cued recall for the first list is then obtained immediately and after a 20-minute delay. Finally, yes–no recognition is measured. Normative data on a variety of learning and memory variables, including consistency of item recall across trials, strength of primacy and recency effects, vulnerability to retroactive and proactive interference, retention of information across delays, enhancement of recall performance by category cueing and recognition testing, and frequency of error types (intrusions, perseverations, and false positives) are provided. Test users should be aware that the normative sample upon which the original CVLT was validated was primarily a highly educated, majority sample; other norms are available for subjects with different educational, racial–ethnic, or cultural backgrounds. Many of these problems have been alleviated, or rendered less serious, with the revision resulting in the CVLT-II.

Nonverbal Memory Tests

A variety of tests using nonverbal stimuli are also available. Some of these tests (Visual Reproduction subtest of the Wechsler Memory Scales; Rey-Osterrieth Complex Figure [Lezak, 1995]) evaluate nonverbal memory by requiring a drawing-from-memory response. The patient's approach to the Rey-Osterrieth figure can be evaluated for the degree of organization (Binder, 1982; Hamby et al., 1993; Stern et al., 1994), and if the separate details of the figure are considered as a list, delayed recall after 20 minutes can be evaluated for primacy and recency effects. It should be emphasized that deficits on drawing-from-memory tests may reflect memory impairment, constructional disability, visuoperceptual dysfunction, or a complex combination of deficits that should be teased apart when interpreting results. For this reason, it is important to test nonverbal memory by including additional tests that do not require a drawing-from-memory response. Benton et al., (1983) and Kaplan (see Milberg et al., 1986) provide multiple-choice alternatives for the Benton VRT and WMS figures, respectively. The WMS-III incorporates a face-learning subtest (using a yes–no recognition format) and has recognition probes for the Visual Reproduction subtest. The Continuous Visual Memory Test (Trahan and Larrabee, 1988) provides a recurring figures type of recognition test with excellent normative data, a visuoperceptual check, and a method for calculating response bias in recognition performance. As indicated above, the WRMT incorporates a forced-choice recognition test for unfamiliar faces.

Tests of Retrograde Amnesia
and Remote Memory

The patient's ability to recall information acquired before the onset of amnesia can be assessed informally by planning an interview containing both autobiographical and public-domain questions. Including the former type of material obviously requires the cooperation of a knowledgeable informant and poses some difficulty in quantification of the severity and temporal parameters of any deficit that emerges. Alternatively, a number of more formal, well-normed assessments of remote memory are available. The Boston Remote Memory Battery (Albert et al., 1979) assesses memory for public events and famous faces, and contains both easy and difficult items from the 1930s to the 1970s. Recent extensions into the most recent decades are available. The test, and others like it, has been used extensively in clinical and experimental research documenting patterns of remote memory impairment in various clinical populations described above, although complications exist with respect to assumptions about when test items were originally learned. That is, one problem with such tests is that, since many items (and faces) are widely accessible to the general public, it is difficult to determine when knowledge about a specific public event or famous personality was actually acquired. This makes interpretation of temporal parameters of remote memory loss very difficult. In an attempt to deal with this problem, Squire and colleagues (Squire, Slater and Chace, 1975) developed a test that assesses memory for television shows broadcast for only one season. This test has been periodically updated and has been used in a variety of studies in Squire's lab and elsewhere. Further refinements of remote memory tests designed to deal with these problems are needed (Mayes et al., 1994a).

It should be noted that tests of retrograde amnesia present substantial methodological and conceptual complexities (Sanders and Warrington, 1971; Squire et al., 1989b). Most of these tests make two important assumptions: (1) that relevant information was learned at about the time it occurred (e.g., that the patient learned in late 1963 about the assassination of President Kennedy), and (2) that all items were learned with approximately equal strength and that forgetting of specific details has proceeded at approximately the same rate since original learning. It is often difficult to determine when a patient learned about a specific event, and it is clear that the method by which the subject learned about the event (e.g., through high school history vs. personal experience) may affect the nature of the memory store tapped by tests of retrograde amnesia.

Specialized Tests of Information Processing

For precise characterization of a patient's memory deficit, several experimental memory tests are available that are designed to evaluate specific aspects of memory-relevant information processing. Tests relevant to encoding ability include Wickens's release from proactive interference procedure (Wickens, 1970), comparison of recall and recognition performance on categorized vs. uncategorized lists, and variations of the levels-of-processing approach of Craik and Lockhart (1972), in which orienting questions at the point of learning direct processing to particular aspects of target stimuli. Rate of forgetting from long-term memory may be evaluated with a variety of recognition paradigms based on the Huppert and Piercy (1979) procedure. The key feature of this approach is to equate initial learning in some meaningful way with a control group, and to then periodically probe recognition accuracy at specified delays after original learning. Retrieval processes are usually evaluated by manipulating cues available during the memory test; comparisons between free recall and recognition, as well as between free and cued recall, are relevant to retrieval explanations of memory disorder. It should be kept in mind, however, that better performance on recognition testing than on recall may not specifically implicate retrieval processes; such a finding is also characteristic of weak memory due to poor initial encoding or a long study–test interval. Other relevant tasks include tests that evaluate memory for temporal order and recency, metamemory, and source amnesia described below.

Effort should also be devoted to documenting domains of spared memory in amnesic patients. Semantic memory can be assessed with general information questions (e.g., Wechsler Adult Intelligence Scale–Revised [WAIS-R] Information subtest; Wechsler, 1981) and with tests of controlled word association (Benton et al., 1983). Performance on indirect tests of memory can be assessed using variants of word-stem completion priming (Graf et al., 1984; Cermak et al., 1997), perceptual identification (Jacoby and Dallas, 1981; Tulving and

Schacter, 1990), motor skill learning (Milner et al., 1968; Willingham, 1998), and other procedures relevant to the specific case.

One issue in evaluating amnesia is determining how to quantify the severity of amnesia in the individual patient. Precise characterization of severity is important in scientific and clinical communication for comparing a given patient with others described in the literature. A commonly used convention is to specify a discrepancy (usually 1 standard deviation [SD] or 15 points) between an omnibus test of memory (e.g., WMS MQ) and a similarly scaled measure of overall cognitive ability (e.g., WAIS IQ; Squire and Shimamura, 1986). One problem with this approach is that the MQ consists of a number of subtests, only some of which measure abilities impaired in amnesia (see Erickson and Scott, 1977; Lezak, 1995). This practice is further complicated by the fact that the WMS–IQ discrepancy was originally formulated when earlier versions of the Wechsler Intelligence Scale were in wide use. Subsequent revisions of the original WMS yield multiple memory indices rather than a single MQ. With all of these options, there is as yet no widely accepted convention for quantitatively representing amnesia severity across laboratories, although the suggestion of Shimamura and Squire (1986) that investigators use a variety of measures with a range of difficulty represents a useful first step. If the lessons of the past are to be learned appropriately, when advancing a particular view of amnesia, it is important to rule out alternative interpretations of the patient's deficit by sufficiently broad neuropsychological analysis. In the documentation of amnesia severity, one must take into account the various restandardizations of the available tests when calculating discrepancy scores.

NEUROPSYCHOLOGICAL ANALYSES OF AMNESIC SYNDROMES

INFORMATION-PROCESSING ACCOUNTS OF AMNESIA

In this section, we shall discuss information-processing accounts of anterograde and retrograde amnesia (Cermak, 1997). Information-processing models assume that complex abilities (e.g., memory) can be subdivided into distinct and more fundamental subprocesses (Klatzky, 1982). This emphasis on process instead of product has stimulated a whole generation of experimental evaluations of the nature of amnesia, often in hopes of disclosing a singular core defect that might account for the range of observed impairments.

Information-processing accounts of amnesia can be grouped into three broad types: (1) those that characterize the defect as impairment in the *acquisition* of new information; (2) those that invoke impaired *maintenance and storage* of information during the retention interval, and (3) those that assert that the amnesic patient has impaired retrieval of information when formally tested (Baddeley, 1982; Squire and Cohen, 1984; Parkin and Leng, 1993; Cermak, 1997). Understandably, proponents of each of these views have tended to rely on certain restricted features of the overall syndrome and to draw largely from a specific patient population. For example, studies favoring an encoding deficit have relied largely on the performance of alcoholic Korsakoff patients, while studies invoking storage deficits as a locus have involved primarily the evaluation of patients with medial temporal lesions.

Researchers who assert that amnesia is the result of an impairment in a specific information-processing ability incur certain formidable responsibilities. As Squire and Cohen (1984) indicate, proponents of this view must demonstrate that such a defect is a cause, rather than a consequence, of amnesia (Mayes et al., 1981). Similarly, when one asserts that amnesia results from the impairment of some information-processing capacity, it is necessary to show that amnesics are differentially affected by manipulations designed to affect that process (the "law of differential deficits"). This has proved to be a demanding task. For example, retrieval explanations of amnesia have relied extensively on the idea that the performance of amnesics on memory tests is influenced more by the method of testing (e.g., cued vs. free recall) than by the method of study. Many studies comparing amnesics to normal subjects on cued recall (Mayes and Meudell, 1981; Wetzel and Squire, 1982) and recognition (Mayes et al., 1980) have shown that the pattern exhibited by amnesics was also shown by normals during the course of natural forgetting. Such findings favor a "weak memory" interpretation of amnesia, rather than a view in which amnesics are disproportionately impaired in retrieval operations. Because of such complexities, growing discomfort has emerged about any view asserting that amnesia results from nothing but encoding, retention, and/or retrieval deficits. Our view is that attempts to localize amnesic defects at specific cognitive loci have been extremely valuable—not as ultimate explanations, but as heuristics in specifying the important ways in which amnesic syndromes may vary.

Amnesia as an Encoding Deficit

The idea that amnesia reflects a deficit that occurs at the time of learning derives mainly from studies showing that certain amnesics, when faced with a memory task, do not organize or encode to-be-learned information in a normal way (Butters and Cermak, 1980). Such studies, mainly involving analysis of the performance of alcoholic Korsakoff patients, have suggested that these patients have difficulty in engaging in deeper, more elaborative levels of information processing, resulting in impoverished stimulus analysis.

Evaluations of encoding deficits as a causative factor in amnesia were stimulated by the levels-of-processing approach to memory introduced by Craik and Lockhart (1972). These authors asserted that memory is the natural result of cognitive operations applied to stimuli at the point of learning, and that deeper, meaning-based, semantic analysis would lead to superior retention compared to that from analysis of the superficial (orthographic or phonemic) characteristics of stimuli. Talland (1965) asserted that the alcoholic Korsakoff patient engaged in a "premature closure of activation" that affected the dynamic processing required for full encoding of to-be-learned stimuli. This laid a foundation for considering Korsakoff amnesia within the context of the levels-of-processing framework. Studies

conducted within this tradition (Cermak and Butters, 1972; Cermak et al., 1973a, 1974, 1976) demonstrated that amnesic Korsakoff patients spontaneously analyze only those features of verbal information that represent superficial levels of processing.

Support for the idea that superficial analysis leads to poor retrieval comes from results of a study (Cermak et al., 1974) using Wickens's (1970) technique of release from proactive interference (PI). In this procedure, three words from the same semantic category are presented. After 20 minutes of distraction, subjects are asked to recall the words. On each subsequent trial, three more words from the same semantic category are presented. As trials proceed, practically all subjects recall fewer and fewer words, until on a later trial, the category to which the words belong is changed. According to Wickens (1970), when a category shift improves performance, this is evidence that the subject must have been encoding information along the shifted dimension (e.g., semantic category membership). When a category switch occurs, normal subjects typically improve their performance because PI is reduced. When this task is given to alcoholic Korsakoff patients, however, the amount of PI release varies with the nature of to-be-learned information. In the Cermak et al. study, normal release was seen when numbers were used as stimuli, but a failure to release from PI was seen with words. Cermak et al. concluded that their retrieval deficit was a direct result of the amnesics' inability to spontaneously analyze words on the basis of their semantic features.

More recent investigations of encoding-deficits theory have shown that, even when alcoholic Korsakoff patients are directed toward semantic analysis via appropriate orienting questions, their retention remains far below normal. This finding, and subsequent results using a variant of Thomson and Tulving's (1970) encoding specificity procedure, has led to a recent modification of the original encoding-deficit theory (Cermak et al., 1980; cf. Verfaellie and Cermak, 1991). In this modification, encoding is redefined as a product of analysis in which subjects cognitively manipulate those features of the information they just analyzed to permit differential storage. By this modified view, amnesics may be able to semantically analyze information, but may not be able to profit from the results of such analysis because they fail to encode its products. Verfaellie and Cermak (1991) assert that this view of encoding (as manipulation and organization of features of information into a more permanent memory) bridges the gap between theories of amnesia that focus on encoding, consolidation, and retrieval deficits. Common to all these theories is the idea that amnesics cannot store new material because they cannot cognitively manipulate the features of the material to permit assimilation into a general knowledge system. Cermak and colleagues (1997) reported that the level of analysis performed at study can affect the unconscious performance of amnesic patients, but that this information is unavailable for conscious retrieval. In this study, participants were asked to analyze study words to either semantic or graphemic instructions. At test time, participants were asked to complete word stems under three different conditions: (1) direct, in which participants were to use the stem as a cue for a studied word; (2) indirect, in which participants were to use the first word that came to mind with no reference to the study list; and (3) oppositional, in which participants were to use the first word that came, as long as it was not from the study list. Cermak et al. found that under all conditions, the amnesic participants completed the word stems with study words more frequently than would be expected by chance, and they were more likely to produce words from the study list that were semantically analyzed during the indirect and oppositional conditions. These findings suggest that amnesics may be unable to endogenously make use of this more detailed encoding.

One problem with encoding-deficit theory, even as modified, is that the abnormal performances it seeks to explain (e.g., failure to release from PI; subnormal performance even when orienting questions direct attention toward semantic features) are not found in all amnesics. For example, normal release from PI after a shift in semantic category was found in patient N.A., patients undergoing bilateral ECT (Squire, 1982b), postencephalitic amnesics (Cermak, 1976), and a patient with amnesia secondary to a left retrosplenial lesion (Valenstein et al., 1986). Also, other studies have suggested that alcoholic Korsakoff patients may show a release from PI effect if they are provided repeated exposure to the new category members (Kinsbourne and Wood, 1975) or if they are forewarned of the impending shift (Winocur et al., 1981).

Cermak and Wong (1999) investigated whether amnesic patients expend less effort toward encoding information, resulting in poor performance. Utilizing a combination of divided attention tasks (word list learning and button pressing) at both encoding and recall, they reported that the amnesic participants were not impaired in the amount of effort expended on the primary task.

Amnesia as a Retention Deficit

Theories that postulate a retention deficit as being responsible for amnesia propose a post-encoding deficit in which memory representations are poorly maintained or poorly elaborated with the passage of time. One such theory was advanced by Milner (1962, 1966), who described a postencoding process called "consolidation" that was presumed to mediate the transition of memory from an unstable short-term memory store to a more permanent and stable long-term store. Retention-deficit views have been based on two main findings: (1) that at least some forms of amnesia show an abnormally rapid rate of forgetting in recognition paradigms, and (2) the same patients tend to display a temporally limited retrograde defect, affecting only those time periods immediately preceding the onset of amnesia.

While encoding-deficit theories have relied primarily on studies of alcoholic Korsakoff patients for supportive data, theories that postulate a deficit in retention and storage have drawn supportive findings primarily from research on patients with damage to medial temporal structures. In Huppert and Piercy's (1979) influential study demonstrating abnormally rapid forgetting in the temporal lobe amnesic, H.M., they found that H.M.'s performance on a memory task was equaled to that of normals by increasing study time, and that H.M.'s performance on a yes–no recognition task was similar to that of controls at a 10-minute delay, but his performance declined when tested 1 and 7 days later. In a similar experiment, Huppert and Piercy presented data suggesting that H.M. also forgot more rapidly than alcoholic Korsakoff patients.

Early studies proposing an association of rapid forgetting with damage to the medial temporal region initially led to the suggestion that forgetting rates (and the retention defect they seemed to indicate) might serve to differentiate medial temporal from diencephalic forms of amnesia (Huppert and Piercy, 1979; Squire, 1982b; Zola-Morgan and Squire, 1982). More recent studies, however, have generally failed to provide support for a link between medial temporal damage and abnormally rapid forgetting (Kopelman, 1985; Freed et al., 1987; McKee and Squire, 1992). These studies will be reviewed in detail below when we consider the possibility that distinct subtypes of amnesia exist.

Squire and colleagues (1984a) suggested that the temporally limited retrograde amnesia said to be typical of patients with medial temporal lobe lesions may result from a defect in consolidation of information. They proposed that consolidation is a gradual process, lasting for months or even years. When this process is interrupted by brain impairment, premorbid memories will be affected, but only for a limited period of time. A network model of consolidation has been recently proposed (Alvarez and Squire, 1994; Squire and Alvarez, 1995). According to this view, the medial temporal system initially stores memory traces. The hippocampal system repeatedly reactivates representations in the neocortex, resulting in the binding between cortical regions and the creation of strong interconnections. After a time, the storage sites become capable of being autonomously activated in a coordinated fashion, after which the medial temporal system is not involved in memory retrieval. At this point, the neocortex becomes capable of being autonomously activated and is able to retrieve memories independent of the hippocampal system. Squire and Alvarez (1995) suggest that the tendency of hippocampal synapses to change quickly permits this structure to store

initial memory traces, until the slower changing neocortical synapses change and allow for the more permanent memory storage. If this process takes place gradually (over a period of years), then retrieval of very remote memories is preserved in individuals with medial temporal amnesia because remote memories are fully consolidated and no longer depend on the activity of the medial temporal system. This view predicts a strong relationship between temporally limited retrograde amnesia and anterograde amnesia, because it suggests that the same mechanism (impairment in the ability of the medial temporal system to mediate time-locked information retrieval prior to the point at which consolidation is complete) may be responsible for both (Squire and Cohen, 1984).

The hypothesis that the process of consolidation ultimately renders the medial temporal system unnecessary for the retrieval of memories has received some criticism (Nadel and Moscovitch, 1997). Noting dissociations within medial temporal lobe retrograde amnesia, such as a lack of temporal gradient for autobiographical information, Nadel and Moscovitch (1997) have argued against the standard model of memory consolidation. Their multiple-trace theory shares a number of features with the standard consolidation model. The main distinction between the models lies in the role of the hippocampus, with the multiple-trace theorists declaring continued involvement of the hippocampal complex in activation and retrieval of memories.

Amnesia as a Retrieval Deficit

The view that amnesia reflects a deficit in information retrieval is based on two main findings: *(1)* that manipulation of testing procedures by providing aids to retrieval in the form of cues or prompts can dramatically improve the memory performance of some amnesic patients, and *(2)* that all amnesics exhibit some form of remote memory loss. Although temporally limited remote memory loss has been explained using a storage metaphor, the idea that more extensive forms of retrograde amnesia must involve a retrieval deficit follows naturally from the assumption that, prior to illness onset, more remote memories must have been encoded and stored in a normal way (Squire and Cohen, 1984).

Retrieval Deficits in Anterograde Amnesia. Warrington and Weiskrantz (1970, 1973) proposed a retrieval-deficit model of amnesia based on findings from studies using the partial information technique. In their initial experiments, amnesic participants were presented on each of five learning trials a series of stimuli that became increasingly less fragmented, until they could identify the stimulus. When the stimuli were re-presented after a 1-day delay, amnesic participants identified them sooner (when stimuli were more fragmented) than on the initial presentation; this finding implies that something was retained from initial stimulus exposure. Despite this facilitation, amnesics showed little evidence of retention on conventional tests of recall and recognition. On the basis of these findings, Warrington and Weiskrantz concluded that retention by amnesics depended more on the method of retrieval than on the method of acquisition. They explained the amnesic deficit as resulting from abnormal susceptibility to interference from competing responses at the point of recall. Because of the emphasis on interference, their model has also been referred to as the *retrieval-interference* model of amnesia.

To provide further support for the presumed effects of interference during retrieval, Warrington and Weiskrantz (1974, 1978) performed a series of experiments using a reversal-learning paradigm. In these experiments, subjects learned two different word lists constructed so that each word on one list began with the same three letters as a word on the second list. Participants studied list 1 once and made multiple attempts to learn list 2. After each trial, retention was assessed with a cued-recall (stem completion) paradigm in which the first three letters of target words were provided. Both healthy controls and amnesics performed well on the list 1 stem completion. Additionally, both groups demonstrated difficulty on the list 2 stem completion, with both groups experiencing interference from list 1. However, while control performance improved with repeated exposure to list 2, amnesics continued to exhibit a high incidence of intrusions from list 1. Warrington and Weiskrantz argued that storage of list 1 had occurred, and that it continued to interfere with retrieval of list 2 words through a process of response competition.

Subsequent research (Warrington and Weiskrantz, 1978) highlighted problems with a strict retrieval-interference interpretation of these data. When the performance of healthy controls and amnesic participants were compared, it was found that the amnesics did not show more susceptibility to interference on the initial list 2 trial, violating the principle of differential deficits. Also, when an attempt was made to reduce response competition (by creating word lists in which each pair of words, one from list 1 and one from list 2, were the only English words beginning with those initial letters) no effect was seen in the amnesic participants' performance. These results led Warrington and Weiskrantz to modify their view and suggest that list 1 responses were so domineering as to actually impede the *learning* of list 2 words. This was an important statement, as it represented the first time that retrieval-deficit theorists conceded the possibility of a deficit in acquisition as being part of their model, thus marking the beginning of an eventual merger between retrieval-deficit and encoding-deficit theories (Winocur et al., 1981; Cermak, 1982; Verfaellie and Cermak, 1991) that characterizes current theory.

Retrieval Deficits in Retrograde Amnesia. Retrieval deficits are more securely invoked in explaining retrograde amnesia. Although temporally limited retrograde amnesia has been attributed to defects in consolidation, this clearly cannot explain the situation in patients whose retrograde amnesia subsides. Thus, the retrograde amnesia that follows closed head injury, which decreases as the post-traumatic anterograde amnesia improves, must be attributed to a reversible retrieval deficit, since memories of events prior to the injury must be present during the amnesia if they are to be recalled afterward. Similarly, patients with transient global amnesia may forget that a relative has died months or years ago, but may recall this clearly after a period of recovery.

As indicated above, the fact that amnesic patients all exhibit some form of remote memory impairment has been taken to mean that a retrieval deficit is involved, since recall of items in remote memory involves memories that were (or should have been) learned prior to the onset of amnesia. A retrieval-deficit view most easily explains decade-nonspecific remote memory impairment, since there would be no basis to suppose that a generalized retrieval deficit would favor certain time periods over others. Such an explanation has, in fact, been advanced to explain remote memory impairment in Huntington's disease (Albert et al., 1981). As indicated above, the shrinking retrograde amnesia seen during recovery of post-traumatic amnesia provides additional strong evidence of a retrieval deficit. After head injury, patients may be amnesic for a period of months or years prior to their injury, but as their anterograde amnesia improves, the retrograde amnesia shrinks to the minutes immediately preceding the injury. This phenomenon may be explained by the patients temporary loss of the ability to retrieve memories within the period of shrinking retrograde amnesia. It is not evident, however, that post-traumatic shrinking retrograde amnesia has the same mechanism as that behind more extensive remote memory deficits seen in other amnesic states.

Some form of retrieval deficit may also explain some of the extensive, temporally graded retrograde amnesia seen in patients with alcoholic Korsakoff's syndrome. It has been argued, however, that this retrograde amnesia may, in fact, result from a progressively severe *acquisition* deficit seen in non-Korsakoff alcoholics (Albert et al., 1980b; Cohen and Squire, 1981). The severity of anterograde learning defects in detoxified non-Korsakoff alcoholics is correlated with the duration of alcohol abuse (Ryan and Butters, 1980a, 1980b). The temporal gradient in the retrograde amnesia of Korsakoff patients may thus reflect the fact that more recent information was never effectively learned. In support of this idea are studies of amnesic patients with acute-onset diencephalic pathology (e.g., stroke, trauma) that generally report relatively mild retrograde amnesia (Cohen and Squire, 1981; Winocur et al., 1984). However, Korsakoff patients, when compared to alcoholic controls, tend to be impaired at *all decades*, even those that predate the onset of abuse-related memory dysfunction (Albert et al., 1980a,b; Cohen and Squire, 1981).

More convincing evidence for a true retrograde amnesia in Korsakoff patients comes from a single case study reported by Butters and Cermak (1986). Patient P.Z., an eminent scientist who had published an autobiography 3 years prior to the onset of Wernicke's encephalopathy in 1982, was studied using remote memory tests. On Albert et al.'s remote memory test, P.Z., like other Korsakoff patients, had significant impairment across all time periods, with some relative sparing of the ability to recognize famous faces from the 1930s and 1940s. Butters and Cermak then devised a remote memory test based on information derived from P.Z.'s autobiography. They found a striking temporal gradient in his memory of autobiographical events, with dramatic and complete impairment of information from the 1960s and 1970s, and relative (though not complete) sparing of very remote memories. The fact that all questions were taken from his own autobiography eliminates the possibility that this information was never learned, although the possibility remains that it was somehow less stable and therefore more difficulty to retrieve for more recent time periods.

These findings led Butters and Miliotis (1985) to propose that the temporally graded retrograde memory impairment in Korsakoff syndrome is the product of two separate factors: (1) an increasingly severe anterograde learning deficit that is gradually acquired through years of alcohol abuse and (2) an impairment of memory retrieval, appearing acutely with the Wernicke stage of the illness that affects all time periods equally. These two superimposed deficits result in the temporally graded retrograde amnesia affecting all time periods.

State-Dependent Learning. Another phenomenon that may illustrate a specific retrieval deficit is state-dependent memory, which is the enhanced ability to recall information when the subject is in the same physiological state as that when learning occurred. For example, the retrieval of information encoded while inebriated may be better recalled after subsequent alcohol ingestion than when sober (Goodwin et al., 1969). State-dependent effects may also be linked to impaired memory for events encoded under stress (Schacter et al., 1996) and may explain some of the effects of aging on conscious recollection (Schramke and Bauer, 1997). A large literature on mood- and state-dependent recall exists; for reviews on this subject see Blaney (1986), Eich (1989), and Eich and Metcalfe (1989).

Summary

Although encoding, retention, and retrieval views all have their merits, it is clear that any view that postulates one (and only one) deficient stage of memory processing cannot explain the variety of deficits seen in amnesia. Instead, it may be better to view encoding, retention, and retrieval as dimensions (or sources of variance) that all contribute in every situation to the strength of a memory trace and that contribute unequally, and in a complex way, to different memory assessment tasks.

MEMORY FUNCTIONS SPARED IN AMNESIA

The studies and formulations just described have largely been designed to explain what is "wrong" with amnesics, in other words, what they cannot do. In the course of examining the scope and limits of amnesic defects, it has become clear that amnesics are not impaired on all memory-related tasks. This behavioral selectivity has had important implications for understanding the way in which memory is organized in the brain, and has had a profound impact on theoretical accounts devised to explain the nature of memory dysfunction in amnesia. Over the past two decades, a substantial literature has developed in the area of memory dissociations, or dissociations between classes of tasks that amnesics can and cannot perform (see Squire, 1987; Schacter et al., 1993; Roediger et al., 1994; Gabrieli, 1998, for reviews). In this section, we first review findings of spared memory function in amnesia, and then discuss theoretical accounts of such dissociations.

Preserved Pre-illness Memory

Although amnesics generally have some form of impairment in memory for events that occurred prior to the onset of amnesia, this loss of memory is not complete. If it were amnesics would be like newborn babies, forced to relearn everything anew. In fact, most amnesics remember more from the time prior to illness onset than they forget. Preserved pre-illness memory can take several forms: intact knowledge structures, preservation of skills, and retained preferences.

Intact Knowledge Structures. The amnesic patient retains substantial intellectual, linguistic, and social skills despite profound impairments in the ability to recall specific information encountered during prior learning episodes. Performance on standardized intellectual tests is frequently normal or near normal. In the pure amnesic, social graces are almost always intact and linguistic skill typically reveals no gross abnormalities; that is, amnesics generally appear to be able to use general knowledge at the same time they have significantly impaired memory and learning skills. One important characteristic of general knowledge that distinguishes it from the type of memory usually impaired in amnesia is that general knowledge is context-free; i.e., its content is devoid of autobiographical information about the time and place in which the information was originally learned. Thus, for example, social and linguistic knowledge is accessed and used without direct reference to the situation in which it was originally learned. This is in contrast to the type of memory manifested in conventional tests of recall and recognition, which refers specifically to a learning experience and involves a directed recollection of information learned at that time.

Motor and Cognitive Skills. In addition to sparing of intellectual, social, and language skill, amnesics frequently show relatively good retention of previously acquired motor and cognitive skills, such as how to ride a bike, play the piano, or use appliances. Evidence that a previously acquired skill can be spared after the onset of amnesia comes from work by Schacter (1983) and Squire and colleagues (1984b). Schacter (1983) provides a fascinating case study of an amnesic who retained his skill at golf, but who became unable to accurately remember his score or his immediately preceding shots on each hole. Moments after teeing off, he would begin to tee another ball, forgetting that he had just taken a shot. (Similar impairments are widely recognized in the general golfing population, with errors tending toward flagrant underestimations of actual scores!) Squire and colleagues taught a mirror-reading skill to depressed psychiatric inpatients prior to a scheduled course of ECT. After treatment was completed, the skill was retained despite marked retrograde amnesia for the training procedure itself.

Preferences. Although very little empirical data are available regarding the effects of memory impairment on personality traits and emotional functioning, Johnson et al. (1985) suggest that feelings and personal preferences may be spared in amnesics to the extent that they are based on memory for general sensory/perceptual features of stimuli and not specific autobiographical memories. Indeed, anecdotal information suggests that many amnesics continue to exhibit personal preferences for such things as favorite color, certain clothes, and food. They continue to like and dislike the people they liked and disliked before even though they may not remember the specific reasons for these feelings. They also retain *general* evaluative responses and emotional reactions. They remember that fire is dangerous and will respond physiologically to previously established fearful stimuli, just as they will appropriately express sadness and joy in response to sad or happy stimuli. Experimental work indicates that memory and emotion are behaviorally and anatomically dissociable; lesions of the hippocampal formation and adjacent cortex affect delayed matching-to-sample (memory) performance but not emotional responsivity, while the opposite pattern is seen after partial or complete lesions of the amygdala (Zola-Mor-

gan et al., 1991). Additional experimental work indicates that food preferences learned prior to hippocampal resection are retained to the extent that they were learned before the operative procedure (Winocur, 1990).

Preserved New Learning Capacities

Most amnesics can learn a wide range of information, even though they have no conscious recollection for the experience upon which the learning is based. Memory without conscious recollective experience has been called *implicit* memory, and is distinguished from *explicit* memory, which entails conscious, deliberate recollection. In general, implicit memory is spared in amnesia, while explicit memory is not (Schacter et al., 1993; Toth, 2000).

Implicit memory is measured using indirect or incidental tasks (Jacoby, 1984; Johnson and Hasher, 1987; Richardson-Klavehn and Bjork, 1988) that make no reference to prior learning episodes at the time of retrieval. Explicit memory is tested directly by asking subjects questions that make specific reference to prior learning (e.g., "Was this word on the list you were shown?"). There is no guarantee, however, that indirect tests measure only implicit memory or that direct tests measure only explicit memory. For example, the normal subject may recall the learning episode and use conscious recall on indirect tests (Kelley and Jacoby, 2000), and the subject may guess or otherwise use nonconscious recollection to succeed on direct tests (Cermak et al., 1997; Verfaellie and Cermak, 1999).

Studies of implicit memory include *(1)* investigations of skill learning, *(2)* studies of repetition priming, *(3)* studies of conditioning and discriminative physiological responses, and *(4)* studies of preference formation.

Skill Learning. Most amnesics are capable of learning new perceptual, cognitive, and motor skills despite a lack of explicit recall of the experiences that lead to such learning (Schacter et al., 1993; Tranel et al., 1994; Rich et al., 1996; Gabrieli, 1998). *How* a skill is learned is generally not accessible to consciousness, even in individuals with intact explicit memory; thus, gradual acquisition of cognitive, perceptual, or motor skills through repetition can occur without conscious or explicit memory.

Milner and colleagues first investigated skill learning in amnesics by studying patient H.M. He demonstrated consistent learning in rotary pursuit and bimanual tracking tasks, despite a lack of memory for having practiced the skill or having previously encountered the apparatus (Corkin, 1968). Similar results have been documented with other amnesics (Starr and Phillips, 1970; Eslinger and Damasio, 1985; Yamashita, 1993). H.M. also improved in daily performance on a mirror-tracing task (Milner, 1962), and he was able to learn a short visual maze and showed significant savings during relearning when tested at various intervals from 1 to 6 days after learning the maze (Milner et al., 1968). Other amnesics have shown practice effects on a variety of complex cognitive skills, such as assembling jigsaw puzzles (Brooks and Baddeley, 1976) and the Tower of Hanoi Puzzle (Cohen, 1984; Squire and Cohen, 1984; Cohen et al., 1985; Saint-Cyr et al., 1988), applying numerical rules (Wood et al., 1982), classifying novel patterns as instances of categories (Knowlton and Squire, 1993; Squire and Knowlton, 1995; Ashby et al., 1998; Reed et al., 1999), and learning stimulus presentation patterns on the serial reaction time task (Nissen and Bullemer, 1987; Reber and Squire, 1998). Several studies have demonstrated that amnesics can gain facility in mirror-reading despite lack of explicit memory for the material (Cohen and Squire, 1980; Verfaellie et al., 1991; Schmidtke et al., 1996). Normal subjects typically show similar degrees of improvement with unfamiliar material, but make greater gains with texts they have seen before, presumably because they can also use explicit memory for previously encountered texts. In many cases, practice effects on skill-learning tasks tend to endure over time, persisting up to 3 months on mirror-reading tasks (Cohen and Squire, 1980) and over a year on the Tower of Hanoi Puzzle (Cohen, 1984).

The skill-learning capacity of amnesic patients has been used in rehabilitative efforts. A number of experiments have demonstrated that amnesics can learn new computer skills (Glisky et al., 1986a; Glisky and Schacter, 1988; Glisky, 1992) and computer-related vocabulary (Glisky et al., 1986b), using the method of vanishing cues, which capitalizes on intact priming capacity in these patients. With this method, amnesics are given increasingly shorter versions of a rule, such as "to save your file, press F10," or of a word, such as "delete" (e.g., "dele__"), until they are able to perform the function or can recall the word without the cue. More will be said about rehabilitative strategies in the concluding section of this chapter.

Recent evidence implicates the cerebellum and basal ganglia in at least some forms of skill learning, and there may be important functional and anatomic differences among different kinds of skill-learning tasks. Rotary pursuit learning is impaired in patients with Huntington's disease (HD) (Heindel et al., 1989; Gabrieli et al., 1997b) and, more variably, in those with Parkinson's disease (PD) (Heindel et al., 1989). Serial reaction time performance is impaired in HD and PD (Knopman and Nissen, 1991; Ferraro et al., 1993). Gabrieli et al. (1997b) showed that performance of HD patients was intact on mirror tracing but impaired on rotary pursuit learning. Patients with cerebellar lesions have been reported to be impaired on mirror tracing (Sanes et al., 1990). Functional imaging studies implicate the motor cortex in rotary pursuit learning (Grafton et al., 1992), while serial reaction time (SRT) learning implicates the basal ganglia (Karni et al., 1995; Doyon et al., 1996; Hazeltine et al., 1997). Behavioral and anatomic dissociations like these suggest that the domain of skill learning is highly complex and must be further subdivided.

Repetition Priming. As indicated above, a series of seminal studies by Warrington and Weiskrantz (1968, 1970, 1974, 1978) demonstrated that amnesics who were severely impaired on tests of recall and recognition could show long-term learning and retention of new information when cued with partial information such as stimulus fragments or word stems. Although findings were interpreted as support for a retrieval-deficit account of amnesia, these results can be construed as the first experimental evidence of intact priming in amnesics.

Repetition priming is the facilitation in the processing of a stimulus that occurs following a prior exposure to the same or related stimulus. Evidence of facilitation is revealed in decreased decision latency, increased accuracy in processing the stimulus, or increased likelihood of generating a previously exposed stimulus in response to a nominal cue. For example, in *lexical decision* tasks, priming is indicated by decreased latency in deciding whether a string of letters represents a real word following the second presentation of the string (Duchek and Neeley, 1989). In *word (perceptual) identification*, priming can be measured by either increased accuracy of identifying previously presented words relative to new words or decreases in exposure time necessary to identify previously exposed items (Jacoby and Dallas, 1981). In *word-stem* or *fragment completion* tasks, priming is reflected by an enhanced tendency to complete fragments, such as "MOT ___ " or "A ___ A ___ IN," with previously studied words (Graf et al., 1982; Tulving et al., 1982). These tasks can be considered indirect tests of memory because no direct reference to the study words is made. Although Warrington and Weiskrantz used a *direct* test (that is, they instructed their subjects to use the cues to recall previously studied items), their amnesic subjects probably used an *implicit* strategy: they treated the memory test as a guessing game. It has subsequently been demonstrated that amnesics perform normally only when indirect instructions are utilized (e.g., "Read this word"; "Generate the first word that comes to mind"; etc.). When *direct* instructions are given, performance by normals is boosted by the use of explicit recollection and amnesic performance may be reduced by a reluctance to guess (Squire et al., 1978; Graf et al., 1984, 1985).

Amnesics have demonstrated facilitated processing of stimuli following previous exposure (study) on *lexical decision tasks* (Moskovitch, 1982; Smith and Oscar Berman, 1990), *object decision tasks* (deciding whether previously shown and novel objects are geometrically possible; see Schacter et al., 1991), *perceptual identification tasks* (Cermak et al., 1998; Verfaellie et al., 1991; Postle and Corkin, 1998), *reading tasks* (Musen et al., 1990; Vaidya et al., 1998), and *word-stem and word-fragment completion tasks* (Diamond and

Rozin, 1984; Shimamura and Squire, 1984; Graf and Schacter, 1985; Graf et al., 1985; Shimamura, 1986; Hamann and Squire, 1996; Cermak et al., 1997).

In the priming literature, an important distinction between perceptual and conceptual forms of priming has been made (Roediger and McDermott, 1993). The examples described above reflect perceptual priming in that processing of stimulus form leads to subsequent facilitation. In conceptual priming, it is processing of word meaning that is important. Examples of conceptual priming tasks are word-association generation (e.g., "What word goes with 'doctor'?" when "nurse" had been studied), and category-exemplar generation (e.g., "Name all the fruits you can" when "apple" had been presented). In some studies, amnesic patients have shown normal conceptual priming on word-association generation (Shimamura and Squire, 1984) and category-exemplar generation (Graf et al., 1985; Cermak et al., 1998; Cermak and Wong, 1998). Korsakoff patients showed normal priming when asked to generate exemplars of categories after having been exposed to a categorized word list, despite being greatly impaired when asked to remember list items in response to category cues (Gardner et al., 1973; Graf et al., 1985; see Kihlstrom, 1980, for similar results with post-hypnotic amnesics). After studying a list of common idioms (e.g., "sour–grapes"), amnesics demonstrated normal priming when asked to freely associate (e.g., "sour–?"), but were impaired when instructed to use the same cues to remember list items (Schacter, 1985). The same finding was observed when the study list consisted of highly related paired associates such as "table–chair" (Shimamura and Squire, 1984). Thus, there is ample evidence that amnesics show conceptual priming, provided that the task allows for implicit retrieval. It should be noted that some failures to demonstrate conceptual priming in amnesia have been reported (Vaidya et al., 1996); the reasons for this are not yet clear.

Psychophysiological and Electrophysiological Correlates. The foregoing studies provide examples of overt behavioral changes that result from prior exposure to stimuli in the absence of a subjective report of remembering. The dissociation between behavioral responses (e.g., generating target items) and conscious verbal report (e.g., remembering target items) represents desynchrony between behavioral and conscious/verbal indicia of memory, and is analogous to similar desynchrony noted frequently among response systems of emotion (Hodgson and Rachman, 1974; Tobias et al., 1992). Lang (1968, 1971) proposed a multiple-system theory of emotion in which verbal, behavioral, and physiological indices were only imperfectly coupled, particularly under states of low arousal.

In the 1980s it was noted that prosopagnosics showed a reliably stronger electrodermal response (EDR) to familiar faces than to nonfamiliar faces in a multiple-choice paradigm, despite their inability to explicitly recognize them as familiar (Bauer, 1984; Tranel and Damasio, 1985; see Chapter 12 in this volume). Schacter (1987a; Schacter et al. 1988) noted the conceptual similarities between sparing of implicit memory in amnesia and spared recognition abilities in agnosia and hemianopia (blindsight). Bauer and Verfaellie (1992) hypothesized that EDR recognition may provide another index of this unconscious form of memory.

In support of this hypothesis, Verfaellie and colleagues (1991) demonstrated that an amnesic patient with a left retrosplenial lesion showed normal EDR to targets despite greatly impaired overt recognition. Verbal recognition and EDR recognition were statistically independent. Similar effects have been demonstrated by Bauer and Verfoillie (1992) in alcoholic Korsakoff patients and patients with early Alzheimer's disease.

Is this form of recognition truly unconscious or does it depend on variables that affect explicit memory? Bauer and Verfaellie (1992) showed that certain variables known to affect explicit memory do not affect EDR, including retention interval (EDR effects persisted up to 4 weeks and were in fact augmented as verbal recognition declined) and levels of processing. Although this supports the hypothesis that EDR recognition more closely resembles implicit phenomena, EDR has been linked to constructs such as orienting, significance detection, metamemory skills, and cognitive effort (e.g., EDR recognition is augmented under conditions of uncertainty), which may correlate with aspects of explicit memory. Further study is needed to define the relationship between EDR (and other measures of autonomic activity) and both implicit and explicit memory.

Recent electrophysiological work using event-related potentials (ERP) has shown evidence that aspects of conscious and unconscious recollection can be manifested in scalp-recorded electroencephalograms (EEG) (Paller et al., 1987; Rugg et al., 1998; Curran, 1999). For example, Rugg et al. (1998) evaluated the ERP correlates of different recognition responses ("new" vs. "old") to studied and unstudied words and found evidence of a response to old words regardless of whether they were recognized. These studies have been of value in further elucidating cognitive components of recollective experience that might contribute to spared memory in amnesia (Paller et al., 1995; Allan et al., 1998; Spencer, 2000; Stenberg, 2000).

Preferences and Other Evaluative Responses. Both anecdotal and formal experimental evidence indicates that emotional responses can be preserved as implicit memories in amnesic patients in the absence of conscious recollection of the experiences on which these reactions are based. The earliest accounts come from observations of alcoholic Korsakoff patients. Korsakoff (1889) observed that a patient expressed fear at the sight of a case for a shock apparatus and thought that the doctor had "probably come to electrify him," even though he did not consciously remember that he had been previously shocked by the apparatus (Schacter, 1987a, p. 512). Korsakoff interpreted this comment as reflecting a memory trace "too weak to enter consciousness." Claparede (1911) surprised a patient by pricking her with a pin hidden in his hand. She later refused to shake hands with him even though her memory for their previous encounter was vague and she could explain her behavior only by stating that "pins are sometimes held in hands." He interpreted the problem as a dissociation between the autobiographical nature of an experience (which he described as "me-ness") and the content of the memory trace it leaves behind (Kihlstrom, 1995; Eustache et al., 1996).

Recent studies have confirmed that amnesics can have preferences despite having no conscious recollection of their basis. Johnson and colleagues (1985) explored this idea formally with a study based on the "mere exposure" effect (Zajonc, 1968). Zajonc had shown that repeated exposure of normal subjects to an object tends to increase judgments of likeability, even if there is no substantive information presented that would support such attitudinal change. This phenomenon occurred even when conscious perception (and therefore overt recognition) was precluded by use of subliminal exposure (Kunst-Wilson and Zajonc, 1980; Zajonc, 1980). In the Johnson et al. study, both Korsakoff patients and controls preferred previously presented Korean melodies over new melodies when asked to choose which of two melodies they preferred. Although normals and amnesics showed equivalent preferences, Korsakoff patients were significantly impaired in their recognition of the old melodies.

In a second study, amnesics and control subjects were shown pictures of two faces, accompanied by fictional biographical information that depicted one positively and the other negatively. When asked 20 days later which of the two they preferred, both groups showed strong preference for the "good guy." Control subjects made this choice 100% of the time and always based their judgment on explicit memory for the accompanying description. The amnesic patients were unable to recall any of the biographical information, yet also showed a strong "good guy" preference (78%). They reported vague reasons for their choice, usually based on the person's physical appearance. This preference was maintained at 1-year follow-up.

Damasio and colleagues (1989) performed a similar experiment with the postencephalitic patient Boswell. It had been observed that Boswell had demonstrated some consistency in seeking out certain staff members (e.g., he would go to a particularly generous staff member when he wanted something) despite his profound inability to consciously recognize people. To examine whether Boswell was able to form new preferences, the experimenters set up an extended series of positive, negative, and neutral encounters with three different confederates. When asked on a forced-choice recognition test to whom he would go for treats, he strongly preferred the positive confederate over the negative one, with the neutral confederate falling in between. This occurred despite his inability to recall anything about any of the people or to demonstrate familiarity with them in any way. These preferences were maintained over a period of years.

These two studies suggest that amnesics can learn new emotional associations of a conceptual nature that persist over long periods of time. They also suggest that emotional responses as reflected by fairly complex behavioral interactions can serve as another measure of spared memory function. This line of research may provide insights on emotional functioning in memory-impaired individuals, about which little is currently known. It has been argued that emotional and mnestic function can be anatomically dissociated within the medial temporal lobe, with emotional functioning depending more on the amygdala, and memory function relying more strongly on the hippocampal system (cf. Zola Morgan et al., 1991).

Classical Conditioning. It has long been known that amnesic patients may show intact classical conditioning of the eyeblink when a conditioned stimulus (CS) (e.g., a tone or light) is paired with an unconditioned stimulus (UCS) (airpuff) applied to the open eye (Weiskrantz and Warrington, 1979). Recent experiments have confirmed that amnesic patients with temporal lobe lesions (including the amnesic H.M.) can readily show both delay (Gabrieli et al., 1995a) and trace conditioning (Woodruff Pak, 1993) and can display the effects of conditioning over long periods of time (Schugens and Daum, 1999), even though they have no general recollection of the CS–UCS relationship or of the general experimental situation. However, one study (McGlinchey Berroth et al., 1997) reported impaired eyeblink conditioning in bitemporal amnesics using the trace-conditioning paradigm. Thus, available results suggest that the hippocampus is not essential for the acquisition of elementary CS–UCS associations in delay eyeblink conditioning. However, it has been demonstrated in at least one other study (McGlinchey Berroth et al., 1999) that the timing of conditioned responses may be abnormal in these patients. Patients with diencephalic damage appear to be impaired in classical eyeblink conditioning (McGlinchey Berroth et al., 1995) using the delay paradigm. A recent study suggested that awareness of the CS–UCS contingency may be critical in successful conditioning within both single-cue (CS+) and differential (CS+ and CS−) trace conditioning, which may help explain some of the discrepancies between delay and trace conditioning (Manns et al., 2000).

Theoretical Accounts of Spared vs. Impaired Learning

A number of theories have been generated to account for the differences between spared and impaired memory functions in amnesia. The most influential of these viewpoints will be discussed below.

Threshold Accounts. Originally, implicit memory was thought to represent a memory trace that was too weak to enter consciousness (Korsakoff, 1889; Prince, 1914; Leibniz, 1916). In this view, implicit memory and explicit memory are qualitatively the same; implicit memory traces are simply not strong enough to reach the threshold of activation necessary for explicit memory, just as some memory traces are strong enough to support recognition but not recall. According to this viewpoint, variables that affect explicit memory performance should have parallel effects on implicit memory, only at a different level of performance. A similar kind of notion has recently been proposed to explain the difference between the subjective states of remembering and knowing (Inoue and Bellezza, 1998). In this model, "remember" judgments reflect stronger traces and more conservative decision-making rules, while "know" judgments reflect weaker traces and more lenient response criteria (Donaldson, 1996; Hirshman and Master, 1997; Toth, 2000).

The idea that explicit memory and implicit memory differ only in sensitivity is contra-

dicted by numerous studies showing that, in normal and amnesic subjects, many variables that affect explicit memory have little or no effect on many forms of implicit memory, and vice versa (see Schacter, 1987a; Richardson-Klavehn and Bjork, 1988; Lewandowsky et al., 1989, for reviews). For example, increased study time or elaborative processing increases explicit memory but often has little effect on indirect tests such as repetition priming (Jacoby and Dallas, 1981). Conversely, manipulations that change perceptual or surface features of stimuli, such as letter case, typeface, or modality of presentation, reduce perceptual repetition priming effects but have little effect on explicit memory (Winnick and Daniel, 1970; Jacoby, 1983b; Blaxton, 1985; Roediger and Weldon, 1987). Other variables, including interference effects (Booker, 1991) and retention intervals (Tulving et al., 1982), have different effects on direct and indirect tests of memory.

Several studies have demonstrated that priming effects in word-fragment completion and mirror reading are statistically ("stochastically") independent of explicit memory (Tulving et al., 1982; Squire et al., 1985). When individual items are analyzed, the stimuli yielding evidence of explicit memory are often different from those yielding evidence of implicit recognition. This is contrary to a threshold account, which would predict that explicitly recognized stimuli would always be implicitly recognized as well.

A recent case study provides further evidence against a threshold account (Fleischman et al., 1997). In this study, a patient with a right temporal lobe excision for epilepsy relief showed normal recall and recognition memory for the modality and font of presented words as well as the words themselves, but showed impaired repetition priming in word identification and visual stem-completion tasks. This dissociation mirrors that usually seen in amnesia, and provides further evidence that implicit and explicit memory are qualitatively distinct.

Taken together, the weight of opposing data suggests that a threshold account of implicit–explicit dissociations is no longer viable.

Multiple Memory Systems Accounts. By far the most popular approach to explaining spared and impaired memory function in amnesia is to postulate the existence of two (or more) memory systems, each responsible for a different type of memory function and each operating according to different parameters (Sherry and Schacter, 1987; Schacter et al., 2000). The "episodic" vs. "semantic" memory distinction (Tulving, 1972, 1983) has been invoked to explain the fact that amnesics, despite profound impairments in establishing new memories, show relative sparing of general semantic knowledge. The distinction between "declarative" and "procedural" (more recently, "nondeclarative") memory (Cohen and Squire, 1980) was originally invoked to explain the relative sparing of skill learning in amnesic subjects. The distinction between "explicit" and "implicit" memory (Graf and Schacter, 1985; Schacter and Graf, 1986a, 1986b) evolved as a more general explanation of spared vs. impaired abilities, and attempted to distinguish between spared and impaired abilities on the basis of recollective experience (aware vs. unaware) and retrieval dynamics (deliberate vs. unintentional). It should be noted that these dichotomies are not mutually exclusive; they each attempt to account for specific findings within this vast literature.

Episodic vs. semantic memory. As indicated above, the amnesic patient retains substantial intellectual, linguistic, and social skill despite profound impairments in the ability to recall specific information encountered in prior learning episodes. Tulving's (1972, 1983) distinction between episodic memory (an autobiographical form of memory for contextually specific events) and semantic memory (general world knowledge, linguistic skill, vocabulary) appears to account for such a dissociation (Kinsbourne and Wood, 1975; Martin and Fedio, 1983; Weingartner et al., 1983; Cermak, 1984; Tulving, 1998). Many authors have argued that amnesia involves a selective impairment in episodic memory, leaving semantic memory largely intact.

Kinsbourne and Wood (1975) were among the first to formally suggest that amnesia could be accounted for in terms of the episodic–semantic distinction. While influential, their report was based largely on clinical observation

and a brief uncontrolled experiment. They asked amnesic patients to define common objects (e.g., "railroad ticket") and to then recall an event from their past in which such an object had been used. They found that the amnesics could provide adequate definitions, but were impaired in recalling specific autobiographical events. Cermak (1984) reported similar findings in a postencephalitic patient.

Cermak (1984) suggested that the episodic–semantic distinction could explain temporally graded retrograde amnesia. As biographical material ages, it becomes progressively more semantic. Through retelling, it becomes incorporated into personal history and becomes part of the personal or family folklore. More recent memories are less likely to have been retold or elaborated, and thus may retain more of an episodic quality. If amnesia reflects a selective impairment in episodic memory, then memories from more remote time periods would be relatively spared as a result of this process. This resembles the consolidation theory of memory, but suggests that cognitive operations, rather than automatic physiological processes, contribute to stable storage of memories in a form that remains accessible to amnesic patients.

If the episodic–semantic distinction reflects a general principle of brain organization, then these domains of memory should show double dissociation in cases of focal brain disease. As indicated above, there is ample evidence that episodic memory can be impaired in the absence of impairment in semantic memory. In addition, there is evidence that developmental amnesia does not preclude the acquisition of factual knowledge or language competence (Vargha-Khadem et al., 1997). There have also been several case reports demonstrating that semantic retrieval can be impaired in the absence of a deficit in episodic/autobiographical retrieval (De Renzi et al., 1987; Grossi et al., 1988; Yasuda et al., 1997).

Indeed, recent evidence suggests that many amnesics suffer impairments of semantic as well as episodic memory (Cermak et al., 1978; Cohen and Squire, 1981; Zola-Morgan et al., 1983; Butters et al., 1987; Verfaellie and Cermak, 1994; Squire and Zola, 1998). For example, Cermak et al. (1978) found that Korsakoff patients had difficulty generating words from what Collins and Loftus (1975) called "conceptual" semantic memory ("Name a fruit that is red"). Butters and colleagues (1987) similarly found Korsakoff amnesics deficient on a verbal fluency task. These results suggest that amnesia (at least the type seen in Korsakoff's syndrome) cannot be described as exclusively episodic in nature.

A more fundamental problem is that episodic and semantic memories are not easily dissociable behaviorally (Squire and Zola, 1998) and seem to involve activation of the same or similar structures in functional imaging studies (Schacter et al., 2000). Not only do they interact in complex ways (for example, episodic learning can have a stimulating effect on semantic search rate (Loftus and Cole, 1974), but also there is no widespread agreement on exactly what makes a memory episodic rather than semantic. This latter problem can be seen in several studies that evaluate the ability of amnesics to acquire new "semantic" knowledge after the onset of their amnesia (Gabrieli et al., 1988; Verfaellie et al., 2000). Squire (1987) suggests reserving the term "episodic" for acts of remembering that are specifically autobiographical.

One recent development of relevance to the episodic–semantic distinction is the finding that amnesic patients can show repetition priming for novel information first encountered after illness onset. The apparent relevance of the episodic–semantic distinction for this kind of dissociation arose from initial findings that normal subjects did not show repetition priming for material (e.g., nonwords) that had no preexisting semantic memory representation (Bentin and Moscovitch, 1988; Kersteen-Tucker, 1991). Initial data suggested that this also held true for amnesics. For example, Cermak and colleagues, (1985) found priming for words but not nonwords in amnesics, consistent with the then-prevailing view that priming reflected activation or modification of semantic memory (Scarborough et al., 1977; Mandler, 1980; Diamond and Rozin, 1984).

However, recent studies have cast doubt on this interpretation by showing normal priming of novel material (e.g., nonwords, novel line patterns and objects) in both normals (Jacoby and Dallas, 1981; Feustel et al., 1983; Jacoby, 1983a; Cermak et al., 1985; 1991; Musen and Treisman, 1991; Rueckl, 1991; Schacter et al., 1991) and amnesics (Smith and Oscar Berman, 1990; Gabrieli et al., 1991; Haist, Schacter et al., 1991; Haist et al., 1992; Musen and Squire, 1992; Bowers and Schacter, 1993; Gooding et al., 1993; Keane et al., 1994, 1995; Postle and Corkin, 1998). These findings suggest the acquisition of new episodic memories, not simply the activation of preexisting representations. As a result, it is now widely believed that amnesics are capable of some forms of episodic learning, but that they are generally unaware of the products of such learning.

In recent years, several cases of focal retrograde amnesia have renewed interest in the relationship between episodic and semantic memory (Kapur et al., 1989, 1992; O'Connor et al., 1992; Hodges and McCarthy, 1995; Hunkin et al., 1995; Carlesimo et al., 1998; Markowitsch et al., 1999). These patients show disproportionate impairment in memory for events and facts encountered prior to illness onset, but show relatively little anterograde memory impairment. In some cases (Markowitsch et al., 1999), a distinction within remote memory has been found in which the patient is impaired in retrieval of general knowledge but unimpaired in retrieval of remote autobiographical events. Available anatomic data suggest that damage to the anterior temporal cortex is involved in most cases of focal retrograde amnesia and that damage to limbic–diencephalic structures contributes to impairment in remote autobiographical memory. However, not all cases of focal retrograde amnesia are clearly suggestive of an episodic–semantic distinction, since careful analysis of the memory loss in many such cases reveals equivalent impairments in remote autobiographical memory as well as factual knowledge, thus implicating both episodic and semantic retrieval deficits (Kapur, 1999).

Declarative vs. procedural (nondeclarative) memory. As indicated above, despite profound impairment in conscious recollection of prior learning episodes, many amnesics show relatively good retention of previously acquired skills and can acquire new skills or procedures that are also dependent on specific learning experiences (Cohen and Squire, 1980; Nissen and Bullemer, 1987; Squire, 1987; Gabrieli et al., 1993; Tranel et al., 1994; Rich et al., 1996; Cohen et al., 1997). Borrowing from the artificial intelligence (Winograd, 1975) and cognitive psychology (Anderson, 1976) literature, Cohen and Squire (1980) suggested that two separate memory systems existed: one dedicated to "declarative" memory (e.g., knowing *that* something was learned), the other dedicated to "procedural" learning (e.g., knowing *how* to perform a skill). Declarative memory includes "the facts, lists, and data of conventional memory experiments and everyday remembering" (Squire, 1987, p. 158), and as such, operates on both episodic and semantic material. Skill learning has been described above. More recently, the term "nondeclarative" has been used in place of "procedural" (cf. Squire, 1987) to encompass skills, priming, conditioning, and other phenomena, in agreement with the classification system proposed earlier by Cermak et al. (1985).

Like the distinction between episodic and semantic memory, the declarative–nondeclarative distinction implies the existence of two separate memory *systems* that differ in their constituent contents and processes. For example, it has been argued that nondeclarative memory entails a knowledge base that cannot be inspected consciously and is not directly reflected in verbal report; in fact, numerous examples (e.g., driving, athletic skill) come to mind in which conscious verbal rehearsal or reflection might actually interfere with the execution of constituent procedures. In contrast, declarative memory entails explicit, verbal retrieval from a well-defined knowledge base; "it includes the facts, lists, and data of conventional memory experiments and everyday remembering" (Squire, 1987, p. 158).

What evidence exists that declarative and nondeclarative memory actually represent distinct memory systems? The behavioral database for this distinction overlaps substantially with that invoked to validate and sustain the distinction between explicit and implicit memory suggested by Graf and Schacter (see below), and consists mainly of demonstrations that amnesics are capable of learning new perceptual and motor skills despite a nearly total lack of explicit recall of experiences that led to such learning (Nissen and Bullemer, 1987; Squire and McKee, 1993; Knowlton et al., 1994; Hamann and Squire, 1995; Reber et al., 1996).

Anatomic evidence for the distinction between procedural and declarative memory comes from work by Zola-Morgan and Squire (1983, 1984) in the macaque. These authors have shown that medial temporal lesions impair declarative memory in the primate as assessed by delayed non-matching to sample. In contrast, these monkeys do not show impaired motor skill learning. They are able to retrieve a Life saver candy threaded onto a thin metal tube that has a right-angle bend at the end, and retain this motor skill over a 1-month interval as well as controls. Available human data also indicate that sensorimotor skill learning is intact in amnesics with basal forebrain lesions (Tranel et al., 1994). In contrast, patients with basal ganglia disease show impaired cognitive and motor skill learning in the absence of severe deficits in declarative memory (Saint-Cyr et al., 1988; Heindel et al., 1989; Knowlton et al., 1996; Westwater et al., 1998). These findings suggests that the memory system involved in declarative learning relies on anatomic structures different from those involved in learning how to perform certain tasks.

Explicit vs. implicit memory. The distinction between explicit and implicit memory has been discussed above. Sherry and Schacter (1987) suggested that separate memory systems may have evolved to efficiently perform functionally incompatible memory processes. The purpose of explicit memory is to represent specific contextual details of events so as to promote conscious, deliberate recollection of unique experiences. Explicit memory is thus highly context-dependent (Tulving and Pearlstone, 1966; Sherry and Schacter, 1987). In contrast, the purpose of implicit memory (which encompasses skill learning, priming, and other indirect forms of memory) is to preserve those aspects of learning situations that tend to recur across specific instances so that processing is facilitated the next time the situation recurs.

Activation Accounts. Activation accounts of memory dissociations have suggested that normal performance on indirect memory tests such as word-stem completion result from temporary, automatic activation of preexisting memory representations (Graf and Mandler, 1984). According to this view, explicit memory requires additional (effortful, elaborative) processing that is selectively impaired in amnesia. The activation view is also relevant to the episodic–semantic memory distinction because priming was initially thought to involve activation of memory representations already resident in semantic memory. Activation views were originally advanced to account for the fact that repetition priming effects tend to dissipate rapidly (Graf et al., 1984; Cermak et al., 1985) and to explain early findings that, in normals and amnesics, priming did not occur for stimuli that had no preexisting memory representations (Scarborough et al., 1977; Diamond and Rozin, 1984; Cermak et al., 1985; Bentin and Moscovitch, 1988; Kersteen-Tucker, 1991).

Two general findings have challenged the activation account. First, priming effects sometimes persist over several weeks or longer (Jacoby and Dallas, 1981; Schacter and Graf, 1986a), which pushes the concept of activation to unacceptable limits. Second, recent studies have shown normal priming of novel material (nonwords, novel line patterns, and new associations) in both normals (Jacoby and Dallas, 1981; Feustel et al., 1983; Jacoby, 1983a; Cermak et al., 1985, 1991; Musen and Triesman, 1990; Schacter et al., 1990; Rueckl, 1991; Goshen-Gottstein et al., 2000) and amnesics (Gabrieli et al., 1990; Schacter et al., 1991; Haist et al., 1992; Musen and Squire, 1992). Haist et al. (1992) found that amnesics showed entirely normal priming for both words and studied nonwords. These findings suggest the acquisition of new memories, not simply the activation of preexisting ones (Gooding et al., 2000).

Further evidence that new learning may underlie at least some forms of priming is provided by recent experiments showing long-lasting priming of novel solutions to complex sentence puzzles (McAndrews et al., 1987), new associations between words (Graf and Schacter, 1985; Schacter, 1985; Schacter and Graf, 1986; Goshen-Gottstein et al., 2000) new

nonverbal patterns (Musen and Squire, 1992), and orthographically illegal nonwords that cannot result from the activation of preexisting orthographic representations (Keane et al., 1995). For example, McAndrews et al. showed a mixed group of amnesic patients a series of difficult-to-comprehend sentences such as "The person was unhappy because the hole closed." Subjects were instructed that the sentence would become comprehensible if they could think of a specific key word or phrase (in this case, "pierced ears"). They had to come up with a solution within 1 minute, and if they did not, the experimenter presented the solution and asked the subject to explain it. Subsequent testing revealed that amnesics were able to generate the key word or phrase needed to solve the sentence puzzles (for periods up to 1 week) after only one exposure to the problem. This convincingly demonstrates that amnesics can implicitly learn and remember the meaning of novel sentences, and suggests that new episodic representations of the sentence–solution relationship can be formed after only a single exposure (Bowers and Schacter, 1993).

In other studies (Graf and Schacter, 1985; Schacter and Graf, 1986), amnesics were exposed to unrelated word pairs (e.g., "window–reason"). In a subsequent test, subjects were presented with the stem of the second word preceded either by the word with which it was studied (e.g., "window-rea___") or with a different word (e.g., "officer-rea___"). Subjects were asked to complete the stem with the first word that came to mind and were told that the preceding word might help them think of a completion. Amnesics with relatively mild memory problems (but not severely amnesic patients) demonstrated more priming when the stem was preceded by the word that originally accompanied it during the study phase than when it was preceded by a different word, thus demonstrating memory for a new association. Although conscious, explicit memory could not account for the findings (since subjects were unable to use the cues to explicitly recall the target words), the fact that priming occurred only in the mildly amnesic patients suggests at least a potential role for residual explicit memory in these effects (Bowers and Schacter, 1993; McKone and Slee, 1997).

Transfer-Appropriate Processing. An influential view of memory dissociations is that direct (e.g., free recall) and indirect (e.g., repetition priming) tasks differentially tap cognitive processes that tend to support explicit vs. implicit memory, respectively. The transfer-appropriate processing (TAP) approach to memory dissociations suggests that memory performance benefits to the extent that the cognitive operations needed to retrieve an item during the memory test overlap with the encoding operations performed during original learning (Blaxton, 1985, 1992, 1995; Roediger and Blaxton, 1987; Roediger et al., 1989, 1994). Most tests of explicit recall allegedly rely on the elaborative, semantic encoding, and have been referred to as reflecting "conceptually driven" processing (Jacoby, 1983a, 1983b). In contrast, most tests of implicit memory (e.g., stem completion, perceptual identification) depend upon the perceptual match between study and test, thus relying on what has been called "data-driven" processing. The resulting account of amnesia suggests that amnesics are capable of extensive data-driven processing, but are impaired in elaborative, conceptually driven processing. Unlike the activation view, the TAP approach views implicit memory effects as episodic in origin, rather than as based on activation of representations already present in semantic memory.

Support for the TAP account has been furnished in a series of experiments that demonstrate the importance of study–test correspondence in cognitive operations (Blaxton, 1985, 1992, 1995; Roediger, 1990; Roediger et al., 1994). Blaxton (1985; experiment 1) found that the relative strength of word-fragment completion and free recall depended on the activities engaged in during the study phase. In this experiment, better word-fragment completion was seen when subjects simply read words ("XXXX-COLD") than when they generated the words from associative cues ("hot-????"). In contrast, better free recall was seen in the generate condition. According to the TAP framework, word-fragment completion depends more on visual processing (which was greater during reading than generating), while free recall depends more on conceptual processing (which was greater during generating

than reading). The TAP approach thus emphasizes the notion of encoding specificity (Tulving and Pearlstone, 1966) and predicts better retrieval when encoding operations are recapitulated during the testing phase.

The TAP approach has encouraged greater specificity regarding the information-processing demands imposed by specific tests of implicit and explicit memory. Although direct tests of memory typically utilize conceptual processes while indirect tests rely more heavily on data-driven processes, both kinds of tests are likely to have both data-driven and conceptually driven components. For example, Blaxton (1985, experiment 2) has shown that certain direct memory tests (e.g., graphemic cued recall, where subjects are cued for a target word ["SUNRISE"] with a graphemically similar word ["SURMISE"]) are heavily data-driven, while certain indirect memory tests (e.g., having subjects study word pairs like "ESPIONAGE–treason," then asking "For what crime were the Rosenbergs executed"?) are conceptually driven. Thus, results of studies that demonstrate parallel effects on explicit and implicit memory may be confounded by the inclusion of conceptual material in an implicit task, or perceptual (data-driven) material in an explicit task.

Although the TAP viewpoint is useful in emphasizing the processing requirements imposed by commonly used tests of memory and in accounting for many of the behavioral dissociations found in the normal literature, there have been some recent findings that have called into question the main assumption that amnesics are deficient only on tasks that demand conceptual processing. In certain situations, amnesics have been shown to display impaired perceptual priming (Cermak et al., 1993; Gabrieli et al., 1994), and in others their performance has been normal on conceptual priming tasks (Keane et al., 1993; Carlesimo, 1994; Cermak et al., 1995). Although there is evidence that the distinction between perceptual and conceptual processing has a basis in functional brain anatomy (Keane et al., 1992; Gabrieli et al., 1995), it is likely that the implicit–explicit distinction may be more useful in the long term in understanding dissociations between what functions are spared and impaired in amnesic patients. Recent data and theory suggest that a combined view that incorporates both the implicit–explicit distinction and the perceptual–conceptual distinction may be most fruitful (Schacter et al., 2000).

Summary. In summarizing this brief review of theoretical accounts of memory dissociations, it is important to recognize that dissociations between implicit and explicit memory are quite diverse and are unlikely to be explained by a single mechanism. For example, activation and processing theories may account for different types of data; some types of implicit memory rely more heavily on activation of preexisting knowledge, whereas others are the result of the laying down of new memory traces based on processing similarities between study and test. The ability to perform indirect tasks that require the laying down of new memory traces may depend on severity of amnesia, while the ability to display activation effects may be less dependent on amnesia severity. In any case, there are clear instances in which amnesics demonstrate priming that depends on the laying down of new traces. To the extent that new traces are laid down, the strength of the nominal cue and type of measure may be critical in determining the duration of the effect.

It has long been known that performance on various direct measures of explicit memory (free recall, cued recall, and recognition) are dissociable; an obvious question for future research is whether indirect (implicit) measures will be similarly dissociated. Recent data on the double dissociation between skill learning and repetition priming in subcortical and cortical dementia (Heindel et al., 1989), and findings of stochastic independence between stem-completion and perceptual identification (Witherspoon and Moscovitch, 1989) suggest that implicit memory may itself be divisible into smaller subsystems (Vaidya et al., 1997).

One key issue that is receiving substantial attention in current literature is the notion that explicit and implicit memory can interact substantially in traditional tasks of memory (cf. Jacoby and Dallas, 1981; Jacoby et al., 1989). Even though a test superficially seems to evaluate explicit memory, performance on it may in part reflect the operation of implicit or un-

conscious processes. For example, Jacoby and Dallas (1981) argued that performance on recognition tests can be based on two relatively independent processes: direct (explicit) recollection, and an unconscious, or implicit, feeling of facilitated processing termed "perceptual fluency." Thus, one may select an item on forced-choice recognition because it is directly remembered or because it seems to "jump off of the page" as a result of perceptual priming or apparent familiarity. Because both explicit memory and implicit memory operate in the same direction (i.e., both would increase the probability of selecting a target item), it has been difficult to specify the relative contribution each has to recognition memory in normals and amnesics. Recently, a "process-dissociation" method has been developed to measure the separate contributions of recollection and fluency or familiarity in memory performances (Jacoby, 1991; Cermak et al., 1992; Kelley and Jacoby, 2000), although this has been criticized with respect to its assumption of two independent processes (Ratcliff et al., 1995; Dodson and Johnson, 1996). It is likely that research in the next decade will lead to increasing specificity with regard to the processes and anatomical substrates of different forms of memory (Schacter et al., 2000).

ANATOMIC CORRELATES OF AMNESIA

The amnesic syndrome can result from focal damage to the medial temporal lobes, the medial thalamus, or the basal forebrain. Anatomically related areas, including the fornix and the retrosplenial cortex, have also been implicated. Anatomic, physiologic, and behavioral studies in nonhuman primates have suggested why these regions may be important for memory. The extensive experimental literature on memory in rats and other non-primates will not be summarized here.

TEMPORAL LOBE

Although there were previous reports of temporal lobe lesions in amnesic patients (von Bechterew, 1900; Grünthal 1947; Glees and Griffith, 1952), the importance of the temporal lobes in memory was established by reports of severe and permanent amnesia after bilateral resections of the medial aspects of the temporal lobes in humans (Scoville, 1954; Scoville and Milner, 1957). The aim of surgery was either to ameliorate psychotic behavior or to treat intractable focal epilepsy. H.M., who was treated for epilepsy, is the best studied of such patients, having been the subject of numerous reports over nearly five decades.

Temporal Lobe Anatomy

H. M.'s intended lesions extended 8 to 9 cm back from the temporal poles, and included the amygdala, the hippocampus, and the parahippocampal region. An understanding of the anatomic connections of these regions is necessary to appreciate the ways in which they may subserve memory. The discussion will focus on the hippocampus and parahippocampal region, since both have been implicated in human and animal studies of amnesia.

The Hippocampus and Parahippocampal Region. The hippocampus is a phylogenetically ancient cortical structure consisting of the dentate gyrus, the sectors of Ammon's horn (cornu Ammonis [CA] 1–4), and subiculum (Fig. 18–1). The internal connections of the hippocampus were identified by Ramón y Cajal and his student Lorrente de Nó (cited by Van Hoesen, 1985), who first described the trisynaptic circuit. Neurons of the entorhinal cortex project via the perforant pathway to synapse on dendrites of granule cells in the dentate gyrus. Granule cell axons project to the dendrites of pyramidal cells in the CA3 region of Ammon's horn (mossy fiber projection). These pyramidal cells have axons that bifurcate, one branch projecting subcortically via the fimbria fornix, and the other to CA1 (Shaffer collateral pathway). CA1 neurons project subcortically via the fimbria, but also to the subiculum, which is the major source of hippocampal efferent projections (Rosene and Van Hoesen, 1977). Efferent fibers from the subiculum project either to subcortical targets (via the fimbria and fornix) or to other cortical regions. The subiculum also projects back to the entorhinal cortex, completing a circuit. The connections described are unidirectional, suggesting an or-

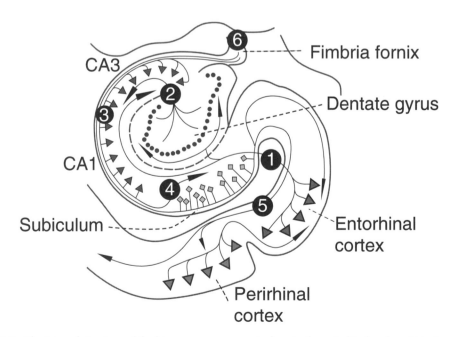

Figure 18–1. The internal structure of the hippocampus. The circled numbers indicate: (1) The perforant pathway; (2) projections from the dentate to CA3; (3) from CA3 to CA1; (4) from CA1 to the subiculum; (5) from the subiculum to the entorhinal and perirhinal cortices, and (6) the subcortical projections of CA3, CA1 and subiculum via the fimbria fornix.

Figure 18–2. The amygdala, hippocampus, and parahippocampal region. The positions of the amygdala (A) and hippocampus (H) are indicated on the left. On the right, the overlying parahippocampal region cortical structures are indicated, namely, the entorhinal cortex (E), perirhinal cortex (P) and parahippocampal cortex (PH).

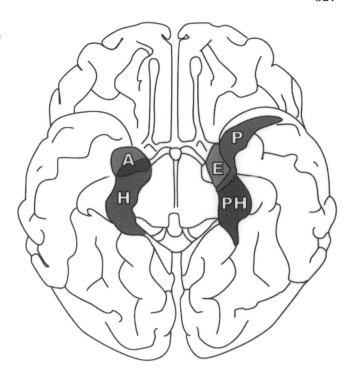

derly progression of information through the hippocampus. The pyramidal cells of CA1 (also called Sommer's sector) are exquisitely sensitive to hypoxia, and loss of these neurons is thought to account for the amnesic syndrome seen in some patients who survive cardiac arrest or other hypoxic events.

Although there are direct cortical connections to the hippocampus proper, for example, cingulate and retrosplenial projections to the subiculum (Mufson and Pandya, 1984; Insuasti et al., 1987a), the majority of hippocampal cortical connections are with the adjacent parahippocampal region. The parahippocampal region consists of rhinal (entorhinal and perirhinal)

cortex, pre- and parasubicular cortex, and parahippocampal cortex (Scharfman et al., 2000) (Fig. 18–2, Table 18–1). The parahippocampal region is hierarchically organized, with the entorhinal cortex being the final common pathway to the hippocampus (Van Hoesen and Pandya, 1975) (Fig. 18–3). The entorhinal cortex receives afferents from perirhinal cortex and the parahippocampal gyrus (Rosene and Van Hoesen, 1977; Van Hoesen et al., 1979; Irle and Markowitsch, 1982; Insausti et al., 1987a). These regions in turn receive projections from polymodal and unimodal association cortex and from supramodal cortices, thus providing entorhinal

Table 18–1. Anatomic Designations

Individual Designations		Collective Designations	
Dentate gyrus			
Ammon's horn (CA1–4)		Hippocampus	
Subiculum			
Presubiculum			
Parasubiculum			
Entorhinal cortex	Rhinal	Parahippocampal region	
Perirhinal cortex	cortex		
Parahippocampal gyrus (areas TH, TF in macaque; post-rhinal cortex in rat)			

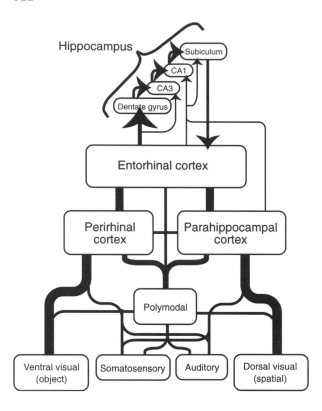

Figure 18–3. Hierarchichal connectivity of the parahippocampal region. The entorhinal cortex is the principal gateway to the hippocampus. Much of the input to entorhinal cortex comes from perirhinal and entorhinal cortices. The visual object stream is preferentially directed to perirhinal cortex, whereas the visual spatial stream is directed to parahippocampal cortex. Lines without arrows indicate bi-directional connections. Adapted from Suzuki and Eichenbaum (2000).

cortex with indirect access to a variety of highly processed information (Van Hoesen et al., 1972; Amaral et al., 1983; Van Hoesen, 1985; Insausti et al., 1987a). Unlike the intrinsic hippocampal connections, which are unidirectional, the connections of the parahippocampal region are reciprocal (Rosene and Van Hoesen, 1977). Both perirhinal and parahippocampal cortices are connected with visual and polymodal cortical regions, and, to a lesser extent, with somatosensory cortex; but only the parahippocampal cortex receives substantial input from parietal polysensory and auditory cortices (see Suzuki and Eichenbaum, 2000).

Subcortical projections from the hippocampus travel in the fornix, a white matter structure that arches through the lateral ventricle and descends medial to the foramen of Munro into the lateral wall of the third ventricle, where it divides at the anterior commissure. Fibers from CA1, CA3, and the subiculum project in the pre-commissural fornix to the lateral septal nucleus (Swanson and Cowan, 1979). Other subicular projections travel in the post-commissural fornix and terminate in either the anterior nuclear complex of the thal-

amus or the mammillary bodies (Swanson and Cowan, 1979; Van Hoesen, 1985). There are also hippocampal projections to the amygdala, nucleus accumbens, and other regions in the basal forebrain, and to the ventromedial hypothalamus (Swanson and Cowan, 1979; Amaral and Insausti, 1990).

The hippocampal → post-commissural fornix → mammillary body projection is evident upon gross inspection of the brain, and was part of the circuit described by Papez in 1937 to explain how emotional expression and feeling, mediated by the hypothalamus, could be coordinated with cognition, mediated by the cortex. The hippocampus projects via the post-commissural fornix to the mammillary bodies, which, in turn, project via the mammillothalamic tract to the anterior nuclei of the thalamus. The circuit is completed by thalamic projections to the cingulate gyrus and cingulate projections, via the cingulate bundle to the hippocampus (Fig. 18–4).

The hippocampus also receives subcortical projections from the basal forebrain (medial septal nucleus and the nucleus of the diagonal band of Broca), from midline, anterior, and lat-

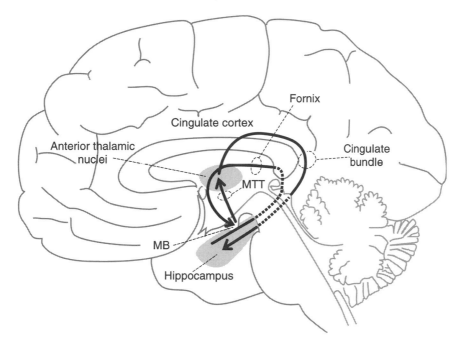

Figure 18–4. Papez' circuit. A schematic drawing of Papez circuit, from the hippocampus via the fornix to the mammillary body (MB) of the hypothalamus; thence via the mamillothalamic tract (MMT) to the anterior thalamic nuclei; thence to the cingulate cortex and via the cingulate bundle to the hippocampus.

erodorsal thalamic nuclei, and from amygdala, hypothalamus, and brainstem, including the central gray, ventral tegmental area, raphé nuclei and locus coeruleus (Herkenham, 1978; Amaral and Cowan, 1980; Van Hoesen, 1985; Insuasti et al., 1987b; Amaral and Insausti, 1990).

The Amygdala. The amygdala is situated immediately anterior to the hippocampus, and deep to the periamygdaloid and perirhinal cortices. It can be broadly conceived as having two parts: a large basolateral group of nuclei, with extensive connections to limbic and association cortex and to dorsomedial thalamus, and a smaller corticomedial segment, which extends into the basal forebrain and has extensive connections with basal forebrain, hypothalamus, and brainstem (DeOlmos, 1990; Heimer and Alheid, 1991; Scott et al., 1991). In a very general sense, the connections of amygdala and hippocampus are similar: both are strongly interconnected with frontal and temporal limbic cortex, and thus have indirect access to polymodal and supramodal neocortical association

areas (Herzog and Van Hoesen, 1976; Rosene and Van Hoesen, 1977). Both project to basal forebrain and hypothalamus. The amygdala and hippocampus also have direct interconnections (Poletti, 1986; Insuausti et al., 1987b; Saunders et al., 1988).

But there are also striking anatomic differences. Although in the brains of higher mammals the amygdala is adjacent to the hippocampus, it differs radically from the hippocampus in structure and derivation. The amygdala is a largely subcortical structure, intimately related to the basal forebrain, and is often classified as one of the basal ganglia. The amygdala is more closely related to limbic and neocortical regions of paleocortical derivation, whereas the hippocampus is archicortical and is more closely related to cortex of archicortical derivation (Pandya and Yeterian, 1990). Thus, the amygdala is more closely related to orbitofrontal and anterior temporal cortex (Porrino et al., 1981), and the hippocampus is more closely related to cingulate cortex. Abnormalities in emotional responsiveness and social interactions are associated with lesions in the amygdala and related anterior temporal and orbitofrontal cortex (Butter and Snyder, 1972).

The subcortical connections of the amygdala also differ from those of the hippocampus. Whereas the hippocampus is related through Papez' circuit with the mammillary bodies and the anterior thalamic nuclei, the amygdala has projections to the dorsomedial nucleus of the thalamus (Nauta, 1961). Basal forebrain connections also differ: the hippocampus is related to more ventral portions of the septal nuclei, and the amygdala has more extensive connections with the bed nucleus of the stria terminalis. Cholinergic projections to the amygdala are from the nucleus basalis of Meynert, whereas the hippocampus receives input from the septal region and diagonal band of Broca (Mesulam et al., 1983). Finally, the amygdala has connections with brainstem autonomic centers (nucleus of the tractus solitarius), providing a direct pathway for limbic–autonomic interaction.

Hippocampal Physiology

Physiological studies reveal cellular mechanisms that could subserve memory in the hippocampus. High-frequency stimulation of the perforant path enhances transmission at synapses in the dentate gyrus. This enhancement, called "long-term potentiation" (LTP), can last weeks (Bliss and Gardner-Medwin, 1973; Lomo, 1971; Bliss and Lomo 1973). Long-term potentiation can be homosynaptic (caused by repetitive firing of one input), heterosynaptic (occurring when two particular inputs to a single neuron fire coincidently), or hebbian (occurring when stimulation of a neuronal afferent occurs when a neuronal cell body is coincidentally depolarized (Bailey et al., 2000). The last two kinds of LTP could represent mechanisms by which two coincident stimuli are associated (see Kennedy, 1989). Further studies have identified cellular mechanisms underlying LTP (see Gustaffsson and Wigstrom, 1988; Kennedy, 1989; Matthies et al., 1990; Bailey et al., 2000). In the experimental setting, drugs that block specific kinds of glutamate receptors may interfere with both LTP and memory (see Izquierdo, 1991). Long-term potentiation is not unique to the hippocampus, however. The access of the hippocampus to highly processed information from many neocortical regions, combined with a mechanism to preserve associations, provides the anatomical and physiologic basis for its putative role in memory.

Behavioral Effects of Temporal Lobe Lesions

Early studies of patients with bilateral temporal lobectomy supported the idea that damage to the hippocampus was necessary for medial temporal lesions to produce amnesia. Scoville and Milner (1957) reviewed 10 patients with bilateral medial temporal resections. Removal of the uncus and amygdala (in one patient) caused no memory loss, but resections that extended posteriorly to involve the hippocampus and parahippocampal gyrus were associated with amnesia. Also, amnesia was more severe with more extensive resections. The relationship between the extent of resection and the severity of amnesia also held for the selective verbal or nonverbal amnesias that followed, respectively, left or right temporal resections (Milner, 1972, 1974; Smith, 1989). Scoville and Milner concluded that amnesia would not occur unless the surgery extended far enough back to involve the hippocampus. The importance of the hippocampus was also supported by Penfield and Milner (1958), who reported two patients with amnesia following unilateral temporal resections. They speculated that preexisting contralateral hippocampal damage explained the severe amnesia after unilateral resection. This was confirmed when one of the patients (P.B.) was found at autopsy to have hippocampal sclerosis in the unoperated temporal lobe, but no damage to other temporal cortical structures or to the amygdala (Penfield and Matheison, 1974).

The case for the importance of the hippocampus in memory was subsequently made even more convincingly by the study of patients who survived cardiopulmonary arrest with well-documented deficits in memory, and whose brains were carefully examined after they died from other causes (Cummings et al., 1984; Zola-Morgan et al., 1986; Victor and Agamanolis, 1990). In each case, damage was restricted almost entirely to the hippocampus, where the pyramidal neurons of CA1, exquisitely sensitive to hypoxia, were selectively destroyed. Global ischemia in the monkey causes similar lesions, with scores on memory tasks comparable to those of monkeys with surgical lesions restricted to the hippocampus (Squire and Zola-Morgan, 1991).

Understanding the anatomic substrate of memory was an obvious target for animal research, since the effects of excision of specific regions could be studied; however, it took nearly two decades after Scoville's original reports before an animal model for human amnesia was developed. In 1978, three influential publications supported widely disparate views. Horel (1978) reviewed the literature available at the time and concluded that the hippocampus was probably not necessary for memory, but that other medial temporal structures, in particular the temporal stem, amygdala, and temporal neocortex, were critical. The temporal stem connected these medial temporal regions with the diencephalon. O'Keefe and Nadel (1978) suggested that the hippocampus, which in rodents could be demonstrated to contain neurons that were activated specifically in relation to an animal's movement through the environment, provided a spatial map. They speculated that in humans an analogous process might serve to record not only spatial but also nonspatial cognitive relationships. This view has recently gained more interest; however, in 1978 it was eclipsed to some degree by studies that established an animal model for human amnesia.

The third view, advanced by Mishkin (1978), suggested that the experimental paradigms for testing memory in animals had simply not been adequate to demonstrate the amnesia that in fact had resulted from medial temporal resections. Gaffan (1974) and Mishkin and Petri (1984) pointed out that recognition memory tests using trial-unique stimuli more nearly approximate the tasks that present problems for human amnesics. Tests that use repeated trials with the same set of stimuli and enable response habits to be formed can be performed well both by human amnesics and animals with medial temporal resections (Mishkin and Petri, 1984). Similarly, both human amnesics and

monkeys with medial temporal lesions can learn new skills (Zola-Morgan and Squire, 1983, 1984). Gaffan (1974) used a delayed matching-to-sample (DMS) task with trial-unique stimuli. The animals were shown a single object, and after a delay this object was presented again along with a new object. The animals were rewarded when they selected the previously shown object. Hundreds of different objects were used so that habitual responses could not develop. Animals with fornix lesions were impaired on this task relative to controls. The delayed non-matching-to-sample (DNMS) task used by Mishkin (1978) was similar except that the animal was rewarded for selecting the new object rather than the previously seen object. This task was learned more readily than the DMS task by normal monkeys, who presumably were drawn to novelty. Monkeys with extensive medial temporal lesions, involving both amygdala and hippocampus, were markedly impaired on the DNMS task. Human amnesics have been tested with the DMS task (Sidman et al., 1968) and the DNMS task (Oscar-Berman and Bonner, 1985; Squire et al., 1988; Zola-Morgan and Squire, 1990a), which they do not perform as well as normal subjects. Other tasks have also been developed that are sensitive to medial temporal lesions in monkeys and that present difficulties for human amnesics (Squire et al., 1988; Zola-Morgan and Squire, 1990a).

The Dual System Theory of Amnesia. The observation that medial temporal lesions involving both the amygdala and the hippocampus produce much more severe deficits on DNMS tasks than lesions that involve either one of these structures alone led to the hypothesis that two parallel systems subserve memory, one involving the hippocampus and the other the amygdala (Mishkin, 1978, 1982; Mishkin and Saunders, 1979; Mishkin et al., 1982). Because either system can subserve memory in large part, lesions in both systems are required to produce severe amnesia. In a series of experiments, Mishkin and colleagues extended their observations to the subcortical projections of these two medial temporal structures. The systems were the two limbic circuits described above: Papez' circuit, involving the hippocampus, fornix, anterior thalamic nuclei, and cingulate cortex, and the lateral limbic circuit involving the anterior temporal cortex and amygdala, amydalofugal pathways, dorsomedial thalamus, and orbitofrontal cortex. Thus lesions that interrupt both the fornix (disrupting Papez' circuit) and the ventral amygdalofugal pathways (disrupting the lateral circuit) cause severe amnesia, whereas lesions restricted to either pathway cause little or no memory disturbance (Bachevalier et al., 1985a, 1985b). Lesions that affect either the posteromedial or anteromedial aspect of the thalamus cause little memory disturbance; but severe amnesia, comparable to that associated with medial temporal ablations, occurs only when *both* anterior and posterior medial thalamic regions are involved (Aggleton and Mishkin, 1983). Finally, lesions that affect the frontal projections of both Papez' circuit (anterior cingulate gyrus) and the lateral circuit (ventromedial frontal lobe) produce greater memory loss than lesions of either alone (Bachevalier and Mishkin, 1986). This series of studies on primates suggests *(1)* that structures within each memory system are highly interdependent, since damage to different parts of each system can cause apparently equivalent deficits; and *(2)* that each system can, to a large extent, carry on the function of the other, since lesions affecting only one system result in little or no memory loss.

This theory had to be modified when it was demonstrated that collateral damage to the perirhinal cortex was responsible for the memory deficits seen after amygdala lesions. Stereotactic lesions of the amygdala sparing perirhinal cortex do not add to the memory deficit of animals with hippocampal and parahippocampal gyrus lesions (Zola-Morgan et al., 1989a). Zola-Morgan et al. (1989b) found that lesions involving both perirhinal and parahippocampal cortex but not the hippocampus cause severe memory impairment in the monkey. This is not explained entirely by interruption of cortical input to the hippocampus, because monkeys with this lesion had *more* severe memory deficits than monkeys with lesions that only involved the hippocampus and parahippocampal gyrus (Zola-Morgan and Squire, 1986; Squire and Zola-Morgan, 1991). Similar findings were re-

ported by Meunier et al. (1993). This suggests that the perirhinal cortex not only conveys information to the hippocampus via entorhinal cortex but contributes to memory in its own right. Because both the amygdala and the perirhinal cortex project to dorsomedial thalamus, the dual system theory could be easily modified by substituting perirhinal cortex for the amygdala.

The Amygdala. Amygdala lesions in nonhuman primates have been associated with impairments in stimulus–reward association (Jones and Mishkin, 1972; Spiegler and Mishkin, 1981) and the association of affect with neutral stimuli (Iwata et al., 1986; Gaffan and Harrison, 1987; LeDoux, 1987; McGaugh et al., 1990), and with defects in social and emotional behavior (Kling and Stecklis, 1976; Zola-Morgan et al., 1989a). In humans, stimulation of the amygdala is particularly likely to result in emotional experiences (Gloor, 1986; see also Chapter 16, this volume). Hippocampal lesions appear to have no effect on the emotional behavior of nonhuman primates (Squire and Zola-Morgan, 1991). The literature cited above suggests that amygdala lesions in primates do not impair performance on standard tests of memory, and that deficits in cross-modal association and memory previously attributed to amygdala lesions resulted from damage to overlying perirhinal cortex.

The literature on human amnesia also sheds little light on the amygdala's function in memory. Narabayashi et al. (1963) reported a series of patients with unilateral or bilateral stereotactic amygdalectomies, many of whom were severely impaired prior to surgery. Although these patients were thought to be free of memory loss postoperatively, specific memory testing was not reported. Milner (1966) reported no deficits in patients with anterior temporal lobe resections that included the amygdala but spared the hippocampus; Andersen (1978) reported inconsistent and relatively mild memory deficits in patients with unilateral stereotactic amygdalotomies. Lee et al. (1988) found no deficits in a patient with bilateral stereotactic amygdalectomies on a cross-modal memory task. Tranel and Hyman (1990) reported memory deficits in a patient with bilateral amygdala calcifications secondary to lipoid proteinosis (Urbach-Wiethe disease); however, microscopic involvement of hippocampus, which may not have been apparent on magnetic resonance (MR) scanning, has been reported in this illness (Holtz, 1962). Thus the contention that amgydala lesions contribute to amnesia in humans remains to be conclusively demonstrated.

It appears, then, that the amygdala is more important for emotion than memory, whereas (despite Papez' prediction) the reverse is true of the hippocampus. Could the amygdala be important in mediating aspects of emotional memory? Damasio et al. (1989) reported that Boswell, a post-encephalitic patient with bilateral temporal and orbitofrontal damage including the amygdala, demonstrated preferences for individuals who had treated him better on the ward, even though he had no explicit memory for these persons or for the incidents that determined his preferences. Baxter and Murray (2002) review evidence that animals with basolateral amygdala lesions express preferences for rewarded stimuli, but fail to modify responses when the reward value of the reinforcer is modified. These animals will perform normally on tasks of learning and memory that do not require them to assign value to a reinforcer, or update the current value of the reinforcer, but they fail to adjust their behavior in response to changes in the reward value of the reinforcer. These are aspects of behavior not usually assessed in standard memory tasks.

Role of Temporal Neocortex vs. Hippocampus. Perirhinal cortical lesions affect performance on DNMS tasks more than hippocampal lesions. In fact, isolated hippocampal lesions in monkeys produce little or no deficit in DNMS performance (Murray et al., 1993; Murray and Mishkin, 1998; but see Alvarez et al., 1995), leading some investigators to question whether there is a role for the hippocampus in memory. Loring et al. (1991) found no difference in verbal memory performance between patients with dominant temporal lobectomies that spared or involved the hippocampus, and Pigott and Milner (1993) found that patients with right temporal lobectomies had visual memory

impairments independent of hippocampal involvement. In animals, lesions of the hippocampus or fornix result in deficits in spatial memory tasks (Mahut and Moss, 1986; Parkinson et al., 1988; Angeli et al., 1993; Malkova et al., 1995; Wan et al., 1999), suggesting that perirhinal cortex and hippocampus may subserve different aspects of memory. Pigott and Milner (1993) found that patients with right temporal resections involving the hippocampus had difficulty recalling object location. There is ample evidence, however, that humans with hippocampal damage, and in particular anoxic injury restricted to CA1, have marked impairment of episodic memory. O'Keefe and Nadel (1978) proposed that episodic memory in humans may make use of brain mechanisms that originally evolved to map spatial relationships. Gaffen has suggested that the relationship between the hippocampal spatial ability and episodic memory is in the ability to associate an object with a specific spatial background, defining an episodic event (Gaffen and Parker, 1996) Spatial information may reach the hippocampus by way of parietal projections to parahippocampal cortex. The parahippocampal gyrus appears to be important for topographic orientation.

The perirhinal cortex, by contrast, can be considered the last link in a chain of visual association cortices in the ventral visual stream critical for object identification. It also has input from other modalities. Murray and Bussey (1999) suggest that perirhinal cortex can encode objects in sufficient complexity as to allow recognition in the most varied circumstances. Monkeys with perirhinal cortical lesions lose the ability to make discriminations on DNMS tasks that they learned preoperatively, but they are nevertheless able to acquire similar discriminations postoperatively (Thorton et al., 1997). Murray and Bussey (1999) postulate that the preoperative discriminations were made on the basis of the most complex analysis of the properties of the object mediated by perirhinal cortex. Postoperatively, the animal can no longer make these kinds of discriminations and fails the task; however, the animal can acquire new discriminations based on less complex analysis mediated by remaining association cortex proximal to the perirhinal cortex. Murray and Bussey propose that perirhinal cortex contributes to networks subserving semantic memory.

This network may involve anterior temporal and inferotemporal neocortex. Lesions of anterior temporal neocortex (temporal pole and portions of the inferotemporal cortex) in monkeys impair performance on DNMS (Spiegler and Mishkin, 1981) and DMS tasks (Horel et al., 1984; Cirillo et al., 1989; George et al., 1989). Horel and colleagues have provided evidence that this cannot be accounted for by impairment in visual discrimination, and they argue that anterior and inferior temporal neocortex contribute to memory (George et al., 1989; see also Horel, 1978). Some patients with anterior unilateral temporal lobectomy sparing the hippocampus have been reported to demonstrate limited memory deficits (Ojemann and Dodrill, 1985; Smith, 1989). Damasio and colleagues (1985, 1987, 1989) suggest that the temporally extensive retrograde amnesia of their postencephalitic patient Boswell might be attributed to anterior temporal neocortical destruction. Boswell's severe retrograde amnesia distinguished him from H.M., whose lesions spared most temporal neocortical areas. Damasio and colleagues propose that anterior temporal neocortex is an area of "convergence zones" in which the unique spatiotemporal complexity of specific events is encoded. Without these convergence zones, Boswell could not reconstruct previous memories or lay down a record to preserve new memories. They suggest that his deficit would have been just as great had the medial temporal structures been spared (Damasio et al., 1989). This, however, is speculative, and it is possible that the severity of his retrograde amnesia reflects instead the co-occurrence of temporal with frontal and/or basal forebrain lesions. Kapur et al. (1992) described severe retrograde amnesia in a woman following closed head injury. Anterograde amnesia cleared nearly completely within 6 months of the injury, but the patient was left with severe retrograde amnesia. Magnetic resonance scans showed bilateral anterior temporal lesions sparing the hippocampus. Head injury, however, typically causes more widespread damage, particularly to subcortical structures. Kapur et al.'s case did have acute frontal white matter changes on MRI. The documentation of severe retrograde amnesia with little or no persisting anterograde amnesia is significant, but localization to anterior temporal requires confirmation. Reed and Squire (1998) described little or no retrograde general or autobiographical memory loss in two patients with moderately severe anterograde amnesia from presumed isolated hippocampal pathology, whereas two patients with postencephalitic amnesia, who had extensive temporal lobe damage not restricted to the hippocampus, had impairments of retrograde as well as anterograde memory.

In summary, the temporal lobes play a significant role in memory; however, the relative contribution of different temporal lobe structures remains to be worked out. At this point, one can argue on the basis of animal models that the hippocampus has a particular role in spatial memory, and that object memory may be more dependent on perirhinal cortex. The hippocampus in humans may subserve episodic memory, and the perirhinal cortex may be necessary to establish semantic memories. The ability of children with hypoxic damage to the hippocampus to acquire semantic information (Vargha-Kardem et al., 1997) and of amnesic patients to acquire new vocabulary words (Verfaellie et al., 2000) suggests some degree of independence between these kinds of memory; however, there is presently not enough evidence to support a neat anatomic parcellation of these functions. A related distinction between episodic recall and recognition memory is made by Aggelton and Brown (1999), who attribute the former to the hippocampal/diencephalic circuit of Papez, and the latter to the perirhinal cortex and dorsomedial thalamus.

PAPEZ' CIRCUIT

The pathologic evidence of mammillary body damage in patients with Wernike-Korsakoff disease combined with the evidence that medial temporal resections result in amnesia led to speculation that Papez' circuit (hippocampus → fornix → mammillary bodies → anterior thalamus → cingulate gyrus → hippocampus) forms the anatomic substrate of memory (Fig. 18–4) (Delay and Brion, 1969). We have already discussed the role of the hippocampus. We will briefly consider the evidence that other components of Papez' circuit are important for memory.

Fornix

It was once widely held that surgical section of the columns of the fornix would not result in memory loss (Dott, 1938; Cairns and Mosberg, 1951; Garcia Bengochea et al., 1954; Woolsey and Nelson, 1975), although there was some early evidence to suggest that memory loss might occur (Hassler and Riechert, 1957; Sweet et al., 1959). Heilman and Sypert (1977) argued that the amnesia experienced by a patient with a tumor near the splenium of the corpus callosum resulted from damage to the fornix. They pointed out that lesions of the fornix posterior to the anterior commissure affect not only fibers destined for the mammillary bodies but also disrupt connections between the hippocampus and the basal forebrain, and direct projections from the hippocampus to the anterior thalamic nuclei (Veazey et al., 1982; Aggleton et al., 1986). They suggested that section of the columns of the fornix ventral to the anterior commissure may not cause amnesia, as it only affects projections to the mammillary bodies. Subsequent experience strongly suggests that fornix damage is usually attended by some degree of amnesia in both animals (Gaffan, 1974; Moss et al., 1981; Owen and Butler, 1981; Carr, 1982; Bachevalier et al., 1985a, 1985; Gaffen, 1993) and humans (Grafman et al., 1985; Gaffan and Gaffan, 1991; Gaffan et al., 1991; Calabrese et al., 1995; D'Esposito et al., 1995b; McMackin et al., 1995; Aggleton et al., 2000; Moudgil et al., 2000; Park et al., 2000). The memory loss that sometimes follows section of the corpus callosum has been attributed to incidental damage to the fornix (Clark and Geffen, 1989). In primates, fornix damage, like hippocampal lesions, impairs spatial memory and memory for objects in a scene, a paradigm that Gaffan (Gaffan and Parker, 1996) suggests is related to episodic memory. In humans, fornix lesions have been found to affect recall more than recognition (familiarity) memory (Aggleton and Brown, 1999), and to cause anterograde but not retrograde amnesia (but see Yasuno et al., 1999).

Mammillary Bodies

The anatomy of mammillary body connections is summarized by Aggleton and Sahgal (1993). This paired hypothalamic nucleus receives substantial input from the hippocampus. There are projections from the subicular complex of the hippocampus through the fornix to the medial mammillary nucleus, which is more affected than the lateral mammillary nucles in Wernicke-Korsakoff disease. There are also hippocampal projections to the lateral mammillary nucleus and tuberomammillary nucleus. These hippocampal–mammillary body connections are not reciprocated. Mamillothalamic projections are also unidirectional. The mammillary bodies also project to the medial septum and midbrain.

The presence of prominent mammillary body damage in Wernicke-Korsakoff syndrome first suggested their importance in memory (Gamper, cited by Victor et al., 1971). Victor and colleagues (1971) examined the mammillary bodies and the dorsomedial thalamic nucleus of 43 alcoholics: 5 had had suffered Wernicke's encephalopathy but had recovered without evidence of memory loss; 38 had Wernicke-Korsakoff disease, with persistent amnesia. At autopsy, all had lesions of the mammillary bodies, but only the 38 patients with persistent memory loss had lesions involving the dorsomedial thalamic nucleus. They concluded that memory loss could not be attributed solely to mammillary body damage, and was more likely to be associated with thalamic lesions. Mair and colleagues (1979) and Mayes et al. (1988) each reported two cases of Wernicke-Korsakoff syndrome with lesions in the thalamus restricted to a thin band of gliosis adjacent to the third ventricle that affected the midline nuclei but not the dorsomedial nucleus. Mair et al. (1979) suggested that the mammillary body lesions (present in each of these patients) may account for the memory loss. Lesions restricted to the mammillary bodies have not been associated with deficits on DNMS tasks in monkeys (Aggleton and Mishkin, 1985); however, deficits have been found on spatial memory tasks in monkeys (Parker and Gaffan, 1997) and in rats (Sziklas and Petrides, 1998). Human cases with selective mammillary body lesions are rare. Dusoir et al. (1990) reported amnesia in a patient with MR evidence of mammillary body lesions following a penetrating injury from a snooker cue (Dusoir et al., 1990). Loesch et al. (1995) reported memory deficits in a patient with a cavernous malformation of the mammillary bodies, and Tanaka et al. (1997) reported memory loss with mammillary body damage following removal of a cystic craniopharyngioma. It is difficult to exclude extramammillary lesions in these cases, especially to adjacent portions of the hypothalamus or basal forebrain

Anterior Thalamic Nuclei

The anterior thalamic nuclei consist of anteromedial (am), anteroventral (av), anterodorsal (ad), and lateral dorsal (ld) nuclei. The medial mammillary nucleus projects ipsilaterally to am and av; whereas the lateral mammillary nucleus projects bilaterally to ad (see Aggleton and Sahgal, 1993). The anterior thalamic nuclei also receive a substantial direct projection from the hippocampus. Pre- and parasubiculum project to av, subiculum to am, and the hippocampus also projects to ld. All of these hippocampal–thalamic projections are reciprocated.

The anterior thalamic nuclei project to the cingulate and retrosplenial cortices, among other locations. The lateral dorsal nucleus projects strongly to retrosplenial cortex, and shows specific degeneration in Alzheimer's disease (Xuereb et al., 1991).

Parker and Gaffen (1997) demonstrated deficits on a delayed matching-to-place task in monkeys with anterior thalamic lesions. Ghika-Schmid and Bogousslavsky (2000) reported a series of 12 patients with anterior thalamic infarcts, all of whom demonstrated anterograde amnesia (verbal with left and nonverbal with right hemisphere lesions) in combination with perseveration, transcortical motor aphasia, apathy, and executive dysfunction. They thought this combination of features was highly suggestive of this localization. The lesions involved the anterior thalamic nuclei and not the dorsomedial or ventrolateral nuclei. They also ex-

tended to involve the mamillothalamic tract and the internal medullary lamina. More often, thalamic lesions in humans associated with severe amnesia spare the anterior thalamic nuclei (see below). The DNMS deficits are reported only with more extensive thalamic involvement

Cingulate and Retrosplenial Cortex

The major cortical connections of the anterior thalamic nuclei are with cingulate gyrus. Bachevalier and Mishkin (1986) suggest that combined lesions of orbitofrontal and anterior cingulate cortex in monkeys damages both memory circuits, the orbitofrontal cortex being connected to the perirhinal–dorsomedial thalamic circuit, and the anterior cingulate to the hippocampal–anterior thalamic circuit. But extensive frontal lesions in humans (Eslinger and Damasio, 1985) do not result in the classical amnesic syndrome. Meunier et al. (1997) described a spatial memory deficit in monkeys with anterior cingulate lesions; studies in rats (Aggleton et al., 1995) suggest that this may be due to damage to the underlying cingulate bundle. The anterior cingulate region appears to play a role in initiating movement, in motivation, and in goal-directed behaviors (Devinsky et al., 1995), but anterior cingulate gyrus lesions have not been associated with amnesia in humans.

The principal projections of the anterior thalamic nuclei, however, are to posterior cingulate cortex, and especially retrosplenial cortex. These cortical regions are also inteconnected with the hippocampus (Morris et al., 1999). Lesions in humans that involve retrosplenial cortex can result in a classical amnesic syndrome (Valenstein et al., 1987), but there remains some debate as to whether the cause of the amnesia is interruption of cingulate/hippocampal connections via the cingulate bundle, damage to the retrosplenial cortex itself, or damage to hippocampal–thalamic, hippocampal–basal forebrain (septal nuclei) or frontal lobe connections traveling in the fornix (Rudge and Warrington, 1991; von Cramon and Shuri, 1992). Additional cases of amnesia with retrosplenial lesions have been reported in the Japanese literature (Takayama et al.,

1991; Katai et al., 1992; Iwasaki et al., 1993; Arita et al., 1995; Yasuda et al., 1997; Sato et al., 1998). Takahashi et al. (1997) reported pure topographic amnesia with a right retrosplenial lesion. Valenstein et al.'s case (1987) was left-sided, and the memory loss was predominately verbal.

THALAMIC AMNESIA

Amnesia associated with tumors in the walls of the third ventricle (Foerster and Gagel, 1933; Lhermitte et al., 1937; Grünthal, 1939; Sprofkin and Sciarra, 1952; Williams and Pennybacker, 1954) provided early evidence that medial thalamic structures may be important in memory. The advent of computed tomographic (CT) and MR imaging made it possible to correlate memory deficits with restricted thalamic lesions in patients with thalamic strokes. Although initial reports appeared to confirm evidence from Wernike-Korsakoff disease cited above that dorsomedial thalamic lesions were associated with memory loss, subsequent studies cast doubt on this. Thus, early reports suggested that N.A., a patient who became amnesic after a fencing foil passed through his nose into the brain (Teuber et al., 1968), had a relatively restricted lesion involving the left dorsomedial thalamic nucleus on CT scan (Squire and Moore, 1979), and that amnesic patients with thalamic strokes had CT evidence of dorsomedial lesions (Speedie and Heilman, 1982; Choi et al., 1983; Bogous-slavsky et al., 1986). High-resolution imaging in N.A., however, revealed that his lesion affected only the ventral aspect of the dorsomedial nucleus, but severely damaged the intralaminar nuclei, mamillothalamic tract, and internal medullary lamina (Squire et al., 1989a). N.A. also had lesions affecting the postcommissural fornix, mammillary bodies, and the right temporal tip. More restricted lesions in patients with thalamic infarctions suggest that thalamic amnesia best correlates with lesions affecting the internal medullary lamina and mamillothalamic tract (Winocur et al., 1984; von Cramon et al., 1985; Gentilini et al., 1987; Graff-Radford et al., 1990; Malamut et al., 1992). More posterior lesions that involve portions of the dorsomedial nucleus but spare the internal medullary lamina and mamillothalamic tract are not associated with amnesia (von Cramon et al., 1985; Kritchevsky et al., 1987; Graff-Radford et al., 1990). The modified dual pathway theory described above suggests that severe and lasting amnesia requires disruption of both Papez' circuit and the perirhinal–dorsomedial thalamic–frontal pathway. Graff-Radford et al. (1990) provided a clear anatomic demonstration in the monkey of the juxtaposition of these two pathways (the mamillothalamic tract and the ventral amygdalofugal pathway) in the internal medullary lamina.

Alternative explanations of thalamic amnesia suggest a role for the midline thalamic nuclei, which include the parataenial, anterior paraventricular, centralis medialis, and reuniens nuclei. These nuclei have connections with the hippocampus (Herkenham, 1978; Amaral and Cowan, 1980; Van Hoesen, 1985; Insuasti et al., 1987b). They are quite consistently damaged in patients with Wernike-Korsakoff disease (Mair et al., 1979; Mayes et al., 1988). Another proposal is that thalamic lesions may disconnect thalamic connections with the frontal lobes. Warrington (Warrington and Weiskrantz, 1982; Warrington, 1985) proposed that restricted thalamic lesions found in their cases of Wernicke-Korsakoff disease (Mair et al., 1979) may disconnect mediodorsal–frontal connections important for coordinating posterior cortical regions subserving semantic memories with frontal structures that impose cognitive structure upon these memories. Kooistra and Heilman (1988) also suggested that thalamofrontal disconnections might contribute to amnesia.

BASAL FOREBRAIN

The basal forebrain is at the junction of the diencephalon and the cerebral hemispheres and has, at minimum, the following components: the septal area, diagonal band of Broca, nucleus accumbens septi, olfactory tubercle, substantia innominata (containing the nucleus basalis of Meynert), bed nucleus of the stria terminalis, and preoptic area (Fig. 18–5). It is the third major region, after the temporal lobes and diencephalon, to be considered essential

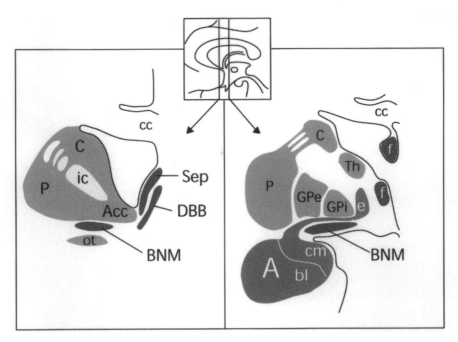

Figure 18–5. The basal forebrain. Two coronal sections through the basal forebrain are shown, as indicated in the mid-sagittal view in the box at the top of the figure. BNM, basal nucleus of Meynert; DBB, diagonal band of Broca; Sep, septal nuclei. The amygdala (A) has basolateral (bl) and centromedial divisions, and it extends into the basal forebrain as the extended amygdala (e). Other structures indicated are the basal ganglia (putamen (P), caudate (C), nucleus accumbens (Acc), and globus pallidus externa (GPe) and interna (GPi). Th, thalamus, and f, fornix, which is sectioned twice.

for normal memory function in humans. It was known for many years that some patients developed memory loss after hemorrhage from aneurysms, particularly after rupture of anterior communicating artery aneurysms (Linqvist and Norlen, 1966; Talland et al., 1967); however, the pathogenesis of this amnesia was not understood. Several lines of evidence suggested that cholinergic neurons in the basal forebrain were involved in memory. Lewis and Shute (1967) documented a cholinergic projection from the medial septal region of the basal forebrain to the hippocampus. For many years, scopolamine, a centrally acting anticholinergic agent, had been used in obstetrics, in conjunction with analgesics, to induce a "twilight" state, after which women would have little recall of their deliveries. Drachman and Leavitt (1974) demonstrated that normal subjects had difficulty with free recall of words when given scopolamine, and that this effect was reversed by physostigmine, a centrally acting anticholinesterase agent that prevents in-

activation of acetylcholine. Mesulam and Van Hoesen (1976) documented a cholinergic projection from the basal nucleus of Meynert, and in subsequent studies Mesulam and colleagues (Mesulam et al., 1983; Mesulam and Mufson, 1984) defined the connections of basal forebrain cholinergic neurons. Neurons in the medial septal nucleus and diagonal band of Broca project strongly to the hippocampus, as had been documented by Lewis and Shute (1967). Cholinergic neurons in the substantia innominata (nucleus basalis of Meynert), however, project widely to limbic and neocortex. In 1981, Whitehouse et al. documented selective loss of neurons in the nucleus basalis of Meynert in patients with Alzheimer's disease. Cell loss in cholinergic neurons of the basal forebrain (Arendt et al., 1983) has also been found in Wernicke-Korsakoff syndrome (Butters, 1985; Butters and Stuss, 1989). All of these lines of evidence suggested a role for the basal forebrain in memory, and more specifically, suggested that the cholinergic projections of the basal forebrain may be of particular importance.

This cholinergic hypothesis (Bartus et al., 1985; Kopelman, 1986) has generated a large volume of research, but the cholinergic hypothesis itself remains to be established (Fibiger, 1991). Cholinergic medication provides a very modest improvement in memory in patients with Alzheimer's disease (Peters and Levin, 1979, 1982; Johns et al., 1983; Thal et al., 1983). It is not surprising, however, that acetylcholine replacment does not have the dramatic effect that dopamine treatment has in Parkinson's disease, since patients with Alzheimer's disease have degeneration in many other areas thought to be of importance in memory, including the target areas of basal forebrain cholinergic projections (the hippocampus, amygdala, and neocortex).

The complexity of basal forebrain anatomy makes it difficult to arrive at firm conclusions about the pathophysiology of amnesia associated with basal forebrain lesions (see Fig. 18–4). In addition to structures containing cholinergic neurons (the substantia innominata, basal nucleus of Meynert, diagonal band of Broca, and septal nuclei), the basal forebrain encompasses pathways and systems that could conceivably participate in memory. The anterior commissure crosses the midline just posterior to the septal nuclei. The columns of the fornix descend through the basal forebrain on their way to the hypothalamus. The ventral amygdalofugal pathway both projects to the basal forebrain and traverses it on its way to the thalamus. Thus basal forebrain lesions, if properly situated, may disrupt one or both of the pathways critical for memory. The medial forebrain bundle, which interconnects brainstem, hypothalamic, and forebrain structures, travels through the lateral hypothalmus and the basal forebrain. Noradrenergic and dopaminergic pathways are represented in the median forebrain bundle. The *extended amygdala* refers to groups of neurons within the basal forebrain, including neurons in the bed nucleus of the stria terminalis and portions of the nucleus accumbens septi, that are anatomically considered to be related to the corticomedial amygdala, with which they are laterally confluent (Heimer and Alheid, 1991). The core of the

nucleus accumbens and the olfactory tubercle closely resemble the caudate-putamen, and form the ventral striatum, which in turn projects to the region of basal forebrain beneath the globus pallidus (the ventral pallidum). It is not known if these areas contribute to memory function. The preoptic area receives projections from amygdala, hippocampus, and other areas of the basal forebrain. It is involved in self-regulatory and species-specific behaviors (Swanson, 1987). It is unknown if it has a role in memory.

Most basal forebrain lesions reported in human cases of amnesia have been large, and they probably affect all or many of the above structures. Often, they also involve areas outside the basal forebrain, such as the orbitofrontal and medial frontal cortices and the caudate nucleus. Irle et al. (1992) studied 30 patients with brain lesions associated with anterior cerebral artery aneurysm rupture and found that severe memory loss was associated with combined lesions in the striatum (caudate) and basal forebrain, whereas lesions restricted to basal forebrain were not associated with memory disturbance. Morris et al. (1992), however, reported a patient with amnesia following removal of a very small glioma in the lamina terminalis, just posterior to the right gyrus rectus. Postoperative MRI scans demonstrated a lesion restricted to the diagonal band of Broca, anterior commissure, nucleus accumbens, and preoptic area. They postulated that destruction of the cholinergic projection to the hippocampus, most of which originates in the nucleus of the diagonal band of Broca, probably accounted for the amnesia, but they could not rule out contributions from other damaged areas. Although the cholinergic hypothesis has been popular, other neurotransmitter pathways may be of importance. Dobkin and Hanlon (1993) report a patient with anterior basal forebrain and caudate nucleus injury whose amnesia improved with treatment with bromocriptine, a selective dopamine agonist. They postulate that damage to dopaminergic pathways coursing through the basal forebrain to the striatum (and elsewhere) may result in memory loss. Bromocriptine had previously been reported to reverse coma in a patient with bilateral hypothalamic damage (Ross and Stewart, 1981), but Dobkin and Hanlon's patient was said to have normal attention. The contribution of dopaminergic pathways to memory remains to be elucidated.

LATERALITY OF LESIONS CAUSING AMNESIA IN HUMANS

Many of the best-studied patients with amnesia have bilateral lesions. When unilateral temporal lobectomy for epilepsy causes severe amnesia, it is usually assumed that there has been prior damage to the contralateral hippocampus. Otherwise, memory deficits are relatively mild, and often are material-specific (verbal for left-sided lesions; visuospatial for right-sided lesions) (Milner, 1972; Jones-Gotman and Milner, 1978; Kaplan et al., 1994). More severe memory disturbances have been described, however, with unilateral lesions. Most often these are left-sided and cause more verbal than nonverbal memory disturbance. This has been reported for left posterior cerebral artery infarctions affecting the medial temporal region (Benson et al., 1974; von Cramon et al., 1988), for left retrosplenial lesions (Valenstein et al., 1987), and for left thalamic lesions (Speedie and Heilman, 1982; Goldenberg et al., 1983; Graff-Radford et al., 1984; Mori et al., 1986). Less often, lesions causing relatively severe amnestic disturbances are right-sided (Graff-Radford et al., 1984; Morris et al., 1992). There are no comparable findings in animals.

SUMMARY OF THE ANATOMY OF MEMORY

It is important to point out that the areas discussed above that are known to be important for normal memory function may not actually contain entire "memory traces." It is considered likely that the parts of the brain that process the information as it is acquired also retain fragmentary traces of experience (Fuster, 1984; Damasio, 1989; Damasio et al., 1989). Damasio (1989) suggests that the hippocampus contributes by recording the context of events in relation to each other and to the person. Thus patients with medial temporal lesions retain general knowledge, but this knowledge lacks contextual complexity necessary for uniqueness or connection to autobiography. Activation of the hippocampus allows for temporally coordinated "retroactivation" of "convergence zones" in temporal cortex which in turn simultaneously activate specifically those neuronal ensembles, widely distributed in primary and association cortices, that were involved in the original experience. He suggests that only with such retroactivation is a memory brought to consciousness. The hippocampus has a limited capacity, and eventually such records are lost or consolidated in different brain areas, so that the hippocampal system is not required for retrieval of remote memories.

It remains unclear how subcortical regions interact with this cortical memory system, but clearly subcortical centers in the basal forebrain and thalamus are critical, since diencephalic amnesics appear not to be able to use their temporal lobes effectively for memory. Cholinergic projections from basal forebrain to neocortex appear to be necessary for cortical plasticity (Jerusalinsky et al., 1997; Kilgard and Merzenich, 1998), and cholinergic projections to hippocampus may have a similar role. Subcortical structures may also provide critical pathways for memory processing, as suggested by the dual system theory, but the unique contribution of different diencephalic and basal forebrain regions to memory function remains to be elucidated.

AMNESIA SUBTYPES: SIMILARITIES AND DIFFERENCES AMONG AMNESICS

These anatomic considerations, together with clinical experience, indicate considerable heterogeneity within the amnesic population. Qualitative performance differences among patients with lesions in different areas would imply that these neuroanatomic regions contribute to memory function in different ways. Over the last three decades, these behavioral and anatomic facts have fueled speculation that there may be several subtypes of amnesia (Lhermitte and Signoret, 1972; Huppert and Piercy, 1979; Squire, 1981).

BITEMPORAL VS. DIENCEPHALIC AMNESIA

Historically, two subtypes have received the most attention: bitemporal amnesia, as exemplified by patient H.M., and diencephalic amnesia, as represented in patients with Alcoholic Korsakoff disease (Victor et al., 1971, 1989; Butters and Cermak, 1980; Butters, 1985) and other patients with discrete thalamic or mammillary body lesions (Mair et al., 1979; Squire and Moore, 1979; Speedie and Heilman, 1982, 1983; Winocur et al., 1984). A third subtype, *basal forebrain amnesia*, has received less study, and will be considered separately.

A key question has been whether these anatomic–descriptive subtypes can be distinguished on behavioral grounds. Data on this issue have come from two main sources: studies evaluating rates of forgetting from long-term memory in diencephalic and bitemporal amnesics, and studies evaluating cognitive deficits specific to diencephalic amnesia, particularly Korsakoff's syndrome.

Rate of Forgetting from Long-Term Memory

One frequently evaluated behavioral dimension is the rate at which information is forgotten once it has been initially learned to some criterion. Using retention intervals from 10 minutes to 7 days, several authors have argued that bitemporal amnesics (H.M., herpes encephalitic, bilateral ECT, and, more controversial, patients with early Alzheimer's disease) may show a more rapid rate of forgetting than diencephalic amnesics or controls (Huppert and Piercy, 1979; Squire, 1981; Martone et al., 1986). In most of these studies, diencephalic patients are given longer stimulus exposures (to counteract an encoding deficit) than those given controls or bitemporals to achieve comparable recognition performance at the shortest delays. This, coupled with faster forgetting for bitemporal patients, initially led to the conclusion that bitemporal amnesia involves a defect in consolidation, while diencephalic amnesia involves an earlier defect in stimulus registration or encoding (Huppert and Piercy, 1979; Squire, 1982a; Winocur, 1984). Once this latter defect is cir-

cumvented, however, by increased exposure to the stimuli, the normal forgetting in diencephalic amnesics has been taken to mean that their consolidation ability is intact.

The widely held view that bitemporal amnesia is distinctively characterized by abnormally rapid forgetting has been questioned by the results of more recent studies. One of the problems with the Huppert and Piercy procedure is that procedures for matching initial recognition levels result in the shortest mean study-to-test interval being longer in the amnesics than in controls (Mayes et al., 1994b). Freed and colleagues (1987) retested H.M.'s recognition memory over intervals of 10 minutes, 24 hours, 72 hours, and 1 week with two recognition paradigms, taking pains to precisely equate his 10-minute recall with that of normals. The first was a modified Huppert and Piercy (1979) rate-of-forgetting paradigm in which H.M. was given increased exposure to pictorial stimuli (10 seconds compared to 1 second for controls) and in which yes–no recognition was probed at the four retention intervals. H.M.'s performance was normal after 10 minutes, but dropped significantly below controls after 24 hours and remained at that level through the 1-week recognition probe. The normal controls continued to forget over the entire week, such that their recognition performance declined to H.M.'s level and was not significantly better than it was at 72 hours or 1 week. Freed et al. suggested that their findings indicated a "normal rate of forgetting over a 1-week delay interval," although as Crosson (1992) has indicated, an alternative explanation of these results is that H.M.'s lowest level of performance for the 1-week interval was raised above previous levels reported by Huppert and Piercy (1979) by virtue of additional stimulus exposure. That is, although Freed et al. focused on the equivalence between H.M. and normals at the 72-hour and 1-week delays, the fact that H.M.'s performance leveled off more rapidly than controls may, in fact, be taken to support rather than refute the notion that bitemporal amnesics forget at an abnormally rapid rate (Crosson, 1992). In the second task reported by Freed et al., forgetting rate was assessed at the same intervals by a forced-choice recognition test rather than by a yes–no recognition test. On this task, H.M.'s performance was not significantly different from controls at any interval and was slightly above that of the controls at 72 hours and 1 week. This is a more convincing demonstration that abnormally rapid forgetting does not necessarily characterize bitemporal amnesia.

McKee and Squire (1992) directly compared rate of forgetting from long-term memory in bitemporal and diencephalic amnesics equated for amnesia severity. Both groups of amnesics received 8 seconds of exposure to each of 120 target pictures, while normal controls received 1 second of exposure. Ten minutes, 2 hours, and 30–32 hours after study, subjects were tested with four different recognition memory tests. On the first, subjects were asked to respond "yes" to a previously studied (old) item and "no" to a new item. The second test required subjects to respond "yes" to a new item and "no" to an old item. In the third test, subjects were asked to point to the one old item in a laterally presented pair (DMS), while in the fourth test, subjects were ask to point to the one new item (DNMS). There were no group differences for any of the recognition tests at any retention interval. Thus, although initial studies differentiated bitemporal and diencephalic amnesia on the basis of long-term forgetting rate, recent studies have tended to emphasize the similarities, rather than the differences, in rate of forgetting in these two groups. Some recent studies suggest that there may be subtle differences in the shape of the forgetting curve when recognition probes are concentrated in the first 30 minutes, but there is little evidence of substantial differences thereafter (Mayes et al., 1994; Downes et al., 1998). McKee and Squire (1992) suggest that, although it is reasonable to suppose that the medial temporal lobe and diencephalic systems should have different contributions to normal memory, "each region might also be an essential component of a larger functional system such that a similar amnesia might result from damage to any portion of that system." The emerging notion that bitemporal and diencephalic amnesia may be more similar than different is consistent with anatomic data comprising the dual system theory described above.

Retrograde Amnesia

Squire (1984) initially suggested that temporally limited retrograde amnesia was due to a defect in consolidation specifically related to dysfunction of the hippocampus (Zola-Morgan and Squire, 1990b). However, Squire et al., (1989b), using an updated version of Cohen and Squire's (1981) remote faces and events tests, found extensive, temporally limited retrograde amnesia in both Korsakoff patients ($n = 7$) and a group of patients with presumed medial temporal pathology secondary to anoxia or ischemia ($n = 3$). Although there were differences in the specific pattern exhibited by individual patients, their retrograde amnesia spanned a period of about 15 years and was not detectable in the more remote time periods. Gade and Mortensen (1990) found graded retrograde memory loss, supposedly typical of patients with bitemporal amnesia, in patients with basal forebrain and diencephalic amnesia (including five patients with Korsakoff's syndrome). It is thus unlikely that differences in the degree or pattern of retrograde amnesia will reliably distinguish among basal forebrain, diencephalic, or medial temporal amnesics, though there may still be reason to distinguish between temporally graded, temporally limited, and decade-nonspecific patterns in the individual case. Some recent clinical and experimental evidence suggests that the degree and pattern of retrograde deficit may depend on concomitant involvement in temporal (Reed and Squire, 1998; Kapur and Brooks, 1999) or frontal (Kopelman, 1991; Kopelman et al., 1999; Winocur and Moscovitch, 1999) cortex that tends to be associated with bitemporal and diencephalic damage.

Deficits Specific to Korsakoff Syndrome

Despite the apparent failure of forgetting rate to consistently distinguish between bitemporal and diencephalic amnesia, other data suggest that certain cognitive abilities might be differentially impaired in diencephalic amnesia, particularly in patients with Korsakoff syndrome. As we shall see, a key issue is whether such impairments are an obligatory part of the amnesia seen in these patients, or whether they result from concomitant frontal involvement.

Defects in Spatiotemporal Aspects of Memory

Memory for temporal order. One such ability concerns the judgment of the temporal order of events—that is, to discriminate when a target item occurred in the study sequence (Huppert and Piercy, 1976; Hirst and Volpe, 1982; McAndrews and Milner, 1991). In a typical temporal order judgment paradigm, subjects are given a list discrimination task in which a target list of stimuli is initially shown, followed after a brief delay by a second target list. During later testing, subjects are asked whether they have seen each stimulus before (recognition judgment) and, if so, whether it belonged to the first or second list (temporal order judgment). In an early study of this phenomenon, Squire et al. (1981a) examined temporal order judgments in bilateral ECT patients, patient N.A., and controls. They found that, although impairments in temporal order judgments were seen in both ECT patients and N.A., recognition judgments were also poor. When recognition performance was subsequently equated with that of normals, no temporal ordering deficit remained. Thus, in these patients, impaired temporal order judgments appeared to be due to poor recognition memory.

However, the impairment in temporal order judgments exhibited by a different amnesic population, patients with alcoholic Korsakoff syndrome, cannot be accounted for on the basis of their poor recognition performance (Squire, 1982b; Meudell et al., 1985; Bowers et al., 1988; Shuren et al., 1997). Several authors (Moscovitch, 1982; Squire, 1982b; Schacter, 1987b) have attributed the temporal ordering impairment in these patients to concomitant frontal lobe pathology known to co-exist with diencephalic damage (Shimamura et al., 1990; Jernigan et al., 1991a, 1991b). Two facts support this interpretation: *(1)* nonamnesic patients with frontal lesions (Corsi, cited in Milner et al., 1991; Shimamura et al., 1990; Johnson et al., 1997) and basal ganglia disease (Sagar et al., 1988) also show impairment in temporal order judgments; and *(2)* deficits in temporal order judgments in amnesics correlate significantly with performance on neuropsychological tests putatively sensitive to frontal pathology such as the Wisconsin Card Sort (Test Squire, 1982b). Although the link to frontal lobe damage has been relatively consistent, there are two reasons to keep the book open on this issue. First, the Wisconsin Card Sort, Test, which is often used to index frontal pathology in reported cases, may not be as specifically sensitive to frontal lobe pathology as originally thought (Anderson et al., 1991). Second, a recent case study of T.R., a densely amnesic patient with a left retrosplenial lesion, suggests that a defect in temporal ordering can exist independent of both recognition ability and frontal lobe function (Bowers et al., 1988). Interestingly, T.R. was dramatically impaired in temporal order judgments for newly acquired information, but had no difficulty judging the temporal order of remote events (see also Parkin and Hunkin, 1993). T.R. performed normally on tests of frontal lobe function, as did a subsequently reported patient with a hypothalamic glioma but no concomitant frontal damage (Parkin and Hunkin, 1993). These findings provide an initial clue that it may be important to distinguish between two kinds of temporal ordering deficits: *(1)* one which is a part of a more general, frontally mediated strategic deficit (as in Korsakoff's syndrome; see Squire, 1982b; Shimamura et al., 1990), and *(2)* another which reflects an anterograde impairment in "time tagging" new information that is independent of frontal pathology (Bowers et al., 1988; Parkin and Hunkin, 1993; Yasuno et al., 1999).

Source monitoring and source amnesia. As indicated above, successful retrieval from episodic memory has an autobiographical quality and is characterized by direct recollection of both the content and source of remembered information (Johnson et al., 1993). The phenomenon of source amnesia illustrates that the content and source of remembered information are potentially dissociable (Shimamura and Squire, 1987). *Source amnesia* refers to a situation in which one remembers some fact or piece of information, but forgets the source of the information. For example, we might remember specific information about a book or movie, but be unable to recollect where that information was learned. Source attributions differentiate autobiographical event memories (from more general knowledge) and source amnesia has been described as a form of memory impairment for spatiotemporal context since it reflects recollection of content devoid of the context (temporal and situational factors) that gives rise to the memory (Shimamura, 1989; Johnson et al., 1992). Schacter et al. (1984) used a paradigm first introduced by Evans and Thorn (1966) to study source amnesia in memory-disordered patients with Alzheimer's disease, closed head injury, and encephalitis. They presented bogus facts (e.g., Bob Hope's father was a fireman) to their patients and then gave a recall test. If a fact was recalled, patients were asked where they had learned it. Many patients demonstrated recall of at least some of the facts, but frequently asserted that they had learned them from a source other than the experimental session. This finding could not be explained by poor memory, since normal subjects whose recall was lowered by a 1-week study–test interval did not commit source errors. Shimamura and Squire (1987) taught obscure (true) facts to a group of Korsakoff patients ($n = 6$) and a group of patients with amnesia secondary to anoxia ($n = 3$). Severe source amnesia, in which recall was attributed to sources other than the experiment, was observed in three of the Korsakoff patients and in one of the anoxic patients. The level of fact memory performance did not predict the degree of source amnesia. Control subjects whose fact memory is reduced by a long delay do not generally exhibit source errors. Furthermore, patients with bitemporal amnesia, including H.M., who display severe defects in fact memory, perform *better* at tests of recency and temporal order than nonamnesic frontal patients (Sagar et al., 1990; Milner et al., 1991).

Some evidence suggests that the severity of source amnesia varies as a function of frontal lobe impairment in amnesic and nonamnesic subjects (Schacter et al., 1984; Janowsky et al., 1989), although some authors (see Johnson et al., 1993) are not willing to rule out important contributions from diencephalic and medial temporal regions. One way of understanding the relative contributions of these various regions is to suggest that source-monitoring tasks make variable demands on cognitive estimation (Shallice and Evans, 1978), reality monitoring

(Johnson, 1991), attribution (Jacoby et al., 1989), and temporal order memory (Hirst and Volpe, 1982; Olton, 1989). It may be that different populations of amnesics are differentially impaired depending on the specific test used to test source monitoring. If this is so, then more precise development of source monitoring assessments may provide a future basis on which such subpopulations may be differentiated (Johnson et al., 1993).

Metamemory and feeling of knowing. Another cognitive domain that appears differentially impaired in alcoholic Korsakoff syndrome has been referred to as *metamemory*. This involves knowledge about (1) one's own memory capabilities, (2) the memory demands of particular tasks or situations, and (3) potentially useful strategies relevant to given tasks or situations (Flavell and Wellman, 1977; Gruneberg, 1983). It encompasses people's beliefs (e.g., "I will [or will not] be able to remember these words") as well as their knowledge about the memory system (e.g., rehearsal strategies that enhance recall). Hirst and Volpe (cited in Hirst, 1982) were among the first to report differentially impaired metamemory in Korsakoff patients when compared to other etiologies of amnesia. On the basis of interviews, they found that Korsakoff patients had less knowledge of mnemonic strategies than patients with amnesia from other causes.

The most widely studied memtamemorial capacity in amnesic patients is the feeling-of-knowing (FOK) phenomenon (cf. Hart, 1965, 1967; Gruneberg and Monks, 1974; Nelson et al., 1982, 1984). In a typical FOK experiment, subjects are asked to freely recall the answers to general information questions of varying difficulty (e.g., "What is the tallest mountain in South America?") until a certain number of failures occur. For these unrecalled items, subjects are then asked to judge the likelihood that they would be able to recognize the correct answer if it was presented along with other likely but incorrect choices. The FOK predictions are then validated by a subsequent recognition test. The general finding in normals is that recognition performance is better for questions eliciting strong FOK than for questions eliciting weak or no FOK.

Shimamura and Squire (1986) evaluated the ability of FOK judgments to predict subsequent recognition performance in patients with Korakoff's syndrome, psychiatric patients undergoing bilateral ECT, a mixed group of amnesics which included N.A., and controls. Using general information questions (study 1) and a sentence memory paradigm that assessed newly learned information (study 2), they found that only the Korsakoff patients displayed impairment in making FOK judgments. From these results, it appears that memtamemory dysfunction is not an obligatory aspect of amnesia, since amnesia can occur without any measurable impairment in FOK. The authors speculated that the disturbed FOK in Korsakoff patients might be a function of their frontal pathology, which would be expected to impair their ability on a variety of judgment and planning tasks.

Summary. It is important to emphasize that deficits in temporal order judgments, source amnesia, and metamemory have frequently been interpreted in the context of frontal lobe pathology, and more generally have been used to distinguish between groups of amnesics with (diencephalic) and without (bitemporal) associated deficits in frontal/executive skills. This distinction has had two very different potential meanings (Schacter, 1987b). The first is that there is a core amnesic syndrome upon which frontal deficits might be nonspecifically superimposed. If this is true, then an important task for neuropsychological research is to distinguish the core from that which is ancillary to amnesia. Arguments of this type are frequently invoked when a cognitive deficit (e.g., failure to release from proactive interference) thought to reflect the nature of the memory disorder in Korsakoff patients is also found to exist in nonamnesic patients with frontal lobe lesions (Moscovitch, 1982). If this is true, such frontal impairments become more of a nuisance to the amnesia researcher than a topic worthy of primary concern. Alternatively, one could suppose that frontal lobe systems have specific memory-related functions (Petrides, 1989). If this is the case, then it becomes important to recognize that patients with frontal-related memory impairment present with a type of

memory disorder that differs from the amnesia associated with lesions to other regions. Indeed, there is growing evidence that the frontal lobes play an important, specific role in mediating temporal context (Stuss et al., 1982; Goldman-Rakic, 1984; Milner et al., 1984; Schacter, 1987b; McAndrews and Milner, 1991), and memory for self-generated responses (Petrides and Milner, 1982), and may contain specific regions that mediate working memory (Goldman-Rakic, 1992) and other important memory-related functions. These findings strongly suggest that specific frontally mediated memory deficits should be admitted into the domain of impairments worthy of study by amnesia researchers.

In this context, it should be noted that recent research has been strongly focused on understanding the neural components of working memory in functional imaging studies that are not linked to the role of this important function in amnesia per se (D'Esposito et al., 1995a; Courtney et al., 1997; Baddeley, 1998; Gabrieli et al., 1998; Smith and Jonides, 1998; Ungerleider et al., 1998). The next important task will be to integrate these findings with evidence from the clinical literature to achieve a better understanding of the clinical relevance of these experimental findings.

BASAL FOREBRAIN AMNESIA

Studies of patients with amnesia from basal forebrain lesions suggest that it is clinically distinctive. As noted above, this form of amnesia most commonly results from vascular lesion or aneurysm surgery in the region of the anterior communicating artery (Okawa et al., 1980; Gade, 1982; Alexander and Freedman, 1983; Damasio et al., 1985b; Vilkki, 1985; Volpe and Hirst, 1983; Phillips et al., 1987; DeLuca and Cicerone, 1989). After basal forebrain damage, the patient exhibits extensive anterograde but variable retrograde amnesia. Temporal gradients similar to that seen in Korsakoff's syndrome have been described (Lindqvist and Norlen, 1966; Gade and Mortensen, 1990). Some authors have also described an impairment in placing memories in proper chronological order (Lindqvist and Norlen, 1966; Talland et al., 1967; Damasio et al., 1985b). Free, and sometimes wild, confabulation appears to be characteristic, particularly in the acute period (Lindqvist and Norlen, 1966; Logue et al., 1968; Talland, et al., 1967; Okawa et al., 1980; Alexander and Freedman, 1983; Damasio et al., 1985b) and may relate to the extent of concomitant orbitofrontal involvement existing along with the memory impairment, particularly in those patients who show spontaneous or unprovoked confabulation (Damasio et al., 1985; Vilkki, 1985; Phillips et al., 1987; DeLuca and Cicerone, 1989; Fischer et al., 1995). Some patients have difficulty distinguishing reality from dreaming. Although these behavioral abnormalities are distinctive, they may not be functionally related to the amnesia: often, basal forebrain amnesia persists after dream–waking confusion and confabulation have subsided (Hashimoto et al., 2000).

Cueing seems to differentially improve memory performance in these patients, and anecdotal evidence suggests that many of these patients can recall specific information in one retrieval attempt, but not the next. These data have led to the general idea that these patients suffer from a problem in accessing information that does exist in long-term memory. However, further data are needed before accepting this proposition confidently. It has frequently been noted that these patients appear apathetic and unconcerned about their memory impairment (Talland et al., 1967; Alexander and Freedman, 1983; Phillips et al., 1987). Interestingly, Talland regarded basal forebrain amnesics as showing striking behavioral similarities to patients with Korsakoff syndrome, and Graff-Radford et al. (1990) saw similarities between these amnesics and those suffering memory loss secondary to paramedian thalamic infarctions. It may be that such similarities arise because the large, vascular lesions that characterize these cases also involve structures or pathways destined for components of the medial temporal or diencephalic memory systems (Gade, 1982; Crosson, 1992). Although these anatomic considerations are important, there are as yet insufficient behavioral data on which to formally compare basal forebrain amnesics with amnesics of diencephalic or bitemporal origin.

CLINICAL PRESENTATION OF DISORDERS ASSOCIATED WITH AMNESIA

Memory loss is a common problem encountered in patients seen by physicians and psychologists. As discussed above, it has considerable localizing significance. It is also a helpful diagnostic finding, since it is a distinguishing feature of several neurological disorders. It is beyond the scope of this book to discuss these illnesses in detail; however, we will provide a brief review of some of the more important disorders.

AGE-ASSOCIATED MEMORY IMPAIRMENT AND BENIGN SENESCENT FORGETFULNESS

Kral (1962) used the term *benign senescent forgetfulness* to describe adults whose memory was poorer than their peers, but who had no other evidence of progressive dementia. Such patients, however, may be difficult to distinguish from patients with early Alzheimer's disease (Welsh et al., 1991). Memory deteriorates with increasing age in normal persons. Normal 70- and 80-year-old persons perform at levels that are 50% below that of young adults on tests of learning and memory (Larrabee et al., 1988). The term *age-associated memory impairment* (AAMI) refers to healthy persons over 50 who are not depressed or demented, who score at least 1 standard deviation below the mean for young adults on tests of memory (Crook et al., 1986; Crook and Larrabee, 1991). A related concept is known as *mild cognitive impairment* (Barker et al., 1995b; Sherwin, 2000). Estimates of the prevalence of AAMI vary widely, depending on the diagnostic criteria employed (Crook and Larrabee, 1991; Youngjohn and Crook, 1993; Larrabee and Crook, 1994; Barker et al., 1995; Larrabee, 1996; Hanninen and Soininen, 1997; Schroder et al., 1998). It is important to note that AAMI as a concept encompasses both objective evidence and subjective report of age-related decline. Failure to include objective measures of decline, or to understand the discrepancy between subjective perception of difficulty and objective age-corrected performance, may lead to an over-estimation of the prevalence of AAMI in the over-50 population (Larrabee, 1996). Many objectively normal adults may complain of memory loss, particularly if they are in intellectually demanding positions, illustrating the importance of subjective report in the AAMI construct.

DEGENERATIVE DISORDERS

Many of the degenerative dementias (such as Pick's, Huntington's, and Parkinson's diseases) eventually affect memory (see Chapter 19), but Alzheimer's disease (AD) typically first manifests with amnesia (Damasio et al., 1989). As discussed above, nearly all of the areas thought to be important in memory are affected by AD, including the medial temporal lobe (Hyman et al., 1984, 1986; Scott et al., 1991), the basal forebrain (Whitehouse et al., 1981), the thalamus (Xuereb et al., 1991), and the neocortex. The memory impairment in advancing AD not only affects new learning but also results in the gradual loss of knowledge structures and semantic memory stores. Eventually, other cognitive domains such as language, visuospatial/perceptual ability, personality, and affect become involved. Thus, the memory loss found in cortical dementia is not as pure as in other forms of amnesia, but takes place in the context of widespread cognitive decline. Recent attempts to examine the relationship between amnesia and dementia with computational modeling have produced promising and interesting results (Murre, 1997, 1999).

VASCULAR DISEASE

Stroke will manifest with amnesia when critical areas are infarcted. The deficits associated with strokes affecting the posterior cerebral artery territory (posterior medial temporal lobe and retrosplenial cortex; Benson et al., 1974), and the thalamic penetrating arteries have been discussed above, as has basal forebrain amnesia from anterior communicating artery aneurysm hemorrhage or surgery. In these cases, the onset of amnesia is abrupt. Improvement is variable, and often patients are left with serious per-manent deficits, even following small infarctions (for example, of the thalamus).

CEREBRAL ANOXIA

Depending upon the degree and duration of ischemia and/or hypoxia, neuronal loss may be widespread or very focal. We have already discussed amnesia following cardiac arrest in which the only pathological feature identified was loss of neurons in field CA1 of the hippocampus (Zola-Morgan et al., 1986). Issues related to characterizing the extent of damage from anoxic or ischemic insults have recently been reviewed (Squire and Zola, 1996).

WERNICKE-KORSAKOFF SYNDROME

Alcoholic Korsakoff syndrome typically develops after years of conjoint alcohol abuse and nutritional deficiency (Butters and Cermak, 1980; Butters, 1984; Victor et al., 1989). Patients first undergo an acute stage of the illness, Wernicke's encephalopathy, in which symptoms of confusion, disorientation, oculomotor dysfunction, and ataxia are present. After this resolves, amnesia can persist as a permanent symptom. Severe anterograde amnesia and an extensive, temporally graded retrograde amnesia are characteristic. Although usually associated with chronic alcohol abuse, Korsakoff syndrome can occur in nonalcoholic patients who suffer chronic avitaminosis secondary to malabsorption syndromes (cf. Becker et al., 1990) or who refuse to eat in the context of a psychiatric disorder (Newman et al., 1998). Lesion location and neuropsychological features related to amnesia are discussed in detail above.

HERPES SIMPLEX ENCEPHALITIS

This disorder causes inflammation and necrosis, particularly in the orbitofrontal and inferior temporal regions. It thus involves limbic structures, including the hippocampus, parahippocampal gyrus, amygdala and overlying cortex, the polar limbic cortex, cingulate gyrus, and the orbitofrontal cortex (Damasio et al., 1989). Patients may present with personality change, confusion, headache, fever, and seizures, and they are often amnestic. Prompt treatment with antiviral agents can control the illness, and full recovery is possible; however, damage to these structures often leaves the patient with severe anterograde and retrograde amnesia. The amnesic syndromes in patient D.R.B. (also known as Boswell; Damasio et al., 1985a) and patient S.S. (Cermak, 1976; Cermak and O'Connor, 1983) have been particularly well characterized. Recent reports indicate that herpes simplex infection can occasionally lead to a syndrome of focal retrograde amnesia (Carlesimo et al., 1998; Fujii et al., 1999; Tanaka et al., 1999).

LIMBIC ENCEPHALITIS

This disorder occurs as a remote effect of carcinoma, and, like herpes encephalitis, affects limbic structures at the base of the forebrain (Corsellis et al., 1968; Khan and Wieser, 1994; Martin et al., 1996). Patients present with personality change, agitation, and amnestic dementia. Amnesia has also been reported in association with Hodgkin's disease (Duyckaerts et al., 1985), probably on the same basis.

TRAUMA

Following closed head injury, patients may have an acute anterograde and retrograde amnesia, the duration of which correlates with the severity of the injury, as measured by the Glasgow Coma Scale, or the duration of unconsciousness (Levin, 1989). The retrograde amnesia typically improves along with improvement in anterograde amnesia, providing evidence that a retrieval deficit is responsible for the portion of the retrograde memory loss that recovers. Residual memory impairment is usually a feature of broader cognitive and attentional impairment, but it can be prominent with severe injuries (Russell and Nathan, 1946; Whitty and Zangwill, 1977). Pathological changes are variable and widespread. Memory dysfunction may be caused by anterior temporal lobe contusions, temporal lobe white matter necrosis, or by more diffuse axonal disruption (Levin, 1989). Cases of focal retrograde amnesia in the relative absence of a new learn-

ing defect have been reported after closed head trauma (Kapur et al., 1992; Hunkin et al., 1995).

TRANSIENT GLOBAL AMNESIA

This distinctive form of amnesia begins suddenly and typically resolves within a day (Fisher and Adams, 1964; Caplan, 1985; Kritchevsky, 1989; Kritchevsky et al., 1988). A severe impairment in new learning and patchy loss of information learned prior to onset are seen. The patient often asks repetitive questions and may be aware of the memory deficit. Fifteen percent of patients complain of headache. After resolution, neuropsychological testing is normal except for amnesia for the episode (Kritchevsky, 1989). Evidence suggests that an episode of transient global amnesia (TGA) does not increase the risk of developing more permanent memory dysfunction. In a recent review of TGA, Kritchevsky (1989) considered the possible etiologic role played by epilepsy (Fisher and Adams, 1958; Fisher, 1982), emotional stress (Oleson and Jørgensen, 1986), occlusive cerebrovascular disease (Heathfield et al., 1973; Shuping et al., 1980), migranous vasospasm (Caplan et al., 1981; Haas and Ross, 1986; Hodges and Warlow, 1990; Tosi and Righetti, 1997; Schmidtke and Ehmsen, 1998) and vertebrobasilar dyscontrol (Caplan, 1985). He found no specific etiology to be convincingly associated with the syndrome, but suggested that transient disturbance in medial temporal and/or diencephalic brain structures appeared to be involved. It is generally believed that, although some form of cerebrovascular disease is frequently invoked to explain TGA, it has no greater incidence in the TGA population than in an age-matched control group (Miller et al., 1987; Hodges and Warlow, 1990), and patients with TGA are equally or less likely to have strokes than a control population (Hodges and Warlow, 1990). However, Moccia and colleagues (1996) found a greater incidence of hypertension and hypercholesterolemia in their patients, and a greater incidence of ischemic damage in patients with longer-duration TGA. Blood flow studies during an episode of TGA have demonstrated reduced flow bitemporally (Stillhard et al., 1990; using PET), or reduced blood flow in the left (more than right) thalamus (Goldenberg et al., 1991), while studies after recovery have either been normal (Fujii et al., 1989), or have demonstrated left temporal hypoperfusion (Laloux et at., 1992).

ELECTROCONVULSIVE THERAPY

Electroconvulsive therapy (ECT) used for relief of depression can produce severe anterograde and temporally limited retrograde amnesia (cf. Miller and Marlin, 1979; Squire, 1984). More severe impairment is seen after bilateral than after unilateral application. The anterograde defect is related in severity to the number of treatments, and is characterized by rapid forgetting and poor delayed recall (Squire, 1984). Substantial, often complete, recovery takes place in the few months after treatment ends (Squire and Chace, 1975; Squire and Slater, 1983). The retrograde amnesia appears to be temporally limited, involving only the few years prior to treatment onset; it too recovers almost completely in the months after treatment (Squire et al., 1976, 1981b). The extent of memory loss appears to be unrelated to therapeutic efficacy (Small et al., 1981; Welch, 1982), although it may be related to the extent of pretreatment cognitive impairment and post-treatment disorientation (Sobin et al., 1995). Although the data are by no means clear, some authors have suggested that ECT-induced memory loss models bilateral temporal lobe disease (Inglis, 1970; Squire, 1984), and several studies have used ECT patients as a contrast for patients with diencephalic pathology.

PSYCHOGENIC AMNESIAS

These disorders are reviewed by Schacter and Kihlstrom (1989). Psychologically induced loss of memory may be normal, as in amnesia for events of childhood (Wetzler and Sweeney, 1986; Usher and Neisser, 1993; Eacott and Crawley, 1999), or for events during sleep (Roth et al., 1988), or they may be pathological, as in the amnesias associated with dissociative states, multiple personality, or with simulated amnesia (Kopelman, 1987; Kessler et al.,

1997; Markowitsch, 1999). A striking loss of autobiographical memory is a hallmark of functional amnesia, and amnesia for one's own name (in the absence of aphasia or severe cognitive dysfunction in other spheres) is seen exclusively in this form of memory loss. Retrograde loss is often disproportionate to anterograde amnesia, and some patients will demonstrate loss of skills or other procedural memories typically retained by organic amnesic patients. Some studies have reported disproportionate loss of personal as opposed to public information taking place during amnestic episodes (Kapur, 1991).

REHABILITATION OF MEMORY DISORDERS

Recently, increased neurobehavioral interest has been devoted to the rehabilitation of patients with memory disorders (Butters et al., 1997). Historically, the field of memory rehabilitation has been guided by practical, rather than theoretical concerns, although there are important recent attempts to formulate an underlying theoretical basis for therapeutic interventions (Baddeley, 1984; Wilson, 1987; Parente and DiCesare, 1991; Sohlberg and Mateer, 1989; Baddeley and Wilson, 1994). As Glisky and Schacter (1987) point out, most rehabilitative interventions have attempted to directly improve memory performance through repetitive practice or exercises (Prigatano et al., 1984) or through the teaching of mnemonic strategies. They refer to this as the "restorative" approach, since its goal is to restore a certain degree of memory skill in these patients, thus improving functional adaptation in real life. Depending on the severity of the memory loss and the nature of material to be learned, some studies have suggested the beneficial effect of rehearsal strategies (Schacter et al., 1985), organizational techniques (Gianutsos and Gianutsos, 1979), and imagery mnemonics (Patten, 1972; Crovitz et al., 1979). Although such techniques have proven useful in individual cases, empirical investigations have generally not supported their efficacy in producing long-term relief of memory impairment, particularly in patients with concomitant deficits in initiation or executive skills (Richardson, 1992; Tate, 1997). A variety of techniques have been used to improve attention (e.g., use of verbal mediation and repetition), encoding (e.g., chunking, PQRST methods for reading and remembering text, imagery mnemonics [Butters et al., 1997]), and retention and retrieval (e.g., spaced retrieval technique [Schacter et al., 1985]). Interested readers should consult recent reviews of cognitive rehabilitation and memory therapy (Wilson and Moffat, 1984; Glisky and Schacter, 1988; Uzzell and Gross, 1986; Meier et al., 1987; Wilson, 1987; Sohlberg and Mateer, 1989; Kreutzer and Wehman, 1991) for information regarding empirical results and specific techniques that may be useful in working with the individual memory-disordered patient.

The alternative compensatory approach seeks to conceptualize the rehabilitation of memory disorders not as a process through which the goal is to restore normal or near-normal memory function, but as a process through which the memory-impaired patient is taught new techniques designed to close the gap between adaptive ability and life demands (Baeckman and Dixon, 1992; Wilson, 2000). This approach has emphasized the use of external memory aids and other assistive technology. For example, the use of electronic timers or personal digital devices (Chute and Bliss, 1994; Kim et al., 1999, 2000), paging systems that remind patients when to perform certain activities (Wilson et al., 1997; Evans et al., 1998), and memory notebooks that serve as tools for organizing information (Sohlberg and Mateer, 1989; Zencius et al., 1991; Burke et al., 1994; Schmitter Edgecombe et al., 1995) have all been used with some degree of effectiveness.

A third approach has been to utilize residual learning capacities in memory-disordered patients as a basis for teaching new facts or skills. Schacter and Glisky (1986) successfully taught memory-disordered patients a computer-related vocabulary using a variant of word-stem completion that they call the "method of vanishing cues" (Glisky et al., 1986b). This technique, in modified form, has also been used successfully in another study designed to teach

computer vocabulary (Hunkin and Parkin, 1995) and in teaching amnesics face–name associations (Thoene and Glisky, 1995), general knowledge facts, names of hospital staff, and how to follow a daily activity schedule (Wilson, 1999).

In related studies, Glisky and colleagues have shown that, using an approach based on skill/procedural learning, memory-disordered patients can be taught functional use of a microcomputer (Glisky et al., 1986a) and that, when enhanced with extensive repetition and direct cueing, such learning could generalize to a real work environment (Glisky and Schacter, 1988). Although such procedures appear to be relatively labor-intensive and may not lead to extensive explicit memory, they do demonstrate that it is possible to obtain generalization of a newly acquired skill to the natural environment; perhaps with further refinement of the technique, such generalization might be made to occur more efficiently. It is important to recognize that the goal of this approach is not to restore or improve memory in any general sense; instead, it is designed to teach a specific skill in hopes of preparing the patient for gainful employment. Glisky and Schacter (1988; see also Schacter and Glisky, 1986) have called this the "domain-specific" approach to distinguish it from the larger body of restorative techniques.

In recent years, the use of "errorless learning" as a rehabilitative technique has received significant attention (Baddeley and Wilson, 1994). Errorless learning is based on the idea that learning from mistakes is largely a process of explicit memory, whereas repeating prior responses is more aligned with implicit memory. Once an error is made, the incorrect response essentially has to be unlearned; otherwise, it may continue to interfere with the execution of correct responses. According to this view, residual implicit memory capabilities might better support the learning of new information if errors are eliminated such that every response is correct (Baddeley and Wilson, 1994). The technique of errorless learning has been used successfully to teach amnesic patients new lists of words (Hunkin et al., 1998), a route through a complex maze (Evans et al., 2000), face–name associations (Komatsu et al., 2000), and tasks of everyday memory functioning (Clare et al., 2000). There is some debate as to whether the benefits of errorless learning accrue from implicit memory (Baddeley and Wilson, 1994) or residual explicit memory (Hunkin et al., 1998), although the available data suggest that this technique is a promising area for future clinical and experimental investigation.

FUNCTIONAL IMAGING STUDIES OF MEMORY

In recent years, an explosion of research in functional imaging of real-time cognitive processing has taken place. Functional imaging techniques make use of the ability to visualize local changes in physiological activity (e.g., cerebral blood flow, glucose utilization, blood oxygenation) while individuals perform specific cognitive tasks. Many studies have examined functional brain activity during declarative (e.g., semantic and episodic; Schacter, 1997; Nyberg et al., 1998; Nyberg and Cabeza, 2000) and nondeclarative (e.g., skills and priming; Passingham, 1997; Schacter and Buckner, 1998) tasks. While a comprehensive review of this vast literature is beyond the scope of this chapter, a brief overview of some of the major findings in this literature will be offered.

Functional imaging studies of episodic memory encoding using positron emission tomography (PET) and functional magnetic resonance imaging (fMRI) have recently been reviewed by Schacter and colleagues (2000). Many early studies of encoding compared brain activity during deep vs. shallow encoding operations that differentially led to high and low levels of subsequent memory, respectively. Results generally found greater activation within left inferior prefrontal cortex (Brodman's Area [BA] 44, 45, 47) during deep encoding (Kapur et al., 1994; Demb et al., 1995; Fletcher et al., 1995). Subsequent studies using event-related MRI have shown greater left inferior frontal activation during the encoding of words that were later recognized (Wagner et al., 1998b). The prefrontal region may play a material-specific role in memory encoding, since at least some studies have shown corresponding right inferior frontal activation during the encoding of nonverbal stimuli (Wagner et al., 1998b). Because lesion studies have clearly highlighted the role of the medial temporal region in episodic memory, functional imaging studies have also focused on the role of the hippocampus and surrounding structures during memory encoding. Many studies have failed to demonstrate medial temporal activations during memory encoding and retrieval, which is regarded by some as a major issue in the field (Tulving and Markowitsch, 1997). However, activations within the medial temporal lobe have been observed under conditions in which exposure to novel stimulus materials is compared to familiar or repeated stimuli (Stern et al., 1996; Tulving et al., 1994). The most recent data suggest greater activation of posterior medial temporal lobe (parahippocampal gyrus) during successfully encoded words or pictures (Gabrieli et al., 1997a; Brewer et al., 1998; Wagner et al., 1998c; Schacter et al., 2000).

Recent functional brain imaging studies have revealed that right prefrontal regions are differentially activated during episodic memory retrieval, an effect that may be linked to monitoring of successfully retrieved items (Ungerleider, 1995; Buckner et al., 1996, 1998b, 1998c; Cabeza et al., 1997). Other studies have shown more bifrontal activation during successful retrieval (Rugg et al., 1996). Additional regions, including anterior cingulate and cerebellum, are more highly activated during recall than recognition, which suggests their role in self-initiated processing (Nyberg and Cabeza, 2000). Several studies have shown that the degree of medial temporal activity may correlate with the level of recall (Nyberg et al., 1996; Fernandez et al., 1998). A significant distinction between retrieval effort and retrieval success may be important in understanding the role of the prefrontal cortex in memory retrieval (Buckner, 1996; Schacter and Buckner, 1998; Wagner et al., 1998a; Buckner et al., 1999; Schacter et al., 2000).

Forms of nondeclarative memory, including priming and skill learning, have also been the subject of recent functional imaging studies. Perceptual priming is revealed by reductions in regional blood flow in extrastriate cortex during visual word-stem and word-fragment completion (Buckner et al., 1995, 1998; Blaxton et al., 1996; Schacter and Buckner, 1998), thus revealing a physiological correlate of performance facilitation seen in behavioral studies. This effect is greater in higher-order visual cortex than in primary regions (Buckner et al., 1998a). In the area of skill learning, the basic finding has been that as skills are learned, alternative pathways or regions become involved in task performance (Grafton et al., 1992; Jenkins et al., 1994; Karni et al., 1995; Krebs et al., 1998; Poldrack et al., 1998). These studies reflect a shift from naive to practiced conditions, with extensive prefrontal or premotor contributions early in the process giving way to other pathways as the task becomes more automatic or practiced.

Taken together, functional imaging studies of memory are consistent with the view that memory performance depends upon a distributed network of cortical and subcortical sites (Fuster, 1997; Nyberg and Cabeza, 2000). The role of specific brain regions and networks likely will be understood at the level of elementary cognitive components of memory that contribute to effective encoding, storage, and retrieval operations. The functional imaging literature is not yet well integrated with the vast literature on lesion-based analysis of memory performance, but it is likely that such integration will be forthcoming with advances in functional imaging technology and with applications of imaging technology to clinical problems of memory.

CONCLUSION

Experimental studies of the amnesic syndrome have provided important information about how memory is normally organized in the brain and have generated new approaches to the clinical study of memory disorders. The sparing of many memory functions has led to structural (systems) and functional (process) distinctions among different types of memory that are only now receiving anatomic verification through behavioral analysis and functional imaging studies. In the next decade, studies of amnesia are likely to benefit substantially from continued interdisciplinary collaboration, owing to the growing availability of sensitive and specific assessment tools and to the development of exciting new technologies.

Four decades of research with amnesic subjects has led to an increased understanding of the role that specific brain regions and brain systems play in normal and disordered memory functions. It could be said that we now have a good understanding of the components, or building blocks, upon which memory performance is based. The focus of the next decade will likely be on building and testing more comprehensive models of memory function at the network level.

Despite remarkable advances in our understanding of the neural basis of memory, definitive answers to some key questions are still not available. Is there a core amnesic syndrome, or are there fundamental differences among patients with lesions to temporal, diencephalic, or basal forebrain components of the distributed memory system?

Which cognitive deficits are necessary and sufficient to produce amnesia? Since amnesic disorders can result from diverse disease processes and may be seen in the context of a variety of cognitive deficits, it seems reasonable to attempt to distinguish between what is causative (central) and what is ancillary to the underlying memory disorder. A prominent example of how this issue complicates contemporary amnesia research is the controversy regarding the role of frontal lobe deficits in the memory impairment of diencephalic (and, perhaps, basal forebrain) amnesics. Traditionally, frontal contributions to memory have been considered to be relatively nonspecific, producing complex disturbances in attention and strategy formation that affect various domains of neuropsychological functioning in addition to memory. However, recent research has revealed that the frontal lobes play specific mnemonic roles, and may mediate complex processes such as working memory and memory for self-generated responses. Thus, frontal contributions to memory are receiving renewed attention, not as nuisance variables, but as aspects of memory functioning worthy of assuming a central place in amnesia research.

How can we best understand distinctions between spared and impaired memory abilities in amnesia? We have considered various ways of viewing these distinctions (e.g., multiple memory systems vs. transfer-appropriate processing) and have suggested that much of the data can be considered supportive of both approaches. That is, the view that memory dissociations support the idea of multiple memory systems and the consideration of such dissociations as being based on differences in cognitive processes applied at study and test are not necessarily mutually exclusive.

What is the relationship between implicit and explicit memory function? It will be important to continue to advance knowledge of the means by which how implicit phenomena (e.g., priming and perceptual fluency) contribute to performances on traditional (explicit) tests of recall and recognition. New strategies for empirically and statistically separating effects of direct recollection (e.g., recall) from the indirect effects of prior stimulus exposure (e.g., perceptual fluency and familiarity) hold significant promise in facilitating this understanding in normal subjects and amnesics.

How will experimental studies of amnesia continue to inform contemporary debates about memory function and dysfunction, including the nature of traumatically induced memory failures (Loftus, 1993; Zola, 1998) or distortions of eyewitness recall in the courtroom (Loftus and Ketcham, 1991; Schacter, 1998)? Understanding of these important topics has already benefited from research on encoding–retrieval interactions, memory for emotional events, and the constructive nature of memory, and will continue to increase as knowledge of normal and abnormal memory phenomena accumulates (Roediger and McDermott, 2000).

The interdisciplinary study of memory and amnesia represents one of the remarkable success stories of contemporary neuropsychology and cognitive neuroscience. Work continues from the clinic to the laboratory, from studies of higher cognitive function to membrane physiology, and from highly controlled experiments to analyses of everyday memory functioning. This remarkable diversity has led to rapid accumulation of important new data and new insights into the complex nature of memory successes and failures. Despite this knowledge, however, less progress has been made in developing effective approaches to the treatment of memory disorders. During the next decade, it is hoped that continuing interdisciplinary activity will provide a sufficient understanding of underlying mechanisms to make the design and implementation of effective interventions and rehabilitative techniques possible.

REFERENCES

Aggleton, J. P., and Brown, M. W. (1999). Episodic memory, amnesia, and the hippocampal–anterior thalamic axis. *Behav. Brain Sci. 22*:425–444.

Aggleton, J. P., Desimone, R., and Mishkin, M. (1986). The origin, course, and termination of the hippocampaothalamic projections in the macaque. *J. Comp. Neurol. 243*:409–421.

Aggleton, J. P., McMackin, D., Carpenter, K., Hornak, J., Kapur, N., Halpin, S., Wiles, C. M., Kamel, H., Brennan, P. Carton, S., and Gaffan, D. (2000). Differential cognitive effects of colloid cysts in the third ventricle that spare or compromise the fornix. *Brain 123*:800–815.

Aggleton, J. P., and Mishkin, M. (1983). Memory impairments following restricted medial thalamic lesions in monkeys. *Exp. Brain Res. 52*:199–209.

Aggleton, J. P., and Mishkin, M. (1985). Mammillary-body lesions and visual recognition in monkeys. *Exp. Brain Res. 58*:190–197.

Aggleton, J. P., Neave, N., Nagle, S., and Sahgal, A. (1995). A comparison of the effects of medial prefrontal, cingulate cortex, and cingulum bundle lesions on tests of spatial memory: evidence of a double dissociation between frontal and cingulum bundle contributions. *J. Neurosci 15*:7270–7281.

Aggleton, J. P., and Sahgal, A. (1993): The contribution of the anterior thalamic nuclei to anterograde amnesia. *Neuropsychologia 31*:1001–1019.

Albert, M. S., Butters, N., and Brandt, J. (1980a). Memory for remote events in alcoholics. *J. Stud. Alcohol 41*:1071–1081.

Albert, M. S., Butters, N., and Brandt, J. (1981). Patterns of remote memory in amnesic and demented patients. *Archives of Neurology, 38*:495–500.

Albert M. S., Butters N., and Levin J. (1979). Temporal gradients in the retrograde amnesia of patients with alcoholic Korsakoff's disease. *Arch. Neurol. 36*:211–216.

Albert, M. S., Butters, N., and Levin, J. (1980b). Memory for remote events in chronic alcoholics and alcoholic Korsakoff patients. *Adv. Exp. Med. Biol.* *126*:719–730.

Alexander, M. P., and Freedman, M. (1983). Amnesia after anterior communicating artery rupture. *Neurology 33(Suppl. 2)*:104.

Allan, K., Wilding, E. L., and Rugg, M. D. (1998). Electrophysiological evidence for dissociable processes contribution to recollection. *Acta Psychol. (Amsterdam) 98*:231–252.

Alvarez, P., and Squire, L. R. (1994). Memory consolidation and the medial temporal-lobe—a simple network model. *Proc. Natl. Acad. Sci. U.S.A. 91*:7041–7045.

Alvarez, P., Zola-Morgan, S., Squire, L. R. (1995). Damage limited to the hippocampal region produces long-lasting memory impairment in monkeys. *J. Neurosci. 15*:3796–3807.

Amaral, D. G., and Cowan, W. M. (1980). Subcortical afferents to the hippocampal formation in the monkey. *J. Comp. Neurol. 189*:573–591.

Amaral, D. G., and Insausti, R. (1990). Hippocampal formation. In *The Human Nervous System*, G. Paxinos (ed.). San Diego: Academic Press, pp. 711–755.

Amaral, D. G., Insausti, R., and Cowan, W. M. (1983). Evidence for a direct projection from the superior temporal gyrus to the entorhinal cortex in the monkey. *Brain Res. 275*:263–277.

Andersen, R. (1978). Cognitive changes after amygdalotomy. *Neuropsychologia 16*:439–451.

Anderson, J. R (1976). *Language, Memory, and Thought*. Hillsdale, NJ: Lawrence Erlbaum Associates.

Anderson, J. R., and Ross, B. H. (1980). Evidence against a semantic–episodic distinction. *J. Exp. Psychol. Hum. Learn. Mem. 6*:441–465.

Anderson, S. W., Damasio, H., Jones, R. D., and Tranel, D. (1991). Wisconsin Card Sorting Test performance as a measure of frontal lobe damage. *J. Clin. Exp. Neuropsychol. 13*:909–922.

Angeli, S. J., Murray, E. A., and Mishkin, M. (1993). Hippocampectomized monkeys can remember one place but not two. *Neuropsychologia 31*:1021–1030.

Arendt, T., Bigl., V., and Arendt, A. (1983). Loss of neurons in the nucleus basalis of Meynert in Alzheimer's disease, paralysis agitans and Korsakoff's disease. *Acta Neuropathol. 61*:101–108.

Arita, K., Uozumi, T., Ogasawara, H., Sugiyama, K., Ohba, S., Pant, B., Kimura, N., and Oshima, H. (1995). A case of pineal germinoma presenting with severe amnesia. *No Shinkei Geka 23*:271–275.

Ashby, F. G., Alfonso Reese, L. A., Turken, A. U., and Waldron, E. M. (1998). A neuropsychological theory of multiple systems in category learning. *Psychol. Rev. 105*:442–481.

Babcock, H. (1930). An experiment in the measurement of mental deterioration. *Arch. Psychol. 117*:105.

Bachevalier, J., and Mishkin, M. (1986). Visual recognition impairment follows ventromedial but not dorsolateral prefrontal lesions in monkeys. *Behav. Brain Res. 20*:249–261.

Bachevalier, J., Parkinson, J. K., and Mishkin, M. (1985a). Visual recognition in monkeys: effects of separate vs. combined transection of fornix and amygdalofugal pathways. *Exp. Brain Res. 57*:554–561.

Bachevalier, J., Saunders, R. C., and Mishkin, M. (1985b). Visual recognition in monkeys: effects of transection of the fornix. *Exp. Brain Res. 57*:547–553.

Baddeley, A. (1984). Memory Theory and Memory Therapy. In *Clinical Management of Memory Disorders*, B. A. Wilson and N. Moffat (eds.). Rockville, MD: Aspen Publications, pp. 5–27.

Baddeley, A. (1998). Recent developments in working memory. *Curr. Opin. Neurobiol. 8*:234–238.

Baddeley, A. D. (1982). Implications of neuropsychological evidence for theories of normal memory. *Philos. Trans. R. Soc. Lond. B Biol. Sci. 298(1089)*:59–72.

Baddeley, A., and Wilson, B. A. (1994). When implicit learning fails: amnesia and the problem of error elimination. *Neuropsychologia 32*:53–68.

Baeckman, L., and Dixon, R. A. (1992). Psychological compensation: a theoretical framework. *Psychol. Bull. 112*:259–283.

Bailey, C. H., Giustetto, M., Huang, Y.-Y., Hawkins, R. D., and Kandel, E. R. (2000). Is heterosynaptic modulation essential for stabilizing Hebbian plasticity and memory? *Nat. Rev. Neurosci. 1*:11–20.

Barker, A., Jones, R., and Jennison, C. (1995a). A prevalence study of age-associated memory impairment. *Br. J. Psychiatry 167*:642–648.

Barker, A., Prior, J., and Jones, R. (1995b). Memory complaint in attenders at a self-referral memory clinic: the role of cognitive factors, affective symptoms and personality. *Int. J. Geriatr. Psychiatry 10*:777–781.

Barr, W. B., Goldberg, E., Wasserstein, J., and Novelly, R. A. (1990). Retrograde amnesia following unilateral temporal lobectomy. *Neuropsychologia 28*:243–255.

Bartus, R. T., Dean, R. L., Beer, B., Ponecorvo, M. J., and Flicker, C. (1985). The cholinergic hypothesis: an historical overview, corrent perspective, and future directions. *Ann. N Y Acad. Sci. 444*:332–358.

Bauer, R. M. (1984). Autonomic recognition of names and faces in prospagnosia: A neuropsychological application of the Guilty Knowledge Test. *Neuropsychologia 22*:457–469.

Bauer, R. M., and Verfallie, M. (1992). Memory dissociations: a cognitive psychophysiology perspective. In L. R. Squire and N. Butters (eds.). *Neuropsychology of Memory* (2nd ed.). pp. 58–71. New York: Guilford Press.

Baxter, M. G., and Murray, E. A. (2002). The amygdala and reward. *Nature Rev. Neurosci. 3*:563–573.

Beaunieux, H., Desgranges, B., Lalevee, C., de la Sayette, V., Lechevalier, B., and Eustache, F. (1998). Preservation of cognitive procedural memory in a case of Korsakoff's syndrome: methodological and theoretical insights. *Percept. Mot. Skills 86(3 Pt 2)*:1267–1287.

Becker J. T., Furman J. M. R., Panisset M., and Smith C. (1990). Characteristics of the memory loss of a patient with Wernicke-Korsakoff's syndrome without alcoholism. *Neuropsychologia 28*:171–179.

Benson, D. F., Marsden, C. D., and Meadows, J. C. (1974). The amnesic syndrome of posterior cerebral artery occlusion. *Acta Neurol. Scand. 50*:133–145.

Bentin, S., and Moscovitch, M. (1988). The time course of repetition effects for words and unfamiliar faces. *J. Exp. Psychol. Gen. 117*:148–160.

Benton, A. L., Hamsher, K. de S., Varney, N. R., and Spreen, O. (1983). *Contributions to Neuropsychological Assessment*. New York: Oxford University Press.

Binder, L. M. (1982). Constructional strategies on Complex Figure drawings after unilateral brain damage. *J. Clin. Neuropsychol. 4*:51–58.

Blaney, P. H. (1986). Affect and memory: a review. *Psychol. Bull. 99*:229–246.

Blaxton, T. A. (1985). Investigating dissociations among memory measures: support for a transfer-appropriate processing framework. *J. Exp. Psychol. Learn. Mem. Cogn. 15*:657–668.

Blaxton, T. A. (1992). Dissociations among memory measures in memory-impaired subjects: evidence for a processing account of memory. *Memory Cogn. 20*:549–562.

Blaxton, T. A. (1995). A process-based view of memory. *J. Int. Neuropsychol. Soc. 1*:112–114.

Blaxton, T. A., Bookheimer, S. Y., Zeffiro, T. A., GFiglozzi, C. M., Gaillard, W. D., and Theodore, W. H. (1996). Functional mapping of human memory using PET: comparisons of perceptual and conceptual tasks. *Can. J. Exp. Psychol. 50*:42–56.

Bliss, T. V. P., and Gardner-Medwin, A. R. (1973). Long-lasting potentiation of synaptic transmission in the dentate area of the unanesthetized rabbit following stimulation of the perforant path. *J. Physiol. 232*:357–374.

Bliss, T. V. P., and Lomo, T. (1973). Long-lasting potentiation of synaptic transmission in the dentate area of the anesthetized rabbit following stimulation of the perforant path. *J. Physiol. 232*:331–356.

Bogousslavsky, J., Regli, F., and Assal, G. (1986). The syndrome of tuberothalamic artery territory infarction. *Stroke 17*:434–441.

Booker, J. (1991). Unpublished dissertation. University of Arizona.

Bowers, D., Verfaellie, M., Valenstein, E., and Heilman, K. M. (1988). Impaired acquisition of temporal order information in amnesia. *Brain Cogn. 8*:47–66.

Bowers, J., and Schacter, D. L. (1993). Priming of novel information in amnesic patients: issues and data. In *Implicit Memory: New Directions in Cognition, Development, and Neuropsychology*, P. Graf and M. E. J. Masson (eds.). Hillsdale, NJ: Lawrence Erlbaum Associates, pp. 303–326.

Brandt, J. (1991). The Hopkins Verbal Learning test: development of a new verbal memory test with six equivalent forms. *Clin. Neuropsychol. 5*:125–142.

Brewer, J. B., Zhao, Z., Desmond, J. E., Glover, G. H., and Gabrieli, J. D. (1998). Making memories: brain activity that predicts how well visual experience will be remembered. *Science 281(5380)*:1185–1187.

Brooks, D. N., Baddeley, A. (1976). What can amnesics learn? *Neuropsychologia 14*:111–122.

Buckner, R. L. (1996). Beyond HERA: contributions of specific prefrontal brain areas to long-term memory retrieval. *Psychonom. Bull. Rev. 3*:149–158.

Buckner, R. L., Goodman, J., Burock, M., Rott, M., Koustaal, W., Schacter, D., Rosen, B., and Dale, A. M. (1998a). Functional–anatomic correlates of object priming in humans revealed by rapid presentation event-related fMRI. *Neuron 20*:285–296.

Buckner, R. L., Kelley, W. M., and Petersen, S. E. (1999). Frontal cortex contributes to human memory formation. *Nat. Neurosci. 2*:311–314.

Buckner, R. L., Koutstaal, W., Schacter, D. L., Dale, A. M., Rotte, M., and Rosen, B. R. (1998b). Functional-anatomic study of episodic retrieval.

II. Selective averaging of event-related fMRI trials to test the retrieval success hypothesis. *Neuroimage* 7(3):163–175.

Buckner, R. L., Koutstaal, W., Schacter, D. L., Wagner, A. D., and Rosen, B. R. (1998c). Functional–anatomic study of episodic retrieval using fMRI. I. Retrieval effort versus retrieval success. *Neuroimage* 7(3):151–162.

Buckner, R. L., Petersen, S. E., Ojemann, G., Miezin, F. M., Squire, L. R., and Raichle, M. E. (1995). Functional anatomical studies of explicit and implicit memory retrieval tasks. *J. Neurosci.* 15:12–29.

Buckner, R. L., Raichle, M. E., Miezin, F. M., and Petersen, S. E. (1996). Functional anatomic studies of memory retrieval for auditory words and visual pictures. *J. Neurosci.* 16:6219–6235.

Burke, J. M., Danick, J. A., Bemis, B., and Durgin, C. J. (1994). A process approach to memory book training for neurological patients. *Brain Inj.* 8:71–81.

Bushke, H., and Fuld, P. A. (1974). Evaluation of storage, retention, and retrieval in disordered memory and learning. *Neurol* 11:1019–1025.

Butter, C. M., and Snyder, D. R. (1972). Alterations in aversive and aggressive behaviors following orbital frontal lesions in rhesus monkeys. *Acta Neurobiol. Exp.* 32:525–565.

Butters, M. A., Soety, E., and Becker, J. T. (1997). Memory rehabilitation. In *Handbook of Neuropsychology and Aging*, P. D. Nussbaum (ed.). New York: Plenum Press, pp. 515–527.

Butters, N. (1984). Alcoholic Korsakoff's syndrome: an update. *Semin. Neurol.* 4:226–244.

Butters, N. (1985). Alcoholic Korsakoff syndrome: some unresolved issues concerning etiology, neuropathology, and cognitive deficits. *J. Clin. Exp. Neuropsychol.* 7:181–210.

Butters N., Cermak, L. S. (1980) *Alcoholic Korsakoff's Syndrome: An Information Processing Approach to Amnesia*. New York: Academic Press.

Butters, N., and Cermak, L. S. (1986). A case study of the forgetting of autobiographical knowledge: implications for the study of retrograde amnesia. In *Autobiographical Memory*, D. Rubin (Ed.). New York: Cambridge University Press, pp. 253–272.

Butters, N., Granholm, E., Salmon, E., Grant, I., and Wolfe, J. (1987). Episodic and semantic memory: a comparison of amnesic and demented patients. *J. Exp. Clin. Neuropsychol.* 9: 479–497.

Butters, N., and Miliotis, P. (1985). Amnesic disorders. In *Clinical Neuropsychology*, (2nd ed.), K. M. Heilman and E. Valenstein (eds.). New York: Oxford University Press, pp. 403–451.

Butters, N., Miliotis, P., Albert, M. S., and Sax, D. S. (1984). Memory assessment: evidence of the heterogeneity of amnesic symptoms. In *Advances in Clinical Neuropsychology, Vol. 1*, G. Goldstein (ed.). New York: Plenum Press, pp. 127–159.

Butters, N., and Stuss, D.T. (1989). Diencephalic amnesia. In *Handbook of Neuropsychology, Vol. 3*, F. Boller and J. Grafman (eds.). L. Squire (section ed.). Amsterdam: Elsevier, pp. 107–148.

Cabeza, R., Grady, C. L., Nyberg, L., McIntosh, A. R., Tulving, E., Kapur, S., Jennings, J. M., Houle, S., and Craik, F. I. (1997). Age-related differences in neural activity during memory encoding and retrieval: a positron emission tomography study. *J. Neurosci.* 17:391–400.

Cairns, H., Mosberg, W. H. (1951). Colloid cyst of the third ventricle. *Surg. Gynecol. Obstet.* 92: 545–570.

Calabrese, P., Markowitsch, H. J., Harders, A. G., Scholz, M., and Gehlen, W. (1995). Fornix damage and memory. A case report. *Cortex* 31:555–564.

Caplan, L. B. (1985). Transient global amnesia. In *Handbook of Clinical Neurology, Vol. 1(45)*, J. A. M. Frederiks (ed.). Amsterdam: Elsevier, pp. 205–218.

Caplan, L., Chedru, F., Lhermitte, F., and Mayman, C. (1981). Transient global amnesia and migraine. *Neurology* 31:1167–1170.

Caramazza, A. (1992). Is cognitive neuropsychology possible? *J. Cogn. Neurosci.* 4:80–95.

Carlesimo, G. A. (1994). Perceptual and conceptual priming in amnesic and alcoholic patients. *Neuropsychologia* 32:903–921.

Carlesimo, G. A., Sabbadini, M., Loasses, A., and Caltagirone, C. (1998). Analysis of the memory impairment in a post-encephalitic patient with focal retrograde amnesia. *Cortex* 34:449–460.

Carr, A. C. (1982). Memory deficit after fornix section. *Neuropsychologia* 20:95–98.

Cermak, L. S. (1976). The encoding capacity of patients with amnesia due to encephalitis. *Neuropsychologia* 14:311–326.

Cermak, L. S. (1982). The long and the short of it in amnesia. In *Human Memory and Amnesia*. L. S. Cermak (ed.). Hillsdale, NJ: Lawrence Erlbaum. pp. 43–59.

Cermak, L. S. (1984). The episodic–semantic distinction in amnesia. In *Neuropsychology of Memory*, L. Squire and N. Butters (eds.). New York: Guilford Press, pp. 55–62.

Cermak, L. S. (1997). A positive approach to viewing processing deficit theories of amnesia. *Memory* 5:89–98.

Cermak, L. S., and Butters, N. (1972). The role of interference and encoding in the short-term memory deficits of Korsakoff Patients. *Neuropsychologia* 10:89–96.

Cermak, L. S., Butters, N., and Gerrein, J. (1973a). The extent of the verbal encoding ability of Korsakoff patients. *Neuropsychologia* 11:85–94.

Cermak, L. S., Butters, N., and Moreines, J. (1974). Some analyses of the verbal encoding deficit of alcoholic Korsakoff patients. *Brain Lang.* 1:141–150.

Cermak, L. S., Hill, R., and Wong, B. (1998). Effects of spacing and repetition on amnesic patients' performance during perceptual identification, stem completion, and category exemplar production. *Neuropsychology* 12:65–77.

Cermak, L. S., Mather, M., and Hill, R. (1997). Unconscious influences on amnesics' word-stem completion. *Neuropsychologia* 35:605–610.

Cermak, L. S., Naus, M., and Reale, L. (1976). Rehearsal and organizational strategies of alcoholic Korsakoff patients. *Brain Lang.* 3:375–385.

Cermak, L. S., and O'Connor, M. (1983). The anterograde and retrograde retrieval ability of a patient with amnesia due to encephalitis. *Neuropsychologia* 21:213–234.

Cermak, L. S., Reale, L., and Baker, E. (1978). Alcoholic Korsakoff patients' retrieval from semantic memory. *Brain Lang.* 5:215–226.

Cermak, L. S., Talbot, N., Chandler, K., and Wolbarst, L. R. (1985). The perceptual priming phenomenon in amnesia. *Neuropsychologia* 23:615–622.

Cermak, L. S., Uhly, B., and Reale, L. (1980). Encoding specificity in the alcoholic Korsakoff patient. *Brain Lang.* 11:119–127.

Cermak, L., Verfaellie, M., and Chase, K. A. (1995). Implicit and explicit memory in amnesia: an analysis of data-driven and conceptually driven processes. *Neuropsychology* 9:281–290.

Cermak, L., Verfaellie, M., and Letourneau, L. (1993). Episodic effects on picture identification for alcoholic Korsakoff patients. *Brain Cogn.* 22:85–97.

Cermak, L. S., Verfaellie, M., Milberg, W., Letourneau, L., and Blackford, S. (1991). A further analysis of perceptual identification priming in alcoholic Korsakoff patients. *Neuropsychologia* 29:725–736.

Cermak, L. S., Verfaellie, M., Sweeney, M., and Jacoby, L. L. (1992). Fluency versus conscious recollection in the word completion performance of amnesic patients. *Brain Cogn.* 20:367–377.

Cermak, L. S., and Wong, B. M. (1998). Amnesic patients' impaired category exemplar production priming. *J. Int. Neuropsychol. Soc.* 4:576–583.

Choi, D., Sudarsky, L., Schachter, S., Biber, M., and Burke, P. (1983). Medial thalamic hemorrhage with amnesia. *Arch. Neurol.* 40:611–613.

Chute, D. L., and Bliss, M. E. (1994). Prosthesis Ware: concepts and caveats for microcomputer-based aids to everyday living. *Exp. Aging Res.* 20:229–238.

Cirillo, R. A., Horel, J. A., and George, P. J. (1989). Lesions of the anterior temporal stem and the performance of delayed match-to-sample and visual discriminations in monkeys. *Behav. Brain Res.* 34:55–69.

Claparede, E. (1911). Recognition and "me-ness" *Arch. Neurol.* 11:79–90. Reprinted in D. Rapoport (Ed.). (1951). Organization and Pathology of Thought, pp. 58–75. New York: Columbia University Press.

Clare, L., Wilson, B. A., Carter, G., Breen, K., Gosses, A., and Hodges, J. R. (2000). Intervening with everyday memory problems in dementia of Alzheimer type: an errorless learning approach. *J. Clin. Exp. Neuropsychol.* 22:132–146.

Clark, C. R., and Geffen, G. M. (1989). Corpus callosum surgery and recent memory. A review. *Brain* 112:165–175.

Cohen, N. J. (1984). Preserved learning capacity in amnesia: evidence for multiple memory systems. In *Neuropsychology of Memory*, L. Squire and N. Butters (eds.). New York: Guilford Press, pp. 83–103.

Cohen, N. J., Eichenbaum, H., Deacedo, B. S., and Corkin, S. (1985). Different memory systems underlying acquisition of procedural and declarative knowledge. *Proc. N. Y. Acad. Sci.* 444:54–71.

Cohen, N. J., Poldrack, R. A., and Eichenbaum, H. (1997). Memory for items and memory for relations in the procedural/declarative memory framework. *Memory* 5:131–178, and in *Theories of Organic Amnesia*, A. R. Mayes and J. J. Downes (eds.). Hove, UK: Psychology Press/Erlbaum (UK) Taylor & Francis, pp. 131–178.

Cohen, N. J., and Squire, L. R. (1980). Preserved learning and retention of pattern analyzing skill in amnesia: Dissociation of knowing how and knowing that. *Science* 210:207–209.

Cohen, N. J., and Squire, L. R. (1981). Retrograde amnesia and remote memory impairment. *Neuropsychologia* 19:337–356.

Collins, A. M., and Loftus, E. F. (1975). A spreading-activation theory of semantic processing. *Psychol. Rev.* 82:407–428.

Corkin, S. (1968). Acquisition of motor skill after bilateral medial temporal lobe excision. *Neuropsychologia* 6:225–265.

Corkin, S. (1984). Lasting consequences of bilateral medial temporal lobectomy: clinical course and experimental findings in H.M. *Semin. Neurol.* 4:249–259.

Corkin, S., Cohen, N. J., and Sagar, H. J. (1983). Memory for remote personal and public events after bilateral medial temporal lobectomy. *Soc. Neurosci. Abstr.* 9:28.

Corsellis, J. A. N., Goldberg, G. J., and Morton, A. R. (1968). Limbic encephalitis and its association with carcinoma. *Brain* 91:481–496.

Corsi, P. M. (1972). *Human Memory and the Medial Temporal Region of the Brain.* Unpublished doctoral dissertation, McGill University.

Courtney, S. M., Ungerleider, L. G., Keil, K., and Haxby, J. V. (1997). Transient and sustained activity in a distributed neural system for human working memory. *Nature* 386(6625):608–611.

Cowan, N. (1988). Evolving conceptions of memory storage, selective attention, and their mutual constraints within the human information-processing system. *Psychol. Bull.* 104:163–191.

Craik, F. I. M., and Lockhart, R. S. (1972). Levels of processing: a framework for memory research. *J. Verbal Learn. Verbal Behav.* 11:671–684.

Crook, T., Bartus, R. T., Ferris, S. H., Whitehouse, P., Cohen, G. D., and Gershon, S. (1986). Age-associated memory impairment: Proposed diagnostic criteria and measures of clinical change. Report of a National Institute of Mental Health work group. *Dev. Neuropsychol.* 2:261–276.

Crook, T. H., and Larrabee, G. J. (1991). Diagnosis, assessment and treatment of age-associated memory impairment. *J. Neural Transm. Suppl.* 33:1–6.

Crosson, B. (1992). *Subcortical Functions in Language and Memory.* New York: Guilford Press.

Crovitz, H. F., Harvey, M. T., and Horn, R. W. (1979). Problems in the acquisition of imaging mnemonics: three brain-damaged cases. *Cortex* 15:225–234.

Cummings, J. L., Tomiyasu, U., Read, S., and Benson, D. F. (1984). Amnesia with hippocampal lesions after cardiopulmonary arrest. *Neurology* 42:263–271.

Curran, T. (1999). The electrophysiology of incidental and intentional retrieval: ERP old/new effects in lexical decision and recognition memory. *Neuropsychologia* 37:771–778.

Damasio, A. R. (1989). Time-locked multiregional retroactivation: a systems-level proposal for the neural substrates of recall and recognition. *Cognition* 33:25–62.

Damasio, A. R., Damasio, H., Tranel, D., Welsh, K., and Brandt, J. (1987). Additional neural and cognitive evidence in patient DRB. *Soc. Neurosci.* 13:1452.

Damasio, A. R., Eslinger, P. J., Damasio, H., Van Hoesen, G. W., and Cornell, S. (1985a). Multimodal amnesic syndrome following bilateral temporal and basal forebrain damage. *Arch. Neurol.* 42:252–259.

Damasio, A. R., Graff-Radford, N. R., Eslinger, P. J., Damasio, H., and Kassell, N. (1985b). Amnesia following basal forebrain lesions. *Arch. Neurol.* 42:263–271.

Damasio, A. R., Tranel, D., and Damasio, H. (1989). Amnesia caused by herpes simplex encephalitis, infarctions in basal forebrain, Alzheimer's disease, and anoxia/ischemia. In *Handbook of Neuropsychology*, F. Boller and J. Grafman (eds.). Amsterdam: Elsevier, pp. 149–166.

Delay, J., and Brion, S. (1969). *Le syndrome de Korsakoff.* Paris: Masson & Cie, 1969.

Delis, D., Kramer, J. H., Kaplan, E., and Ober, B. A. (2000). *California Verbal Learning Test (2nd Edition).* San Antonio TX: The Psychological Condition.

Delis, D. (1989). Neuropsychological assessment of learning and memory. In F. Boller and J. Grafman (ed.). *Handbook of Neuropsychology (Vol. 3)*, pp. 3–33. Amsterdam: Elsevier.

DeLuca, J., and Cicerone, K. (1989). Cognitive impairments following anterior communicating artery aneurysm. *J. Clin. Exp. Neuropsychol.* 11:47.

Demb, J. B., Desmond, J. E., Wagner, A. D., Vaidya, C. J., Glover, G. H., and Gabrieli, J. D. (1995). Semantic encoding and retrieval in the left inferior prefrontal cortex: a functional MRI study of task difficulty and process specificity. *J. Neurosci.* 15:5870–5878.

DeOlmos, J. S. (1990). Amygdala. In *The Human Nervous System*, G. Paxinos (ed.). San Diego: Academic Press, pp. 583–710.

De Renzi, E., Liotti, M., and Nichelli, P. (1987). Semantic amnesia with preservation of autobiographic memory. A case report. *Cortex* 23:575–597.

D'Esposito, M., Detre, J. A., Alsop, D. C., Shin, R. K., Atlas, S., and Grossman, M. (1995a). The neural basis of the central executive system of working memory. *Nature* 378(6554):279–281.

D'Esposito, M., Verfaellie, M., Alexander, M. P., and Katz, D. I. (1995b). Amnesia following traumatic ilateral fornix transection. *Neurology* 45:1546–1550.

Devinsky, O., Morrell, M. J., and Vogt, B. A. (1995).

Contributions of anterior cingulate cortex to behaviour. *Brain* 118:279–306.

Diamond, R., and Rozin, P. (1984). Activation of existing memories in the amnesic syndrome. *J. Abnorm. Psychol.* 93:98–105.

Dobkin, B. H., and Hanlon, R. (1993). Dopamine agonist treatment of antegrade amnesia from a mediobasal forebrain injury. *Ann. Neurol.* 33:313–316.

Dodson, C. S., and Johnson, M. K. (1996). Some problems with the process–dissociation approach to memory. *J. Exp. Psychol. Gen.* 125:181–194.

Donaldson, W. (1996). The role of decision processes in remembering and knowing. *Memory Cogn.* 24:523–533.

Dott, N. M. (1938). Surgical aspects of the hypothalamus. In *The Hypothalamus: Morphological, Functional, Clinical and Surgical Aspects*, W. E. Clark, le G., J. Beattie, G. Riddoch, and N. M. Dott. (eds.). Edinburgh: Oliver and Boyd, pp. 131–185.

Downes, J. J., Holdstock, J. S., Symons, V., and Mayes, A. R. (1998). Do amnesics forget colours pathologically fast? *Cortex* 34:337–355.

Doyon, J., Owen, A. M., Petrides, M., Sziklas, V., and Evans, A. C. (1996). Functional anatomy of visuomotor skill learning in human subjects examined with positron emission tomography. *Eur. J. Neurosci.* 8:637–648.

Drachman, D. A., and Arbit, J. (1966). Memory and the hippocampal complex. *Arch. Neurol.* 15:52–61.

Drachman, D. A., and Leavitt, J. (1974). Human memory and the cholinergic system. A relationship to aging? *Arch. Neurol.* 30.113–121.

Duchek, J. M., and Neeley, J. H. (1989). A dissociative word-frequency × levels of processing interaction in episodic recognition and lexical decision tasks. *Memory Cogn.* 17:148–162.

Dusoir, H., Kapur, N., Byrnes, D. P., McKinstry, S., and Hoare, R. D. (1990). The role of diencephalic pathoogy in human memory disorder. Evidence from a penetrating paranasal brain injury. *Brain* 113:1695–1706.

Duyckaerts, C., Derouesne, C., Signoret, J. L., Gray, F., Escourolle, R., and Castaigne, P. (1985). Bilateral and limited amygdala-hippocampal lesions causing a pure amnesic syndrome. *Ann. Neurol.* 18:314–319.

Eacott, M. J., and Crawley, R. A. (1999). Childhood amnesia: on answering questions about very early life events. *Memory* 7:279–292.

Eich, E. (1989). Theoretical issues in state dependent memory. In *Varieties of Memory and Consciousness: Essays in Honour of Endel Tulving*, H. L. Roediger and F. I. M. Craik (eds.). Hillsdale, NJ: Lawrence Erlbaum Associates, pp. 331–354.

Eich, E., and Metcalfe, J. (1989). Mood dependent memory for internal versus external events. *J. Exp. Psychol. Learn. Mem. Cogn.* 15:443–455.

Erickson, R. C. and Scott, M. L. (1977). Clinical memory testing: A review. *Psychol Bull* 84:1130–1149.

Eslinger, P. J., and Damasio, A. R. (1985). Severe disturbance of higher cognition after bilateral frontal lobe ablation: patient EVR. *Neurology* 35:1731–1741.

Eustache, F., Desgranges, B., and Messerli, P. (1996). Edouard Claparede and human memory [in French]. *Rev. Neurol. (Paris)* 152:602–610.

Evans, F. J., and Thorn, W. A. F. (1966). Two types of posthypnotic amnesia: recall amnesia and source amnesia. *Int. J. Clin. Exp. Hypn.* 14:162–179.

Evans, J. J., Emslie, H., and Wilson, B. A. (1998). External cueing systems in the rehabilitation of executive impairments of action. *J. Int. Neuropsychol. Soc.* 4:399–408.

Evans, J. J., Winson, B. A., Schuri, U., Andrade, J., Baddeley, A., Bruna, O., Canavan, T., Della Sala, S., Green, R., Laaksonen, R., Lorenzi, L., and Taussik, I. (2000). A comparison of "errorless" and "trial-and-error" learning methods for teaching individuals with acquired memory deficits. *Neuropsychol. Rehabil.* 10:67–101.

Fernandez, G., Weyerts, H., Schrader Bolsche, M., Tendolkar, I., Smid, H. G., Tempelmann, C., Hinrichs, H., Scheich, H., Elger, C. E., Mangun, G. R., and Heinze, H. J. (1998). Successful verbal encoding into episodic memory engages the posterior hippocampus: a parametrically analyzed functional magnetic resonance imaging study. *J. Neurosci.* 18:1841–1847.

Ferraro, I. R., Balota, D. A., and Connor, T. (1993). Implicit memory and the formation of new associations in nondemented Parkinson's disease individuals and individuals with senile dementia of the Alzheimer type: a serial reaction time (SRT) investigation. *Brain Cogn.* 21:163–180.

Feustel, T. C., Shiffrin, R. M., and Salasoo, A. (1983). Episodic and lexical contributions to the repetition effect in word identification. *J. Exp. Psychol. Gen.* 112:309–346.

Fibiger, H. C. (1991). Cholinergic mechanisms in learning, memory and dementia: a review of recent evidence. *Trends Neurosci.* 14:220–223.

Fischer, R. S., Alexander, M. P., D'Esposito, M., and Otto, R. (1995). Neuropsychological and neuroanatomical correlates of confabulation. *J. Clin. Exp. Neuropsychol. 17*:20–28.

Fisher, C. M. (1982). Transient global amnesia: precipitating activities and other observations. *Arch. Neurol. 39*:605–608.

Fisher, C. M., and Adams, R. D. (1958). Transient global amnesia. *Trans. Am. Neurol. Assoc. 83*: 143–145.

Flavell, J. H., and Wellman, H. M. (1977). Metamemory. In *Perspectives on the Development of Memory and Cognition*, R. V. Kail and J. W. Hagen (eds.). Hillsdale, NJ: Lawrence Erlbaum Associates, pp. 3–33.

Fleischman, D. A., Vaidya, C. J., Lange, K. L., and Gabrieli, J. D. (1997). A dissociation between perceptual explicit and implicit memory processes. *Brain Cogn. 35*:42–57.

Fletcher, P. C., Frith, C. D., Grasby, P. M., Shallice, T., Frackowiak, R. S., and Dolan, R. J. (1995). Brain systems for encoding and retrieval of auditory–verbal memory. An in vivo study in humans. *Brain 118(Pt 2)*:401–416.

Foerster, O. and Gagel, O. (1933). Ein Fall von Ependymcyste des III Ventrikels. Ein Beitrag zur Frage der Beziehungen psychischer Störungen zum Hirnstamm. *Z. Gesamte Neurol. Psychiatie 149*:312–344.

Freed, D. M., Corkin, S., and Cohen, N. J. (1987). Forgetting in H.M.: a second look. *Neuropsychologia 25*:461–471.

Fujii, T., Yamadori, A., Endo, K., Suzuki, K., and Fukatsu, R. (1999). Disproportionate retrograde amnesia in a patient with herpes simplex encephalitis. *Cortex 35*:599–614.

Fujii, K., Sadoshima, S., Ishitsuka, T., Kusuda, K., Kuwabara, Y., Ichiya, Y., Fujishima, M. (1989). Regional cerebral blood flow and metabolism in patients with transient global amnesia: a positron emission tomography study. *J. Neurol. Neurosurg. Psychiatr. 52*:622–630.

Funahashi, S., Bruce, C. J., and Goldman-Rakic, P. S. (1989). Mnemonic coding of visual space in the monkey's dorsolateral prefrontal cortex. *J. Neurophysiol. 61*:1–19.

Fuster, J. M. (1984). The cortical substrate of memory. In *Neuropsychology of Memory*, L. R. Squires and N. Butters (eds.). New York: Guilford Press, pp. 279–286.

Fuster, J. M. (1997). Network memory. *Trends Neurosci. 20*:451–459.

Gabrieli, J. D. (1998). Cognitive neuroscience of human memory. *Annu. Rev. Psychol. 49*:87–115.

Gabrieli, J. D., Cohen, N. J., and Corkin, S. (1988). The impaired learning of semantic knowledge following bilateral medial temporal-lobe resection. *Brain Cogn. 7*:157–177.

Gabrieli, J. D., Corkin, S., Mickel, S. F., and Growdon, J. H. (1993). Intact acquisition and long-term retention of mirror-tracing skill in Alzheimer's disease and in global amnesia. *Behav. Neurosci. 107*:899–910.

Gabrieli, J. D., McGlinchey Berroth, R., Carrillo, M. C., Gluck, M. A., Cermak, L. S., and Disterhoft, J. F. (1995a). Intact delay-eyeblink classical conditioning in amnesia. *Behav. Neurosci. 109*:819–827.

Gabrieli, J. D., Milberg, W., Keane, M. M., and Corkin, S. (1990). Intact priming of patterns despite impaired memory. *Neuropsychologia 28*: 417–427.

Gabrieli, J. D., Poldrack, R. A., and Desmond, J. E. (1998). The role of left prefrontal cortex in language and memory. *Proc. Natl. Acad. Sci. U.S.A. 95*:906–913.

Gabrieli, J. D. E., Brewer, J. B., Desmond, J. E., and Glover, G. H. (1997). Separate neural bases of two fundamental memory processes in the human medial temporal lobe. *Science 276(5310)*: 264–266.

Gabrieli, J. D. E., Fleischman, D. A., Keane, M. M., Reminger, S. L., and Morrell, F. (1995b). Double dissociation between memory systems underlying explicit and implicit memory in the human brain. *Psychol. Sci. 6*:76–82.

Gabrieli, J. D. E., Keane, M. M., Stanger, B. Z., Kjelgaard, M. M., Corkin, S., and Growdon, J. H. (1994). Dissociations among structural–perceptual, lexical–semantic, and event–fact memory systems in amnsic, Alzheimer's and normal subjects. *Cortex 30*:75–103.

Gabrieli, J. D. E., Stebbins, G. T., Singh, J., Willingham, D. B., and Goetz, C. G. (1997b). Intact mirror tracing and impaired rotary-pursuit skill learning in patients with Huntington's disease: evidence for dissociable memory systems in skill learning. *Neuropsychology 11*:272–281.

Gade, A. (1982). Amnesia after operations on aneurysms of the anterior communicating artery. *Surg. Neurol. 18*:46–49.

Gade, A., and Mortensen, E. L. (1990). Temporal gradient in the remote memory impairment of amnesic patients with lesions in the basal forebrain. *Neuropsychologia 28*:985–1001.

Gaffan, D. (1974). Recognition impaired and association intact in the memory of monkeys after transection of the fornix. *J. Comp. Physiol. Psychol. 86*:1100–1109.

Gaffan, D. (1993). Additive effects of forgetting and fornix transection in the temporal gradient of retrograde amnesia. *Neuropsychologia 31*:1055–1066.

Gaffan, D., and Gaffan, E. A. (1991). Amnesia in

man following transection of the fornix: a review. *Brain* 114:2611–2618.

Gaffan, D., and Harrison, S. (1987). Amygdalectomy and disconnection in visual learning for auditory secondary reinforcment by monkeys. *J. Neurosci.* 7:2285–2292.

Gaffan, D., and Parker, A. (1996). Interaction of perirhinal cortex with the fornix-fimbria: memory for objects and "object-in-place" memory. *J. Neurosci.* 16:5864–5869.

Gaffan, E. A., Gaffan, D., and Hodges, J. R. (1991). Amnesia following damage to the left fornix and to other sites: a comparative study. *Brain* 114: 1297–1313.

Garcia Bencochea, F., De La Torre, O., Esquivel, O., Vieta, R., and Fernandec, C. (1954). The section of the fornix in the surgical treatment of certain epilepsies: a preliminary report. *Trans. Am. Neurol. Assoc.* 79:176–178.

Gardner, H., Boller, F., Moreines, J., and Butters, N. (1973). Retrieving information from Korsakoff patients. Effects of categorical cues and reference to the task. *Cortex* 9:165–175.

Gentilini, M., DeRenzi, E. and Crisi, G. (1987). Bilateral paramedian thalamic artery infarcts: report of eight cases. *J Neurol. Neurosurg. Psychiatry* 50:900–909.

George, P. J., Horel, J. A., and Cirillo, R. A. (1989). Reversible cold lesions of the parahippocampal gyrus in monkeys result in deficits on the delayed match-to-sample and other visual tasks. *Behav. Brain Res.* 34:163–178.

Ghika-Schmid, F., and Bogousslavsky, J. (2000). The acute behavioral syndrome of anterior thalamic infarction: a prospective study of 12 cases. *Ann. Neurol.*, 48:220–227.

Gianutsos, R. and Gianutsos, J. (1979). Rehabilitating the verbal recall of brain damaged patients by mnemonic training: an experimental demonstration using single-case methodology. *J Clin Neuropsychol* 1:117–135.

Glees, P., and Griffith, H. B. (1952). Bilateral destruction of the hippocampus (cornu ammonis) in a case of dementia. *Psychiatr. Neurol. Med. Psychol.* 123:193–204.

Glisky, E. L. (1992). Acquisition and transfer of declarative and procedural knowledge by memory-impaired patients: a computer data-entry task. *Neuropsychologia* 30:899–910.

Glisky, E. L., and Schacter, D. L. (1988). Long-term retention of computer learning by patients with memory disorders. *Neuropsychologia* 26:173–178.

Glisky, E. L., Schacter, D. L., and Tulving, E. (1986a). Computer learning by memory-impaired patients: acquisition and retention of complex knowledge. *Neuropsychologia* 24:313–328.

Glisky, E. L., Schacter, D. L., and Tulving, E. (1986b). Learning and retention of computer-related vocabulary in memory-impaired patients: method of vanishing cues. *J. Clin. Exp. Neuropsychol.* 8:292–312.

Gloor, P. (1986). Role of the human limbic system in perception, memory, and affect: lessons from temporal lobe epilepsy. In *The Limbic System: Functional Organization and Clinical Disorders*, B. K. Doane and K. E. Livingston (eds.). New York: Raven Press, pp.159–169.

Goldenberg, G., Wimmer, A., and Maly, J. (1983). Amnesic syndrome with a unilateral thalamic lesion: a case report. *J. Neurol.* 229:79–86.

Goldenberg, G., Podreka, I., Pfaffelmeyer, N., Wessely, P., and Deecke, L. (1991). Thalamic ischemia in transient global amnesia: a SPECT Study. *Neurology* 41:1748–1752.

Goldman-Rakic, P. S. (1984). Modular organization of the prefrontal cortex. *Trends Neurosci.* 7:419–424.

Goldman-Rakic, P. S. (1992). Prefrontal cortical dysfunction in schizophrenia: the relevance of working memory. In *Psychopathology and the Brain*, B. Carroll (ed.). New York: Raven Press.

Gooding, P. A., Mayes, A. R., and van Eijk, R. (2000). A meta-analysis of indirect memory tests for novel material in organic amnesics. *Neuropsychologia* 38:666–676.

Gooding, P. A., van Eijk, R., Mayes, A. R., and Meudell, P. (1993). Preserved pattern completion priming for novel, abstract geometric shapes in amnesics of several aetiologies. *Neuropsychologia* 31:789–810.

Goodwin, D. W., Powell, B., Bremer, D., Hoine, H., and Stern, J. (1969). Alcohol and recall: state dependent effects in man. *Science* 163:1358–1360.

Goshen-Gottstein, Y., Moscovitch, M., and Melo, B. (2000). Intact implicit memory for newly formed verbal associations in amnesic patients following single study trials. *Neuropsychology* 14:570–578.

Graf, P., and Mandler, G. (1984). Activation makes words more accessible, but not necessarily more retrievable. *J Verb Learn Verb Behav* 23:553–568.

Graf, P., Mandler, G., and Haden, P. E. (1982). Simulating amnesic symptoms in normal subjects. *Science* 218(4578):1243–1244.

Graf, P., and Schacter, D. L. (1985). Implicit and explicit memory for new associations in normal and amnesic subjects. *J. Exp. Psychol. Learn. Mem. Cogn.* 11:501–518.

Graf, P., Shimamura, A. P., and Squire, L. R. (1985). Priming across modalities and priming across category levels: extending the domain of preserved function in amnesia. *J. Exp. Psychol. Learn. Mem. Cogn.* 11:386–396.

Graf, P., Squire, L. R., and Mandler, G. (1984). The information that amnesic patients do not forget. *J. Exp. Psychol: Learn. Mem. Cogn.* 10:164–178.

Graff-Radford, N. R., Damasio, H., Yamada, T., Eslinger, P. J., and Damasio, A. R. (1985). Non-haemmorhagic thalamic infarction: clinical, neuropsychological, and electrophysiological findings in four anatomical groups defined by computerized tomography. *Brain* 108:458–516.

Graff-Radford, N. R., Eslinger, P. J., Damasio, A. R., and Yamada, T. (1984). Nonhemmorhagic infarction of the thalamus: behavioral, anatomic, and physiological correlates. *Neurology* 34: 14–23.

Graff-Radford, N. R., Tranel, D., Van Hoesen, G. W., and Brandt, J. P. (1990). Diencephalic amnesia. *Brain* 113:1–25.

Grafman, J., Salazar, A. M., Weingartner, J., Vance, S. C., and Ludlow, C. (1985). Isolated impairment of memory following a penetrating lesion of the fornix cerebri. *Arch. Neurol.* 42:1162–1168.

Grafton, S. T., Mzaaiotta, J. C., Presty, S., Friston, K. J., Frackowiak, R. S. J., and Phelps, M. E. (1992). Functional anatomy of human procedural learning determined with regional cerebral blood flow and PET. *J. Neurosci.* 12:2242–2248.

Grossi, D., Trojano, L., Grasso, A., and Orsini, A. (1988). Selective "semantic amnesia" after closed-head injury. A case report. *Cortex* 24:457–464.

Gruneberg, M. M. (1983). Memory processes unique to humans. In *Memory in Animals and Man*, A. Mayes (ed.). London: Von Nortrand, pp. 253–281.

Gruneberg, M. M., and Monks, J. (1974). Feeling of knowing and cued recall. *Acta Psychol.* 41: 257–265.

Grünthal, E. (1939). Über das Corpus mamillare und den Korsakowshcen Symptomenkomplex. *Confin. Neurol.* 2:64–95.

Grünthal, E. (1947). Über das klinische Bild nach umschriebenem beiderseitigem Ausfall der Ammonshornrinde. *Monatsschr. Psychiatr. Neurol.* 113:1–6.

Gustafsson, B. and Wigstrom, H. (1988). Physiological mechanisms underlying long-term potentiation. *Trends Neurosci.* 11:156–162.

Haas, D. C., and Ross, G. S. (1986). Transient global amnesia triggered by mild head trauma. *Brain* 109:251–257.

Haist, F., Musen, G., and Squire, L. R. (1991). Intact priming of words and nonwords in amnesia. *Psychobiology* 19:275–285.

Hamann, S. B., and Squire, L. R. (1995). On the acquisition of new declarative knowledge in amnesia. *Behav. Neurosci.* 109:1027–1044.

Hamann, S. B., and Squire, L. R. (1996). Level-of-processing effects in word-completion priming: a neuropsychological study. *J. Exp. Psychol. Learn. Mem. Cogn.* 22:933–947.

Hamann, S. B., and Squire, L. R. (1997). Intact perceptual memory in the absence of conscious memory. *Behav. Neurosci.* 111:850–854.

Hamby, S. L., Wilkins, J. W., and Barry, N. S. (1993). Organizational quality on the Rey-Osterrieth and Taylor Complex Figure tests: a new scoring system. *Psychol. Assess.* 5:27–33.

Hanninen, T., and Soininen, H. (1997). Age-associated memory impairment. Normal aging or warning of dementia? *Drugs Aging* 11:480–489.

Hart, J. T. (1965). Memory and the feeling-of-knowing experience. *J. Ed. Psychol.* 56:208–216.

Hart, J. T. (1967). Memory and the memory-monitoring process. *J. Verbal Learn. Verbal Behav.* 6:685–691.

Hashimoto, R., Tanaka, Y., and Nakano, I. (2000). Amnesic confabulatory syndrome after focal basal forebrain damage. *Neurology* 54:978–980.

Hassler, R., and Riechert, T. (1957). Über einen Fall von doppelseitiger Fornicotomie bei sogenannter temporaler Epilepsie. *Acta Neurocuir. (Wien)* 5:330–340.

Hazeltine, E., Grafton, S. T., and Ivry, R. (1997). Attention and stimulus characteristics determine the locus of motor-sequence encoding: a PET study. *Brain* 120:123–140.

Heathfield, K. W. G., Croft, P. B., and Swash, M. (1973). The syndrome of transient global amnesia. *Brain* 96:729–736.

Heilman, K. M., and Sypert, G. W. (1977). Korsakoff's syndrome resulting from bilateral fornix lesions. *Neurology* 27:490–493.

Heimer, L., and Alheid, G. F. (1991). Piecing together the puzzle of basal forebrain anatomy. In *The Basal Forebrain*, T. C. Napier, P. W. Kalivas, and I. Hanin (eds.). New York: Plenum Press [referenced by Medline as *Adv. Exp. Med. Biol.* 295:1–42, 1991].

Heindel, W. C., Salmon, D. P., Shults, C. W., Walicke, P. A., and Butters, N. (1989). Neuropsychological evicence for multiple implicit memory systems: a comparison of Alzheimer's, Huntington's, and Parkinson's disease patients. *J. Neurosci.* 9:582–587.

Herkenham, M. (1978). The connections of the nucleus reuniens thalami: evidence for a direct thalmo-hippocampal pathway in the rat. *J. Comp. Neurol.* 177:589–610.

Herzog, A. G., and Van Hoesen, G. W. (1976). Temporal neocortical afferent connections to the amygdala in the rhesus monkey. *Brain Res.* 115: 57–69.

Hirshman, E., and Master, S. (1997). Modeling the conscious correlates of recognition memory: reflections on the remember-know paradigm. *Mem. Cogn.* 25:345–351.

Hirst, W. (1982). The amnesic syndrome: descriptions of explanations. *Psychol. Bull.* 91:435–462.

Hirst, W., and Volpe, B. T. (1982). Temporal order judgements with amnesia. *Brain Cogn.* 1:294–306.

Hodges, J. R., and McCarthy, R. A. (1995). Loss of remote memory: a cognitive neuropsychological perspective. *Curr. Opin. Neurobiol.* 5:178–183.

Hodges, J. R., and Warlow, C. P. (1990). The aetiology of transient global amnesia. A case control study of 114 cases with prospective follow-up. *Brain* 113:639–657.

Hodgson, R., and Rachman, S. (1977). Desynchrony in measures of fear. *Behav. Res. Ther.* 12:319–326.

Holtz, K. H. (1962). Über Gehirn- und Augenveränderunge bei Hyalinosis cutis et mucosae (lipoid Proteinose) mit Autopsiebefund. *Arch. Klin. Exp. Dermatol.* 214:289–306.

Horel, J. A. (1978). The neuroanatomy of amnesia. A critique of the hippocampal memory hypothesis. *Brain* 101:403–445.

Horel, J. A., Voytko, M. L., and Salsbury, K. (1984). Visual learning suppressed by cooling of the temporal lobe. *Behav. Neurosci.* 98:310–324.

Hunkin, N. M., and Parkin, A. J. (1995). The method of vanishing cues: an evaluation of its effectiveness in teaching memory-impaired individuals. *Neuropsychologia* 33:1255–1279.

Hunkin, N. M., Parkin, A. J., Bradley, V. A., Burrows, E. H., Aldrich, F. K., Jansari, A., and Burdon-Cooper, C. (1995). Focal retrograde amnesia following closed head injury: a case study and theoretical account. *Neuropsychologia* 33:509–523.

Hunkin, N. M., Squires, E. J., Parkin, A. J., and Tidy, J. A. (1998). Are the benefits of errorless learning dependent on implicit memory? *Neuropsychologia* 36:25–36.

Huppert, F. A., and Piercy, M. (1976). Recognition memory in amnesic patients: effect of temporal context and familiarity of material. *Cortex* 12:3–20.

Huppert, F. A., and Piercy, M. (1979). Normal and abnormal forgetting in organic amnesia: effect of locus of lesion. *Cortex* 15:385–390.

Hyman, B. T., Van Hoesen, G. W., Kromer, J. J., and Damasio, A. R. (1986). Perforant pathway changes and the memory impairment of Alzheimer's disease. *Ann. Neurol.* 20:472–481.

Hyman, B. T., Van Hoesen, G. W., Damasio, A. R., and Barnes, C. L. (1984). Cell-specific pathology isolates the hippocampal formation in Alzheimer's disease. *Science* 225:1168–1170.

Inglis, J. (1970). Shock, surgery, and cerebral asymmetry. *Br. J. Psychiatry* 117:143–148.

Inoue, C., and Bellezza, F. S. (1998). The detection model of recognition using know and remember judgments. *Mem. Cogn.* 26:299–308.

Insausti, R., Amaral, D. G., and Cowan, W. M. (1987a). The entorhinal cortex of the monkey: II. Cortical afferents. *J. Comp. Neurol.* 264:356–395.

Insausti, R., Amaral, D. G., and Cowan, W. M. (1987b). The entorhinal cortex of the monkey: III. Subcortical afferents. *J. Comp. Neurol.* 264:396–408.

Irle, E., and Markowitsch, H. J. (1982). Widespread cortical projections of the hippocampal formation in the cat. *Neuroscience* 7:2637–2647.

Irle, E., Wowra, B., and Kunert, H., (1992). Memory disturbances following anterior communicating artery rupture. *Ann. Neurol.* 31:473–480.

Iwasaki, S., Arihara, T., Torii, H., Hiraguti, M., Kitamoto, F., Nakagawa, A., Nakagawa, H., Fujiki, S., Nakamura, T., and Kurauchi, M. (1993). A case of splenial astrocytoma with various neuropsychological symptoms. *No To Shinkei* 45:1067–1073.

Iwata, J., LeDoux, J. E., Meeley, M. P., Arneric, S., and Reis, D. J. (1986). Intrinsic neurons in amygdaloid field projected to by the medial geniculate body mediate emotional responses conditioned to acoustic stimuli. *Brain Res.* 383:195–214.

Izquierdo, I. (1991). Role of NMDA receptors in memory. *Trends Pharmacol. Sci.* 12:128–129.

Jacoby, L. L. (1983a). Analyzing interactive processes in reading. *J. Verbal Learn. Verbal Behav.* 22:485–508.

Jacoby, L. L. (1983b). Perceptual enhancement: persistent effects of an experience. *J. Exp. Psychol. Learn. Mem. Cogn.* 9:21–38.

Jacoby, L. L. (1984). Incidental versus intentional retrieval: remembering and awareness as separate issues. In *Neuropsychology of Memory*, L. R. Squire and N. Butters (eds.). New York: Guilford Press, pp. 145–156.

Jacoby, L. L. (1991). A process dissociation framework: separating automatic from intentional uses of memory. *J. Mem. Lang.* 30:513–541.

Jacoby, L. L., and Dallas, M. (1981). On the relationship between autobiographical memory and perceptual learning. *J. Exp. Psychol. Gen.* 3:306–340.

Jacoby, L. L., and Kelly, C. (1992). Unconscious influences of memory: dissociations and automaticity. In *Neuropsychology of Consciousness*,

A. D. Milner and M. Rugg (eds.). New York: Academic Press, pp. 201–233.

Jacoby, L. L., Kelly, C. M., and Dywan, J. (1989). Memory attributions. In *Varieties of Memory and Consciousness: Essays in Honour of Endel Tulving*, H. L. Roediger and F. I. M. Craik (eds.). Hillsdale, NJ: Lawrence Erlbaum Associates, pp. 391–422.

Janowsky, J. S., Shimamura, A. P., and Squire, L. R. (1989). Memory and metamemory: comparisons between patients with frontal lobe lesions and amnesic patients. *Psychobiology* 17:3–11.

Jenkins, I. H., Brooks, D. J., Nixon, P. D., Frackowiak, R. S. J., and Passingham, R. E. (1994). Motor sequence learning: a study with positron emoission tomography. *J. Neurosci.* 18:5026–5034.

Jernigan, T. L., Butters, N., DiTraglia, G., Schafer, K., Smith, T., Irwin, M., Grant, I., Schuckit, M., and Cermak, L. S. (1991a). Reduced cerebral grey matter observed in alcoholics using magnetic resonance imaging. *Alcohol Clin. Exp. Res.* 15:418–427.

Jernigan, T. L., Schafer, K., Butters, N., and Cermak, L. S. (1991b). Magnetic resonance imaging of alcoholic Korsakoff patients. *Neuropsychopharmacology* 4:175–186.

Jerusalinsky, D., Kornisiuk, E., and Izquierdo, I. (1997). Cholinergic neurotransmission and synaptic plasticity concerning memory processing. *Neurochem Res.* 22:507–515.

Johns, C. A., Greenwald, B. S., Mohs, R. C., and Davis, K. L. (1983). The cholinergic treatment strategy in ageing and senile dementia. *Psychopharmacol. Bull.* 19:185–197.

Johnson, M. K. (1991). Reality monitoring: evidence from confabulation in organic brain disease patients. In *Awareness of Deficit After Brain Injury*, G. Prigatano and D. L. Schacter (eds.). New York: Oxford University Press, pp. 176–197.

Johnson, M. K., and Hasher, L. (1987). Human learning and memory. In M. R. Rosenzweig and L. W. Porter (eds.) *Annual Review of Psychology*, 38. Palo Alto CA: Annual Reviews. Inc., pp. 631–688.

Johnson, M. K., Hashtroudi, S., and Lindsay, D. S. (1993). Source monitoring. *Psychol. Bull.* 114: 3–28.

Johnson, M. K., Kim, J. K., and Risse, G. (1985). Do alcoholic Korsakoff's patients acquire affective reactions? *J. Exp. Psychol. Learn. Mem. Cogn.* 11:22–36.

Johnson, M. K., O'Connor, M., and Cantor, J. (1997). Confabulation, memory deficits, and frontal dysfunction. *Brain Cogn.* 34:189–206.

Jones, B., and Mishkin, M. (1972). Limbic lesions and the problem of stimulus-reinforcement associations. *Exp. Neurol.* 36:362–377.

Jones-Gotman, M., and Milner, B. (1978). Right temporal-lobe contribution to image-mediated verbal learning. *Neuropsychologia* 16:61–71.

Kaplan, E. F., Fein, D., Morris, R., and Delis, D. (1991). WAIS-R as a neuropsychological instrument. San Antonio, TX: Psychological Corporation.

Kaplan, R. F., Meadows, M. E., Verfaellie, M., Kwan, E., Ehrenberg, B. L., Bromfield, E. B., and Cohen, R. A. (1994). Lateralization of memory for the visual attributes of objects: evidence from the posterior cerebral artery amobarbital test. *Neurology* 44:1069–1073.

Kapur, N. (1991). Amnesia in relation to fugue states—distinguishing a neurological from a psychogenic basis. *Br. J. Psychiatry* 159:872–877.

Kapur, N. (1999). Syndromes of retrograde amnesia: a conceptual and empirical synthesis. *Psychol. Bull.* 125:800–825.

Kapur, N., and Brooks, D. J. (1999). Temporally specific retrograde amnesia in two cases of discrete bilateral hippocampal pathology. *Hippocampus* 9:247–254.

Kapur, N., and Butters, N. (1977). Visuoperceptive deficits in long-term alcoholics with Korsakoff's psychosis. *J. Stud. Alcohol* 38:2025–2035.

Kapur, S., Craik, F. I., Tulving, E., Wilson, A. A., Houle, S., and Brown, G. M. (1994). Neuroanatomical correlates of encoding in episodic memory: levels of processing effect. *Proc. Natl. Acad. Sci. U. S. A.* 91:2008–2011.

Kapur, N., Ellison, D., Smith, M. P., McLellan, D. L., and Burrows, E. H. (1992). Focal retrograde amnesia following bilateral temporal lobe pathology. A neuropsychological and magnetic resonance study. *Brain* 115 Pt 1:73–85.

Kapur, N., Young, A., Bateman, D., and Kennedy, P. (1989). Focal retrograde amnesia: a long-term clinical and neuropsychological follow-up. *Cortex* 25:387–402.

Karni, A., Meyer, G., Jezzard, P., Adams, M. M., Turner, R., and Ungerleider, L. G. (1995). Functional MRI evidence for adult motor cortex plasticity during motor skill learning. *Nature* 377: 155–158.

Katai, S., Maruyama, T., Hashimoto, T., and Yanagisawa, N. (1992). A case of cerebral infarction presenting as retrospinal amnesia. *Rinsho Shinkeigaku* 32:1281–1287.

Keane, M. M., Clarke, H., and Corkin, S. (1992). Impaired perceptual priming and intact conceptual priming in a patient with bilateral posterior cerebral lesions. *Soc. Neurosci. Abstr.* 18:386.

Keane, M. M., Gabrieli, J. D., Growdon, J. H., and Corkin, S. (1994). Priming in perceptual identification of pseudowords is normal in Alzheimer's disease. *Neuropsychologia* 32:343–356.

Keane, M. M., Gabrieli, J. D. E., Monti, L. A., Cantor, J. M., and Noland, J. S. (1993). Amnesic patients show normal priming and a normal depth-of-processing effect in a conceptually driven implicit memory task. *Soc. Neurosci. Abstr.* 19:1079.

Keane, M. M., Gabrieli, J. D., Noland, J. S., and McNealy, S. I. (1995). Normal perceptual priming of orthographically illegal nonwords in amnesia. *J. Int. Neuropsychol. Soc.* 1:425–433.

Kelley, C. M., and Jacoby, L. L. (2000). Recollection and familiarity: process-dissociation. In *The Oxford Handbook of Memory*, E. Tulving and F. I. M. Craik (eds.). New York: Oxford University Press, pp. 215–228.

Kennedy, M. B. (1989). Regulation of synaptic transmission in the central nervous system: Long-term potentiation. *Cell* 59:777–787.

Kersteen-Tucker, Z. (1991). Long-term repetition priming with symmetrical polygons and words. *Mem. Cogn.* 19:37–43.

Kessler, J., Markowitsch, H. J., Huber, M., Kalbe, E., Weber-Luxenburger, G., and Kock, P. (1997). Massive and persistent anterograde amnesia in the absence of detectable brain damage: anterograde psychogenic amnesia or gross reduction in sustained effort? *J. Clin. Exp. Neuropsychol.* 19:604–614.

Khan, N., and Wieser, II. G. (1994). Limbic encephalitis: a case report. *Epilepsy Res.* 17:175–181.

Kihlstrom, J. F. (1980). Posthypnotic amnesia for recently learned materials: Interactions with "episodie" and "semantic" memory. *Cognitive Psychology* 12:227–251.

Kihlstrom, J. F. (1995). Memory and consciousness: an appreciation of Claparede and recognition et moiite. *Conscious Cogn.* 4:379–386.

Kilgard, M. P., and Merzenich, M. M. (1998). Cortical map reorganization enabled by nucleus basalis activity. *Science* 279:1714–1718.

Kim, H. J., Burke, D. T., Dowds, M. M., and George, J. (1999). Utility of a microcomputer as an external memory aid for a memory-impaired head injury patient during in-patient rehabilitation. *Brain Inj.* 13:147–150.

Kim, H. J., Burke, D. T., Dowds, M. M., Jr., Boone, K. A., and Park, G. J. (2000). Electronic memory aids for outpatient brain injury: follow-up findings. *Brain Inj.* 14:187–196.

Kinsbourne, M., and Wood, F. (1975). Short-term memory processes and the amnesic syndrome. In *Short-Term Memory*, D. Deutsch and J. A. Deutsch (eds.). New York: Academic Press, pp. 258–291.

Klatzky, R. L. (1982). *Human Memory*, 2nd ed. San Francisco: W.H. Freeman.

Kling, A., and Steklis, H. D. (1976). A neural substrate for affiliative behavior in non-human primates. *Brain Behav. Evol.* 13:216–238.

Knopman, D., and Nissen, M. J. (1991). Procedural learning is impaired in Huntington's disease: evidence from the serial reaction time task. *Neuropsychologia* 29:245–254.

Knowlton, B. J., Mangels, J. A., and Squire, L. R. (1996). A neostriatal habit learning system in humans. *Science* 273(5280):1399–1402.

Knowlton, B. J., and Squire, L. R. (1993). The learning of categories: parallel brain systems for item memory and category knowledge. *Science* 262(5140):1747–1749.

Knowlton, B. J., Squire, L. R., and Gluck, M. A. (1994). Probabilistic classification learning in amnesia. *Learn. Mem.* 1:106–120.

Komatsu, S., Mimura, M., Kato, M., Wakamatsu, N., and Kashima, H. (2000). Errorless and effortful processes involved in the learning of face–name associations by patients with alcoholic Korsakoff's syndrome. *Neuropsychol. Rehabil.* 10:113–132.

Kooistra, C. A. and Heilman, K. M. (1988). Memory loss from a subcortical white matter infarct. *J. Neurol. Neurosurg. Psychiatry* 51:866–869.

Kopelman, M. D. (1985). Rates of forgetting in Alzheimer-type dementia and Korsakoff's syndrome. *Neuropsychologia* 23:623–638.

Kopelman, M. D. (1986). The cholinergic neurotransmitter system in human memory and dementia: a review. *Q. J. Exp. Psychol.* 38A:535–573.

Kopelman, M. D. (1987). Amnesia: organic and psychogenic. *Br J Psychiatry* 150:428–442.

Kopelman, M. D. (1991). Frontal dysfunction and memory deficits in the alcoholic Korsakoff syndrome and Alzheimer-type dementia. *Brain* 114(Pt 1A):117–137.

Kopelman, M. D. (1995). The Korsakoff syndrome. *Br. J. Psychiatry* 166:154–173.

Kopelman, M. D., Stanhope, N., and Kingsley, D. (1999). Retrograde amnesia in patients with diencephalic, temporal lobe or frontal lesions. *Neuropsychologia* 37:939–958.

Korsakoff, S. S. (1889). Etude mèdico-psychologique sur une forme des maladies de la mémoire. *Rev. Philosophique* 28:501–530.

Kosslyn, S. M., and Intriligator, J. R. (1992). Is cognitive neuropsychology plausible? The perils of sitting on a one-legged stool. *J. Cogn. Neurosci.* 4:96–106.

Kosslyn, S. M., and Koenig, O. (1992). *Wet Mind: The New Cognitive Neuroscience*. New York: Free Press.

Kral, V. A. (1962). Senescent forgetfulness: Benign and malignant. *J. Can. Med. Assoc.* 86:251–260.

Krebs, H., Brasherskrug, T., Rauch, S., Savage, C., Hogan, N., Rubin, R., Fischman, A., and Alpert, N. (1998). Robot-aided functional imaging: application to a motor learning study. *Hum. Brain Mapping* 6:59–72.

Kreutzer, J. S., and Wehman, P. H. (ed.). (1991). *Cognitive Rehabilitation for Persons with Traumatic Brain Injury*. Baltimore, MD: Paul H. Brooks Publishing Company.

Kritchevsky, M. (1989). Transient global amnesia. In *Handbook of Neuropsychology, Vol. 3*, F. Boller and J. Grafman (eds.). Amsterdam: Elsevier, pp. 167–182.

Kritchevsky, M., Graff-Radford, N. R., and Damasio, A. R. (1987). Normal memory after damage to medial thalamus. *Arch. Neurol.* 44:959–962.

Kritchevsky, M., Squire, L. R., and Zouzounis, J. A. (1988). Transient global amnesia: characterization of anterograde and retrograde amnesia. *Neurology* 38:213–219.

Kunst-Wilson, W. R., and Zajonc, R. B. (1980). Affective discrimination of stimuli that cannot be recognized. *Science* 207:557–558.

Laloux, P., Brichant, C., Cauwe, F., Decoster, P. (1992). Technetium-99m HM-PAO single photon computed tomography imaging in transient global amnesia. *Arch. Neurol.* 49:543–546.

Lang, P. J. (1968). Fear reduction and fear behavior: Problems in treating a construct. In J. M. Schein (ed.). Research in Psychotherapy. pp. 90–103. Washington DC: American Psychological Association.

Lang, P. J. (1971). The application of psychophysiological methods to the study of psychotherapy and behavior modification. In A. E. Bergin and S. L. Garfield (eds.). Handbook of Psychotherapy and Behavior Change: An Empirical Analysis, pp. 75–125. New York: Wiley.

Larrabee, G. J. (1996). Age-associated memory impairment: definition and psychometric characteristics. *Aging Neuropsychol. Cogn.* 3:118–131.

Larrabee, G. J., and Crook, T. H. (1994). Estimated prevalence of age-associated memory impairment derived from standardized tests of memory function. *Int. Psychogeriatr.* 6:95–104.

Larrabee, G. J., and Crook, T. H., III. (1995). Assessment of learning and memory. In *Clinical Neuropsychological Assessment: A Cognitive Approach*, R. L. Mapou and J. Spector (eds.). New York: Plenum Press, pp. 185–213.

Larrabee, G. J., Trahan, D. E., Curtiss, G., and Levin, H. S. (1988). Normative data for the Selective Reminding Test. *Neuropsychology* 2:173–182.

LeDoux, J. E. (1987). Emotion. In *Handbook of Physiology, Vol. 5*, V. B. Mountcastle, F. Plum, and S. R. Geiger (eds.). Bethesda: American Physiological Society, pp. 419–460.

Lee, G. P., Meador, K. J., Smith, J. R., Loring, D. W., and Flanigin, H. F. (1988). Preserved crossmodal association following bilateral amygdalotomy in man. *Int. J. Neurosci.* 40:47–55.

Leibniz, G. W. (1916). New Essays Concerning Human Understanding. Chicago: Open Court.

Levin, H. S. (1989). Memory deficit after closed head injury. In *Handbook of Neuropsychology, Vol. 3*, F. Boller and J. Grafman (eds.). Amsterdam: Elsevier, pp. 183–207.

Lewandowsky, S., Dunn, J. C., and Kirsner, K. (1989). *Implicit Memory, Theoretical Issues*. Hillsdale, NJ: Lawrence Erlbaum.

Lewis, P. R., and Shute, C. C. D. (1967). The cholinergic limbic system: projections of the hippocampal formation, medial cortex, nuclei of the ascending cholinergic reticular system, and the subfornical organ and supra-optic crest. *Brain* 90:521–540.

Lezak, M. D. (1995). *Neuropsychological Assessment, 3rd ed*. New York: Oxford University Press.

Lhermitte, J., Doussinet, P., and Ajuriaguerra, J. (1937). Une observation de la forme Korsakowienne des tumeurs du 3ᵉ ventricule. *Rev. Neurol. (Paris)* 68:709–711.

Lhermitte, F., and Signoret, J.-L. (1972). Analyse neuropsychologique et differenciation des syndromes amnesiques. *Rev. Neurol. (Paris) 126:* 161–178.

Lindqvist, G., and Norlen, G. (1966). Korsakoff's syndrome after operation on ruptured aneurysm of the anterior communicating artery. *Acta Psychiatr. Scand.* 42:24–34.

Loesch, D. V., Gilman S., Del Dotto, J., and Rosenblum, M. L. (1995). Cavernous malformation of the mammillary bodies: neuropsychological implications. Case report. *J. Neurosurg.* 83:354–358.

Loftus, E. F. (1993). The reality of repressed memories. *Am. Psychol.* 48:516–537.

Loftus, E. F., and Cole, W. (1974). Retrieving attribute and name information from semantic memory. *J. Exp. Psychol.* 102:1116–1122.

Loftus, E. F., and Ketcham, K. (1991). *Witness for the Defense: The Accused, the Eyewitness, and the Expert who Puts Memory on Trial*. New York: St. Martin's.

Logue, V., Durward, M., Pratt, R. T. C., Piercy, M., and Nixon, W. L. B. (1968). The quality of survival after rupture of an anterior cerebral aneurysm. *Br. J. Psychiatry 114:*137–160.

Lomo, T. (1971). Patterns of activation in a monsynaptic cortical pathway: the perforant path input to the dentate areas of the hipocampal formation. *Exp. Brain Res. 12:*18–45.

Loring, D. W., Lee, G. P., Meador, K. J. et al. (1991). Hippocampal contribution to verbal memory following dominant-hemisphere temporal lobectomy. *J. Clin. Exp. Neuropsychol. 13:*575–586.

Loring, D. W., and Papanicolaou, A. C. (1987). Memory assessment in neuropsychology: Theoretical considerations and practical utility. *J. Clin. Exp. Neuropsychol. 9:*340–358.

Mahut, H., and Moss, M. (1986). The monkey and the sea horse. In: *The Hippocampus*, R. L. Isaacson, and K. H. Pripram, (eds.). New York: Plenum Press, pp. 241–279.

Mair, W. G. P., Warrington, E. K., and Weiskrantz, L. (1979). Memory disorder in Korsakoff's psychosis: A neuropathological and neuropsychological investigation of two cases. *Brain 102:*749–783.

Malamut, B. L., Graff-Radford, N., Chawluk, J., Grossman, R. I., and Gur, R.C. (1992). Memory in a case of bilateral thalamic infarction. *Neurology 42:*163–169.

Malkova, L., Mishkin, M., and Bachevalier, J. (1995). Long-term effects of selective neonatal temporal lobe lesions on learning and memory in monkeys. *Behav. Neurosci. 109:*212–226.

Mandler, G. (1980). Recognizing: the judgement of previous occurrence. *Psychol. Rev. 87:*252–271.

Manns, J. R., Clark, R. E., and Squire, L. R. (2000). Awareness predicts the magnitude of single-cue trace eyeblink conditioning. *Hippocampus 10:*181–186.

Markowitsch, H. J. (1999). Functional neuroimaging correlates of functional amnesia. *Memory 7:*561–583.

Markowitsch, H. J., Calabrese, P., Neufeld, H., Gehlen, W., and Durwen, H. F. (1999). Retrograde amnesia for world knowledge and preserved memory for autobiographic events. A case report. *Cortex 35:*243–252.

Marslen-Wilson, W. D., and Teuber, H.-L. (1974). Memory for remote events in anterograde amnesia: recognition of public figures from newsphotographs. *Neuropsychologia 13:*353–364.

Martin, A., and Fedio, P. (1983). Word production and comprehension in Alzheimer's disease: the breakdown of semantic knowledge. *Brain Lang. 19:*124–141.

Martin, R. C., Haut, M. W., Goeta Kreisler, K., and Blumenthal, D. (1996). Neuropsychological functioning in a patient with paraneoplastic limbic encephalitis. *J. Int. Neuropsychol. Soc. 2:* 460–466.

Martone, M., Butters, N., and Trauner, D. (1986). Some analyses of forgetting pictorial material in amnesic and demented patients. *J. Clin. Exp. Neuropsychol. 8:*161–178.

Matthies, H., Frey, U., Reymann, K., Krug, M., Jork, R., and Schroeder, H. (1990). Different mechanisms and multiple stages of LTP. In *Excitatory Amino Acids and Neuronal Plasticity*, Ben-Ari Y. (ed.). New York: Plenum Press, pp. 359–368.

Mayes, A. R., Downes, J. J., McDonald, C., Poole, V., Rooke, S., Sagar, H. J., and Meudell, P. R. (1994a). Two tests for assessing remote public knowledge: a tool for assessing retrograde amnesia. *Memory 2:*183–210.

Mayes, A. R., Downes, J. J., Symons, V., and Shoqeirat, M. (1994b). Do amnesics forget faces pathologically fast? *Cortex 30:*543–563.

Mayes, A. R., and Meudell, P. (1981). How similar is immediate memory in amnesic patients to delayed memory in normal subjects? A replication, extension and reassessment of the amnesic cueing effect. *Neuropsychologia 18:*527–540.

Mayes, A. R., Meudell, P. R., Mann, D., and Pickering, A. (1988). Location of lesions in Korsakoff's syndrome: neuropsychological and neuropathological data on two patients. *Cortex 24:*367–388.

Mayes, A. R., Meudell, P. R., and Neary, D. (1980). Do amnesics adopt inefficient encoding strategies with faces and random shapes? *Neuropsychologia 18.*527–540.

Mayes, A., Meudell, P., and Som, S. (1981). Further similarities between amnesia and normal attenuated memory: Effects of paired-associate learning and contextual shifts. *Neuropsychologia 18:*655–664.

McAndrews, M. P., Glisky, E. L., and Schacter, D. L. (1987). When priming persists: long-lasting implicit memory for a single episode in amnesic patients. *Neuropsychologia 25:*497–506.

McAndrews, M. P., and Milner, B. (1991). The frontal cortex and memory for temporal order. *Neuropsychologia 29:*849–859.

McGaugh, J. L., Introini-Collison, I. B., Nagahara, A. H., Cahill, L., Brioni, J. D., and Castellano, C. (1990). Involvement of the amygdaloid complex in neuromodulatory influences on memory storage. *Neurosci. Biobehav. Rev. 14:*425–431.

McGlinchey Berroth, R., Brawn, C., and Disterhoft, J. F. (1999). Temporal discrimination learning in severe amnesic patients reveals an alteration in the timing of eyeblink conditioned responses. *Behav. Neurosci. 113:*10–18.

McGlinchey Berroth, R., Carrillo, M. C., Gabrieli, J. D., Brawn, C. M., and Disterhoft, J. F. (1997). Impaired trace eyeblink conditioning in bilateral, medial-temporal lobe amnesia. *Behav. Neurosci. 111:*873–882.

McGlinchey Berroth, R., Cermak, L. S., Carrillo, M. C., Armfield, S., Gabrieli, J. D., and Disterhoft, J. F. (1995). Impaired delay eyeblink conditioning in amnesic Korsakoff's patients and recovered alcoholics. *Alcohol Clin. Exp. Res. 19:* 1127–1132.

McKee, R. D., and Squire, L. R. (1992). Both hippocampal and diencephalic amnesia result in normal forgetting for complex visual material. *J. Clin. Exp. Neuropsychol. 14:*103.

McKone, E., and Slee, J. A. (1997). Explicit contamination in "implicit" memory for new associations. *Mem. Cogn. 25:*352–366.

McKoon, G., Ratcliff, R., and Dell, G. S. (1986). A critical evaluation of the semantic-episodic distinction. *J. Exp. Psychol. Learn. Mem. Cogn. 12:* 295–306.

McMackin, D., Cockburn, J., Anslow, P., and Gaffan, D. (1995). Correlation of fornix damage with memory impairment in six cases of colloid cyst removal. *Acta Neurochir. (Wien) 135:* 12–18.

Meier, M. J., Benton, A. L., and Diller, L. (1987). *Neuropsychological Rehabilitation.* New York: Guilford Press.

Mesulam, M.-M. and Mufson, E. J. (1984). Neural inputs into the nucleus basalis of the substantia innominata (Ch4) in the resus monkey. *Brain 107:*253–274.

Mesulam, M.-M., Mufson, E. J., Levey, E. J., and Wainer, B. H. (1983). Cholinergic innervation of cortex by the basal forebrain: cytochemistry and cortical connections of the septal area, diagonal band nuclei, nucleus basalis (substantia innominata) and hypothalmus in the rhesus monkey. *J. Comp. Neurol. 214:*170–197.

Mesulam, M.-M. and Van Hoesen, G. W. (1976). Acetylcholinesterase containing basal forebrain neurons in the rhesus monkey project to neocortex. *Brain Res. 109:*152–157.

Meudell, P., and Mayes, A. (1981). The Claparede phenomenon: a further example in amnesics, a demonstration of a similar effect in normal people with attenuated memory, and a reinterpretation. *Curr. Psychol. Res. 1:*75–88.

Meudell, P. R., Northern, B., Snowden, J. S., and Neary, D. (1980). Long-term memory for fa-

mous voices in amnesic and normal subjects. *Neuropsychologia 18:*133–139.

Meunier, M., Bachevalier, J., Mishkin, M., and Murray, E. A. (1993). Effects on visual recognition of combined and separate ablations of the entorhinal and perirhinal cortex in rhesus monkeys. *J. Neurosci. 13:*5418–5432.

Meunier, M., Bachevalier, J., and Mishkin, M. (1997). Effects of orbitofrontal and anterior cingulate lesions on object and spatial memory in rhesus monkeys. *Neuropsychologia 35:*999–1016.

Milberg, W. P., Hebber, N., and Kaplan, E. (1986). The Boston process approach to neuropsychological assessment. In I. Grant and K. M. Adams (eds.). *Neuropsychological Assessment of Neuropsychiatric Disorders.* New York: Oxford University Press.

Miller, E. (1973). Short and long-term memory in patients with presenile dementia (Alzheimers disease). *Psychol. Med. 3:*221–224.

Miller, R. R., and Marlin, N. A. (1979). Amnesia following electroconvulsive shock. In J. F. Kilstrohm and F. J. Evans (eds.). *Functional Disorders of Memory,* pp. 143–178. Hillsdale, NJ: Lawrence Erlbaum.

Miller, J. W., Petersen, R.C., Metter, E. J., Millikan, C. H., and Yanagihara, T. (1987). Transient global amnesia: clinical characteristics and prognosis. *Neurology 37:*733–737.

Milner, B. (1962). Les troubles de la memoire accompagnant des lesions hippocampiques bilaterales. In *Physiologie de l'hippocampe,* P. Passouant (ed.). Paris: Centre National de la Recherche Scientifique.

Milner, B. (1966). Amnesia following operation on the temporal lobes. In *Amnesia,* C. W. M. Whitty and O. L. Zangwill (eds.). London: Butterworths.

Milner, B. (1972). Disorders of learning and memory after temporal lobe lesions in man. *Clin. Neurosurg. 19:*421–446.

Milner, B. (1974). Hemispheric specialization: scope and limits. In *The Neurosciences: Third Study Program,* F. O. Schmitt, and F. G. Worden, (eds.). Cambridge, MA: MIT Press, pp. 75–89.

Milner, B., Corkin, S., and Teuber, H.-L. (1968). Further analysis of the hippocampal amnesic syndrome: 14-year follow-up study of H.M. *Neuropsychologia 6:*215–234.

Milner, B., Corsi, P. M., Leonard, G. (1991). Frontal-lobe contributions to recency judgments. *Neuropsychologia 29:*601–618.

Milner, B., and Petrides, M. (1984). Behavioural effects of frontal-lobe lesions in man. *Trends Neurosci. 7:*403–407.

Mishkin, M. (1978). Memory in monkeys severely impaired by combined but not separate removal of the amygdala and hippocampus. *Nature* 273:297–298.

Mishkin, M. (1982). A memory system in the monkey. *Phil. Trans. R. Soc. Lond.* 298:85–95.

Mishkin, M., and Petri H. L. (1984). Memories and habits: some implications for the analysis of learning and retention. In *Neuropsychology of Memory*, L. R. Squire and N. Butters (eds.). New York: Guilford Press, pp. 287–296.

Mishkin, M., and Saunders, R. C. (1979). Degree of memory impairment in monkeys related to amount of conjoint damage to amygdaloid and hippocampal systems. *Soc. Neurosci. Abstr.* 5:320.

Mishkin, M., Spiegler, B. J., Saunders, R. C., and Malamut, B. L. (1982). An animal model of global amnesia. In *Alzheimer's Disease: A Report of Progress*, S. Corkin, et al. (eds.). New York: Raven Press, pp. 235–247.

Moccia, F., Aramini, A., Montobbio, P., Altomonte, F., and Greco, G. (1996). Transient global amnesia: disease or syndrome? *Ital. J. Neurol. Sci.* 17:211–214.

Mori, E., Yamadori, A., and Mitani, Y. (1986). Left thalamic infarction and disturbance of verbal memory: a clinicoanatomical study with a new method of computed tomographic stereotaxic lesion localization. *Ann. Neurol.* 20:671–676.

Morris, M. K., Bowers, D., Chatterjee, A., and Heilman, K. M. (1992). Amnesia following a discrete basal forebrain lesion. *Brain* 115:1827–1847.

Morris, R., Petrides, M., and Pandya, D. N. (1999). Architecture and connections of retrosplenial area 30 in the rhesus monkey (*Macaca mulatta*). *Eur. J. Neurosci.* 11:2506–2518.

Moscovitch, M. (1982). Multiple dissociations of function in amnesia. In *Human Memory and Amnesia*, L.S. Cermak (ed.). Hillsdale, NJ: Lawrence Erlbaum Associates, pp. 337–370.

Moss, M., Mahut, H., Zola-Morgan, S. (1981). Concurrent discrimination learning of monkeys after hippocampal, entorhinal, or fornix lesions. *J. Neurosci.* 1:227–240.

Moudgil, S. S., Azzouz, M., Al-Azzaz, A., Haut, M., and Guttmann, L. (2000). Amnesia due to fornix infarction. *Stroke* 31:1418–1419.

Mufson, E. J., and Pandya, D. N. (1984). Some observations on the course and composition of the cingulum bundle in the rhesus monkey. *J. Comp. Neurol.* 225:31–43.

Murray, E. A. and Bussey, T. J. (1999). Perceptual-mnemonic functions of the perirhinal cortex. *Trends Cogn. Sci.* 3:142–151.

Murray, E. A., Gaffan, D., and Mishkin, M. (1993). Neural substrates of visual stimulus-stimulus association in rhesus monkeys. *J. Neurosci.* 13:4549–4561.

Murray, E. A., and Mishkin, M. (1998). Object recognition and location memory in monkeys with excitotoxic lesions of the amygdala and hippocampus. *J. Neurosci.* 18:6568–6582.

Murre, J. M. (1997). Implicit and explicit memory in amnesia: some explanations and predictions by the TraceLink model. *Memory* 5:213–232.

Murre, J. M. (1999). Interaction of cortex and hippocampus in a model of amnesia and semantic dementia. *Rev. Neurosci.* 10:267–278.

Musen, G., and Squire, L. R. (1992). Nonverbal priming in amnesia. *Mem. Cogn.* 20:441–448.

Musen, G., Shimamura, A. P., and Squire, L. R. (1990). Intact text-specific reading skill in amnesia. *J. Exp. Psychol. Learn. Mem. Cogn.* 16:1068–1076.

Musen, G., and Triesman, A. (1990). Implicit and explicit memory for visual patterns. *J. Exp. Psychol. Learn. Mem. Cogn.* 16:127–137.

Nadel, L., and Moskovitch, M. (1997). Memory consolidation, retrograde amnesia, and the hippocampal complex. *Curr. Opin. Neurobiol.* 7:217–227.

Narabayashi, H., Nagao, T., Saito, Y., Yoshida, M., and Nagahata, M. (1963). Stereotaxic amygdalotomy for behavior disorders. *Arch. Neurol.* 9:1–16.

Nauta, W. J. H. (1961). Fibre degeneration following lesions of the amygdaloid complex in the monkey. *J. Anat.* 95:515–531.

Nelson, T. O., Gerler, D., and Narens, L. (1984). Accuracy of feeling-of-knowing judgements for predicting perceptual identification and relearning. *J. Exp. Psychol. Gen.* 113:282–300.

Nelson, T. O., Leonesio, R. J., Shimamura, A. P., Landwehr, R. F., and Narens, L. (1982). Overlearning and the feeling of knowing. *J. Exp. Psychol. Learn. Mem. Cogn.* 8:279–288.

Newman, M. E., Adityanjee, E., Sobolewski, E., and Jampala, V. C. (1998). Wernicke-Korsakoff amnestic syndrome secondary to malnutrition in a patient with schizoaffective disorder. *Neuropsychiatry Neuropsychol. Behav. Neurol.* 11:241–244.

Nissen, M. J., and Bullemer, P. (1987). Attentional requirements of learning: evidence from performance measures. *Cogn. Psychol.* 19:1–32.

Nyberg, L., and Cabeza, R. (2000). Brain imaging of memory. In *The Oxford Handbook of Memory*, E. Tulving and F. I. M. Craik (eds.). New York: Oxford University Press, pp. 501–519.

Nyberg, L., McIntosh, A. R., Cabeza, R., Nilsson,

L. G., Houle, S., Habib, R., and Tulving, E. (1996). Network analysis of positron emission tomography regional cerebral blood flow data: ensemble inhibition during episodic memory retrieval. *J. Neurosci.* 16:3753–3759.

Nyberg, L., McIntosh, A. R., and Tulving, E. (1998). Functional brain imaging of episodic and semantic memory with positron emission tomography. *J. Mol. Med.* 76:48–53.

O'Connor, M., Butters, N., Miliotis, P., Eslinger, P., and Cermak, L. S. (1992). The dissociation of anterograde and retrograde amnesia in a patient with herpes encephalitis. *J. Clin. Exp. Neuropsychol.* 14:159–178.

Ojemann, G. A., and Dodrill, C. B. (1985). Verbal memory deficits after left temporal lobectomy for epilepsy. *J. Neurosurg.* 62:101–107.

Okawa, M., Maeda, S., Nukui, H., and Kawafuchi, J. (1980). Psychiatric symptoms in ruptured anterior communicating aneurysms: social prognosis. *Acta Psychiatr. Scand.* 61:306–312.

O'Keefe, J., and Nadel, L. (1978). *The Hippocampus as a Cognitive Map.* London: Oxford University Press.

Olesen, J., and Jørgensen, M. B. (1986). Leao's spreading depression in the hippocampus explains transient global amnesia: a hypothesis. *Acta Neurol. Scand.* 73:219–220.

Olton, D. S. (1989). Inferring psychological dissociations from experimental dissociations: the temporal context of episodic memory. In *Varieties of Memory and consciousness: Essays in Honour of Endel Tulving*, H. L. Roediger and F. I. M. Craik (eds.). Hillsdale NJ: Lawrence Erlbaum Associates, pp. 161–177.

Oscar-Berman, M., and Bonner R.T. (1985). Matching- and delayed matching-to-sample performance as measures of visual processing, selective attention, and memory in aging and alcoholic individuals. *Neuropsychologia* 23:639–651.

Owen, M. J., and Butler, S. R. (1981). Amnesia after transection of the fornix in monkeys: long-term memory imparied, short-term memory intact. *Behav. Brain Res.* 3:115–123.

Paller, K. A., Kutas, M., and Mayes, A. R. (1987). Neural correlates of encoding in an incidental learning paradigm. *Electroencephalogr. Clin. Neurophysiol.* 67:360–371.

Paller, K. A., Kutas, M., and McIsaac, H. K. (1995). Monitoring conscious recollection via the electrical activity of the brain. *Psychol. Sci.* 6:107–111.

Pandya, D. N., and Yeterian, E. H. (1990). Architecture and connections of cerebral cortex: im-

plications for brain evolution and function. In *Neurobiology of Higher Cognitive Function*, A. B. Scheibel and A. F. Wechsler (eds.). New York: The Guilford Press, pp. 53–84.

Parente, R., and DiCesare, A. (1991). Retraining memory: theory, evaluation and applications. In *Cognitive Rehabilitation for Persons with Traumatic Brain Injury*, J. S. Kreutzer and P. H. Wehman (eds.). Paul H. Brooks Publishing Company: Baltimore, MD. pp. 147–162.

Park, S. A., Hahn, J. H., Kim, J. I., Na, D. L., and Huh, K. (2000). Memory deficits after bilateral anterior fornix infarction. *Neurology* 54:1379–1382.

Parker, A., and Gaffan, D. (1997). Mammillary body lesions in monkeys impair object-in-place memory: functional unity of the fornix-mammillary system. *J. Cogn. Neurosci.* 9:512–521.

Parkin, A. J., and Hunkin, N. M. (1993). Impaired temporal context memory on anterograde but not retrograde tests in the absence of frontal pathology. *Cortex* 29:267–280.

Parkinson, J. K., Murray, E. A., Mishkin, M. (1988). A selective mnemonic role for the hippocampus in monkeys: memory for the location of objects. *J. Neurosci.* 8:4159–4167.

Passingham, R. (1997). Functional organization of the motor system. In *Human Brain Function*, R. S. J. Frackowiak, K. J. Friston, C. D. Frith, R. J. Dolan, and J. C. Mazziota (eds.). Toronto: Academic Press, pp. 243–274.

Patten, B. M. (1972). The ancient art of memory: Usefulness in treatment. *Arch Neurol* 26:25–31.

Penfield, W., and Mathieson, G. (1974). Memory. Autopsy findings and comments on the role of hippocampus in experiential recall. *Arch. Neurol.* 31:145–154.

Penfield, W., and Milner, B. (1958). Memory deficit produced by bilateral lesions in the hippocampal zone. *Arch. Neurol. Psychiatry* 79:475–497.

Peters, B. H., and Levin, H. S. (1979). Effects of physostigmine and lecithin on memory in Alzheimer disease. *Ann. Neurol.* 6:219–221.

Peters, B. H., and Levin, H. S. (1982). Chronic oral physostigmine and lecithin administraiton in memory disorders of aging. In *Alzheimer's Disease: A Report of Progress in Research*, S. Corkin, J. H. Davis, E. Growdon, and R. J. Writman (eds.). New York: Raven Press, pp. 421–426.

Petrides, M. (1989). Frontal lobes and memory. In F. Boller and J. Grafman (eds.). *Handbook of Neuropsychology (Vol. 3).*, pp. 75–90. Amsterdam: Elsevier.

Petrides, M., and Milner, B. (1982). Deficits on subject-ordered tasks after frontal- and temporal-lobe lesions in man. *Neuropsychologia 20*:249–262.

Phillips, S., Sangalang, V., and Sterns, G. (1987). Basal forebrain infarction: a clinicopathologic correlation. *Arch. Neurol. 44*:1134–1138.

Pigott, S., and Milner, B. (1993). Memory for different aspects of complex visual scenese after unilateral temporal or frontal lobe resection. *Neuropsychologia 31*:1–15.

Poldrack, R., Desmond, J., Glover, G., and Gabrieli, J. (1998). The neural basis of visual skill learning: an fMRI study of mirror reading. *Cereb. Cortex 8*:1–10.

Poletti, C. E. (1986) Is the limbic system a limbic system? Studies of hippocampal efferents: their functional and clinical implications. In *The Limbic System: Functional Organization and Clinical Disorders*, B. K. Doane and K. E. Livingston (eds.). New York: Raven Press, pp. 79–94.

Porrino, L. J., Crane, A. M., and Goldman-Rakic, P. S. (1981). Direct and indirect pathways from the amygdala to the frontal lobe in rhesus monkeys. *J. Comp. Neurol. 198*:121–136.

Postle, B. R., and Corkin, S. (1998). Impaired word-stem completion priming but intact perceptual identification priming with novel words: evidence from the amnesic patient H.M. *Neuropsychologia 36*:421–440.

Prigatano, G. P., Fordyce, D. J., Zeiner, H. K., Roueche, J. R., Pepping, M., and Wood, B. C. (1984). Neuropsychological rehabilitation after closed head injury in young adults. *J. Neurol. Neurosurg. Psychiat. 47*:505–513.

Prince, M. (1914). *The Unconscious*. New York: Macmillan.

Randt, C. T., and Brown, E. R. (1983). Randt Memory Test. Bayport, NY: Life Science Associates.

Ratcliff, R., Van Zandt, T., and McKoon, G. (1995). Process dissociation, single-process theories, and recognition memory. *J. Exp. Psychol. Gen. 124*:352–374.

Reber, P. J., Knowlton, B. J., and Squire, L. R. (1996). Dissociable properties of memory systems: differences in the flexibility of declarative and nondeclarative knowledge. *Behav. Neurosci. 110*:861–871.

Reber, P. J., and Squire, L. R. (1998). Encapsulation of implicit and explicit memory in sequence learning. *J. Cogn. Neurosci. 10*:248–263.

Reed, J. M., and Squire, L. R. (1998). Retrograde amnesia for facts and events: findings from four new cases. *J. Neurosci. 18*:3943–3954.

Reed, J. M., Squire, L. R., Patalano, A. L., Smith, E. E., and Jonides, J. (1999). Learning about categories that are defined by object-like stimuli despite impaired declarative memory. *Behav. Neurosci. 113*:411–419.

Rich, J. B., Bylsma, F. W., and Brandt, J. (1996). Item priming and skill learning in amnesia. *J. Clin. Exp. Neuropsychol. 18*:148–158.

Richardson, J.T. (1992). Imagery mnemonics and memory remediation. *Neurology 42*:283–286.

Richardson-Klavehn, A., and Bjork, R. A. (1988). Measures of memory. *Ann. Rev. Psychol. 39*:475–543.

Roediger, H. L. (1990). Implicit memory: retention without remembering. *Am. Psychol. 45*:1043–1056.

Roediger, H. L., and Blaxton, T. A. (1987). Effects of varying modality, surface features, and retention interval on priming in word fragment completion. *Mem. Cogn. 15*:379–388.

Roediger, H. L., III, Guynn, M. J., and Jones, T. C. (1994). Implicit memory: a tutorial review. In *Perspectives on Psychological Science, Vol. 2. The State of the Art* G. D'Ydewalle, and P. Eelen (eds.). Hove, England, UK: Lawrence Erlbaum Associates, pp. 67–94.

Roediger, H. L., and McDermott, K. B. (1993). Implicit memory in normal human subjects. In *Handbook of Neuropsychology, Vol. 8*, F. Boller and J. Grafman (eds.). New York: Elsevier, pp. 63–131.

Roediger, H. L., and McDermott, K. B. (2000). Distortions of memory. In *The Oxford Handbook of Memory*, E. Tulving and F. I. M. Craik (eds.). New York: Oxford University Press, pp. 149–162.

Roediger, H. L., and Weldon, M. S. (1987). Reversing the picture superiority effect. In *Imagery and related mnemonic processes: theory, individual differences, and applications*. M. A. McDaniel and M. Pressley (eds.). New York: Springer, pp. 151–174.

Roediger, H. L., Weldon, M. S., and Challis, B. H. (1989). Explaining dissociations between implicit and explicit measures of retention: a processing account. In *Varieties of Memory: Essays in Honour of Endel Tulving*, H. L. Roediger and F. I. M. Craik (eds.). Hillsdale, NJ: Lawrence Erlbaum Associates, pp. 3–41.

Rosene, D. L., and Van Hoesen, G. W. (1977). Hippocampal efferents reach widespread areas of cerebral cortex and amygdala in the rhesus monkey. *Science 198*:315–317.

Ross, E. D. (1980a). Sensory-specific and fractional disorders of recent memory in man. I: Isolated loss of visual recent memory. *Arc. Neurol. 37*:193–200.

Ross, E. D. (1980b). Sensory-specific and fractional disorders of recent memory in man. II. Unilateral loss of tactile recent memory. *Arch. Neurol.* 37:267–272.

Ross, E. D. (1982). Disorders of recent memory in humans. *Trends Neurosci.* 5:170–172.

Ross, E. D., and Stewart, R. M. (1981). Akinetic mutism from hypothalamic damage: successful treatment with dopamine agonists. *Neurology* 31:1435–1439.

Roth, T., Roehrs, T., Zwyghuizen Doorenbos, A., Stepanski, E., and Wittig, R. (1988). Sleep and memory. *Psychopharmacol. Ser.* 6:140–145.

Rudge, P., and Warrington, E. K. (1991). Selective impairment of memory and visual perception in splenial tumours. *Brain* 114:349–360.

Rueckl, J. G. (1991). Similarity effects in word and pseudoword repetition priming. *J. Exp. Psychol. Learn. Mem. Cogn.* 16:374–391.

Rugg, M. D., Fletcher, P. C., Frith, C. D., Frackowiak, R. S., and Dolan, R. J. (1996). Differential activation of the prefrontal cortex in successful and unsuccessful memory retrieval. *Brain* 119:2073–2083.

Rugg, M. D., Mark, R. E., Walla, P., Schloerscheidt, A. M., Burch, C. S., and Allan, K. (1998). Dissociation of the neural corelates of implicit and explicit memory. *Nature* 392:595–598.

Russell, E. W. (1981). The pathology and clinical examination of memory. In *Handbook of Clinical Neuropsychology*, S. B. Filskov and T. J. Boll (eds.). New York: John Wiley and Sons, pp. 287–319.

Russell, W. R., and Nathan, P. W. (1946). Traumatic amnesia. *Brain* 69:290–300.

Ryan, C., and Butters, N. (1980a). Further evidence for a continuum of impairment encompassing male alcoholic Korsakoff patients and chronic alcoholic men. *Alcohol. Clin. Exp. Res.* 4:190–197.

Ryan, C., and Butters, N. (1980b). Learning and memory impairments in young and old alcoholics: evidence for the premature-aging hypothesis. *Alcohol. Clin. Exp. Res.* 4:288–293.

Sagar, H. J., Sullivan, E. V., Gabrieli, J. D. E., Corkin, S., and Growden, J. H. (1988). Temporal ordering and short term memory deficits in Parkinson's disease. *Brain* 111:525–539.

Sagar, H. J., Gabrieli, J. D. E., Sullivan, E. V., and Corkin, S. (1990). Recency and frequency discrimination in the amnesic patient H.M. *Brain* 113:581–602.

Saint-Cyr, J. A., Taylor, A. E., and Lang, A. E. (1988). Procedural learning and neostriatal dysfunction in man. *Brain* 111:941–959.

Sanders, H. I., and Warrington, E. K. (1971). Memory for remote events in amnesic patients. *Brain* 94:661–668.

Sanes, J. N., Dimitrov, B., and Hallett, M. (1990). Motor learning in patients with cerebellar dysfunction. *Brain* 113:103–120.

Sato, K., Sakajiri, K., Komai, K., and Takamori, M. (1998). *No To Shinkei* 50:69–73.

Saunders, R. C., Rosene, D. L., and Van Hoesen, G. W. (1988). Comparison of the efferents of the amygdala and the hippocampal formation in the rhesus monkey: II. Reciprocal and non-reciprocal connections. *J. Comp. Neurol.* 271:185–207.

Scarborough, D. L., Cortese, C., and Scarborough, H. S. (1977). Frequency and repetition effects in lexical memory. *J. Exp. Psychol. Hum. Percep. Perform.*, 3:1–17.

Schacter, D. (1983). Amnesia observed: remembering and forgetting in a natural environment. *J. Abnorm. Psychol.* 92:236–242.

Schacter, D. L. (1985). Priming of old and new knowledge in amnesic patients and normal subjects. *Ann. N Y Acad. Sci.* 444:41–53.

Schacter, D. L. (1987a). Implicit memory: history and current status. *J. Exp. Psychol. Learn. Mem. Cogn.* 13:501–518.

Schacter, D. L. (1987b). Memory, amnesia, and frontal lobe dysfunction: a critique and interpretation. *Psychobiology* 15:21–36.

Schacter, D. L. (1989a). Memory. In *Foundations of Cognitive Science*, M. I. Posner (ed.). Cambridge, MA: MIT Press, pp. 683–725.

Schacter, D. L. (1989b). On the relation between memory and consciousness: dissociable interactions and conscious experience. In *Varieties of Memory and Consciousness: Essays in Honour of Endel Tulving*, H. L. Roediger and F. I. M. Craik (eds.). Hillsdale, NJ: Lawrence Erlbaum Associates, pp. 355–389.

Schacter, D. L. (1997). The cognitive neuroscience of memory: perspectives from neuroimaging research. *Phil. Trans. R. Soc. Lond. B Biol. Sci.*, 352(1362):1689–1695.

Schacter, D. L. (1998). Illusory memories: a cognitive neuroscience analysis. In *Metacognition and Cognitive Neuropsychology: Monitoring and Control Processes*, G. Mazzoni and T. O. Nelson (eds.). Mahwah, NJ: Lawrence Erlbaum Associates, pp. 119–138.

Schacter, D. L., and Buckner, R. L. (1998). On the relations among priming, conscious recollection, and intentional retrieval: evidence from neuroimaging research. *Neurobiol. Learn. Mem.* 70:284–303.

Schacter, D. L., Chiu, C. Y. P., and Ochsner, K. N. (1993). Implicit memory: a selective review. *Ann. Rev. Neurosci.* 16:159–182.

Schacter, D. L., Cooper, L. A., and Delaney, S. M. (1990). Implicit memory for unfamiliar objects depends on access to structural descriptions. *J. Exp. Psychol. Gen.* 119:5–24.

Schacter, D. L., Cooper, L. A., Tharan, M., and Rubens, A. B. (1991). Preserved priming of novel objects in patients with memory disorders. *J. Cogn. Neurosci.* 3:118–131.

Schacter, D., McAndrews, M. P., and Moskovitch, M. (1988). Access to consciousness: Dissociations between implicit and explicit knowledge in neuropsychological syndromes. In L. Weiskrantz (ed.). *Thought without Language*, pp. 242–278. New York: Oxford University Press.

Schacter, D. L., and Glisky, E. L. (1986). Memory remediation, restoration, alleviation, and the acquisition of domain-specific knowledge. In B. Uzzell and Y. Gross (eds.). Clinical Neuropsychology of Intervention. Boston: Martinus Nijhoff.

Schacter, D. L., and Graf, P. (1986a). Effects of elaborative processing on implicit and explicit memory for new associations. *J. Exp. Psychol. Learn. Mem.* 12:432–444.

Schacter, D. L., and Graf, P. (1986b). Preserved learning in amnesic patients: perspectives from research on direct priming. *J. Clin. Exp. Neuropsychol.* 8:727–743.

Schacter, D. L., Harbluck, J., and McLachlan, D. (1984). Retrieval without recollection. An experimental analysis of source amnesia. *J. Verbal Learn. Verbal Behav.* 23:593–611.

Schacter, D L. and Kihlstrom, J. F. (1989). Functional amnesia. F. Boller and J. Grafman (Eds.) *Handbook of Neuropsychology* (Vol. 3), pp. 209–231. Amsterdam: Elsevier.

Schacter, D. L., Koutstaal, W., and Norman, K. A. (1996). Can cognitive neuroscience illuminate the nature of traumatic childhood memories? *Curr. Opin. Neurobiol.* 6:207–214.

Schacter, D. L., Norman, K. A., and Koutstaal, W. (1998). The cognitive neuroscience of constructive memory. *Annu. Rev. Psychol.* 49:289–318.

Schacter, D. L., Rich, S. A., and Stampp, M. S. (1985). Remediation of memory disorders: experimental evaluation of the spaced-retrieval technique. *J. Clin. Exp. Neuropsychol.* 7:79–96.

Schacter, D. L., Wagner, A. D., and Buckner, R. L. (2000). Memory systems of 1999. In *The Oxford Handbook of Memory*, E. Tulving and F. I. M. Craik (eds.). New York: Oxford University Press, pp. 627–643.

Scharfman, H. E., Witter, M. P., and Schwarcz, R. (2000). Preface. *The Parahippocampal Region. Implications for Neurological and Psychiatric Diseases*, Scharfman, H. E., Witter, M. P., and R. Schwarcz (eds.). *Ann. N. Y. Acad. Sci., Vol. 911*, pp. ix–xii.

Schmidtke, K., and Ehmsen, L. (1998). Transient global amnesia and migraine. A case–control study. *Eur. Neurol.* 40:9–14.

Schmidtke, K., Handschu, R., and Vollmer, H. (1996). Cognitive procedural learning in amnesia. *Brain Cogn.* 32:441–467.

Schmitter Edgecombe, M., Fahy, J. F., Whelan, J. P., and Long, C. J. (1995). Memory remediation after severe closed head injury: notebook training versus supportive therapy. *J. Consult. Clin. Psychol.* 63:484–489.

Schramke, C. J., and Bauer, R. M. (1997). State-dependent learning in older and younger adults. *Psychol. Aging* 12:255–262.

Schroder, J., Kratz, B., Pantel, J., Minnemann, E., Lehr, U., and Sauer, H. (1998). Prevalence of mild cognitive impairment in an elderly community sample. *J. Neural Transm. Suppl.* 54:51–59.

Schugens, M. M., and Daum, I. (1999). Long-term retention of classical eyeblink conditioning in amnesia. *Neuroreport* 10:149–152.

Scott, S. A., DeKosky, S. T., and Scheff, S. W. (1991). Volumetric atrophy of the amygdala in Alzheimer's disease: quantitative serial reconstruction. *Neurology* 41:351–356.

Scoville, W. B. (1954). The limbic lobe in man. *J. Neurosurg* 11:64–66.

Scoville, W. B., and Milner, B. (1957). Loss of recent memory after bilateral hippocampal lesions. *J. Neurol. Neurosurg. Psychiatry* 20:11–21.

Seltzer, B., and Benson, D. F. (1974). The temporal pattern of retrograde amnesia in Korsakoff's disease. *Neurology* 24:527–530.

Shallice, T., and Evans, M. E. (1978). The involvement of the frontal lobes in cognitive estimation. *Cortex* 14:294–303.

Sherry, D. F., and Schacter, D. L. (1987). The evolution of multiple memory systems. *Psychol. Rev.* 94:439–454.

Sherwin, B. B. (2000). Mild cognitive impairment: potential pharmacological treatment options. *J. Am. Geriatr. Soc.* 48:431–441.

Shimamura, A. P. (1986). Priming effects in amnesia: evidence for a dissociable memory function. *Q. J. Exp. Psychol.* 38A:619–644.

Shimamura, A. P. (1989). Disorders of memory: the cognitive science perspective. In *Handbook of Neuropsychology, Vol. 3*, F. Boller and J. Grafman (eds.). Amsterdam: Elsevier, pp. 35–73.

Shimamura, A. P., Janowsky, J. S., and Squire, L. R. (1990). Memory for the temporal order of events in patients with frontal lobe lesions and amnesic patients. *Neuropsychologia* 28:803–813.

Shimamura, A. P., Jernigan, T. L., and Squire, L. R. (1988). Korsakoff's syndrome: radiologic (CT) findings and neuropsychological correlates. *J. Neurosci.* 8:4400–4410.

Shimamura, A. P., and Squire, L. R. (1984). Paired-associate learning and priming effects in amnesia: a neuropsychological study. *J. Exp. Psychol. Gen.* 113:556–570.

Shimamura, A. P., and Squire, L. R. (1986). Memory and metamemory: a study of the feeling-of-knowing phenomenon in amnesic patients. *J. Exp. Psychol. Learn. Mem. Cogn.* 12:452–460.

Shimamura, A. P., and Squire, L. R. (1987). A neuropsychological study of fact memory and source amnesia. *J. Exp. Psychol. Learn. Mem. Cogn.* 13:464–473.

Shuping, J. R., Rollinson, R. D., and Toole, J. F. (1980). Transient global amnesia. *Ann. Neurol.* 7:281–285.

Shuren, J. E., Jacobs, D. H., and Heilman, K. M. (1997). Diencephalic temporal order amnesia. *J. Neurol. Neurosurg. Psychiatry* 62:163–168.

Sidman, M., Stoddard, L. T., and Mohr, J. P. (1968). Some additional observations of immediate meory in a patient iwth bilateral hippocampal lesions. *Neuropsychologia* 6:245–254.

Small, I. F., Milstein, V., and Small, J. G. (1981). Relationship between clinical and cognitive change with bilateral and unilateral ECT. *Biol. Psychiatry* 16:793–794.

Smith, E. E., and Jonides, J. (1998). Neuroimaging analyses of human working memory. *Proc. Natl. Acad. Sci. U. S. A.* 95:12061–12068.

Smith, M. E., and Oscar Berman, M. (1990). Repetition priming of words and pseudowords in divided attention and in amnesia. *J. Exp. Psychol. Learn. Mem. Cogn.* 16:1033–1042.

Smith, M. L. (1989). Memory disorders associated with temporal-lobe lesions. In *Handbook of Neuropsychology, Vol. 3*, Boller, F. and Grafman J. (eds.). Amsterdam: Elsevier, pp. 91–106.

Sobin, C., Sackeim, H. A., Prudic, J., Devanand, D. P., Moody, B. J., and McElhiney, M. C. (1995). Predictors of retrograde amnesia following ECT. *Am. J. Psychiatry* 152:995–1001.

Sohlberg, M. M., and Mateer, C. A. (1989). Training use of compensatory memory books: a three-stage behavioral approach. *J. Clin. Exp. Neuropsychol.* 11:871–891.

Speedie, L., and Heilman, K. M. (1982). Amnesic disturbance following infarction of the left dorsomedial nucleus of the thalamus. *Neuropsychologia* 20:597–604.

Speedie, L., and Heilman, K. M. (1983). Anterograde memory deficits for visuospatial material after infarction of the right thalamus. *Arch. Neurol.* 40:183–186.

Spencer, K. M. (2000). On the search for the neurophysiological manifestation of recollective experience. *Psychophysiology* 37:494–506.

Spiegler, B. J. and Mishkin, M. (1981). Evidence for the sequential participation of inferior temporal cortex and amygdala in the acquisition of stimulus–reward associations. *Behav. Brain Res.* 3:303–317.

Sprofkin, B. E. and Sciarra, D. (1952). Korsakoff's psychosis associated with cerebral tumors. *Neurology* 2:427–434.

Squire, L. R. (1981). Two forms of human amnesia: an analysis of forgetting. *J. Neurosci.* 1:635–640.

Squire, L. R. (1982a). The neuropsychology of human memory. *Ann. Rev. Neurosci.* 5:241–273.

Squire, L. R. (1982b). Comparison between forms of amnesia: some deficits are unique to Korsakoff syndrome. *J. Exp. Psychol. Learn. Mem. Cogn.* 8:560–571.

Squire, L. R. (1984). ECT and memory dysfunction. In *ECT: Basic Mechanisms*, B. Lerer, R. D. Weiner, and R. H. Belmaker (eds.). Washington, DC: American Psychiatric Press, pp. 156–163.

Squire, L. R. (1987). *Memory and Brain*. New York: Oxford University Press.

Squire, L. R., and Alvarez, P. (1995). Retrograde amnesia and memory consolidation: a neurobiological perspective. *Curr. Opin. Neurobiol.* 5:169–177.

Squire, L. R., Amaral, D. G., Zola-Morgan, S., Kritchevsky, M., and Press, G. (1989a). Description of brain injury in the amnesic patient N.A. based on magnetic resonance imaging. *Exp. Neurol.* 105:23–35.

Squire, L. R., and Chace, P. M. (1975). Memory functions six to nine months after electroconvulsive therapy. *Arch. Gen. Psychiatry* 32:1157–1164.

Squire, L. R., Chace, P. M., and Slater, P. C. (1976). Retrograde amnesia following electroconvulsive therapy. *Nature* 260:775–777.

Squire, L. R., and Cohen, N. J. (1984). Human memory and amnesia. In *Neurobiology of Learning and Memory*, G. Lynch, J. L. McGaugh, and N. M. Weinberger (eds.). pp. 3–64.

Squire, L. R., Cohen, N. J., and Nadel, L. (1984a). The medial temporal region and memory consolidation: A new hypothesis. In *Memory Consolidation*, H. Weingartner and E. Parker (eds.). Hillsdale NJ: Lawrence Erlbaum Associates.

Squire, L. R., Cohen, N. J., and Zouzounis, J. A. (1984b). Preserved memory in retrograde amnesia: sparing of a recently acquired skill. *Neuropsychologia* 22:145–152.

Squire, L. R., and Fox, M. M. (1980). Assessment

of remote memory: validation of the television test by repeated testing during a seven-day period. *Behav. Res. Methods Instrum. 12*:583–586.

Squire, L. R., Haist, F., and Shimamura, A. P. (1989b). The neurology of memory: quantitative assessment of retrograde amnesia in two groups of amnesic patients. *J. Neurosci. 9*:828–839.

Squire, L. R., and Knowlton, B. J. (1995). Learning about categories in the absence of memory. *Proc. Natl. Acad. Sci. U.S.A. 92*:12470–12474.

Squire, L. R., and McKee, R. D. (1993). Declarative and nondeclarative memory in opposition: when prior events influence amnesic patients more than normal subjects. *Mem. Cogn. 21*:424–430.

Squire, L. R., and Moore, R. Y. (1979). Dorsal thalamic lesion in a noted case of chronic memory dysfunction. *Ann. Neurol. 6*:503–506.

Squire, L. R., Nadel, L., and Slater, P. C. (1981a). Anterograde amnesia and memory for temporal order. *Neuropsychologia 19*:141–145.

Squire, L. R., and Shimamura, A. P. (1986). Characterizing amnesic patients for neurobehavioral study. *Behav. Neurosci. 100*:866–877.

Squire, L. R., Shimamura, A. P., and Graf, P. (1985). Strength and duration of priming effects in normal subjects and amnesic patients. *Neuropsychologia 25*:195–210.

Squire, L. R., and Slater, P. C. (1975). Forgetting in very long-term memory as assessed by an improved questionnaire technique. *J Exp Psychol: Hum Learn Mem 1*:50–54.

Squire, L. R., and Slater, P. C. (1983). Electroconvulsive therapy and complaints of memory dysfunction: a prospective three-year follow-up study. *Br. J. Psychiatry 142*:1–8.

Squire, L. R., Slater, P., and Chace, P. M. (1975). Retrograde amnesia: temporal gradient in very long-term memory following electroconvulsive therapy. *Science 187*:77–79.

Squire, L. R., Slater, P. C., and Miller, P. (1981b). Retrograde amnesia following ECT: long-term follow-up studies. *Arch. Gen. Psychiatry 38*:89–95.

Squire, L. R., Wetzel, C. D., and Slater, P. C. (1978). Anterograde amnesia following ECT: an analysis of the beneficial effect of partial information. *Neuropsychologia 16*:339–347.

Squire, L. R., and Zola, S. M. (1996). Ischemic brain damage and memory impairment: a commentary. *Hippocampus 6*:546–552.

Squire, L. R., and Zola, S. M. (1998). Episodic memory, semantic memory, and amnesia. *Hippocampus 8*:205–211.

Squire, L. R., and Zola-Morgan, S. (1991). The medial temporal lobe memory system. *Science 253*:1380–1386.

Squire, L. R., Zola-Morgan, S., and Chen, K. (1988). Human amnesia and animal models of amnesia: performance of amnesic patients on tests designed for the monkey. *Behav. Neurosci. 102*:210–211.

Stenberg, G. (2000). Semantic processing without conscious identification: evidence from event-related potentials. *J. Exp. Psychol. Learn. Mem. Cogn. 26*:973–1004.

Starr, A. and Phillips, L. (1970). Verbal and motor memory in the amnestic syndrome. *Neuropsychologia 8*:75–88.

Stern, C. E., Corkin, S., Gonzalez, R. G., Guimaraes, A. R., Baker, J. R., Jennings, P. J., Carr, C. A., Sugiura, R. M., Vedantham, V., and Rosen, B. R. (1996). The hippocampal formation participates in novel picture encoding: evidence from functional magnetic resonance imaging. *Proc. Natl. Acad. Sci. U.S.A. 93*:8660–8665.

Stern, R. A., Singer, E. A., Duke, L. M., Singer, N. G. (1994). The Boston Qualitative Scoring System for the Rey-Osterrieth Complex Figure: description and interrater reliability. *Clin. Neuropsychol. 8*:309–322.

Stillhard, G., Landis, T., Schiess, R., Regard, M., Sialer, G. (1990). Bitemporal hypoperfusion in transient global amnesia: 99m-Tc-HM-PAO SPECT and neuropsychological findings during and after an attack. *J. Neurol. Neurosurg. Psychiat. 53*:339–342.

Stuss, D. T., Kaplan, E. F., Benson, D. F., Weir, W. S., Chiulli, S., and Sarazin, F. F. (1982). Evidence for the involvement of orbitofrontal cortex in memory functions: an interference effect. *J. Comp. Physiol. Psychol. 96*:913–925.

Suzuki, W. I, and Eichenbaum, H. (2000). The neurophysiology of memory. In *Ann. N. Y. Acad. Sci. 911*:175–191.

Swanson, L. (1987). The hypothalamus. In *Handbook of Chemical Neuroanatomy: Integrate Systems of the CNS. Part I—Hypothalamus, Hippocampus, Amygdala, Retina. Vol. 5*, (A. Bjorklund, T. Hokfelt, and L. Swanson, (eds.). Amsterdam: Elsevier, pp. 1–124.

Swanson, L. W., and Cowan, W. M. (1979). An autoradiographic study of the organization of the efferent connections of the hippocampal formation in the rat. *J. Comp. Neurol. 172*:49–84.

Sweet, W. H., Talland, G. A., and Ervin, F. R. (1959). Loss of recent memory following section of fornix. *Trans. Am. Neurol. Assoc. 84*:76–82.

Sziklas, V., and Petrides, M. (1998). Memory and the region of the mammillary bodies. *Prog. Neurobiol. 54*:55–70.

Takahashi, N., Kawamura, M., Shiota, J., Kasahata, N., Hirayama, K. (1997). *Neurology 49*:464–469.

Takayama, Y., Kamo, H., Ohkawa, Y., Akiguchi, I., and Kimura, J. (1991). A case of retrosplenial amnesia. *Rinsho Shinkeigaku 31*:331–333.

Talland, G. (1965). *Deranged Memory*. New York: Academic Press.

Talland, G., Sweet, W. H., and Ballantine, H. T. (1967). Amnesic syndrome with anterior communicating artery aneurysm. *J. Nerv. Ment. Dis. 145*:179–192.

Tanaka, Y., Miyazawa, Y., Akaoka, F., and Yamada, T. (1997). Amnesia following damage to the mammillary bodies. *Neurology 48*:160–165.

Tanaka, Y., Miyazawa, Y., Hashimoto, R., Nakano, I., and Obayashi, T. (1999). Postencephalitic focal retrograde amnesia after bilateral anterior temporal lobe damage. *Neurology 53*:344–350.

Tate, R. L. (1997). Beyond one-bun, two-shoe: recent advances in the psychological rehabilitation of memory disorders after acquired brain injury. *Brain Inj. 11*:907–918.

Teuber, H.-L., Milner, B., and Vaughan, H. G. (1968). Persistent anterograde amnesia after stab wound to the basal brain. *Neuropsychologia 6*:267–282.

Thal, L. J., Fuld, P. A., Masure, D. M., and Sharpless, S. (1983). Oral physostigmine and lecithin improves memory in Alzheimer's disease. *Ann. Neurol. 113*:491–496.

Thoene, A. I., and Glisky, E. L. (1995). Learning of name-face associations in memory impaired patients: a comparison of different training procedures. *J. Int. Neuropsychol. Soc. 1*:29–38.

Thomson, D. M., and Tulving, E. (1970). Associateive encoding and retrieval: weak and strong cues. *J. Exp. Psychol. 86*:255–262.

Thornton, J. A., Rothblat, L. A., and Murray, E. A. (1997). Rhinal cortex removal produces amnesia for preoperatively learned discrimination problems but fails to disrupt postoperative acquisition and retention in rhesus monkeys. *J. Neurosci. 17*:8536–8549.

Tobias, B. A., Kihlstrom, J. F., and Schacter, D. L. (1992). Emotion and implicit memory. In S. A. Christianson (ed.). *Handbook of Emotion and Memory*. Hillsdale, NJ: Lawrence Erlbaum.

Tosi, L., and Righetti, C. A. (1997). Transient global amnesia and migraine in young people. *Clin. Neurol. Neurosurg. 99*:63–65.

Toth, J. P. (2000). Nonconscious forms of human memory. In *The Oxford Handbook of Memory*, E. Tulving and F. I. M. Craik (eds.). New York: Oxford University Press, pp. 245–261.

Trahan, D. E. and Larrabee, G. J. (1986). *Continu-ous Visual Memory Test*. Odessa, FL: Psychological Assessment Resources.

Tranel, D., and Damasio, A. R. (1985). Knowledge without awareness: an autonomic index of facial recognition by prosopagnosics. *Science 228*: 1453–1454.

Tranel, D. and Hyman, B. T. (1990). Neuropsychological correlates of bilateral amygdala damage. *Arch. Neurol. 47*:349–355.

Tranel, D., Damasio, A. R., Damasio, H., and Brandt, J. P. (1994). Sensorimotor skill learning in amnesia: additional evidence for the neural basis of nondeclarative memory. *Learn. Mem. 1*:165–179.

Tulving, E. (1972). Episodic and semantic memory. In *Organization of Memory*, E. Tulving and W. Donaldson (eds.). New York: Academic Press, pp. 381–403.

Tulving, E. (1983). *Elements of Episodic Memory*. New York: Oxford University Press.

Tulving, E. (1998). Neurocognitive processes of human memory. In *Basic Mechanisms in Cognition and Language*, C. von Euler, I. Lundberg, and R. Llinas (eds.). Amsterdam: Elsevier, pp. 261–281.

Tulving, E., and Markowitsch, H. J. (1997). Memory beyond the hippocampus. *Curr. Opin. Neurobiol. 7*:209–216.

Tulving, E., Markowitsch, H. J., Kapur, S., Habib, R., and Houle, S. (1994). Novelty encoding networks in the human brain: positron emission tomography data. *Neuroreport 5*:2525–2528.

Tulving, E., and Pearlstone, Z. (1966). Availability versus acessability of information in memory for words. *J. Verbal Learn. Behav. 5*:381–391.

Tulving, E., and Schacter, D. L. (1990). Priming and human memory systems. *Science 247(4940)*: 301–306.

Tulving, E., Schacter, D., and Stark, H. A. (1982). Priming effects in word-fragment completion are independent of recognition memory. *J. Exp. Psychol. Learn. Mem. Cogn. 8*:336–342.

Ungerleider, L. G. (1995). Functional brain imaging studies of cortical mechanisms for memory. *Science 270(5237)*:769–775.

Ungerleider, L. G., Courtney, S. M., and Haxby, J. V. (1998). A neural system for human visual working memory. *Proc. Natl. Acad. Sci. U.S.A. 95*:883–890.

Usher, J. A., and Neisser, U. (1993). Childhood amnesia and the beginnings of memory for four early life events. *J. Exp. Psychol. Gen. 122*:155–165.

Uzzell, B. and Gross, Y. (1986). (Eds.). *Clinical Neuropsychology of Intervention*. Boston: Martinus Nijhoff.

Vaidya, C. J., Gabrieli, J. D. E., Demb, J. B., Keane, M. M., and Wetzel, L. C. (1996). Impaired priming on the general knowledge task in amnesia. *Neuropsychology* 10:529–537.

Vaidya, C. J., Gabrieli, J. D. E., Keane, M. M., Monti, L. A., Gutierrez-Rivas, H., and Zarella, M. M. (1997). Evidence for multiple mechanisms of conceptual priming on implicit memory tests. *J. Exp. Psychol. Learn. Mem. Cogn.* 23:1324–1343.

Vaidya, C. J., Gabrieli, J. D., Verfaellie, M., Fleischman, D., and Askari, N. (1998). Font-specific priming following global amnesia and occipital lobe damage. *Neuropsychology* 12:183–192.

Valenstein, E., Bowers, D., Verfaellie, M., Heilman, K. M., Day, A., and Watson, R. T. (1987). Retrosplenial amnesia. *Brain* 110:1631–1646.

Van Hoesen, G. W. (1985). Neural systems of the non-human primate forebrain implicated in memory. *Ann. N. Y. Acad. Sci.* 444:97–112.

Van Hoesen, G. W., and Pandya, D. N. (1975). Some connections of the entorhinal (area 28) and perirhinal (area 35) cortices of the rhesus monkey. I. Temporal lobe afferents. *Brain Res.* 95:25–38.

Van Hoesen, G. W., Pandya, D. N., and Butters, N. (1972). Cortical afferents to the entorhinal cortex of the rhesus monkey. *Science* 175:1471–1473.

Van Hoesen, G. W., Rosene, D. L. and Mesulam, M.-M. (1979). Subicular input from temporal cortex in the rhesus monkey. *Science* 205:608–610.

Vargha-Khadem, F., Gadian, D. G., Watkins, K. E., Connelly, A., Van Paesschen, W., and Mishkin, M. (1997). Differential effects of early hippocampal pathology on episodic and semantic memory. *Science* 277(5324):376–380.

Veazey, R. B., Amaral, D. G., and Cowan, W. M. (1982). The morphology and connections of the posterior hypothalamus in the cynomolgus monkey (*Maccaca fascicularis*). II. Efferent connections. *J. Comp. Neurol.* 207:135–156.

Verfaellie, M., Bauer, R. M., and Bowers, D. (1991). Autonomic and behavioral evidence of 'implicit' memory in amnesia. *Brain Cogn.* 15:10–25.

Verfaellie, M., and Cermak, L. S. (1991). Neuropsychological issues in amnesia. In *Learning and Memory: A Biological View (2nd ed.)*. J. L. Martinez and R. P. Kesner (eds.). San Diego, CA: Academic Press, pp. 467–497.

Verfaellie, M., and Cermak, L. S. (1994). Acquisition of generic memory in amnesia. *Cortex* 30:293–303.

Verfaellie, M., and Cermak, L. S. (1999). Perceptual fluency as a cue for recognition judgments in amnesia. *Neuropsychology* 13:198–205.

Verfaellie, M., Koseff, P., and Alexander, M. P. (2000). Acquisition of novel semantic information in amnesia: effects of lesion location. *Neuropsychologia* 38:484–492.

Victor, M., Adams, R. D., and Collins, G. H. (1971). *The Wernicke-Korsakoff Syndrome*. Philadelphia: F. A. Davis.

Victor, M., Adams, R. D., and Collins, G. H. (1989). *The Wernicke-Korsakoff Syndrome and Related Neurologic Disorders Due to Alcoholism and Malnutrition, 2nd ed.* Philadelphia: F. A. Davis.

Victor, M., and Agamanolis, D. (1990). Amnesia due to lesions confined to the hippocampus: a clinical–pathologic study. *J. Cogn. Neurosci.* 2:246–257.

Vilkki, J. (1985) Amnesic syndromes after surgery of anterior communicating artery aneurysms. *Cortex* 21:431–444.

Volpe, B. T., and Hirst, W. (1983). Amnesia following the rupture and repair of an anterior communicating artery aneurysm. *J. Neurol. Neurosurg. Psychiatry* 46:704–709.

von Bechterew, W. (1900). Demonstration eines Gehirns mit Zerstörung der vorderen und inneren Theile der Hirnrinde beider Schläfenlappen. *Neurol. Zentralbl.* 19:990–991.

von Cramon, D. Y., Hebel, N., and Schuri, U. (1985). A contribution to the anatomical basis of thalamic amnesia. *Brain* 108:993–1008.

von Cramon, D. Y., Hebel, N., and Schuri, U. (1988). Verbal memory and learning in unilateral posterior cerebral infarction. A report on 30 cases. *Brain* 111:1061–1077.

von Cramon, D.Y., and Schuri, U. (1992). The septohippocampal pathways and their relevance to human memory: a case report. *Cortex* 28:411–422.

Wagner, A. D., Desmond, J. E., Glover, G. H., and Gabrieli, J. D. (1998a). Prefrontal cortex and recognition memory. Functional-MRI evidence for context-dependent retrieval processes. *Brain,* 121(Pt 10):1985–2002.

Wagner, A. D., Poldrack, R. A., Eldridge, L. L., Desmond, J. E., Glover, G. H., and Gabrieli, J. D. (1998b). Material-specific lateralization of prefrontal activation during episodic encoding and retrieval. *Neuroreport* 9:3711–3717.

Wagner, A. D., Schacter, D. L., Rotte, M., Koutstaal, W., Maril, A., Dale, A. M., Rosen, B. R., and Buckner, R. L. (1998c). Verbal memory encoding: brain activity predicts subsequent remembering and forgetting. *Science* 281:1188–1191.

Wan, H., Aggleton, J. P., and Brown, M. W. (1999). Different contributions of the hippocampus and perirhinal cortex to recognition memory. *J. Neurosci. 19*:1142–1148.

Warrington, E. K., and Weiskrantz, L. (1970). The amnesic syndrome: consolidation or retrieval? *Nature 228*:628–630.

Warrington, E. K., and Weiskrantz, L. (1973). An analysis of short-term and long-term memory defects in man. In *The Physiological Basis of Memory*, J. A. Deutsch (ed.), New York: Academic Press.

Warrington, E. K., and Weiskrantz, L. (1974). The effect of prior learning on subsequent retention in amnesic patients. *Neuropsychologia 12*:419–428.

Warrington, E. K., and Weiskrantz, L. (1978). Further analysis of the prior learning effect in amnesic patients. *Neuropsychologia 16*:169–177.

Warrington, E.K., and Weiskrantz, L. (1982). Amnesia: a disconnection syndrome? *Neuropsychologia 20*:233–248.

Warrington, E. K. (1984). *Recognition Memory Test*. Windsor, UK: NFER-Nelson.

Warrington, E. K. (1985). A disconnection analysis of amnesia. *Ann. N. Y. Acad. Sci. 444*:72–77.

Wechsler, D. (1945). A standardized memory scale for clinical use. *J. Psychol. 19*:87–95.

Wechsler, D. (1981). *WAIS-R Manual*. New York: Psychological Corporation.

Wechsler, D. (1987). *Wechsler Memory Scale-Revised Manual*. San Antonio, TX: Psychological Corporation.

Weinberg, J., Diller, L., Gerstman, L., and Schulman, P. (1972). Digit span in right and left hemiplegics. *J. Clin. Psychol. 28*:361.

Weingartner, H., Grafman, J., Boutelle, W., Kaye, W., and Martin, P. (1983). Forms of cognitive failure. *Science 221*:380–382.

Weiskrantz, L., and Warrington, E. K. (1979). Conditioning in amnesic patients. *Neuropsychologia 17*:187–194.

Welch, C. A. (1982). The relative efficacy of unilateral nondominant and bilateral stimulation. *Psychopharmacol. Bull. 18*:68–70.

Welsh, K., Butters, N., Hughes, J., Mohs, R., and Heyman, A. (1991). Detection of abnormal memory decline in mild cases of Alzheimer's disease using CERAD neuropsychological measures. *Arch. Neurol. 48*:278–281.

Westwater, H., McDowall, J., Siegert, R., Mossman, S., and Abernethy, D. (1998). Implicit learning in Parkinson's disease: evidence from a verbal version of the serial reaction time task. *J. Clin. Exp. Neuropsychol. 20*:413–418.

Wetzel, C. D., and Squire, L. R. (1982). Cued recall in anterograde amnesia. *Brain Lang. 15*:70–81.

Wetzler, S. E., and Sweeney, J. A. (1986). Childhood amnesia: a conceptualization in cognitive-psychological terms. *J. Am. Psychoanal. Assoc. 34*:663–685.

Whitehouse, P. J., Price, D. L., Clark, A. W., Coyle, J. T., and DeLong, M. R. (1981). Alzheimer disease: evidence for selective loss of cholinergic neurons in the nucleus baslis. *Ann. Neurol. 10*:122–126.

Whitty, C. D., and Zangwill, O. L. (eds.). (1977). *Amnesia*. London: Butterworths.

Wickelgren, W. A. (1979). Chunking and consolidation: a theoretical synthesis of semantic networks, configuring in condition, S-R versus cognitive learning, normal forgetting, the amnesic syndrome, and the hippocampal arousal system. *Psychol. Rev. 86*:44–60.

Wickens, D. D. (1970). Encoding strategies of words: an empirical approach to meaning. *Psychol. Rev. 22*:1–15.

Williams, M., and Pennybacker, J. (1954). Memory disturbances in third ventricle tumours. *J. Neurol. Neurosurg. Psychiatry 17*:115–123.

Willingham, D. B. (1998). A neuropsychological theory of motor skill learning. *Psychol. Rev. 105*:558–584.

Wilson, B. A (1987). *Rehabilitation of Memory*. New York: Guilford Press.

Wilson, B. A. (1999). Memory rehabilitation in brain-injured people. In *Cognitive Neurorehabilitation*, D. T. Stuss and G. Winocur (eds.). New York: Cambridge University Press, pp. 333–346.

Wilson, B. A. (2000). Compensating for cognitive deficits following brain injury. *Neuropsychol. Rev. 10*:233–243.

Wilson, B. A., Evans, J. J., Emslie, H., and Malinek, V. (1997). Evaluation of NeuroPage: a new memory aid. *J. Neurol. Neurosurg. Psychiatry 63*:113–115.

Wilson, B. A., and Moffat, N. (Eds.) (1984). *Clinical Management of Memory Problems*. Rockville, MD: Aspen Publications.

Winnick, W. A., and Daniel, S. A. (1970). Two kinds of response priming in tachishscopic recognition. *J. Exp. Psychol. 84*:74–81.

Winocur, G. (1984). Memory localization in the brain. In *Neuropsychology of Memory*, L. R. Squire and N. Butters (eds.). New York: Guilford Press, pp. 122–133.

Winocur, G. (1990). Anterograde and retrograde amnesia in rats with dorsal hippocampal or dorsomedial thalamic lesions. *Behav. Brain Res. 38*:145–154.

Winocur, G., Kinsbourne, M., and Moscovitch, M. (1981). The effect of cueing on release from proactive interference in Korsakoff amnesic patients. *J. Exp. Psychol. Hum. Learn. Mem. 7*:56–65.

Winocur, G., and Moscovitch, M. (1999). Anterograde and retrograde amnesia after lesions to frontal cortex in rats. *J. Neurosci. 19*:9611–9617.

Winocur, G., Oxbury, S., Roberts, R., Agnetti, V., and Davis, C. (1984). Amnesia in a patient with bilateral lesions to the thalamus. *Neuropsychologia 22*:123–143.

Winograd, T. (1975). Understanding natural language. In D. Bobrow and A. Collins (eds.). *Representation and Understanding*. New York: Academic Press.

Witherspoon, D. and Moscovitch, M. (1989). Stochastic independence between two implicit memory tests. *J. Exp. Psychol. Learn. Mem. Cogn. 15*:22–30.

Wood, F., Ebert, V., and Kinsbourne, M. (1982). The episodic-semantic memory distinction in memory and amnesia: clinical and experimental observations. In *Human Memory and Amnesia*, L. S. Cermak (ed.). Hillsdale, NJ: Lawrence Erlbaum Associates, pp. 167–194.

Woodruff Pak, D. S. (1993). Eyeblink classical conditioning in H.M.: delay and trace paradigms. *Behav. Neurosci. 107*:911–925.

Woolsey, R. M., and Nelson, J. S. (1975). Asymptomatic destruction of the fornix in man. *Arch. Neurol. 32*:566–568.

Xuereb, J. H., Perry, R. H., Candy, J. M., Perry, E. K., Marshall, E., and Bonham, J. R. (1991). Nerve cell loss in the thalamus in Alzheimer's disease and Parkinson's disease. *Brain 114*: 1363–1379.

Yamashita, H. (1993). Perceptual-motor learning in amnesic patients with medial temporal lobe lesions. *Percept. Mot. Skills 77(3 Pt 2)*:1311–1314.

Yasuda, K., Watanabe, O., and Ono, Y. (1997). Dissociation between semantic and autobiographic memory: a case report. *Cortex 33*:623–638.

Yasuno, F., Hirata, M., Takimoto, H., Taniguchi, M., Nakagawa, Y., Ikejiri, Y., Nishikawa, T., Shinozaki, K., Tanabe, H., Sugita, Y., and Takeda, M. (1999). Retrograde temporal order amnesia resulting from damage to the fornix. *J. Neurol. Neurosurg. Psychiatry 67*:102–105.

Youngjohn, J. R., and Crook, T. H. (1993). Stability of everyday memory in age-associated memory impairment: a longitudinal study. *Neuropsychology 7*:406–416.

Zajonc, R. B. (1968). Attitudinal effects of mere exposure. *J. Pers. Soc. Psychol. 9*:1–27.

Zajonc, R. B. (1980). Feeling and thinking: Preferences need no inferences. *American Psychologist 35*:151–175.

Zencius, A., Wesolowski, M. D., Krankowski, T., and Burke, W. H. (1991). Memory notebook training with traumatically brain-injured clients. *Brain Inj. 5*:321–325.

Zola, S. M. (1998). Memory, amnesia, and the issue of recovered memory: neurobiological aspects. *Clin. Psychol. Rev. 18*:915–932.

Zola-Morgan, S., Cohen, N. J., and Squire, L. R. (1983). Recall of remote episodic memory in amnesia. *Neuropsychologia 21*:487–500.

Zola-Morgan, S., and Squire, L. R. (1983). Intact perceptuo-motor skill learning in monkeys with medial temporal lobe lesions. *Soc. Neurosci. Abstr. 9*:27.

Zola-Morgan S., and Squire, L. R. (1984). Preserved learning in monkeys with medial temporal lesions: sparing of motor and cognitive skills. *J. Neurosci. 4*:1072–1085.

Zola-Morgan, S. and Squire, L. R. (1986). Memory impairment in monkeys following lesions restricted to the hippocampus. *Behav. Neurosci. 100*:155–160.

Zola-Morgan, S., and Squire, L. R. (1990a). The neuropsychology of memory: parallel findings in human and nonhuman primates. *Ann. N.Y. Acad. Sci. 608*:434–450.

Zola-Morgan, S., and Squire, L. R. (1990b). The primate hippocampal formation: evidence for a time-limited role in memory storage. *Science 250*:288–290.

Zola-Morgan, S., Squire, L. R., and Amaral, D. G. (1986). Human amnesia and the medial temporal region: enduring memory impairment following a bilateral lesion limited to field CA1 of the hippocampus. *J. Neurosci. 6*:2950–2967.

Zola-Morgan, S., Squire, L. R., and Amaral, D. G. (1989a). Lesions of the amygdala that spare adjacent cortical regions do not impair memory or exacerbate the impairment following lesions of the hippocampal formation. *J. Neurosci. 9*:1922–1936.

Zola-Morgan, S., Squire, L. R., Amaral, D. G., and Suzuki, W. A. (1989b). Lesions of perirhinal and parahippocampal cortex that spare the amygdala and hippocampal formation produce severe memory impairment. *J. Neurosci. 9*:4355–4370.

Zola Morgan, S., Squire, L. R., Alvarez Royo, P., and Clower, R. P. (1991). Independence of memory functions and emotional behavior: separate contributions of the hippocampal formation and the amygdala. *Hippocampus 1*:207–220.

19

Neuropsychology of Dementia

DAVID KNOPMAN AND OLA SELNES

Dementia is a syndrome defined by a non-acute decline in cognition that interferes with functioning in everyday living (American Psychiatric Association, 1994). Dementia, in contrast to disorders defined by deficits in only one cognitive or behavioral domain, is diagnosed when there are deficits in multiple domains. Memory dysfunction, abnormalities in speech and/or language, abnormalities in visuospatial function, deficits in abstract reasoning and executive function, and mood or personality changes are the principal manifestations of the dementia syndrome. The most common dementia, Alzheimer's disease (AD), almost invariably includes striking deficits in new learning and recent memory. Alzheimer's disease has an insidious onset and virtually always exhibits a declining course. Other common disorders in the dementia family may have prominent dysfunction in other cognitive domains, but typically also lead to functional deterioration. We would prefer to restrict the term *dementia* to conditions that are progressive, and use the term *static encephalopathy* to refer to the cognitive impairment states associated with a cerebral infarction, anoxic encephalopathy, traumatic brain injury, or other monophasic, nonprogressive brain insults.

HISTORICAL CONTEXT

Decline in intellectual function as a disorder of the elderly was recognized in antiquity. Throughout most of history, the disorder that we now think of as dementia was viewed as an inevitable consequence of aging (Berchtold and Cotman, 1998). The distinction between the aging process and dementia is a recent conceptual development. The term *dementia* was first used in a clinical context similar to its current form in the eighteenth century by Pinel and Esquirol (Cummings and Benson, 1992; Berchtold and Cotman, 1998). The linkage of a neuropathological state and a clinical dementia was first made by Alois Alzheimer in 1907. However, Blessed and colleagues (1968), in their landmark article on the quantitative relationships between the histopathological findings and cognition in AD, also deserve credit for opening the modern study of dementia. Since their 1968 report, the field of dementia went from a backwater to one of the premier areas of neuroscientific investigation. The cognitive methodology that Blessed et al. used to make their seminal observations represents the foundation of a rich collaboration between cognitive neuroscientists and clinicians. The fundamental principles established by these pioneers—that components of cognitive function important to dementia can be identified and that these components can be quantitated—are the basis of this chapter.

DIAGNOSIS OF DEMENTIA

The diagnostic formulations of dementia that are the most widely used in North America are based on definitions contained in National Institute of Neurologic, Communicative Disorders and Stroke-Alzheimer's Disease and Related Disorders Association (NINCDS-ADRDA) and the *Diagnostic and Statistical Manual of Mental Disorders*, 4th ed. (DSM-IV). The two definitions are given in Table 19–1. The International Classification of Diseases, 10th revision (ICD-10) (World Health Organization, 1992) offers a slightly different formulation that is not used widely in clinical practice or research in North America.

The DSM-IV definition of dementia requires that the deficits be "sufficiently severe to cause impairment in social or occupational functioning," regardless of the level of cognitive function. Many clinicians who view cognitive dysfunction as the sine qua non of the diagnosis of dementia find that this requirement decreases diagnostic sensitivity. However, decline in social and occupational function from a previously higher level can be viewed as the ultimate validation of the diagnosis.

The second core aspect of the diagnosis of dementia is the pattern of cognitive impairment. Dementia involves dysfunction in multiple domains. Both the DSM-IV and NINCDS-ADRDA definitions of dementia are somewhat overly Alzheimer-centric in their specification of memory impairment as required for diagnosis. A more general definition of dementia, such as that proposed by Cummings and Benson (1992), requires impairment in three of the five major domains (memory, language, visuospatial, executive, and affective-personality). Later in this chapter, dementia syndromes that feature disproportionate impairment of one of these domains will be considered in detail.

The third core component of the diagnosis of dementia is the exclusions, in particular, delirium. The temporal profile of dementia is that of a gradually appearing condition, and one in which symptoms steadily worsen.

In community-based ambulatory settings, the diagnosis of dementia is moderately reliable (Fratiglioni et al., 1992; Graham et al., 1996; Larson et al., 1998). Both Fratiglioni et al. and Graham et al. noted that the diagnostic problems with the definition of dementia arise mainly with cases that are neither clearly

Table 19–1. Definitions of Dementia

DSM-IV Criteria for Dementia (American Psychiatric Association, 1994)

1. Development of multiple cognitive deficits (pp. 134, 142) manifested by Memory impairment (impaired ability to learn new information *or* recall previously learned information), and at least one of the following:
Aphasia (language disturbance)
Apraxia (impaired ability to carry out motor activities despite intact motor function)
Agnosia (failure to recognize or identify objects despite intact sensory functions)
Disturbance in executive functioning (i.e., planning organization, sequencing, abstracting).
2. Cognitive deficits must be sufficiently severe to cause impairment in occupational or social function and must represent a decline from a previously higher level of functioning (p. 135).
3. Deficits do not exclusively occur during the course of a delirium.

NINCDS-ADRDA Criteria for Clinical Diagnosis of Alzheimer's Disease (McKhann et al., 1984)

"A decline in memory and other cognitive functions in comparison with the patient's previous level of function as determined by a history of decline in performance and by abnormalities noted from clinical examination and neuropsychological tests. A diagnosis of dementia cannot be made when consciousness is impaired by delirium, drowsiness, stupor or coma or when other clinical abnormalities prevent adequate evaluation of mental status. Dementia is a diagnosis based on behavior."

normal nor clearly demented. These latter individuals typically exhibit a discordance between cognitive or neuropsychologically derived evidence regarding their cognitive status and informant-based assessments of their daily functioning (Pittman et al., 1992; Herlitz et al., 1997). In clinical situations, typical aging and mild cognitive impairment pose important diagnostic challenges, but in acute care situations in particular, depression, delirium, and psychosis are also important conditions to distinguish from dementia.

EPIDEMIOLOGY OF DEMENTIA

DIAGNOSTIC COMPOSITION OF DEMENTIA IN POPULATION SAMPLES

Findings from autopsy studies (Wade et al., 1987; Joachim et al., 1988; Boller et al., 1989; Galasko et al., 1994; Holmes et al., 1999; Lim et al., 1999), clinical series (Larson et al., 1985; Thal et al., 1988) and population-based surveys (Evans et al., 1989; Kokmen et al., 1989; Bachman et al., 1992, Canadian Study of Health and Aging, 1994; Hendrie et al., 1995; Graves et al., 1996; White et al., 1996; Hofman et al., 1997; Fillenbaum et al., 1998) indicate that AD is the most common dementia in North America and Europe. At least 50% to as many as 80% of dementia patients have AD. Both the epidemiological and neuropathological studies indicate that a substantial fraction of AD patients also have secondary diagnoses. Vascular dementia is the second most common disorder in dementia samples, while dementia with parkinsonism (a clinical diagnosis) or dementia with Lewy bodies (a pathological diagnosis emerging as a clinical diagnosis) is the next most common form of dementia.

PREVALENCE

Dementia is largely but not exclusively a diagnosis of the elderly. The prevalence of dementia and AD increases with advancing age (Pfeffer et al., 1987; Evans et al., 1989; Kokmen et al., 1989; Bachman et al., 1992, Canadian Study of Health and Aging, 1994; Hen-

drie et al., 1995; Ott et al., 1995; Graves et al., 1996; White et al., 1996; Hofman et al., 1997; Fillenbaum et al., 1998). There is considerable consistency across recent prevalence surveys in North America and Europe, especially when case-finding methods for mild dementia are similar. In 65- to 70-year-olds the prevalence of dementia is approximately 1 per 100 individuals. With each subsequent 5-year increment, the prevalence of dementia and AD doubles. Over age 85 years, estimates of the prevalence of dementia vary between 20% to nearly 50% (Pfeffer et al., 1987; Evans et al., 1989; Kokmen et al., 1989; Bachman et al., 1992, 1993; Hendrie et al., 1995; Ott et al., 1995; Graves et al., 1996; White et al., 1996; Hofman et al., 1997; Fillenbaum et al., 1998). Beyond age 85, it appears that dementia prevalence continues to rise. Some earlier studies found a decrease above this age, but most recent studies have confirmed that the proportion of individuals with dementia continues to rise over this age. At the younger end of the age spectrum, dementia is quite rare in terms of numbers of cases in the population, but dementia in young and middle-aged adults nonetheless represents an important group of diseases for neuropsychologists.

INCIDENCE

The number of newly diagnosed cases of dementia also rises dramatically with advancing age (Bachman et al., 1993; Stern et al., 1994b; Hebert et al., 1995; Fillenbaum et al., 1998; Gao et al., 1998; Jorm and Jolley, 1998; Ott et al., 1998a; Rocca et al., 1998). The number of new cases of dementia, mainly AD, begins to exceed one per hundred individuals per year as early as the early 70's to the early 80's. It is not until the late 70's or mid-80's that the rate of new cases reaches two per hundred individuals per year. The differences in definitions of dementia account for the variability in estimates of incidence rates among studies, with those studies using definitions that admit milder cases showing the higher incidence rates. Because patients with dementia tend to live for several years to as long as a decade or more beyond disease onset, incidence rates are considerably lower than prevalence rates.

RISK FACTORS FOR DEMENTIA AND ALZHEIMER'S DISEASE

Conditions Associated with Increased Risk

Despite a large number of studies devoted to the detection of risk factors for dementia, only a few characteristics clearly increase an individual's risk for developing dementia. The two most prominent risk factors are advancing age and a family history of dementia.

Family history is an important risk factor for AD (Lautenschlager et al., 1996) and other forms of dementia. In AD, the apolipoprotein E (APOE) genotype is a major element of genetic risk for AD, with onset occurring between roughly age 50 and age 75 (Farrer et al., 1997). There are three genes associated with early-onset AD: the Alzheimer precursor protein gene on chromosome 21, the presenilin 1 gene on chromosome 14, and the presenilin 2 gene on chromosome 1. Interestingly, other than age of onset, there are no consistent clinical differences between familial and nonfamilial AD (Swearer et al., 1992; Farlow et al., 1994; Campion et al., 1995; Lopera et al., 1997).

Very low educational achievement (less than eighth grade education) has been a consistently observed, modestly potent risk factor that increases a person's odds of developing AD by two to three times (Zhang et al., 1990; Friedland, 1993; Katzman, 1993; Stern et al., 1994b, 1995; Cobb et al., 1995; Ott et al., 1995; Callahan et al., 1996). There may be a threshold effect for education so that studies that do not include large numbers of subjects with less than an eighth grade education may not detect the association (Beard et al., 1992). Even when diagnostic methods are specifically modified to reduce educational or cultural biases, the education effect remains (Stern et al., 1995).

Snowdon and colleagues (1996) have shown that cognitive performance at age 20 years was predictive of the subsequent development of dementia roughly 50 years later. Their hypothesis is that early life experiences and environment contribute to the development of brain reserve. Better childhood brain "nurturing" presumably leads to better brain function, which in turn acts as a buffer in ameliorating the deleterious effects of AD pathology later in life. In general, enriched childhood environments will be associated with higher educational attainment, but in Snowdon's view it is the sum of all enriching experiences, not the least of which is good childhood nutrition, that protects individuals from the subsequent development of dementia.

Head injury in the remote past may be a risk factor for AD (French et al., 1985; Chandra et al., 1989; Graves et al., 1990; Mortimer et al., 1991), but concerns about recall bias have not been refuted. A prospective study that enrolled nondemented subjects found no association between minor head injuries and the subsequent development of AD (Mehta et al., 1999). However, because of the link between boxing and AD (Roberts et al., 1990; Jordan et al., 1997), the importance of non–sport-related head trauma to AD seems plausible. Mayeux and colleagues (1995) have proposed that the risk of head trauma for AD is mediated by APOE $\epsilon4$ genotype, but this association was not seen in the one available study of newly diagnosed dementia patients in a prospective study (Mehta et al., 1999).

Cardiovascular disease confers a small to moderate increased risk for subsequent cognitive impairment (Elias et al., 1993; Prince et al., 1994; Launer et al., 1995; Kalmijn et al., 1996; Carmelli et al., 1998) or AD (Hofman et al., 1997). The cardiovascular risk factors associated with AD include atherosclerosis broadly defined, history of stroke, history of mid-life hypertension, and carotid artery disease. Diabetes mellitus is prominently associated with vascular dementia (Leibson et al., 1997), as is hypertension (Prince et al., 1994; Rockwood et al., 1997).

PROTECTIVE FACTORS

Two protective factors that have been observed prospectively include estrogen replacement therapy (ERT) (Brenner et al., 1994; Paganini-Hill and Henderson, 1996; Tang et al., 1996; Kawas et al., 1997; Jacobs et al., 1998) and the use of nonsteroidal anti-inflammatory drugs (NSAIDs) (Breitner et al., 1994; Andersen et al., 1995; McGeer et al., 1996; Stewart et al., 1997; Prince et al., 1998). However, epidemiological associations do not prove causality. Estrogen replacement therapy or NSAID use could have been associated with some other factors that actually mediated the risk of AD. The compelling element of both the ERT and the NSAID stories is that neuropathological observations also support a biologically relevant role for estrogen (Luine, 1985; McEwen et al., 1997) and inflammation (McGeer and Rogers, 1992; Lue et al., 1996; Rogers et al., 1996) in AD pathogenesis. The use of statin-type cholesterol lowering drug has also been associated with a lower risk for AD (Jick et al., 2000; Wolozin et al., 2000).

Cigarette smoking has appeared in most studies as a protective factor for AD (Graves et al., 1991; Hebert et al., 1992; Brenner et al., 1993; Ford et al., 1996), although in other studies it has been a risk factor (Prince et al., 1996; Galanis et al., 1997; Ott et al., 1998b). Intuitively, it would appear more likely to be a risk factor because of its association with vascular disease. However, the putative mechanism by which smoking could be protective is via stimulation of nicotinic receptors in the brain. Nicotinic receptors on cholinergic neurons might mediate the production of trophic factors that promote survival of key neuronal populations in AD (Whitehouse and Kalaria, 1995).

DISTINGUISHING DEMENTIA FROM OTHER SYNDROMES

As a first step in the diagnostic process, the syndrome of dementia must be distinguished from other states. Traditionally, delirium, focal neurological syndromes, depression, and psychosis dominated this list. We would add aging, mild cognitive impairment, and auditory or visual deficits to this list.

AGING

Beliefs about the cognitive changes that occur with aging make early diagnosis of dementia difficult. Recognizing that a patient is experiencing lapses in memory, visuospatial function, judgment, or language that are outside the normal variability of everyday life is a challenge for both lay people and health-care professionals. Dementia is underdiagnosed (Callahan et al., 1995; Eefsting et al., 1996; Ross et al., 1997); "normal" aging is often the explanation given for the failure to diagnose it.

The distinction between cognitive aging and dementia is a challenging one. Genuine declines in mental speed occur even in optimally healthy elderly people. In cross-sectional studies, a small number of individuals with undiagnosed incipient dementia will be present (Sliwinski et al., 1996; Wilson et al., 1999). Thus, unselected samples of elders perform less well than comparison groups who are in their 20's. In longitudinal studies and in studies in which only the healthiest of elderly people were studied, the only consistent finding across the age spectrum (at least up to about age 75) was slowing of performance (Schaie, 1989a). Several longitudinal studies of individuals over age 65 have demonstrated only slight declines of cognition in large population samples of nondemented elderly (Colsher and Wallace, 1991; Ganguli et al., 1996; Haan et al., 1999; Wilson et al., 1999). In one of the few studies that longitudinally examined nondemented individuals over age 75, persons who were over 75 declined more on cognitive testing than did 65- to 75-year-olds (Brayne et al., 1999).

The domains of learning and memory are usually considered to show the greatest changes with typical aging (Small et al., 1999). Decline in learning with aging might be mediated by slowing of cognitive processing, but the end result is impaired new learning. There are several types of learning and memory that come into play in day-to-day affairs, but rote retention of something like a phone number for less than a minute and longer-term retention of a several-sentence message are two prototypical memory tasks. On tasks that involve immediate recall of a large number of items (e.g., 7 or more words or digits), older adults have a lower learning rate. Performance by older adults on verbal learning tasks from the neuropsychology laboratory offers insights into those functions (Geffen et al., 1990; Mitrushina et al., 1991; Petersen et al., 1992). In a test such as the Auditory Verbal Learning Task, the subject is asked to learn a list of 15 words over five trials and then recall them 30 minutes later. In the learning phase, older adults are clearly less successful as the length of the list of items to be remembered increases (Geffen et al., 1990). On delayed recall, however, older individuals are nearly as effective as younger individuals in recalling words after a delay, as a percentage of words successfully learned initially. Delayed-recall performance in healthy elders is preserved into the tenth decade (Petersen et al., 1992). Delayed-recall performance is severely impaired in AD patients, in contrast.

Many language functions decline very little with normal aging (Schaie, 1989a; Howieson et al., 1993). Once people reach middle age, vocabulary levels remain stable. Naming and comprehension abilities also change very little over the lifespan well into the eighth or ninth decades of life. Even verbal fluency declines only slightly with age when speed of processing is taken into account (Schaie, 1989b).

In contrast, abstract reasoning declines with normal aging (Schaie, 1989a, 1989b; Albert et al., 1990; Howieson et al., 1993). As mental speed drops, healthy elders may be less adept at performing concentration-demanding tasks without the benefit of paper and pencil. Consequently, typical elders do worse on tests of abstract reasoning than younger individuals. However, the declines that are evident in the laboratory setting may not be obvious in daily affairs because individuals are able to compensate for reduced mental speed by experience and acumen acquired over a lifetime. Just as in memory disorder, when deficits in abstract reasoning appear, brain disease rather than normal aging is, by far, the likely etiology.

An axiom of assessment of mental function in the elderly is that cognitive decline from a previously higher level is simply not compatible with a diagnosis of normal aging. In general, low cognitive performance (without respect to whether decline has been documented) is also suggestive of dementia rather than typical aging. However, the possibility that life-long intellectual disability is the cause of poor memory and abstract reasoning abilities must first be ruled out.

MILD COGNITIVE IMPAIRMENT WITHOUT IMPAIRMENT IN SOCIAL AND OCCUPATIONAL FUNCTION

A commonly encountered scenario occurs when a patient exhibits mild but definite cognitive impairment on mental status tests or neuropsychological assessments, but neither the patient nor family informants are willing to state that the patient has any difficulties in daily affairs (functional impairment). The DSM-IV and NINCDS-ADRDA criteria for dementia do not provide an operational approach for dealing with this discrepancy. The DSM-IV definition of dementia requires that the deficits be "sufficiently severe to cause impairment in social or occupational functioning," regardless of the premorbid level of cognitive function. Thus, according to the DSM-IV definition of dementia, if no impairment in social and occupational functioning can be established, the diagnosis of dementia should not be made.

Such patients are common, and it is incorrect to diagnose them as normal. Several researchers have recognized that individuals with cognitive impairment but allegedly normal daily function are common in population-based studies. In the Honolulu-Asia Aging study (White et al., 1996), 20% of subjects who met cognitive criteria for dementia did not meet the functional impairment criteria. In the Canadian Study (Graham et al., 1996), a similar proportion (17%) of cases with neuropsychologically based diagnosis of dementia lacked confirmation of impairment from an informant. Pittman et al. (1992) found that 35% of subjects with a dementia diagnosis by neuropsychological assessment were not diagnosed as demented by clinicians, presumably because of the absence of informant-based reports of functional impairment. Petersen et al. (1995) have shown that after excluding persons with known prior brain injuries, individuals with mild cognitive impairment have an increased risk of developing dementia. Many other groups (Masur et al., 1994; Jacobs et al., 1995; Linn et al., 1995; Tierney et al., 1996b; Herlitz et al., 1997; Fabrigoule et al., 1998) have observed that poorer performance on cognitive tests predicts the subsequent development of dementia. Other investigators (Morris et al.,

1996; Rubin et al., 1998) have taken a stronger stand in claiming that individuals who present with mild cognitive impairment in the form of poor recent memory without documentation of impairment in daily function almost invariably turn out to have AD. However, in population-based studies, cognitive impairment without functional decline is likely to include a mixture of both patients with static encephalopathies, such as survivors of traumatic brain injury, cardiac arrest, depression, psychiatric conditions, and mental retardation, and incipient dementia patients (Graham et al., 1997).

At the present time, there is no consensus on how to diagnose the patient with mild cognitive impairment and no functional impairment. One proposed definition of mild cognitive impairment states that the patient should have normal daily function, normal non-memory cognitive function, and impairment of delayed free recall in the AD range (Petersen et al., 1995). This definition of mild cognitive impairment is currently being applied in clinical trials meant to forestall the development of diagnosable AD.

We prefer to avoid the term *age-associated memory impairment* because it implies that the deficits could be normal and carry no negative prognostic implications, something that the longitudinal study of such patients shows to be clearly untrue. Patients with mild cognitive impairment should be told of the caveats regarding the diagnosis and the risk for subsequently developing dementia, and be encouraged to return for reassessment in 6 months to 1 year.

FOCAL CEREBRAL LESIONS

Patients with focal right hemisphere lesions such as infarctions (Mesulam et al., 1976) may develop delirium acutely that can sometimes evolve into a clinical state that mimics dementia. Similarly, patients who sustain lesions in other cognitively eloquent locations in the brain such as the left parietal lobe (Devinsky et al., 1988), thalamus (Graff-Radford et al., 1990), or hippocampus (Zola-Morgan et al., 1986; Ott and Saver, 1993) may have cognitive impairment in more than one domain in a pattern that overlaps with the dementia syndrome. Cerebrovascular lesions in these locations

should present with acute changes in function, which should distinguish these lesions from dementia due to AD, dementia with Lewy bodies, or frontotemporal dementia.

VISUAL AND AUDITORY DEFICITS

Visual loss and impaired hearing adversely affect function especially in the elderly (Keller et al., 1999). Sensory deficits may not affect cognition per se, but they can lead to decline in independence in daily living abilities in a way that may mimic dementia.

Visual changes in the elderly are very common (Rahmani et al., 1996). Glaucoma, cataracts, and macular degeneration affect a large proportion of elderly individuals. The consequences of visual loss include social isolation, visual misperceptions, and dependence on others that can mimic some of the manifestations of dementia. When assessing a patient with apparent functional impairment, it is essential to ask whether degraded vision could account for some or all of the deficits.

Similarly, hearing loss (Ives et al., 1995; Jerger et al., 1995) is common in the elderly and may also lead to social isolation. In addition, hearing loss can mimic memory loss by giving the appearance of inattentiveness or failure to recall conversations. As with visual loss, loss of auditory acuity at levels that interfere with processing ordinary conversations should be considered part of the evaluation of a patient with memory loss. Unlike cognitively normal elders who typically have peripheral hearing loss with good compensatory abilities, patients with mild dementia also have evidence of central auditory dysfunction, where functional hearing is worse than expected based on pure tone hearing loss (Gates et al., 1995).

DELIRIUM

Delirium by definition is acute in onset, occurring over hours to days. Delirium is a common disorder in hospitalized elderly patients (Francis et al., 1990; Inouye and Charpentier, 1996). While dementia may not be commonly mistaken for delirium, delirium (also referred to as *acute confusional state*) may be misdiagnosed as dementia if the clinician fails to appreciate the onset and progression of the cognitive disorder. Delirium and dementia are also distinguished by the impairment of level of arousal and attention in delirium, and its relative preservation in dementia. Patients with delirium experience fluctuations in their levels of consciousness and also have impaired attention and concentration. Dementia patients, in contrast, do not have fluctuations in their level of consciousness and often have virtually normal attention and concentration in the mild stages of the illness. A simple but underutilized bedside tool for detecting delirium is writing. Perhaps because writing involves multiple functions—language, visuoconstructional ability, and the ability to plan and initiate action—it is particularly sensitive to global cognitive impairment (Chedru and Geschwind, 1972). A patient who is mildly to moderately demented but not delirious may still be able to compose and write a sentence on command.

When the two disorders overlap, diagnosis may be more difficult. Dementia patients are at greater risk for delirium in the setting of acute medical illnesses (Francis et al., 1990; Lerner et al., 1997). Longitudinal follow-up studies of patients who experience delirium have shown that they do not always have a complete cognitive recovery (Murray et al., 1993), perhaps because the episode of delirium unmasked incipient or unrecognized dementia. Thus, dementia should be a consideration to be addressed during post hospitalization follow-up in an elderly patient who experiences delirium. Delaying assessment until several weeks after resolution of the acute illness is advisable, so that the patient's performance is not adversely affected by a resolving delirium.

DEPRESSION

Dementia and depression often overlap (Yesavage, 1993). Patients with depression without dementia may have complaints of impaired memory and concentration, but they typically perform better than expected on mental status testing. Patients with pure depression are more likely than dementia patients to complain spontaneously of memory problems, but that difference is not always a reliable discriminator. Depressed patients will volunteer

that they are sad or despondent, but spontaneous or elicited complaints of being sad do not rule out dementia either. Objective cognitive impairment, usually but not always, differentiates dementia from depression (La Rue, 1989; Bieliauskas, 1993). Competent bedside mental status or neuropsychological assessment is necessary to characterize cognitive function adequately to make a diagnosis in a patient with depression and cognitive complaints.

Low mood, apathy, and loss of initiative may be presenting symptoms of dementia (Kramer and Reifler, 1992; Oppenheim, 1994). Even when patients are thought to have depression as their primary diagnosis, the new onset of depression in late life carries an increased risk for subsequently developing dementia. In the experience of practioners at one dementia clinic (Reding et al., 1985), 57% of individuals who were initially diagnosed with depression later went on to develop dementia. In other studies the rate of the development of dementia may not be quite as high (Pearlson et al., 1989). Nonetheless, an elderly person who develops depression is at high risk for subsequently developing dementia (Alexopoulos and Chester, 1992; Berger et al., 1999).

PSYCHOSIS

When psychotic symptoms such as hallucinations, delusions, paranoia, or bizarre behaviors occur in late middle-aged or elderly individuals who have no prior history of psychiatric disease, it is highly likely that these behaviors are manifestations of an underlying dementing disorder. Thus, schizophrenia should not be a serious diagnostic consideration in older patients with new-onset psychotic symptoms.

ACQUIRED BUT STABLE COGNITIVE DEFICITS

We use the term *static encephalopathy* to identify the syndrome of cognitive deficits in multiple domains that occur and persist as a result of a single event, such as an episode of anoxic–ischemic encephalopathy, a stroke, a serious central nervous system infection, head trauma, or any of a number of other monophasic neurological illnesses. In principle, with a good history, the prognosis for these patients should be readily distinguished from that of the dementia of AD by virtue of the existence of the inciting neurological event. In population studies, patients with static encephalopathies and cognitive dysfunction are common (Graham et al., 1997).

NEUROPSYCHOLOGICAL AND CLINICAL ASSESSMENT IN DEMENTIA IN THE ELDERLY

INFORMATION FROM THE INFORMANT

The historical and functional information needed to diagnose dementia is gained by querying a knowledgeable informant and performing a cognitive assessment of the patient. Instruments that have been validated for informant interviews for diagnosing dementia include the Dementia Questionnaire (DQ) (Kawas et al., 1994; Ellis et al., 1998), the Informant Questionnaire on Cognitive Decline in the Elderly (IQCODE) (Jorm, 1994), and the Functional Activities Questionnaire (FAQ) (Pfeffer et al., 1982). The Clinical Dementia Rating Scale (Hughes et al., 1982; Morris, 1993) also includes a semistructured interview that covers most of the major domains that are queried with informants.

Informant input for determining impairment in social function will provide greater specificity of the diagnosis of dementia than that from a diagnosis based solely on neuropsychological criteria (Pittman et al., 1992; Callahan et al., 1996). Particularly for individuals with low educational achievement, informant histories provide an external validation of the cognitive assessments. Cognitive test norms might not be valid when culturally and educationally diverse populations are being evaluated. The trade-off is that informants may overlook substantial impairment in social and occupational functioning on the part of the patient, which will result in loss of sensitivity, particularly for mild dementia. For the practicing clinician, the interpretation of the history as reported by informants must be subjected to the same critical scrutiny as the cognitive testing

data. Clinicians must weigh all sources of data in drawing diagnostic conclusions.

BEDSIDE COGNITIVE ASSESSMENT TOOLS

Cognitive assessments that have been validated for bedside use include the Mini-Mental State examination (MMSE) (Folstein et al., 1975), the modified Mini-Mental State (3MS) (Teng and Chui, 1987), the Orientation-Memory-Concentration test (Katzman et al., 1983), the Short Test of Mental Status (Kokmen et al., 1991), the Neurobehavioral Cognitive Screening test (Kiernan et al., 1987), and others.

It is beyond the scope of this chapter to consider the composition of mental status examinations in detail. They all contain questions about orientation, but beyond that common feature, there is quite a range of coverage of different cognitive domains. Bedside cognitive assessments such as the MMSE have imperfect sensitivity as stand-alone instruments (Anthony et al., 1982; O'Connor et al., 1989, Kukull et al., 1994). For the diagnosis of dementia, a test like the MMSE is overweighted for language testing and underweighted for recent memory and executive function assessments. The three-word recall task in the MMSE may be useful for screening, but it is imperfectly correlated with neuropsychologically validated tests of recent memory (Cullum et al., 1993). The Orientation-Memory-Concentration test (Katzman et al., 1983) provides somewhat greater weight for memory dysfunction and executive dysfunction. The "months backwards" item of this instrument may provide a sensitive measure of the constructs of mental agility and working memory that we have included under the category of executive function (Ball et al., 1999).

A stand-alone battery of items sensitive to executive function has also been developed (Royall et al., 1992), and is intended to be used in conjunction with a standard mental status instrument. The bedside battery of executive function includes such tasks as imitating sequences of hand movements ("fist-edge-palm"), echopraxia avoidance (inhibiting certain behaviors despite implicit prompts to do so), and other activities requiring sustained attention such as reciting the months backwards or generating a list of words of a particular semantic category or first letter (word fluency).

A collection of several tests suitable for administration at the bedside such as the Seven Minute Screen (Solomon et al., 1998) is, in principle, much better for early dementia detection because it includes tasks known to be sensitive to the earliest deficits: a 16-item memory task, a verbal fluency task, and clock drawing. Its advantages over shorter instruments for dementia detection have not been evaluated in a head-to-head comparison in an unselected sample of subjects.

For patients who are not native English speakers, analysis of performance on these tests administered through an interpreter must be conducted with considerable caution. In addition, educational and occupational background affects performance on these tests and diagnosis (Kittner et al., 1986; Crum et al., 1993; Evans et al., 1993; Wiederholt et al., 1993; Kukull et al., 1994; Tangalos et al., 1996; Elias et al., 1997). Both low socioeconomic status (Pittman et al., 1992) and very high prior intellectual achievement (Inouye et al., 1993) present challenges to diagnosis.

Mental status examinations are also moderately correlated with assessments of daily functioning in dementia (Pfeffer et al., 1982; Galasko et al., 1997; Gelinas et al., 1999). The remarkable degree of relationship between synaptic density in AD (DeKosky and Scheff, 1990; Terry et al., 1991) and mental status previously mentioned, and the relationship between functional measures and mental status are powerful validators of bedside cognitive assessment.

LABORATORY COGNITIVE NEUROPSYCHOLOGICAL ASSESSMENT

In patients with mild symptoms, those with possible dysexecutive syndrome, and those in whom depression might play a role, neuropsychological testing is a necessary part of the evaluation for suspected dementia. Bedside testing of executive functions, memory function, or visuospatial function is usually not as informative, discriminating, or reliable as laboratory-based tests. Neuropsychological testing can evaluate the severity of impairment in different cognitive domains with greater precision than can bedside tests and thus establish specific patterns or profiles of cognitive impairment (Pasquier, 1999). Even though no cognitive profiles are perfectly specific or sensitive to a given dementia diagnosis, establishing a profile that is *consistent* with a given dementia subtype is quite helpful. For example, in a patient with prominent behavioral disturbances such as agitation and disinhibition that might point to a frontotemporal dementia, a neuropsychological test profile that documents severe recent memory and visuospatial disturbances would keep AD in the differential diagnosis.

Alternatively, formal neuropsychological testing may not be necessary in situations where the informant's information is diagnostic and where skilled clinicians can make use of bedside clinical tools (Stuss et al., 1996). Consider a patient with a 3-year history of memory impairment and no complaints of depression who scores below 20/30 on the MMSE (and who has less than ninth 9th grade education): such a patient may not need neuropsychological assessment. Mental status examinations, particularly if they are supplemented at the bedside by additional tasks, can approximate the diagnostic value of longer tests in many instances.

A number of studies have examined the role of neuropsychological assessment in the diagnosis of dementia, compared to clinical diagnoses (Pittman et al., 1992; Monsch et al., 1995; Stuss et al., 1996; Tierney et al., 1996b; Herlitz et al., 1997). These studies used expert clinicians to generate the clinical diagnoses. Consequently, the fact that neuropsychological assessment had relatively modest additional value above and beyond a skilled clinician's assessment in these studies does not generalize to routine practice. The value of neuropsychological testing in routine clinical practice may be quite high for physicians who have little training in cognitive assessment beyond screening examinations. Neurologists and other physicians with less experience and expertise in bedside cognitive assessment skills should make broader use of neuropsychological consultations. Those physicians who are comfortable with and skilled in bedside cognitive assessment may have more selective uses for neuropsychological assessments.

Memory

The neuropsychological assessment of recent verbal memory has definite advantages over bedside testing. The key features of neuropsychological assessment of memory in dementia evaluations include the use of supraspan length material, appropriate learning format (either multiple learning trials or elaborative encoding), delayed free recall, and delayed recognition. The widely used laboratory tests, such as the Auditory Verbal Learning Test (Geffen et al., 1990; Crossen and Wiens, 1994; Lezak, 1995), the California Verbal Learning Test (Delis et al., 1988; Crossen and Wiens, 1994; Elwood, 1995; Lezak, 1995), the Wechsler Memory Scale, Revised or 3rd Edition Logical Memory subtest, the Consortium to Establish a Registry for Alzheimer's Disease (CERAD) word recall test (Welsh et al., 1994; Mohs et al., 1997), or the Free and Cued Recall (Grober et al., 1988), allow for much better separation of normal and abnormal performance. Confounding effects of immediate recall are also minimized with longer delay intervals and longer lists. For patients in whom bedside assessment of recent memory function yields conflicting or inconclusive data, neuropsychological assessment of recent memory is very useful. The usefulness of visual memory testing is uncertain. While some authors have found it to be useful in differentiating dementia patients from normals (Eslinger et al., 1985), others have noted that on some tests, visual memory deficits (at least those measured by the Wechsler Memory Scale-Revised Visual Memory subtests) may be confounded by visuoconstructional deficits (Leonberger et al., 1991).

Language Functions

Quantitation of performance on naming to confrontation and comprehension of spoken language are important reasons for neuropsychological consultation in dementia patients. The Boston Naming Test is widely used in North America for assessing confrontation naming. The Token Test is widely used for formal assessment of auditory comprehension (De Renzi and Vignolo, 1982).

Verbal fluency is a frequently used task that assesses both verbal expressive abilities and ex-

ecutive functions. Several studies have shown that category or letter fluency is useful in early detection of dementia due to AD (Monsch et al., 1992; Welsh et al., 1994). Moreover, verbal fluency tests are useful for diagnosing patients with frontotemporal dementia (FTD) and progressive supranuclear palsy (PSP).

Assessment of vocabulary level and other measures of verbal ability can be particularly useful in estimating a patient's premorbid level of cognitive function. The Vocabulary subtest of the Wechsler Adult Intelligence Scale–Revised (WAIS-R) or WAIS-III are useful for evaluating premorbid verbal abilities. The National Adult Reading Test–Revised (NART-R) has also been used for the purpose of estimating premorbid verbal intelligence. Its advantage over the WAIS Vocabulary test in this context is that the NART simply requires correct pronunciation of the test words. In contrast, the vocabulary test requires not only recognizing the test word but also explaining its meaning, a function that may be impaired even in early dementia (Maddrey et al., 1996).

Visuospatial Function

Testing of visuospatial function with tests such as the Block Design subtest of the WAIS-R (Wechsler, 1981; Lezak, 1995) in the neuropsychological laboratory is considerably more detailed than is feasible with bedside testing. Other tests used include copying, and then later drawing from memory, the Rey-Osterreith Figure.

Visuospatial function is abnormal in many forms of dementia, even when patients are able to copy intersecting pentagons or draw a clock. Furthermore, bedside testing of visuospatial function usually requires intact dominant limb function. In patients with hemiparesis or other causes of dysfunction of the dominant hand or arm, neuropsychological tests such as Benton Judgement of Line Orientation (Lezak, 1995) may be used to evaluate visuospatial reasoning with minimal need for limb-motor function. Another test of visuospatial abilities that requires little motor input is the Raven's Standard Progressive Matrices Test. Pfeffer et al. (1981) found this task useful in screening for dementia, although Knopman and Ryberg (1989) found considerable overlap between probable AD patients and normally elderly controls. Other tests described in the next section, such as Trailmaking, Porteus Mazes, and Wisconsin Card Sort, all require visuospatial processing for successful performance.

Frontal Lobe Function, Executive Function, and Abstract Reasoning

Brain regions anterior to the motor cortex are involved with attention, working memory, and the categorization of contingent relationships. In non–brain-damaged individuals the separate frontal regions are interconnected and act cooperatively to support reasoning and decision making. We use the term *executive function* to encompass broadly the functions that are supported by the frontal lobes. The neuropsychology laboratory assessment of executive function—mental agility, foresight, planning, freedom from distraction, ability to shift mental set—has several advantages over the kinds of executive tasks that can be assessed with bedside techniques. The laboratory tests utilize specialized test materials. The instruments used to assess executive function take considerable time to administer. Because they are intensely demanding of concentration, testing situations that are optimally quiet and free from distractions are necessary.

Widely used tests include the Word Fluency task, Stroop tests, Wisconsin Card Sorting Test (Anderson et al., 1991), the Trailmaking Test, and the Porteus Mazes (Lezak, 1995). In interpreting the results of these assessments, it is important to be aware that not all frontal lobe lesions produce impairment on executive tests (Anderson et al., 1991; Rahman et al., 1999), and that impaired performance on tests of executive function does not always signify a frontal lobe lesion. Patients with low educational achievement typically score worse on tests of executive function (Kittner et al., 1986; Ganguli et al., 1991; Welsh et al., 1994; Cerhan et al., 1998) than do patients with depression (Beats et al., 1996). Patients with prominent visuospatial deficits will do poorly on the Wisconsin Card Sorting Test, Porteus Mazes, and Trailmaking Test because those tasks are visually based.

CONFOUNDING EFFECTS OF EDUCATION ON COGNITIVE ASSESSMENT

Low educational achievement has important effects on cognitive assessment in cases of suspected dementia. Low educational achievement usually implies that a subject was never exposed to the kinds of cognitive assessment experiences that become increasingly rigorous from elementary education to secondary education to post-secondary educational experiences. Many procedures used in both bedside and laboratory assessment of cognition utilize procedures and materials that are very similar to those used in aptitude testing for post-secondary education. As a consequence, individuals with less than ninth grade education may simply not have experience with some test procedures that are commonplace for college-educated individuals. In addition, educational achievement is a proxy for innate intelligence. Although the correlation is grossly imperfect, there is a relationship between educational achievement, the educational achievement of one's parents, the occupation of one's parents, the socioeconomic circumstances of one's childhood and adulthood, and other factors that affect health status in general and cognition in particular. While these topics are beyond the scope of this chapter, they are directly relevant in considering the diagnosis of dementia from a cognitive assessment perspective.

In normal individuals, prior educational achievement has a powerful effect on cognitive performance (Scherr et al., 1988; Ganguli et al., 1991; Stern et al., 1992; Crum et al., 1993; Inouye et al., 1993; Welsh et al., 1994; Cerhan et al., 1998). For example, in a very large population-based sample from the Atherosclerosis Risk in Communities study (Cerhan et al., 1998), there was almost a twofold difference in the number of symbols completed on the Digit Symbol Substitution Subtest of the WAIS-R between individuals with less than ninth grade education and those with at least some college education. The difference was observed in both men and women, and in individuals between the ages of 45–59 as well as 60–69. A similar phenomenon was observed on the word fluency test.

Educational achievement also had an impact on word recall in the 10-word Delayed Word Recall task, but the difference between those with less than ninth grade education and at least some college education was smaller, with the better-educated individuals performing at most only 25% better than the lower-educated subgroup.

In attempting to create criterion-based diagnoses of dementia based on neuropsychological (Stern et al., 1992; Welsh et al., 1994) or bedside mental status assessments (Crum et al., 1993), the education effect on test scores creates considerable difficulty. Dividing subjects into low-, middle-, and high-education strata allows the test criteria to be applied in a strata-specific manner. Others have attempted to apply more sophisticated correlational procedures to score corrections for education (Kittner et al., 1986). Both approaches have merit, but the stratification procedure is somewhat easier to apply in clinical settings. Yet, because the explanatory relationship between educational level and cognitive function is only moderate, any form of education-based correction of raw test scores may worsen diagnostic accuracy rather than improve it.

OTHER DEMENTIA ASSESSMENT TOOLS

Increasingly, clinicians have come to rely on standardized assessment instruments for diagnosis and management of dementia patients. The MMSE and other standardized mental status exams have already been discussed. There are other aspects of dementia that are equally important to capture quantitatively, such as behavior, function, and staging of the disease.

Behavior

A wide variety of neuropsychiatric symptoms occur in AD and other dementias. These behaviors may be challenging to quantitate because the symptoms may vary in frequency and severity. Rare behaviors may be catastrophically severe, whereas frequent behaviors may be minor nuisances. The Neuropsychiatric Inventory (Cummings et al., 1994) rates 12 behaviors that are common in AD and other dementias. Another test used for assessment of behavior in dementia is known at the Behav-

ioral Pathology in Alzheimer's Disease Rating Scale (Reisberg et al., 1987).

Function

Activities of daily living (ADL) as they relate to dementia can be conveniently divided into two categories, basic and instrumental. Basic activities of daily living (Lawton and Brody, 1969) are included as queries. Basic ADLs are typically impaired in more severely demented patients. Pfeffer et al. (1982) developed a questionnaire for instrumental daily living activities that is particularly useful for the assessment of patients with mild dementia. The Pfeffer tool is not useful for moderately demented individuals. Galasko et al. (1997) have developed a scale for use in clinical trials that has a broad range of performance. Other scales that have been used in AD clinical trials include the Interview for Deterioration in Daily Functioning Activities in Dementia (IDDD) (Teunisse et al., 1991), which contains 33 items, of which 17 involve complex or instrumental activities, and the Disability Assessment in Dementia (DAD) (Gelinas et al., 1999).

Global Disease Severity Scales

The Clinical Dementia Rating (CDR) Scale (Hughes et al., 1982; Morris, 1993) is one that includes most aspects of dementia and also provides explicit descriptions of each stage. Six different domains are rated separately: orientation, memory, judgment/problem-solving, function in home/hobbies, function in community affairs, and basic ADLs. Each domain is rated on a 5-point scale. A scoring algorithm (Morris, 1993) allows derivation of an overall rating. Another scale that is also widely used is the Global Deterioration Scale (Reisberg et al., 1982). It uses 8 rating points, ranging from normal through the various stages of severity.

LONGITUDINAL FOLLOW-UP OF COGNITIVE DECLINE IN DEMENTIA

In typical practice situations, clinicians rely on bedside mental status examinations and serial discussions with caregivers to determine rate of progression of dementia and to make predictions about future problems. In AD patients, the rate of change on the MMSE is about 3 ± 4 points per year (Katzman et al., 1988; Ortof and Crystal, 1989; Salmon et al., 1990; van Belle et al., 1990; Galasko et al., 1991; Schneider, 1992; Kraemer et al., 1994). Although that small amount of change may strike some clinicians as insensitive, the rate of change on the MMSE is probably a reasonable reflection of the global decline of an AD patient. At some times, the MMSE seems even too sensitive. On an individual level, the rate of decline over one 6-month or 1-year period does not predict the rate over the next interval (Salmon et al., 1990).

The rate of decline in patients with typical AD depends on where the patient performs on initial assessment. Although there is tremendous interindividual variability, cognitive decline on a test like the MMSE or an expanded instrument like the Alzheimer's Disease Assessment Scale, cognitive portion (ADAS-cog) (Rosen et al., 1984) exhibits a curvilinear relationship between baseline cognitive status and rate of decline over 6 months to 1 year (Morris et al., 1993; Stern et al., 1994a). The smallest changes occur at the mildest and more severe ends of the spectrum. The reasons for this pattern could relate to the properties of the tests or could relate to the disease progression itself. It is nearly impossible to distinguish which explanation is correct. The point may be an academic one, because from a clinical perspective, the observation of less decline in milder or more severe patients has been repeatedly observed.

Bedside mental status examinations are usually well suited for longitudinal follow-up, with some exceptions. For AD patients whose disease is not very mild, the MMSE functions quite well for detecting change over the course of the disease. In some circumstances, a test like the MMSE may be inadequate for longitudinal follow-up. Patients with mild FTD, for example, may score near perfect on the MMSE, and fail to show decline on a test that correlates performance with global decline. Patients with progressive aphasia may also not be the best candidates for the use of a test like the MMSE. In these instances, individual selection of cognitive measures, such as tests of verbal fluency or tests of reasoning and mental agility, may be more valuable. Similarly, in patients with the visual variant of AD, additional drawing and construction tasks should be used.

NEUROPSYCHOLOGICAL SYNDROMIC SUBTYPES OF DEMENTIA

There are a few major clinical–neuropsychological patterns in the dementias that correspond to the principal domains of dysfunction. The predominance of one particular domain of impairment may be of use diagnostically.

The *anterograde amnesic syndrome* is the most common, and AD is its prototypical example. Patients with AD almost always have other cognitive deficits, but typically, the symptoms of memory loss and forgetfulness stand out. Many of the non-AD dementias such as vascular dementia may, on occasion, feature anterograde amnesia as the dominant symptom, so that this syndrome is not specific for AD. The hippocampal system is the anatomic region implicated by anterograde amnesia in dementia, but the fact that the pathology of AD includes both hippocampal as well as neocortical regions makes the link with AD and anterograde amnesia more of a clinical–diagnostic link rather than a clinical association with a discrete anatomic region.

The syndrome of disproportionate abnormalities in executive cognitive dysfunction and behavioral dysregulation is termed *frontotemporal dementia* (FTD) (Neary et al., 1988). Frontotemporal dementia is usually not due to AD. However, AD patients may have prominent executive deficits along with equally intense anterograde amnesia. The neuropsychological syndrome of FTD is usually associated with pathology in prefrontal and anterior temporal neocortical regions. However, lesions in subcortical regions such as the thalamus, the neostriatum, or the white matter pathways linking them to the prefrontal and anterior temporal regions may also produce a similar pattern of cognitive and behavioral deficits. The term *frontotemporal dementia* seems firmly ensconced in current usage; we prefer to refer to the cognitive deficits that occur in this syndrome as *executive deficits*.

Disturbances of language function may also occur out of proportion to other cognitive deficits (Mesulam, 1982). They may be of two subtypes. When prominent anomia and comprehension difficulty are the form that the language disorder takes, the syndrome is referred to as *semantic dementia*, whereas when there are prominent expressive difficulties, the syndrome is referred to as *primary progressive aphasia*. As with FTD, these disorders are usually due to non-AD pathology in the dominant frontal lobes (when there are expressive difficulties) and temporal lobes (when anomia and comprehension deficits are dominant).

When *visuospatial impairment* is the principal or presenting symptomatology, the brunt of the pathology, usually of the AD type, is seen in the parietal and occipital lobes. Clinically, the syndrome is sometimes referred to as *posterior cerebral cortical atrophy* or the *visual variant of AD*, the former being preferred because non-AD dementias are also occasionally seen in patients with prominent visuospatial impairment (Victoroff et al., 1994).

Finally, there are several dementias in which prominent motor and psychomotor slowing occurs in the setting of relative preservation of cortical functions such as language, calculation, and praxis. This pattern of *dementia with psychomotor slowing* occurs in a subset of patients with human immunodeficiency virus (HIV) infection (Navia et al., 1986) and in degenerative disorders such as progressive supranuclear palsy or Huntington's disease. The pattern of cognitive dysfunction in a condition such as HIV dementia is distinguished from FTD on the basis of prominence of cognitive slowing compared to impaired judgment. HIV dementia occurs only during the late stages of AIDS, and modern antiretroviral therapies have reduced the incidence of this dementia.

NEUROPSYCHOLOGICAL ASPECTS OF ALZHEIMER'S DISEASE

Cognitive function in AD, as measured by a test such as the MMSE, is remarkably well correlated with pathological markers of the disease. In a study that involved a brain biopsy 1 day after the MMSE had been administered, the number of synapses counted in electron microscopic sections had a correlation coefficient of 0.77 with the MMSE (DeKosky and Scheff, 1990). An autopsy-based study that used mental status examinations performed 2 weeks to 3 years prior to death showed a similarly very high correlation between synaptic density and mental status examinations (Terry et al., 1991). From diagnostic and management perspectives, evaluation of specific cognitive domains adds considerable information beyond what can be obtained from a global assessment.

Prospective neuropsychological studies (Masur et al., 1994; Jacobs et al., 1995; Linn et al., 1995; Petersen et al., 1995; Tierney et al., 1996b; Herlitz et al., 1997; Fabrigoule et al., 1998) have shown that individuals destined to develop AD experience subclinical declines in cognition within a few years of the point that the illness becomes clinically manifest. Impairment in recent memory is the most likely preclinical abnormality to be seen, but poorer performance in multiple domains may also be seen.

COGNITIVE DOMAINS

Patients with AD by definition (Table 19–2) have deficits in multiple cognitive domains. The cognitive deficits are typically evident on mental status examination and are readily deduced from the descriptions of the patient's symptoms provided by a caregiver. Analyses of large series of AD patients suggests that three subtypes of AD can be identified according to the degree of impairment of language function and visuospatial function (Fisher et al., 1999). About equal numbers in a large referral population had greater language impairment or greater visuospatial impairment or equal dysfunction in both domains.

DECLARATIVE MEMORY AND EXPLICIT LEARNING

Both the NINCDS-ADRDA and DSM-IV definitions require memory impairment for a diagnosis of dementia. The deficit in "memory" in AD is best characterized as a deficit in new learning and encoding of information where there is the intention to learn (Storandt et al.,

Table 19–2. Essentials of NINCDS-ADRDA Criteria for Clinical Diagnosis of Alzheimer's Disease

Criteria for Clinical Diagnosis of Probable Alzheimer's Disease

Dementia established by clinical examination and documented (by mental status tests) and confirmed by
   neuropsychological tests
Deficits in two or more areas of cognition
Progressive worsening of memory and other cognitive functions
No disturbances in consciousness
Onset between ages 40 and 90
Absence of systemic disorders or other brain disease that in and of themselves could account for progressive deficits in
   memory and cognition

Features that Make Alzheimer's Disease Uncertain or Unlikely

Sudden, apoplectic onset
Focal neurological findings such as hemiparesis, sensory loss, visual field deficits, and incoordination early in the course
   of the illness
Seizures or gait disturbances at the onset or very early in the course of the illness

Criteria for Clinical Diagnosis of Possible Alzheimer's Disease

May be made on the basis of the dementia syndrome, in the absence of other neurological, psychiatric, or systemic
   disorders sufficient to cause dementia, and in the presence of variations in the onset, presentation, or clinical course
May be made in the presence of a second systemic or brain disorder sufficient to produce dementia, which is not
   considered to be *the* cause of the dementia
When a single, gradually progressive severe cognitive deficit is identified in the absence of other identifiable causes

Source: McKhann et al. (1984).

1984; Knopman and Ryberg, 1989; Welsh et al., 1991; Petersen et al., 1994; Herlitz et al., 1995; Tierney et al., 1996; Grober and Kawas, 1997).

The DSM-IV criteria include both new learning and remote memory under the heading of memory. The anatomic and cognitive basis of remote memory is distinct from that of recent memory function. Remote autobiographical and worldly memories are part of semantic memory, which, while impaired in AD patients, is not as profoundly impaired as new learning (Kopelman et al., 1989; Greene et al., 1995). In many mildly demented AD patients, retrieval of information from the remote past is minimally impaired (Storandt et al., 1998). In the Canadian Study of Health and Aging, the deletion of the requirement for deficits in "remote" memory nearly doubled the number of subjects considered to have a memory problem (Erkinjuntti et al., 1997). Moreover, quantitative evaluation of "previously learned material" (remote memory, or information acquired years before) is difficult in many mildly or even moderately demented individuals.

The memory disorder in AD is best demonstrated on list-learning tasks, such as the Auditory Verbal Learning Task, the California Verbal Learning Test (see below), or the CERAD 10-word list (Welsh et al., 1992; Mohs et al., 1997), that involve learning new material and testing by free recall after a delay of 20 to 60 minutes. During the earliest stages of AD, acquisition of new information may be relatively normal, but delayed recall will nonetheless be impaired (Fox et al., 1998). In slightly more impaired patients with mild AD, there is impaired initial learning of supraspan length material, impairment in free recall after a delay of 30 minutes, impairment in cued recall, and to a lesser extent, impairment in recognition memory. Patients with AD exhibit much more impairment for items at the beginning of the list (reduced primacy effect) than at the end of the list (less impairment of "recency" effect) (Martin et al., 1985). On subsequent trials they show a flatter learning curve than normals in that they learn fewer additional words.

Another paradigm that captures other aspects of the memory impairment in AD (Kopelman, 1985) involves the presentation of three numbers or words followed by free recall after delays of 0, 2, 5, 10, and 15 seconds (a variant of the Brown Peterson paradigm).

The delay interval is filled with a distractor task, usually counting backwards by 2's or 3's. Compared to normals, who ordinarily exhibit a 50% decay in recall after 15 seconds, AD patients are at that level within 5 seconds and have virtually no recall at 15 seconds. Even though the material is subspan in quantity, i.e., three items, the imposition of a distractor task substantially interferes with recall in AD patients.

Learning and free recall are most useful for diagnosis of mild AD, but are less useful for defining the different stages of AD. Learning and recall performance descend to very low levels as patients move into the moderate stages of the disease (Welsh et al., 1992; Mohs et al., 1997). Recognition memory, by contrast, which is often nearly intact in patients with mild AD, declines more slowly over the course of the disease (Welsh et al., 1992).

It is widely accepted that the memory deficit in AD patients can be accounted for by the neuropathological changes involving the hippocampus, subiculum and entorhinal cortex (Hyman et al., 1990). All three regions are heavily involved early in the disease. Magnetic resonance (MR) scanning studies confirm that brain atrophy in the hippocampal regions is often observable at the time of diagnosis (Jack et al., 1997) and is correlated with the degree of memory impairment (Petersen et al., 2000). The relationship between the learning deficits (impaired primacy effect, flat learning curve, impaired delayed recall) and the pathology in the hippocampal system in AD is entirely consistent with our understanding from other disease states of the anatomic basis of learning.

The cholinergic projection neurons in the nucleus basalis, diagonal band, and septum are almost always subjected to neurofibrillary tangle formation (Saper et al., 1985). Dysfunction in cholinergic input to the hippocampus probably also plays a role in the memory disorder of AD (Hyman et al., 1987). There is a moderately strong correlation between performance on mental status examinations and the degree of cholinergic dysfunction (Francis et al., 1985; DeKosky et al., 1992). There are no studies that have evaluated the relationship of memory function specifically to cholinergic markers, however.

IMPLICIT LEARNING

Over the past two decades, unaware learning of certain tasks in the presence of dense anterograde amnesia has been recognized. Several paradigms have been devised to tap into this function, such as various types of semantic priming tasks (Gabrieli et al., 1994; Heindel et al., 1997) and several motor learning tasks (Grafman et al., 1990b; Knopman, 1991; Willingham et al., 1997). Although there is some controversy as to the relationship between dementia severity and the preservation of implicit learning, it appears that some learning without awareness can occur in AD patients.

ORIENTATION

Orientation is impaired in patients with AD, although not invariably in patients with mild disease (Katzman et al., 1983; Klein et al., 1985; Fillenbaum et al., 1987; Huff et al., 1987; Galasko et al., 1990; Koss et al., 1996). Orientation for time and place is mediated by memory, attention, language, visual function, and even executive functions; its impairment is a proxy for dysfunction in one or more of those domains. Orientation is virtually always impaired in dementia patients eventually.

LANGUAGE

Disturbances of language function are recognized as part of the core symptomatology of AD. While empiric studies confirm subtle language impairment even in the mild stages of AD, frank aphasia typically occurs only during the later stages of the illness most of the time. On rare occasions, patients with AD may present initially with symptoms of aphasia out of proportion to other cognitive symptoms. These patients may be incorrectly classified as having primary progressive aphasia (Mesulam, 1982; Faber-Langendoen et al., 1988; Green et al., 1990; Snowden and Neary, 1993). Several research groups have made the observation that patients with early-onset AD may have greater impairment of language than late-onset patients (Breitner and Folstein, 1984; Imamura et al., 1998); this perhaps reflects a biological difference in the spread of AD pathology in the neocortex as a function of age.

By far the most common language abnormality during early stages of dementia is word-finding difficulty, or dysnomia. The dysnomia is sensitive to word frequency (Shuttleworth and Huber, 1988). A deficit in semantic processing is thought to be in part responsible for naming deficit in Alzheimer's disease (Goldstein et al., 1992; Salmon et al., 1999), but studies examining naming errors in AD suggest that lexical access problems and impaired activation of output phonology may be contributory (Nicholas et al., 1996). Category-specific naming deficits are not typically seen with AD. Comprehension of conversational speech is thought to be relatively preserved during early stages of the disease, although formal testing may reveal some deficits even in patients with milder disease (Grossman and White-Devine, 1998; Croot et al., 1999).

Disorders of writing tend to occur relatively early in patients with AD, consistent with relatively early involvement of the parietal lobes (Croisile, 1999). The degree of writing impairment correlates with dementia severity in AD (Horner et al., 1988). Poor performance of writing by AD patients probably arises from multiple sources, including impairment in lexicosemantic systems (Rapcsak et al., 1989b; Lambert et al., 1996) as well as perseveration, executive dysfunction, and apraxia (Glosser et al., 1999).

Reduction in the number of words produced in tasks of verbal fluency is highly discriminating for mild AD (Monsch et al., 1992; Welsh et al., 1992). Verbal fluency continues to deteriorate with increasing severity of AD. This verbal task is typically thought of as a measure of executive function. Repetition deficits do not occur in mild AD; the function tends to be preserved until later stages of the disease.

In contrast, some language tasks are relatively resistant to dysfunction in mild or even moderate AD. Longitudinal studies suggest that language functions such as reading are relatively preserved (Paque and Warrington, 1995). Tests of reading of uncommon, irregularly spelled words, such as the New Adult Reading Test, can be used to determine premorbid intellectual levels in AD (Willshire et al., 1991; Maddrey et al., 1996).

VISUOSPATIAL FUNCTION

Disturbances of visuospatial function commonly occur in AD. In rare cases, the dominant presentation of the dementia is a gradually developing Balint's syndrome (Crystal et al., 1982; Hof et al., 1990; Mendez et al., 1990; Graff-Radford et al., 1993; Levine et al., 1993; Victoroff et al., 1994; Binetti et al., 1998; Giannakopoulos et al., 1999).

Unfortunately, visuospatial function is one area where the standard definitions of AD lack clarity. The DSM-IV criteria include *agnosia*, which is a severe disturbance of visual recognition rarely present in early stages of AD or other types of dementia. There is no specific reference to milder dysfunction of higher visual and spatial functions. The NINCDS-ADRDA criteria (McKhann et al., 1984) refers to visual perception and to "praxis" but describes the latter as visual constructional ability.

There is little evidence of impairment at the level of elemental visual perception during the early stages. Patients with early AD tend not to have difficulties with identifying the common objects in line drawings such as on the Boston Naming Test. However, the perception of spatial relationships on a measure such as the Judgement of Line Orientation can be impaired relatively early (Finton et al., 1998).

In mild AD, tests of visual constructions that involve copying of simple figures may not be substantially impaired (Welsh et al., 1992). Patients with AD as well as patients with vascular dementia or dementia with Lewy Bodies of mild or greater severity tend to be impaired on more complex tests of visuoconstruction, such as clock drawing (Esteban-Santillan et al., 1998; Cahn-Weiner et al., 1999), the Rey Complex Figure, or Block Design from the WAIS-III. With progression of the disease, more severe forms of visuospatial synthesis, such as difficulties recognizing familiar faces or familiar environments, begin to emerge. It is therefore not surprising that patients with AD have difficulty with tasks that combine perception of spatial relationships with numbers, such as clock drawing and perception of time from analog clocks. Patients with AD are impaired on tasks that involve figure–ground discriminations or discrimination of complex visual scenes (Mendez et al., 1990). As would be expected, visuospatial deficits in AD are generally related to right hemisphere dysfunction (Haxby et al., 1990; Cahn-Weiner et al., 1999).

EXECUTIVE FUNCTIONS

Early in the dementia of AD, executive deficits are readily apparent, and distinguish patients with mild AD from normals (Kopelman, 1991; Welsh et al., 1992; Lafleche and Albert, 1995; Mohs et al., 1997; Collette et al., 1999). Judgment and abstract reasoning are invariably affected even in mildly demented patients and by the moderate stages of AD, may be untestable. Verbal fluency, trailmaking, maze-solving, or card-sorting tasks all demonstrate these findings. In a subset of AD patients, executive deficits are very prominent (Johnson et al., 1999). Patients with AD are generally impaired on measures of competency. Their ability to understand the consequences of medical decisions tends to correlate with several cognitive measures, including executive function tasks (Marson et al., 1996, 1999). The NINCDS-ADRDA definition of AD refers to "problem-solving" in citing executive function.

More specifically, working memory, mental agility, and set-shifting are prominently impaired (Perry and Hodges, 1999). On tests measuring sustained or divided attention (Greene et al., 1995; Johannsen et al., 1999; Perry and Hodges, 1999) or habituation and inhibition (Langley et al., 1998), AD patients show substantial impairment. For example, experiments that require patients to divide attention between two tasks show that this manipulation results in more dysfunction for AD patients than does sustaining attention on one task (Johannsen et al., 1999). Because attention is an important component of the performance of many neuropsychological tests, impaired attention may result in poor results in other cognitive domains. Disproportionately poor performance on simple tests of attention, such as digit span, may indicate that the patient is suffering from delirium rather than dementia.

Simpler tasks that can be used at the bedside, such as reciting the months of the year backwards, solving arithmetic problems (for someone with known prior basic arithmetic skills), clock drawing, or testing verbal similarities and differences, also bring out executive deficits in AD patients. Ability to inhibit inappropriate actions and to carry out two cognitive tasks simultaneously (holding the result of one calculation in one's mind while carrying out a second calculation, and then adding the result together) may be two of the most important underlying executive functions to be impaired in AD (Collette et al., 1999).

Deficits in executive function can influence performance in multiple cognitive domains. For example, poor organizational strategies on tests of verbal learning and lack of a consistent strategy on tests of visuoconstructionalies abilities have been reported with frontal lobe dysfunction. Retrieval of remote memories may also be compromised with frontal lobe involvement (Kopelman, 1991). Executive functions depend on integration of prefrontal and subcortical activity (Cummings, 1993).

In contrast to AD, the frontotemporal dementias have executive dysfunction as their principle deficits (see below). In addition, dementias without hippocampal involvement but with predominant striatal, thalamic, or white matter (subcortical) involvement, such as progressive supranuclear palsy, HIV-dementia, and vascular dementia, tend to be characterized by disproportionate executive dysfunction (see below).

APRAXIA

Clinically significant ideomotor apraxia is often inapparent or modest in mild AD (Della Sala et al., 1987; Rapcsak et al., 1989a; Travniczek-Marterer et al., 1993; Mohs et al., 1997). Limb-transitive actions (e.g., "Show me how you would use a comb") elicit the greatest impairment in AD patients (Rapcsak et al., 1989a). Patients with AD present with symptoms of apraxia as the earliest symptoms extremely rarely (Green et al., 1995). The role of apraxia as a symptom of dementia has been confounded by imprecision in the use of the term. In the DSM-IV definition of dementia, ideomotor apraxia is specified. The NINCDS-ADRDA criteria broadened the meaning of the word *apraxia* to include visuoconstructional deficits, but we would prefer to maintain the traditional use of the word *apraxia*. There is some evidence that measuring response latency for executing gestures may provide a more sensitive measure of early (subclinical) apraxia in AD (Willis et al., 1998). It has also been suggested that imitation of meaningless gestures may be a more sensitive measure of early apraxia in AD than the traditional approach using purposeful actions (Dobigny-Roman et al., 1998). Ideomotor apraxia observed in some patients with AD is unrelated to impaired motor learning skills on tasks such as the Rotor Pursuit Task (tracking a moving target on a spinning disk) (Jacobs et al., 1999).

Even though ideational apraxia was first described in patients with dementia and confusional states, only a few contemporary studies have compared ideational and ideomotor praxis. Ochipa et al. (1992) found that ideational praxis, as defined by tool–action relationships and tool–object associations, could be disturbed in some AD patients who had relatively preserved ideomotor praxis and relatively preserved language function. Rapczak et al. (1989a), who used tasks composed of serial actions as a measure of ideational apraxia, found that scores for performance on ideomotor and ideational praxis tasks were highly correlated in AD.

Apraxia is not a more prominent symptom in patients with early-onset familial Alzheimer's disease than in late-onset sporadic AD (Swearer et al., 1992).

MOTOR AND PSYCHOMOTOR

While performance on tests of simple motor function, such as finger tapping, pegboard, or reaction time, may be mildly slowed in patients with AD compared with that in neurologically intact individuals (Goldman et al., 1999), these deficits are nonetheless very mild when compared with the changes in memory and other cognitive functions. By contrast, patients with dementias of predominantly subcortical involvement, such as Parkinson's disease, HIV dementia, and cerebrovascular dementia, tend to have early and more prominent impairment in areas of motor and psychomotor speed. Therefore, tests of motor speed are very important for distinguishing cortical dementias from subcortical dementias.

ANOSOGNOSIA

Anosognosia, or unawareness of disability, is nearly universal among individuals with AD (Lopez et al., 1994; Seltzer et al., 1997). The anosognosia for the memory problems and other disabilities is not complete, in that occasional patients will readily admit to their problems (Grut et al., 1993), although these individuals are almost never able to act on their concerns. Most patients tend to dismiss or minimize memory failures, errors in judgment, or other lapses when queried about them by family or physicians. The patient's lack of motivation to seek medical attention is one of the major impediments to the diagnosis, since the burden falls on others to recognize the problem, decide to act on it, and then convince the patient to accede.

BEHAVIORAL AND AFFECTIVE CHANGES

Disturbances of behavior or changes in comportment are among the core symptoms of AD (Oppenheim, 1994), but behavioral abnormalities also occur in FTD (Neary et al., 1988, 1998; Gustafson, 1993), Lewy body dementia (Hansen et al., 1990; McKeith et al., 1996; Salmon et al., 1996), and vascular dementia. The spectrum of changes is protean in AD, ranging from increased apathy and social withdrawal to disinhibition or irritability (Reisberg et al., 1987; Teri et al., 1988; Mega et al., 1996a; Reichman et al., 1996; Devanand et al., 1997; Gilley et al., 1997; Patterson et al., 1997). Mega et al. (1996a) found that apathy was the most common neuropsychiatric symptom in their series of AD patients, followed by agitation, anxiety, irritability, and depression.

NEUROPSYCHOLOGICAL ASPECTS OF OTHER DEMENTIAS

VASCULAR DEMENTIA

The cognitive deficits in vascular dementia are varied, reflecting the diversity of pathology that is currently included under the heading of vascular dementia. Usually, but not always, patients with vascular dementia have other typical symptoms and signs of cerebrovascular disease, such as hemiparesis or hemianopia. Patients with cerebrovascular disease may develop the syndrome of dementia in the presence of cerebral infarctions with single strategically placed lesions in such regions as the hippocampus, thalamus, or parietal lobes. Vascular dementia can also be seen in patients with multiple large vessel cortical infarctions or smaller vessel, deep, lacunar-type infarctions. Patients with cerebrovascular disease often have cognitive deficits that are too mild to be characterized as dementia; their presence in the spectrum of cerebrovascular disease and cognitive dysfunction is important to recognize (Hachinski, 1994).

Longitudinal studies have shown that stroke is a risk factor for cognitive decline and dementia (Tatemichi et al., 1990, 1992, 1994; Kokmen et al., 1996; Kuller et al., 1998; Longstreth et al., 1998). Furthermore, cerebrovascular pathology in a patient with slowly evolving dementia plays an important supporting role behind AD pathology (Snowdon et al., 1997; Heyman et al., 1998).

Most commonly, however, dementia in the setting of vascular disease is associated with a mixture of AD neuropathological changes and infarctions (Wade et al., 1987; Galasko et al., 1994; Victoroff et al., 1995; Holmes et al., 1999; Lim et al., 1999). Pure vascular pathology sufficient to account for dementia is only approximately half as common as vascular pathology mixed with AD (Holmes et al., 1999; Lim et al., 1999). Thus, while it is appropriate to consider the diagnosis of pure vascular dementia, referred to as "probable vascular dementia" by recent criteria (Chui et al., 1992; Roman et al., 1993), the numerically more common circumstance is AD combined with vascular disease. Patients with both AD and vascular pathology are referred to under various labels, such as "AD with cerebrovascular disease," "possible AD," or "possible vascular dementia."

Given the variability inherent in the diagnostic criteria for vascular dementia, it is not surprising that a diagnostic neuropsychological pattern for vascular dementia has yet to be identified (Looi and Sachdev, 1999). Dementia due to a series of large cortical infarctions will have substantially different clinical manifestations than dementia due to lacunar infarctions in the striatum and thalamus. Multiple lacunar infarctions may produce a pattern of cognitive impairment that is similar to FTD, as a result of deafferentation and deefferentation of prefrontal regions by the subcortical infarctions (Wolfe et al., 1990).

Recent reviews of the neuropsychological characteristics of vascular dementia have emphasized motor and psychomotor slowing, executive deficits, visuoconstructional abnormalities, and less prominent involvement of functions such as language and calculations (Desmond, 1996). In group comparisons, the most robust neuropsychological distinguishing feature of vascular dementia has been the greater deficits in the executive domain than those in AD patients (Looi and Sachdev, 1999). Although patients with vascular dementia do not differ from patients with AD in their performance on tests of new verbal learning, recognition memory is frequently better preserved than free recall (Cummings, 1994), which is consistent with the more prominent executive dysfunction seen in vascular dementia. The overal gestalt of the cognitive profile of vascular dementia is closer to a subcortical–frontal profile than an cortical–amnesic profile of impairment.

Neuropsychologists who encounter patients with dementia and vascular disease should be aware that clinical diagnostic criteria for vascular dementia have low predictive accuracy (Wade et al., 1987; Galasko et al., 1994; Victoroff et al., 1995; Holmes et al., 1999; Lim et al., 1999). Hence, vascular dementia patients in clinical studies will have substantial variability in their underlying pathology. Comparisons between vascular dementia and other dementias are also limited by the fact that not all studies evaluated all relevant cognitive domains. For example, only 1 of the 27 studies analyzed by Looi and Sachdev (1999) included a measure of motor speed. More meaningful studies of the neuropsychological characteristics of vascular dementia must await more refined and validated clinical diagnostic criteria as well as better definition of vascular dementia subtypes.

CLINICAL SYNDROME OF DEMENTIA WITH LEWY BODIES

In the past decade, the distinctive dementia that occurs in parkinsonian patients has become better appreciated. Clinicopathological studies documented the existence of a subset of individuals with AD pathology who also had profuse cortical Lewy bodies. Retrospective analysis of the clinical protocols of such patients revealed a number of distinctive features. Diagnostic criteria for dementia with Lewy bodies (DLB) (McKeith et al., 1996) were subsequently proposed to identify such individuals antemortem. These criteria include gait and balance disturbances, dementia, prominent visual hallucinations and delusions, fluctuations in cognitive status or arousal, sensitivity to dopaminergic blocking drugs such as first-generation antipsychotics, and other less consistently seen symptoms and signs. Unfortunately, the sensitivity of the McKeith et al. criteria for DLB is poor, even though the specificity is good (Mega et al., 1996b; Litvan et al., 1998b; Holmes et al., 1999; Luis et al., 1999). Dementia with Lewy bodies should be considered whenever a patient with dementia exhibits fluctuating confusion, falls, or unexplained syncope.

The cognitive disorder of DLB is similar to that of AD with a few exceptions (Hansen et al., 1990; Salmon et al., 1996; Ferman et al., 1999). Thus, it is difficult to distinguish DLB and AD with certainty on neurocognitive grounds, particularly in more severely demented patients. Patients with DLB have slightly better memory performance (Heyman et al., 1999) but somewhat worse executive functions than do AD patients. For example, DLB patients are likely to do worse on word fluency tasks than AD patients at the same global severity level. Patients with DLB have

some of the cognitive deficits seen in frontotemporal dementias, including lack of initiative and apathy. Both AD and DLB have impairment of visuospatial processing and constructions, but these symptoms may appear earlier in DLB patients and may be somewhat worse. The visual hallucinations in DLB patients are dramatic, elaborate, and often quite outrageous. Delusional thinking often occurs. Psychomotor and motor slowing tends to be more prominent in DLB than in AD (Salmon et al., 1996).

The combination of parkinsonism and dementia confers a worse prognosis than that associated with typical AD. Several studies, using different methods of case identification, have shown that patients with extrapyramidal features and dementia progress more rapidly than patients with dementia due to AD alone (Chui et al., 1994; Olichney et al., 1998).

Dementia with Lewy bodies represents a mixture of AD and Lewy body pathology at autopsy (Hansen et al., 1993; Hulette et al., 1995; Hansen and Samuel, 1997; Heyman et al., 1999). Given this overlap and heterogeneity, it should be expected that the clinical manifestations of DLB patients overlap with those of patients with AD. In general, patients with Lewy body pathology have less intense neurofibrillary tangle pathology than patients with pure AD. At the far end of the spectrum, there is a subset of patients with DLB who have no AD pathology (Hely et al., 1996; Hansen and Samuel, 1997), but these patients cannot be differentiated clinically from DLB patients with concomitant AD. The link between neurochemical (Sabbagh et al., 1999) and neuropathological markers (Samuel et al., 1997) on the one hand, and cognition on the other, in DLB is weaker than in AD.

CLINICAL SYNDROME OF FRONTOTEMPORAL DEMENTIA

Frontotemporal dementia (FTD) as a syndrome differs from the syndrome of anterograde amnesia in the disproportionate impairment of judgment and reasoning compared to recent memory. The term *dysexecutive syndrome* has been applied to the cognitive syndrome of patients with FTD who have grossly disturbed abstract reasoning, poor judgment and reduced mental flexibility (Neary et al., 1988; Gustafson, 1993, Lund and Manchester Groups, 1994). In many instances, FTD patients can recall minute details of recent events and conversations, even though they cannot use the memories in socially appropriate or functionally productive ways. Yet, caregivers complain that the patient's day-to-day memory functioning is impaired. Inattention, inability to focus on one task, and easy distractibility may account for the impairment of memory in daily activities ("strategic failure" rather than "amnesic failure" in Neary and Snowden's terms) (Neary and Snowden, 1991).

Patients with FTD have a disturbance of personality, behavioral control, comportment, and social awareness that is as intense or exceeds the magnitude of the cognitive deficits. Patients may become socially inappropriate, excessively ebullient, or inappropriately aggressive or may get themselves into trouble because of grossly impaired judgment. Loss of insight and disinhibition contribute to the burden that these patients pose to caregivers. These deficits also highlight the functions of the prefrontal and anterior temporal lobes by showing the consequences of pathology in these regions. The behavioral disturbances are often initially attributed to primary psychiatric diseases such as mania or psychosis. Alternatively, in patients who demonstrate primarily apathy and inertia, their social withdrawal may lead to a diagnosis of depression, but no improvement on antidepressants.

Motor deficits in patients with the syndrome of FTD are variable. In some patients, FTD is associated with corticobasal degeneration, and unilateral limb apraxia may result. In other patients who may later prove to have progressive supranuclear palsy or DLB pathologically, rigidity and bradykinesia may be prominent. Some patients with FTD will have buccofacial apraxia relatively early in their illness (Tyrrell et al., 1991).

Although AD pathology may on rare occasion produce a pattern of grossly impaired judgment, disturbed behavior, and relatively preserved recent memory, the FTD syndrome will prove to be due to non-AD pathology in most instances. The prototypical pathological disease that produces a FTD is Pick's disease. However, recent investigations have shown that Pick's disease (defined by the presence of Pick bodies in cortical and hippocampal neurons) is only one member of a larger group of disorders (Neary, 1990, 1997; Brun, 1993; Kertesz and Munoz, 1998). Some show distinctive pathology such as Pick cells (also known as swollen chromatolytic neurons) and many show no distinctive histological features. In all of these disorders, the brunt of the gross pathology in the FTDs is in the neocortex of the frontal and anterior temporal lobes. Variations in the severity of pathology can be seen between right and left hemispheres and between frontal and anterior temporal loci. Moreover, in rare instances, the pathology is purely in subcortical gray matter structures; this pattern has been called "progressive subcortical gliosis" (Neumann and Cohn, 1967). Many of these entities have been linked to pathological alterations in the tau protein, a major microtubule-associated protein (Feany and Dickson, 1996; Spillantini and Goedert, 1998). The major distinction between FTD and progressive aphasia may simply be in the preponderance of right vs. left hemisphere involvement. The distinction between frontal and temporal pathology, however, does not have identifiable clinical differences.

Diagnostic criteria for FTD were published from a consensus conference (Neary et al., 1998). The diagnostic criteria reflect the cognitive and behavioral characteristics of FTD observed in pathologically verified cases. The current criteria (Neary et al., 1998) and those of an earlier version (Lund and Manchester Groups, 1994) have been subjected to clinical pathological analysis. Unfortunately, although there are clear differences in the typical clinical presentations of patients with neuropathological AD and patients with neuropathological Pick's disease and its close relatives, there is considerable overlap (Miller et al., 1997; Varma et al., 1999).

Psychometric testing plays an essential role in the diagnosis of FTD because the bedside mental status examination lacks sensitivity for early signs of executive dysfunction. Patients with FTD may be fully oriented and score in the nominally normal range on a test such as the MMSE. At the time of presentation, the typical patient with FTD will show either no impairment or mild impairment on tests of recent memory. For example, an FTD patient may recall between 6 and 9 words on a 15-word list-learning task after a 30-minute delay. The patient may similarly perform at or just below the normal range on tests such as the Block Design subtest of the WAIS-R, and may have no difficulty with copying figures such as the intersecting pentagons of the MMSE. In contrast, the same patient may be able to produce fewer than 5 words per letter in a letter fluency task over 60 seconds. The FTD patient may score poorly on the digit symbol substitution task, be unable to perform Part B of the Trailmaking Task, be able to solve only the simplest of mazes, and be unable to complete even one category on the Wisconsin Card Sorting Task.

Neuroimaging may show evidence of frontal or anterior temporal atrophy, though not in all cases, especially early in the disease (Knopman et al., 1990). Functional imaging with SPECT or PET may be more sensitive for the early diagnosis of FTD (Kamo et al., 1987; Miller et al., 1991; Friedland et al., 1993; Read et al., 1995; Talbot et al., 1998), but there are still limited data on the actual clinical utility of functional imaging in the differential diagnosis of dementia and FTD.

DEMENTIAS WITH PROMINENT LANGUAGE DISTURBANCES

The distinctive features of primary progressive aphasia, the more common of the dementias with language disturbance, are the relative excess of dysfunction of expressive language-related functions and the relative paucity of anterograde amnesia in contrast to AD (Snowden and Neary, 1993; Kertesz et al., 1994; Snowdon et al., 1996). Conversational speech is nonfluent and hesitant, with frequent pauses for word finding. A rarer form of language disturbance, semantic dementia, is characterized by normally articulated, fluent speech, but marked deficits in production and comprehension of single words. It may be due to AD (Green et al., 1990), but some cases of semantic dementia with nonspecific histology have

been reported (Hodges et al., 1992; Schwarz et al., 1998)

Cognitive functions other than language may be relatively spared during the early stages of primary progressive aphasia. The evaluation of memory and other non-language cognitive domains in patients with progressive aphasia requires prudent choice of tests to minimize the potential confounding effects of verbal skills. The mental status examination and the history of deficits are pivotal in the diagnosis of primary progressive aphasia. Age of onset is typically relatively young, with fewer cases with onset after age 70 (Westbury and Bub, 1997). Personality and insight are frequently preserved until later stages of the illness. Progressive aphasia patients may remain independent in their activities of daily living. There is variability in the extent to which progressive aphasia progresses to global dementia. Progression to global dementia as an outcome of primary progressive aphasia is not a certainty, but it is likely.

Neuropsychologically, patients with progressive aphasia may present with any type of aphasia. In addition to the most common presentation of anomic aphasia, cases of progressive dysarthria (Selnes et al., 1996) and progressive conduction aphasia (Hachisuka et al., 1999) have also been described. The relative preservation of auditory comprehension in patients with progressive aphasia helps to differentiate them from patients with semantic dementia. Reading tends to be relatively preserved in progressive aphasia, while disturbances of writing often mirror the degree of impairment in verbal production. Repetition tends to be spared until later stages of the illness. There are few quantitative data available on large series of progressive aphasia to evaluate neuropsychological performance in cognitive domains such as memory and visuospatial and executive-type functions (Westbury and Bub, 1997). Nonetheless, results of meta-analysis of cases dating back to 1982 provide some guidance as to which specific neuropsychological tests can help differentiate progressive aphasia from dementia with speech and language disorders (Zakzanis, 1999). In addition to relatively preserved visuospatial functions, patients with primary progressive aphasia also tend to have relatively preserved nonverbal memory performance. The differentiation of primary progressive aphasia from AD can best be made by longitudinal assessment.

Patients with semantic dementia differ from those with primary progressive aphasia in that their speech is fluent and their comprehension is often quite poor (Hodges et al., 1992; Schwarz et al., 1998). Patients with semantic dementia are similar to progressive aphasia patients in their poor expressive naming abilities and their tendency to show the behavioral features of FTD. They may also exhibit evolution to a more pervasive dementing disorder.

As with FTDs, patients with progressive aphasia may show focal atrophy on structural imaging, especially of the dominant hemisphere's inferior frontal and insular regions. In semantic dementia, the atrophy tends to be more focussed on the temporal lobe. Similarly, functional imaging may detect hypometabolism in either region. Neither structural nor functional imaging confirmation of focal atrophy is necessary for the diagnosis, however, as both progressive aphasia and semantic dementia are clinical diagnoses.

PROGRESSIVE SUPRANUCLEAR PALSY AND CORTICOBASAL DEGENERATION

Progressive supranuclear palsy (PSP) was first labeled as a subcortical dementia (Albert et al., 1974) because PSP patients had somewhat better recent memory than AD patients but very poor executive function, apathy, and loss of initiative (Albert et al., 1974; Gearing et al., 1994; Grafman et al., 1995; Litvan et al., 1996, 1998a). Patients with PSP also have substantial motoric deficits, including the diagnostic vertical eye movement disorder, extrapyramidal signs, and brainstem nuclear motor dysfunction. While they often show profound deficits on such tasks as verbal fluency, trailmaking, or digit symbol substitution, PSP patients perform in only a mildly impaired range on tests of recall and language (Milberg and Albert, 1989; Grafman et al., 1990a; Pillon et al., 1994).

A related disorder, corticobasal degeneration, exhibits a similar pattern of prominent executive deficits (Pillon et al., 1995; Bergeron et

al., 1998). Unilateral ideomotor apraxia, limb dystonia, myoclonus, and cortical sensory deficits are important features of corticobasal degeneration (Rinne et al., 1994; Litvan et al., 1997). One comparative study noted that patients with corticobasal degeneration are more likely than PSP patients to experience depression than apathy (Litvan et al., 1998a).

Corticobasal degeneration patients may exhibit progressive aphasia (Clark et al., 1986) or exhibit a typical FTD syndrome (Kertesz, 1997). Recent clinicopathological studies have suggested that the overlap between the movement disorder disease of corticobasal degeneration and the dementing disorder with swollen chromatolytic neurons is considerable (Boeve et al., 1999; Grimes et al., 1999).

HUNTINGTON'S DISEASE

Huntington's disease (HD) is the most common autosomal dominant neurological disease of adults. It is a disorder whose gene mutation involves an excessive number of trinucleotide repeats. The gene for Huntington's disease, *IT15*, is located on chromosome 4 and codes for a protein known as huntingtin (Reddy et al., 1999).

The disorder may occur prior to age 20, but most cases occur between the ages of 20 and 40 years. The movement disorder and the cognitive disorder usually have onset more or less simultaneously, but they may be dissociated. Huntington's disease is also complicated by multiple psychiatric symptoms including mood disorders, psychotic behavior, anxiety, irritabilty, and aggression. Some observers have commented on the association between affective disturbances in HD patients and the disordered family environments that so often occur in the disease (Mindham et al., 1985; Folstein, 1991). The neuropathology of HD appears to be limited to the caudate and putamen, with the cerebral cortex only mildly affected (Vonsattel and DiFiglia, 1998).

The cognitive disorder of HD is another of the disorders to which the term *subcortical dementia* was applied to draw attention to the cognitive and behavioral distinctions between HD and AD. Indeed, HD patients have predominantly subcortical pathology (Vonsattel and DiFiglia, 1998), but growing understanding of the relationship between the caudate nucleus and the frontal lobes (Cummings, 1993) provides an alternative and unifying account of the dysexecutive deficits in HD. Patients with HD tend to exhibit cognitive slowing that is proportionately worse than their recent memory disturbance (Brandt et al., 1988; Bamford et al., 1989, 1995; Jason et al., 1997). They also show substantial dysexecutive deficits (Lange et al., 1995). Such deficits may also be seen in asymptomatic individuals who are carriers of the abnormal HD gene (Lawrence et al., 1998). The behavioral correlates of the dysexecutive syndrome in HD are well known; some HD patients exhibit poor judgment, socially inappropriate behavior, and impulsiveness, while other are apathetic and abulic (Caine et al., 1978). Language functions deteriorate only very late in the course of HD, and may be unaffected in early HD.

HIV-RELATED DEMENTIA

HIV-related dementia, also known as AIDS dementia complex, is a complication of HIV infection that occurs in the setting of severe immunosuppresion during advanced HIV disease. The incidence of HIV-related dementia has been estimated at approximately 7% per year after the first AIDS-defining illness (McArthur et al., 1993). A milder form of HIV-related dementia has been designated "HIV-1 associated minor cognitive/motor deficit." Definitional criteria for both of these conditions have been provided by the American Academy of Neurology AIDS Task Force (1991). The exact prevalence and clinical significance of the milder forms of HIV-related cognitive impairment have been controversial. Early studies with small sample sizes found evidence of a high frequency of cognitive impairment during the early, asymptomatic stages of HIV infection (Grant et al., 1987). However, larger cohort studies did not report significant differences in neuropsychological test performance between asymptomatic HIV-infected patients and seronegative controls (Selnes et al., 1990).

Although there is some variability in the neuropsychological test profile associated with early HIV-related dementia, certain key neuropsychological features can help determine whether the cognitive changes are likely to be HIV related or not. The principal feature is psychomotor and motor slowing. On measures such as the Grooved Pegboard, the slowing is typically most pronounced in the nondominant hand. The second feature is a mild–moderate memory disturbance. Although free recall may be moderately impaired, recognition memory tends to be relatively preserved during the early stages. Mild to moderate constructional impairment on tasks such as copying a three-dimensional cube, a clock, or the Rey Complex Figure, is a third feature. A relative absence of significant dysnomia, dyscalculia, or other parietal lobe findings is also characteristic of the subcortical dementia of HIV. The HIV Dementia Scale is a screening test designed to be particularly sensitive to this subcortical profile (Power et al., 1995; Berghuis et al., 1999).

Cognitive dysfunction and brain atrophy, particularly of the caudate nucleus, are related (Hall et al., 1996; Kieburtz et al., 1996; Stout et al., 1998). Neuropathologically, findings are somewhat bland given the severity of the clinical deficits. Multinucleated giant cells are seen in multiple brain regions, as are microglial nodules containing macrophages, lymphocytes, and microglia. Perivascular inflammation, cortical spongiform changes, and synaptic loss occur (Price et al., 1988). The details of the pathophysiology of HIV dementia are still being worked out. The virus gains entry to the central nervous system soon after infection, but the dementia develops only after years of progressive immunosuppression. There is increasing evidence that the brain injury is due to the indirect effects of immune activation rather than primary infection of neurons by the HIV virus (Zink et al., 1999).

Most of the information about the pattern of neuropsychological abnormalities associated with HIV dementia have been collected in relatively young individuals. When evaluating older HIV-infected patients, it is important to consider other causes of a predominantly dysexecutive or subcortical pattern of cognitive impairment, such as vascular dementia or FTD.

REFERENCES

Albert, M. L., Feldman, R. G., and Willis, A. L. (1974). The 'subcortical dementia' of progressive supranuclear palsy. *J. Neurol. Neurosurg. Psychiatry* 37:121–130.

Albert, M. S., Wolfe, J., and Lafleche, G. (1990). Differences in abstraction ability with age. *Psychol. Aging* 5:94–100.

Alexopoulos, G. S. and Chester, J. G. (1992). Outcomes of geriatric depression. *Clin. Geriatr. Med.* 8:363–376.

American Academy of Neurology (1991). Nomenclature and research case definitions for neurologic manifestations of human immunodeficiency virus-type 1 (HIV-1) infection. Report of a Working Group of the American Academy of Neurology AIDS Task Force. *Neurology* 41:778–785.

American Academy of Neurology (1996). Assessment: neuropsychological testing of adults. Considerations for neurologists. Report of the Therapeutics and Technology Assessment Subcommittee of the American Academy of Neurology. *Neurology* 47:592–599.

American Psychiatric Association (1994). *Diagnostic and Statistical Manual of Mental Disorders,* (Fourth Edition). Washington DC, American Psychiatric Association.

Andersen, K., Launer, L. J., Ott, A., Hoes, A. W., Breteler, M. M., and Hofman, A. (1995). Do nonsteroidal anti-inflammatory drugs decrease the risk for Alzheimer's disease? The Rotterdam Study. *Neurology* 45:1441–1445.

Anderson, S. W., Damasio, H., Jones, R. D., and Tranel, D. (1991). Wisconsin Card Sorting Test performance as a measure of frontal lobe damage. *J. Clin. Exp. Neuropsychol.* 13:909–922.

Anthony, J. C., LeResche, L., Niaz, U., von Korff, M. R., and Folstein, M. F. (1982). Limits of the 'Mini-Mental State' as a screening test for dementia and delirium among hospital patients. *Psychol. Med.* 12:397–408.

Bachman, D. L., Wolf, P. A., Linn, R., Knoefel, J. E., Cobb, J., Belanger, A., et al. (1992). Prevalence of dementia and probable senile dementia of the Alzheimer type in the Framingham Study. *Neurology* 42:115–119.

Bachman, D. L., Wolf, P. A., Linn, R. T., Knoefel, J. E., Cobb, J. L., Belanger, A. J. et al., (1993). Incidence of dementia and probable Alzheimer's disease in a general population: the Framingham Study. *Neurology* 43:515–519.

Ball, L. J., Bisher, G. B., and Birge, S. J. (1999). A simple test of central processing speed: an ex-

tension of the Short Blessed Test. *J. Am. Geriatr. Soc.* 47:1359–1363.

Bamford, K. A., Caine, E. D., Kido, D. K., Cox, C., and Shoulson, I. (1995). A prospective evaluation of cognitive decline in early Huntington's disease: functional and radiographic correlates. *Neurology* 45:1867–1873.

Bamford, K. A., Caine, E. D., Kido, D. K., Plassche, W. M., and Shoulson, I. (1989). Clinical–pathologic correlation in Huntington's disease: a neuropsychological and computed tomography study. *Neurology* 39:796–801.

Beard, C. M., Kokmen, E., Offord, K. P., and Kurland, L. T. (1992). Lack of association between Alzheimer's disease and education, occupation, marital status, or living arrangement. *Neurology* 42:2063–2068.

Beats, B. C., Sahakian, B. J., and Levy, R. (1996). Cognitive performance in tests sensitive to frontal lobe dysfunction in the elderly depressed. *Psychol. Med.* 26:591–603.

Berchtold, N. C., and Cotman, C. W. (1998). Evolution in the conceptualization of dementia and Alzheimer's disease: Greco-Roman period to the 1960s. *Neurobiol. Aging* 19:173–189.

Berger, A. K., Fratiglioni, L., Forsell, Y., Winblad, B., and Backman, L. (1999). The occurrence of depressive symptoms in the preclinical phase of AD: a population-based study. *Neurology* 53: 1998–2002.

Bergeron, C., Davis, A., and Lang, A. E. (1998). Corticobasal ganglionic degeneration and progressive supranuclear palsy presenting with cognitive decline. *Brain Pathol.* 8:355–365.

Berghuis, J. P., Uldall, K. K., and Lalonde, B. (1999). Validity of two scales in identifying HIV-associated dementia. *J. Acquir. Immune Defic. Syndr.* 21:134–140.

Bieliauskas, L. A. (1993). Depressed or not depressed? That is the question. *J. Clin. Exp. Neuropsychol.* 15:119–134.

Binetti, G., Cappa, S. F., Magni, E., Padovani, A., Bianchetti, A., and Trabucchi, M. (1998). Visual and spatial perception in the early phase of Alzheimer's disease. *Neuropsychology* 12:29–33.

Blessed, G., Tomlinson, B. E., and Roth, M. (1968). The association between quantitative measures of dementia and of senile change in the cerebral grey matter of elderly subjects. *Br. J. Psychiatry* 114:797–811.

Boeve, B. F., Maraganore, D. M., Parisi, J. E., Ahlskog, J. E., Graff-Radford, N., Caselli, R. J., et al. (1999). Pathologic heterogeneity in clinically diagnosed corticobasal degeneration. *Neurology* 53:795–800.

Boller, F., Lopez, O. L., and Moossy, J. (1989). Diagnosis of dementia: clinicopathologic correlations. *Neurology* 39:76–79.

Brandt, J., Folstein, S. E., and Folstein, M. F. (1988). Differential cognitive impairment in Alzheimer's disease and Huntington's disease. *Ann. Neurol.* 23:555–561.

Brayne, C., Spiegelhalter, D. J., Dufouil, C., Chi, L. Y., Dening, T. R., Paykel, E. S., et al. (1999). Estimating the true extent of cognitive decline in the old old. *J. Am. Geriatr. Soc.* 47:1283–1288.

Breitner, J. C., and Folstein, M. F. (1984). Familial Alzheimer dementia: a prevalent disorder with specific clinical features. *Psychol. Med.* 14: 63–80.

Breitner, J. C., Gau, B. A., Welsh, K. A., Plassman, B. L., McDonald, W. M., Helms, M. J., et al. (1994). Inverse association of anti-inflammatory treatments and Alzheimer's disease: initial results of a co-twin control study. *Neurology* 44:227–232.

Brenner, D. E., Kukull, W. A., Stergachis, A., van Belle, G., Bowen, J. D., McCormick, W. C., et al. (1994). Postmenopausal estrogen replacement therapy and the risk of Alzheimer's disease: a population-based case-control study. *Am. J. Epidemiol.* 140:262–267.

Brenner, D. E., Kukull, W. A., van Belle, G., Bowen, J. D., McCormick, W. C., Teri, L., et al. (1993). Relationship between cigarette smoking and Alzheimer's disease in a population-based case–control study. *Neurology* 43:293–300.

Brun, A. (1993). Frontal lobe degeneration of non-Alzheimer type revisited. *Dementia* 4:126–131.

Cahn-Weiner, D. A., Sullivan, E. V., Shear, P. K., Fama, R., Lim, K. O., Yesavage, J. A. et al. (1999). Brain structural and cognitive correlates of clock drawing performance in Alzheimer's disease. *J. Int. Neuropsychol. Soc.* 5:502–509.

Caine, E. D., Hunt, R. D., Weingartner, H., and Ebert, M. H. (1978). Huntington's dementia. Clinical and neuropsychological features. *Arch. Gen. Psychiatry* 35:377–384.

Callahan, C. M., Hall, K. S., Hui, S. L., Musick, B. S., Unverzagt, F. W., and Hendrie, H. C. (1996). Relationship of age, education, and occupation with dementia among a community-based sample of African Americans. *Arch. Neurol.* 53:134–140.

Callahan, C. M., Hendrie, H. C., and Tierney, W. M. (1995). Documentation and evaluation of cognitive impairment in elderly primary care patients. *Ann. Intern. Med.* 122:422–429.

Campion, D., Brice, A., Hannequin, D., Tardieu, S., Dubois, B., Calenda, A., et al. (1995). A large pedigree with early-onset Alzheimer's disease: clinical, neuropathologic, and genetic characterization. *Neurology* 45:80–85.

Canadian Study of Health and Aging. (1994). Canadian study of health and aging: study methods and prevalence of dementia. *CMAJ* 150:899–913.

Carmelli, D., Swan, G. E., Reed, T., Miller, B., Wolf, P. A., Jarvik, G. P., et al. (1998). Midlife cardiovascular risk factors, ApoE, and cognitive decline in elderly male twins. *Neurology* 50:1580–1585.

Cerhan, J. R., Folsom, A. R., Mortimer, J. A., Shahar, E., Knopman, D. S., McGovern, P. G., et al. (1998). Correlates of cognitive function in middle-aged adults. Atherosclerosis Risk in Communities (ARIC) Study investigators. *Gerontology* 44:95–105.

Chandra, V., Kokmen, E., Schoenberg, B. S., and Beard, C. M. (1989). Head trauma with loss of consciousness as a risk factor for Alzheimer's disease. *Neurology* 39:1576–1578.

Chedru, F., and Geschwind, N. (1972). Writing disturbances in acute confusional states. *Neuropsychologia* 10:343–353.

Chui, H. C., Lyness, S. A., Sobel, E., and Schneider, L. S. (1994). Extrapyramidal signs and psychiatric symptoms predict faster cognitive decline in Alzheimer's disease. *Arch. Neurol.* 51:676–681.

Chui, H. C., Victoroff, J. I., Margolin, D., Jagust, W., Shankle, R., and Katzman, R. (1992). Criteria for the diagnosis of ischemic vascular dementia proposed by the State of California Alzheimer's Disease Diagnostic and Treatment Centers. *Neurology* 42:473–480.

Clark, A. W., Manz, H. J., White, C. L. D., Lehmann, J., Miller, D., and Coyle, J. T. (1986). Cortical degeneration with swollen chromatolytic neurons: its relationship to Pick's disease. *J. Neuropathol. Exp. Neurol.* 45:268–284.

Cobb, J. L., Wolf, P. A., Au R., White, R., and D'Agostino, R. B. (1995). The effect of education on the incidence of dementia and Alzheimer's disease in the Framingham Study. *Neurology* 45:1707–1712.

Collette, F., Van der Linden, M., and Salmon, E. (1999). Executive dysfunction in Alzheimer's disease. *Cortex* 35:57–72.

Colsher, P. L., and Wallace, R. B. (1991). Longitudinal application of cognitive function measures in a defined population of community-dwelling elders. *Ann. Epidemiol.* 1:215–230.

Croisile, B. (1999). Agraphia in Alzheimer's disease. *Dement. Geriatr. Cogn. Disord.* 10:226–230.

Croot, K., Hodges, J. R., and Patterson, K. (1999).

Evidence for impaired sentence comprehension in early Alzheimer's disease. *J. Int. Neuropsychol. Soc.* 5:393–404.

Crossen, J. R., and Wiens, A. N. (1994). Comparison of the Auditory–Verbal Learning Test (AVLT) and California Verbal Learning Test (CVLT) in a sample of normal subjects. *J. Clin. Exp. Neuropsychol.* 16:190–194.

Crum, R. M., Anthony, J. C., Bassett, S. S., and Folstein, M. F. (1993). Population-based norms for the Mini-Mental State Examination by age and educational level. *JAMA* 269:2386–2391.

Crystal, H. A., Horoupian, D. S., Katzman, R., and Jotkowitz, S. (1982). Biopsy-proved Alzheimer disease presenting as a right parietal lobe syndrome. *Ann. Neurol.* 12:186–188.

Cullum, C. M., Thompson, L. L., and Smernoff, E. N. (1993). Three word recall as a measure of memory. *J. Clin. Exp. Neuropsychol.* 15:321–329.

Cummings, J. L. (1993). Frontal–subcortical circuits and human behavior. *Arch. Neurol.* 50:873–880.

Cummings, J. L. (1994). Vascular subcortical dementias: clinical aspects. *Dementia* 5:177–180.

Cummings, J. L., and Benson, D. F. (1992). *Dementia: A Clinical Approach.* Boston: Butterworths.

Cummings, J. L., Mega, M., Gray, K., Rosenberg-Thompson, S., Carusi, D. A., and Gornbein, J. (1994). The Neuropsychiatric Inventory: comprehensive assessment of psychopathology in dementia. *Neurology* 44:2308–2314.

DeKosky, S. T., Harbaugh, R. E., Schmitt, F. A., Bakay, R. A., Chui, H. C., Knopman, D. S., et al. (1992). Cortical biopsy in Alzheimer's disease: diagnostic accuracy and neurochemical, neuropathological, and cognitive correlations. Intraventricular Bethanecol Study Group. *Ann. Neurol.* 32:625–632.

DeKosky, S. T., and Scheff, S. W. (1990). Synapse loss in frontal cortex biopsies in Alzheimer's disease: correlation with cognitive severity. *Ann. Neurol.* 27:457–464.

Delis, D. C., Freeland, J., Kramer, J. H., and Kaplan, E. (1988). Integrating clinical assessment with cognitive neuroscience: construct validation of the California Verbal Learning Test. *J. Consult. Clin. Psychol.* 56:123–130.

Della Sala, S., Lucchelli, F., and Spinnler, H. (1987). Ideomotor apraxia in patients with dementia of Alzheimer type. *J. Neurol.* 234:91–93.

De Renzi, E., and Vignolo, L. A. (1982). The Token Test: a sensitive test to detect receptive disturbances in aphasics. *Brain* 103:337–350.

Desmond, D. W. (1996). Vascular dementia: a construct in evolution. *Cerebrovasc. Brain Metab. Rev.* 8:296–325.

Devanand, D. P., Jacobs, D. M., Tang, M. X., Del Castillo-Castaneda, C., Sano, M., Marder, K. et al. (1997). The course of psychopathologic features in mild to moderate Alzheimer disease. *Arch. Gen. Psychiatry* 54:257–263.

Devinsky, O., Bear, D., and Volpe, B. T. (1988). Confusional states following posterior cerebral artery infarction. *Arch. Neurol.* 45:160–163.

Dobigny-Roman, N., Dieudonne-Moinet, B., Tortrat, D., Verny, M., and Forette, B. (1998). Ideomotor apraxia test: a new test of imitation of gestures for elderly people. *Eur. J. Neurol.* 5:571–578.

Eefsting, J. A., Boersma, F., Van den Brink, W., and Van Tilburg, W. (1996). Differences in prevalence of dementia based on community survey and general practitioner recognition. *Psychol. Med.* 26:1223–1230.

Elias, M. F., Elias, P. K., D'Agostino, R. B., Silbershatz, H., and Wolf, P. A. (1997). Role of age, education, and gender on cognitive performance in the Framingham Heart Study: community-based norms. *Exp. Aging Res.* 23:201–235.

Elias, M. F., Wolf, P. A., D'Agostino, R. B., Cobb, J., and White, L. R. (1993). Untreated blood pressure level is inversely related to cognitive functioning: the Framingham Study. *Am. J. Epidemiol.* 138:353–364.

Ellis, R. J., Jan, K., Kawas, C., Koller, W. C., Lyons, K. E., Jeste, D. V., et al. (1998). Diagnostic validity of the dementia questionnaire for Alzheimer disease. *Arch. Neurol.* 55:360–365.

Elwood, R. W. (1995). The California Verbal Learning Test: psychometric characteristics and clinical application. *Neuropsychol. Rev.* 5:173–201.

Erkinjuntti, T., Ostbye, T., Steenhuis, R., and Hachinski, V. (1997). The effect of different diagnostic criteria on the prevalence of dementia. *N. Engl. J. Med.* 337:1667–1674.

Eslinger, P. J., Damasio, A. R., Benton, A. L., and Van Allen, M. (1985). Neuropsychologic detection of abnormal mental decline in older persons. *JAMA* 253:670–674.

Esteban-Santillan, C., Praditsuwan, R., Ueda, H., and Geldmacher, D. S. (1978). Clock drawing test in very mild Alzheimer's disease. *J. Am. Geriatr. Soc.* 46:1266–1269.

Evans, D. A., Beckett, L. A., Albert, M. S., Hebert, L. E., Scherr, P. A., Funkenstein, H. H., et al. (1993). Level of education and change in cognitive function in a community population of older persons. *Ann. Epidemiol.* 3:71–77.

Evans, D. A., Funkenstein, H. H., Albert, M. S.,

Scherr, P. A., Cook, N. R., Chown, M. J., et al. (1989). Prevalence of Alzheimer's disease in a community population of older persons. Higher than previously reported. *JAMA* 262:2551–2556.

Faber-Langendoen, K., Morris, J. C., Knesevich, J. W., LaBarge, E., Miller, J. P., and Berg, L. (1988). Aphasia in senile dementia of the Alzheimer type. *Ann. Neurol.* 23:365–370.

Fabrigoule, C., Rouch, I., Taberly, A., Letenneur, L., Commenges, D., Mazaux, J. M., et al. (1998). Cognitive process in preclinical phase of dementia. *Brain* 121:135–141.

Farlow, M., Murrell, J., Ghetti, B., Unverzagt, F., Zeldenrust, S., and Benson, M. (1994). Clinical characteristics in a kindred with early-onset Alzheimer's disease and their linkage to a G → T change at position 2149 of the amyloid precursor protein gene. *Neurology* 44:105–111.

Farrer, L. A., Cupples, L. A., Haines, J. L., Hyman, B., Kukull, W. A., Mayeux, R., et al. (1997). Effects of age, sex, and ethnicity on the association between apolipoprotein E genotype and Alzheimer disease. A meta-analysis. APOE and Alzheimer Disease Meta-analysis Consortium. *JAMA* 278:1349–1356.

Feany, M. B., and Dickson, D. W. (1996). Neurodegenerative disorders with extensive tau pathology: a comparative study and review. *Ann. Neurol.* 40:139–148.

Ferman, T. J., Boeve, B. F., Smith, G. E., Silber, M. H., Kokmen, E., Petersen, R. C., Ivnik, R. J. (1999). REM sleep behavior disorder and dementia: cognitive differences when compared with AD. *Neurology* 52:951–957.

Fillenbaum, G. G., Heyman, A., Huber, M. S., Woodbury, M. A., Leiss, J., Schmader, K. E., et al. (1998). The prevalence and 3-year incidence of dementia in older black and white community residents. *J. Clin. Epidemiol.* 51:587–595.

Fillenbaum, G. G., Heyman, A., Wilkinson, W. E., and Haynes, C. S. (1987). Comparison of two screening tests in Alzheimer's disease. The correlation and reliability of the Mini-Mental State Examination and the modified Blessed test. *Arch. Neurol.* 44:924–947.

Finton, M. J., Lucas, J. A., Graff-Radford, N. R., and Uitti, R. J. (1998). Analysis of visuospatial errors in patients with Alzheimer's disease or Parkinson's disease. *J. Clin. Exp. Neuropsychol.* 20: 186–193.

Fisher, N. J., Rourke, B. P., and Bieliauskas, L. A. (1999). Neuropsychological subgroups of patients with Alzheimer's disease: an examination of the first 10 years of CERAD data. *J. Clin. Exp. Neuropsychol.* 21:488–518.

Folstein, M. F., Folstein, S. E., and McHugh, P. R. (1975). "Mini-mental state". A practical method for grading the cognitive state of patients for the clinician. *J. Psychiatr. Res.* 12:189–198.

Folstein, S. E. (1991). The psychopathology of Huntington's disease. *Res. Publ. Assoc. Res. Nerv. Ment. Dis.* 69:181–191.

Ford, A. B., Mefrouche, Z., Friedland, R. P., and Debanne, S. M. (1996). Smoking and cognitive impairment: a population-based study. *J. Am. Geriatr. Soc.* 44:905–909.

Fox, N. C., Warrington, E. K., Seiffer, A. L., Agnew, S. K., and Rossor, M. N. (1998). Presymptomatic cognitive deficits in individuals at risk of familial Alzheimer's disease. A longitudinal prospective study. *Brain* 121:1631–1639.

Francis, J., Martin, D., and Kapoor, W. N. (1990). A prospective study of delirium in hospitalized elderly. *JAMA* 263:1097–1101.

Francis, P. T., Palmer, A. M., Sims, N. R., Bowen, D. M., Davison, A. N., Esiri, M. M., et al. (1985). Neurochemical studies of early-onset Alzheimer's disease. Possible influence on treatment. *N. Engl. J. Med.* 313:7–11.

Fratiglioni, L., Grut, M., Forsell, Y., Viitanen, M., and Winblad, B. (1992). Clinical diagnosis of Alzheimer's disease and other dementias in a population survey. Agreement and causes of disagreement in applying *Diagnostic and Statistical Manual of Mental Disorders, Revised Third Edition*, criteria. *Arch. Neurol.* 49:927–932.

French, L. R., Schuman, L. M., Mortimer, J. A., Hutton, J. T., Boatman, R. A., and Christians, B. (1985). A case–control study of dementia of the Alzheimer type. *Am. J. Epidemiol.* 121:414–421.

Friedland, R. P. (1993). Epidemiology, education, and the ecology of Alzheimer's disease. *Neurology* 43:246–249.

Friedland, R. P., Koss, E., Lerner, A., Hedera, P., Ellis, W., Dronkers, N., et al. (1993). Functional imaging, the frontal lobes, and dementia. *Dementia* 4:192–203.

Gabrieli, J. D., Keane, M. M., Stanger, B. Z., Kjelgaard, M. M., Corkin, S., and Growdon, J. H. (1994). Dissociations among structural–perceptual, lexical–semantic, and event–fact memory systems in Alzheimer, amnesic, and normal subjects. *Cortex* 30:75–103.

Galanis, D. J., Petrovitch, H., Launer, L. J., Harris, T. B., Foley, D. J., and White, L. R. (1997). Smoking history in middle age and subsequent cognitive performance in elderly Japanese-American men. The Honolulu-Asia Aging Study. *Am. J. Epidemiol.* 145:507–515.

Galasko, D., Bennett, D., Sano, M., Ernesto, C.,

Thomas, R., Grundman, M., et al. (1997). An inventory to assess activities of daily living for clinical trials in Alzheimer's disease. The Alzheimer's Disease Cooperative Study. *Alzheimer Dis. Assoc. Disord.* 11 Suppl 2:S33–S39.

Galasko, D., Corey-Bloom, J., and Thal, L. J. (1991). Monitoring progression in Alzheimer's disease. *J. Am. Geriatr. Soc.* 39:932–941.

Galasko, D., Hansen, L. A., Katzman, R., Wiederholt, W., Masliah, E., Terry, R., et al. (1994). Clinical–neuropathological correlations in Alzheimer's disease and related dementias. *Arch. Neurol.* 51:888–895.

Galasko, D., Klauber, M. R., Hofstetter, C. R., Salmon, D. P., Lasker, B., and Thal, L. J. (1990). The Mini-Mental State Examination in the early diagnosis of Alzheimer's disease. *Arch. Neurol.* 47:49–52.

Ganguli, M., Ratcliff, G., Huff, F. J., Belle, S., Kancel, M. J., Fischer, L., et al. (1991). Effects of age, gender, and education on cognitive tests in a rural elderly community sample: norms from the Monongahela Valley Independent Elders Survey. *Neuroepidemiology* 10:42–52.

Ganguli, M., Seaberg, E. C., Ratcliff, G. G., Belle, S. H., and DeKosky, S. T. (1996). Cognitive stability over 2 years in a rural elderly population: the MoVIES project. *Neuroepidemiology* 15:42–50.

Gao, S., Hendrie, H. C., Hall, K. S., and Hui, S. (1998). The relationships between age, sex, and the incidence of dementia and Alzheimer disease: a meta-analysis. *Arch. Gen. Psychiatry* 55:809–815.

Gates, G. A., Karzon, R. K., Garcia, P., Peterein, J., Storandt, M., Morris, J. C., et al. (1995). Auditory dysfunction in aging and senile dementia of the Alzheimer's type. *Arch. Neurol.* 52:626–634.

Geffen, G., Moar, K. J., O'Hanlon, A. P., Clark, C. R., and Geffen, L. B. (1990). Performance measures of 16- to 86-year-old males and females on the Auditory Verbal Learning Test. *Clin. Neuropsychol.* 4:45–63.

Gelinas, I., Gauthier, L., McIntyre, M., and Gauthier, S. (1999). Development of a functional measure for persons with Alzheimer's disease: the disability assessment for dementia. *Am. J. Occup. Ther.* 53:471–481.

Giannakopoulos, P., Gold, G., Duc, M., Michel, J. P., Hof, P. R., and Bouras, C. (1999). Neuroanatomic correlates of visual agnosia in Alzheimer's disease: a clinicopathologic study. *Neurology* 52:71–77.

Gilley, D. W., Wilson, R. S., Beckett, L. A., and Evans, D. A. (1997). Psychotic symptoms and physically aggressive behavior in Alzheimer's disease. *J. Am. Geriatr. Soc.* 45:1074–1079.

Glosser, G., Kohn, S. E., Sands, L., Grugan, P. K., and Friedman, R. B. (1999). Impaired spelling in Alzheimer's disease: a linguistic deficit? *Neuropsychologia* 37:807–815.

Goldman, W. P., Baty, J. D., Buckles, V. D., Sahrmann, S., and Morris, J. C. (1999). Motor dysfunction in mildly demented AD individuals without extrapyramidal signs. *Neurology* 53:956–962.

Goldstein, F. C., Green, J., Presley, R., and Green, R. C. (1992). Dysnomia in Alzheimer's disease: an evaluation of neurobehavioral subtypes. *Brain Lang.* 43:308–322.

Graff-Radford, N. R., Bolling, J. P., Earnest, F. T., Shuster, E. A., Caselli, R. J., and Brazis, P. W. (1993). Simultanagnosia as the initial sign of degenerative dementia. *Mayo Clin. Proc.* 68:955–964.

Graff-Radford, N. R., Tranel, D., Van Hoesen, G. W., and Brandt, J. P. (1990). Diencephalic amnesia. *Brain* 113:1–25.

Grafman, J., Litvan, I., Gomez, C., and Chase, T. N. (1990a). Frontal lobe function in progressive supranuclear palsy. *Arch. Neurol.* 47:553–558.

Grafman, J., Litvan, I., and Stark, M. (1995). Neuropsychological features of progressive supranuclear palsy. *Brain Cogn.* 28:311–320.

Grafman, J., Weingartner, H., Newhouse, P. A., Thompson, K., Lalonde, F., Litvan, I., et al. (1990b). Implicit learning in patients with Alzheimer's disease. *Pharmacopsychiatry* 23:94–101.

Graham, J. E., Rockwood, K., Beattie, B. L., Eastwood, R., Gauthier, S., Tuokko, H., et al. (1997). Prevalence and severity of cognitive impairment with and without dementia in an elderly population. *Lancet* 349:1793–1796.

Graham, J. E., Rockwood, K., Beattie, B. L., McDowell, I., Eastwood, R., and Gauthier, S. (1996). Standardization of the diagnosis of dementia in the Canadian Study of Health and Aging. *Neuroepidemiology* 15:246–256.

Grant, I., Atkinson, J. H., Hesselink, J. R., Kennedy, C. J., Richman, D. D., Spector, S. A., et al. (1987). Evidence for early central nervous system involvement in the acquired immunodeficiency syndrome (AIDS) and other human immunodeficiency virus (HIV) infections. Studies with neuropsychologic testing and magnetic resonance imaging [published erratum appears in *Ann. Intern. Med.* 1988;*108(3)*:496]. *Ann. Intern. Med. 107*:828–836.

Graves, A. B., Larson, E. B., Edland, S. D., Bowen, J. D., McCormick, W. C., McCurry, S. M., et al. (1996). Prevalence of dementia and its subtypes in the Japanese American population of King County, Washington State. The Kame Project. *Am. J. Epidemiol. 144*:760–771.

Graves, A. B., van Duijn, C. M., Chandra, V., Fratiglioni, L., Heyman, A., Jorm, A. F., et al. (1991). Alcohol and tobacco consumption as risk factors for Alzheimer's disease: a collaborative re-analysis of case–control studies. EURODEM Risk Factors Research Group. *Int. J. Epidemiol. 20(Suppl 2)*:S48–S57.

Graves, A. B., White, E., Koepsell, T. D., Reifler, B. V., van Belle, G., Larson, E. B., et al. (1990). The association between head trauma and Alzheimer's disease. *Am. J. Epidemiol. 131*:491–501.

Green, J., Morris, J. C., Sandson, J., McKeel, D. W., Jr., and Miller, J. W. (1990). Progressive aphasia: a precursor of global dementia? *Neurology 40*:423–429.

Green, R. C., Goldstein, F. C., Mirra, S. S., Alazraki, N. P., Baxt, J. L., and Bakay, R. A. (1995). Slowly progressive apraxia in Alzheimer's disease. *J. Neurol. Neurosurg. Psychiatry 59*:312–315.

Greene, J. D., Hodges, J. R., and Baddeley, A. D. (1995). Autobiographical memory and executive function in early dementia of Alzheimer type. *Neuropsychologia 33*:1647–1670.

Grimes, D. A., Lang, A. E., and Bergeron, C. B. (1999). Dementia as the most common presentation of cortical–basal ganglionic degeneration. *Neurology 53*:1969–1974.

Grober, E., Buschke, H., Crystal, H., Bang, S., and Dresner, R. (1988). Screening for dementia by memory testing. *Neurology 38*:900–903.

Grober, E., and Kawas, C. (1997). Learning and retention in preclinical and early Alzheimer's disease. *Psychol. Aging 12*:183–188.

Grossman, M., and White-Devine, T. (1998). Sentence comprehension in Alzheimer's disease. *Brain Lang. 62*:186–201.

Grut, M., Jorm, A. F., Fratiglioni, L., Forsell, Y., Viitanen, M., and Winblad, B. (1993). Memory complaints of elderly people in a population survey: variation according to dementia stage and depression. *J. Am. Geriatr. Soc. 41*:1295–1300.

Gustafson, L. (1993). Clinical picture of frontal lobe degeneration of non-Alzheimer type. *Dementia 4*:143–148.

Haan, M. N., Shemanski, L., Jagust, W. J., Mano-

lio, T. A., and Kuller, L. (1999). The role of APOE epsilon4 in modulating effects of other risk factors for cognitive decline in elderly persons. *JAMA 282*:40–46.

Hachinski, V. (1994). Vascular dementia: a radical redefinition. *Dementia 5*:130–132.

Hachisuka, K., Uchida, M., Nozaki, Y., Hashiguchi, S., and Sasaki, M. (1999). Primary progressive aphasia presenting as conduction aphasia. *J. Neurol. Sci. 167*:137–141.

Hall, M., Whaley, R., Robertson, K., Hamby, S., Wilkins, J., and Hall, C. (1996). The correlation between neuropsychological and neuroanatomic changes over time in asymptomatic and symptomatic HIV-1-infected individuals. *Neurology 46*:1697–1702.

Hansen, L., Salmon, D., Galasko, D., Masliah, E., Katzman, R., DeTeresa, R., et al. (1990). The Lewy body variant of Alzheimer's disease: a clinical and pathologic entity. *Neurology 40*:1–8.

Hansen, L. A., Masliah, E., Galasko, D., and Terry, R. D. (1993). Plaque-only Alzheimer disease is usually the Lewy body variant, and vice versa. *J. Neuropathol. Exp. Neurol. 52*:648–654.

Hansen, L. A., and Samuel, W. (1997). Criteria for Alzheimer's disease and the nosology of dementia with Lewy bodies. *Neurology 48*:126–132.

Haxby, J. V., Grady, C. L., Koss, E., Horwitz, B., Heston, L., Schapiro, M., et al. (1990). Longitudinal study of cerebral metabolic asymmetries and associated neuropsychological patterns in early dementia of the Alzheimer type. *Arch. Neurol. 47*:753–760.

Hebert, L. E., Scherr, P. A., Beckett, L. A., Albert, M. S., Pilgrim, D. M., Chown, M. J., et al. (1995). Age-specific incidence of Alzheimer's disease in a community population. *JAMA 273*:1354–1359.

Hebert, L. E., Scherr, P. A., Beckett, L. A., Funkenstein, H. H., Albert, M. S., Chown, M. J., et al. (1992). Relation of smoking and alcohol consumption to incident Alzheimer's disease. *Am. J. Epidemiol. 135*:347–355.

Heindel, W. C., Cahn, D. A., and Salmon, D. P. (1997). Non-associative lexical priming is impaired in Alzheimer's disease. *Neuropsychologia 35*:1365–1372.

Hely, M. A., Reid, W. G., Halliday, G. M., McRitchie, D. A., Leicester, J., Joffe, R., et al. (1996). Diffuse Lewy body disease: clinical features in nine cases without coexistent Alzheimer's disease. *J. Neurol. Neurosurg. Psychiatry 60*:531–538.

Hendrie, H. C., Osuntokun, B. O., Hall, K. S., Ogunniyi, A. O., Hui, S. L., Unverzagt, F. W., et al. (1995). Prevalence of Alzheimer's disease and dementia in two communities: Nigerian Africans and African Americans. *Am. J. Psychiatry 152*:1485–1492.

Herlitz, A., Hill, R. D., Fratiglioni, L., and Backman, L. (1995). Episodic memory and visuospatial ability in detecting and staging dementia in a community-based sample of very old adults. *J. Gerontol. A Biol. Sci. Med. Sci. 50*:M107–M113.

Herlitz, A., Small, B. J., Fratiglioni, L., Almkvist, O., Viitanen, M., and Backman, L. (1997). Detection of mild dementia in community surveys. Is it possible to increase the accuracy of our diagnostic instruments? *Arch. Neurol. 54*:319–324.

Heyman, A., Fillenbaum, G. G., Gearing, M., Mirra, S. S., Welsh-Bohmer, K. A., Peterson, B., et al. (1999). Comparison of Lewy body variant of Alzheimer's disease with pure Alzheimer's disease: Consortium to Establish a Registry for Alzheimer's Disease, Part XIX. *Neurology 52*:1839–1844.

Heyman, A., Fillenbaum, G. G., Welsh-Bohmer, K. A., Gearing, M., Mirra, S. S., Mohs, R. C., et al. (1998). Cerebral infarcts in patients with autopsy-proven Alzheimer's disease: CERAD, part XVIII. Consortium to Establish a Registry for Alzheimer's Disease. *Neurology 51*:159–162.

Hodges, J. R., Patterson, K., Oxbury, S., and Funnell, E. (1992). Semantic dementia. Progressive fluent aphasia with temporal lobe atrophy. *Brain 115*:1783–1806.

Hof, P. R., Bouras, C., Constantinidis, J., and Morrison, J. H. (1990). Selective disconnection of specific visual association pathways in cases of Alzheimer's disease presenting with Balint's syndrome. *J. Neuropathol. Exp. Neurol. 49*:168–184.

Hofman, A., Ott, A., Breteler, M. M., Bots, M. L., Slooter, A. J., van Harskamp, F., et al. (1997). Atherosclerosis, apolipoprotein E, and prevalence of dementia and Alzheimer's disease in the Rotterdam Study. *Lancet 349*:151–154.

Holmes, C., Cairns, N., Lantos, P., and Mann, A. (1999). Validity of current clinical criteria for Alzheimer's disease, vascular dementia and dementia with Lewy bodies. *Br. J. Psychiatry 174*:45–50.

Horner, J., Heyman, A., Dawson, D., and Rogers, H. (1998). The relationship of agraphia to the severity of dementia in Alzheimer's disease. *Arch. Neurol. 45*:760–763.

Howieson, D. B., Holm, L. A., Kaye, J. A., Oken, B. S., and Howieson, J. (1993). Neurologic function in the optimally healthy oldest old. Neuropsychological evaluation. *Neurology 43*:1882–1886.

Huff, F. J., Becker, J. T., Belle, S. H., Nebes, R. D.,

Holland, A. L., and Boller, F. (1987). Cognitive deficits and clinical diagnosis of Alzheimer's disease. *Neurology 37*:1119–1124.

Hughes, C. P., Berg, L., Danziger, W. L., Coben, L. A., and Martin, R. L. (1982). A new clinical scale for the staging of dementia. *Br. J. Psychiatry 140*:566–572.

Hulette, C., Mirra, S., Wilkinson, W., Heyman, A., Fillenbaum, G., and Clark, C. (1995). The Consortium to Establish a Registry for Alzheimer's Disease (CERAD). Part IX. A prospective cliniconeuropathologic study of Parkinson's features in Alzheimer's disease. *Neurology 45*:1991–1995.

Hyman, B. T., Kromer, L. J., and Van Hoesen, G. W. (1987). Reinnervation of the hippocampal perforant pathway zone in Alzheimer's disease. *Ann. Neurol. 21*:259–267.

Hyman, B. T., Van Hoesen, G. W., and Damasio, A. R. (1990). Memory-related neural systems in Alzheimer's disease: an anatomic study. *Neurology 40*:1721–1730.

Imamura, T., Takatsuki, Y., Fujimori, M., Hirono, N., Ikejiri, Y., Shimomura, T., et al. (1998). Age at onset and language disturbances in Alzheimer's disease. *Neuropsychologia 36*:945–949.

Inouye, S. K., Albert, M. S., Mohs, R., Sun, K., and Berkman, L. F. (1993). Cognitive performance in a high-functioning community-dwelling elderly population. *J. Gerontol. 48*:M146–M151.

Inouye, S. K., and Charpentier, P. A. (1996). Precipitating factors for delirium in hospitalized elderly persons. Predictive model and interrelationship with baseline vulnerability. *JAMA 275*:852–857.

Ives, D. G., Bonino, P., Traven, N. D., and Kuller, L. H. (1995). Characteristics and comorbidities of rural older adults with hearing impairment. *J. Am. Geriatr. Soc. 43*:803–806.

Jack, C. R., Jr., Petersen, R. C., Xu, Y. C., Waring, S. C., O'Brien, P. C., Tangalos, E. G., et al. (1997). Medial temporal atrophy on MRI in normal aging and very mild Alzheimer's disease. *Neurology 49*:786–794.

Jacobs, D. H., Adair, J. C., Williamson, D. J., Na, D. L., Gold, M., Foundas, A. L., et al. (1999). Apraxia and motor-skill acquisition in Alzheimer's disease are dissociable. *Neuropsychologia 37*:875–880.

Jacobs, D. M., Sano, M., Dooneief, G., Marder, K., Bell, K. L., and Stern, Y. (1995). Neuropsychological detection and characterization of preclinical Alzheimer's disease. *Neurology 45*:957–962.

Jacobs, D. M., Tang, M. X., Stern, Y., Sano, M.,

Marder, K., Bell, K. L., et al. (1998). Cognitive function in nondemented older women who took estrogen after menopause. *Neurology* 50:368–373.

Jason, G. W., Suchowersky, O., Pajurkova, E. M., Graham, L., Klimek, M. L., Garber, A. T., et al. (1997). Cognitive manifestations of Huntington disease in relation to genetic structure and clinical onset. *Arch. Neurol.* 54:1081–1088.

Jerger, J., Chmiel, R., Wilson, N., and Luchi, R. (1995). Hearing impairment in older adults: new concepts. *J. Am. Geriatr. Soc.* 43:928–935.

Jick, H., Zomberg, G. L., Jick, S. S., Seshadri, S., Drachman, D. A. (2000). Statins and the risk of dementia. *Lancet* 356:1627–1631.

Joachim, C. L., Morris, J. H., and Selkoe, D. J. (1988). Clinically diagnosed Alzheimer's disease: autopsy results in 150 cases. *Ann. Neurol.* 24:50–56.

Johannsen, P., Jakobsen, J., Bruhn, P., and Gjedde, A. (1999). Cortical responses to sustained and divided attention in Alzheimer's disease. *Neuroimage* 10:269–281.

Johnson, J. K., Head, E., Kim, R., Starr, A., and Cotman, C. W. (1999). Clinical and pathological evidence for a frontal variant of Alzheimer disease. *Arch. Neurol.* 56:1233–1239.

Jordan, B. D., Relkin, N. R., Ravdin, L. D., Jacobs, A. R., Bennett, A., and Gandy, S. (1997). Apolipoprotein E epsilon4 associated with chronic traumatic brain injury in boxing. *JAMA* 278:136–140.

Jorm, A. F. (1994). A short form of the Informant Questionnaire on Cognitive Decline in the Elderly (IQCODE): development and cross-validation. *Psychol. Med.* 24:145–153.

Jorm, A. F., and Jolley, D. (1998). The incidence of dementia: a meta-analysis. *Neurology* 51:728–733.

Kalmijn, S., Feskens, E. J., Launer, L. J., and Kromhout, D. (1996). Cerebrovascular disease, the apolipoprotein e4 allele, and cognitive decline in a community-based study of elderly men. *Stroke* 27:2230–2235.

Kamo, H., McGeer, P. L., Harrop, R., McGeer, E. G., Calne, D. B., Martin, W. R., et al. (1987). Positron emission tomography and histopathology in Pick's disease. *Neurology* 37:439–445.

Katzman, R. (1993). Education and the prevalence of dementia and Alzheimer's disease. *Neurology* 43:13–20.

Katzman, R., Brown, T., Fuld, P., Peck, A., Schechter, R., and Schimmel, H. (1983). Validation of a short Orientation-Memory-Concentration Test of cognitive impairment. *Am. J. Psychiatry* 140:734–739.

Katzman, R., Brown, T., Thal, L. J., Fuld, P. A., Aronson, M., Butters, N., et al. (1988). Comparison of rate of annual change of mental status score in four independent studies of patients with Alzheimer's disease. *Ann. Neurol.* 24:384–389.

Kawas, C., Resnick, S., Morrison, A., Brookmeyer, R., Corrada, M., Zonderman, A., et al. (1997). A prospective study of estrogen replacement therapy and the risk of developing Alzheimer's disease: the Baltimore Longitudinal Study of Aging. *Neurology* 48:1517–1521.

Kawas, C., Segal, J., Stewart, W. F., Corrada, M., and Thal, L. J. (1994). A validation study of the Dementia Questionnaire. *Arch. Neurol.* 51:901–906.

Keller, B. K., Morton, J. L., Thomas, V. S., and Potter, J. F. (1999). The effect of visual and hearing impairments on functional status. *J. Am. Geriatr. Soc.* 47:1319–1325.

Kertesz, A. (1997). Frontotemporal dementia, Pick disease, and corticobasal degeneration. One entity or 3? 1. *Arch. Neurol.* 54:1427–1429.

Kertesz, A., Hudson, L., Mackenzie, I. R., and Munoz, D. G. (1994). The pathology and nosology of primary progressive aphasia. *Neurology* 44:2065–2072.

Kertesz, A., and Munoz, D. (1998). Pick's disease, frontotemporal dementia, and Pick complex: emerging concepts. *Arch. Neurol.* 55:302–304.

Kieburtz, K., Ketonen, L., Cox, C., Grossman, H., Holloway, R., Booth, H., et al. (1996). Cognitive performance and regional brain volume in human immunodeficiency virus type 1 infection. *Arch. Neurol.* 53:155–158.

Kiernan, R. J., Mueller, J., Langston, J. W., and Van Dyke, C. (1987). The Neurobehavioral Cognitive Status Examination: a brief but quantitative approach to cognitive assessment. *Ann. Intern. Med.* 107:481–485.

Kittner, S. J., White, L. R., Farmer, M. E., Wolz, M., Kaplan, E., Moes, E., et al. (1986). Methodological issues in screening for dementia: the problem of education adjustment. *J. Chron. Dis.* 39:163–170.

Klein, L. E., Roca, R. P., McArthur, J., Vogelsang, G., Klein, G. B., Kirby, S. M., et al. (1985). Diagnosing dementia. Univariate and multivariate analyses of the mental status examination. *J. Am. Geriatr. Soc.* 33:483–488.

Knopman, D. (1991) Long-term retention of implicitly acquired learning in patients with Alzheimer's disease. *J. Clin. Exp. Neuropsychol.* 13:880–894.

Knopman, D. S., Mastri, A. R., Frey, W. H., Sung,

J. H., and Rustan, T. (1990). Dementia lacking distinctive histologic features: a common non-Alzheimer degenerative dementia. *Neurology* 40:251–256.

Knopman, D. S., and Ryberg, S. (1989). A verbal memory test with high predictive accuracy for dementia of the Alzheimer type. *Arch. Neurol.* 46:141–145.

Kokmen, E., Beard, C. M., Offord, K. P., and Kurland, L. T. (1989). Prevalence of medically diagnosed dementia in a defined United States population: Rochester, Minnesota, January 1, 1975. *Neurology* 39:773–776.

Kokmen, E., Smith, G. E., Petersen, R. C., Tangalos, E., and Ivnik, R. C. (1991). The short test of mental status. Correlations with standardized psychometric testing. *Arch. Neurol.* 48:725–728.

Kokmen, E., Whisnant, J. P., O'Fallon, W. M., Chu, C. P., and Beard, C. M. (1996). Dementia after ischemic stroke: a population-based study in Rochester, Minnesota (1960–1984). *Neurology* 46:154–159.

Kopelman, M. D. (1985). Rates of forgetting in Alzheimer-type dementia and Korsakoff's syndrome. *Neuropsychologia* 23:623–638.

Kopelman, M. D. (1991). Frontal dysfunction and memory deficits in the alcoholic Korsakoff syndrome and Alzheimer-type dementia. *Brain* 114: 117–137.

Kopelman, M. D., Wilson, B. A., and Baddeley, A. D. (1989). The autobiographical memory interview: a new assessment of autobiographical and personal semantic memory in amnesic patients. *J. Clin. Exp. Neuropsychol.* 11:724–744.

Koss, E., Edland, S., Fillenbaum, G., Mohs, R., Clark, C., Galasko, D., et al. (1996). Clinical and neuropsychological differences between patients with earlier and later onset of Alzheimer's disease: a CERAD analysis, Part XII. *Neurology* 46:136–141.

Kraemer, H. C., Tinklenberg, J., and Yesavage, J. A. (1994). 'How far' vs 'how fast' in Alzheimer's disease. The question revisited. *Arch. Neurol.* 51:275–279.

Kramer, S. I., and Reifler, B. V. (1992). Depression, dementia, and reversible dementia. *Clin. Geriatr. Med.* 8:289–297.

Kukull, W. A., Larson, E. B., Teri, L., Bowen, J., McCormick, W., and Pfanschmidt, M. L. (1994). The Mini-Mental State Examination score and the clinical diagnosis of dementia. *J. Clin. Epidemiol.* 47:1061–1067.

Kuller, L. H., Shemanski, L., Manolio, T., Haan, M., Fried, L., Bryan, N., et al. (1998). Relationship between ApoE, MRI findings, and cognitive

function in the Cardiovascular Health Study. *Stroke* 29:388–398.

Lafleche, G., and Albert, M. S. (1995). Executive function deficits in mild Alzheimer's disease. *Neuropsychology* 9:313–320.

Lambert, J., Eustache, F., Viader, F., Dary, M., Rioux, P., Lechevalier, B., et al. (1996). Agraphia in Alzheimer's disease: an independent lexical impairment. *Brain Lang.* 53:222–233.

Lange, K. W., Sahakian, B. J., Quinn, N. P., Marsden, C. D., and Robbins, T. W. (1995). Comparison of executive and visuospatial memory function in Huntington's disease and dementia of Alzheimer type matched for degree of dementia. *J. Neurol. Neurosurg. Psychiatry* 58:598–606.

Langley, L. K., Overmier, J. B., Knopman, D. S., and Prod'Homme, M. M. (1998). Inhibition and habituation: preserved mechanisms of attentional selection in aging and Alzheimer's disease. *Neuropsychology* 12:353–366.

Larson, E. B., McCurry, S. M., Graves, A. B., Bowen, J. D., Rice, M. M., and McCormick, W. C. (1998). Standardization of the clinical diagnosis of the dementia syndrome and its subtypes in a cross-sectional study: the Ni-Hon-Sea experience. *J. Gerontol. A Biol. Sci. Med. Sci.* 53A: M313–M319.

Larson, E. B., Reifler, B. V., Sumi, S. M., Canfield, C. G., and Chinn, N. M. (1985). Diagnostic evaluation of 200 elderly outpatients with suspected dementia. *J. Gerontol.* 40:536–543.

La Rue, A. (1989). Patterns of performance on the Fuld Object Memory Evaluation in elderly inpatients with depression or dementia. *J. Clin. Exp. Neuropsychol.* 11:409–422.

Launer, L. J., Masaki, K., Petrovitch, H., Foley, D., and Havlik, R. J. (1995). The association between midlife blood pressure levels and late-life cognitive function. The Honolulu-Asia Aging Study. *JAMA* 274:1846–1851.

Lautenschlager, N. T., Cupples, L. A., Rao, V. S., Auerbach, S. A., Becker, R., Burke, J., et al. (1996). Risk of dementia among relatives of Alzheimer's disease patients in the MIRAGE study: what is in store for the oldest old? *Neurology* 46:641–650.

Lawrence, A. D., Hodges, J. R., Rosser, A. E., Kershaw, A., ffrench-Constant, C., Rubinsztein, D. C., et al. (1998). Evidence for specific cognitive deficits in preclinical Huntington's disease. *Brain* 121:1329–1341.

Lawton, M. P., and Brody, E. M. (1969). Assessment of older people: self-maintaining and instrumental activities of daily living. *Gerontologist* 9:179–186.

Leibson, C. L., Rocca, W. A., Hanson, V. A., Cha, R., Kokmen, E., O'Brien, P. C., et al. (1997). Risk of dementia among persons with diabetes mellitus: a population-based cohort study. *Am. J. Epidemiol.* 145:301–308.

Leonberger, T. F., Nicks, S. D., Goldfader, P. R., and Munz, D. C. (1991). Factor analysis of the Wechsler Memory Scale-Revised and the Halstead-Reitan Neuropsychological Battery. *Clin. Neuropsychol.* 5:83–88.

Lerner, A. J., Hedera, P., Koss, E., Stuckey, J., and Friedland, R. P. (1997). Delirium in Alzheimer disease. *Alzheimer Dis. Assoc. Disord.* 11:16–20.

Levine, D. N., Lee, J. M., and Fisher, C. M. (1993). The visual variant of Alzheimer's disease: a clinicopathologic case study. *Neurology* 43:305–313.

Lezak, M. D. (1995). *Neuropsychological Assessment*. New York: Oxford University Press.

Lim, A., Tsuang, D., Kukull, W., Nochlin, D., Leverenz, J., McCormick, W., et al. (1999). Clinico-neuropathological correlation of Alzheimer's disease in a community-based case series. *J. Am. Geriatr. Soc.* 47:564–569.

Linn, R. T., Wolf, P. A., Bachman, D. L., Knoefel, J. E., Cobb, J. L., Belanger, A. J., et al. (1995). The 'preclinical phase' of probable Alzheimer's disease. A 13-year prospective study of the Framingham cohort. *Arch. Neurol.* 52:485–490.

Litvan, I., Agid, Y., Goetz, C., Jankovic, J., Wenning, G. K., Brandel, J. P., et al. (1997). Accuracy of the clinical diagnosis of corticobasal degeneration: a clinicopathologic study. *Neurology* 48:119–125.

Litvan, I., Cummings, J. L., and Mega, M. (1998a). Neuropsychiatric features of corticobasal degeneration. *J. Neurol. Neurosurg. Psychiatry* 65:717–721.

Litvan, I., MacIntyre, A., Goetz, C. G., Wenning, G. K., Jellinger, K., Verny, M., et al. (1998b) Accuracy of the clinical diagnoses of Lewy body disease, Parkinson disease, and dementia with Lewy bodies: a clinicopathologic study. *Arch. Neurol.* 55:969–978.

Litvan, I., Mega, M. S., Cummings, J. L., and Fairbanks, L. (1996). Neuropsychiatric aspects of progressive supranuclear palsy. *Neurology* 47:1184–1189.

Longstreth, W. T., Jr., Bernick, C., Manolio, T. A., Bryan, N., Jungreis, C. A., and Price, T. R. (1998). Lacunar infarcts defined by magnetic resonance imaging of 3660 elderly people: the Cardiovascular Health Study. *Arch. Neurol.* 55:1217–1225.

Looi, J. C., and Sachdev, P. S. (1999). Differentiation of vascular dementia from AD on neuropsychological tests. *Neurology* 53:670–678.

Lopera, F., Ardilla, A., Martinez, A., Madrigal, L., Arango-Viana, J. C., Lemere, C. A., et al. (1997). Clinical features of early-onset Alzheimer disease in a large kindred with an E280A presenilin-1 mutation. *JAMA* 277:793–799.

Lopez, O. L., Becker, J. T., Somsak, D., Dew, M. A., and DeKosky, S. T. (1994). Awareness of cognitive deficits and anosognosia in probable Alzheimer's disease. *Eur. Neurol.* 34:277–282.

Lue, L. F., Brachova, L., Civin, W. H., and Rogers, J. (1996). Inflammation, A beta deposition, and neurofibrillary tangle formation as correlates of Alzheimer's disease neurodegeneration. *J. Neuropathol. Exp. Neurol.* 55:1083–1088.

Luine, V. N. (1985). Estradiol increases choline acetyltransferase activity in specific basal forebrain nuclei and projection areas of female rats. *Exp. Neurol.* 89:484–490.

Luis, C. A., Barker, W. W., Gajaraj, K., Harwood, D., Petersen, R., Kashuba, A., et al. (1999). Sensitivity and specificity of three clinical criteria for dementia with Lewy bodies in an autopsy-verified sample. *Int. J. Geriatr. Psychiatry* 14:526–533.

Lund and Manchester Groups. (1994). Clinical and neuropathological criteria for frontotemporal dementia. The Lund and Manchester Groups. *J. Neurol. Neurosurg. Psychiatry* 57:416–418.

Maddrey, A. M., Cullum, C. M., Weiner, M. F., and Filley, C. M. (1996). Premorbid intelligence estimation and level of dementia in Alzheimer's disease. *J. Int. Neuropsychol. Soc.* 2:551–555.

Marson, D. C., Annis, S. M., McInturff, B., Bartolucci, A., and Harrell, L. E. (1999). Error behaviors associated with loss of competency in Alzheimer's disease. *Neurology* 53:1983–1992.

Marson, D. C., Chatterjee, A., Ingram, K. K., and Harrell, L. E. (1996). Toward a neurologic model of competency: cognitive predictors of capacity to consent in Alzheimer's disease using three different legal standards. *Neurology* 46:666–672.

Martin, A., Brouwers, P., Cox, C., and Fedio, P. (1985). On the nature of the verbal memory deficit in Alzheimer's disease. *Brain Lang.* 25:323–341.

Masur, D. M., Sliwinski, M., Lipton, R. B., Blau, A. D., and Crystal, H. A. (1994). Neuropsychological prediction of dementia and the absence of dementia in healthy elderly persons. *Neurology* 44:1427–1432.

Mayeux, R., Ottman, R., Maestre, G., Ngai, C., Tang, M. X., Ginsberg, H., et al. (1995). Synergistic effects of traumatic head injury and apolipoprotein-epsilon 4 in patients with Alzheimer's disease. *Neurology* 45:555–557.

McArthur, J. C., Hoover, D. R., Bacellar, H., Miller, E. N., Cohen, B. A., Becker, J. T., et al. (1993). Dementia in AIDS patients: incidence and risk factors. Multicenter AIDS Cohort Study. *Neurology* 43:2245–2252.

McEwen, B. S., Alves, S. E., Bulloch, K., and Weiland, N. G. (1997). Ovarian steroids and the brain: implications for cognition and aging. *Neurology* 48:S8–S15.

McGeer, P. L., and Rogers, J. (1992). Anti-inflammatory agents as a therapeutic approach to Alzheimer's disease. *Neurology* 42:447–449.

McGeer, P. L., Schulzer, M., and McGeer, E. G. (1996). Arthritis and anti-inflammatory agents as possible protective factors for Alzheimer's disease: a review of 17 epidemiologic studies. *Neurology* 47:425–432.

McKeith, I. G., Galasko, D., Kosaka, K., Perry, E. K., Dickson, D. W., Hansen, L. A., et al. (1996). Consensus guidelines for the clinical and pathologic diagnosis of dementia with Lewy bodies (DLB): report of the Consortium on DLB International Workshop. *Neurology* 47:1113–1124.

McKhann, G., Drachman, D., Folstein, M., Katzman, R., Price, D., and Stadlan, E. M. (1984). Clinical diagnosis of Alzheimer's disease: report of the NINCDS-ADRDA Work Group under the auspices of Department of Health and Human Services Task Force on Alzheimer's Disease. *Neurology* 34:939–944.

Mega, M. S., Cummings, J. L., Fiorello, T., and Gornbein, J. (1996a). The spectrum of behavioral changes in Alzheimer's disease. *Neurology* 46:130–135.

Mega, M. S., Masterman, D. L., Benson, D. F., Vinters, H. V., Tomiyasu, U., Craig, A. H., et al. (1996b). Dementia with Lewy bodies: reliability and validity of clinical and pathologic criteria. *Neurology* 47:1403–1409.

Mehta, K. M., Ott, A., Kalmijn, S., Slooter, A. J., van Duijn, C. M., Hofman, A., et al. (1999). Head trauma and risk of dementia and Alzheimer's disease: The Rotterdam Study. *Neurology* 53:1959–1962.

Mendez, M. F., Mendez, M. A., Martin, R., Smyth, K. A., and Whitehouse, P. J. (1990). Complex visual disturbances in Alzheimer's disease. *Neurology* 40:439–443.

Mesulam, M. M. (1982). Slowly progressive aphasia without generalized dementia. *Ann. Neurol. 11:* 592–598.

Mesulam, M. M., Waxman, S. G., Geschwind, N., and Sabin, T. D. (1976). Acute confusional states with right middle cerebral artery infarctions. *J. Neurol. Neurosurg. Psychiatry* 39:84–89.

Milberg, W., and Albert, M. (1989). Cognitive differences between patients with progressive supranuclear palsy and Alzheimer's disease. *J. Clin. Exp. Neuropsychol.* 11:605–614.

Miller, B. L., Cummings, J. L., Villanueva-Meyer, J., Boone, K., Mehringer, C. M., Lesser, I. M., et al. (1991). Frontal lobe degeneration: clinical, neuropsychological, and SPECT characteristics. *Neurology* 41:1374–382.

Miller, B. L., Ikonte, C., Ponton, M., Levy, M., Boone, K., Darby, A., et al. (1997). A study of the Lund-Manchester research criteria for frontotemporal dementia: clinical and single-photon emission CT correlations. *Neurology* 48:937–942.

Mindham, R. H., Steele, C., Folstein, M. F., and Lucas, J. (1985). A comparison of the frequency of major affective disorder in Huntington's disease and Alzheimer's disease. *J. Neurol. Neurosurg. Psychiatry* 48:1172–1174.

Mitrushina, M., Satz, P., Chervinsky, A., and D'Elia, L. (1991). Performance of four age groups of normal elderly on the Rey Auditory-Verbal Learning Test. *J. Clin. Psychol.* 47:351–357.

Mohs, R. C., Knopman, D., Petersen, R. C., Ferris, S. H., Ernesto, C., Grundman, M., et al. (1997). Development of cognitive instruments for use in clinical trials of antidementia drugs: additions to the Alzheimer's Disease Assessment Scale that broaden its scope. The Alzheimer's Disease Cooperative Study. *Alzheimer Dis. Assoc. Disord. 11 Suppl 2:*S13–S21.

Monsch, A. U., Bondi, M. W., Butters, N., Salmon, D. P., Katzman, R., and Thal, L. J. (1992). Comparisons of verbal fluency tasks in the detection of dementia of the Alzheimer type. *Arch. Neurol.* 49:1253–1258.

Monsch, A. U., Bondi, M. W., Salmon, D. P., Butters, N., Thal, L. J., Hansen, L. A., et al. (1995). Clinical validity of the Mattis Dementia Rating Scale in detecting Dementia of the Alzheimer type. A double cross-validation and application to a community-dwelling sample. *Arch. Neurol.* 52:899–904.

Morris, J. C. (1993). The Clinical Dementia Rating (CDR): current version and scoring rules. *Neurology* 43:2412–2414.

Morris, J. C., Edland, S., Clark, C., Galasko, D., Koss, E., Mohs, R., et al. (1993). The consortium to establish a registry for Alzheimer's disease (CERAD). Part IV. Rates of cognitive change in the longitudinal assessment of probable Alzheimer's disease. *Neurology* 43:2457–2465.

Morris, J. C., Storandt, M., McKeel, D. W., Jr., Rubin, E. H., Price, J. L., Grant, E. A., et al. (1996).

Cerebral amyloid deposition and diffuse plaques in "normal" aging: evidence for presymptomatic and very mild Alzheimer's disease. *Neurology* 46:707–719.

Mortimer, J. A., van Duijn, C. M., Chandra, V., Fratiglioni, L., Graves, A. B., Heyman, A. et al. (1991). Head trauma as a risk factor for Alzheimer's disease: a collaborative re-analysis of case–control studies. EURODEM Risk Factors Research Group. *Int. J. Epidemiol. 20 Suppl* 2:S28–S35.

Murray, A. M., Levkoff, S. E., Wetle, T. T., Beckett, L., Cleary, P. D., Schor, J. D., et al. (1993). Acute delirium and functional decline in the hospitalized elderly patient. *J. Gerontol. 48:* M181–M186.

Navia, B. A., Jordan, B. D., and Price, R. W. (1986). The AIDS dementia complex: I. Clinical features. *Ann. Neurol. 19:*517–524.

Neary, D. (1990). Non-Alzheimer's disease forms of cerebral atrophy. *J. Neurol. Neurosurg. Psychiatry* 53:929–931.

Neary, D. (1997). Frontotemporal degeneration, Pick disease, and corticobasal degeneration. One entity or 3? 3. *Arch. Neurol.* 54:1425–1427.

Neary, D., and Snowden, J. S. (1991). Dementia of the frontal lobe type. In *Frontal Lobe Function and Dysfunction*, H. S. Levin, H. Eisenberg, and A. L. Benton (eds.). New York: Oxford University Press, pp. 304–317.

Neary, D., Snowden, J. S., Gustafson, L., Passant, U., Stuss, D., Black, S., et al. (1998). Frontotemporal lobar degeneration: a consensus on clinical diagnostic criteria. *Neurology* 51:1546–1554.

Neary, D., Snowden, J. S., Northen, B., and Goulding, P. (1988). Dementia of frontal lobe type. *J. Neurol. Neurosurg. Psychiatry* 51:353–361.

Neumann, M. A., and Cohn, R. (1967). Progressive subcortical gliosis, a rare form of presenile dementia. *Brain 90:*405–418.

Nicholas, M., Obler, L. K., Au, R., and Albert, M. L. (1996). On the nature of naming errors in aging and dementia: a study of semantic relatedness. *Brain Lang 54:*184–195.

Ochipa, C., Rothi, L. J., and Heilman, K. M. (1992). Conceptual apraxia in Alzheimer's disease. *Brain* 115:1061–1071.

O'Connor, D. W., Pollitt, P. A., Hyde, J. B., Fellows, J. L., Miller, N. D., Brook, C. P., et al. (1989). The reliability and validity of the Mini-Mental State in a British community survey. *J. Psychiatr. Res.* 23:87–96.

Olichney, J. M., Galasko, D., Salmon, D. P., Hofstetter, C. R., Hansen, L. A., Katzman, R., et al. (1998). Cognitive decline is faster in Lewy body variant than in Alzheimer's disease. *Neurology* 51:351–357.

Oppenheim, G. (1994). The earliest signs of Alzheimer's disease. *J. Geriatr. Psychiatry Neurol.* 7:116–120.

Ortof, E., and Crystal, H. A. (1989). Rate of progression of Alzheimer's disease. *J. Am. Geriatr. Soc.* 37:511–514.

Ott, A., Breteler, M. M., van Harskamp, F., Claus, J. J., van der Cammen, T. J., Grobbee, D. E., et al. (1995). Prevalence of Alzheimer's disease and vascular dementia: association with education. The Rotterdam Study. *BMJ 310:*970–973.

Ott, A., Breteler, M. M., van Harskamp, F., Stijnen, T., and Hofman, A. (1988a). Incidence and risk of dementia. The Rotterdam Study. *Am. J. Epidemiol. 147:*574–580.

Ott, A., Slooter, A. J., Hofman, A., van Harskamp, F., Witteman, J. C., Van Broeckhoven, C., et al. (1998b). Smoking and risk of dementia and Alzheimer's disease in a population-based cohort study: The Rotterdam Study. *Lancet 351:*1840–1843.

Ott, B. R., and Saver, J. L. (1993). Unilateral amnesic stroke. Six new cases and a review of the literature. *Stroke 24:*1033–1042.

Paganini-Hill, A., and Henderson, V. W. (1996). Estrogen replacement therapy and risk of Alzheimer disease. *Arch. Intern. Med.* 156:2213–2217.

Paque, L., and Warrington, E. K. (1995). A longitudinal study of reading ability in patients suffering from dementia. *J. Int. Neuropsychol. Soc.* 1:517–524.

Pasquier, F. (1999). Early diagnosis of dementia: neuropsychology. *J. Neurol.* 246:6–15.

Patterson, M. B., Mack, J. L., Mackell, J. A., Thomas, R., Tariot, P., Weiner, M., et al. (1997). A longitudinal study of behavioral pathology across five levels of dementia severity in Alzheimer's disease: the CERAD Behavior Rating Scale for Dementia. The Alzheimer's Disease Cooperative Study. *Alzheimer Dis. Assoc. Disord. 11 Suppl 2:*S40–S44.

Pearlson, G. D., Rabins, P. V., Kim, W. S., Speedie, L. J., Moberg, P. J., Burns, A., et al. (1989). Structural brain CT changes and cognitive deficits in elderly depressives with and without reversible dementia ('pseudodementia'). *Psychol. Med. 19:*573–584.

Perry, R. J., and Hodges, J. R. (1999). Attention and executive deficits in Alzheimer's disease. A critical review. *Brain* 122:383–404.

Petersen, R. C., Jack, C. R., Jr., Xu, Y. C., Waring, S. C., O'Brien, P. C., Smith, G. E., et al. (2000).

Memory and MRI-based hippocampal volumes in aging and AD. *Neurology* 54:581–587.

Petersen, R. C., Smith, G., Kokmen, E., Ivnik, R. J., and Tangalos, E. G. (1992). Memory function in normal aging. *Neurology* 42:396–401.

Petersen, R. C., Smith, G. E., Ivnik, R. J., Kokmen, E., and Tangalos, E. G. (1994). Memory function in very early Alzheimer's disease. *Neurology* 44:867–872.

Petersen, R. C., Smith, G. E., Ivnik, R. J., Tangalos, E. G., Schaid, D. J., Thibodeau, S. N., et al. (1995). Apolipoprotein E status as a predictor of the development of Alzheimer's disease in memory-impaired individuals. *JAMA* 273:1274–1278.

Pfeffer, R. I., Afifi, A. A., and Chance, J. M. (1987). Prevalence of Alzheimer's disease in a retirement community. *Am. J. Epidemiol.* 125:420–436.

Pfeffer, R. I., Kurosaki, T. T., Harrah, C. H., Jr., Chance, J. M., Bates, D., Detels, R., et al. (1981). A survey diagnostic tool for senile dementia. *Am. J. Epidemiol.* 114:515–527.

Pfeffer, R. I., Kurosaki, T. T., Harrah, C. H., Jr., Chance, J. M., and Filos, S. (1982). Measurement of functional activities in older adults in the community. *J. Gerontol.* 37:323–329.

Pillon, B., Blin, J., Vidailhet, M., Deweer, B., Sirigu, A., Dubois, B., et al. (1995). The neuropsychological pattern of corticobasal degeneration: comparison with progressive supranuclear palsy and Alzheimer's disease. *Neurology* 45:1477–1483.

Pillon, B., Deweer, B., Michon, A., Malapani, C., Agid, Y., and Dubois, B. (1994). Are explicit memory disorders of progressive supranuclear palsy related to damage to striatofrontal circuits? Comparison with Alzheimer's, Parkinson's, and Huntington's diseases. *Neurology* 44:1264–12670.

Pittman, J., Andrews, H., Tatemichi, T., Link, B., Struening, E., Stern, Y., et al. (1992). Diagnosis of dementia in a heterogeneous population. A comparison of paradigm-based diagnosis and physician's diagnosis. *Arch. Neurol.* 49:461–467.

Power, C., Selnes, O. A., Grim, J. A., and McArthur, J. C. (1995). HIV Dementia Scale: a rapid screening test. *J. Acquir. Immune Defic. Syndr. Hum. Retrovirol.* 8:273–278.

Price, R. W., Brew, B., Sidtis, J., Rosenblum, M., Scheck, A. C., and Cleary, P. (1988). The brain in AIDS: central nervous system HIV-1 infection and AIDS dementia complex. *Science* 239:586–592.

Prince, M., Cullen, M., and Mann, A. (1994). Risk factors for Alzheimer's disease and dementia: a case–control study based on the MRC elderly hypertension trial. *Neurology* 44:97–104.

Prince, M., Lewis, G., Bird, A., Blizard, R., and Mann, A. (1996). A longitudinal study of factors predicting change in cognitive test scores over time, in an older hypertensive population. *Psychol. Med.* 26:555–568.

Prince, M., Rabe-Hesketh, S., and Brennan, P. (1998). Do antiarthritic drugs decrease the risk for cognitive decline? An analysis based on data from the MRC treatment trial of hypertension in older adults. *Neurology* 50:374–379.

Rahman, S., Sahakian, B. J., Hodges, J. R., Rogers, R. D., and Robbins, T. W. (1999). Specific cognitive deficits in mild frontal variant frontotemporal dementia. *Brain* 122:1469–1493.

Rahmani, B., Tielsch, J. M., Katz, J., Gottsch, J., Quigley, H., Javitt, J., et al. (1996). The cause-specific prevalence of visual impairment in an urban population. The Baltimore Eye Survey. *Ophthalmology* 103:1721–1726.

Rapcsak, S. Z., Croswell, S. C., and Rubens, A. B. (1989a). Apraxia in Alzheimer's disease. *Neurology* 39:664–668.

Rapcsak, S. Z., Kentros, M., and Rubens, A. B. (1989b). Impaired recognition of meaningful sounds in Alzheimer's disease. *Arch. Neurol.* 46:1298–1300.

Read, S. L., Miller, B. L., Mena, I., Kim, R., Itabashi, H., and Darby, A. (1995). SPECT in dementia: clinical and pathological correlation. *J. Am. Geriatr. Soc.* 43:1243–1247.

Reddy, P. H., Williams, M., and Tagle, D. A. (1999). Recent advances in understanding the pathogenesis of Huntington's disease. *Trends Neurosci.* 22:248–255.

Reding, M., Haycox, J., and Blass, J. (1985). Depression in patients referred to a dementia clinic. A three-year prospective study. *Arch. Neurol.* 42:894–896.

Reichman, W. E., Coyne, A. C., Amirneni, S., Molino, B., Jr., and Egan, S. (1996). Negative symptoms in Alzheimer's disease. *Am. J. Psychiatry* 153:424–426.

Reisberg, B., Borenstein, J., Salob, S. P., Ferris, S. H., Franssen, E., and Georgotas, A. (1987). Behavioral symptoms in Alzheimer's disease: phenomenology and treatment. *J. Clin. Psychiatry* 48(Suppl):9–15.

Reisberg, B., Ferris, S. H., de Leon, M. J., and Crook, T. (1982). The Global Deterioration Scale for assessment of primary degenerative dementia. *Am. J. Psychiatry* 139:1136–1139.

Rinne, J. O., Lee, M. S., Thompson, P. D., and Marsden, C. D. (1994). Corticobasal degeneration. A clinical study of 36 cases. *Brain 117:* 1183–1196.

Roberts, G. W., Allsop, D., and Bruton, C. (1990). The occult aftermath of boxing. *J. Neurol. Neurosurg. Psychiatry 53:*373–378.

Rocca, W. A., Cha, R. H., Waring, S. C., and Kokmen, E. (1998). Incidence of dementia and Alzheimer's disease: a reanalysis of data from Rochester, Minnesota, 1975–1984. *Am. J. Epidemiol. 148:*51–62.

Rockwood, K., Ebly, E., Hachinski, V., and Hogan, D. (1997). Presence and treatment of vascular risk factors in patients with vascular cognitive impairment. *Arch. Neurol. 54:*33–39.

Rogers, J., Webster, S., Lue, L. F., Brachova, L., Civin, W. H., Emmerling, M., et al. (1996). Inflammation and Alzheimer's disease pathogenesis. *Neurobiol. Aging 17:*681–686.

Roman, G. C., Tatemichi, T. K., Erkinjuntti, T., Cummings, J. L., Masdeu, J. C., Garcia, J. H., et al. (1993). Vascular dementia: diagnostic criteria for research studies. Report of the NINDS-AIREN International Workshop. *Neurology 43:*250–260.

Rosen, W. G., Mohs, R. C., and Davis, K. L. (1984). A new rating scale for Alzheimer's disease. *Am. J. Psychiatry 141:*1356–1364.

Ross, G. W., Abbott, R. D., Petrovitch, H., Masaki, K. H., Murdaugh, C., Trockman, C., et al. (1997). Frequency and characteristics of silent dementia among elderly Japanese-American men. The Honolulu-Asia Aging Study. *JAMA 277:*800–805.

Royall, D. R., Mahurin, R. K., and Gray, K. F. (1992). Bedside assessment of executive cognitive impairment: the executive interview. *J. Am. Geriatr. Soc. 40:*1221–1226.

Rubin, E. H., Storandt, M., Miller, J. P., Kinscherf, D. A., Grant, E. A., Morris, J. C., et al. (1998). A prospective study of cognitive function and onset of dementia in cognitively healthy elders. *Arch. Neurol. 55:*395–401.

Sabbagh, M. N., Corey-Bloom, J., Tiraboschi, P., Thomas, R., Masliah, E., and Thal, L. J. (1999). Neurochemical markers do not correlate with cognitive decline in the Lewy body variant of Alzheimer disease. *Arch. Neurol. 56:*1458–1461.

Salmon, D. P., Butters, N., and Chan, A. S. (1999). The deterioration of semantic memory in Alzheimer's disease. *Can. J. Exp. Psychol. 53:*108–117.

Salmon, D. P., Galasko, D., Hansen, L. A., Masliah, E., Butters, N., Thal, L. J., et al. (1996). Neuropsychological deficits associated with diffuse Lewy body disease. *Brain Cogn. 31:*148–165.

Salmon, D. P., Thal, L. J., Butters, N., and Heindel, W. C. (1990). Longitudinal evaluation of dementia of the Alzheimer type: a comparison of 3 standardized mental status examinations. *Neurology 40:*1225–1230.

Samuel, W., Alford, M., Hofstetter, C. R., and Hansen, L. (1997). Dementia with Lewy bodies versus pure Alzheimer disease: differences in cognition, neuropathology, cholinergic dysfunction, and synapse density. *J. Neuropathol. Exp. Neurol. 56:*499–508.

Saper, C. B., German, D. C., and White, C. L. D. (1985). Neuronal pathology in the nucleus basalis and associated cell groups in senile dementia of the Alzheimer's type: possible role in cell loss. *Neurology 35:*1089–1095.

Schaie, K. W. (1989a). The hazards of cognitive aging. *Gerontologist 29:*484–493.

Schaie, K. W. (1989b). Perceptual speed in adulthood: cross-sectional and longitudinal studies. *Psychol. Aging 4:*443–453.

Scherr, P. A., Albert, M. S., Funkenstein, H. H., Cook, N. R., Hennekens, C. H., Branch, L. G., et al. (1988). Correlates of cognitive function in an elderly community population. *Am. J. Epidemiol. 128:*1084–1101.

Schneider, L. S. (1992). Tracking dementia by the IMC and the MMSE. *J. Am. Geriatr. Soc. 40:*537–538.

Schwarz, M., De Bleser, R., Poeck, K., and Weis, J. (1998). A case of primary progressive aphasia. A 14-year follow-up study with neuropathological findings. *Brain 121:*115–126.

Selnes, O. A., Holcomb, H. H., and Gordon, B. (1996). Images in neuroscience. Progressive dysarthria: structural and brain correlations. *Am. J. Psychiatry 153:*309–310.

Selnes, O. A., Miller, E., McArthur, J., Gordon, B., Munoz, A., Sheridan, K., et al. (1990). HIV-1 infection: no evidence of cognitive decline during the asymptomatic stages. The Multicenter AIDS Cohort Study. *Neurology 40:*204–208.

Seltzer, B., Vasterling, J. J., Yoder, J. A., and Thompson, K. A. (1997). Awareness of deficit in Alzheimer's disease: relation to caregiver burden. *Gerontologist 37:*20–24.

Shuttleworth, E. C., and Huber, S. J. (1988). The naming disorder of dementia of Alzheimer type. *Brain Lang. 34:*222–234.

Sliwinski, M., Lipton, R. B., Buschke, H., and Stewart, W. (1996). The effects of preclinical dementia on estimates of normal cognitive functioning in aging. *J. Gerontol. B Psychol. Sci. Soc. Sci. 51:*217–225.

Small, S. A., Stern, Y., Tang, M., and Mayeux, R.

(1999). Selective decline in memory function among healthy elderly. *Neurology* 52:1392–1396.

Snowden, J. S., and Neary, D. (1993). Progressive language dysfunction and lobar atrophy. *Dementia* 4:226–231.

Snowdon, D. A., Greiner, L. H., Mortimer, J. A., Riley, K. P., Greiner, P. A., and Markesbery, W. R. (1997). Brain infarction and the clinical expression of Alzheimer disease. The Nun Study. *JAMA* 277:813–817.

Snowdon, D. A., Kemper, S. J., Mortimer, J. A., Greiner, L. H., Wekstein, D. R., and Markesbery, W. R. (1996). Linguistic ability in early life and cognitive function and Alzheimer's disease in late life. Findings from the Nun Study. *JAMA* 275:528–532.

Solomon, P. R., Hirschoff, A., Kelly, B., Relin, M., Brush, M., DeVeaux, R. D., et al. (1998). A 7 minute neurocognitive screening battery highly sensitive to Alzheimer's disease. *Arch. Neurol.* 55:349–355.

Spillantini, M. G., and Goedert, M. (1998). Tau protein pathology in neurodegenerative diseases. *Trends Neurosci.* 21:428–433.

Stern, R. G., Mohs, R. C., Davidson, M., Schmeidler, J., Silverman, J., Kramer-Ginsberg, E., et al. (1994a). A longitudinal study of Alzheimer's disease: measurement, rate, and predictors of cognitive deterioration. *Am. J. Psychiatry* 151:390–396.

Stern, Y., Andrews, H., Pittman, J., Sano, M., Tatemichi, T., Lantigua, R., et al. (1992). Diagnosis of dementia in a heterogeneous population. Development of a neuropsychological paradigm-based diagnosis of dementia and quantified correction for the effects of education. *Arch. Neurol.* 49:453–460.

Stern, Y., Gurland, B., Tatemichi, T. K., Tang, M. X., Wilder, D., and Mayeux, R. (1994b). Influence of education and occupation on the incidence of Alzheimer's disease. *JAMA* 271:1004–1010.

Stern, Y., Tang, M. X., Denaro, J., and Mayeux, R. (1995). Increased risk of mortality in Alzheimer's disease patients with more advanced educational and occupational attainment. *Ann. Neurol.* 37:590–595.

Stewart, W. F., Kawas, C., Corrada, M., and Metter, E. J. (1997). Risk of Alzheimer's disease and duration of NSAID use. *Neurology* 48:626–632.

Storandt, M., Botwinick, J., Danziger, W. L., Berg, L., and Hughes, C. P. (1984). Psychometric differentiation of mild senile dementia of the Alzheimer type. *Arch. Neurol.* 41:497–499.

Storandt, M., Kaskie, B., and Von Dras, D. D. (1998). Temporal memory for remote events in healthy aging and dementia. *Psychol. Aging* 13:4–7.

Stout, J. C., Ellis, R. J., Jernigan, T. L., Archibald, S. L., Abramson, I., Wolfson, T., et al. (1998). Progressive cerebral volume loss in human immunodeficiency virus infection: a longitudinal volumetric magnetic resonance imaging study. HIV Neurobehavioral Research Center Group. *Arch. Neurol.* 55:161–168.

Stuss, D. T., Meiran, N., Guzman, D. A., Lafleche, G., and Willmer, J. (1996). Do long tests yield a more accurate diagnosis of dementia than short tests? A comparison of 5 neuropsychological tests. *Arch. Neurol.* 53:1033–1039.

Swearer, J. M., O'Donnell, B. F., Drachman, D. A., and Woodward, B. M. (1992). Neuropsychological features of familial Alzheimer's disease. *Ann. Neurol.* 32:687–694.

Talbot, P. R., Lloyd, J. J., Snowden, J. S., Neary, D., and Testa, H. J. (1998). A clinical role for 99mTc-HMPAO SPECT in the investigation of dementia? *J. Neurol. Neurosurg. Psychiatry* 64:306–313.

Tang, M. X., Jacobs, D., Stern, Y., Marder, K., Schofield, P., Gurland, B., et al. (1996). Effect of oestrogen during menopause on risk and age at onset of Alzheimer's disease. *Lancet* 348:429–432.

Tangalos, E. G., Smith, G. E., Ivnik, R. J., Petersen, R. C., Kokmen, E., Kurland, L. T., et al. (1996). The Mini-Mental State Examination in general medical practice: clinical utility and acceptance. *Mayo Clin. Proc.* 71:829–837.

Tatemichi, T. K., Desmond, D. W., Mayeux, R., Paik, M., Stern, Y., Sano, M., et al. (1992). Dementia after stroke: baseline frequency, risks, and clinical features in a hospitalized cohort. *Neurology* 42:1185–1193.

Tatemichi, T. K., Foulkes, M. A., Mohr, J. P., Hewitt, J. R., Hier, D. B., Price, T. R., et al. (1990). Dementia in stroke survivors in the Stroke Data Bank cohort. Prevalence, incidence, risk factors, and computed tomographic findings. *Stroke* 21:858–866.

Tatemichi, T. K., Paik, M., Bagiella, E., Desmond, D. W., Stern, Y., Sano, M., et al. (1994). Risk of dementia after stroke in a hospitalized cohort: results of a longitudinal study. *Neurology* 44:1885–1891.

Teng, E. L., and Chui, H. C. (1987). The Modified Mini-Mental State (3MS) examination. *J. Clin. Psychiatry* 48:314–318.

Teri, L., Larson, E. B., and Reifler, B. V. (1988).

Behavioral disturbance in dementia of the Alzheimer's type. *J. Am. Geriatr. Soc.* 36:1–6.

Terry, R. D., Masliah, E., Salmon, D. P., Butters, N., DeTeresa, R., Hill, R., et al. (1991). Physical basis of cognitive alterations in Alzheimer's disease: synapse loss is the major correlate of cognitive impairment. *Ann. Neurol.* 30:572–580.

Teunisse, S., Derix, M. M., and van Crevel, H. (1991). Assessing the severity of dementia. Patient and caregiver. *Arch. Neurol.* 48:274–277.

Thal, L. J., Grundman, M., and Klauber, M. R. (1988). Dementia: characteristics of a referral population and factors associated with progression. *Neurology* 38:1083–1090.

Tierney, M. C., Szalai, J. P., Snow, W. G., and Fisher, R. H. (1996a). The prediction of Alzheimer disease. The role of patient and informant perceptions of cognitive deficits. *Arch. Neurol.* 53:423–427.

Tierney, M. C., Szalai, J. P., Snow, W. G., Fisher, R. H., Nores, A., Nadon, G., et al. (1996b). Prediction of probable Alzheimer's disease in memory-impaired patients: a prospective longitudinal study. *Neurology* 46:661–665.

Travniczek-Marterer, A., Danielczyk, W., Simanyi, M., and Fischer, P. (1993). Ideomotor apraxia in Alzheimer's disease. *Acta Neurol. Scand.* 88:1–4.

Tyrrell, P. J., Kartsounis, L. D., Frackowiak, R. S., Findley, L. J., and Rossor, M. N. (1991). Progressive loss of speech output and orofacial dyspraxia associated with frontal lobe hypometabolism. *J. Neurol. Neurosurg. Psychiatry* 54:351–357.

van Belle, G., Uhlmann, R. F., Hughes, J. P., and Larson, E. B. (1990). Reliability of estimates of changes in mental status test performance in senile dementia of the Alzheimer type. *J. Clin. Epidemiol.* 43:589–595.

Varma, A. R., Snowden, J. S., Lloyd, J. J., Talbot, P. R., Mann, D. M., and Neary, D. (1999). Evaluation of the NINCDS-ADRDA criteria in the differentiation of Alzheimer's disease and frontotemporal dementia. *J. Neurol. Neurosurg. Psychiatry* 66:184–188.

Victoroff, J., Mack, W. J., Lyness, S. A., and Chui, H. C. (1995). Multicenter clinicopathological correlation in dementia. *Am. J. Psychiatry* 152:1476–1484.

Victoroff, J., Ross, G. W., Benson, D. F., Verity, M. A., and Vinters, H. V. (1994). Posterior cortical atrophy. Neuropathologic correlations. *Arch. Neurol.* 51:269–274.

Vonsattel, J. P., and DiFiglia, M. (1998). Huntington disease. *J. Neuropathol. Exp. Neurol.* 57:369–384.

Wade, J. P., Mirsen, T. R., Hachinski, V. C., Fisman, M., Lau, C., and Merskey, H. (1987). The clinical diagnosis of Alzheimer's disease. *Arch. Neurol.* 44:24–29.

Wechsler, D. (1981). *Wechsler Adult Intelligence Scale–Revised (WAIS-R)*. New York: The Psychological Corporation.

Welsh, K., Butters, N., Hughes, J., Mohs, R., and Heyman, A. (1991). Detection of abnormal memory decline in mild cases of Alzheimer's disease using CERAD neuropsychological measures. *Arch. Neurol.* 48:278–281.

Welsh, K. A., Butters, N., Hughes, J. P., Mohs, R. C., and Heyman, A. (1992). Detection and staging of dementia in Alzheimer's disease. Use of the neuropsychological measures developed for the Consortium to Establish a Registry for Alzheimer's Disease. *Arch. Neurol.* 49:448–452.

Welsh, K. A., Butters, N., Mohs, R. C., Beekly, D., Edland, S., Fillenbaum, G., et al. (1994). The Consortium to Establish a Registry for Alzheimer's Disease (CERAD). Part V. A normative study of the neuropsychological battery. *Neurology* 44:609–614.

Westbury, C., and Bub, D. (1997). Primary progressive aphasia: a review of 112 cases. *Brain Lang.* 60:381–406.

White, L., Petrovitch, H., Ross, G. W., Masaki, K. H., Abbott, R. D., Teng, E. L., et al. (1996). Prevalence of dementia in older Japanese-American men in Hawaii: the Honolulu-Asia Aging Study. *JAMA* 276:955–960.

Whitehouse, P. J., and Kalaria, R. N. (1995). Nicotinic receptors and neurodegenerative dementing diseases: basic research and clinical implications. *Alzheimer Dis. Assoc. Disord.* 9 Suppl 2:3–5.

Wiederholt, W. C., Cahn, D., Butters, N. M., Salmon, D. P., Kritz-Silverstein, D., and Barrett-Connor, E. (1993). Effects of age, gender and education on selected neuropsychological tests in an elderly community cohort. *J. Am. Geriatr. Soc.* 41:639–647.

Willingham, D. B., Peterson, E. W., Manning, C., and Brashear, H. R. (1997). Patients with Alzheimer's disease who cannot perform some motor skills show normal learning of other motor skills. *Neuropsychology* 11:261–271.

Willis, L., Behrens, M., Mack, W., and Chui, H. (1998). Ideomotor apraxia in early Alzheimer's disease: time and accuracy measures. *Brain Cogn.* 38:220–233.

Willshire, D., Kinsella, G., and Prior, M. (1991). Estimating WAIS-R IQ from the National Adult Reading Test: a cross-validation. *J. Clin. Exp. Neuropsychol.* 13:204–216.

Wilson, R. S., Beckett, L. A., Bennett, D. A., Albert, M. S., and Evans, D. A. (1999). Change in cognitive function in older persons from a community population: relation to age and Alzheimer disease. *Arch. Neurol. 56*:1274–1279.

Wolfe, N., Linn, R., Babikian, V. L., Knoefel, J. E., and Albert, M. L. (1990). Frontal systems impairment following multiple lacunar infarcts. *Arch. Neurol. 47*:129–132.

Wolozin, B., Kellman, W., Ruosseau, P., Celesia, G. G., Siegel, G. (2000). Decreased prevalence of Alzheimer disease associated with 3-hydroxyl-3 methyl-glutaryl coenzyme reductase inhibitors. *Arch Neurol. 57*:1439–1443.

World Health Organization (1992). Mental and behavioral disorders (F00–F99). In *The International Classification of Diseases, 10th Revision: ICD-10*. Geneva: World Health Organization, pp. 311–388.

Yesavage, J. (1993). Differential diagnosis between depression and dementia. *Am. J. Med. 94*:23S–28S.

Zakzanis, K. K. (1999). The neuropsychological signature of primary progressive aphasia. *Brain Lang. 70*:70–85.

Zhang, M. Y., Katzman, R., Salmon, D., Jin, H., Cai, G. J., Wang, Z. Y., et al. (1990). The prevalence of dementia and Alzheimer's disease in Shanghai, China: impact of age, gender, and education. *Ann. Neurol. 27*:428–437.

Zink, W. E., Zheng, J., Persidsky, Y., Poluektova, L., and Gendelman, H. E. (1999). The neuropathogenesis of HIV-1 infection. *FEMS Immunol. Med. Microbiol. 26*:233–241.

Zola-Morgan, S., Squire, L. R., and Amaral, D. G. (1986). Human amnesia and the medial temporal region: enduring memory impairment following a bilateral lesion limited to field CA1 of the hippocampus. *J. Neurosci. 6*:2950–2967.

20

Recovery of Cognition

ANDREW KERTESZ AND BRIAN T. GOLD

Recent advances in technology, especially in functional imaging and evoked potentials, have contributed substantially to our understanding of mechanisms and patterns of cognitive recovery in patients. Considerable progress has been made in the basic neurobiology of recovery using cell cultures, gene expression, grafting, and neural transplantation techniques. In this chapter, we shall deal with recovery at the neural systems level that is clinically, anatomically, and physiologically accessible. The study of recovery is more than just a practical consideration for the clinician to provide prognosis, or a baseline for therapy. It is also important because of the theoretical implications for cerebral reorganization. The study of clinical recovery in the human central nervous system (CNS) has been difficult because it requires that patients be followed for months or years. Clinicians observing patients in the acute state often do not have the opportunity to follow them for a long time, and rehabilitation specialists rarely see them during the early stages of their illness. Assessment of the efficacy of treatment is complicated by the difficulty of finding matching controls to determine the extent of spontaneous recovery. Those interested primarily in clinical and pathological diagnosis often disregard changes in performance and tend to view the neuropsychological deficit as

stable. Despite these pitfalls, a considerable body of information has accumulated on the recovery of cognitive functions. There are several reviews of various aspects of recovery (Finger et al., 1988; Kolb, 1995; Wilson, 1998; Johansson, 2000).

The mechanisms underlying recovery of cognitive, or for that matter, other CNS functions are incompletely understood. Before discussing the patterns of recovery in specific clinical situations, it is worthwhile to review briefly the major theories proposed to explain recovery of function, as well as some of the experimental evidence supporting these theories.

THEORIES OF RECOVERY OF FUNCTION

FIRST-STAGE RECOVERY

Recovery from brain damage due to stroke or trauma can be divided into two stages. The first stage is related to recovery from the acute effects of metabolic and membrane failure, ionic and transmitter imbalance, hemorrhage, cellular reaction, and edema. In stroke, the reestablishment of the circulation in the area of partial ischemia or "ischemic penumbra" (Kohlmeyer, 1976; Astrup et al., 1981), and reperfusion after thrombolysis (Zivin et al., 1985) are possible early mechanisms of recovery. The ischemic threshold of cerebral perfusion for membrane failure is around 8 ml/100 g brain tissue/minute, in contrast to the normal blood flow of 20 ml/100 g/minute. Therefore, damage can be reversed if blood flow can be elevated above anoxic values. The rapid recovery from neurological deficit after a stroke is often attributed to the recovery of function of the cells in this area of ischemic penumbra. The size of the ischemic penumbra has been estimated using measures of cerebral oxygenation and more recently by comparing magnetic resonance imaging (MRI) changes reflecting core infarct size with the larger areas of ischemia that include the ischemic penumbra demonstrated by diffusion-weighted images (DWI) and perfusion-weighted images (PWI). Many of the new neuroprotective agents attempt to minimize brain damage by protecting cells in the ischemic penumbra until oxygenation can be restored. Thrombolysis with newly developed biologicals such as tissue plasminogen activator (TPA) can produce dramatic recovery by reopening occluded arteries (reperfusion).

Alterations in tissue water and electrolytes, such as the development of edema in trauma and ischemia, are responsible for some of the early changes in the acute phase of injury and in the first stage of recovery. Some of the pharmacological treatments of initial trauma attempt to control cerebral edema. Use of corticosteroids, although undoubtedly valuable in treating the vasogenic edema associated with brain tumor, is controversial for treating trauma and is contraindicated for stroke because the brain edema that accompanies stroke is cytotoxic rather than vasomotor. Hyperosmolar agents such as mannitol and glycerol reduce brain volume and increase cerebral blood flow, but unfortunately have only a temporary effect, and may even produce rebound edema.

One of the important electrolyte changes in acute ischemia and trauma is the increase of intracellular calcium (Ca), which inhibits mitochondrial respiration. Calcium activates phospholipase and other lysosomal enzymes that destroy mitochondria and the cytoskeleton. Impaired membrane permeability in-creases Ca influx, which seriously interferes with neuronal functioning. Calcium channel antagonists not only inhibit Ca influx but also prevent the postischemic reduction of cerebral blood flow and reduce mortality in experimental animals. Some excitatory amino acids, particularly glutamate, influence Ca channels and, since Ca influx is considered a major mechanism of injury, pharmacological agents inhibiting the glutamate cascade and the opening of Ca channels may promote early recovery (Gelmers et al., 1988; Stevens and Yaksh, 1990).

Another mechanism of damage is the accumulation of free radicals. Various antioxidants and agents, called "lazaroids," mop these up, and may therefore promote early recovery (Tazaki et al., 1988). The restoration of high-energy phosphates depleted by ischemia also contributes to early recovery (Argentino et al., 1989).

The first few days and weeks after the onset of a stroke or trauma may be a critical time of regrowth, when partially damaged neurons start to regenerate injured parts and other neurons form new connections to compensate for ones that have been lost.

Feeney and Sutton (1987) suggested that a depression of the catecholamine neurotransmitter system might contribute to behavioral deficits following a stroke. Amphetamines, which increase catecholamine transmission, produced lasting improvement in animal stroke models.

Many of the neuroprotectives or recovery-enhancing pharmaceuticals are based on basic neurological and neurochemical research as described above. Neuropharmacological agents are often tried in both stroke and trauma. Several clinical trials are in progress for medications that have passed the scrutiny of animal experiments.

SECOND-STAGE RECOVERY

This chapter will focus on second-stage recovery of cognitive function. This stage takes place months or even years after injury. Second-stage recovery mechanisms remain largely unknown. A significant amount of physiological and functional recovery in this stage probably results from intact structures compensating for the functional loss. Axonal regrowth and collateral sprouting are important mechanisms in the peripheral nervous system and, in certain instances, in the CNS. However, in humans with large lesions that cause focal cognitive loss, compensation is likely effected by *(a)* ipsilateral physiologically and anatomically connected structures; *(b)* contralateral homologous cortical areas, or *(c)* subcortical systems hierarchically related to the damaged structures. Some of the theories of how cognitive recovery takes place will be summarized below.

Theory of Equipotentiality and the Embryogenetic Analogy

The observation that recovery occurs after destruction of a brain area leads to the conclusion that a particular function cannot be localized to a portion of the brain and contradicts the idea of rigid localization of function in the nervous system. One of the earliest opponents of cortical localization was Flourens (1824), who demonstrated recovery after ablative experiments in pigeons and chickens. Lashley (1938) based his well-known theory of equipotentiality on similar extensive ablations in rats. He also found 18 cases in the clinical literature in which he could correlate the degree of recovery from motor aphasia with the estimated magnitude of lesions in the frontal lobe. He considered this analogous to the finding that learning in brain-lesioned animals was positively correlated with the amount of remaining intact cortical tissue, and negatively with the extent of ablation. Lashley compared the plasticity of cerebral cortex to the embryogenetic capacitiy of the organism to develop fully from a fertilized ovum. Therefore, recovery may represent a continuation of the growth capacity of the organism that it manifested in its earlier development. Lashley also reviewed the evidence that there are certain basic areas of the cerebral cortex that are required to remain intact for compensation to take place. One of the prime examples of the concept of essential cortex is the visual striate cortex.

Diaschisis

Von Monakow (1914), who established the principle of diaschisis to explain second-stage recovery, used aphasia as the most obvious model for studying recovery. His theory of diaschisis stipulated that acute damage to the nervous system such as in stroke deprives the surrounding, functionally connected tissues from innervation, therefore, they become inactivated, similar to the previously well-known phenomenon of "spinal shock." As innervation is regained from uninjured areas, function returns to these undamaged structures. The phenomenon of diaschisis has been widely accepted and subsequently elaborated, with biochemical and physiological supporting evidence.

Even before Von Monakow's diaschisis theory, it was noted that sudden lesions produced more deficit than slowly growing ones. Dax (1865) suggested that left hemisphere lesions may not result in aphasia if the lesion develops gradually. Subsequent animal experimentation confirmed this "serial lesion" effect (Ades and Raab, 1946). Incremental, serial lesions adding up to the same size as a single lesion in one experiment created much less deficit and sometimes no deficit at all, as the animal compensated well after each smaller lesion. Small strokes often remain silent, and tumors may slowly grow to astonishingly large size without symptoms.

Regeneration and Plasticity

Whereas at one time it was thought that regeneration primarily occurred only in the peripheral nervous system, in the past several decades studies have shown regeneration in the CNS. Axonal regrowth has been demonstrated in ascending catecholaminergic fibers; growing zones tend to invade vacant terminal spaces (Schneider, 1973). In addition, neighboring neurons may sprout and send fibers to synapse on vacant terminals, a phenomenon called "collateral sprouting" (Liu and Chambers, 1958). Both regenerative and collateral sprouting have been demonstrated by Moore (1974) in the mammalian nervous system. Collateral sprouting appears to be more important, whether from intact axons or from collaterals of the damaged ones. Denervation hypersensitivity may explain why some central structures become more responsive to stimulation after damage (Stavraky, 1961). The remaining fibers from the damaged area may produce a greater effect on the denervated region, thereby promoting recovery. The opposite effect, however, has also been argued. The initial hypersensitivity could induce inhibition of function (diaschisis), and the appearance of collateral sprouting might reduce the denervation and the accompanying inhibition (Goldberger, 1974).

Neuronal plasticity following lesions has been shown to occur extensively in animals (Merzenich et al., 1983). Changes in cortical maps can occur with training or with experience (Pascual-Leone et al., 1994; Hallett, 1999). Cortical reorganization may be related in part to long-term potentiation of neurons (Bear and Malenka, 1994). Nerve growth factors, glutamate cascade and GABA inhibition, noradrenalin, and nitric oxide systems have all been found to be regulators of synaptic reorganization. There is increasing evidence that astrocytes take an active part in synaptic plasticity. Changes in membrane excitability, growth of new connections, and increase in dendritic spines have been demonstrated to result from enriched environment and training, and are likely to be mechanisms of second-stage CNS recovery (Johansson, 2000).

Redundancy and Vicariation

A somewhat different theory implies that there is a biological protective mechanism built into the organism, anticipating injury. Redundancy provides structures that can substitute for the damaged functions. The idea that some neuronal structures can take over functions that they were not associated with previously is called "vicarious functioning." This theory was first proposed by Fritsch and Hitzig (1870) and subsequently promoted by Munk (1881), who thought that regions of the brain previously "not occupied" could assume certain functions. Pavlov also argued for vicarious functioning and a large factor of redundancy, stating that there were many potential conditioned reflex

paths that are never used by the normal organism. Lashley (1938), however, thought that preservation of a part of a system concerned with the same function is necessary. Bucy (1934) performed "reverse ablations," removing areas first that were shown previously to be necessary for recovery and finding no deficits, which indicated that areas needed for recovery do not necessarily contribute to normal function. Clinically, it is evident that right hemisphere lesions do not cause aphasia in most people, even though the right hemisphere subserves some language functions, and may play a role in recovery.

Jackson (1873) promoted the idea that the nervous system is organized hierarchically, with higher levels controlling lower ones. Function is re-represented at several levels. Damage at higher levels releases lower ones from inhibition and leads to "compensation." Geschwind (1974) cited examples of neuronal systems that could take over function when released by destruction of higher centers: the spinal cord innervation of the diaphragm, which occurs when brainstem structures are damaged is one such system. Often mentioned examples of hierarchical representation are the existence of several cortical sensory systems (Woolsey and Van der Loos, 1970) or two visual systems with rostrocaudal connection in the occipital cortex and brainstem.

Hemispheric Substitution

Fritsch and Hitzig (1870) observed dogs after unilateral cortical lesioning and proposed that the opposite hemisphere was taking over motor function for the injured hemisphere. In adult animals, however, destruction of an analogous area in the opposite hemisphere did not interrupt recovery. In humans, observations of patients with hemispherectomies (Smith, 1966) and callosal sections (Gazzaniga, 1970) provided evidence that the right hemisphere is capable of assuming some speech functions, such as comprehension (nouns better than verbs) and automatic nonpropositional speech. Kinsbourne (1971) argued that the right hemisphere may be the source of some aphasic speech because right carotid sodium amytal injection produced aphasia in patients who had recovered from aphasia caused by left hemisphere strokes. In the adult, however, the extent to which this recovery occurs is finite, both in cases of hemispherectomy and in global aphasics. The language function of global aphasics with extensive perisylvian infarction is very similar to that of patients hemispherectomized on the left as adults. This suggests that the remaining language function in global aphasia is probably subserved entirely by the right hemisphere. That the restitution of speech is often due to the activity of the opposite hemisphere is known as *Henschen's axiom*. Henschen (1922) gave credit to Wernicke and other contemporaries for this principle. Nielsen (1946) further advocated the idea that the variable extent of recovery is related to the variable capacity of the right hemisphere to substitute speech. Geschwind (1969) also believed that there is a considerable amount of individual variation in hemispheric substitution. Some individuals can make use of certain commissural connections and can activate some cortical mechanisms in the right hemisphere more than others. Further discussion of hemispheric substitution takes place in the section Functional Imaging and Recovery (below).

Functional Compensation

Functional compensation explains recovery with a behavioral rather than a neural model. Instead of rerouting connections, the brain-damaged organism develops new solutions to problems using residual structures. Substitute maneuvers have been observed in various experimental situations. Luria (1970) formulated one of the theories of retraining called "dynamic reorganization," which explains how changes in the nervous system are affected by physiological shifts of function.

Motivational factors, which affect post-lesion behavior in animals, are even more important in humans. The experiments of Franz and Oden (1917), in which subjects were forced to use paralyzed limbs, provided evidence that intense motivation is effective. Stoicheff (1960) demonstrated the effect of positive and negative verbal comments on the performance of aphasics. Improvement was promoted by positive reinforcement, and worsening was observed with negative reinforcement. Many patients develop functional disorders superimposed on their organic deficit. A passive attitude and depression are particularly likely to impede recovery (Robinson and Benson, 1981). Depression following stroke is relatively common and will be discussed in the stroke section of the chapter.

RECOVERY FROM SPECIFIC COGNITIVE DEFICITS

FACTORS AFFECTING RECOVERY FROM APHASIA

Initially, most long-term studies of aphasic patients concerned patients in therapy. Vignolo (1964) was the first to include the objective assessment of untreated patients at various intervals. Subsequent studies of spontaneous recovery have been performed by Culton (1969), Sarno et al. (1970a, 1970b), Sarno and Levita (1971), Hagen (1973), Basso et al. (1975), and Kertesz and McCabe (1977). These studies are difficult to compare, because the methods of evaluation differed. The patient populations were not comparable, with some authors restricting their study to severe aphasics (Sarno et al., 1970a, 1970b; Sarno and Levita 1971) and others trying to look at an unselected population (Kertesz and McCabe, 1977).

Aphasia Type

Head (1926) recognized that some types of aphasia improve more rapidly than others. Different classification systems were used to group patients. Hagen (1973), for example, used Schuell's system (Schuell et al., 1964), whereas Basso et al. (1975) divided their patients into only two categories—Broca's and Wernicke's aphasics. Weisenburg and McBride (1935), Butfield and Zangwill (1946), Messerli et al. (1976), and Kertesz and McCabe (1977) considered Broca's or "expressive" aphasics to improve most; Vignolo (1964) considered expressive disorders to have a poor prognosis, but he did not separate Broca's from global aphasics, and the severely affected global patients influenced the results. Basso et al. (1975) did not find any difference between the recovery of fluent and nonfluent aphasic patients. The variability of conclusions, in part, reflects problems in classification. For example, an expressive disorder is found in many different kinds of aphasias, and the expressive–receptive dichotomy itself is misleading. Some studies only dealt with the recovery of certain symptoms rather than the overall aphasic deficits (Selnes et al., 1983; Knopman et al., 1983). The interval between follow-up examinations and the methods of assessment differed from study to study. In spite of these differences, several important factors in the recovery of treated and untreated patients emerge.

We assessed the recovery of 47 patients with aphasia following stroke who had both an initial examination with the Western Aphasia Battery (WAB) (Kertesz and McCabe, 1977) in the acute stages of illness and a follow-up test performed 3 months, 6 months, and 1 year later. The outcome was categorized on the basis of the aphasia quotient (AQ), a summary score of the WAB at 1 year post-stroke. Many of the global aphasics remained severely impaired. Although some regained comprehension, most remained nonfluent. Broca's and Wernicke's aphasics showed a wider range of outcome. Some patients with Wernicke's aphasia retained fluent jargon for many months. After a while, however, they lost their phonemic paraphasias and their language deficit consisted of verbal substitutions and anomia. Broca's aphasics had an intermediate outlook, just about evenly divided between fair and good recovery. Anomic, conduction, and transcortical aphasics had a uniformly good prognosis, with most of the cases showing excellent spontaneous recovery. To define recovery from aphasia, we used a conservative cutoff AQ of 93.8, which was the actual mean score of a standardization group of brain-damaged patients who were judged clinically not to be aphasic (Kertesz and Poole, 1974). This increases the specificity, but decreases the sensitivity of the total score. A cutoff of 100 would increase sensitivity, but decrease specificity for aphasic impairment. Final AQs indicated that 12 anomic, 5 conduction, 2 transcortical sensory, and 1 transcortical motor aphasic reached the criterion of recovery. Although this represents only 21% of the

93 patients having aphasias with various etiologies (Kertesz and McCabe, 1977), it represents 62.5% of the conduction, 50% of the transcortical, and 48% of the anomic patients. The overall prognosis, regardless of aphasia type, for the 47 patients followed for a year was as follows: poor for 28%, fair for 19%, good for 13%, and excellent for 40%. A significant number of patients who recovered by 3 months were not included in this analysis. Adding these would raise excellent prognosis to more than 50%.

We also studied the evolution of aphasic syndromes, which Leischner (1976) called "Syndromenwandeln." We documented the patterns of transformation from one clinically distinct aphasic type to another, as defined by subscores on subsequent examinations using the WAB (Kertesz and McCabe, 1977). We found that anomic aphasia is a common end stage of evolution, in addition to being a common aphasic syndrome de novo. Four of 13 Wernicke's, 4 of 8 transcortical, 4 of 17 Broca's, 2 of 8 conduction, and 1 of 22 global aphasias evolved into anomic aphasia. Reversal of the usual direction of evolution of aphasic patterns should make the clinician suspect that a new lesion has appeared, such as a degenerative condition, an extension of a stroke, or a tumor. Thus, for example, an anomic aphasic of a vascular etiology should not in the course of recovery become nonfluent, nor should the patient develop fluent paraphasic or neologistic jargon. A dissolution of language in dementia, however, may produce this kind of reversal of the pattern of evolution in vascular aphasia. There are some patients with Alzheimer's disease who have anomic aphasia initially, then subsequently develop a picture of transcortical sensory or Wernicke's aphasia (Kertesz et al., 1986). Most patients with primary progressive aphasia have pathology related to Pick's disease (Kertesz and Munoz, 1998).

Severity

The initial severity of the aphasia is closely tied to the type of aphasia, and it is considered to be highly predictive of outcome (Godfrey and Douglass, 1959; Schuell et al., 1964; Sands et al., 1969; Sarno et al., 1970a, 1970b; Gloning et al., 1976; Kertesz and McCabe, 1977). Unfortunately, it is not always considered in studies of recovery. The most severely affected patients show poor outcome, whether treated or not (Sarno et al., 1970b). Mildly affected patients, by contrast, more often recover completely (Kertesz and McCabe, 1977). Initial severity affects recovery rates in a complex paradoxical fashion, because patients with initially low scores may have more room to improve than those with high scores, who have reached "ceiling." Treated patients tend to be selected from the less severe groups and unless initial severity is controlled, studies of treatment should not be considered reliable. There are various methods of controlling for initial severity, such as analysis of covariance, using outcome measures instead of recovery rates or the change expressed as percentage of initial severity, or comparing patients who have the same degree of impairment.

Age

Transfer of function occurs more easily in the immature nervous system. Kennard (1936) became famous for demonstrating that unilateral precentral lesions in immature animals have minimal effects when compared with similar lesions in adults. In children, recovery from aphasia acquired before the age of 10 to 12 is excellent (Basser, 1962; Hécaen, 1976). Maturation of the left hemisphere appears to inhibit the language abilities of the right hemisphere. Lesions in the left speech area early in life, before this inhibition can develop facilitate the transfer of function (Milner, 1974). It has been proposed that the functional plasticity of the young may depend on the adaptability of Golgi type II cells (Hirsch and Jacobson, 1974). These cells remain adaptive, whereas cells with long axons responsible for the major transmission of information in and out of the CNS are under early and exacting genetic specification and control. In humans, the flexibility of these neurons may be terminated in the teens by hormonal changes. This may explain the age limit on the functional plasticity of the brain. It is of interest that acquisition of a foreign language without an accent also appears to be limited by puberty. Although comparisons between

species are risky, there appears to be an analogous effect of hormone levels on bird song acquisition (Nottebohm, 1970).

The influence of age is controversial in the adult population. There is a clinical impression that younger patients recover better (Eisenson, 1949; Wepman, 1951; Vignolo, 1964). Some of these studies include younger post-traumatic patients, contaminating the age factor with etiology. We demonstrated an inverse correlation between age and initial recovery rates (from 0 to 3 months), but when we excluded the post-traumatic group whose mean age was well below that of the patients with infarction, the trend just missed being significant (Kertesz and McCabe, 1977). Others have failed to show any correlation between age and recovery in etiologically homogenous populations such as those with stroke (Culton, 1971; Sarno, 1971; Smith et al., 1972).

Sex and Handedness

Specific sex differences in cognition between men and women have been shown primarily in spatial orientation and mathematical tasks, which are better performed by males. Normal males and females perform similarly on intelligence tests, and claims for sexual dimorphism in the brain, although numerous, have not been supported unequivocally. The larger size of the male brain, which on the average weighs 200 g more than the female brain, does not appear to be advantageous to recovery. Recent studies have shown sex differences in cortical density of neurons. Males have relatively less overproduction of neurons during gestation than females and this would explain their earlier vulnerability to injury, but later they may have more protection from injury because of higher neuronal density (de Courten-Myers, 1999). It was also assumed that females may have more bilaterally distributed language, therefore they would recover better from aphasia than males, but we did not find any sex differences in aphasia recovery (Kertesz, 1988). More recent studies also confirmed the relative sex equality in functional processing using positron emission tomography (PET) and functional magnetic resonance imaging (fMRI) (Frost et al., 1999), and found no sex difference in recovery (Pedersen et al., 1995).

The data from Subirana (1969) and Gloning et al. (1969) indicate that left-handers recover better from aphasias than right-handers. Gloning et al. (1969) also suggested that left-handers are likely to become aphasic regardless of which hemisphere is damaged. Right-handers with a history of left-handedness among parents, siblings, or children were said to recover better than right-handers without such a family history (Geschwind, 1974). The evidence for this is largely anecdotal. We looked at the few left-handers in our population and they showed a variable rate of recovery, not significantly different from the right-handed group. A larger population study could not demonstrate an effect of handedness or stroke laterality (Pedersen et al., 1995).

Anatomical and Functional Variations

The anatomy of the speech areas is variable, so that lesions of similar size may affect language differently in different patients. In addition, there may be some variability in the degree to which language is lateralized. Some studies, discussed above, assumed that left-handers are more likely to have language function in both hemispheres. Recently, attempts were made to correlate the in vivo measurement of anatomical asymmetries, particularly of language areas, with functional differences (Kertesz et al., 1990). Anatomical asymmetries, as measured on computed tomography (CT) scans, were correlated with recovery (Pieniadz et al., 1983). Global aphasics who had atypical asymmetries, indicating more bilateral or reverse distribution of language function, appeared to recover better. We have studied a wider range of fluent and nonfluent aphasics and could not confirm these observations (Kertesz, 1988). Anatomical asymmetries are complex variables interacting with the multifactorial recovery phenomenon, and more sophisticated multivariate analysis will be required to detect any effect. It could be that anatomical asymmetries, as we measure them, relate more to a handedness variable rather than language distribution, as suggested by some of our studies in normals (Kertesz et al., 1990), and this is

why we are not seeing an effect on language recovery. The individual variations in the intra- and interhemispheric distribution of various functional components may contribute to an important extent to the ability of the mature brain to compensate after a single nonprogressive lesion.

Intelligence, Education, and Health

Darley (1972) considered premorbid intelligence, health, and social milieu to have significant influence on recovery. Although intellectual and educational level influence what the patient and family consider satisfying recovery, Keenan and Brassel's (1974) study indicated that health, employment, and age had little, if any, prognostic value when compared with factors such as listening and motor speech (comprehension and fluency). Sarno et al. (1970a) similarly showed that recovery in severe aphasia was not influenced by age, gender, education, occupational status, pre-illness language proficiency, or current living environment. Other pathological variations, such as repeated stroke insults, cerebral atrophy, intercurrent latent dementia, etc., remain factors to be considered or even studied directly, although they are usually controlled by exclusion in most studies.

Time Course for Recovery

There is a considerable amount of agreement about the time course of recovery. A large number of stroke patients recover a great deal in the first 2 weeks (Kohlmeyer, 1976). The greatest amount of improvement from aphasia occurs in the first 2 or 3 months after onset (Vignolo, 1964; Culton, 1969; Sarno and Levita, 1971; Basso et al., 1975; Kertesz and McCabe, 1977). After 6 months, the rate of recovery significantly drops (Butfield and Zangwill, 1946; Vignolo, 1964; Sands et al., 1969; Kertesz and McCabe, 1977). In the majority of cases, spontaneous recovery does not seem to occur after a year (Culton, 1969; Kertesz and McCabe, 1977); however, there are reports of improvement in cases receiving therapy many years after the stroke (Marks et al., 1957; Schuell et al., 1964; Smith et al., 1972; Broida, 1977; Naeser et al., 1990).

Linguistic Features of Recovery

Various language components recover differently, contributing to the differences of recovery among patients with different aphasia types. Alajouanine (1956) distinguished four stages of recovery in severe expressive aphasia: (1) differentiation by intonation, (2) decreased automatic utterances, (3) less-rigid stereotypic utterances, and (4) volitional, slow, agrammatical speech. Kertesz and Benson (1970) pointed out the predictable pattern of linguistic recovery in jargon aphasia. Copious neologistic or phonemic jargon is replaced by verbal paraphasias or semantic jargon, and eventually anomia, or more rarely a "pure" word deafness, develops. The fact that overproduction of jargon is replaced by anomic gaps or circumlocutions indicates that there is recovery of regulatory or inhibitory systems. There are numerous language features that have been tested longitudinally. Kriendler and Fradis (1968) found that naming, oral imitation, and comprehension of nouns showed the most improvement. In the study of Broca's aphasics by Kenin and Swisher (1972), gains were greater in comprehension than in expressive language, but no such difference was found by Sarno and Levita (1971). Hagen (1973) found improvement in language formulation, auditory retention, visual comprehension, and visual motor abilities in a 3- to 6-month period after the onset of symptoms. Ludlow (1977) detected greatest improvement in digit repetition backwards, identification by sentence, and word fluency in fluent aphasics; while digit repetition forward, sentence comprehension, and tactile naming improved most in Broca's aphasics. Both groups showed the greatest gains in mean sentence length, grammaticability index, and sentence production index in the second month after onset of symptoms. We studied various language components in four groups of 31 untreated aphasics (Lomas and Kertesz, 1978). Comprehension of yes–no questions, sequential commands, and repetition were the most improved components, and word fluency (generation of words in a semantic category) improved least. In fact, word fluency remained impaired while all other language factors improved, indicating that the test of word gener-

ation measures a nonlanguage factor often assumed to be a frontal, executive function (see Recovery and Functional Imaging, below). This is corroborated by the observation that word fluency is often impaired in nonaphasic demented subjects (Kertesz et al., 1986). The highest overall recovery scores were attained by the low-fluency, high-comprehension group (mostly Broca's aphasia). The groups with low initial comprehension showed recovery in yes–no comprehension and repetition tasks, and patients with high comprehension recovered in all tasks except word fluency.

Lesion Size and Location in Recovery

The importance of lesion size has been discussed already in conjunction with theories of equipotentiality. Clinicians have repeatedly observed that recovery was proportional to lesion size (Kertesz et al., 1979; Knopman et al., 1983; Selnes et al., 1983). However, lesion size by itself does not account for all the variability in recovery, and lesion location is also a major factor that interacts with lesion size.

Our studies demonstrated the importance of structures that surround the lesion areas in the recovery process. Those left hemisphere structures that are connected with the opercular and anterior insular regions play a crucial role in recovery from Broca's aphasia (Kertesz, 1988). Patients with damage to adjacent areas, especially the inferior portion of the precentral gyrus and the anterior parietal region, have less recovery than those where these areas are spared, which suggests a role of these areas in compensation.

Similarly, in Wernicke's aphasia the second temporal gyrus, the insular region, and the supramarginal gyrus that surround the superior temporal area are instrumental in recovery (Kertesz et al., 1989). Damage to these areas results in persisting Wernicke's aphasia. Larger posterior lesions may destroy cortex that has access to a potential right hemisphere comprehension process. Certain subcortical white matter structures such as the temporal isthmus and the arcuate fasciculus are often involved in Wernicke's aphasia, and the temporal isthmus involvement correlates significantly with outcome in our study. Naeser et al. (1987) also found the temporal isthmus to be significant, but not the posterior structures. Selnes et al. (1983) concluded that the reversal of the suppression of left posterior temporal and inferior parietal region function by transsynaptic mechanisms appeared to be the most plausible explanation for recovery of auditory comprehension.

Lesion size is undoubtedly the most significant factor in the extent of recovery. However, important exceptions are seen in certain crucial areas in the left hemisphere that are more important for prognosis than others. Motor and premotor phonemic assembly mechanisms are elaborated by a cortical–subcortical network that can be partially damaged with good recovery. However, if both cortical and subcortical components of the network are impaired, recovery is much less likely. A similar complex integration of various structures takes place for the mechanisms of language comprehension, although interhemispheric connections seem to be playing a larger role in comprehension than in motor output. It seems that a restricted deficit in the dominant hemisphere auditory association area, the posterior superior temporal gyrus, and the planum temporale can be compensated for by the opposite or homologous hemispheric structures, or by surrounding structures in the temporal and inferior parietal regions and in the insula. However, when either of these compensating structures is affected, or when the lesion is large and precludes access to right hemisphere areas with potential language capacity, recovery is not as likely.

RECOVERY FROM COGNITIVE DEFICITS OTHER THAN APHASIA

Recovery from Alexia

Recovery from alexia is scantily documented. Newcombe et al. (1976) drew recovery curves for the performance of two patients who were followed—one for 6 months and one for 4 years—after removal of occipital lesions (abscess and meningioma). Without language therapy, the rate of recovery of the ability to read word lists was maximal initially and decelerated until 8 to 10 weeks after surgery, at which time a lower rate was achieved. Newcombe et al. (1976) classified linguistic errors

as (1) visual confusions (beg → leg), (2) failure of grapheme–phoneme translation (of → off), (3) semantic substitutions (berry → grape), and (4) combinations of these. "Pure dyslexics" tended to make visual errors, and patients with dysphasic symptoms showed more grapheme–phoneme mistranslations; semantic errors were rare. Mixed errors were numerous initially, with many neologistic errors occurring. In the residual phase the visual errors seemed independent of the syntactic class of words, but in cases of persistent aphasia, syntax had a marked effect; nouns were easier to read than verbs or adjectives. A study of recovery of phonological alexia is discussed in Recovery and Functional Imaging (below).

Whole word recognition can be selectively impaired due to brain damage and compensation occurs by a strategy of letter-by-letter reading (Patterson and Kay, 1982). This form of alexia is often seen without any language impairment. It was first described by Desjerine as pure alexia without agraphia, although its association with agraphia is frequent. There have been several attempts to treat these patients. The results are variable and the prognosis for spontaneous recovery is considered poor (Rothi and Moss, 1992).

Recovery of Nonverbal Function in Aphasics

Studies of aphasic patients have shown that performance on nonverbal intelligence tests is also impaired, with some interesting dissociations. Culton (1969) used Raven's Standard Progressive Matrices in testing aphasics and found that considerable recovery of nonverbal performance occurred after 2 months; no further recovery occurred after 11 months. Our own analysis of Raven's Coloured Progressive Matrices (RCPM) performance in aphasic patients suggested that, of all the subtests in the aphasia battery, language comprehension correlated best with performance on the RCPM (Kertesz, 1979).

Recovery of Neglect and Visuospatial Impairment

Lawson (1962) emphasized that unawareness of left unilateral neglect retards recovery and that active treatment is needed to overcome it. Campbell and Oxbury (1976) examined the performance of right hemisphere–damaged patients 3 to 4 weeks and then 6 months after a stroke, on verbal and nonverbal tasks, including block design and matrices. Those who demonstrated neglect on the initial drawing tests remained impaired on visuospatial tests 6 months later, in spite of the resolution of neglect. Other reports describe unilateral neglect remaining up to 12 years after onset. Visual neglect and the inability to scan the environment has been the target of rehabilitation by Weinberg et al. (1977). This was a controlled study of right hemisphere stroke patients using reading, written arithmetic, cancellation of letters, matching of faces, double simultaneous stimulation, and the Performance subtest of the Wechsler Adult Intelligence Scale (WAIS). The rehabilitation efforts included anchoring points on the left side, encouraging leftward head turning, decreasing the density of stimuli, and pacing visual tracking to prevent drifts to the right. The pharmacotherapy of neglect is based on the reversal of neglect by dopamine agonists and epinephrine in animals and humans (Fleet et al., 1987). Levine et al. (1986) found that recovery of neglect correlated negatively with sulcal atrophy. Although they did not find one particular area of the right hemisphere responsible for recovery, they thought that any of the multiple critical areas may have limited the duration of neglect. (*For a further discussion of neglect see Chapter 13*).

Cortical Blindness and Visual Agnosia

Recovery from cortical blindness and related syndromes of the parietal and occipital lobes has been described by Gloning et al. (1968). There appear to be regular stages of progression from cortical blindness through visual agnosia and partially impaired perceptual function to recovery. Sometimes syndromes of visual agnosia remain persistent (Kertesz, 1979).

Recovery of Memory

The etiology of the most frequently studied memory loss is trauma. The prognosis of post-traumatic memory impairment has been correlated with the duration of post-traumatic amnesia by Russell (1971): 82% of his patients returned to full duty, 92% of these in less than 3 weeks. Learning capacity may continue to be impaired after the acute amnesia has subsided (the post-concussional syndrome). The phenomenon of shrinking retrograde amnesia seen with head trauma (Russell and Nathan, 1946; Benson and Geschwind, 1967) suggests that during the amnestic period memories are not lost but rather cannot be activated (retrieved). Recent monographs on memory rehabilitation reflect the increase in the treatment of head-injured adults, funded by compensation schemes in industrialized countries (Prigitano, 1985; Sohlberg and Mateer, 1989).

Memory loss secondary to alcoholic, postinfectious, and toxic causes, when severe, tends to persist (Talland, 1965), whereas electroconvulsive therapy (ECT)-induced memory loss is rarely permanent (Williams, 1966). The acute amnestic confabulatory syndrome (Wernicke's encephalopathy) often subsides within weeks, becoming a more chronic state of Korsakoff's psychosis. Korsakoff, himself, was optimistic about the prognosis but did not have reliable reports beyond the acute stage. Later clinicians denied seeing complete remissions. Victor and Adams (1953) arrived at a more hopeful conclusion but noted that "complete restoration of memory is . . . unusual when the defect is severe." Amnestic symptoms from unilateral infarctions subside in a few months, but more lasting deficit occurs with bilateral posterior cerebral artery involvement (Benson et al., 1975).

RECOVERY ACCORDING TO ETIOLOGY

Much of what we know of first- and second-stage recovery from focal lesions originates from the study of stroke models in animals and patients. The role of etiology in recovery is considerable, therefore, each of the major forms of brain injury, such as stroke, trauma, and inflammation, will be separately discussed.

Recovery from Stroke

Stroke outcome has been extensively studied, some of it with population-based methods.

However, it seems the larger the study the less specific the conclusions. There is a great deal of variation, depending on the location, size, and nature of the stroke. Fatality varies from 15% to 50% at 28 days (Wolfe et al., 1999). Large-scale stroke recovery studies pointed out that early recovery in the first week is a good predictor of final outcome (Jørgensen et al., 1999). One of the common outcomes is dependency measured by the Barthel Index. This is a simple scale often used in stroke outcome research because it is so easily administered even by telephone. Another outcome measure, which is considered more sensitive than the Barthel Index, is the Functional Independence Measure, which samples more items in more detail. It also includes measures of communication and cognition, which are important components of post-stroke function (Keith et al., 1987). The Rankin Scale is an observer-related global measure of handicap which uses only five grades.

Depression plays an important negative role in stroke recovery. Although initially depression was considered to be more common with left-sided lesions, most studies show no difference between the two hemispheres. The incidence of depressive symptoms was 22% at 1 year in the Sunnybrook Stroke Study (Hermann et al., 1998). There is a relationship between the extent of neurological impairment and depressive symptoms, and also correlation with functional outcome. It is generally accepted that although these causes are interrelated, the treatment of depression is important in optimizing recovery.

The parallels between recovery of neuropsychological function and motor function are significant enough that a working knowledge of the principles is essential. There is an extensive body of information on the interaction between motor and neuropsychological recovery. The testing of hemiplegia is a more uniform procedure than the testing of neuropsychological disorders, and in spite of the variability, there is general agreement about many aspects. For example, recovery of the upper extremity is not as good as that of the lower extremity. Motion returns proximally and then recovers in the more distal portions of the arm. A study by Van Buskirk (1955) concluded that restitution of

function occurs chiefly in the first 2 months and appears to be a spontaneous process. When full recovery occurs, initial motion begins within 2 weeks and full recovery usually occurs within 3 months. About 45% of patients recover full motion, 40% recover partial motion, and 15% do not recover function of the upper extremity (when followed for more than 7 months). In a study of the role of cerebral dominance in the recovery of ambulation, right hemiplegics recovered independent ambulation more often and faster than left hemiplegics. The spatial–perceptual deficiencies of left hemiplegics were considered to be more resistant to recovery and hampered recovery of ambulation (Cassvan et al., 1976).

Encephalitis

Recovery after encephalitis depends on the etiology and the severity of the infection. Of all the encephalitidies, herpes simplex virus encephalitis (HSVE) is the most common. In the past the prognosis in this illness was uniformly poor, but this has been altered by treatment with acyclovir in the acute phase, especially if it is started less than 4 days after the first mental symptoms (Kaplan and Bain, 1999). The HSVE patients seem to be more severely affected than those with other forms of encephalitis (Hokkanen et al., 1996). Bilateral lesions tend to show less recovery. Many cases of encephalitis do not have definite etiology and there is an overlap between various types of viruses causing cognitive impairment. The frequency of pronounced memory impairment or dementia was approximately 13% in another study (Hokkanen and Launes, 1997). At times, intractable epilepsy compounds the picture, contributing to cognitive deterioration in some cases.

Traumatic Brain Injury

Penetrating head injury is considerably different from closed head injury. Furthermore, there is variation in the speed and path of penetrating missiles and in the severity of concussion. Post-traumatic recovery is therefore even more heterogenous than recovery from vascular insults.

Patients with post-traumatic aphasia recover better than patients with aphasia following stroke (Butfield and Zangwill, 1946; Wepman, 1951; Marks et al., 1957; Godfrey and Douglass, 1959; Luria, 1970). Complete recovery was seen in more than half of our post-traumatic cases (Kertesz and McCabe, 1977). Dramatic spontaneous recovery, such as global aphasia improving to a mild anomic state, occurred after closed head injury but not in patients with vascular lesions with a similar degree of initial impairment. Even though patients with traumatic aphasia recover quickly compared to those with stroke, severe persisting dysarthria often disrupts communication. A study by Ludlow et al. (1986) on Vietnam veterans showed that the lesions that produced persisting asyntactic or Broca's aphasia are large and involve subcortical structures and the parietal area in addition to Broca's area.

Performance skills on the WAIS took longer to recover than verbal intelligence in patients with traumatic brain injuries (Bond, 1975). The most rapid recovery occurred during the first 6 months; recovery then slowly reached a maximum at 24 months. Psychosocial outcome, which was affected by intellectual and personality changes, correlated negatively with the duration of post-traumatic amnesia.

Levin et al. (1982) have provided data concerning the relationship between the duration of post-traumatic coma and prognosis in closed head injury. A recent review by Levin (1998) of the outcomes in cognitive function after traumatic brain injury summarizes the investigation of cognitive recovery utilizing experimental cognitive tasks, including measures of executive function and discourse processing, in addition to reviewing neuroimaging and the potential for rehabilitation. A moderate to severe traumatic brain injury group was examined with neuropsychological, psychosocial, and vocational measures in three groups of Glasgow Outcome Scale (GOS) (Satz et al., 1998). Neuropsychological test performance negatively correlated with GOS with increased prevalence of depression and unemployability. The prognostic value of the severity of acute injury and the duration of post-traumatic amnesia (PTA) for recovery was examined in mild to moderate head injury with a Glasgow Coma Score (GCS) of 9 to 14 (van der Naalt et al., 1999). The PTA was assessed prospectively and outcome was determined by the GOS. Even though most patients still reported complaints, more than two-thirds resumed previous work. The most frequent complaints were headache, irritability, forgetfulness, and poor concentration. Behavioral problems were even more likely than cognitive ones to interfere with return to work. Outcome correlated better with the duration of PTA than with the GCS. The authors suggested that a more detailed outcome scale will increase the accuracy in predicting recovery.

Neurophysiological techniques have utilized event-related potentials as an index to cognitive function during recovery from head injury (Keren et al., 1998). The auditory P300 waves generated by unexpected auditory stimuli were analyzed including the latencies and amplitudes of P3, P2, N2, and N1 components. Increased P3 latencies were seen in more severely injured groups and shortening of the P3 latencies were observed with recovery. Similar shortening of latencies in recovery were found for the N2 component. These physiological changes were correlated with improvement in neuropsychological tests scores for short-term and long-term story recall and for word recall, particularly in the P3 component, which seemed to correlate best with recovery from closed head injury.

Mild head injury (MHI) or the post concussive syndrome (PCS) recovers in a variable fashion. The involvement of insurance claims, litigation, and the expense of rehabilitation makes this area very contentious. At times, poor correlation appears between subjective complaints and objective measures of impairment (Bernstein, 1999). There are many methodological problems in the objective evaluation of recovery in MHI. The base rates of many symptoms are high in the noninjured population and there is generally a failure to match controls to MHI subjects on demographic and motivational factors. Well-conducted studies usually show good long-term neuropsychological recovery. Unfortunately, there is poor specificity for the so-called post-concussion symptoms that occur frequently in non–brain-damaged controls (Larrabee, 1997). Persistent post-concussive symptoms are more difficult to explain but many consider them to be a function of litigation or somatization (Alexander, 1997). Traumatic brain injury in children and adolescents shows a similar pattern of recovery with sometimes unexplained persistence of symptoms. The shaken infant syndrome can produce severe shearing injury that is unique to small children (Guthrie et al., 1999). Adolescent athletes have received special attention because they suffer from concussion frequently and recovery tends to be taken for granted, even though there is often some residual cognitive deficit. Recovery is particularly difficult to measure in this cohort of developing individuals because return to baseline from an impaired state may not be sufficient, considering controls may show increased performance in the interval during which recovery is observed (Daniel et al., 1999).

Recovery from Subarachnoid Hemorrhage

Subarachnoid hemorrhage accounts for approximately 5% of strokes, and it tends to occur in younger individuals. The outcomes are variable depending on how much brain infarction or brain destruction occurs from the hemorrhage. Some patients recover remarkably even from severe coma if the hemorrhage has not caused significant destruction in the brain, sudden increased intracranial pressure with herniation, or cerebral infarction secondary to vasoconstriction. A follow-up study of a general subarachnoid hemorrhage population showed 40% cognitive impairment, and 50% had not returned to full-time work, for some because of physical disability (Dombovy et al., 1998). The rupture of anterior communicating artery aneurysms (ACA) has a particular tendency to impair memory. Some patients have severe anterograde amnesia and others, an associated executive impairment. The retrograde amnesia often shows a temporal gradient, which tends to attenuate with time as recovery takes place. Patients with more severe executive impairments have more extensive bilateral frontal lesions and less recovery (D'Esposito et al., 1996).

Aphasias resulting from subarachnoid hemorrhage have shown a wide variation in rate of recovery (Kertesz and McCabe, 1977). This variability is presumably related to the extent of hemorrhage and to the variable presence of infarction or tissue destruction. To some extent, the prognosis is predictable from the initial severity of the aphasia. It is of interest that some of the worst jargon and global aphasias have been seen following ruptured middle cerebral artery aneurysms. Rubens (1977) pointed out that the dramatic recovery from thalamic hemorrhage in one patient was caused by the distortion of neural structures by the hemorrhage, rather than by their destruction. Although hemorrhages can initially be devastating, the subsequent recovery can be rapid and surprisingly complete. Therefore, recovery studies should distinguish intracerebral hemorrhage from infarcts.

Anoxic Hypotensive Brain Injury

The cognitive sequelae of anoxic hypotensive brain injury following cardiac arrest is variable and good cognitive function can be seen despite initially severe coma. Therefore, good recovery was not predicted by initial GCS in individual case reports (Kaplan, 1999). Sustained coma for several days carries a bad prognosis. An exception to this, however, has also been published (Hopkins et al., 1995). This study also emphasized that similar admission GCS can result in different outcome. Cardiac arrest survivors recover from cognitive impairment to a variable degree. Time to post-arrest awakening is the most reliable predictor of long-term cognitive functioning. About one-third of the patients have delayed memory deficit on 6-month follow-up (Sauve et al., 1996).

RECOVERY AND FUNCTIONAL IMAGING

Investigations of cognitive recovery using functional neuroimaging can generally be divided into studies examining brain metabolic or cerebral blood (CBF) flow processes of patients at rest, and those examining brain activation patterns associated with the performance of some cognitive task. A wide variety of isotopes and imaging technologies have been used in each kind of research. Resting metabolic and CBF studies have used single photon emission computed tomography (SPECT), Xenon 133 (133-Xe) with detector probes, and fludeoxyglucose (FDG) or oxygen 15–labeled water ($H_2^{15}O$) with PET. Cognitive activation studies have also used SPECT, 133-Xe, PET, and, more recently, fMRI. Detection of cortical activation in functional neuroimaging depends on a multiplicity of complex physiological and technical factors. Physiological factors include the extent of adaptation, the balance of activation and inhibition, and anatomical and physiological variability. Technical factors influencing the results include the spatial resolution of the imaging technique, the field of view being imaged, and signal-to-noise ratio.

Primary candidates that have been proposed to support functional recovery are ipsilateral structures surrounding the infarct, and contralateral homologous regions. Thus far, resting metabolic studies have favored the ipsilateral network hypothesis. Using the 133-Xe intraarterial method, Nagata et al. (1986) reported that patients with good recovery of language showed a mean CBF of 60.4% of the normal hemispheric flow value. Good recovery of speech was correlated with the degree of regional CBF in the ischemic area in patients with non-embolic cerebral infarction (but not in hemorrhage patients). Similarly, both Metter et al. (1987) and Karbe et al. (1989) showed that language performance in post-stroke aphasia is related significantly to glucose metabolism in the left temporoparietal region of the dominant hemisphere.

Several early resting metabolism studies showed increase in right hemisphere regional CBF (rCBF) in patients demonstrating some recovery from aphasia, and interpreted the results as evidence for right hemispheric compensation (Knopman et al., 1984; Demeurisse and Capon, 1987). However, the results of subsequent studies using more sophisticated three-dimensional methodologies have suggested that diffuse right hemisphere CBF seen in early studies may reflect nonspecific activation and not actual cognitive compensation (Heiss et al., 1993; Iglesias et al., 1996). Iglesias et al. (1996) studied 19 patients suffering their first ischemic stroke. Cerebral metabolic

rate using PET and a full neurological profile was obtained within the first 18 hours following stroke, and again 15 to 30 days post-onset. The authors found no correlation between oxygen metabolism in the contralateral hemisphere and early neurological recovery. Heiss et al. (1993) used PET to examine the regional glucose metabolism of 26 patients following first ischemic stroke. Only the glucose value of the entire left hemisphere had a significant effect on the residual variance of the Token Test regression equation. Another metabolic study found glucose metabolism in specific left hemisphere loci, particularly the temporoparietal cortex, predictive of recovery of language comprehension 2 years post-onset (Karbe et al., 1995).

More recently, neuroimaging studies of cognitive recovery have examined dynamic patterns of cerebral activation during the performance of various cognitive tasks. These activation studies have attempted to pinpoint cerebral regions supporting the restitution of cognitive function following stroke or other cerebrovascular accidents (CVA). At the systems level, functional activation neuroimaging techniques attempt to fractionate language and other mental functions to establish various components of the processes, both in input and output modalities. Timing of the experiment, the connectivity of functioning (inhibition and excitation), and regional anatomical differences contribute to the complexity of these studies. The statistical evaluation can also be crucial in the results. The actual cognitive process under study is often accompanied by more generalized or strategic processing involved in searching, problem solving, effort, and other executive functions not specific for the target process. For example, in neuroimaging studies of language recovery, activation may represent more peripheral functions such as articulation rather than the actual associative process under investigation. To isolate the function being examined, activation resulting from the target process is compared with activation resulting from control conditions, which include nonessential cognitive and motor processes inherent in the target task. Functional PET and MRI use multiple single-subject analyses to study the mechanisms of recovery.

Cognitive activation studies provide further support for the ipsilateral hypothesis, with some evidence for right hemisphere contribution to recovery for select processes. Weiller et al. (1995) compare the rCBF patterns of six recovered aphasic patients with left posterior perisylvian lesions and six control subjects during verb generation and repetition. Compared to a rest state, control subjects activated the left posterior, superior, and middle temporal gyrus (Wernicke's area) and Broca's area during the verb generation and repetition tasks, and additional lateral prefrontal regions during verb generation. Control subjects showed only weak right hemisphere activation during verb generation and repetition compared to the resting baseline. Recovered patients demonstrated similar left frontal activation to that of control subjects in each comparison. However, patients also showed significant activation in right superior temporal and lateral prefrontal regions homologous to left hemisphere sites activated by controls. Weiller et al. (1995) concluded that recovery of language comprehension is mediated by a bilateral network of areas, including frontotemporal regions of the right hemisphere.

Different results were obtained by Heiss et al. (1997) who used PET to compare the rCBF of six aphasic subjects during word repetition and rest conditions. Activation experiments and language assessments took place at 4 weeks and 12–18 months following stroke. The three patients with eventual improvement in language scores showed significantly greater activation of left hemispheric speech areas, especially the left superior temporal gyrus, resulting from the repetition–rest comparison, than those without improved language scores. Heiss et al. (1997) concluded that recovery from aphasia depends greatly on the degree of functional integrity of speech areas of the dominant hemisphere. Right hemisphere activation was interpreted as a nonspecific involvement of the network activation in an effort to perform a complex task.

Warburton et al. (1999) examined the rCBF patterns of six patients with left hemisphere lesions who showed partial recovery of language and nine normal control subjects, during verb retrieval. The experimental task required subjects to generate verbs associated with heard nouns. Compared to a rest control condition, both patients and controls demonstrated activation of the anterior cingulate, medial premotor, and dorsolateral frontal regions of the left hemisphere during verb generation. Activation of the cingulate gyrus was attributed to attentional components of the activation task. All normal subjects and five of the six patients showed activation in the inferolateral temporal cortex. The one patient who did not show significant left inferolateral temporal activation performed very poorly on the verb retrieval task. Three of the six patients showed additional activation of right dorsolateral frontal areas. Importantly, however, similar regions were activated by four of the nine normal subjects. Thus, this study found that the rCBF patterns of recovered patients during cued verb generation were largely indistinguishable from those of normal controls except in the lesioned area, in which case activations were perilesional. The recovery of word retrieval after a left hemispheric lesion was dependent on the responsiveness of peri infarct tissue and not on a laterality shift of function. Warburton et al. (1999) emphasized the variable degree of lateralization of rCBF in other areas of the cortex, depending on the subject, calling attention to the importance of single-subject analysis for patient studies.

Thiel et al. (2001) compared PET activity during verb generation and comprehension (saying a verb in response to a noun) with resting activity in a population of patients with left hemisphere tumors. They concluded that compensation was associated with increased activation in left hemisphere regions outside the language areas. Leff et al. (2002) used a more specific listening task to words at different rates in a group of patients with left superior temporal region infarcts. Their results, also using PET, suggested a laterality shift, indicating compensation for word perception in homologous right superior temporal regions. This continuing controversy points out the technical and methodological complexities of these studies, including the paradigms used in functional activation studies, as well as the variability of the lesions. The difficulty evaluating the methodology and results of functional activation studies emphasizes the need for caution in interpreting results, especially if they are not supported by lesion evidence.

Functional MRI studies of recovery are as yet few. Miura et al. (1999) used fMRI study recovery of speech of a patient with Broca's aphasia. Two weeks after the onset of infarction, the fMRI signal was absent from the left frontal lobe during verbal tasks. Symptomatic improvement 4 weeks later was accompanied by an increased fMRI signal. Finally, 7 month's post-onset, when recovery was complete, the blood oxygen level–dependent signal had returned to levels similar to those observed in normal subjects during speech tasks.

A study by Small et al. (1998) suggests that it may be possible to use fMRI to assess changes in brain physiology associated with the successful adoption of novel cognitive strategies following language rehabilitation. The authors examined brain activation patterns of a patient with phonological dyslexia during reading before and after therapy. Before therapy, the primary focus of her activation during reading, compared to viewing false fonts, was in the left angular gyrus. The patient was then trained on a decompositional reading strategy emphasizing grapheme-to-phoneme correspondences. Following successful therapy and the adoption of a decompositional reading strategy, the fMRI experiment was repeated. The main focus of the patient's activation in the second fMRI experiment was in the left lingual gyrus, which suggests that successful language rehabilitation was based on the recruitment of a novel functional pathway.

We have used fMRI to study the partial recovery of semantic processing of visual words of a patient with a global aphasia (Gold and Kertesz, 2000). In a semantic task, the patient and a control subject matched on the basis of age, sex, handedness, and education background decided which of two visual words shared a closer semantic relationship with a third target word. In an orthographic control task, the subjects viewed the same words from the semantic task and made decisions about spelling. Although their performance was equal, indicating full task engagement by the patient, they showed strikingly different functional activation patterns resulting from the semantic–orthographic comparison. The con-

trol recruited a network of left hemisphere regions extending from the temporo-occipito-parietal junction through the middle temporal gyrus to the inferior frontal gyrus. In the patient, the same comparison activated a network of right hemisphere regions approximately homologous to left hemisphere sites recruited by the control and activated by non–brain-damaged subjects in other neuroimaging studies of semantic processing. The late age of onset of the patient's left hemisphere stroke resulting in a global aphasia and lack of any prior brain damage suggested normal lateralization of language processes in this strongly right-handed man. Results from the patient demonstrated the right hemisphere's ability for partial and selective takeover of visual lexicosemantic processing.

Evidence for similar right hemisphere contribution to recovery of visual language comprehension has been documented by Thulborn et al. (1999). These authors compared fMRI signal intensities in two patients with left-sided lesions shortly after CVA and again approximately 6 months post-onset. Patients read silently simple sentences (in an experimental task) and stared at a central fixation in a control task. Six males without neurological disorder also completed the fMRI paradigm. Compared to the central fixation control task, the sentence comprehension task activated a large bilateral network in the normal control subjects. When functional maps were averaged across control subjects, regions activated significantly by the reading–rest comparison were the inferior frontal gyri, posterior superior temporal gyri, intraparietal sulci, dorsolateral prefrontal areas (superior and inferior frontal eye fields), and the visual cortices. As expected, stronger left hemisphere fMRI signal in the control subjects was seen in the inferior frontal and posterior superior temporal areas, corresponding to Broca's area and Wernicke's area, respectively. In the two patients, the reading–rest comparison activated a bilateral network of regions generally similar to that observed in control subjects. However, over time, each patient showed increased activation of right hemisphere areas homologous to lesioned areas. Patient 1's fMRI signal in the inferior frontal cortex during reading, which was bilateral shortly following CVA, was lateralized to a right hemisphere homologue of Broca's area 6 months post-onset. Similarly, patient 2 showed increased recruitment of a right hemisphere homologue of Wernicke's area, and concomitant decreased response in Wernicke's area itself, from before CVA to 3 months post-onset and from 3 to 9 months post-onset.

In general, functional neuroimaging research suggests that the recovery of cognition following CVA is dependent on the responsiveness of peri-infarct tissue and not on a laterality shift of function. The degree of importance of the right hemisphere in recovery appears to be specific to some cognitive processes in which that hemisphere plays a role in the normal network, with some evidence for the influence of the contralateral hemisphere in the restitution of auditory and visual comprehension of language. Recent research with functional neuroimaging suggests exciting possibilities for the examination of physiological change accompanying successful rehabilitation. Future imaging studies of recovery will need to address issues of individual differences in degrees of laterality, age, education, and IQ.

REFERENCES

Ades, H. W., and Raab, D. H. (1946). Recovery of motor function after two-stage extirpation of area 4 in monkeys. *J. Neurophysiol.* 9:55–60.

Alajouanine, T. (1956). Verbal realization in aphasia. *Brain* 79:1–28.

Alexander, M. P. (1997). Minor traumatic brain injury: a review of physiogenesis and psychogenesis. *Semin. Clin. Neuropsychiatry* 2:177–187.

Argentino, C., Sacchetti, M. L., Toni, D., et al. (1989). GM_1 ganglioside therapy in acute ischemic stroke. *Stroke* 20:1143–1149.

Astrup, J., Siesjo, B. K., and Symon, L. (1981). Thresholds in cerebral ischemia—the ischemia penumbra. *Stroke* 12:723–725.

Basser, L. S. (1962). Hemiplegia of early onset and the faculty of speech with special reference to the effects of hemispherectomy. *Brain* 85:427–460.

Basso, A., Faglioni, P., and Vignolo, L. A. (1975). Etude controlee de la reeducation of language dans l'aphasie: comparaison entre aphasiques traites et non-traitee. *Rev. Neurol. (Paris) 131:* 607–614.

Bear, M. F., and Malenka, R. C. (1994). Synaptic plasticity: LTP and LTD. *Curr. Opin. Neurobiol.* 4:389–399.

Benson, D. F., and Geschwind, N. (1967). Shrinking retrograde amnesia. *J. Neurol. Neurosurg. Psychiatry* 30:539–544.

Benson, D. F., Marsden, C. D., and Meadows, J. C. (1975). The amnesic syndrome of posterior cerebral artery occlusion. *Acta Neurol. Scand.* 50:133–145.

Bernstein, D. M. (1999). Recovery from mild head injury. *Brain Inj.* 13:151–172.

Bond, M. R. (1975). Assessment of the psychosocial outcome after severe head injury. *Ciba Found Symp 34:*141–157.

Broida, H. (1977). Language therapy effects in long-term aphasia. *Arch. Phys. Med. Rehabil.* 58:248–253.

Bucy, P. C. (1934). The relation of the premotor cortex to motor activity. *J. Nerv. Ment. Dis.* 79:621–630.

Butfield, E., and Zangwill, O. L. (1946). Re-education in aphasia. A review of 70 cases. *J. Neurol. Neurosurg. Psychiatry* 9:75–79.

Campbell, D. C., and Oxbury, J. M. (1976). Recovery from unilateral visuospatial neglect. *Cortex* 12:303–312.

Cassvan, A., Ross, P. L., Dyer, P. R., and Zane, L. (1976). Lateralization in stroke syndromes as a factor in ambulation. *Arch. Phys. Med. Rehabil.* 57:583–587.

Culton, G. L. (1969). Spontaneous recovery from aphasia. *J. Speech Hear. Res.* 12:825–832.

Culton, G. L. (1971). Reaction to age as a factor in chronic aphasia in stroke patients. *J. Speech Hear. Disord.* 36:563–564.

Daniel, J. C., Olesniewicz, M. H., Reeves, D. L., Tam, D., Bleiberg, J., Thatcher, R., and Salazar, A. (1999). Repeated measures of cognitive processing efficiency in adolescent athletes: implications for monitoring recovery from concussion. *Neuropsychiatry Neuropsychol. Behav. Neurol.* 12:167–169.

Darley, F. L. (1972). The efficacy of language rehabilitation in aphasia. *J. Speech Hear. Disord.* 30:3–22.

Dax, M. (1865). Lesions de la moitie gauche de l'encephale coincivant avec l'oubli des signes de la pensee. Paris: *Gaz. Hebd. Med. Chir.*

Dax, M. (1865). Lésions de la moitié gauche de l'encephale coincivant avec l'oubli des signes de la pensée. *Gaz Hebd. Med. Chir:* 2éme série 2.

de Courten-Myers, G. M. (1999). The human cerebral cortex: gender differences in structure and function. *J. Neuropathol. Exp. Neurol.* 58:217–226.

Demeurisse, G., and Capon, A. (1987). Language recovery in aphasic stroke patients: clinical, CT and CBF studies. *Aphasiology* 1:301–315.

D'Esposito, M., Alexander, M. P., Fischer, R., McGlinchey-Berroth, R., and O'Connor, M. (1996). Recovery of memory and executive function following anterior communicating artery aneurysm rupture. *J. Int. Neuropsychol. Soc.* 2:565–570.

Dombovy, M. L., Drew-Cates, J., and Serdans, R. (1998). Recovery and rehabilitation following subarachnoid haemorrhage: part II. Long-term follow-up. *Brain Inj.* 12:887–894.

Eisenson, J. (1949). Prognostic factors related to language rehabilitation in aphasic patients. *J. Speech Hear. Disord.* 14:262–264.

Feeney, D. M., and Sutton, R. L. (1987). Pharmacotherapy for recovery of function after brain injury. *CRC Crit. Rev. Neurobiol.* 3:135–197.

Finger, S., LeVere, T. E., Almli, C. R., and Stein, D. G. (1988). *Brain Injury and Recovery: Theoretical and Controversial Issues*. New York: Plenum Press.

Fleet, W. S., Valenstein, E., Watson, R. T., and Heilman, K. M. (1987). Dopamine agonist therapy for neglect in humans. *Neurology* 37:1765–1771.

Flourens, P. (1824). *Recherches Experimentales sur les Proprietes et les Fonctions du Systeme Nerveux dans les Animaux Vertebres*. Paris: Cervot.

Franz, S. I., and Oden, R. (1917). On cerebral motor control: the recovery from experimentally produced hemiplegia. *Psychobiology* 1:3–18.

Fritsch, G., and Hitzig, E. (1870). Uber die elektrische Erregbarkeit des Grosshirns. *Arch. Anat. Physiol. (Leipzig)* 37:300–332.

Frost, J. A., Binder, J. R., Springer, J. A., Hammeke, T. A., Bellgowan, P. S. F., Rao, S. M., and Cox, R. W. (1999). Language processing is strongly left lateralized in both sexes. Evidence from functional MRI. *Brain* 122:199–208.

Gazzaniga, M. S. (1970). *The Bissected Brain*. New York: Appleton.

Gelmers, H. J., Gorter, K., DeWeerdt, C. J., and Wiezer, H. J. A. (1988). A controlled trial of nimodopine in acute ischemic stroke. *N. Engl. J. Med.* 318:203–207.

Geschwind, N. (1969). Problems in the anatomical understanding of the aphasias. In *Contributions to Clinical Neuropsychology*, A. Benton (ed.). Chicago: Aldine, pp. 107–128.

Geschwind, N. (1974). Late changes in the nervous system: an overview. In *Plasticity and Recovery of Function in the Central Nervous System*, D. Stein, J. Rosen, and N. Butters (eds.). New York: Academic Press, pp. 467–508.

Gloning, I., Gloning, K., and Haff, H. (1968). *Neuropsychological Symptoms and Syndromes in Lesions of the Occipital Lobes and Adjacent Areas*. Paris: Gauthier-Villars.

Gloning, I., Gloning, K., Haub, G., and Quatember, R. (1969). Comparison of verbal behavior in right-handed and non–right-handed patients with anatomically verified lesion of one hemisphere. *Cortex* 5:43–52.

Gloning, K., Trappl, R., Heiss, W. D., and Quatember, R. (eds.). (1976). *Prognosis and Speech Therapy in Aphasia in Neurolinguistics. 4. Recovery in Aphasics*. Amsterdam: Swets & Zeitlinger.

Godfrey, C. M., and Douglass, E. (1959). The recovery process in aphasia. *CMAJ* 80:618–624.

Gold, B. T., and Kertesz, A. (2000). Right hemisphere semantic processing of visual words in an aphasic patient: an fMRI study. *Brain Lang.* 73:456–465.

Goldberger, M. E. (1974). Recovery of movement after CNS lesions in monkeys. In *Plasticity and Recovery of Function in the Central Nervous System*, D. Stein, J. Rosen, and N. Butters (eds.). New York: Academic Press, pp. 265–237.

Guthrie, E., Mast, J., Richards, P., McQuaid, M., and Pavlakis, S. (1999). Traumatic brain injury in children and adolescents. *Child Adolesc. Psychiatr. Clin. North Am.* 8:807–826.

Hagen, C. (1973). Communication abilities in hemiplegia: effect of speech therapy. *Arch. Phys. Med. Rehabil.* 54:454–463.

Hallett, M. (1999). Plasticity in the human motor system. *Neuroscientist* 5:324–332.

Head, H. (1926). *Aphasia and Kindred Disorders of Speech*. Cambridge, UK: Cambridge University Press.

Hécaen, H. (1976). Acquired aphasia in children and the ontogenesis of hemispheric functional specialization. *Brain Lang.* 3:114–134.

Heiss, W.-D., Karbe, H., Weber-Luxenburger, G., Herholz, K., Kessler, J., Pietrzyk, U., and Pawlik, G. (1997). Speech-induced cerebral metabolic activation reflects recovery from aphasia. *J. Neurol. Sci.* 145:213–217.

Heiss, W.-D., Kessler, J., Karbe, H., Fink, G. R., and Pawlik, G. (1993). Cerebral glucose metabolism as a predictor of recovery from aphasia in ischemic stroke. *Arch. Neurol.* 50:958–964.

Henschen, S. E. (1922). *Klinische und anatomische Beitrage zur Pathologie des Gehirns, Vols. 5, 6, 7*. Stockholm: Nordiska Bokhandelin.

Hermann, N., Black, S. E., Lawrence, J., Szekely, C., and Szalai, J. P. (1998). The Sunnybrook Stroke Study: a prospective study of depressive symptoms and functional outcome. *Stroke* 29:618–624.

Hirsch, H. V. B., and Jacobson, M. (1974). The perfect brain. In *Fundamentals of Psychobiology*, M. S. Gazzaniga and C. B. Blakemore (eds.). New York: Academic Press.

Hokkanen, L., and Launes, J. (1997). Cognitive recovery instead of decline after acute encephalitis: a prospective follow-up study. *J. Neurol. Neurosurg. Psychiatry 63*:222–227.

Hokkanen, L., Poutiainen, E., Valanne, L., Salonen, O., Iivanainen, M., and Launes, J. (1996). Cognitive impairment after acute encephalitis: comparison of herpes simplex and other aetiologies. *J. Neurol. Neurosurg. Psychiatry 61*:478–484.

Hopkins, R. O., Gale, S. D., Johnson, S. C., Anderson, C. V., Bigler, E. D., Blatter, D. D., and Weaver, L. K. (1995). Severe anoxia with and without concomitant brain atrophy and neuropsychological impairments. *J. Int. Neuropsychol. Soc. 1*:501–509.

Iglesias, S., Marchal, G., Rioux, P., et al. (1996). Do changes in oxygen metabolism in the unaffected cerebral hemisphere underlie early neurological recovery after stroke? A positron emission tomography study. *Stroke 27*:1192–1199.

Jackson, J. H. (1873). On the anatomical and physiological localization of movements in the brain. *Lancet 1*:84–85, 162–164, 232–234.

Johansson, B. B. (2000). Brain plasticity and stroke rehabilitation: The Willis Lecture. *Stroke 31*:223–230.

Jørgensen, H. S., Reith, J., Nakayama, H., Kammersgaard, L. P., Raaschou, H. O., and Skyhøj Olsen, T. (1999). What determines good recovery in patients with the most severe strokes? The Copenhagen Stroke Study. *Stroke 30*:2008–2012.

Kaplan, C. P. (1999). Anoxic–hypotensive brain injury: neuropsychological performance at 1 month as an indicator of recovery. *Brain Inj. 13*:304–310.

Kaplan C. P., and Bain, K. P. (1999). Cognitive outcome after emergent treatment of acute herpes simplex encephalitis with acyclovir. *Brain Inj. 13*:935–941.

Karbe, H., Herholz, K., Szelies, B., Pawlik, G., Wienhard, K., and Heiss, W. D. (1989). Regional metabolic correlates of Token test results in cortical and subcortical left hemispheric infarction. *Neurology 39*:1083–1088.

Karbe, H., Kessler, J., Herholz, K., Fink, G. R., and Heiss, W.-D. (1995). Long-term prognosis of poststroke aphasia studied with positron emission tomography. *Arch. Neurol. 52*:186–190.

Keenan, S. S., and Brassel, E. G. (1974). A study of factors related to prognosis for individual aphasic patients. *J. Speech Hear. Disord. 39*:257–269.

Keith, R. A., Granger, C. V., Hamilton, B. B., and Sherwin, F. S. (1987). The Functional Independence Measure: a new tool for rehabilitation. In: *Advances in Clinical Rehabilitation*, M. G. Eisenberg and R. C. Grzesiak (eds.). New York: Springer-Verlag, pp. 6–18.

Kenin, M., and Swisher, L. (1972). A study of pattern of recovery in aphasia. *Cortex 8*:56–68.

Kennard, M. A. (1936). Age and other factors in motor recovery from precentral lesions in monkeys. *Am. J. Physiol. 115*:138–146.

Keren O., Ben-Dror, S., Stern, M. J., Golberg, G., and Groswasser, Z. (1998). Event-related potentials as an index of cognitive function during recovery from severe closed head injury. *J. Head. Trauma Rehabil. 13*:15–30.

Kertesz, A. (1979). *Aphasia and Associated Disorders: Taxonomy, Localization and Recovery*. New York: Grune & Stratton.

Kertesz, A. (1988). What do we learn from aphasia? In *Advances in Neurology, Vol. 47: Functional Recovery in Neurological Disease*, S. G. Waxman (ed.). New York: Raven Press, pp. 277–292.

Kertesz, A.; Appell, J., and Fisman, M. (1986). The dissolution of language in Alzheimer's disease. *Can. J. Neurol. Sci. 13*:415–418.

Kertesz, A., and Benson, D. F. (1970). Neologistic jargon: a clinicopathological study. *Cortex 6*: 362–387.

Kertesz, A., Dennis, S., Polk, M., and McCabe, P. (1989). The structural determinants of recovery in Wernicke's aphasia. *Neurology 39(Suppl 1)*: 177.

Kertesz, A., Harlock, W., and Coates, R. (1979). Computer tomographic localization, lesion size and prognosis in aphasia. *Brain Lang. 3*:34–50.

Kertesz, A., and McCabe, P. (1977). Recovery patterns and prognosis in aphasia. *Brain 100*:1–18.

Kertsz, A., and Munoz, D. G. (1998). *Pick's Disease and Pick Complex*. New York: Wiley-Liss.

Kertesz, A., Polk, M., Black, S. E., and Howell, J. (1990). Sex, handedness, and the morphometry of cerebral asymmetries on magnetic resonance imaging. *Brain Res. 530*:40–48.

Kertesz, A., and Poole, E. (1974). The aphasia quotient: the taxonomic approach to measurement of aphasic disability. *Can. J. Neurol. Sci. 1*:7–16.

Kinsbourne, M. (1971), The minor cerebral hemisphere as a source of aphasic speech. *Arch. Neurol. 25*:302–306.

Knopman, D. S., Rubens, A. B., Selnes, O. R.,

Klassen, A. C., et al. (1984). Mechanisms of recovery from aphasia: evidence from serial xenon 133 cerebral blood flow studies. *Ann. Neurol.* 15:530–535.

Knopman, D. S., Selnes, O. A., Niccum, N., Rubens, A. B., Yock, D., and Larson, D. (1983). A longitudinal study of speech fluency in aphasia: CT correlates of recovery and persistent nonfluency. *Neurology* 33:1170–1178.

Kohlmeyer, K. (1976). Aphasia due to focal disorders of cerebral circulation: some aspects of localization and of spontaneous recovery. In *Neurolinguistics. 4. Recovery in Aphasics.* Y. Lebrun and R. Hoops (eds). Amsterdam: Swets & Zeitlinger, pp. 79–95.

Kolb, B. (1995). *Plasticity and Behaviour.* Hillsdale, NJ: Lawrence Erlbaum Associates.

Kreindler, A., and Fradis, A. (1968). *Performances in Aphasia: A Neurodynamical, Diagnostic and Psychological Study.* Paris: Gauthier-Villars.

Larrabee, G. J. (1997). Neuropsychological outcome, post-concussion symptoms, and forensic considerations in mild closed head trauma. *Semin. Clin. Neuropsychiatry* 2:196–206.

Lashley, K. S. (1938). Factors limiting recovery after central nervous lesions. *J. Nerv. Ment. Dis.* 88:733–755.

Lawson, I. R. (1962). Visual–spatial neglect in lesions of the right cerebral hemisphere: a study in recovery. *Neurology* 12:23–33.

Leff, A., Crinion, J., Scott, S., Turkheimer, F., Howard, D., and Wise, R. (2002). A physiological change in the homotopic cortex following left posterior temporal lobe infarction. *Ann. Neurol.* 51:553–558.

Leischner, A. (1976). *Aptitude of Aphasics for Language Treatment in Neurolinguistics. 4. Recovery of Aphasics.* Amsterdam: Swets and Zeitlinger.

Levin, H. S. (1998). Cognitive function outcomes after traumatic brain injury. *Curr. Opin. Neurol.* 11:643–646.

Levin, H. S., Benton, A. L., and Grossman, R. G. (1982). *Neurobehavioral Consequences of Closed Head Injury.* Oxford: Oxford University Press.

Levine, D. N., Warach, J. D., Benowitz, L., and Calvanio, R. (1986). Left spatial neglect: effects of lesion size and premorbid brain atrophy on severity and recovery following right cerebral infarction. *Neurology* 36:362–366.

Liu, C. N., and Chambers, W. W. (1958). Intraspinal sprouting of dorsal root axons. *Arch. Neurol.* 79:46–61.

Lomas, J., and Kertesz, A. (1978). Patterns of spontaneous recovery in aphasic groups: a study of adult stroke patients. *Brain Lang.* 5:388–401.

Ludlow, C. (1977). Recovery from aphasia: a foundation for treatment. In *Rationale for Adult Aphasia Therapy*, M. A. Sullivan and M. S. Kommers (eds.). Nebraska: University of Nebraska Medical Center, pp. 97–134.

Ludlow, C., Rosenberg, J., Fair, C., Buck, D., Schesselman, S., and Salazar, A. (1986). Brain lesions associated with nonfluent aphasia fifteen years following penetrating head injury. *Brain* 109:55–80.

Luria, A. R. (1970). *Traumatic Aphasia.* The Hague: Mouton.

Marks, M. M., Taylor, M. L., and Rusk, L. A. (1957). Rehabilitation of the aphasic patient: a survey of three years' experience in a rehabilitation setting. *Neurology* 7:837–843.

Merzenich, M. M., Kaas, J. H., Wall, J. T., Nelson, R. J., Sur, M., and Felleman, D. (1983). Topographic reorganization of somatosensory cortical areas 3b and 1 in adult monkeys following restricted deafferentation. *Neuroscience* 8:33–55.

Messerli, P., Tissot, A., and Rodrigues, J. (1976). Recovery from aphasia: some factors of prognosis. In *Neurolinguistics. 4. Recovery in Aphasics.* Y. Lebrun and R. Hoops (eds). Amsterdam: Swets & Zeitlinger, pp. 124–135.

Metter, E. J., Kempler, D., Jackson, C. A., et al. (1987). Cerebellar glucose metabolism in chronic aphasia. *Neurology* 37:1599–1606.

Milner, B. (1974). Hemispheric specialization: scope and limits. In *The Neurosciences: Third Study Program*, F. O. Schmitt, and F. G. Worden (eds.). Cambridge, MA: MIT Press, pp. 75–89.

Miura, K., Nakamura, Y., Miura, F., Yamada, I., Takahashi, M., Yoshikawa, A., and Mizobata, T. (1999). Functional magnetic resonance imaging to word generation task in a patient with Broca's aphasia. *J. Neurol.* 246:939–942.

Moore, R. Y. (1974). Central regeneration and recovery of function: the problem of collateral reinnervation. In *Plasticity and Recovery of Function in the Central Nervous System.* D. G. Stein, J. J. Rosen, and N. Butters (eds.). New York: Academic Press, pp. 111–128.

Munk, H. (1881). *Ueber die Funktionen der Grosshirnrinde, Gesammelte Mitteilungen aus den Jahren 1877–1880.* Berlin: Hirshwald.

Naeser, M. A., Gaddie, A., Palumbo, C. L., and Stiassny-Eder, D. (1990). Late recovery of auditory comprehension in global aphasia: improved recovery observed with subcortical temporal isthmus lesion versus Wernicke's cortical area lesion. *Arch. Neurol.* 47:425–432.

Naeser, M. A., Helm-Estabrooks, N., Haas, G.,

Auerbach, S., and Srinivasan, M. (1987). Relationship between lesion extent in Wernicke's area on computed tomographic scan and predicting recovery of comprehension in Wernicke's aphasia. *Arch. Neurol. 44*:73–82.

Nagata, K., Yunoki, K., Kabe, S., Suzuki, A., and Araki, G. (1986). Regional cerebral flow correlates of aphasia outcome in cerebral hemorrhage and cerebral infarction. *Stroke 17*:417–423.

Newcombe, F., Hions, R. W., and Marshall, J. C. (1976). Acquired dyslexia: recovery and retraining. In *Neurolinguistics. 4. Recovery in Aphasics*, Y. Lebrun and R. Hoops (eds.). Amsterdam: Swets & Zeitlinger, pp. 146–162.

Nielsen, J. M. (1946). *Agnosia, Apraxia, Aphasia.* New York: Hoeber.

Nottebohm, F. (1970). Ontogeny of bird song. *Science 167*:950–956.

Pascual-Leone, A., Grafman, J., and Hallett, M. (1994). Modulation of cortical motor output maps during development of implicit and explicit knowledge. *Science 263*:1287–1289.

Patterson, K., and Kay, K. (1982). Letter-by-letter reading: Psychological descriptions of a neurological description of a neurological syndrome. *Q. J. Exp. Psychol. 34A*:411–441.

Pedersen, P. M., Jørgensen, H. S., Nakayama, H., Raaschou, H. O., and Olsen, T. S. (1995). Aphasia in acute stroke: incidence, determinants, and recovery. *Ann. Neurol. 38*:659–666.

Pieniadz, J. M., Naeser, M. A., KIoff, E., and Levine, H. L. (1983). CT scan cerebral hemispheric asymmetry measurements in stroke cases with global aphasia: atypical asymmetries associated with improved recovery. *Cortex 19*:371–391.

Prigitano, G. (1985). *Neuropsychological Rehabilitation After Brain Injury.* Baltimore: Johns Hopkins University Press.

Robinson, R. G., and Benson, D. F. (1981). Depression in aphasic patients: frequency, severity and clinical pathological correlations. *Brain Lang. 14*:610–614.

Rothi, L. J. G., and Moss, S. (1992). Alexia without agraphia: Potential for model assisted therapy. *Commun. Dis. 2*:11–18.

Rubens, A. (1977). The role of changes within the central nervous system during recovery from aphasia. In *Rationale for Adult Aphasia Therapy*, M. A. Sullivan and M. S. Kommers (eds.). Nebraska: University of Nebraska Medical Center, pp. 28–43.

Russell, W. R. (1971). *The Traumatic Amnesias.* London: Oxford University Press.

Russell, W. R., and Nathan, P. W. (1946). Traumatic amnesia. *Brain 69*:280–300.

Sands, E., Sarno, M. T., and Shankweiler, D. (1969). Long-term assessment of language function in aphasia due to stroke. *Arch. Phys. Med. Rehabil. 50*:202–222.

Sarno, M. T., and Levita, E. (1971). Natural course of recovery in severe aphasia. *Arch. Phys. Med. Rehabil. 52*:175–179.

Sarno, M. T., Silverman, M., and Levita, E. (1970a). Psychosocial factors and recovery in geriatric patients with severe aphasia. *J. Am. Geriatr. Soc. 18*:405–409.

Sarno, M. T., Silverman, M., and Levita, E. (1970b). Speech therapy and language recovery in severe aphasia. *J. Speech Hear. Res. 13*:607–623.

Satz, P., Zaucha, K., Forney, D. L., McCleary, C., Asarnow, R. F., Light, R., et al. (1998). Neuropsychological, psychosocial and vocational correlates of the Glasgow Outcome Scale at 6 months post-injury: a study of moderate to severe traumatic brain injury patients. *Brain Inj. 12*:555–567.

Sauve, M. J., Walker, J. A., Massa, S. M., Winkle, R. A., Scheinman, M. M. (1996). Patterns of cognitive recovery in sudden cardiac arrest survivors: the pilot study. *Heart Lung 25*:172–181.

Schneider, G. E. (1073). Early lesions of superior colliculus: factors affecting the formation of abnormal retinal projections. *Brain Behav. Evol. 8*:73–109.

Schuell, A., Jenkins, J. J., and Jimenez-Pabon, E. (1964). *Aphasia in Adults.* New York: Harper & Row.

Selnes, O. A., Knopman, D. S., Niccum, N., and Rubens, A. B. (1983). CT scan correlates of auditory comprehension deficits in aphasia: a prospective recovery study. *Ann. Neurol. 13*: 558–566.

Small, S. L., Kendall Flores, D., and Noll, D. C. (1998). Different neural circuits subserve reading before and after therapy for acquired dyslexia. *Brain Lang. 62*:298–308.

Smith, A. (1966). Speech and other functions after left (dominant) hemispherectomy. *J. Neurol. Neurosurg. Psychiatry 29*:467–471.

Smith, A., Chamoux, R., Leri, J., London, R., and Muraski, A. (1972). *Diagnosis, Intelligence and Rehabilitation of Chronic Aphasics.* Ann Arbor: University of Michigan Department of Physical Medicine and Rehabilitation.

Sohlberg, M., and Mateer, C. (1989). *Introduction to Cognitive Rehabilitation.* Mississauga: Gilford Press.

Stavraky, G. W. (1961). *Supersensitivity Following Lesions of the Nervous System.* Toronto: University of Toronto Press.

Stevens, M. K., and Yaksh, T. L. (1990). Systemic studies on the effects of the NMDA receptor antagonist MK-801 on cerebral blood flow and responsivity, EEG, and blood–brain barrier following complete reversible cerebral ischemia. *J. Cereb. Blood Flow Metab.* 10:77–88.

Stoicheff, M. L. (1960). Motivating instructions and language performance of dysphasic subjects. *J. Speech Hear. Res.* 3:75–85.

Subirana, A. (1969). Handedness and cerebral dominance. In *Handbook of Clinical Neurology*, P. J. Vinken and G. W. Bruyn (eds.). Amsterdam: North Holland, pp. 248–273.

Tazaki, Y., Sakai, F., Otomo, E., et al. (1988). Treatment of cerebral infarction with a choline precursor in a multi-center double blind placebo-controlled study. *Stroke* 19:211–216.

Talland, G. A. (1965). *Deranged Memory*. New York: Academic Press.

Thiel, A., Herholz, K., Koyuncu, A., et al. (2001). Plasticity of language networks in patients with brain tumors: A positron emission tomography activation study. *Ann. Neurol.* 50:620–629.

Thulborn K. R., Carpenter, P. A., and Just, M. A. (1999). Plasticity of language-related brain function during recovery from stroke. *Stroke* 30:749–754.

Van Buskirk, C. (1955). Prognostic value of sensory defect in rehabilitation of hemiplegics. *Neurology* 6:407–411.

van der Naalt, J., van Zomeren, A. H., Sluiter, W. J., and Minderhoud, J. M. (1999). One year outcome in mild to moderate head injury: the predictive value of acute injury characteristics related to complaints and return to work. *J. Neurol. Neurosurg. Psychiatry* 66:207–213.

Victor, M., and Adams, R. D. (1958). The effect of alcohol on the nervous system. *Proc. Assoc. Res. Nerv. Ment. Dis.* 32:526–573.

Vignolo, L. A. (1964). Evolution of aphasia and language rehabilitation. A retrospective exploratory study. *Cortex* 1:344–367.

Von Monakow, C. (1914). *Die lokalisation im Grosshirn und der Abbau funktionen durch corticale Herde*. Wiesbaden: Bergmann.

Warburton, E., Price, C. J., Swinburn, K., and Wise, F. J. S. (1999). Mechanisms of recovery from aphasia: evidence from positron emission tomography studies. *J. Neurol. Neurosurg. Psychiatry* 66:155–161.

Weinberg, J., Diller, L., Gordon, W. A., Gerstman, L. J., Lieberman, A., Lakin, P., et al. (1977). Visual scanning training effect on reading-related tasks in acquired right brain damage. *Arch. Phys. Med. Rehabil.* 58:479–486.

Weisenburg, T., and McBride, K. E. (1935). *Aphasia: A Clinical and Psychological Study*. New York: Commonwealth Fund.

Weiller, C., Isensee, C., Rijntjes, M., Huber, W., Müller, S., Bier, D., et al. (1995). Recovery from Wernicke's aphasia: a positron emission tomographic study. *Ann. Neurol.* 37:723–732.

Wepman, J. M. (1951). *Recovery from Aphasia*. New York: Ronald Press.

Williams, M. (1966). Memory disorders associated with electroconvulsive therapy. In *Amnesia*. C. W. M. Whitby and O. L. Zangweill (eds.). London: Butterworths, pp. 134–149.

Wilson, B. (1998). Recovery of cognitive functions following nonprogressive brain injury. *Curr. Opin. Neurobiol.* 8:281–287.

Wolfe, C. D. A., Tilling, K., Beech, R., and Rudd, A. G. (1999). Variations in case fatality and dependency from stroke in Western and Central Europe. *Stroke* 30:350–356.

Woolsey, T., and Van der Loos, H. (1970). The structural organization of layer IV in the somatosensory region (S1) of mouse cerebral cortex. *Brain Res.* 17:205–242.

Zivin, J. A., Fisher, M., DeGirolami, J., Hemenway, C. C., and Stashak, J. A. (1985). Tissue plasminogen activator reduces neurological damage after cerebral embolism. *Science* 230:1289–1292.

21

Pharmacotherapy of Cognition

PATRICK McNAMARA AND MARTIN L. ALBERT

Treatment of cognitive disorders with drugs that modulate forebrain neurotransmitter systems is still in the early, experimental stage. Well-controlled studies of potential therapeutic agents are the exception rather than the rule, and clinicians generally are not familiar with the results of the studies that have been performed. This situation is unfortunate, as existing research indicates that pharmacologic approaches to restoration of cognitive function may be effective, especially when combined with behavioral and cognitive techniques. In this chapter we review selected topics in the pharmacology of cognition with the aim of increasing the pace and quality of research in the field.

METHODOLOGIC ISSUES

Identification and study of potentially useful drugs that can help restore cognitive function after brain injury are difficult and have often been a haphazard enterprise (Stahl et al., 1987; Pryse-Phillips et al., 2001). Methodologic and practical problems abound. First, properly controlled studies of potentially useful agents are expensive and time-consuming. Often there are not enough patients who share a given profile of deficit to achieve adequate statistical

power. Even when adequate power is achieved, dropout rates are often high. Second, there is little consensus on exactly what endpoint measures to use to demonstrate reliable, consistent, and functional restoration of cognitive function. In the realm of language processes alone, for example, researchers can choose from an array of measures that sample fluency, syntax, naming, repetition, comprehension, pragmatics, discourse, and so on (Goodglass and Kaplan, 1983). The large number of neurocognitive measures relative to the small number of subjects increases the probability of detecting statistically significant changes on outcome measures simply on the basis of chance alone. Finally, it is exceedingly difficult in studies of human cognition to control possible confounding factors that are known to influence recovery. Potential confounding variables include subject-related factors such as age, gender, handedness, premorbid intelligence, overall health status, and post-injury social support systems; lesion-related variables such as size, type, and site of lesion; and treatment-related variables such as side effects from the target drug and dose effects, as well as confounding effects of concomitant cognitive and behavioral therapies. No single study has yet been able to constrain all potential confounding variables. However, some attempt should be made to control them, and when full control is not possible, some attempt should be made to disentangle effects of these variables from effects of the drug.

Spontaneous recovery of function is another potential confounding factor that frequently is not addressed in studies of pharmacotherapy for cognition. Virtually all patients without degenerative disorder who sustain a brain injury show some amount of recovery of function after the initial injury. Although the rate of spontaneous recovery tends to plateau some months after injury, slower but real recovery can continue years after the initial injury.

Despite these obstacles to performing well-designed studies of cognitive pharmacotherapy, useful facts have nevertheless been collected concerning modulation of forebrain neurotransmitter systems that can affect cognition. We will focus here on the catecholaminergic and cholinergic systems, as these have been the most intensely studied. The serotoninergic system is known to affect certain aspects of cognition as well (Spoont, 1992; Robert et al., 1999), but these effects appear to be most pronounced in the areas of mood, anti-nociception, and arousal states rather than cognition per se. Similarly, the inhibitory cortical neurotransmitter gamma aminobutyric acid (GABA) and the excitatory transmitters, such as glutamate, histamine, and aspartate, are known to influence cognition (Meador, 1997; Fernandez-Novoa and Cacabelow, 2001), but study of drugs that selectively or predominantly influence these transmitters are still rare.

In this chapter we shall review the chemical and functional neuroanatomy of the acetylcholine (Ach), dopamine (DA), and noradrenergic (NE) systems in so far as they might influence higher cognitive functioning. We next review studies of effects of these neurochemical systems on fundamental cognitive operations, such as activation of selective brain regions, working and long-term memory, attention, and speed of cognitive processing. We will then focus on specific pharmacotherapeutic efforts to improve selected neuropsychologic deficits such as executive cognitive function deficits, the memory disorder associated with Alzheimer's disease, nonfluent aphasia, and unilateral spatial neglect. We will conclude with a short discussion of general principles of pharmacotherapy of cognition and a comment on clinical lessons learned from research to date.

NEUROANATOMY OF ACETYLCHOLINE, DOPAMINE, AND NOREPINEPHRINE

ACETYLCHOLINE

Forebrain nuclei such as the nucleus basalis of Meynert and the substantia inominata appear to be primary sources of cortical cholinergic innervation (Mesulam, 1988; Hasselmo and Linster, 1999). The nucleus basalis of Meynert also projects onto the amygdala. Mesulam (1995) also showed that the cholinergic medial septal nucleus and nuclei of the diagonal band send cholinergic projections to the hippocampal formation, cingulate cortex, and certain hypothalamic sites. While most basal forebrain cholinergic neurons project diffusely throughout the cortex, they *receive* inputs from only a few major areas, including the reticular activating system (RAS), the limbic system, and orbitofrontal cortex (Mesulam, 1988; Oscar-Berman et al., 1991). In nonhuman primates, Ach fibers densely innervate motor, premotor, and temporal association cortices. Antidromic activation studies have shown that Ach cells projecting into temporal association cortex are physiologically heterogeneous, exhibiting diverse rates and patterns of firing and discharge (Foote and Morrison, 1987). Target areas of these Ach fibers may therefore be more controlled by individual Ach neurons, as compared to other modulatory transmitters that exhibit a less diverse set of modulatory controls than Ach neurons. Acetylcholine also interacts with two major classes of receptors in cortical target areas: muscarinic and nicotinic. Muscarinic receptors use G proteins for signal transduction and are metabotropic, while nicotinic receptors are ionotropic.

Cholinergic activity may also be greater on the left in human brain. Amaducci et al. (1981) reported greater cholinacetyltransferase (CAT) activity in the left than in the right temporal lobes in postmortem human brain. Glick et al. (1982) found evidence for greater CAT activity in the left than in the right globus pallidus in postmortem human brain.

DOPAMINE

Dopamine is manufactured in the pigmented neurons of the substantia nigra (SN) and the ventral tegmental area (VTA). There are three major ascending dopaminergic systems: the nigro-striatal tract, which ascends from the SN to the corpus striatum; the mesolimbic system, which ascends from the SN and medial VTA to limbic sites including the cingulate gyrus; and the mesocortical system, which ascends from the anteromedial tegmentum and VTA to neocortical sites including supplementary motor area (SMA) and prefrontal cortex (Goldman-Rakic, 1987; Le Moal and Simon, 1991; Lewis, 1992; Randolph Swartz, 1999).

Forebrain DA innervation decreases in a rostrocaudal gradient such that only trace amounts of DA are found in occipital areas. The primary motor cortex exhibits the most dense innervation pattern, with supplementary motor area and prefrontal and inferior parietal areas following close behind. Sensory regions and layer IV neurons are sparsely innervated by dopaminergic fibers. In summary, DA fibers preferentially innervate prefrontal, motor, and association areas in the cortex. Large numbers of DA receptors (mainly D1 receptor types) are found on the spines of pyramidal cells in layer III. These neurons are projection neurons allowing for communication between association areas of the cortex. D1 receptors in the striatum and cortex modulate glutaminergic input to cortical pyramidal cells through structures called "triads," in which a dopaminergic and a glutaminergic terminal synapse onto pyramidal projection neurons. This anatomical arrangement allows DA to influence cortical-to-cortical processing via its input into pyramidal firing patterns.

NOREPINEPHRINE

Noradrenergic innervation of the neocortex arises from the locus coeruleus (LC) in the pontine brainstem (Foote and Morrison, 1987;

Lewis, 1992; Coull, 1994; Arnsten, 1998). Despite the relatively small number of neurons, the LC innervates every major region of the forebrain. Like DA, NE fibers run primarily in an anteroposterior plane. Individual neurons give off numerous collaterals innervating many different cortical regions. The primary somatosensory and motor regions are densely innervated in all six layers, but temporal and primary visual cortex are more sparsely innervated. Note that this pattern complements that of Ach fibers that project primarily to temporal and orbitofrontal cortex. Lesions of the dorsolateral prefrontal cortex are known to disinhibit firing of LC neurons and to impair regulation of the LC. Indeed, the prefrontal cortex may supply the only cortical afferents to the LC (Arnsten and Goldman-Rakic, 1985; Sara and Herve-Minville, 1995; Arnsten, 1998). This anatomical arrangement suggests that the prefrontal cortex and the ascending noradrenergic system mutually influence one another's processing properties. An impairment in the functioning of one will affect the functioning of the other. Pharmacologic agents that influence LC noradrenergic activity will also influence prefrontal functions.

NEUROMODULATOR INTERACTIONS

Cognitive functions are very likely not the result of single neurotransmitter effects. Rather, neuromodulators probably exert their effects via activation of relatively large regional brain systems and then modulation of specific neural circuits within those regions. These kinds of modulatory effects can only be accomplished via interactions among two or more modulatory substances. Some of the important neuromodulator interactions affecting cognitive performance involve cholinergic–dopaminergic interactions, and cholinergic–noradrenergic interactions (D'Esposito and Albert, 1991; Levin et al., 1992). For example, the combination of the noradrenergic agent clonidine and the anticholinesterase physostigmine enhances memory performance in aged monkeys to a greater degree than either drug alone (Terry et al., 1993). The complementary effects of DA and Ach systems on cognition are now commonplace and easily demonstrated. Radial maze memory deficits in rats, for example, due to cholinergic blockade can be reversed by depletion of DA stores but not by depletion of other neurotransmitter systems. Conversely, deficits induced by dopaminergic blockade on avoidance learning tasks in rats can be reversed by cholinergic blockade but not by depletion of other transmitter systems (Levin et al., 1992). Clearly these neurotransmitter systems act in concert to support cognitive functions, and any drug given to influence one system will necessarily affect complementary systems. Thus, whenever we measure effects of a given drug on a cognitive system we have to assume that the drug is affecting more than one neurotransmitter system even if the drug is considered to be a "selective" pharmacologic agent.

NEUROMODULATORY INFLUENCES ON FUNDAMENTAL COGNITIVE OPERATIONS

MEMORY

Human memory systems can be usefully analyzed into two broad, ecologically valid categories: procedural and declarative (Cermak, 1987). *Procedural memories* are classified as unconscious motor habits supported by neural circuits of the basal ganglia, while typical *declarative memories* are conceived to be verbally reportable personal episodes, supported by forebrain neural structures. Declarative memories are further subdivided into episodic and semantic variants, and episodic memory is further subdivided into aware vs. unaware memory. The most studied portion of aware memory, in turn, is commonly called "working memory." Each of these memory types is associated with a particular neuroanatomy that, when disrupted, results in impairment of the given memory type. Episodic (but not semantic) memories, for example, tend to be impaired after medial temporal and diencephalic lesions, while semantic (but not episodic) memories tend to be impaired after posterior cortical lesions. Acetylcholine appears to be crucially involved in all memory types. The catecholamines play a central role in procedural memory and in working memory.

Acetylcholine

Forebrain cholinergic activity appears to influence both memory capacity and memory formation (Drachman and Leavitt, 1974; Drachman, 1977; Bartus et al., 1987; Callaway et al., 1992; Winkler et al., 1995). Anticholinergics (for example, the antagonist scopolamine) impair initial memory formation, and therefore affect free recall as well (Bartus et al., 1987; Callaway et al., 1992). Once a memory is formed, however, retention is unaffected by anticholinergic agents. In contrast, cholinomimetics (e.g., the anticholinesterases and nicotine) can enhance memory processes. Scopolamine-induced memory deficits are ameliorated by the anticholinesterase physostigmine but not by a benzodiazepine antagonist. We will have more to say about Ach and memory when we discuss pharmacotherapy for Alzheimer's disease.

Dopamine

Williams and Goldman-Rakic (1995) have investigated the role of DA in modulation of what they call "memory fields" in the cortex. It has been known for some time that selected neurons in the sulcus principalis of the monkey become active during the delay period of delayed-response tasks. If these "memory neurons" are prevented (through lesioning or freezing) from firing during the delay period, the monkey cannot perform the delayed-response task (Fuster, 1989). *Memory fields* are defined as the maximal firing of a memory neuron to a memory representation of a visual target that had appeared in various locations of the visual field. The cells increase firing when the tested animals must retain the location of the target during a delay period between target presentation and time of response. These memory field neurons appear to depend selectively on DA. Iontophoretic application of DA to the prefrontal cortex during performance of a delayed-response task induces an increase in memory neuron firing during the delay period

(Sawaguchi et al., 1991; Arnsten, 1998). Depletion of DA from this region of prefrontal cortex induces cognitive deficit as measured by delayed-response type tasks (Brozoski et al., 1979). Measurement of DA concentration within the prefrontal cortex of monkeys before and during performance of the delayed-response task shows a significant increase in DA levels while the animals are engaged in the delay period. Injections of selective D1 receptor antagonists and nonselective D1 antagonists such as haloperidol (but not cholinergic or serotoninergic antagonists) to the monkey's prefrontal cortex induces deficits in the delayed-response task that are dose-dependent. The higher the dose the worse the performance. Thus, DA appears to regulate directly one aspect of working memory capacity in the monkey (Watanabe et al., 1997). Dopamine enhances working memory only within a certain limited concentration range, however. Higher or lower doses are associated with functional impairment (Gotham et al., 1988; Arnsten, 1998). Recent studies have also shown that semantic memory networks and spatial cues in humans can be modulated by dopaminergic stimulation (Kischka et al., 1996; Luciana and Collins, 1997).

Norepinephrine

Antereograde memory in patients with alcoholic Korsakoff syndrome is enhanced by clonidine (an alpha-2 adrenergic agonist) and by NE precursors (McEntee et al., 1984; Mair and McEntee, 1986). Clonidine also enhances memory functions in aged monkeys (Arnsten and Goldman-Rakic, 1985; Arnsten et al., 1996). Interestingly, clonidine improves performance on the spatial delayed-response task in monkeys after lesions to the prefrontal cortex (Cai et al., 1993).

ATTENTION

Acetylcholine

The anticholinergic drug scopolamine abnormally prolongs the event-related potential (ERP) P300 wave (an index of attention) and slows reaction time (Callaway et al., 1992; Meador, 1997). Anticholinergics impair performance on a variety of vigilance tasks like the continuous performance test, while cholinomimetics have the opposite effect (Rusted and Warburton, 1989). Cholinergic modulation of attentional switching and of vigilance is generally thought to be mediated by muscarinic receptors.

Norepinephrine

Discharge rates of LC neurons are increased by arousal and attentiveness (Foote and Morison, 1987). Electrical stimulation of the LC produces a suppression of ongoing background cortical activity, thereby enhancing stimulus evoked activity, resulting in enhanced signal-to-noise ratios in neuronal processing. The LC appears to be preferentially activated by novel stimuli. Once a novel or significant stimulus is detected, neuronal firing to non-novel stimuli are attenuated or suppressed, thereby focusing attention on task-relevant behaviors. As mentioned above, lesions of the prefrontal cortex are known to disinhibit firing of LC neurons and to impair regulation of the LC (Sara and Herve-Minville, 1995; Arnsten et al., 1996; Arnsten, 1998). This finding suggests that voluntary control of attentional switching may be mediated in part by descending fibers from prefrontal cortex onto noradrenergic neurons of the LC. Conversely, ascending noradrenergic fibers to prefrontal cortex may mediate processes of attentional switching, such as the rate at which attention is disengaged from the current task and then applied to the next task. The cognitive consequences of prefrontal dysfunction should therefore be associated with attentional dysfunction or with inability to suppress distracting or irrelevant stimuli. Drugs (such as clonidine or ritalin) that activate prefrontal cortex should indirectly (through its effects on LC regulation) improve attentional function.

Clinical studies of Parkinson's disease (PD) suggest that cortical NE influences attentional switching (Stern et al., 1984; Mayeux et al., 1987; Cools et al., 1995; Riekkenen et al., 1998). Postmortem studies of cortical NE and methoxyhydroxyphenethyleneglycol (MHPG;

the major metabolite of NE), consistently report decrements of these chemical indices in PD patients with attentional dysfunction (Kuipers and Wolters, 1995). Stern and colleagues (1984) found significant correlations between NE metabolite levels in PD patients with performance on reaction time tasks and continuous performance tasks that measure attention and vigilance. More recently, Riekkinen et al. (1998) reported significant correlations between measures of cerebrospinal fluid (CSF) NE levels and attentional cognitive performance in PD.

Dopamine

Dopamine neurons of the VTA and SN have long been associated with both the attentional and reward systems of the brain (Le Moal and Simon, 1991; Lewis, 1992; Schultz et al., 1995; Koob and Le Moal, 1997; Joyce and Hutton, 1998; Randolph Swartz, 1999). Virtually all of the known substance addictions exert their addictive actions, in part, by prolonging the influence of DA on target neurons (Koob and Le Moal, 1997). The VTA DA neuron responses appear to be necessary to facilitate formation of associations between attended stimuli that predict reward and behavioral responses that obtain reward (Schultz et al., 1995). The optimal stimuli for activating DA neurons are unexpected appetitive rewards. These stimuli most effectively capture attention (Schultz et al., 1995).

Studies of attentional function in PD suggest that forebrain DA, in addition to cortical NE, is crucially involved in attentional switching (Cools et al., 1995; Lange et al., 1995; Taylor and Saint-Cyr, 1995). There is, for example, a well-established PD attentional switching deficit on category alternation paradigms in which patients are required to generate names in one category for about a minute and then switch to another category (Downes et al., 1993; Cools et al., 1995). Patients with PD find it difficult to generate an adequate number of names after switching categories. Administration of the dopaminergic drug levodopa protects against this switching deficit for many patients who exhibit the deficit (Lange et al., 1992, 1995).

PROCESSING RATES OR SPEED OF COGNITIVE PROCESSING

Speed of cognitive processing represents a fundamental measure of cognitive performance in cognitive psychology and related fields of inquiry (Sternberg, 1975; Cerella et al., 1993). Cognitive slowing in aging and in age-related disorders is associated with cognitive dysfunction such as deficits in memory, language comprehension, calculation, planning, and working memory (see papers in Cerella et al., 1993). Speed of cognitive processing can be influenced by pharmacologic agents and the cognitive disorders related to cognitive slowing can be ameliorated with appropriate pharmacotherapy.

Dopamine

Dopamine may be particularly important for regulation of speed of cognitive processing. Much of the clinical evidence comes from work with patients with parkinsonian syndromes and bradyphrenia. Patients with PD and patients with progressive supranuclear palsy frequently evidence frontal dysfunction, and slowed mental operations or bradyphrenia (Wilson et al., 1980; Stern et al., 1984; Rogers, 1986; Mayeux et al., 1987; Rogers et al., 1987; Dubois et al., 1988; Pillon et al., 1989; Wolfe et al., 1990; Powe et al., 1991; Dubois and Pillon, 1992). Both the frontal dysfunction and the bradyphrenia are correlated with concentrations of catecholamine metabolites in CSF (Agid et al., 1987; Mayeux et al., 1987; Wolfe et al., 1990). Using the Sternberg (1975) memory scanning paradigm to measure cognitive slowing in PD patients, Wilson et al. (1980) found evidence for cognitive slowing in elderly PD patients. Using the same paradigm, Powe et al. (1991) found evidence of relatively normal memory scanning time in PD patients only when on levodopa medicine. Like Gotham et al. (1988), they speculate that overstimulation of DA receptors in less denervated frontal–caudate neuronal loops could lead to dysfunction in these neurocognitive circuits. Nevertheless, the bradyphrenia associated with progres-sive supranuclear palsy is less responsive to dopaminergic replacement therapy than the bradyphrenia noted in some PD patients (Dubois et al., 1988). This suggests that cognitive slowing may also involve non-dopaminergic systems as well.

Norepinephrine

Rammsayer et al. (2001) found that temporal discrimination was improved (relative to placebo) in healthy volunteers after 2 mg of reboxetine (an NE reuptake inhibitor).

Acetylcholine

Pillon and colleagues (1989) administered a timed visual discrimination task (15 superimposed images of everyday objects, e.g., a lamp) to 70 patients with moderate to severe PD. The 15-objects test performance did not correlate with akinesia scores in patients withdrawn from dopaminergic medications, but did correlate with the parkinsonian disability score, which is a measure of residual axial motor function not usually affected by dopaminergic treatment. The authors suggested that bradyphrenia, as measured by the 15-objects test, is not significantly related to DA systems, rather Ach is more likely implicated. Reinspection of their data, however, reveals that the time needed to identify 12 of the 15 objects increased by 58% in 70 patients while off levodopa and almost half (32 patients) of the patients improved their performance while on levodopa. Thus, both cholinergic and dopaminergic mechanisms may influence performance on tasks measuring extent and degree of bradyphrenia.

PHARMACOTHERAPY FOR SELECTED NEUROPSYCHOLOGICAL SYNDROMES

DEFICITS IN EXECUTIVE COGNITIVE FUNCTIONS

Executive cognitive functions refer broadly to cognitive activity involving the planning, initiation, monitoring, and adjustment of nonroutine and goal-directed behaviors and are disproportionately impaired in traumatic brain injury, attention-deficit hyperactivity disorder, schizophrenia, PD and in most disorders asso-

ciated with prefrontal dysfunction (Fuster, 1989; Taylor and Saint-Cyr, 1991; Elias and Treland, 1999). Antidopaminergic antipsychotics such as haloperidol are known to affect executive cognitive functions adversely in some patients with schizophrenia (Friedman et al., 1999). The atypical neuroleptics risperidone and clozapine have been shown to improve executive functions as measured by verbal fluency tasks (McGurk, 1999), the Digit Span Distractibility test (Green et al., 1997), and the Trails-B Test (McGurk et al., 1997). Atypical neuroleptics may increase DA by antagonizing 5-HT_{2A} receptors which in turn activate dopaminergic neurons in the VTA. Interestingly, apart from verbal fluency, long-term administration of clozapine does not appear to improve executive cognitive functions in schizophrenics (Buchanan et al., 1994; Hoff et al., 1996). Long-term administration of clozapine may result in excessive prefrontal cortical levels of DA, as clozapine is known to induce an increase in extracellular concentration of DA in the prefrontal cortex (Murphy et al., 1996; Friedman et al., 1999).

Optimal dosing with the noradrenergic agonist clonidine has been reported to improve executive cognitive functions in a variety of disorders (Cai et al., 1993; Coull, 1994; Arnsten, 1998). For example, Cai et al. found that reserpine-induced spatial working memory deficits in nonhuman primates could be reversed with clonidine.

Levodopa, a dopaminergic drug used to treat PD, has been shown to significantly enhance performance of PD patients on executive cognitive functions tests such as the Wisconsin Card Sort Test, the Tower of London Planning Test, verbal fluency tasks, and some forms of visual–spatial functioning linked to executive cognitive functions (Gotham et al., 1988; Lange et al., 1992, 1995; Kulisevsky et al., 1996; Cools et al., 2002; Mattay et al., 2002). Lange et al. (1992; 1995) found that PD patients were dramatically impaired on frontal or executive function tests (Tower of London Task, set shifting, working memory, and spatial attention span) only when withdrawn from levodopa medication. Performance on nonfrontally mediated tests such as visual memory tests was not impaired when patients were off levodopa. However, conflicting results abound in the research literature. For example, Gotham et al. (1988) assessed the performance of PD patients on four executive cognitive function tests that are known to be sensitive to prefrontal cortical dysfunction: (1) the Wisconsin Card Sort Test; (2) verbal fluency, including alternating between categories; (3) a self-ordered pointing task in which the patient was presented with a card depicting 12 figures and then required to point to a different figure on each trial; and (4) a task that involved learning to match abstract figures with particular colors. The patients were tested while on levodopa medication, and then while off the medication. Verbal fluency was within normal limits while on levodopa but declined significantly (at least with the alternation task) while off levodopa. Wisconsin Card Sort Test performance was impaired both on and off levodopa. Patients showed largely normal performance on the two remaining tasks while off levodopa, but they were significantly impaired while on it. The authors speculate that overstimulation of DA receptors in less denervated frontal–caudate neuronal loops could lead to dysfunction in these neurocognitive circuits. There is, in fact, evidence that excessive levels of DA in prefrontal cortex can impair prefrontal cognitive functions (Murphy et al., 1996; Arnsten, 1998; Friedman et al., 1999). Kulisevsky et al. (1996) found significant decrements in executive functions (including the Wisconsin Card Sort Test) of a group of PD patients displaying major medication-related fluctuations in motor control compared with those showing a good response to therapy. The decrements occurred when off levodopa.

ALZHEIMER'S DISEASE

Alzheimer's disease (AD) has been linked to a loss of cholinergic neurons in the nucleus basalis of Meynert, and other cholinergic sites that project to the medial temporal lobe, such as the diagonal band of Broca and the septal nucleus, have also been implicated (Whitehouse et al., 1981). However, early attempts to treat the dementia of AD by pharmacologically increasing cholinergic activity met with only modest success (Bartus et al., 1987; Davis et

al., 1992; Farlow and Evans, 1998; DeKosky, 1999). This should not be surprising since several neurotransmitter systems are affected in AD (Meador, 1997). More recent attempts utilizing cholinesterase inhibitors have met with greater success. Unlike other areas under investigation in the pharmacotherapy of cognition, methodologic and experimental design issues in the study of AD, such as the choice of objective outcome measures and recruitment of adequate numbers of research patients, have been frequently addressed, at least with respect to investigations of the effectiveness of anticholinesterase agents. A small number of large, multicenter, double-blind, placebo-controlled clinical trials have been conducted with these agents.

To establish drug efficacy in the treatment of AD, an improvement of approximately 4 points on the cognitive subscale of the Alzheimer's Disease Assessment Scale (ADAS-Cog; Rosen et al., 1984, but see Demers et al., 2000) is required. This test assesses memory, spatial orientation, language, and praxis on a 70-point scale. While clinical trials of various anticholinesterases generally show mildly improved cognitive scores on this test, it is not clear whether these improvements translate into better patient functioning in daily life. There is as yet no consensus on the best instrument to use to assess drug effects on activities of daily living, and very few studies have shown positive effects on these daily activities despite mildly improved cognitive test scores. A small number of double-blind, placebo-controlled trials have been conducted with the anticholinesterase tacrine hydrochloride (Davis et al., 1992; Farlow et al., 1992; Knapp et al., 1994). Positive treatment effects were achieved in the range of 160 mg/day and were generally modest, although statistically significant by the 4-point ADAS-Cog standard. Dropout rates in these trials were quite high because of the hepatotoxicity of tacrine hydrochloride and its cholinergic side effects. Another anticholinesterase agent, donepezil, produces less severe side effects at therapeutic doses and as yet no hepatotoxicity, but treatment effects did not reach the 4-point ADAS-Cog criterion (Rogers et al., 1998). Rivastigmine is a cholinesterase inhibitor that has been shown to produce significant cognitive improvement by the ADAS-Cog criterion at relatively high doses of 6 to 12 mg/day (Rosler et al., 1999). Cholinergic side effects were noted but were relatively well tolerated. In Rosler et al.'s study, 65% of patients in the high-dose group completed the study. In general, studies of cholinesterase inhibitors have revealed that pharmacotherapeutic efforts may be effective by accepted research criteria, but the magnitude of cognitive improvement and the proportion of patients who respond to the drugs have both been modest. Individual differences in patients (e.g., degree of AchE inhibition achieved with the drug, stage of disease, comorbidities) likely contribute to the variability of response.

SPEECH AND LANGUAGE FUNCTIONS

Speech Initiation and Speech Fluency

Neurochemical, neurophysiological, and neuroanatomical studies define a widely distributed neural network that supports speech initiation and speech fluency (Deacon, 1992). This network, which includes supplementary motor area (SMA), the anterior cingulate gyrus, and the periaqeductal gray (PAG) matter, is modulated, in part, by dopaminergic pharmacosystems (Rosenberger, 1980). The anterior cingulate gyrus, which sends efferents directly onto the periaqueductal central gray, appears to influence the initiation and voluntary control of vocalization. Electrical stimulation of the periaqueductal central gray substance in the midbrain and upper pons elicits species-specific vocalizations in humans and other mammals. Destruction of the central gray substance can cause mutism, among other clinical phenomena. Patients with bilateral lesions within the cingulate area often undergo a period of mutism followed by slow recovery during which speech is aprosodic and initiation of speech is rare. The anterior cingulate gyrus receives efferents from the dopamine-rich SMA in the cortex (see Goldberg, 1987; Deacon, 1992, for review).

Regional cerebral blood flow studies have demonstrated dramatic activation of SMA associated with both inner speech (silent counting) and automatic speech production (counting aloud). Activation was seen in both left and right SMAs. The SMA lesions in humans are associated with transcortical motor aphasia as well as transient mutism. Thus SMA appears to regulate, through its network connections with the anterior cingulate and PAG, both initiation of speech and its maintenance. Recent studies also point to a role of the insula in speech and language functions (Dronkers, 1996). Dopamine appears to be the facilitatory transmitter for the network. There is considerable evidence that dopaminergic pathways innervate the SMA and the insula as well as inferior prefrontal regions of the brain responsible for speech initiation and fluency (Le Moal and Simon, 1991; Lewis, 1992). There is also evidence that dopaminergic activity is greater on the left in human brain. Oke et al. (1978) and Glick et al. (1982) found greater catecholaminergic activity in left forebrain sites than in right-sided sites in postmortem human brain.

Language Functions in Parkinson's Disease

One way to investigate the chemical anatomy of speech and language functions is to examine these functions in patients with PD, since PD is associated with relatively specific forebrain catecholaminergic dysfunction (Lang and Lozano, 1998; McNamara and Durso, 2000). With regard to speech and language production, PD patients often exhibit fluency and motor speech disorders (Critchley, 1981; Illes et al., 1988; Illes, 1989), word-finding difficulties (Matison et al., 1982; Auriacombe et al., 1993), and grammatical difficulties. They tend, for example, to use simplified sentence structures with an increase in the ratio of open-class items (nouns, verbs, adjectives) to closed-class items (determiners, auxiliaries, prepositions, etc.) as well as an increase in the frequency and duration of hesitations and pauses (Illes et al., 1988; Illes, 1989; McNamara et al., 1992) at critical sites in a sentence.

With regard to language comprehension, these patients often exhibit what appears to be a mild to moderate syntactic comprehension deficit (Lieberman et al., 1990, 1992; Grossman et al., 1991; Natsopoulos et al., 1991; Mc-Namara et al., 1996; Grossman, 1999). Preliminary data suggest that some memory-related aspects of the comprehension deficit in PD may be linked to catecholaminergic mechanisms (McNamara et al., 1996; Grossman, 1999; Grossman et al., 2001). For example, McNamara et al. (1996) studied eight patients with mild to severe PD who were tested both on and off levodopa, using queries to test for working memory–based comprehension of orally presented target sentences. They found that comprehension declined in the off state relative to the on state for all sentence types probed except direct-object sentences. Grossman et al. (2001) found that comprehension of grammatically complex sentences declined (relative to less complex but equally long sentences) when PD patients were "off" levodopa.

Clinical Pharmacotherapeutic Studies of Aphasia

Several recent critical reviews have appeared on this topic (Small, 1994; Mimura et al., 1995; Walker-Batson, 1998), so we will only briefly summarize studies that demonstrated some positive effect of pharmacotherapy. One important result of these reviews suggests that optimal recovery across aphasia types appears to occur when pharmacotherapy is combined with traditional cognitive-behavioral and speech therapy regimens. For example, McNeil et al. (1995) found that dextroamphetamine alone did not significantly improve lexical–semantic deficits in a patient with primary progressive aphasia. When combined with behavioral therapy, however, these deficits were significantly ameliorated relative to either drug or behavioral therapy alone. More recently, Walker-Batson (1998) reported similar findings. The potentiation of recovery through combination treatments with pharmacologic agents plus behavioral regimens is consistent with results from research on animals. Feeney and Hovda (1985), for example, found that loss of binocular rivalry and depth perception in the cat after bilateral ablation of visual cortex could be reversed only when cats were treated with both visual experience and dextroamphetamine.

There is some evidence that amphetamine is effective for treatment of nonfluent aphasia. Benson (1970) used a double-blind, placebo-controlled design ($n = 10$ patients) to study the effects of amphetamine on aphasia. Results from early (2–3 months after stroke) and late (6 or more months after stroke) treatment regimens were compared. A beneficial effect on both verbal and nonverbal measures was observed in the early-treated but not the late-treated patients. Walker-Batson (1998) later replicated these findings in a group of 11 mixed aphasics. Overall recovery, with scores on the Porch Index of Communicative Abilities as indices of recovery, was accelerated in the 6-month post-onset period by a fixed dose of amphetamine administration begun within 30 days of the stroke.

Dopaminergic agents may be effective for nonfluent aphasia and cholinergic agents for fluent varieties. Albert et al. (1988), using an on–off design, reported improved fluency and naming scores in a patient with nonfluent aphasia treated with bromocriptine. Fluency and naming scores returned to baseline after the drug was discontinued. Gupta and Mlcoch (1992) replicated the effect of improved fluency scores after bromocriptine treatment in two aphasic patients but Sabe et al. (1995) and MacLennan et al. (1991) could not document any improvement in speech and language scores in nonfluent aphasics who were treated with bromocriptine late in the recovery process. More recently, Tanaka et al. (2000) conducted a double-blind, crossover study with bromocriptine. They administered the drug (5–7.5 mg/day for 4 weeks) to 10 patients with a Broca-type aphasia. Statistically significant improvement (pre- to post-treatment) on naming and fluency scores was documented in the mild aphasics, but not in the severely impaired aphasics. Previously, Tanaka and colleagues (1997) had documented naming and comprehension improvement in fluent aphasics using the cholinergic agent bifemelane. They built on the work of Moscowitch and colleagues (1991), who reported that an anticholinesterase agent improved language performance in eight fluent "semantic" aphasics. Using the anticholinesterase agent physostigmine, Jacobs et al. (1996) found improved confrontation naming ability in persons with anomia. Albert (2000) provides an in-depth discussion of dopaminergic influences on nonfluent aphasia and cholinergic influences on fluent aphasia.

These clinical studies of pharmacotherapy for aphasia suggest that the timing of drug administration relative to the time of onset of the brain injury may be critical. Also, pharmacotherapy seems to be potentiated by concomitant cognitive or speech therapy.

UNILATERAL SPATIAL NEGLECT

When patients with unilateral cerebral lesions fail to detect or respond to stimuli in the contralateral hemispace, they are said to exhibit unilateral neglect (Heilman and Van Den Abell, 1980; Heilman et al., 1993). Because lesions of ascending DA projections in rats and monkeys can cause long-lasting contralateral neglect (Pycock, 1980), some investigators have studied effects of dopaminergic stimulation on neglect in humans (Valenstein et al., 1980; Fleet et al., 1987; Barret et al., 1997; Grujic et al., 1998; Diamond, 2001). Fleet et al. demonstrated an improvement of neglect symptoms in two patients treated (for 3 and 4 weeks) with the DA agonist bromocriptine. Grujic et al. (1998) evaluated the effects of bromocriptine on visual search in a sample of seven consecutive patients with right hemisphere lesions. Patients were tested before and after treatment with bromocriptine on a computerized visual search task. Like most patients with right hemisphere–associated attentional dysfunction, patients at baseline were less accurate and had slower reaction times for target detection in the contralateral left hemifield. After bromocriptine was administered, however, patients tended to spend more time exploring the ipsilesional hemispace and therefore increased the relative neglect of the contralesional left hemispace. However, target detection accuracy did not change. The authors concluded that bromocriptine may worsen some aspects of hemispatial neglect in patients with lesions that include the postsynaptic components of ascending dopaminergic pathways (see also Barret et al., 1997). In such patients, dopaminergic stimulation could influence the intact hemisphere, causing a further shift of visual search away from the contralesional hemispace.

CONCLUSIONS

Contemporary cognitive neuroscience has largely disposed of earlier notions of one-to-one correspondence between brain anatomy and complex behaviors (Robbins and Brown, 1990; Cohen and Servan-Schrieber, 1992; Posner and Dehaene, 1994). Equally for chemicocognitive correlations, complex cognitive systems cannot be reduced to fluctuations in a single neurochemically active substance (Lister and Weingartner, 1987; Stahl et al., 1987; Servan-Schreiber et al., 1998). It is likely that a single neurochemical substance, being widely distributed, would be implicated in many (but not all) complex behaviors, whereas a single behavioral act would be influenced by many (but not all) chemical systems. Thus, modifications in many chemical systems should be implicated in every cognitive act, and, consequently, a comprehensive neurochemistry of cognition remains a dream for future realization. Nevertheless, our review of the literature suggests that broad correlations between neurochemical systems and neurocognitive systems can be identified: cholinergic systems are important for selective activation of neurocognitive systems associated with orbitofrontal and temporal lobes, while the catecholaminergic systems appear preferentially to activate striatal and prefrontal neurocognitive networks (Oscar-Berman et al. 1991). Dopaminergic systems support processes related to motoric and verbal fluency such as initiation of action or initiation and maintenance of vocalization. Cholinergic systems are crucial for regulating capacity and allocation of resources in verbal memory. Interactions between DA and Ach circuits may regulate rates of processing for those functions localized to perisylvian and anterior temporal/insular sites.

While it is clear that selective cognitive changes are reliably associated with distinct neurochemical profiles, it is less clear *how* neurotransmitter activity supports complex cognitive functions. In their neural network simulations of DA's effects on cognition, Servan-

Schreiber et al. (1998) suggest that DA's effects can be modeled by increasing the gain parameter on the network's activation function for all units in areas of the brain network where DA is presumed to function. The gain parameter controls the sensitivity of the network's activation/inhibition responsivity. Similarly, Geschwind and Galaburda (1985) have suggested that neurotransmitters more generally might perform an *activation* function. Brain regions are considered to be essentially silent unless and until they are activated by release of the appropriate transmitter from terminals synapsing in the region. Rusted and Warburton (1989) have suggested that neurotransmitters might alter resource allocation or the *memory capacity* of a given system. Just and Carpenter (1992) have pointed out that capacity constraints may influence the extent to which cognitive systems can be considered to be modular; the potential for two systems to interact may depend on available capacity. Rusted and Warburton (1989) argued that neurotransmitters would influence *attentional switching*, or the ability to attend appropriately to more than one source of information. Finally, neurotransmitters might influence cognitive operations by regulating the *speed* of those operations. Our review has shown that each of these mechanisms—activation, capacity constraints, attentional switching, and processing rates—can be manipulated pharmacologically.

Although the science of pharmacotherapy for cognitive disorders is still in its infancy, a set of facts has been established from experimental work with humans and nonhuman animals that can guide further clinical study. First and most important, loss of certain cognitive functions after brain damage can be partially restored in some patients with selective pharmacologic intervention. That is, pharmacotherapy for cognition can be effective. Second, the timing of drug administration relative to the time of injury may be critical. Some agents, such as the amphetamines, seem to exert their beneficial effects only when given during an early window of opportunity. Third, many drugs exhibit dose–response curves on selected cognitive functions. Inverted U-response curves are common in which the drug exerts beneficial effects only at optimal doses and is either ineffective or harmful at lower or higher doses. Fourth, some potentiation of effect occurs when two complementary pharmacosystems (e.g., dopaminergic and cholinergic) interact, yet few or no pharmacotherapeutic interventions are currently aimed at producing such interactions. Finally, for most (though not all) pharmacotherapeutic agents, optimal recovery seems to occur when pharmacotherapy is combined with behavioral therapy.

REFERENCES

Albert, M. L. (2000). Towards a neurochemistry of naming and anomia. In *Language and the Brain*, Y. Grodzinsky, L. Shapiro, and D. Swinney (eds.). San Diego: Academic Press, pp. 157–165.

Albert, M. L., Bachman, D. L., Morgan, A., and Helm-Estabrooks, N. (1988). Pharmacotherapy for aphasia. *Neurology* 38:877–879.

Amaducci, L., Sorbi, S., Albanese, A., and Gainotti, G. (1981). Choline acetyltranserferase (ChAT) activity differs in right and left human temporal lobes. *Neurology* 31:799–805.

Arnsten, A. F. T. (1998). Catecholamine modulation of prefrontal cortical cognitive function. *Trends Cogn. Sci.* 2:436–447.

Arnsten, A. F. T., and Goldman-Rakic, P. S. (1985). Alpha adrenergic mechanisms in prefrontal cortex associated with cognitive decline in aged non-human primates. *Science* 230:1273–1276.

Arnsten, A. F. T., Steere, J. C., and Hunt, R. D. (1996). The contribuition of alpha-2 noradrenergic mechaisms to prefrontal cortical cognitive function. *Arch. Gen. Psychiatry* 53:448–455.

Auriacombe, S., Grossman, M., Carvell, S., Gollomp, S., Stern, M., and Hurtig, H. (1993). Verbal fluency deficits in Parkinson's disease. *Neuropsychologia* 7:182–192.

Barrett, A., Crucian, G., Schwartz, R., et al. (1997). Dopamine agonist therapy worsens motor-intentional neglect. *Neurology* 48:A374.

Bartus, R. T., Dean, R. L., and Flicker, C., (1987). Cholinergic psychopharmacology: an integration of human and animal research on memory. In: *Psychopharmacology: The Third Generation of Progress*, H. Y. Meltzer, (ed.). New York: Raven Press, pp. 219–232.

Benson, D. F. (1970). Presentation 10. In *Behavioral Changes in Cerebrovascular Disease*, A. L. Benton (ed.). New York: Harper and Row, p. 77.

Brozoski, T., Brown, R., Rosvold, H., and Goldman, P. (1979). Cognitive deficit caused by regional depletion of dopamine in prefrontal cortex of rhesus monkey. *Science* 205:929–931.

Buchanan, R. W., Holstein, C., and Breier, A. (1994). The comparative efficacy and long-term effect of clozapine treatment on neuropsychological test performance. *Biol. Psychiatry 36:* 717–725.

Cai, J. X., Ma, Y., Xu, L., and Hu, X. (1993). Reserpine impairs spatial working memory performance in monkeys: reversal by the alpha-2 adrenergic agonist clonidine. *Brain Res. 614:* 191–196.

Callaway, E., Halliday, R., and Naylor, H. (1992). Cholinergic activity and constraints on information processing. *Biol. Psychiatry 33:*1–22.

Cerella, J., Rybash, J., Hoyer, W., and Commons, M. L. (eds). (1993). *Adult Information Processing: Limits on Loss*. New York: Academic Press.

Cermak, L. S. (1987). Models of memory loss in Korsakoff and alcoholic patients. In *Neuropsychology of Alcoholism*, O. A. Parsons, N. Butters, and P. E. Nathan (eds.). New York: Guilford Press, pp. 207–226.

Cohen, J., and Servan-Schreiber, D. (1992). Context, cortex, and dopamine: a connectionist approach to behavior and biology in schizophrenia. *Psychol. Rev. 99:*45–77.

Cools, A., Berger, H., Buytenhuijs, E., Horstink, M., and Van Spaendonck, K. (1995). Manifestations of switching disorders in animals and man with dopamine deficits in A_{10} and/or A_9 circuitries. In *Mental Dysfunction in Parkinson's Disease*, E. Wolters and P. Scheltens (eds.). ICG, pp. 49–68.

Cools, R., Stefona, E., Barker, R. A., Robbins, T. W., and Owen, A. M. (2002). Dopaminergic modulation of high-level cognition in Parkinson's disease: The role of the prefrontal cortex revealed by PET. *Brain 125:*584–594.

Coull, J. T. (1994). Pharmacological manipulations of the alpha-2 noradrenergic system: effects on cognition. *Drugs Aging 5:*116–126.

Critchley, E. (1981). Speech disorders of parkinsonism: a review. *J. Neurol. Neurosurg. Psychiatry 44:*751–758.

Davis, K. L., Thal, L. J., Gamzu, E. R., Davis, C. R., Woolson, R. F., Gracon, S. I., Drachman, D. A., Schneider, L. S., Whitehouse, P. J., Hoover, T. M., et al. (1992). A double-blind, placebo-controlled multicenter study of tacrine for Alzhemer's disease. *N. Engl. J. Med. 327:*1253–1259.

Deacon, T. (1992). The neural circuitry underlying primate calls and human language. In *Language Origins: A Multidisciplinary Approach,* J. Wind, B. Chiarelli, B. Bichakjian, and A. Nocentini, (eds.). Proceedings of NATO Advanced Institute, Corona, Italy, Amsterdam: Kluwer, pp. 121–162.

DeKosky, S.T. (1999). Treatment of cognitive impairments in Alzheimer's disease. In *Pharmacology of Cognition*, Education Program Syllabus, American Academy of Neurology, 51st Annual Meeting Toronto, Ontario, Canada, pp. 2PC.005-1–2PC.005-13.

D'Esposito, M., and Albert, M. L. (1991). Pharmacology of memory. In: *Memoire et Vieillissement*, Paris: Maloine Editeur, pp. 247–252.

Diamond, P. T. (2001). Rehabilitative management of post-stroke visuospatial inattention. *Disability Rehabilitation 23:*407–412.

Downes, J., Sharp, H., Costall, B., Sagar, H., and Howe, J. (1993). Alternating fluency in Parkinson's disease: an evaluation of the attentional control theory of cognitive impairment. *Brain 116:*887–902.

Drachman, D. (1977). Memory and cognitive function in man. Does the cholinergic system have a specific role? *Neuroloy 27:*783–790.

Drachman, D. A., and Leavitt, J. (1974). Human memory and the cholinergic system. *Arch. Neurol. 30.*113–121.

Dronkers, N. F. (1996). A new brain region for coordinating speech articulation. *Nature 384(6605):* 159–161.

Elias, J. W., and Treland, J. E. (1999). Executive function in Parkinson's disease and subcortical disorders. *Semin. Clin. Neuropsychiatry 4:*34–40.

Farlow, M. R., and Evans, R. M. (1998). Pharmacologic treatment of cognition in Alzheimer's dementia. *Neurology 51(Suppl. 1):*S36–S44.

Farlow, M., Gracon, S. I., Hershey, L. A., et al., (1992). A controlled trial of tacrine in Alzheimer's Disease. *JAMA 268:*2523–2529.

Feeney, D. M., and Hovda, D. A. (1985). Reinstatement of binocular depth perception by amphetamine and visual experience after visual cortex ablation. *Brain Res. 342:*352–356.

Fernandez-Novoa, L., and Cacabelow, R. (2001). Histamine function in brain disorders. *Behav. Brain Res. 124:*213–233.

Fleet, W. S., Valenstein, E., Watson, R. T., et al. (1987). Dopamine agonist therapy for neglect in humans. *Neurology 37:*1765–1770.

Foote, S., and Morrison, J. (1987). Extrathalamic modulation of cortical function. *Ann. Rev. Neurosci. 10:*67–95.

Friedman, J. I., Temporini, H., and Davis, K. L. (1999). Pharmacologic strategies for augmenting cognitive performance in schizophrenia. *Biol. Psychiatry 45:*1–16.

Fuster, J. M. (1989). *The Prefrontal Cortex. Anatomy, Physiology and Neuropsychology of the Frontal Lobe*, 2nd ed. New York: Raven Press.

Geschwind, N., and Galaburda, A. (1985). Cerebral lateralization: biological mechanisms, associations and pathology. *Arch. Neurol. 42*:428–458, 521–532.

Glick, S., Ross, D., and Hough, L. (1982). Lateral asymmetry of neurotransmitters in human brain. *Brain Res. 234*:53–63.

Goldberg, G. (1987). From intent to action. Evolution and function of the premotor systems of the frontal lobe. In *The Frontal Lobes Revisited*, E. Perceman (ed.). New York: IRBN Press, pp. 273–306.

Goldman-Rakic, P. (1987). Circuitry of primate prefrontal cortex and regulation of behavior by representational memory. In *Higher Cortical Function, Handbook of Physiology*, V. Mountcastle and F. Plum (eds.). Bethesda, MD: American Physiological Society, pp. 373–417.

Goodglass, H., and Kaplan, E. (1983). *The Assessment of Aphasia and Related Disorders*, 2nd ed. Philadelphia: Lea and Febiger.

Gotham, A., Brown, R., and Marsden, C. (1988). "Frontal" cognitive functions in patients with Parkinson's disease "on" and "off" levodopa. *Brain 111*:299–321.

Green, M., Marshall, B., Wirshing, W., et al. (1997). Does risperidone improve verbal working memory in treatment resistant schizophrenia? *Am. J. Psychiatry 154*:799–804.

Grossman, M. (1999). Sentence comprehension in Parkinson's disease. *Brain Cogn. 40*:387–413.

Grossman, M., Carvell, S., Gollomp, S., Stern, M., Vernon, G., and Hurtig, H. (1991). Sentence comprehension and praxis deficits in Parkinson's disease. *Neurology 41*:1620–1626.

Grossman, M., Glosser, G., Kalmanson, J., Morris, J., Stern, M. B., and Hurtig, H. I. (2001). Dopamine supports sentence comprehension in Parkinson's Disease. *J. Neurol. Sci. 184(2)*:123–130.

Grujic, Z., Mapstone, M., Gitelman, D. R., Johnson, N., Weintraub, S., Hays, A., Kwasnica, C., Harvey, R., Mesulam, M.-M. (1998). Dopamine agonists reorient visual exploration away from the neglected hemispace. *Neurology 51*:1395–1398.

Gupta, S. R., and Mlcoch, A. G. (1992). Bromocriptine treatment of nonfluent aphasia. *Arch. Phys. Med. Rehabil. 73*:373–376.

Hasselmo, M. E., and Linster, C. (1999). Acetylcholine and frontal cortex "signal to noise ratio". In: B. L. Miller and J. L. Cummings (Eds), *The Human Frontal Lobes: Functions and Disorders*. New York: The Guilford Press, 139–158.

Heilman, K. M., and Van Den Abell, T. (1980). Right hemisphere dominance for attention: the mechanism underlying hemispheric asymmetries of inattention (neglect). *Neurology 30*:327–330.

Heilman, K. M., and Valenstein, E. (1993). Neglect and related disorders. In K. Heilman and E. Valenstein (Eds) *Clinical Neuropsychology 3rd Edition*, NY: Oxford University Press.

Hoff, A., Faustman, W., Wieneke, M., et al. (1996). The effect of clozapine on symptom reduction, neurocognitive function and clinical management in treatment refractory state hospital schizophrenic inpatients. *Neuropsychopharmacology 15*:361–369.

Illes, J. (1989). Neurolinguistic features of spontaneous language production dissociate three forms of neurodegenerative disease: Alzheimer's, Huntington's, and Parkinson's. *Brain Lang. 37*:628–642.

Illes, J., Metter, E., Hanson, W., and Iritani, S. (1988). Language production in Parkinson's disease: acoustic and linguistic considerations. *Brain Lang. 33*:146–160.

Jacobs, D. H., Shuren, J., Gold, M., et al. (1996). Physostigmine pharmacotherapy for anomia. *Neurocase 2*:83–91.

Joyce, E., and Hutton, S. (1998). The behavioral pharmacology of brain dopamine systems: implication for the cognitive pharmacotherapy of schizophrenia. In: *Disorders of Brain and Mind*, M. A. Ron and A. S. David (eds.). Cambridge, UK: Cambridge University Press, pp. 84–122.

Just, M., and Carpenter, P. (1992). A capacity theory of comprehension: individual differences in working memory. *Psychol. Rev. 1*:122–149.

Kischka, U., Kammer, Th., Maier, S., Weisbrod, M., Thimm, M., and Spitzer, M. (1996). Dopaminergic modulation of semantic network activation. *Neuropsychologia 34*:1107–1113.

Koob, G., and Le Moal, M. (1997). Drug abuse: hedonic homeostatic dysregulation. *Science 278*:52–58.

Knapp, M., Knopman, D., Solomon, P., Pendlebury, W. W., Davis, C. S., and Gracon, S. (1994). A 30-week randomized controlled trial of high dose tacrine in patients with Alzheimer's disease. *JAMA 271*:985–991.

Kuiper, M. A., and Wolters, E. Ch. (1995). CSF biochemistry in Parkinson's disease patients with mental dysfunction. In: *Mental Dysfunction in Parkinson's Disease*. E. Wolters and Scheltens, P. (eds.). ICG, pp. 163–176.

Kulisevsky, J., Avial, A., Barbanoj, M., Antonijoan, R., Berthier, M. L., and Gironell, A. (1996).

Acute effects of levodopa on neuropsychological performance in stable and fluctuating Parkinson's disease patients at different levodopa plasma levels. *Brain 119*:2121–2132.

Lang, A. E., and Lozano, A. M. (1998). Medical progress: Parkinson's disease. *N. Engl. J. Med. 339*:1130–1143.

Lange, K. W., Paul, G. M., Naumann, M., and Gesell, W. (1995). Dopaminergic effects on cognitive performance in patients with Parkinson's disease. *J. Neural Transm. Suppl. 46*:423–432.

Lange, K. W., Robbins, T. W., Marsden, C. D., James, M., Owen, A. M., and Paul, G. M. (1992). L-dopa withdrawal in Parkinson's disease selectively impairs cognitive performance in tests sensitive to frontal lobe dysfunction. *Psychopharmacology 107*:394–404.

Le Moal, M., and Simon, H. (1991). Mesocorticolimbic dopaminergic network: functional and regulatory roles. *Physiol. Rev. 71*:155–234.

Levin, E. D., Decker, M. W., and Butcher, L. L. (eds.). (1992). *Neurotransmitter Interactions and Cognitive Function*. Boston: Birkhauser.

Lewis, D. A. (1992). The catecholaminergic innervation of primate prefrontal cortex. *J. Neural Transm. Suppl. 36*:179–200.

Lieberman, P., Friedman, J., and Feldman, L. (1990). Syntax comprehension in Parkinson's disease. *J. Nerv. Ment. Dis. 178*:360–366.

Lieberman, P., Kako, E., Friedman, J., Tajchman, G., Feldman, L., and Jiminez, E. (1992). Speech production, syntax comprehension, and cognitive deficits in Parkinson's disease. *Brain Lang. 43*:169–189.

Lister, R. G., and Weingartner, H. J. (1987). Neuropharmacological strategies for understanding psychobiological determinants of cognition. *Hum. Neurobiol. 6*:119–127.

Luciana, M., and Collins, P. (1997). Dopaminergic modulation of working memory for spatial but not object cues in normal humans. *J. Cogn. Neurosci. 9*:330–347.

MacLennan, D. L., Nicholas, L. E., Morley, G. K., et al., (1991). The effects of bromocriptine on speech and language function in a man with transcortical motor aphasia. *Clin. Aphasiol. 21*:145–155.

Mair, R. G., and McEntee, W. J. (1986). Cognitive enhancement in Korsakoff's psychosis by clonidine: a comparison with L-dopa and epehdrine. *Psychopharmacology (Berl.) 88*:374–380.

Matison, R., Mayeux, R., Rosen, J., and Fahn, S. (1982). "Tip of the tongue" phenomenon in Parkinson's disease. *Neurology 32*:567–570.

Mattay, V. S., Tessitore, A., Callicott, J. H.,

Bertolino, A., Goldberg, T. E., Chase, T. N., Hyde, T. M., and Weinberger, D. R. (2002). Dopaminergic modulation of cortical function in patients with Parkinson's disease. *Ann. Neurol. 51*:156–164.

Mayeux, R., Stern, Y., Sano, M., Cote, L., and Williams, J. B. W. (1987). Clinical and biochemical correlates of bradyphrenia in Parkinson's disease. *Neurology 37*:1130–1134.

McEntee, W. J., Mair, R. G., and Langlis, P. J. (1984). Neurochemical pathology in Korsakoff psychosis: implications for other cognitive disorders. *Neurology 34*:648–652.

McGurk, S. R. (1999). The effects of clozapine on cognitive functioning in schizophrenia. *J. Clin. Psychiatry 6(Suppl. 12)*:24–30.

McGurk, S., Green, M., Wirshing, W., et al. (1997). The effects of risperidone vs haloperidol in treatment-resistant schizophrenia: the Trailmaking Test. *CNS Spectrums 2*:60–64.

McNamara, P., and Durso, R. (2000). Language functions in Parkinson's disease: evidence for a neurochemistry of language. In: *Neurobehavior of Language and Cognition: Studies of Normal Aging and Brain Damage*, L. Obler, and L. T. Connor, (eds.). New York: Kluwer Academic Publishers, pp. 201–212.

McNamara, P., Krueger, M., O'Quin, K., Clark, J., and Durso, R. (1996). Grammaticality judgments and sentence comprehension in Parkinson's disease: a comparison with Broca's aphasia. *Int. J. Neurosci. 86*:151–166.

McNamara, P., Obler, L. K., Au, R., Durso, R., and Albert, M. (1992). Speech monitoring skills in Alzheimer's disease, Parkinson's disease and normal aging. *Brain Lang. 42*:38–51.

McNeil, M. R., Small, S. L., Masterson, R. J., and Fossett, T. (1995). Behavioral and pharmacological treatment of lexical-semantic deficits in case of primary progressive aphasia. *Am. J. Speech Lang. Pathol. 4*:76–87.

Meador, K. J. (1997). An overview of neurotransmitters in cognitive function. In *Pharmcology of Cognition*. Half Day Course, American Academy of Neurology, 49th Annual meeting, Boston, pp. 337–381.

Mesulam, M.-M. (1988). Central cholinergic pathways: neuroanatomy and some behavioral implications. In: *Neurotransmitters and Cortical Functions*. M. Anoli, T. A. Reader, R. W. Dykes, and P. Gloor (eds.). New York, Plenum Press, pp. 237–260.

Mesulam, M.-M. (1995). Structure and function of cholinergic pathways in the cerebral cortex, limbic system, basal ganglia, and thalamus of the human brain. In *Psychopharmacology: The Fourth Generation of Progress*. F. E. Bloom and D. J. Kupfer (eds.). New York: Raven Press, pp. 135–146.

Mimura, M., McNamara, P., and Albert, M. (1995). Towards a pharmacotherapy for aphasia. In *Handbook of Neurological Speech and Language Disorders*, H. Kirshner (ed.). New York: Marcel Dekker, pp. 465–482.

Moscowitch, L., McNamara, P., and Albert, M. L. (1991). Neurochemical correlates of aphasia. *Neurology 41(suppl. 1)*:410.

Murphy, B., Arnsten, A. F. T., Goldman-Rakic, P. S., and Roth, R. H. (1996). Increased dopamine turnover in the prefrontal cortex impairs spatial working memory performance in rats and monkeys. *Proc. Natl. Acad. Sci. U.S.A. 93*:1325–1329.

Natsopoulos, D., Katsarou, Z., Bostantzopoulos, S., Grouios, G., Mentenopoulos, G., and Logothetis J. (1991). Strategies in comprehension of relative clauses in Parkinsonian patients. *Cortex 27*:255–268.

Oke, A., Keller, R., Mefford, I., and Adams, R. (1978). Lateralization of norepinephrine in human thalamus. *Science 200*:1411–1413.

Oscar-Berman, M., McNamara, P., and Freedman, M. (1991). Delayed response tasks: parallels between experimental ablation studies and findings in patients with frontal lesions. In: *Frontal Lobe Function and Injury*, H. S. Levin and H. M. Eisenberg (eds). San Diego: Academic Press, pp. 230–255.

Pillon, B., Dubois, F., Bonnet, A., Esteguy, M., Guimaraes, J., Vigouret, J., Lhermitte, F., and Agid, Y. (1989). Cognitive "slowing" in Parkinson's disease fails to respond to levodopa treatment: "the 15 objects test." *Neurology 39*:762–768.

Powe, W., Berger, W., Benke, Th., and Schelosky, L. (1991). High speed memory scanning in Parkinson's disease: adverse effects of levodopa. *Ann. Neurol. 29*:670–673.

Posner, M., and Dehaene, S. (1994). Attentional networks. *Trends Neurosci. 17*:75–79.

Pryse-Phillips, W., Sternberg, S., Rochon, P., Naglie, G., Strong, H., and Feightner, J. (2001). The use of medications for cognitive enhancement. *Can. J. Neurol. Sci.*, Suppl. 1:S108–S114.

Pycock, C. J. (1980). Turning behavior in animals. *Neuroscience 5*:461–514.

Rammsayer, T. H., Hennig, J., Haag, A., and Lange, N. (2001). Effects of noradrenergic activity on temporal information processing in humans. *Q. J. Exp. Psychol. B 54*:247–258.

Randolph Swartz, J. (1999). Dopamine projections and frontal systems function. In *The Human Frontal Lobes: Functions and Disorders*, B. L. Miller and J. L. Cummings (eds.). New York: The Guilford Press, pp. 159–173.

Riekkinen, M., Kejonen, K., Jakala, P., Soininen, H., and Riekkinen, P., Jr. (1998). Reduction of noradrenaline impairs attention and dopamine depletion slows responses in Parkinson's disease. *Eur. J. Neurosci. 10(4)*:1429–1435.

Robbins, T., and Brown, V. (1990). The role of the striatum in the mental chronometry of action: a theoretical review. *Rev. Neurosci. 2*:181–213.

Robert, P. H., Aubin-Brunet, V., and Darcourt, G. (1999). Serotonin and the frontal lobes. In: *The Human Frontal Lobes: Functions and Disorders*, B. L. Miller and J. L. Cummings (eds.). New York: The Guilford Press, pp. 125–138.

Rogers, D. (1986). Bradyphrenia in parkinsonism: a historical review. *Psychol. Med. 16*:257–265.

Rogers, D., Lees, A., Smith, E., Trimble, M., and Stern, G. (1987). Bradyphrenia in Parkinson's disease and psychomotor retardation in depressive illness: an experimental study. *Brain 110*:761–776.

Rogers, S. L., Farlow, M. R., Doody, R. S., Mohs, R., and Friedhoff, L. T. (1998). A 24-week double-blind, placebo-controlled trial of donepzil in patients with Alzheimer's disease. Donepzil Study group. *Neurology 50*:136–145.

Rosen, W. G., Mohs, R. C., and Davis, K. L. (1984). A new rating scale for Alzheimer's disease. *Am. J. Psychiatry 141*:1356–1364.

Rosenberger, P. B. (1980). Dopaminergic systems and speech fluency. *J. Fluency Disord. 5*:255–267.

Rosler, M., Anand, R., Cicin-Sain, A., et al. (1999). Efficacy and safety of rivastigmine in patients with Alzheimer's disease: international randomized controlled trial. *BMJ 318*:633–640.

Rusted, J. M., and Warburton, D. M. (1989). Cognitive models and cholinergic drugs. *Neuropsychobiology 21*:31–36.

Sabe, L., Salvarezza, F., Garcia Cuerva, A., Leiguarda, R., and Starkstein, S. (1995). A randomized double-blind placebo controlled study of bromocriptine in non-fluent aphasia. *Neurology 45*:2272–2274.

Sara, S. J., and Herve-Minville, A. (1995). Inhibitory influence of frontal cortex on locus coeruleus. *Proc. Natl. Acad. Sci. U.S.A. 92*:6032–6036.

Sawaguchi, T., and Goldman-Rakic, P. S. (1991). D1 dopamine receptor in prefrontal cortex: Involvement in working memory. *Science 251*:947–950.

Schultz, W., Romo, R., Ljungberg, T., Mirenowicz,

J., Hollerman, J., and Dickinson, A. (1995). Reward-related signals carried by dopamine neurons. In *Models of Information Processing in the Basal Ganglia*, J. Houk, J. Davis, and D. Beiser, (eds.). Cambridge, MA: MIT Press, pp. 233–248.

Servan-Schreiber, D., Carter, C. S., Bruno, R. M., and Cohen, J. D. (1998). Dopamine and the mechanisms of cognition: Part II. D-amphetamine effects in human subjects performing a selective attention task. *Biol. Psychiatry 43:*723–729.

Small, S. L. (1994). Pharmacotherapy of aphasia: a critical review. *Stroke 25:*1282–1289.

Spoont, M. (1992). Modulatory role of serotonin in neural information processing: implications for human psychopathology. *Psychol. Bull. 112:*330–350.

Stahl, S. M., Iverson, S. D., and Goodman, E. C. (eds.). (1987). *Cognitive Neurochemistry.* New York: Oxford University Press.

Stern, Y., Mayeaux, R., and Cote, L. (1984). Reaction time and vigilance in Parkinson's disease. Possible role of altered norepinephrine metabolism. *Arch. Neurol. 41:*1086–1089.

Sternberg, S. (1975). Memory scanning: new findings and current controversies. *Q. J. Exp. Psychol. 27:*1–32.

Tanaka, Y., Albert, M. L., Hujita, K., et al. (2000). Dopamine agonist improves speech output in non-fluent aphasia. Presented at American Academy of Neurology, 2000.

Tanaka, Y., Miyazaki, M., and Albert, M. L. (1997). Effects of increased cholinergic activity on naming in aphasia. *Lancet 350:*116–117.

Taylor, A., and Saint-Cyr, J. (1991). Executive function. In: *Parkinson's Disease: A Neurobiological Perspective* S. Huber and J. Cummings (eds.). Oxford: Oxford University Press, pp. 74–85.

Taylor, A., and Saint-Cyr, J. (1995). The neuropsychology of Parkinson's disease. *Brain Cogn. 28:*281–296.

Terry, A. V., Jackson, W. J., and Buccafusco, J. J. (1993). Effects of concomitant cholinergic and adrenergic stimulation on learning and memory performance by young and aged monkeys. *Cereb. Cortex 3:*304–312.

Valenstein, E., Van Den Abell, T., Tankle, R., Heilman, K. M. (1980). Apomorphine-induced turning after recovery from neglect induced by cortical lesions. *Neurology 30:*358.

Walker-Batson, D. (1998). Pharmacotherapy in the treatment of aphasia. In *Restorative Neurology: Advances in Pharmacotherapy for Recovery after Stroke.* L. B. Goldstein (ed.). Armonk, NY: Futura Publishing, pp. 257–270.

Watanabe M., Kodama, T., and Hikosaka, K. (1997). Increase in extracellular dopamine in the primate prefrontal cortex during a working memory task. *J. Neurophysiol. 78:*2795–2798.

Whitehouse, P. J., Price, D. L., Clark, A. W., Coyle, J. T., and DeLong, J. T. (1981). Alzheimer's disease: evidence for a selective loss of cholinergic neurons in the nucleus basalis. *Ann. Neurol. 10:*122–126.

Williams, G. V., and Goldman-Rakic, P. S. (1995). Modulation of memory fields by dopamine D1 receptors in prefrontal cortex. *Nature 376:*572–575.

Wilson, R. S., Kaszniak, A. W., Klawans, H. L., and Garron, D. C. (1980). High speed memory scanning in parkinsonism. *Cortex 16:*67–72.

Winkler, J., Suhr, S., Gage, F., Thal, L., and Fisher, L. (1995). Essential role of neocortical acetylcholine in spatial memory. *Nature 375:*484–487.

Wolfe, N., Katz, D. I., Albert, M. L., Almozolino, A., Durso, R., Smith, M. C., and Volicer, L. (1990). Neuropsychological profile linked to low dopamine in Alzheimer's disease, major depression and Parkinson's disease. *J. Neurol. Neurosurg. Psychiatry 53:*516–519.

Subject Index

Author Index